Principles of Pediatric and Neonatal Emergencies

Principles of Pediatric and Neonatal Emergencies

4th Edition

Editor-in-Chief

Piyush Gupta
MD FIAP FNNF FAMS
Professor and Head
Department of Pediatrics
University College of Medical Sciences and Guru Teg Bahadur Hospital
New Delhi, India
President-Elect, Indian Academy of Pediatrics 2020

Chief Academic Editors

Arvind Bagga
MD FIAP FAMS FISN
Professor
Division of Nephrology
Department of Pediatrics
All India Institute of Medical Sciences
New Delhi, India

Siddarth Ramji
MD FNNF
Director-Professsor
Department of Neonatology
Maulana Azad Medical College
and Associated Lok Nayak Hospital
New Delhi, India

Academic Editors

Krishan Chugh
MD MNAMS FISCCM
Director and Head
Department of Pediatrics and
Pediatric Intensive Care Unit
Fortis Memorial Research Institute
Gurugram, Haryana, India

Rakesh Lodha
MD
Professor
Department of Pediatrics
All India Institute of Medical
Sciences
New Delhi, India

Executive Editors

Pooja Dewan
MD MNAMS FIAP
Professor
Division of Hemato-Oncology
Department of Pediatrics
University College of Medical Sciences
New Delhi, India

Jaya Shankar Kaushik
MD DNB DM
Associate Professor
Department of Pediatrics
Pandit Bhagwat Dayal Sharma
Postgraduate Institute of Medical Sciences
Rohtak, Haryana, India

Managing Editor

Dheeraj Shah
MD FIAP MNAMS
Professor
Department of Pediatrics
University College of Medical Sciences
and Guru Teg Bahadur Hospital
New Delhi, India

Forewords

Digant D Shastri, Bakul Jayant Parekh

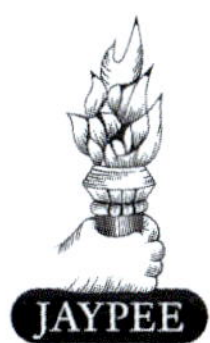

JAYPEE BROTHERS MEDICAL PUBLISHERS
The Health Sciences Publisher
New Delhi | London

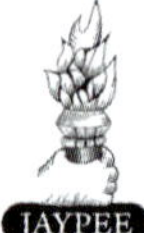

Jaypee Brothers Medical Publishers (P) Ltd

Headquarters
EMCA House, 23/23-B
Ansari Road, Daryaganj
New Delhi 110 002, India
Landline: +91-11-23272143, +91-11-23272703
+91-11-23282021, +91-11-23245672
e-mail: jaypee@jaypeebrothers.com

Corporate Office
4838/24, Ansari Road, Daryaganj
New Delhi 110 002, India
Phone: +91-11-43574357
Fax: +91-11-43574314
e-mail: jaypee@jaypeebrothers.com

Overseas Office
JP Medical Ltd.
83, Victoria Street, London
SW1H 0HW (UK)
Phone: +44-20 3170 8910
e-mail: info@jpmedpub.com

EU GPSR Authorised Representative
Logos Europe, 9 rue Nicolas Poussin
17000, La Rochelle, France
Phone: +33 (0) 6 67 93 73 78
e-mail: contact@logoseurope.eu

Website: www.jaypeebrothers.com
Website: www.jaypeedigital.com

Principles of Pediatric and Neonatal Emergencies

First Edition: 1994
Second Edition: 2004
Third Edition: 2011
Fourth Edition: 2020, **Reprint: 2026**

ISBN: 978-93-89587-20-3

Printed at: Samrat Offset Pvt. Ltd.

Contributing Authors

Aashay A Shah MD
Senior Resident and Fellow
Department of Pediatrics
Gastroenterology and Hepatology
and Nutrition
Medanta—The Medicity
Gurugram, Haryana, India

Abhay K Shah MD DPed FIAP
Senior Consultant Pediatrician and
Infectious Diseases Specialist
Director
Dr Abhay K Shah Children Hospital
Maninagar
Ahmedabad, Gujarat, India

Abhijeet Saha MD
Professor
Department of Pediatrics
Lady Hardinge Medical College and
Associated Kalawati Saran Children's
Hospital, New Delhi, India

Aditi Sinha MD
Assistant Professor
Division of Nephrology
Department of Pediatrics
All India Institute of Medical Sciences
New Delhi, India

Ajay N Gangopadhyay MBBS MS MCh
Ex-Professor
Department of Pediatric Surgery
Institute of Medical Sciences
Banaras Hindu University
Varanasi, Uttar Pradesh, India

Aman Elwadhi MD
Senior Resident
Department of Pediatrics
Lady Hardinge Medical College and
Associated
Kalawati Saran Children's Hospital
New Delhi, India

Amber Kumar MD FNB
Assistant Professor
Department of Pediatrics
All India Institute of Medical Sciences
Bhopal, Madhya Pradesh, India

Amir Maroof Khan MD
Associate Professor
Department of Community Medicine
University College of Medical Sciences
New Delhi, India

Amit Kumar Satapathy MD
Assistant Professor
Department of Pediatrics
All India Institute of Medical Sciences
Bhubaneswar, Odisha, India

Amitabh Singh MD
Assistant Professor
Department of Pediatrics
Vardhman Mahavir Medical College and
Safdarjung Hospital
New Delhi, India

Anil Sachdev MD
Director
Pediatric Emergency
Critical Care and Pulmonology
Sir Ganga Ram Hospital
New Delhi, India

Anil Vasudevan MD
Professor and Head
Department of Pediatric Nephrology
St John's Medical College Hospital
Bengaluru, Karnataka, India

Aniruddha Ghosh MD DNB
Senior Resident
Department of Pediatrics
Institute of Child Health
Kolkata, West Bengal, India

Anita Saxena MD DM FACC
Professor
Department of Cardiology
All India Institute of Medical Sciences
New Delhi, India

Anju Seth MD
Director Professor
Department of Pediatrics
Lady Hardinge Medical College and
Associated
Kalawati Saran Children's Hospital
New Delhi, India

Anju Virmani MD DNB
Associate Director
Pediatric Endocrinology
Max Smart Superspecialty Hospital
Saket, New Delhi
Pentamed Hospital and Rainbow
Hospital, New Delhi and
Max Hospital, Gurugram, Haryana, India

Ankit Vishwani MD
Senior Resident
Department of ENT
University College of Medical Sciences
and Guru Teg Bahadur Hospital
New Delhi, India

Ankita Goel Sharma MD
Associate Professor
Department of Pediatrics
Lady Hardinge Medical College and
Associated Kalawati Saran Children's
Hospital
New Delhi, India

Anshu Srivastava MD DM
Professor
Department of Pediatric Gastroenterology
Sanjay Gandhi Postgraduate Institute of
Medical Sciences
Lucknow, Uttar Pradesh, India

Anup Mohta MS MCh FAMS
Director-Professor
Department of Surgery
Lady Hardinge Medical College
New Delhi, India

Anurag Agarwal MD
Associate Professor
Department of Pediatrics
Maulana Azad Medical College
New Delhi, India

Anuva Bansal MD
Senior Resident
Department of Dermatology and
Sexually Transmitted Diseases
Maulana Azad Medical College and
Associated Lok Nayak Hospital and
GB Pant Hospital
New Delhi, India

Aparajita Mitra MS MCh Post-doctoral Fellowship in Pediatric Urology
Assistant Professor
Department of Pediatric Surgery
All India Institute of Medical Sciences
New Delhi, India

Arohi Gupta MBBS MD
Senior Resident
Department of Pediatrics
Lady Hardinge Medical College and Associated Kalawati Saran Children's Hospital
New Delhi, India

Arpana Iyengar MD
Professor
Department of Pediatric Nephrology
St John's Medical College Hospital
Bengaluru, Karnataka, India

Arun Goel MD
Consultant Plastic Surgeon and Unit Head
Department of Burns and Plastic Surgery
Maulana Azad Medical College and Associated Lok Nayak Hospital
New Delhi, India

Arun Kumar MD MRCP FRCPCH
Consultant Pediatrician
Croydon University Hospital
Surrey, UK

Arushi Gahlot Saini MD DM
Assistant Professor
Pediatric Neurology Unit
Department of Pediatrics
Postgraduate Institute of Medical Education and Research
Chandigarh, India

Arvind Bagga MD FIAP FAMS FISN
Professor
Division of Nephrology
Department of Pediatrics
All India Institute of Medical Sciences
New Delhi, India

Ashish Suri MBBS MCh DNB MNAMS
Professor and Unit Head
Department of Neurosurgery
All India Institute of Medical Sciences
New Delhi, India

Ashok K Patwari MD MNAMS FIAP FAMS
Former Director Professor Pediatrics
Lady Hardinge Medical College
New Delhi
Former Research Professor
International Health
Boston University School of Public Health
Boston, USA

Ashutosh Yajurvedi Dch Fellowship in Neonatology
Consultant Pediatrician, Yajurvedi Hospital
Solapur, Maharashtra, India

Atul Kulkarni MD
Assistant Professor
Department of Pediatrics
Ashwini Rural Medical College
Solapur, Maharashtra, India

Atul Mohan Kochhar MD DNB MNAMS FAAD
Professor and Consultant
Department of Dermatology and Sexually Transmitted Diseases,
Lok Nayak Hospital and associated MAMC and GB Pant Hospital
New Delhi, India

Baljeet Maini MD
Professor
Department of Pediatrics
Teerthankar Mahaveer Medical College and Research Center
Teerthankar Mahaveer University
Moradabad, Uttar Pradesh, India

Bharat Choudhary MD FPEM
Fellow of Academic College of Emergency Experts (FACEE)
Assistant Professor
Trauma and Emergency (Pediatrics)
All India Institute of Medical Sciences
Jodhpur, Rajasthan, India

Bharat Mehra MD
Fellow
Pediatric Intensive Care Unit
Sir Ganga Ram Hospital
New Delhi, India

Bhavna Dhingra MD DNB
Additional Professor
Department of Pediatrics
All India Institute of Medical Sciences
Bhopal, Madhya Pradesh, India

Bhupeshwari Patel MD FACEE
Assistant Professor
Department of Pediatrics
All India Institute of Medical Sciences
Bhopal, Madhya Pradesh, India

Bhushan Sagade MS
Clinical Associate
Department of Pediatric Orthopedics
BJ Wadia Hospital for Children
Mumbai, Maharashtra, India

Bilal Khan MD
Attending Consultant
Pediatric Intensive Care Unit
Fortis Memorial Research Institute
Gurugram, Haryana, India

Bindiya Gupta MD MAMS FICOG
Associate Professor
Department of Obstetrics and Gynecology
University College of Medical Sciences and Guru Teg Bahadur Hospital
New Delhi, India

Bipin Jose MD MRCPCH
Consultant Pediatric Intensivist
Rajagiri Hospital
Kochi, Kerala, India

Biraj Parjauli MD DM
Fellow, Pediatric Critical Care
Division of Pediatric Emergency and Intensive Care
Advanced Pediatrics Center
Postgraduate Institute of Medical Education and Research
Chandigarh, India

Chandra Mohan Kumar MD PGDAP MAMS
Professor
Department of Pediatrics and Adolescent Medicine
Hamdard Institute of Medical Sciences and Research
New Delhi, India

Chhaya Sambharya Prasad MD
Developmental Pediatrician
Director
Accredited Social Health Activist
Center for Autism and Intellectual Developmental Disorders
Chandigarh, India

Christy Cathreen Thomas MD
Fellow
Division of Nephrology
Department of Pediatrics
All India Institute of Medical Sciences
New Delhi, India

Daniel Krich MD
Fellow in Pediatric Pulmonology
New York Medical College
Maria Fareri Children's Hospital at
Westchester Medical Center
New York, USA

Deepak K Gupta MBBS MS MCh
Professor
Department of Neurosurgery
Neurosciences Center and Associated
JPN Apex Trauma Center
All India Institute of Medical Sciences
New Delhi, India

Deepak Kumar MD
Assistant Professor
Department of Pediatrics
Maulana Azad Medical College
New Delhi, India

Deepak Sharma MD
Consultant
Department of Neonatology
Fernandez Hospital
Hyderabad, Telangana, India

Deepika Harit MD
Associate Professor
Department of Pediatrics
University College of Medical Sciences
and Guru Teg Bahadur Hospital
New Delhi, India

Dheeraj Shah MD FIAP MNAMS
Professor
Department of Pediatrics
University College of Medical Sciences
and Guru Teg Bahadur Hospital
New Delhi, India

Dhiren Gupta MD
Co-Director
Pediatric Intensive Care
Sir Ganga Ram Hospital
New Delhi, India

Dinesh Raj MD
Associate Consultant
Department of Pediatrics
Holy Family Hospital
New Delhi, India

Dipen Vasudev Patel MD
Professor
Department of Pediatrics
Pramukhswami Medical College
Anand, Gujarat, India

Dipti Kapoor MD
Associate Professor
Department of Pediatrics
Lady Hardinge Medical College and
Associated Kalawati Saran Children's
Hospital
New Delhi, India

Divya Chauhan MD
Senior Resident
Department of Obstetrics and Gynecology
University College of Medical Sciences
and Guru Teg Bahadur Hospital
New Delhi, India

G Kalra MDS
Reader
Sardar Patel PG Institute of Dental and
Medical Sciences
Lucknow, Uttar Pradesh, India

Garima Gupta MD
Assistant Professor
Department of Pediatrics
North Delhi Municipal Corporation
Medical College
New Delhi, India

Girish Chandra Bhatt MD MAMS
Associate Professor
Department of Pediatrics
All India Institute of Medical Sciences
Bhopal, Madhya Pradesh, India

HPS Sachdev MD FAMS
Senior Consultant
Department of Pediatrics and Clinical
Epidemiology
Sitaram Bhartia Institute of Science
and Research
New Delhi, India

Indumathy Santhanam MD DCH
Professor and Head
Department of Pediatric Emergency
Medicine
Institute of Child Health
Madras Medical College
Chennai, Tamil Nadu, India

Javed Ismail MD DM
Consultant
Pediatric Critical Care
Apollo KH Hospitals
Vellore, Tamil Nadu, India

Jaya Shankar Kaushik MD DNB DM
Associate Professor
Department of Pediatrics
Pandit Bhagwat Dayal Sharma
Postgraduate Institute of Medical
Sciences
Rohtak, Haryana, India

Jayashree M MD FIAP FICCM
Professor and Chief
Division of Pediatric Emergency and
Intensive Care
Advanced Pediatrics Center
Postgraduate Institute of Medical
Education and Research
Chandigarh, India

Jayendra Seetharaman MD
Senior Resident
Department of Pediatric
Gastroenterology
Sanjay Gandhi Postgraduate Institute of
Medical Sciences
Lucknow, Uttar Pradesh, India

Jhuma Sankar MD
Associate Professor
Department of Pediatrics
All India Institute of Medical
Sciences
New Delhi, India

Jitendra Meena MD
Senior Resident
Division of Nephrology
Department of Pediatrics
All India Institute of Medical
Sciences
New Delhi, India

JK Dhillon MDS
Ex-Associate Professor
Department of Pedodontics and Preventive Dentistry
Maulana Azad Institute of Dental Sciences
New Delhi, India

Jogender Kumar DM
Assistant Professor
Newborn Unit
Department of Pediatrics
Postgraduate Institute of Medical Education and Research
Chandigarh, India

Joseph John MD DNB
Additional Professor and Head
Department of Pediatrics
All India Institute of Medical Sciences
Bhubaneswar, Odisha, India

Joseph L Mathew MD PhD Fellow (Ped Respirology)
Professor
Division of Pediatric Pulmonology
Advanced Pediatrics Center
Postgraduate Institute of Medical Education and Research
Chandigarh, India

Kana Ram Jat MD
Associate Professor
Division of Pediatric Pulmonology
Department of Pediatrics
All India Institute of Medical Sciences
New Delhi, India

Kausalya Raghuraman MD
Senior Resident
Department of Microbiology
Pandit Bhagwat Dayal Sharma
Postgraduate Institute of Medical Sciences
Rohtak, Haryana, India

Kavitha TK MD
Fellow, Pediatric Critical Care
Division of Pediatric Emergency and Intensive Care
Advanced Pediatrics Center
Postgraduate Institute of Medical Education and Research
Chandigarh, India

Krishan Chugh MD MNAMS FISCCM
Director and Head
Department of Pediatrics and Pediatric Intensive Care Unit
Fortis Memorial Research Institute
Gurugram, Haryana, India

Krishna Mohan Gulla MD DM
Assistant Professor
Department of Pediatrics
Advanced Pediatric Center
Postgraduate Institute of Medical Education and Research
Chandigarh, India

Kuntal Roy Chowdhuri MS MCh
Associate Consultant
Department of Cardiothoracic and Vascular Surgery
BM Birla Heart Research Center
Kolkata, West Bengal, India

Lalitha Janakiraman MD DCH
Senior Consultant Pediatrician
Kanchi Kamakoti CHILDS Trust Hospital and
The CHILDS Trust Medical Research Foundation
Chennai, Tamil Nadu, India

Lokesh Guglani MD FAAP
Associate Professor
Division of Pulmonology
Allergy/Immunology
Cystic Fibrosis and Sleep
Department of Pediatrics
Emory University School of Medicine
Children's Healthcare of Atlanta-Egleston
Atlanta, Georgia, USA

Madhuradhar Chegondi MBBS MD FAAP
Consultant
Division of Critical Care Medicine Stead Family Children's Hospital
Assistant Professor
Department of Pediatrics
University of Iowa
Carver College of Medicine
Iowa City, Iowa, USA

Mahesh Kamate MD DM
Professor
Department of Pediatric Neurology
KAHER's Jawaharlal Nehru Medical College
Belagavi, Karnataka, India

Mahesh Maheshwari MD
Associate Professor
Department of Pediatrics
All India Institute of Medical Sciences
Bhopal, Madhya Pradesh, India

Mandar Agashe MS
Consultant Pediatric Orthopedic Surgeon
Director
Agashe's Pediatric Superspecialty Care
Kurla, Mumbai
Assistant Honorary Consultant
BJ Wadia Hospital for Children
Mumbai, Maharashtra, India

Maninder Dhaliwal DNB
Associate Director
Pediatric Critical Care Unit
Department of Pediatrics
Medanta—The Medicity
Gurugram, Haryana, India

Manish Kori MD
Consultant
Pediatric Intensive Care Unit
Fortis Memorial Research Institute
Gurugram, Haryana, India

Mehak Bansal MBBS DNB IDPCCM
Clinical Fellow (Pediatric Intensive Care Unit), Great Ormond Street Hospital
London, UK

Mukta Mantan MD DNB
Professor
Department of Pediatrics
Maulana Azad Medical College and Associated Hospitals
New Delhi, India

Nandkishor S Kabra MD DNB DM
Director, Neonatal Intensive Care Unit
Department of Neonatology
Surya Hospitals
Mumbai, Maharashtra, India

Narendra Kumar Bagri MD
Assistant Professor
Division of Rheumatology
Department of Pediatrics
All India Institute of Medical Sciences
New Delhi, India

Naveen Sankhyan MD DM
Additional Professor
Pediatric Neurology Unit
Department of Pediatrics
Postgraduate Institute of Medical
Education and Research
Chandigarh, India

Neelam Mohan MD
Director
Department of Pediatric
Gastroenterology
Hepatology and Liver Transplantation
Medanta—The Medicity
Gurugram, Haryana, India

Neelima Gupta MD
Director Professor
Department of ENT
University College of Medical Sciences
and Guru Teg Bahadur Hospital
New Delhi, India

Neeraj Gupta MD DM
Additional Professor
Department of Neonatology
All India Institute of Medical Sciences
Jodhpur, Rajasthan, India

Neha Rastogi MD
Consultant
Department of Pediatric Hematology
Oncology and Bone Marrow
Transplantation
Cancer Institute
Medanta—The Medicity
Gurugram, Haryana, India

Neha Thakur MD FACEE
Assistant Professor
Department of Pediatrics
Dr Ram Manohar Lohia Institute of
Medical Sciences
Lucknow, Uttar Pradesh, India

Nidhi Bedi MD
Assistant Professor
Department of Pediatrics
Hamdard Institute of Medical Sciences
and Research
New Delhi, India

P Ramesh Menon MD
Assistant Professor (Neonatology)
Department of Pediatrics
All India Institute of Medical Sciences
New Delhi, India

Parvathi U Iyer MD
Director
Pediatric Cardiac Intensive Care
Fortis Escorts Heart Institute
New Delhi, India

Payal Gupta DNB
Fellow in Pediatric Ophthalmology
Sadguru Netra Chikitsalaya
Chitrakoot, Madhya Pradesh, India

Peeyush Jain MD
Senior Consultant
Department of Pediatrics
Hindu Rao Hospital and North Delhi
Municipal Corporation Medical College
New Delhi, India

Pinky Meena MD
Senior Resident
Department of Pediatrics
University College of Medical Sciences
New Delhi, India

Piyush Gupta MD FIAP FNNF FAMS
Professor and Head
Department of Pediatrics
University College of Medical
Sciences and Guru Teg Bahadur
Hospital
New Delhi, India

Pooja Dewan MD MNAMS FIAP
Professor
Division of Hemato-Oncology
Department of Pediatrics
University College of Medical Sciences
New Delhi, India

Pooja P Mallya DNB
Junior Consultant
Pediatric Hematology
Oncology and Blood and Marrow
Transplantation
Mazumdar Shaw Cancer Center
Narayana Health City
Bengaluru, Karnataka, India

Pranav Gupta MBBS DNB MRCPCH
Consultant
Department of Pediatrics
Tirath Ram Shah Hospital
New Delhi, India

Praveen Khilnani MD
Senior Consultant Pediatric
Pulmonology and Critical Care
Clinical Director
Madhukar Rainbow Children's Hospital
New Delhi, India

Parveen Kumar Antil MD
Senior Resident
Department of Pediatrics
Maharishi Markandeshwar Institute
of Medical Sciences and Research
Ambala, Haryana, India

Praveen Kumar MD DM
Professor and Head
Division of Neonatology
Department of Pediatrics
Postgraduate Institute of Medical
Education and Research
Chandigarh, India

Praveen Kumar MD
Director Professor
Department of Pediatrics
Lady Hardinge Medical College and
Associated
Kalawati Saran Children's Hospital
New Delhi, India

Preeti Anand MBBS DNB
Consultant
Pediatrics and Pediatric Intensive Care
Max Smart Superspecialty Hospital
Saket, New Delhi, India

Preeti Jain MD
Professor
Department of Physiology
Maulana Azad Medical College
New Delhi, India

Preeti Singh MD
Assistant Professor
Department of Pediatrics
Lady Hardinge Medical College and Associated
Kalawati Saran Children's Hospital
New Delhi, India

Prerna Batra MD MNAMS FACEE
Professor
Department of Pediatrics
University College of Medical Sciences
and Guru Teg Bahadur Hospital
New Delhi, India

Priyanka Aggarwal MD
Assistant Professor
Division of Pediatric Hematology Oncology
Department of Pediatrics
Institute of Medical Sciences
Banaras Hindu University
Varanasi, Uttar Pradesh, India

Priyanka Madaan MD DM
Senior Research Associate
Pediatric Neurology Unit
Department of Pediatrics
Postgraduate Institute of Medical Education and Research
Chandigarh, India

R Ganesh MBBS DNB MNAMS MRCPCH PhD
Senior Consultant Pediatrician
Rainbow Children's Hospital
Chennai, Tamil Nadu, India

Rachna Pasi DCH DNB MNAMS (PhD)
Assistant Professor
Department of Pediatrics
Himalayan Institute of Medical Sciences
Dehradun, Uttarakhand, India

Rachna Bhargava PhD
Additional Professor of Clinical Psychology
National Drug Dependence Treatment Center
Department of Psychiatry
All India Institute of Medical Sciences
New Delhi, India

Rachna Seth MD
Professor
Division of Pediatric Oncology
Chair
InPoG Late Effects Subcommittee
Department of Pediatrics
All India Institute of Medical Sciences
New Delhi, India

Rajeshwari Nataraj DNB
Senior Consultant
Pediatric Intensive Care Unit
and Cardiothoracic Intensive Care Unit
Apollo Children's Hospital
Chennai, Tamil Nadu, India

Rajniti Prasad MD
Professor and Head
Department of Pediatrics
Institute of Medical Sciences
Banaras Hindu University
Varanasi, Uttar Pradesh, India

Rakesh Lodha MD
Professor
Department of Pediatrics
All India Institute of Medical Sciences
New Delhi, India

Raman Deep MD
Additional Professor of Psychiatry
Department of Psychiatry
All India Institute of Medical Sciences
New Delhi, India

Rangan Srinivasaraghavan MD
Assistant Professor
Developmental Pediatrics Unit
Department of Child Health
Christian Medical College
Vellore, Tamil Nadu, India

Ranjith Kumar Manokaran MD DM
Assistant Professor
Pediatric Neurology
Sri Ramachandra Medical College
Chennai, Tamil Nadu, India

Reshma Aramanadka MD DM
Fellow, Pediatric Critical Care
Division of Pediatric Emergency and Intensive Care
Advanced Pediatrics Center
Postgraduate Institute of Medical Education and Research
Chandigarh, India

Rhishikesh P Thakre DCH MD DNB DM FCPS FIAP
Director
Neo Clinic and Hospital
Aurangabad, Maharashtra, India

Rishi Bolia MD DM
Assistant Professor
Division of Pediatric Gastroenterology
Department of Gastroenterology
Postgraduate Institute of Medical Education and Research
Chandigarh, India

Ritabrata Kundu MD FIAP
Professor
Department of Pediatrics
Institute of Child Health
Kolkata, West Bengal, India

Ruchi Rai MD
Professor
Department of Neonatology-Maternal and Reproductive Health
Superspecialty Pediatric Hospital and Postgraduate Teaching Institute
NOIDA, Uttar Pradesh, India

S Mahadevan MD PhD MNAMS
Professor and Head
Department of Pediatrics
Women and Children Hospital
Jawaharlal Institute of Postgraduate Medical Education and Research
Puducherry, India

Samriti Gupta MD
Assistant Professor
Department of Pediatrics
Dr Rajendra Prasad Government Medical College
Kangra, Himachal Pradesh, India

Sandeep Kumar Kanwal MD PDCDM
Consultant
Division of Pediatric Intensive Care Unit
Department of Pediatrics
Lady Hardinge Medical College and Associated Kalawati Saran Children's Hospital
New Delhi, India

Sangeetha Yoganathan MD DNB DM
Professor
Department of Neurological Sciences
Christian Medical College
Vellore, Tamil Nadu, India

Sankaran Krishnan MPH FAAP
Associate Professor of Pediatrics and Clinical Public Health
Associate Program Director
Pediatric Pulmonology
New York Medical College
Maria Fareri Children's Hospital at Westchester Medical Center
New York, USA

Satinder Aneja MD
Professor
Department of Pediatrics
School of Medical Sciences and Research
Sharda University
Greater Noida, Uttar Pradesh, India

Satish Kumar Aggarwal MS MCh
Chairman
Pediatric Surgery
Sir Ganga Ram Hospital
Formerly Director Professor of Pediatric Surgery
Maulana Azad Medical College and Associated Lok Nayak and GB Pant Hospitals
New Delhi, India

Satvik Bansal MD Fellowships in Neonatology
Assistant Professor
Department of Pediatrics
Gajra Raja Medical College
Gwalior, Madhya Pradesh, India

Shalu Gupta MD DM
Professor
Department of Pediatrics
Lady Hardinge Medical College and Associated Kalawati Saran Children's Hospital
New Delhi, India

Shalu Jain DNB
Senior Resident
Department of Pediatrics
University College of Medical Sciences and Guru Teg Bahadur Hospital
New Delhi, India

Sharmila B Mukherjee MD
Professor
Department of Pediatrics
Lady Hardinge Medical College and Associated Kalawati Saran Children's Hospital
New Delhi, India

Sharada Sathish Kumar DCH DNB FPEM
Consultant
Emergency Medicine Unit
Mehta's Children's Hospital
Chennai, Tamil Nadu, India

Shashi Kant Dhir MD
Senior Resident
Division of Neonatology
Department of Pediatrics
Postgraduate Institute of Medical Education and Research
Chandigarh, India

Sheffali Gulati MD FAMS
Professor
DM Pediatric Neurology Program
Faculty In-Charge
Center of Excellence and Advanced Research on Childhood Neurodevelopmental Disorders
Chief
Child Neurology Division
Department of Pediatrics
All India Institute of Medical Sciences
New Delhi, India

Shipra Agrawal MD
Senior Resident
Department of Pediatrics
Maulana Azad Medical College and Associated Hospitals
New Delhi, India

Shiv Sajan Saini MD DM
Assistant Professor
Division of Neonatology
Department of Pediatrics
Postgraduate Institute of Medical Education and Research
Chandigarh, India

Shweta Kedia
MBBS MS MCh
Associate Professor
Department of Neurosurgery
All India Institute of Medical Sciences
New Delhi, India

Siddarth Ramji MD FNNF
Director-Professsor
Department of Neonatology
Maulana Azad Medical College and Associated Lok Nayak Hospital
New Delhi, India

SK Kabra MD FIAP FAMS
Professor
Department of Pediatrics
All India Institute of Medical Sciences
New Delhi, India

Somashekar M Nimbalkar MD
Professor
Department of Pediatrics
Pramukhswami Medical College
Anand, Gujarat, India

Sonali Ghosh MD
Associate Consultant
Pediatric Intensive Care Unit
Fortis Memorial Research Institute
Gurugram, Haryana, India

Soonu Udani MD
Medical Director and Head
Critical Care and Emergency Services
SRCC Children's Hospital Managed by Narayana Health
Mumbai, Maharashtra, India

Sourabh Dutta PhD MD
Professor
Newborn Unit
Department of Pediatrics
Postgraduate Institute of Medical Education and Research
Chandigarh, India

Srikant Das MD
Assistant Professor
Department of Pediatrics
Director of Pediatric Electrophysiology
University of Arkansas for Medical Sciences
Little Rock, Arkansas, USA

Srinivas Murki MD DM
Chief Neonatologist
Paramitha Children's Hospital
Hyderabad, Telangana, India

Suchitra Ranjit MD FCCM
Consultant In-Charge
Pediatric Intensive Care Unit
Apollo Children's Hospital
Chennai, Tamil Nadu, India

Sumaira Khalil DNB
Pediatric Specialist
Vardhman Mahavir Medical College and
Safdarjung Hospital
New Delhi, India

Sunil Bhat MD FNB
Director and Clinical Lead
Pediatric Hematology, Oncology and
Blood and Marrow Transplantation
Narayana Health Network Hospitals
SRCC NH Children's Hospital
Mumbai, India
Mazumdar Shaw Cancer Center
Narayana Health City
Bengaluru, Karnataka, India

Sunita Bijarnia-Mahay DCH DNB FGMM
Senior Consultant
Institute of Medical Genetics and
Genomics
Associate Professor
Ganga Ram Institute of Postgraduate
Medical Education and Research
Sir Ganga Ram Hospital
New Delhi, India

Surender K Yachha MD DM
Head
Department of Pediatric
Gastroenterology
Hepatology and Liver Transplant
Sakra World Hospital
Bengaluru, Karnataka, India

Suresh Gupta MD
Senior Consultant
Pediatric Emergency and Critical Care
Institute of Child Health
Sir Ganga Ram Hospital
New Delhi, India

Suresh Kumar Angurana
MD DM MNAMS FIMSA FCCP
Assistant Professor
Division of Pediatric Critical Care
Department of Pediatrics
Advanced Pediatrics Center
Postgraduate Institute of Medical
Education and Research
Chandigarh, India

Swathi Chacham MBBS MD DM MAMS
Additional Professor
Former Head
Department of Pediatrics
All India Institute of Medical Sciences
Rishikesh, Uttarakhand, India

Tsering Sandup MCh
Senior Resident
Cardiothoracic and Vascular Surgery
All India Institute of Medical Sciences
New Delhi, India

Ujjal Poddar MD DNB DM
Professor and Head
Department of Pediatric Gastroenterology
Sanjay Gandhi Postgraduate Institute of
Medical Sciences
Lucknow, Uttar Pradesh, India

Urmila Jhamb MD
Director-Professor and Head
Department of Pediatrics
Maulana Azad Medical College
New Delhi, India

Utpal Kant Singh MD
Professor
Department of Pediatrics
Nalanda Medical College
Patna, Bihar, India

Utkarsh Kohli MD
Assistant Professor of Pediatrics
Director
Pediatric Cardiac Electrophysiology
Laboratory
Division of Pediatric Cardiology
Department of Pediatrics
The University of Chicago Pritzker School
of Medicine
Chicago, Illinois, USA

Vaibhav Pandey MBBS MS MCh
Associate Professor
Department of Pediatric Surgery
Institute of Medical Sciences
Banaras Hindu University
Varanasi, Uttar Pradesh, India

Vineeta Gupta MD
Professor and In-Charge
Division of Pediatric Hematology
Oncology
Department of Pediatrics
Institute of Medical Sciences
Banaras Hindu University
Varanasi, Uttar Pradesh, India

Vivek Chaturvedi DM
Senior Consultant
Cardiology and Director Cardiac
Electrophysiology and Pacing
Narayana Superspecialty Hospital
Gurugram, Haryana, India

VP Mathur MDS
Professor and Head
Department of Pedodontics and
Preventive Dentistry
Center for Dental Education and
Research
All India Institute of Medical Sciences
New Delhi, India

Vyom Aggarwal MD DNB FRCPCH
Senior Consultant
Department of Pediatrics
Tirath Ram Shah Hospital
New Delhi, India

Foreword

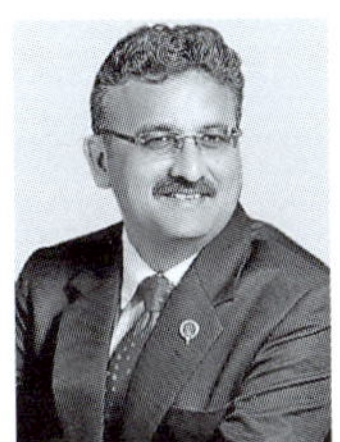

It is indeed a proud pleasure for me to write the "Foreword" for the 4th edition of the textbook on *Principles of Pediatric and Neonatal Emergencies.*

India is the second most populous country in the world and will soon overtake China in being "numero uno". There is a growing disparity between the numbers of patients per doctor as well as a definite deficit of Emergency Physicians. By and large in most of the hospitals the doctors working in the casualty department or the emergency room are mostly resident/intern or medical officer who evaluates the patient and calls what they determine is the relevant specialty to take over the case. Their job is not just limited to primary evaluation, first aid and calling the specialist, but they need to initiate the emergency management also. In view of these, there is the need for a book on emergency management in Indian context which can be of help to these workforce who work in situations where each second is precious.

The Indian Academy of Pediatrics is constantly working towards improving child health in our country and to achieve its mission statement, it works through knowledge update of doctors. Apart from conducting conferences and CMEs, it also publishes journals and textbooks. This textbook on *Principles of Pediatric and Neonatal Emergencies* is a venture of Indian Pediatrics, Journal of the Indian Academy of Pediatrics, can be of great help as reference manual for not only the people who are working in casualty/emergency room but also to primary care pediatricians.

This multi-author book has been extremely well planned with eight sections under which through 91 chapters, all aspects of pediatric emergency care are very well covered. Common pediatric and neonatal emergencies have been authored by leading experts in their subspecialty. This ensures that all the recent advances in respective sub-specialties have been updated. Apart from sections on pediatric and neonatal medical emergencies, the book has many new facets including organization of emergency department, initial stabilization, and pediatric surgical emergencies that are often overlooked otherwise. Section on emergency procedures have been outlined very well and will be very useful to residents in training. The two Annexures on pediatric drug dosage and reference values surely proved to be great usefulness for the clinicians in routine emergency care.

The book has simple tables, algorithms and flowcharts for a quick view. This book covers almost everything that would be required to provide care for sick children and my compliments to all the members of the editorial board lead by a great teacher and writer Dr Piyush Gupta for their untiring efforts.

This comprehensive textbook with excellent illustrations would motivate young budding residents and will be very useful to them. I am sure this book will serve as a ready reference for every pediatrician providing emergency services to children. Apart from its place on the bookshelves of fellow pediatricians, this book must be present in every pediatric emergency for ready reference. This would ensure that we provide the best of care with updated knowledge.

My best wishes and regards.

Digant D Shastri
President, Indian Academy of Pediatrics 2019

Foreword

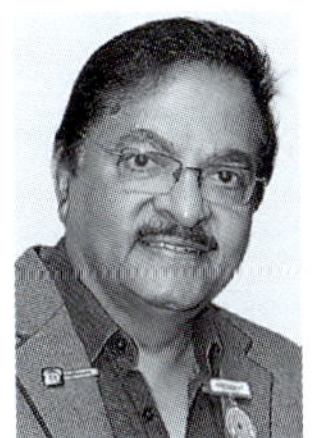

I am delighted to write the foreword for the fourth edition of *Principles of Pediatric and Neonatal Emergencies*. The first edition was published in 1994 under the editorship of Dr Sachdev, Dr Puri, Dr Bagga and Dr Panna Choudhury. In fact, this first edition was also built upon on an earlier venture "Pediatric and Neonatal Emergencies". We recognized early on the need for the various principles regarding Pediatric and Neonatal Emergencies. Dr Sachdev and his associate editors have met that need, representing many disciplines that IAP serves, and all having contributed to the evolution of the science behind pediatric and neonatal emergencies. The first edition was very well received, having been through several printings! This prompted Dr Sachdev and his team come out with the second edition in 2004 and subsequently a third edition in 2011 was published by the very eminent Dr Panna, Dr Bagga, Dr S Ramji, Dr RK Puri and Dr Piyush Gupta. Now, eight years later, Dr Piyush Gupta and his able editorial team have completely updated and revised version with several new chapters and sections using the same multidisciplinary approach that has been the hallmark of success of the previous models.

In addition to providing a practical resource containing the core science of pediatric and neonatal emergencies principles, it is designed to serve as:

1. A companion resource for the practicing pediatrician;
2. A valuable clinical resource for the generalist; and
3. An interdisciplinary document that recognizes both the common body of knowledge and the unique skills that each member of the multidisciplinary team possesses.

All pediatricians, neonatologists and especially intensivists require a proper knowledge of pediatric and neonatal emergencies, which forms our target audience. It has covered various topics, which are of relevance in our day-to-day practice and also for the postgraduates very effectively and in detailed descriptions.

Each chapter contains evidence-based background information emphasizing core science, intended for the professional who already possesses a basic understanding of the basic principles. The fourth edition reflects new guidelines that have evolved in various disciplines, and benefits from a new formal definition along with the closure of several gaps pointed out by clinicians and reviewers. The flow of information has improved tremendously.

It is my hope and expectation that this book will provide an enhanced learning experience and referenced resource for all health professionals caring for infants and children, leading to improved patient care.

Bakul Jayant Parekh
President, Indian Academy of Pediatrics 2020

Preface to the Fourth Edition

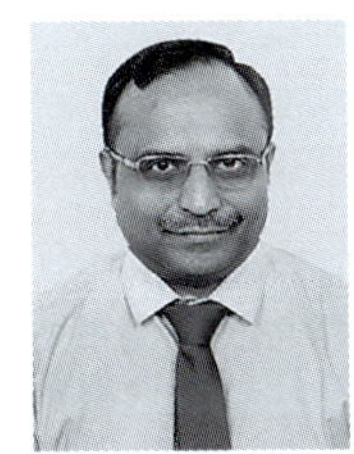

We are delighted to present this completely revised fourth edition of *Principles of Pediatric and Neonatal Emergencies*, a flagship publication of Indian Pediatrics. We hope that this treatise will cater to the needs of not only general pediatricians and neonatologists, but also of all physicians involved in immediate care of children with acute illnesses. For the first time, the book has a pleasing color format with high quality paper, which will result in better visual appeal and understanding. With its focus on management of acute illnesses in emergency settings, especially in low- and middle-income settings, the book will be highly relevant to the needs of pediatricians working in developing countries.

This book continues to have the privilege of scholarly writings from illustrious authors, across the country. In the last decade, there have been major developments in various pediatric subspecialties, which have now become integral part of the broad specialty of Pediatrics. With several pediatric subspecialty courses and fellowship programs running in country, we have taken care to involve several authors who are well trained and experienced in these subspecialties, simultaneously retaining the simplicity of the presentation for benefit of general pediatricians. We express our gratitude for all old and new authors for their valuable contribution to this edition. Most chapters have been completely rewritten, incorporating latest consensus guidelines of management by various academic bodies and incorporating flowcharts and key points. The emphasis continues to be on initial management of common and important emergencies affecting children. Detailed discussions on etiology and pathophysiology have been avoided.

We hope that this textbook shall be extremely valuable for pediatricians, physicians, resident doctors and other trainees, and will be an essential part of shelf in all pediatric emergency units. As before, all the royalties generated from the sale of the book shall pass onto the journal *Indian Pediatrics.*

We are grateful to M/s Jaypee Brothers Medical Publishers (P) Ltd., New Delhi, India for their meticulous typesetting, heeding to all our requests, and expeditious publication.

Dheeraj Shah
Editor-in-Chief, Indian Pediatrics (2014–2019)
on behalf of the Editorial Team of the Book

Preface to the First Edition

For the practitioners of pediatric care, emergencies in children and neonates are an inescapable fact in their daily routine. Better understanding of pathophysiology and drug metabolism and availability of newer investigative and diagnostic facilities have led to the creation of new frontiers in this important subject. Prompt recognition and appropriate management of these emergencies make the difference between life and death. A variety of traditional western textbooks provide information on this topic. However, this updated knowledge is often not relevant for the developing world situation.

Inspired by the success of its earlier venture titled *Pediatric and Neonatal Emergencies,* Indian Pediatrics—the official journal of the Indian Academy of Pediatrics, took up the formidable challenge of providing comprehensive state-of-the-art information on the subject which would also be pertinent in the Indian milieu. The present publication has been extensively updated and enlarged from the earlier experiment, which now appears like a distant cousin. Guidelines have also been incorporated for organization of pediatric intensive care units.

We are indebted to the group of distinguished contributors who promptly responded to our call, despite constraints of their busy schedules.

This volume is intended for the pediatricians and physicians sharing initial contact with emergencies in children and neonates as well as those responsible for the subsequent critical and intensive care. Postgraduate students should find it of particular help. The book should also prove invaluable for all current and intended pediatric emergency care units.

The editors share of financial benefits from the royalties would accrue to the Indian Pediatrics in an attempt to make the journal self-sufficient. We are grateful to the publishers for ensuring the high quality of the book as well as its expeditious publication.

This volume is dedicated to the memory of late Dr Man Mohan, an active associate in the earlier venture.

HPS Sachdev
RK Puri
A Bagga
P Choudhury

New Delhi
February, 1994

Contents

SECTION 3 Pediatric Medical Emergencies

Section Editors: *Rakesh Lodha, Arvind Bagga, Jaya Shankar Kaushik*
Dheeraj Shah, Pooja Dewan, Piyush Gupta

SECTION 4 Environmental Problems

Section Editor: *Dheeraj Shah*

SECTION 5 Toxicological Emergencies

Section Editor: *Rakesh Lodha*

SECTION 6 Neonatal Emergencies

Section Editor: *Siddarth Ramji*

SECTION 7 Pediatric Surgical Emergencies

Section Editor: Piyush Gupta

SECTION 8 Emergency Procedures

Section Editor: *Jaya Shankar Kaushik*

Annexures

Section Editor: *Piyush Gupta*

SECTION 1

Organization of Emergency Department

Section Editor: *Krishan Chugh*

CHAPTER

1

Approach to Child in Emergency Department

Krishan Chugh, Sonali Ghosh

PEDIATRICIAN'S CONTACT WITH THE SICK CHILD

The anxious family members bring children to the physician as soon as they perceive that the child has a serious illness or injury. No matter where the pediatrician is, the responsibilities go far beyond just providing the immediate medical attention to the sick child. Many a times, the family is totally unaware about the illness of the child or its true seriousness because the child may only be crying inconsolably or conversely be very lethargic. The infant may not be able to communicate at all to the parents and their anxiety, and often guilt, create a situation whereby the "family is the patient" and not just the child. At such a time the pediatrician has to give a look of confidence and competence while simultaneously showing understanding and empathy. Hence, the importance of initial encounter of the pediatrician with the sick child and his family cannot be overemphasized.

The pediatrician has to understand the anxieties and fears of sick children and their families when they come to him (**Table 1**). The fears of the parents and the family may be different from that of the child. He has to formulate an approach to the child and the family taking into consideration those factors within the limits of the time and facilities available. The following basic principles facilitate the examination and treatment of the sick children:[1,2]

1. Remain calm and confident.
2. Establish rapport with the parent and the child.
3. Be direct and honest.
4. Do not separate the parent and the child.
5. Make as many observations as possible without touching the child.
6. Be flexible in the order and method of examination. It is not absolutely necessary to examine the child in the order taught in undergraduate teaching days. The information gathered in any practical way can later on be synthesized into a systematic outline.
7. Examination that produces pain or discomfort should be performed last of all, e.g. examination of throat with a spatula or examination of ears.
8. Keep the child and caretaker informed.
9. Be kind and provide feedback and reassurance. When applying these principles to an Indian context, the family scenario of "elders" accompanying the child

Table 1: Fears of the family and the child

Fears of the family
1. Fear of death of the child
2. Fear of serious illness
3. Fear of incurable illness
4. Fear of the unknown: What next?
5. Fear of separation of child for examination/procedure/treatment
6. Fear of unknown and possibly not fully competent staff caring for the child
7. Fear of unfamiliar environment
8. Fear of machines/instruments
9. Fear of being told "sickness is because of your negligence"
10. Fear of economic loss because of child's illness
Fears of the child (are age dependent)
1. Stranger anxiety
2. Separation from parents
3. Pain
4. Fear of the unknown
5. Fear of unfamiliar environment

must be taken into account. It must be remembered that often they and not the parents of the child are decision makers. Similarly, the importance of an individual who spends maximum time with the child as a caregiver should not be forgotten when eliciting a history.

AGE-RELATED APPROACH

Optimum physical examination of an infant or child requires his cooperation. All efforts should be made to gain the confidence and trust of the child so that he is not struggling during the examination. The few extra minutes required for this purpose may not be available in a critically ill patient in whom measures for resuscitation must be instituted immediately.[3]

While every pediatrician develops his own methods and "tricks" for overcoming the initial resistance of the child, some general recommendations can be made. These techniques are based on an understanding of the age-related fears and the important developmental issues at that age. This developmental approach to pediatric emergency patient (**Table 2**) has been found quite useful.

Pre-school children are generally the most difficult patients. Their fears of separation and pain are particularly strong. However, they can be won over by encouraging fantasy, play and participation in examination. Simple explanation of the procedure being performed is helpful. School age children want to participate in their own care. Thus, they should be given choices. For example, when auscultating chest, the child may be asked whether he would prefer examination lying down or sitting. Each step must be explained to them and then their cooperation can be sought more easily.

In contrast to these age groups, the two extremes of pediatric age groups are easier to examine. For neonates, a comfortable environment and warm hand are all that is required. Over the next few months the infants can be engaged by sounds produced by the examiner or some bright colored objects or toys shown to them. Similarly, adolescents do not offer any difficulty in examination provided they are assured of confidentiality and autonomy. Respect for their privacy must be fully honored. If the pediatrician's gender is not same as that of the adolescent, it may be a good idea to have a paraclinical worker or a colleague of the adolescent patient's gender to be inside the examination room. Choice of having the parents inside should be left to the adolescent patient.

At all other ages, it is preferable to have the parents/caregivers around when the patient is being examined. In fact, as much of the examination as possible should be performed with the child in the mother's custody. At times it may become necessary to examine a restless child when being given breast feed. For this, it is our duty to provide privacy to the mother.

COMPLETE PHYSICAL EXAMINATION

The importance of a complete head to toe examination in the emergency room must be appreciated by all those working there (**Table 3**). This is true even when an obvious diagnosis has been made and the patient is apparently improving on the immediate treatment provided. For example, a toddler has been brought for high fever and irritability. On examination, clear evidence of upper respiratory tract infection is found. Antipyretics (which also have analgesic effects) are given along with tepid

Table 2: Development approach in pediatric emergency

Age	*Important development issues*	*Fears*	*Useful techniques*
Infancy 0–1	Minimal language: Feel an extension of parents, sensitive to physical environment	Stranger anxiety	Keep parents in sight and touch, avoid hunger, use warm hands, keep room warm
Toddler 1–3	Receptive language more advanced than expressive, see themselves as individuals, assertive will	Brief separation, pain	Maintain verbal communication, examine in parent's lap, allow some choices when possible
Pre-school 3–5	Excellent expressive skills for thoughts and feelings, rich fantasy life, magical thinking, strong concept of self	Long separation, pain	Allow expression, encourage fantasy and play, encourage participation in care
School age 5–10	Fully developed language, understanding of body structure and function, able to reason and compromise experience with self control, incomplete understanding of death	Disfigurement, loss of function, death	Explain procedures, explain pathophysiology and treatment, project positive outcome, stress child's ability to master situation, respect physical modesty
Adolescence 10–19	Self–determination decision making, peer group important, realistic view of death	Loss of autonomy, loss of peer acceptance, death	Allow choices and control stress, acceptance by peers, respect autonomy, stress confidentiality

Table 3: Commonly missed areas in a complete examination

Area	*Examples*
1. Ear: otoscopic examination	Otitis media
2. Genitalia	Torsion testis
3. Anal region	Anal fissure
4. Pupils	Poisoning
5. Blood pressure	Shock, hypertensive crisis
6. Femoral pulses	Coarctation of aorta
7. Skin covered by undergarments	Petechiae

sponging. Child's fever comes down. He is not restless anymore and is sent home. Such a child is likely to return if the associated acute otitis media was missed.

Following the ABCDENTTT checklist (**Box 1**), pediatric patient can be assessed from head to toe. Unclothing the child is an important step to facilitate examination of the covered areas, especially the genitalia. Again, for such an examination, especially for adolescents, adequate privacy must be provided.

There is a general tendency of the parents to over clothe their young children, more so during winter months. This could hinder optimum examination of even the chest or the abdomen.

A 6-month-old child was brought to the casualty department for fever and excessive crying. He had "neck-stiffness". All arrangements for performing a lumbar puncture were made. Child's high-neck pullover was removed for doing the lumbar puncture and he suddenly stopped crying and became cheerful. Gone was his "neck-stiffness."

Many a times, a complete examination is not possible during the first attempt. The child may be uncooperative or he may be having a problem that needs immediate attention, e.g. a convulsing child. Obviously, the pediatrician must return to this patient at another appropriate occasion to complete the examination.

There are other occasions when a complete examination has indeed been performed but a re-check after a few minutes may be necessary. For example, a child may have apparent tachycardia with fever raising doubts about say myocarditis. One hour later when his fever has been controlled tachycardia may settle down completely. Thus, repeated examinations may be required in some children to get the complete picture.

Box 1: ABCDENTTT checklist for head to toe examination

General	Behavior- normal/lively/irritable/lethargic
Airway	Stridor Noisy breathing Drooling
Breathing	Recession/accessory muscles Respiratory rate Auscultation Oxygen saturations
Circulation	Peripheral temperature and color Pulse Capillary refill Blood pressure
Disability	Alert Voice only Pain only Unresponsive
ENT	Ears and throat
Temperature	Tympanic or axillary
Tummy	Abdominal examination

IDENTIFICATION OF AN ACUTELY ILL CHILD

Experience as well as statistics show that a large number of patients coming to the emergency department do not have any life-threatening problem. Emergency departments (EDs) are for sick or injured children and not necessarily for dying children. However, at times ED personnel may fail to respond with appropriate speed and urgency when a patient requiring say cardiopulmonary resuscitation, arrives in the ED. Thus, it is important to train all those involved in the care of acutely sick children to recognize life-threatening situations. A "**Recognition Bundle**" can be created by the institution and followed for early recognition resulting in improved outcomes. There should also be "**Resuscitation Bundle**", "**Stabilization Bundle**" and finally a "**Performance Bundle**" to audit the performance of the laid down Bundle interventions and make appropriate corrections to overcome the barriers in implementation.[4]

The Pediatric Assessment Triangle (PAT) is an important aspect during initial assessment of a sick child. It is used by PALS, APLS and many other courses and has been proven to identify those patients having more serious illness.[5] The triangle is simplified approach for evaluation of a child. Its basis is visual and auditory clues. There are three arms of the triangle; each of these elements is further divided into certain parameters. By assessing these parameters, the healthcare providers can identify the underlying physiological abnormality of the child.

1. Appearance
   - Look
   - Consolability
   - Interactivity
   - Tone
   - Speech/cry
2. Breathing effort
   - Retractions
   - Nasal flaring
   - Breath sounds abnormality
   - Abnormal positioning
3. Circulation
   - Pallor
   - Cyanosis
   - Bleeding
   - Skin mottling.

These abnormalities help the healthcare provider to categorize the sick child into: shock—compensated or decompensated, cardiopulmonary arrest, respiratory distress, respiratory failure, primary brain dysfunction, or other systemic abnormality. The measures of resuscitation are instituted accordingly.

Observe the general behavior and color. It can be assessed even from a distance. Record what the child is actually doing. Respiratory rate can be counted. Look for any rash, recession or nasal flaring before touching the child. Listen for abnormal respiratory sounds such as audible wheeze, stridor or grunting.

Change in behavior of the child or his response to stimuli given by the parents or the examiner during an examination and observation period can provide important clues to the overall degree of sickness of the child. Consolability of a child who is irritable is an example. If the child who was crying and fussing as his first response on contact with a doctor can be quietened down and made to submit to an examination would indicate a normal behavioral response and would generally go against a serious illness demanding immediate intervention. However, it must be remembered that the expected response would vary according to the age of the child. Certain observational scales have been developed and validated to identify serious illness in febrile children. One such scale[6] takes six items into consideration, viz., quality of cry, reaction to parent stimulation, variation in state of wakefulness and sleep, color, hydration and response to social overtures.

Another set of criteria[7] has been found to be useful in evaluating children with fever and petechiae. These criteria were: irritability (inconsolable crying or screaming), lethargy (as determined subjectively by the caregiver, nursing or medical staff), shock (capillary refill time greater than 2 seconds and/or hypotension),abnormality of the peripheral blood white cells count (<5,000 or >15,000 per cu mm) and elevation of C-reactive protein (CRP) (>5 mg/L). These criteria were labeled as "ILL- criteria" (irritability, lethargy, low capillary refill) and were found to have a high sensitivity for identifying children with positive blood cultures. Sensitivity was good even when CRP was not included. It has been shown in several earlier studies that taken individually these criteria have limitations.[8-10]

Children can deteriorate very quickly. Raised heart rate and respiratory rate should raise an alarm. So one should be familiar with the values at different ages (**Table 4**). Pulse oximeters has been found to be very useful in assessing an acutely ill child.

Age considerations in assessing a child with fever are also important. Thus, febrile young infants less than 3 months age are more likely to have serious illness than an older child. Although it is well known that the common viral fever can also cause high fever, generally the risk of bacteremia increases as the degree of fever increases, but even at >40°C the risk is only 7%.[11]

CPR IN EMERGENCY DEPARTMENT

Cardiopulmonary resuscitation (CPR) performed in a child who has already had cardiac arrest is a labor intensive, tension producing procedure that more often than not is a frustrating exercise. Chances of intact survival are abysmally low.[11-15] Thus, it is very important to recognize life-threatening illness immediately. A focused history and quick examination should be done. It is better to have a structured approach. The standard alphabetical order of A for airway, B for breathing and C for circulation is the most appropriate method. These are followed by D for disability prevention and E for exposure (**Table 5**).

THE DEATH OF A CHILD IN THE EMERGENCY DEPARTMENT

After the death of a child, emergency physician again plays an important role. The transition is from treating the now dead patient to a caregiver for the other surviving patients in the emergency waiting his attention. Its success depends on many factors: number of patients in emergency who require attention, skill and experience of the physician, notification of death to proper authorities in case of child maltreatment or violent death, discussion of postmortem

Table 4: Respiratory rate and heart rate at different ages

Age (years)	*Respiratory rate (breaths per minute)*	*Heart rate (beats per minute)*	*Systolic BP (mm Hg)*
Neonate	60	160	70
<1	35–45	110–160	75
1–5	25–35	95–140	80–90
5–12	20–25	80–120	90–110
>12	15–20	60–110	100–120

Table 5: Pediatric primary survey and resuscitation measures

A. Airway/Cervical Spine Control
- Assess airway patency
  - If patient conscious—maintain position of comfort
  - If compromised—position, suction oral airway
  - If unmaintainable—oral endotracheal intubation
- Maintain cervical spine in neutral position with manual immobilization, if head/facial trauma or high- risk injury

B. Breathing
- Assess respiratory rate, color, work of breathing, mental status
- If respiratory effort adequate—administer high-flow supplemental oxygen
- If respiratory effort inadequate—bag-valve-mask ventilation with 100% oxygen, naso/orogastric tube, consider endotracheal intubation or LMA

C. Circulation/Hemorrhage Control
- Assess heart rate, pulse quality, color, skin signs, mental status
- If perfusion adequate—apply cardiac monitor, establish IV access, direct pressure to bleeding sites
- If signs of shock—establish vascular access (IV/IO), isotonic fluid bolus, baseline laboratory studies, cardiac monitor, urinary catheter
- If ongoing hemorrhage suspected and continued signs of shock—blood transfusion and surgical consultation

D. Disability (Neurologic Status)
- Assess pupillary function, mental status (AVPU)
- If decreased level of consciousness—reassess and optimize oxygenation, ventilation, circulation
- If increased ICP suspected—elevate head of bed, consider mild hyperventilation, neurosurgical consultation

E. Exposure
- Remove clothing for complete evaluation. Prevent heat loss with blankets, heat lamps, radiant warmer

(AVPU: alertness, response to voice, response to pain, unresponsive; ICP: intracranial pressure; IO: intraosseous; IV: intravenous)

examination or raising request for organ donation. If possible during resuscitation, the physician should speak to the family and prepare them for eventualities.[16] If the family arrives after the patient has been pronounced dead, the physician should inform them compassionately about the child's death. He may also give details of the resuscitative efforts that were done. No conflicting information should be given to the family by the emergency care team.

Family Presence in Resuscitations

Family presence in the ED has been defined as "the presence of family in the patient care area, in a location that affords visual or physical contact with the patient during invasive procedures or resuscitation events". A study of family presence during resuscitation attempts showed that 67% thought their presence was a benefit to the patient, 76% believed their grieving was made easier, 97% would choose to witness it again, and 100% felt confident that everything possible had been done to save their family member.[17] The joint policy statement from the AAP, ACEP and ENA recommends that all EDs caring for children should have a written policy regarding family presence.[18,19] Some healthcare providers may feel uneasy when family members are around. ED staff should give option to the family if they want to be present or not.

Notification of Death

Before declaring the death of a child, a physician should introduce himself to the family members. He should try to be with the family. Also, some support personnel should be accompanying. The physician should prepare himself what needs to be communicated before breaking the bad news. Death should be clearly communicated to the family avoiding euphemisms like "passed on", "didn't make it" or "is with God now" as these may be misunderstood. Avoid language that sounds harsh or creates confusion in the family members or may create suspicion regarding the credibility of medical staff. Inclusion of the word "death" during the conversation at this stage is recommended for unambiguously communicating what has happened.

If the child is alive on arrival in the ED, but is very sick, family should be updated about the patient's condition frequently. More importantly, if the child is expected to die, family should be counseled that resuscitative efforts are continued but the child is not expected to survive.[20] Allow grief response and facilitate grief. The physician can also give physical support (hold hands, touch the shoulder) to family members.

According to a survey,[21] the following family interventions after unexpected death of an infant were found useful:

1. Accept family's grief reactions openly.
2. Family should be given an opportunity to express their feelings.
3. Allow the family to hold or to be in the room alone with their dead infant.
4. Clarify misconceptions.
5. Provide as clear an explanation as possible for the cause of the death in a way that would minimize their guilt.
6. All help should be provided for transporting the dead body for the funeral.
7. Arrange a private place for the family to gather.

Individualized family-centered care during the death of a child is a priority and should be handled with compassion and tactfulness. Emergency physician can promote personal grieving and healing of the family of the dead child even as he continues to provide the best care to survivors.

KEY MESSAGES

- The pediatrician has to allay the anxiety of the parents and the sick child while taking care of the latter in an emergency room.
- A complete head to toe examination is a must even though the pediatrician is confident about his diagnosis.
- Age related approach for a child helps to build a rapport with the child.
- Emphasis should be on training all those involved in taking care of a sick child and also to recognize life-threatening situations.

REFERENCES

1. Seidel JS, Henderson DP. Approach to the pediatric patient in the emergency department. In: Barkin RM, editor. Pediatric Emergency Medicine: Concepts and Clinical Practice. St. Louis: Mosby; 1997. p. 1-7.
2. Friday JH, Henretig FM. Techniques for examining the fearful child. In: Fleisher GR, Ludwig S, editors. Textbook of Pediatric Emergency Medicine. Baltimore: William and Wilkins; 1993. p. 74-92.
3. Dacey MJ. Managing the unstable patient. The first ten minutes often set the course. Postgrad Med J. 1999;105:69-72.
4. American College of Critical Care Medicine. Clinical Practice Parameters for Hemodynamic Support of Pediatric and Neonatal Septic Shock. Crit Care Med. 2017;45:1061-93.
5. Fernandez A, Benito J, Mintegi S. Is this child sick? Usefulness of the Pediatric Assessment Triangle in emergency settings. Jornal de Pediatria (Versão em Português). 2017;93:60-7.
6. Mc Carthy PL, Shape MR, Spiesel SZ. Observation scales to identify serious illness in febrile children. Pediatrics. 1982;70: 802-11.
7. Brogan PA, Raffles A. The management of fever and petechiae: Making sense of rash decisions. Arch Dis Child. 2000;83:506-7.
8. Marzouk O, Bestwic K, Thomson AP, *et al.* Variation in serum C-reactive protein across the clinical spectrum of meningococcal disease. Acta Pediatr. 1993;82:729-33.
9. Kuppermann N, Malley R, Inkelis SH, *et al.* Clinical and hematological features do not reliably identify children with unsuspected meningococcal disease. Pediatrics. 1999;103: 20-2.
10. Polard AJ, DeMunter C, Nadel S, *et al.* Abandoning empirical antibiotics for febrile children. Lancet. 1997;350:811-22.
11. McCarthy PL. Evaluation of the sick child in office and clinic. In: Behrman RE, Kliegman RM, Janson HB, editors. Nelson's Textbook of Pediatrics. Philadelphia: WB Saunders Co; 2000. p. 228-31.
12. Lewis JK, Minter MG, Eshelman SJ, *et al.* Outcome of pediatric resuscitation. Ann Emerg Med. 1983;12:297-99.
13. O' Rourke PP. Outcome of children who are apneic and pulseless in the emergency room. Crit Care Med. 1986;14:466-8.
14. Zaritsky A. Selected concepts and controversies in pediatric cardiopulmonary resuscitation. Crit Care Clin. 1988;4:735-54.
15. Spandorfer PR, Alessandrini EA, Shaw KN, *et al.* Pediatric emergency medicine research: A critical evaluation. Pediatr Emerg Care. 2003;19:293-301.
16. Resuscitation Council (UK). Bereavement. In: Resuscitation Council UK, editor. Advanced Life Support Course Manual. London, United Kingdom: Resuscitation Council (UK); 1998.
17. Doyle CJ, Post H, Burney RE, *et al.* Family participation during resuscitation: An option. Ann Emerg Med. 1987;16:673-5.
18. O'Malley PJ, Brown K, Krug SE. Committee on Pediatric Emergency Medicine. Patient and family-centered care of children in the emergency department. Pediatrics. 2008;122.
19. American College of Emergency Physicians. Patient- and family-centered care and the role of the emergency physician providing care to a child in the emergency department [reaffirmed April 2012]. Irving, TX: American College of Emergency Physicians; 2006.
20. Boie ET, Moore BP, Brummett C, *et al.* Do parents want to be present during invasive procedures performed on their children in the emergency department? A survey of 400 parents. Ann Emerg Med. 1999;34:70-4.
21. Smialek Z. Observations on immediate reactions of families to sudden infant death. Pediatrics. 1978;62:160-5.

CHAPTER

2

Ethical and Legal Issues in Emergency Care

Krishan Chugh, Bilal Khan

ETHICS

Ethics has been defined as moral beliefs and rules about right and wrong. It is important to consider the ethical issues because values of patients, families, doctors, other health care professionals and those of the society as a whole have profound influence on the practice of pediatric emergency medicine.

Medical Ethics is based on Sound Principles

There are four fundamental principles of medical ethics:

1. *Beneficence (Do well)*: The care that the physician provides should benefit the patient.
2. *Non-maleficence (First do no harm)*: Under this principle the physician should ensure that his actions would not harm the patient.
3. *Respect autonomy*: All individuals are not alike. They may differ in their beliefs and respond differently to the same situation. Thus, the patient and his family should be allowed to decide what is good for them.
4. *Justice (Be just and fair)*: The physician should not deny or institute treatment on the basis of factors (e.g. paying capacity) other than the actual medical condition of the patient.

All attempts should be made by the physician to follow these principles at all stages of care in the pediatric emergency department. In order to properly care for patients, the emergency physician has an obligation to understand ethical principles and the reasoning process one must go through to resolve an ethical dilemma. Emergency physicians face such complex decisions on a routine basis. Ethical reasoning skills are obviously a core competence in emergency medicine, even if easy answers are elusive.[1]

The ethical dimensions of the jurisprudence in emergency medicine care system are founded on and integral to the principle of the "Right to Life and Dignity" enshrined in Article 21 of the Constitution of India.

In India, over past few years violations of patient's rights have escalated into a widespread phenomenon on account of the low political priority given to public health in policy and planning. There is a growing consensus at national and international level that all patients must enjoy certain basic rights. In other words, the patient is entitled to certain amount of protection to be ensured by physicians, healthcare providers and the State, which have been codified in various societies and countries in the form of Charters of Patient's Rights. In India, there are various legal provisions related to Patient's Rights which are scattered across different legal documents, e.g. The Constitution of India, Article 21; Indian Medical Council (Professional Conduct, Etiquette and Ethics) Regulations 2002; The Consumer Protection Act 1986; Drugs and Cosmetic Act 1940; Clinical Establishment Act 2010. At present Ministry of health and family welfare, Government of India is in the process of finalization of the draft of "Charters of Patient Rights" prepared by National Human Rights Commission which includes 17 provisions and is available at website of Ministry of Health and Family Welfare.[2]

CURRENT STATE OF HEALTH CARE IN INDIA

India is now the world's third largest economy in terms of its Gross National Income with the potential to develop more equitably. Despite years of strong economic growth and increased health spending by the Government in recent years the Government spending on healthcare in India is only 1.02% of GDP (2015-2016) and rest comes from the private sector (Total 4.02%).[3]

India does not have a centralized body which provides guidelines for training and operation of emergency medical services (EMS). Emergency medical services are fragmented and not accessible in many parts of the country. Most people do not know the number to call in case of an emergency; services such as Dial 108/102/1298 for Ambulances. Considering the constraints in the resources, we as physicians require a focused understanding of the principles of distributive justice and resource allocation and need to balance between appropriate public health interventions such as vaccination and ensuring access to primary care with the resource intensive idea of emergency and critical care.[4]

LEGAL RESPONSIBILITIES

Preserving life is an "absolute and non-negotiable" duty of medical professional under Article 21 of the Constitution of India. In the process of providing emergency medical service to a patient, pediatrician has to keep in mind his legal duties towards the patient. The basic principles are:[5]

1. Physician cannot refuse emergency treatment to a patient, irrespective of his cast, creed, geographical placement, ability to pay, etc. However for good reason, when a patient is suffering from an ailment which is not within the range of experience of the treating physician, it is necessary to arrange for transfer to another hospital or medical practitioner, who can stabilize the person and provide further medical treatment.[6] This is in contrast to the practice of medicine in his clinic in a non-emergency situation where the physician can choose his patients, say according to their capacity to pay his fee.
2. The physician may still be held responsible for not having provided the emergency treatment even when the patient (in pediatrics, the parents of the child patient) refused to be treated by him. The argument runs that the patient would not have refused treatment had he understood the seriousness of his illness. Thus, recording of vital signs and general condition remains the responsibility of the emergency department physician even if the patient is waiting for a senior doctor or his private doctor to arrive.
3. Patience and delicacy should characterize the physician. Confidences concerning individual or domestic life entrusted by patients to a physician and defects in the disposition or character of patients observed during medical attendance should never be revealed unless their revelation is required by the laws of the State, like:
    - In a court of law under orders of the Presiding Judge
    - In circumstances where there is a serious and identified risk to a specific person and/or community
    - Notifiable diseases. In case of communicable/notifiable diseases, concerned public health authorities should be informed immediately
4. The physician should neither exaggerate nor minimize the gravity of a patient's condition. He should ensure himself that the patient, his relatives or his responsible friends have such knowledge of the patient's condition as will serve the best interests of the patient and the family.
5. In case of serious illness and in doubtful or difficult conditions, the physician should request consultation, but under any circumstances such consultation should be justifiable and in the interest of the patient only and not for any other consideration.
6. Every physician should prescribe drugs with generic names legibly and preferably in capital letters and he/she shall ensure that there is a rational prescription and use of drugs.
7. When an individual brings a case against a physician, it is the responsibility of that individual (the plaintiff) to prove negligence, etc. by the physician (defendant).
8. It is the responsibility of the emergency physician to ensure that the patient gets definitive care after the emergency care. Thus if, the emergency physician terminates the physician-patient relationship without the patient's consent and without giving the patient sufficient opportunity to secure the services of another competent physician, it will be considered as a case of abandonment. This also applies to transfer of the patient from one emergency department to another.

TYPES OF LEGAL RISKS

Both civil and criminal cases may be brought against the emergency pediatrician. Civil suits generally are brought for procuring compensation for a death or disability caused during treatment. Criminal charges may be leveled against the physician for negligence resulting in death or disability. If found guilty, the physician may have to serve a term in jail.

The individual suing the physician has to first prove that the physician did not follow the "standard of care." This would amount to negligence. Then, it has to be established that this negligence was the cause of the injury or disability suffered by the patient.

LEGAL RISK FACTORS

Pediatricians who care for children requiring emergency treatment are at a greater risk for being dragged to the court by the family. This is because of several reasons:

1. Chance of death or permanent disability is more in children brought to the emergency department by virtue of greater seriousness of the illness.
2. The medical problems brought to the emergency physician are complex. Often, he is working under stress, may be for long hours and under inadequate conditions, e.g. too much noise and disturbance, too many serious patients to be looked after simultaneously, etc. These factors increase the chances of error.
3. There is no previous, ongoing patient-doctor relationship before the emergency encounter. Thus, the family may not have the same "faith" in the emergency pediatrician, which it has in the regular pediatrician. In fact, in general the specialty of emergency medicine and the emergency medical specialist is not well understood by our patients.[7]
4. The family members are under stress and they may have a guilt complex. They may feel responsible for their child's critical condition. This provokes them to retaliate and put the blame on the most obvious person across, i.e. the physician.
5. The parents may have waited for long before the physician could attend to them as he was looking after other seriously ill patients. The anger is directed towards the physician. Thus, it is important for the nurses and other paramedical staff to recognize a critically ill child as soon as he is brought to the emergency department or even a pediatrician's clinic so that he gets top priority.
6. The courts may allow large sum of money as compensation to the family taking into consideration the long years that the child may have lived. This fact may also induce the parents to proceed against the pediatrician in the court.

LEGAL AND ETHICAL ISSUES IN CONSENT

When a patient approaches a physician, consent for physical examination is implied, provided this does not harm the patient. Thus, when a child is brought to the emergency pediatrician, he goes ahead and performs a physical examination without getting a signed consent. A written consent, however, becomes necessary when the physician is going to perform a procedure or hospitalize the child. Generally, blanket consent is not considered sufficient legally, nor is it ethical. Thus "I am willing for the hospitalization and treatment, including diagnostic and therapeutic procedures on my child" is not a complete consent. These words did not name the procedure nor did they explain the risks involved. Insufficient information invalidates the consent.

From such discussions, concept of "informed consent" took birth. The quality of the consent given by the parents or guardian became the focus of attention. Patient's parents have to be regarded as informed consumers. An informed consent is expected to cover the following:

- Diagnosis
- Nature and purpose of proposed procedure or treatment
- Risks, side effects and consequence of the proposed procedure
- Reasonably available alternatives and their risks
- Expected outcome without the procedure.

Such a consent form would obviously be quite long. But, it should not contain any technical language and medical terms, which an ordinary person cannot understand. Further, an informed consent should be in the language that the patient's parents can understand.

Consent can be given/signed by any one of the parents and in their absence by the guardian. The guardian may be a relative, a neighbor, a teacher or the child's in-charge in the daycare center. However, it is essential that the person giving the consent should be an adult. Minors cannot give consent– neither for themselves nor for others.

In a life-threatening situation, the physician may not wait for a formal consent and may institute the essential measures immediately. In such a situation the pediatrician is more likely to be sued for withholding the life saving treatment rather than for providing them without parental consent.

An informed consent has four essential features: Competency, information, understanding and voluntariness.[8] Competency implies that the person giving consent has medical decisional capacity. Disagreement with the physician's decisions does not necessarily mean incompetency. Thus, a reasonably intelligent father who is not under the effect of alcohol/drugs, who refuses a lumbar puncture to "rule out" meningitis in a child with seizures and fever is not incompetent.

Once it is presumed that the parent is competent, his consent is based mainly on the information provided regarding the disease, procedures, risks, side effects and need of the procedure. The information may need to be presented repeatedly or even in an audiovisual form.[9]

It has been found that physicians generally overestimate the capability of their patients to fully understand the information provided.[10] It is the duty of the physician to be reasonably sure that the parent understands and comprehends the information provided to him regarding his child's treatment.

Finally, the consent should not be given under any direct or indirect pressure from the physician to accept the treatment that is the physician's favorite when other equally good alternatives exist. The parents should be given sufficient time to understand and digest the information provided. However, time may be a constraint in some acute emergencies.

ETHICAL AND LEGAL ISSUES IN TRAINING AND RESEARCH

Unique situations are encountered in the pediatric emergency department with regard to ethical conduct of research.[11] There are fears in the minds of many parents and relatives that their child is being made a subject of some experiment when being treated in a large hospital, especially, a teaching hospital. This indeed may be true. However, the important issue is somewhat different: Are the child's interests being harmed by being enrolled in the "study" or the "experiment" (in the parent's language). If the answer to this question is in the affirmative an ethical wrong is being done—the harm may be only financial. Thus, no patient can be denied a treatment or a procedure that is the "standard of care" in similar circumstances in other institutions. Yes, an additional mode of treatment may be given to some and denied to others. Here too, this treatment should be reasonably safe.

The senior doctors often encourage their junior colleagues to "practice" procedures in dead or dying patients. Endotracheal intubation is one such example. It is agreed by all that the newcomers have to be given "hands on training" and a recently dead patient provides such an opportunity. However, the sensitivities of the family should be taken into consideration even at this stage. It must been sure that they are not watching the "trials" by a new resident doctor on their child's dead body directly or through a window or a displaced curtain.

The issue of using a dying (but not dead) patient for a similar purpose is more complex. A new inexperienced resident doctor may be assigned the duty of inserting a central venous catheter in a child who is dying and has no reasonable chance of survival. Again, the sensitivities of the family should be respected and the procedure performed only under direct supervision of the experienced senior physician.

The emergence of technological innovation in medical education has the potential to address ethical dilemmas in the education of trainees and simultaneously improve how we train the next generation of physicians. These technological advances (virtual reality, simulation, and e-learning) have the potential of allowing trainees to become proficient in skills before performing them on patients.

Biomedical research involving children is also needed for the benefit of future generations of humanity. Research leads to advances in medical care which can potentially improve the health and quality of life of children. There are diseases which affect only children, for example, hyaline membrane disease, birth asphyxia, neonatal hyperbilirubinemia, extrahepatic biliary atresia, infantile spasms, infantile tremor syndrome, Kawasaki disease, etc. Such diseases have no adult counterparts and therefore, it is necessary to carry out research in children to advance our knowledge of these diseases. Additionally, even if the same disease affects both children and adults, the pathophysiology and responses to treatment in children may differ from those in adults. Hence, we cannot simply extrapolate the medications approved for adults to children. Some diseases such as nephrotic syndrome, hypertension and rheumatoid arthritis affect both adults and children, but the pathophysiological basis and clinical approach is very different in the two.

Indian Council of Medical Research (ICMR) has revised guidelines in 2017 for biomedical research in newborn and children. Adequate information about the research is given in simple and unambiguous language in a document known as the informed consent form to participant/parent/legally accepted representative (LAR). Research involving children in emergency situations should be carried out only when it is scientifically justified and cannot be carried out outside this setting; examples include research in resuscitation, life threatening emergencies, etc. All principles of ethical research need to be followed and there are no exceptions for obtaining consent. In emergency situations when no surrogate consents can be taken, as the parents/care givers/LAR may not be in a situation to give consent, once the child has been stabilized, a deferred/delayed consent is a must. In case the parents refuse the deferred consent, the child should not be included in the research, and no further research related procedures/data collection should be done from the patient.[12]

Ethically, it is agreed that training must occur and education must go on. Otherwise, after a period of time we would have no trained personnel at all. Benefits of an academic program are tremendous to the patient community also. But we must ensure that concerns of the family in this regard are adequately addressed.

ETHICAL AND LEGAL ISSUES IN CPR

Cardiopulmonary resuscitation (CPR) in a patient who has suffered cardiorespiratory arrest is a very difficult area from ethical and legal angles. Decisions must be made rapidly and often must be based on suboptimal levels of information available at the time.[13] When a child is "brought dead", i.e. heartbeats are not audible and there is no respiration, should the emergency pediatrician carry out CPR in every single case? The body may be cold, suggesting long delay; CPR is likely to be futile. However, the body may be cold because of exposure to cold environment or drowning in cold water. Next, should the treating physician ask almost whole of his team to come and participate in CPR even when there are more easily salvageable patients needing immediate attention in the emergency ward. Further, once CPR has been started, how long should it be continued if there is no response at all. And, what about the situation where momentarily an apparently perfusing cardiac rhythm appears repeatedly. Well, most studies show that continuation of CPR beyond 25 minutes is futile in such circumstances.[14]

During CPR or as it is being started it is advisable to keep the family informed as best as possible. There have been instances where parents have blamed the CPR for their child's death. A few minutes spent in explaining why and how of CPR by one of the medical staff members will virtually eliminate the chances of such an occurrence.

ETHICAL AND LEGAL ISSUES IN WITHHOLDING LIFE SUPPORT

Doctor is expected to "give life" and not "take it away". Hence, physicians are inclined to continue life support measures even when chance of survival is virtually zero. Law does not empower the physician to withhold or withdraw life support. However on specific occasion like a brain dead child, the question of withdrawing supporting devices to sustain cardiopulmonary function even after brain death shall be decided only by a team of doctors and not merely by the treating physician alone. A team of doctors shall declare withdrawal of support system and such team shall consist of the doctors in accordance with the provisions of the Transplantation of Human Organ Act, 1994.[5] Till this stage, the decisions to be made by the physician are based on clear enunciation. But, beyond this the lines get blurred. What should the answer be to the question of such a child's father: "Should I take the child home". Best way out is to discuss all the aspects with the family members, give them time to again think over the matter in the light of the discussion and again sit down with the family to help them understand that there is no such provision in Indian law.

ETHICAL AND LEGAL ISSUES IN DEATH

Organ transplant has raised several legal and ethical issues related to death in the hospital or to patients brought dead to the hospitals. In our country law is silent regarding withdrawal of life support in a patient who is brain dead. However, ethically it is considered fair. But, all attempts should be made to explain the circumstance to the parents and make them a part of the decision making.[15] Once they are convinced the subject of organ donation can be broached. Only when the parents are willing can the subject be discussed any further. It is generally agreed that physicians are not making sufficient efforts to get the parents of dying and dead children to donate the organs of their child.

HOSPITAL ETHICS COMMITTEES

Most large hospitals have their own ethics committees which help in providing guidelines about the "gray areas" of medical practice. The assumption is that the emergency physician by virtue of basic human nature and because of direct involvement in a particular situation may get carried away and make a biased decision. On the other hand a group of dispassionate but well-informed individuals who constitute the ethics committee can guide that individual through the difficult situations. Such committees develop consensus on contentious issues. In recent years their functions have been evaluated in USA. It has been observed that they have decreased the problem of undertreatment and replaced it by the problem of over treatment.[16,17]

THE MEDICAL RECORD

The case sheet, as the medical record is often called, is an important document for the treatment of the child in the emergency department as well as in the court of law, should a legal dispute arise. The record should have the name, address, father's name and the hospital number on each page. All entries should be dated and timed. The condition of a seriously ill child changes quite rapidly and the medical record should be able to reflect that clearly. Sweeping statements like on examination nothing abnormal diagnosed (O/E-NAD) in seriously ill child give an impression of being careless in both examining the child as well as recording. Some important positive as well as negative findings should always be recorded. The physician's notes should not be at variance with that of the nurse or of another physician/specialist. All major events during the patient's stay in the emergency department should be recorded with time and date clearly mentioned. In a busy emergency department it is acceptable to write a detailed note at periodic intervals in which all that has been observed and done is noted with time of each action and observation clearly recorded.

Every physician shall maintain the medical records pertaining to his/her indoor patients for a period of 3 years from the date of commencement of the treatment in a standard proforma laid down by the Medical Council of India and if any request is made for medical records either by the patients/authorized attendant or legal authorities involved, the same may be duly acknowledged and documents shall be issued within the period of 72 hours.

In the court of law, the battle is fought almost entirely on the basis of the entries made in the medical record. Hence, its legal importance cannot be overemphasized. It has been said that a good medical record is the physician's best defence. Indeed, the law suit may be filed several months or even years later and the physician may remember very little about the case. Even the plaintiff's lawyer is likely to look at the case record and then decide whether there are enough lacunae for him to offer a reasonable chance of success to his client. A complete, well documented record that convincingly gives the diagnosis and records actions which are appropriate for the diagnosis and the clinical condition of the patient suggests to the lawyer not to proceed any further.

No attempt should be made to "doctor"or "enhance", i.e. change, add or delete entries in the record at a later stage. The judges tend to take this seriously. The lawyers argue that only the guilty conscience would attempt to alter the record. Even at the time when physician was writing the record in the emergency department any "corrections" should be neatly made. The part/word to be deleted should be struck off by one single line only and no attempt should be made to completely conceal what was originally written.

KEY MESSAGES

- Follow the three D's carefully—duty, dialogue (communication with the patient's family) and documentation.
- Keep yourself informed about the legal aspects of medicine.
- Perform chart review with pre-established medical and legal criteria.
- Know how to contact the administrator and a lawyer 24 hours a day, 7 days a week.
- Know how to obtain a court order 24 hours a day 7 days a week or what to do if an order cannot be obtained.

REFERENCES

1. Geiderman JM. Ethics seminars: Consent and refusal in urban American emergency department: Two case studies. Acad Em Med. 2001;8:278-81.

2. Ministry of Health and Family Welfare. "Charters of patient rights". Available from: *http://www.mohfw.gov.in.* Accessed July 24, 2019.
3. Ministry of Health and Family Welfare. Situation analysis-Backdrop to the National Health Policy 2017. Available from: *http://www.mohfw.gov.in.* Accessed July 24, 2019.
4. Murthy S, Chugh K, Musa N, *et al.* Pediatric critical care in low-resource settings: A call to action. Front Pediatr. doi: 10.3389/fped.2019.00080
5. Medical Council of India. Indian Medical Council (professional conduct, etiquette and Ethics) Regulations, 2002 (amended up to 8th October 2016). Available from: *http://www.mciindia.org.* Accessed July 24, 2019.
6. Law Commission of India; 201st report, August 2006. Available from: *www.lawcommissionofindia.nic.in/.* Accessed July 24, 2019.
7. Olsen JC, Johnson BC, Brown AM, *et al.* Patient perceptions of the specialty of emergency medicine. Am J Emerg Med. 2000; 18:278-81.
8. Frader J, Thompson A. Ethical issues in the pediatric intensive care unit. Pediatric Clin N Am. 1994;41:1405-21.
9. Lidz CW, Appelbaum DS, Meisel A. Two models of implementing informed consent. Arch Intern Med. 1988;148:1385-7.
10. Meisel A, Roth LH. What we do and do not know about informed consent. JAMA. 1981;246:2473-4.
11. Fish SS. Research ethics in emergency medicine. Emerg Med Clin N Am. 1999;17:461-74.
12. ICMR. 2017. National ethical guidelines for biomedical research involving children. Available from: *http://www.icmr.nic.in.* Accessed July 24, 2019.
13. Macro CA. Ethical issues of resuscitation. Emerg Med Clin N Am. 1999;17:527-38.
14. Schindler MB, Bohn D, Cox PN, *et al.* Outcome of out of hospital cardiac or respiratory arrest in children. New Eng J Med. 1996;335:1473-9.
15. Farrell MM, Levin DL. Brain death in the pediatric patient: Historical, sociologic, medical, religious, cultural, legal and ethical considerations. Critical Care Med. 1993;21:1951-8.
16. Mahowald MB. Baby Doe Committee: A critical evaluation. Clin Perinatal. 1988;15:789-806.
17. Weisbard A. Defensive law: A new perspective of informed consent. Arch Int Med. 1986;146:860-4.

CHAPTER

3 Organization of Pediatric Emergency Services

Krishan Chugh, Manish Kori

Emergency medical service for children is an all-encompassing, multidisciplinary system that includes parents, primary care providers, prehospital care providers and transport system, community hospital care and tertiary care referral center emergency departments, and pediatric in-patient units including critical care facilities.[1]

Assessment of emergency medical care in New Delhi[2] and Chennai[3] in India confirmed the general impression that the organized prehospital care is scanty and that the development of emergency medicine is still in its early stages.[1]

CHALLENGES IN COMMON EMERGENCY ROOMS[4]

It is crucial that children receive the same level of care available to adults. Specific needs of children should be addressed. This can be achieved by simple measures like availability of dedicated equipment, coordination between pediatric and general emergency staff and provision of a lead physician for children. Other challenges important to care of children include-lack of facilities for mother and child; lack of hospital beds suitable for children; poor preparation for pediatric emergency conditions; insufficient equipment when needed; and availability of cross specialty services at odd hours.

Lack of well-organized pediatric emergency services has been shown to directly impact 24–48-hour mortality.[5] Organization of such comprehensive pediatric emergency services at a national level or community level is a task that requires planning, resources, manpower and political will. Many models are available from the western countries, which can be adopted for our country with suitable modifications. However, for the present, limitation of resources would not permit us to take any such exercise at a large scale. But an attempt can be made to interconnect and link the centers where such facilities are available with each other and with other smaller centers in the peripheral places so as to provide a better service to people within the given resources. Thus, large hospitals with well-equipped pediatric emergency departments can be encouraged to form linkages with the smaller centers as well as individual private practices within their area. Referral from them, especially during 'non-working hours' and nights can serve as the admission base of the larger hospital. This will be a welcome step for the large private sector hospitals whose pediatric departments rarely have a high bed occupancy ratio.

While the organization of pediatric emergency services at the national level will have to be done by the health administrators, all pediatricians have a role to play in the development of these services within their own institutions.

PEDIATRIC EMERGENCY SERVICE IN A GENERAL/PEDIATRIC HOSPITAL

The services to be provided by an emergency department (ED) should be planned according to the needs of the community that it proposes to serve. Thus, it is important to study the epidemiology of diseases in the area. The size of population is a determinant of the expected patient number. Sociocultural factors, customs and beliefs of the population should also be taken into consideration when planning a pediatric emergency department.[6] There are very few hospitals where services are provided exclusively to children. Such hospitals are the centers where an "ideal" pediatric emergency department can be set up. It can be safely assumed that pediatricians, who have adequate training in pediatrics, will manage medical services in such a hospital and its emergency department. However, that may not be enough. The medical personnel directly involved in the care of sick children should have a special training in pediatric emergency management and in pediatric advanced life support (PALS). Core knowledge for these can be obtained from standardized courses like PALS course of the American Heart Association or the APLS (Advanced Pediatric Life Support) course of the American Academy of Pediatrics and the American College of Emergency Physicians. These courses also provide an opportunity to practice the skills required in the emergency departments on manikins. Having acquired the core knowledge and the skills, these pediatricians can further improve their performance by an analysis of the management they provided when dealing with emergencies in their own department. These specialists should take recertification in such courses at recommended intervals to maintain their skills and be aware of the latest developments in this field.

Training of Personnel

While a dedicated team should continue to "man" the emergency department twenty-four hours, it is understandable that new resident doctors and postgraduate students will be added at regular intervals in such institutions. These students and residents should be fully supervised at least in the initial weeks of their posting in the ED. Ongoing educational sessions should be a regular feature in the department. They should be taught the skills like endotracheal intubation etc., within the first few days of their posting. Till they are reasonably well trained the senior, more skilled pediatricians should continue to perform the lifesaving procedures themselves.

Nurses are the most important personnel in any emergency department since they are involved in the care of sick children in the ED at all stages. Indeed, they may be the first ones to look at the sick child and start providing the care till the pediatrician arrives. Hence, it is equally important that they are well trained in important lifesaving procedures. They may not have the skills to do endotracheal intubation but they should certainly be able to clear the airway and maintain it clear by head tilt-chin lift or jaw-thrust maneuvers and perform the bag-valve mask ventilation. These should be taught to them and the knowledge and skills be renewed at frequent intervals.

However, more important is to identify an acutely ill child, especially the one with respiratory, cardiac or neurologic life-threatening problems. Recording of vital signs like pulse, respiration, blood pressure and temperature is done quite meticulously by all nurses. However, they are often not trained to react appropriately to abnormalities in these parameters. Again, some new nurses will come on their rotation/posting. They should be adequately supervised during their initial weeks in the ED, especially when dealing with life-threatening situations.

Besides the medical staff, other helping and non-clinical staff is on duty in the ED. They are often not well educated and have no training what-so-ever in medicine. They can also be trained to recognize some of the life-threatening situations. Sometimes, in a busy ED all the trained personnel may be busy looking after the sick children and there may be many more waiting. If in such a situation another new patient arrives who has a life-threatening disorder these helpers should be able to gauge the gravity of the situation to the extent that they can inform the pediatrician about it. American College of Critical Care Medicine in its recent guidelines[7] has encouraged all institutions to follow their own institution developed trigger tools to recognize septic shock at the earliest and definitely in the pre-designated time frame so as to start the appropriate resuscitative measures quickly and get better outcomes. The set of interventions used for this purpose have been named as "**Recognition Bundle**".

Needs of Children are Different

There are other important issues in the working of pediatric emergency department in general hospitals. As a rule in a general hospital, adult patient gets more importance than children do and the pediatric patient does not get the same quality of service as an adult visiting the emergency department does. Often there is a common emergency department of adult and children. This is quite natural for a general hospital.

However, the needs of children are different in the ED compared to adults.[8] Thus, the equipment, the training of medical and paramedical staff, etc., is very different. For these reasons, it has been recommended that there should be a designated area within the general ED for pediatric patients. Further at all times adequate staff with pediatric training should be available for pediatric patients (**Table 1**).[9] Since medical staff in the general ED can change often, it is advisable to have written policies and protocols for the care of pediatric patient.

PEDIATRIC EMERGENCY SERVICES IN THE CLINIC

The pediatrician's office/clinic/outpatient (OPD) is generally a lively place where not only sick children come for advice, but even normal cheerful children visit for their regular checks and immunizations. It appears an unlikely place where a critically ill child will come. However, this can happen occasionally. It is important to train staff at the reception even in a clinic to recognize a critically ill child so that the pediatrician can be informed immediately. The pediatrician also should not ignore the request by parents who insist on being attended early because their child is "very sick". One way can be for the pediatrician to send his nurse or go himself and have a quick look at that patient so that at least a life-threatening situation is not missed.

It is mandatory for the pediatrician to have adequate equipment and supplies of disposables and drugs for treatment of a child who is critically ill and requires immediate resuscitative measures (**Table 2**).[10] The responsibilities of the pediatrician in such a situation include providing CPR and other treatment. Further, he has to ensure safe transfer of such a child to a suitable treatment center.[11]

Table 1: Pediatric equipment guidelines for emergency department

The following supplies and equipment are recommended by the American College of Emergency Physicians for Pediatric Patients in a general emergency department (ED)	An emergency cart or other system to house supplies, equipment, and drugs for a designated pediatric resuscitation area should be available
Monitoring devices	*Medications*
Blood pressure cuffs (neonatal, infant, child, adult-arm, thigh) ECG monitor—defibrillation/cardioverter with pediatric and adult-sized paddles and hard copy recording capability	Activated charcoal Adenosine *Antidotes immediately available:* • Cyanide kit • Flumazenil • Methylene blue
End-tidal PCO_2 monitor and/or pediatric CO_2 detector otoscope/ophthalmoscope/stethoscope	• Naloxone
Pediatric monitor, pulse oximeter with pediatric adapter sphygmomanometer and Doppler ultrasound blood pressure devices	Antipyretics Atropine
Thermometer (hypothermia)	Barbiturates
Central venous pressure monitoring equipment	Benzodiazepines
Vascular access supplies and equipment Arm boards (infant, child, and adult sizes)	Beta-agonist (commonly albuterol) for inhalation
Blood gas kits	Beta-blockers
Butterfly needles (19–25 G)	Bretylium
Catheter-over-needle devices (16–24 G)	Calcium chloride
Central venous catheters (3–8 Fr)	Dextrose
Infusion pumps, drip or volumetric, with microinfusion capability, with appropriate tubing and connectors	Dexamethasone Dopamine Epinephrine (1:1,000 and 1:10,000)
Intra-osseous needles (16, 18 G)	Furosemide
IV administration sets and extension tubing	Glucagon
IV fluid/blood warmer	Hydrocortisone
IV solutions: In addition to standard solutions, the following should be readily available to the ED for the care of pediatric patients	Insulin Isoproterenol Lidocaine
D10W	Magnesium sulfate
D5W 0.2% NS	Mannitol
Umbilical vein catheters (feeding tubes size 5 Fr may be used)	Methylprednisolone Narcotics

Contd...

Contd...

Vascular access supplies utilizing the Seldinger technique	Neuromuscular blocking agents
Respiratory equipment and supplies	*Medications*
Bag-valve-mask resuscitator, self-inflating (child and adult)	• Succinylcholine • Pancuronium and/or vecuronium
Clear oxygen masks	Potassium chloride
Standard and non-rebreathing (neonatal, infant, child, adult)	Phenytoin Procainamide
Oral airways	Racemic epinephrine for inhalation
Sizes : 0,1,2,3,4,5	Sodium bicarbonate
Suction catheters	Verapamil
Sizes: 6, 8, 10, 12, 14, 16 Fr	Related supplies/equipment
Tracheostomy tubes Shiley tube sizes: 00, 0, 1, 2, 3, 4, 6	Medication chart, tape, or other system to assure ready access to information on proper per-kilogram dose for resuscitation drugs and equipment sizes
Endotracheal tubes	
Uncuffed sizes: 2.5, 3.0, 3.5, 4.0, 4.5, 5.0 mm Cuffed sizes: 5.5, 6.0, 6.5, 7.0, 7.5, 8.0-mm Stylets for endotracheal tubes (pediatric and adult)	
Laryngoscope handle (pediatric)	*Miscellaneous equipment*
Laryngoscope blades	
Curved: 2, 3	Infant scale and older child scale
Straight or Miller: 0, 1, 2, 3 Pediatric Magill forceps	Infant formulas, dextrose in water with various nipple sizes
Sizes: 12, 16, 20, 24, 28, 30 Fr Nasal cannulae (child and adult) NG tubes Sizes: 6, 8, 10, 12, 14, 16 Fr	Heating source, overhead warmer preferred
Medical photography capability	Tube thoracostomy and water seal drainage
Oral rehydrating solution, such as Pedialyte, Ricelyte	Thoracotomy tray with chest tubesq
	Sizes: 8–40 Fr
Pediatric restraining devices	
Specialized pediatric trays	Urinary catheterization Sizes: 5–12 Fr
Cricothyrotomy including needle cricothyrotomy Lumbar puncture	Venous cutdown
Newborn kit	*Fracture management devices*
Umbilical vessel cannulation supplies	Femur splint (child and adult)
Meconium aspirator	Semi-rigid neck collars (child and adult)
Obstetric pack	Spinal immobilization board
Peritoneal lavage	
Adapted from reference 10.	

Documentation of all that the pediatrician has observed and done is absolutely essential for optimum treatment to continue as well as for legal purposes.

PHYSICAL DESIGN OF EMERGENCY DEPARTMENT

When the hospital building is at a planning stage, the architect, administrators and a physician who is well informed about the needs and working of a pediatric emergency department should interact with each other. The area to be allocated to the ED would depend on the number of patients expected to visit the ED every day. The total area has to be divided into many smaller areas/ cubicles/rooms according to the services planned to be provided in the ED. Information which would assist in the planning of an emergency department include:

- Annual census and trends
- Average daily census with peak patient volumes
- Triage categories of patient presentations
- Admission/transfer rate, including the number of cases requiring monitoring
- Average length of stay
- Turnaround times for radiology and pathology
- Additional information which pertain to the role delineation of the department, i.e. trauma service, regional referral service.

Total Size

The total internal area of the emergency department, excluding observation ward and internal medical imaging area if present, should be at least 50 m^2/1000 yearly attendances or 145 m^2/1000 yearly admissions, whichever size is greater. The minimum size of a functional emergency department that can incorporate all of the major areas is 700 m^2. These figures are based upon access block being minimal. Emergency departments may take extended amounts of time from conception to completion, therefore allowances for future growth and development must be made in the design process.

Total Number of Treatment Areas

The total number of patient treatment areas should be at least 1/1100 yearly attendances or 1/400 yearly admissions,

Table 2: Pediatric emergency equipment in clinics

Respiratory equipment	*Monitoring*
Oxygen cylinder with flowmeter	Blood pressure cuffs—infant, child, adult
Oxygen masks—neonate, infant, child, adult size	Sphygmomanometer
Bag-valve-mask resuscitator, with reservoir	Cardiac monitor
Suction machine	Pulse oximeter with infant and pediatric probe
Yankauer suction tip	ECG monitor/defibrillator with pediatric paddles
Suction catheters-8F, 10F, 14F	*Cardiac arrest board*
Feeding tubes-5F, 8F	*Medication*
Laryngeal mask airway (LMA)	Resuscitation
Intubation equipment	Epinephrine—1:1,000, 1:10,000
Laryngoscope handle with	Atropine
Straight blade 0, 1, 2	Sodium bicarbonate - 4.2%, 8.4%
Straight or curved blade 2, 3	Glucose - 25% solution
Endotracheal tubes	Anticonvulsant
Uncuffed 3.0, 3.5, 4.0, 4.5, 5.0, 5.5 mm ID	Lorazepam, midazolam, diazepam
Cuffed 6.0, 7.0 mm ID	Phenobarbital, levetiracetam
Stylets—infant, adult	Antibiotics, parenteral
Disposable end-tidal CO_2 detector	Poisoning
Nebulizer	Ipecac
Fluid management	Activated charcoal
IV catheters, short, over the needle - 16, 18, 20, 22, 24 gauge	Respiratory/allergic
Butterfly needles - 21, 23, 25 gauge	Salbutamol for inhalation
IV boards, tape, povidone-iodine and alcohol swabs, tourniquet	Epinephrine - 1:1,000
Pediatric infusion set/volume control device	Methylprednisolone/prednisolone
Intraosseous needles—15–18 gauge	Diphenhydramine, parenteral
Isotonic fluids (normal saline and lactated Ringer solution and Albumin)	Miscellaneous
	Naloxone

whichever is greater in number. Areas such as procedure, plaster and interview rooms are not considered as treatment areas nor are holding bays or observation unit beds for admitted patients. The number of resuscitation areas should be no less than 1/15,000 yearly attendances or 1/5,000 yearly admissions and at least 1/2 of the total number of treatment areas should have physiological monitoring.

Functional Relationships

There are described in **Box 1**.

Bed spacing: In the acute treatment area, there should be at least 2.4 meters of clear floor space between beds. The minimum length should be 3 meters.

Lighting: It is essential that a high standard focused examination light is available in all treatment areas. Each examination light should have a power output of 30,000 lux, illuminate a field size of at least 150 mm and be of robust construction. Clinical care areas should have exposure to daylight wherever possible to minimize patient and staff disorientation. Lighting should conform to acceptable standards.

Sound control: Clinical care areas should be designed so as to minimize the transmission of sound between adjacent treatment areas and sound levels should conform to the World Health Organization guidelines. Distressed relatives/Interview rooms and selected offices should have a high level of sound control to ensure privacy.

Service Panels

Service panels should be minimally equipped as follows:

- *Resuscitation room* (for each patient space)
  - 3 × oxygen outlets
  - 2 × medical air outlets
  - 3 × suction outlets
  - 16 × GPOs in at least two separate panels
  - 1 × nitrous oxide outlet (optional)
  - 1 × scavenging unit.
- *Acute treatment bed*
  - 2 × oxygen outlets
  - 1 × medical air outlet
  - 2 × suction outlets
  - 8 × GPOs in two separate panels
  - 1 × nitrous oxide outlet (optional)
  - 1 × scavenging unit.
- *Procedure room/suture room/plaster room*
  - 2 × oxygen outlets
  - 1 × medical air outlet
  - 1 × suction outlets
  - 8 × GPOs in two separate panels
  - 1 × nitrous oxide outlet
  - 1 × scavenging unit.
- *Consultation room*
  - 1 × oxygen outlet
  - 1 × suction outlet
  - 4 × GPOs.
- *External service panels*
  - 3 × oxygen outlets
  - 2 × medical air outlets
  - 2 × suction outlets
  - 12 × GPOs in at least two separate panels
  - 1 × nitrous oxide outlet (optional)
  - 1 × scavenging unit.

Physiological Monitors

Each acute treatment area bed should have access to a physiological monitor. Central monitoring is recommended. Monitors should have printing and monitoring functions for ECG, NIBP, temperature, and SpO_2.

UTILIZATION OF SPACE

Space determinants revolve around the major functional areas of the department. These may be divided broadly into:

1. *Reception area*: All patients arriving in the ED should pass by the reception. The seriously ill patients should be carried/wheeled in to the ED directly without stopping

Box 1: Functional access to emergency department from other areas

Direct access	*Ready access*	*Access*
Ambulance Medical imaging Short stay unit	Car parking Helipad (if applicable) Coronary care unit Intensive care unit Operating rooms Pathology/Transfusion service Medical records	Inpatient wards Pharmacy Outpatients Mortuary

at the reception. One of the relatives can stop at the reception to make required records. This area should have appropriate registers for making manual entries as well as the computer to make electronic records.

2. A *waiting hall* for the patients who are waiting for their turn to be seen by the ED nurse and doctor should be located in between the reception and the nurse's desk. Another waiting or rest area is required to provide space for the relatives of children who are being looked after inside. We must remember that it is customary in our country for a child to be accompanied by several relatives, neighbors and friends when he is brought to the ED with a serious illness. These people are often worried, tired and even agitated. A suitable place for them to sit and relax is essential. The waiting area must be of a total size of at least 5.0 m^2/1000 yearly attendances in area, that includes seating, telephones, vending machines, display for literature, public toilets and circulation space. The waiting room should include one seat per 1000 yearly attendances.
3. The *patient area* should be divided into two distinct sections. One for children who are not seriously ill but need to be observed for next few hours, for example, a child with high fever or a child with diarrhea and vomiting who is being given oral rehydration solution (ORS). Indeed, if the number of patients with diarrhea and dehydration is high, a separate ward/unit (the diarrhea treatment unit) may be required.

   The second section of the patient area can be designated for those children who are seriously ill and require intensive treatment, for example, a child with hypovolemic shock who is being given intravenous fluid boluses. This area should be fitted with electronic monitors, at least the pulse oximeters. When a number of interventions are being performed on a critically ill child, a lot of space is required all around the child. This should be provided for. Similarly, a child who needs cardiopulmonary resuscitation (CPR) also requires extra working space. With all the emergency staff working around this patient, it is not a pleasant sight for the rest of the patients and their relatives in the ED. Hence, some privacy is required. Curtains and screens can be used.

   The patient area should be connected with the hospital wards and the pediatric intensive care unit (PICU) through a separate door so that the patients who are admitted to the hospital from the ED do not have to pass through the reception again.[12]
4. *Procedure room*: Separate room for procedures like lumbar puncture, tube thoracostomy, thoracentesis, abdominal paracentesis, bladder catheterization, suturing, etc. is essential. There should be adequate space around the patient's bed for the paramedical staff and the equipment required. It requires noise insulation and must be at least 2.0 m^2 in size.

   Minimal equipment and fittings include:
   - Service panel as above
   - Operating theater light suspended from the ceiling with minimum 80,000 lux
   - X-ray viewing box/digital imaging system
   - Monitoring equipment—NIBP, SpO_2, ECG with access to resuscitation equipment.
5. *Nebulization area*: Just as separate designated area is recommended for diarrhea treatment, an area where the child can sit with the mother for receiving nebulized medication is desirable.
6. Central oxygen and suction should be available in all areas, which are regularly used for patient care. In fact, even those areas, which are only seldom used for patient care, should have supply of central oxygen and suction.
7. Side lab and radiology are also desirable in the emergency department itself.
8. Nursing station and resident doctor's work area should be open areas from where they can observe all the patients in the emergency department. Retirement rooms should be provided for them, especially if they are expected to work for long hours. It must be remembered that tired, exhausted, stressed medical staff cannot be expected to make judgments correctly and quickly.
9. Amenities like telephone for the public should be available within or just outside the ED. A play area for children is also recommended by experts.
10. *Resuscitation room/bay*: This room is used for the resuscitation and treatment of critically ill or injured patients. It has the following requirements:
    - Minimum size for a single bed resuscitation room is 3.5 m^2 or 2.5 m^2 for each bed space if in a multibedded room (not including storage area).
    - Area to fit a specialized uninterrupted resuscitation bed.
    - Space to ensure 360° access to all parts of the patient for procedures.
    - Circulation space to allow movement of staff and equipment around the work area.

- Space for equipment, monitors, storage, wash up and disposal facilities.
- Appropriate lighting, equipment to hang IV fluids, etc.
- Maximum possible visual and auditory privacy for the occupants of the room and other patients and relatives.

11. *Acute treatment area*: This area is used for the management of patients with acute illnesses. The requirements are:
    - Area to fit a standard mobile bed.
    - Storage space for essential equipment, e.g. oxygen masks.
    - Space to allow monitoring equipment to be housed.
    - Minimum space between beds is 2.4 meters.
    - Each treatment area must be at least 12 m^2 in area.

COMPUTERS IN THE EMERGENCY DEPARTMENT

In this information age, computers are being used in all walks of life. They have invaded every area and department of the hospitals also. However, their application in patient care has not yet reached the optimum potential. The emergency department is an area where computers can be very helpful. Besides keeping records, accounts and transporting laboratory data ("the data nets") computers are a source of knowledge bank (a kind of medical library) within the ED ("the knowledge nets"). Thus, textbooks, rare medical conditions, etc. are available at the click of a mouse. The Internet makes much more information available almost at the bedside. The information is particularly useful when caring for children with poisoning. 'Computerized diagnostic referencing' is an application of computers that can provide real short cuts to difficult diagnostic problems. Software's are available which incorporate the latest knowledge in the medical field that can be applied to patient care directly. Computer is a tool that can help the pediatrician meet the expectations of the parents who think their emergency pediatrician is providing them the best and the latest in medical knowledge.

It has been suggested that in the setting of emergency, information needs to be delivered quickly to those who provide care. Thus, immediate information should be accessible within 15 seconds, further information within three minutes and a digest of some detail in around 10 minutes.[13] Further, this information should be "evidence based", informed by the most valid clinical research available. Some Internet sites use "critically appraised topics" (CATs) in a structured abstract form, which can be easily accessed without payment.[14]

SIMULATION BASED TRAINING IN PEDIATRIC EMERGENCY DEPARTMENTS

Skill development of residents and fellows in pediatric emergency scenario is a challenge. It is a well-accepted fact that safe and effective pediatric patient care requires properly trained care providers. Reduction in exposure to critical time sensitive procedures has been found in various pediatric emergency training programs.[15] This is even more important for crucial procedures like endotracheal intubation. In a retrospective review in an emergency department, success rate of first pass intubation was found to be as low as 52%.[16] Various reasons cited have been duty hour limitations, continuous strive to eliminate medical errors and reduction in total number of pediatric critical care events.[17]

To overcome these limitations, simulation based training can provide opportunities for skill development in a safe environment.[18] In a study in US, use of simulation in training of pediatric emergency fellows, most of the pediatric emergency fellowship program directors recognized the role of high-fidelity simulation in enhancing clinical exposure and help training in procedural skills.[19] Implementation of high-fidelity simulation along with debriefing helps trainees with targeted performance feedback.[20] In a survey of various pediatric emergency fellowship programs in US, frequent use of simulation in pediatric emergency medicine was found to enhance skills. The percentage of programs using simulation was increased as compared to previous studies. Simulation is being used to train in improving decision making, technical skills and communication. It is also being used to assess pediatric emergency medicine trainee competency and help improve procedural training and complex decision-making skills.[18] However, patient outcomes in real life cases and cost effectiveness remain to be proven.

QUALITY IMPROVEMENT IN PEDIATRIC EMERGENCY DEPARTMENT

Quality in health care has been historically defined as "the degree to which health services for individuals and populations increase the likelihood of desired health outcomes and are consistent with current professional knowledge".[21] WHO definition adds that "in order to achieve this, health care must be safe, effective, timely, efficient, equitable and people-centered".[22] Various challenges to assessing healthcare quality in children are attributed to their unique needs. Four specific areas of challenge identified in this regard are 1. Development, 2. Dependency, 3. Different epidemiology, 4. Demographics.[23] A systemic process was used to identify and develop evidence-based quality indicators for pediatric emergency conditions and the authors identified condition based specific quality indicators.[24]

It is understood that quality measures require significant resources and rely on updated electronic medical records. Retrieving quality measures in emergency departments which do not have full electronic medical record back-up is highly resource intensive as it relies on sampling and manual review of medical records.[25] It is believed that for continuous quality improvement in the future, focus must be on effective provider training, availability and effective utilization of resources and measurement of quality of healthcare delivery.[26]

SCORING SYSTEMS IN EMERGENCY DEPARTMENT

Although there are scoring systems like PRISM (pediatric risk of mortality), SOFA, qSOFA and PIM (Pediatric Index of Mortality); they are designed to be used in a Pediatric Intensive Care Unit setting and include physical as well as laboratory variables. Scoring systems more suited to the emergency department have been studied and proposed to facilitate early identification of severity of illness and appropriate management. The "TOPRS" score (temperature, oxygen saturation, pulse rate, respiratory rate, sensorium and seizures) was studied in the emergency department of a teaching hospital in northern India. The score consisted of only physical variables. Increase in the number of abnormal variables was associated with statistically significant increase in mortality.[27] The "CLARIPED" tool was assessed in Brazil for risk classification in pediatric emergencies.[28] Another score based on physical criteria- the SICK score (Signs of Inflammation in Children that Kill) has been used in resource limited settings. It is based on the physical variables of SIRS (Systemic Inflammatory Response Syndrome). This score has the advantage of being immediately applicable on arrival to emergency, not requiring laboratory results or specialized training for implementation.[29] The Pediatric Early Warning Score (PEWS) developed by Monaghan[30] has been studied in pediatric emergency departments. Mixed results have been obtained.[31]

REDUCING THE BURDEN IN EMERGENCY

To reduce wait times and emergency department length of stay, many emergency department front-end models have been described.[32,33] Front-end has been defined as the patient care processes from the time of patient's arrival in emergency department to the time an ED healthcare provider assumes formal responsibility for management. Suggested steps include immediate bedding, bedside registration, triage based case protocols, physician at triage, tracking systems, resource based triage systems, waiting room design enhancements, full/surge capacity protocols, time to evaluation guarantee and referral to next care center. Role of triage nurse ordering has been studied in improving emergency department quality parameters like length of stay, physician initial assessment, etc. It was found to reduce emergency department length of stay, particularly in patients suspected to have fractures. The applicability of this concept should be studied in pediatric emergency department scenario.[34]

COST OF EMERGENCY CARE

Pediatric emergency care is expensive to the state (in government run institutions) or to the individual family (in privately run institutions). In recent past costs of medical treatment, especially the emergency care has received a lot of attention in USA. Their answer has been "managed care". Managed care is defined as the delivery of health care with a focus on quality and cost efficiency and places importance on preventive care. Managed care aims at limiting services to "true emergencies" with follow-up directed at network care providers.[15] However, such networks do not exist in our country and we will have to find our own answers to cost problems.

Finally, in our efforts to provide the efficient, technology based, cost-effective services to pediatric emergency patients we must not forget the 'human-touch'. It is the lack of human touch because of poor communication that leads to dissatisfaction in the doctor-patient-family relationship.[35]

KEY MESSAGES

- Needs for pediatric critical care are very different from that of adults and, thus, critically ill children are best managed in a separate Emergency Department (ED) and PICU by personnel specially trained to manage such children.
- Though the setting up and running of pediatric emergency care facilities in developing countries is a difficult and challenging task, the very exigencies of developing countries necessitate such establishment.
- High incidence of infections, malnutrition, chronic diseases, etc. necessitates a robust pediatric emergency and intensive care infrastructure.

REFERENCES

1. Baker MD, Anwer JR. Prehospital care. In: Fleisher GR, Ludwig S, editors. Textbook of Pediatric Emergency Medicine. Baltimore: William and Wilkins; 1993. p. 74-92.
2. PoSaw LL, Aggarwal P, Bernstein SL. Emergency medicine in New Delhi area, India. Annals Emerg Med. 1998;32:609-15.
3. Alagappan K, Cherukuri K, Narang V, *et al.* Early development of emergency medicine in Chennai (Madras), India. Annals Emer Med. 1998;32:604-8.
4. International Federation for Emergency Medicine. 2012 International Standards of Care for Children in Emergency Departments. Available from: *https://www.ifem.cc/resources/ifem-policies-guidelines/*. Accessed 21 March 2019.
5. Molyneux E. Improving triage and emergency care for children reduces inpatient mortality in a resource-constrained setting. Bull WHO. 2006;2006:314-9.
6. Mellick LB, Asch SM. Pediatric emergency department environment. In: Barkin RM, editor. Pediatric Emergency Medicine: Concepts and Clinical Practice. St. Louis: Mosby; 1997. p. 8-14.
7. American College of Critical Care Medicine. Clinical practice parameters for hemodynamic support of pediatric and neonatal septic shock. Crit Care Med. 2017;45:1061-93.
8. Tsai A, Kallssen G. Epidemiology of pediatric prehospital care. Ann Emerg Care. 1987;16:284-91.
9. Brownstein DR, Rivara FP. Emergency medical services for children. In: Behrman RE, Kliegman RM, Jenson HB, editors. Nelson Textbook of Pediatrics. Philadelphia: WB Saunders Co.; 2000. p. 237-45.
10. American College of Emergency Physicians: Pediatric equipment guidelines. Ann Emerg Med. 1995;25:307-21.
11. Flores G, Weinstock DJ. The preparedness of pediatrician for emergency in the office. Arch Pediatr Adolesc Med. 1996;150: 249-51.
12. Recommendation. Consensus guidelines for pediatric intensive care unit in India. Indian Pediatr. 2002;39.1165-74.
13. Simon JE. Computerized diagnostic referencing in pediatric emergency medicine. Pediatric Clin N Am. 1992;39:1165-74.
14. Hodge Dee. Managed care and the pediatric emergency department. Pediatr Clin N Am. 1999;46:1329-40.
15. Chen E, Cho C, Shofer F, *et al.* Resident exposure to critical patients in a pediatric emergency department. Pediatr Emerg Care. 2007;23:774-8.
16. Kerrey B, Rinderknecht A, Geis G, *et al.* Rapid sequence intubation for pediatric emergency patients: Higher frequency of failed attempts and adverse effects found by video review. Annals Emerg Med. 2012;60:251-9.
17. Doughty C, Kessler D, Zuckerbraun N, *et al.* Simulation in pediatric emergency medicine fellowships. Pediatrics. 2015;136:e152-e8.
18. Barry Issenberg S, Mcgaghie W, Petrusa E, *et al.* Features and uses of high-fidelity medical simulations that lead to effective learning: A BEME systematic review. Medical Teacher. 2005;27:10-28.
19. Eppich W, Nypaver M, Mahajan P, *et al.* The role of high-fidelity simulation in training pediatric emergency medicine fellows in the United States and Canada. Pediat Emerg Care. 2013;29:1-7.
20. Anderson J, Aylor M, Leonard D. Instructional design dogma: Creating planned learning experiences in simulation. J Crit Care. 2008;23:595-602.
21. Lohr K, Schroeder S. A strategy for quality assurance in Medicare. New Engl J Med. 1990;322:707-12.
22. World Health Organization. 2019. What is Quality of Care and why is it important? Available from: *https://www.who.int/maternal_child_adolescent/topics/quality-of-care/definition/en/*. Accessed July 24, 2019.
23. Beal AC, Co JPT, Dougherty D. Quality measures for children's health care. Pediatrics. 2004;113 (Suppl. 1):199-209.
24. Stang A, Straus S, Crotts J, *et al.* Quality indicators for high acuity pediatric conditions. Pediatrics. 2013;132:752-62.
25. Borland M, Shepherd M. Quality in paediatric emergency medicine: Measurement and reporting. J Paediatr Child Health. 2016;52:131-6.
26. Macias CG. Quality improvement in pediatric emergency medicine. Acad Pediatr. 2013;13 (6 Suppl.):S61-8.
27. Bains HS, Soni RK. A simple clinical score "TORPS" to predict outcome in pediatric emergency department in a tertiary hospital in India. Iran J Pediatr. 2012;22:97-101.
28. Magalhães-Barbosa M, Prata-Barbosa A, Cunha A, *et al.* CLARIPED: A new tool for risk classification in pediatric emergencies. Rev Paul Pediatr. 2016;34:254-62.
29. Gupta M, Chakrabarty A, Halstead R, *et al.* Validation of "Signs of Inflammation in Children that Kill" (SICK) score for immediate non-invasive assessment of severity of illness. Italian J Pediatr. 2010;36:35.
30. Monaghan A. Detecting and managing deterioration in children. Paediatr Nurs. 2005;17:32-35.
31. Gold D, Mihalov L, Cohen D. Evaluating the Pediatric Early Warning Score (PEWS) system for admitted patients in the pediatric emergency department. Acad Emer Med. 2014;21: 1249-56.
32. Wiler J, Gentle C, Halfpenny J, *et al.* Optimizing emergency department front end operations. Annals Emer Med. 2010; 55:142-60.
33. Rowe B, Villa-Roel C, Guo X, *et al.* The role of triage nurse ordering on mitigating overcrowding in emergency departments: A systematic review. Acad Emer Med. 2011;18: 1349-57.
34. Chan T, Killeen J, Kelly D, *et al.* Impact of rapid entry and accelerated care at triage on reducing emergency department patient wait times, lengths of stay, and rate of left without being seen. Annals Emer Med. 2015;46:491-7.
35. Simpson M, Buchman R, Stewart M. Doctor-patient communication: The Toronto consensus statement. BMJ. 1991; 303:1385-8.

CHAPTER

4

Transport of a Sick Child

P Ramesh Menon, Tsering Sandup

INTRODUCTION

The standardized model of "transfer of a sick child" has a motto of "the right patient is taken at the right time, by the right people, to the right place by the right form of transport and receives the right care throughout". It is based on the "ACCEPT" approach [A-Assessment, C-Control, C-Communication, E-Evaluation, P-Preparation, Packaging, Pre-departure checks, T-Transport]. A brief framework including history and development is discussed here.

HISTORICAL BACKGROUND[1,2]

Centralization of critical care for the sickest patient including children in leading healthcare centers and intensive care units has become the norm in healthcare in the new millennium. This has led to the development of the science of time-critical transfer of a sick child by specialist-teams and related outcomes in the developed world with insurance-based healthcare services.

Military beginnings—Initially, the experience developed was in the transfer of sick and injured in the war for the military (during world wars); then terrorist attacks and civil unrest and strife became a major burden. The focus was on immediate stabilization and rapid evacuation of the critically injured enabling survival of immediate injury. These programs began to be applied to road/traffic accidents, cardiac and neurological emergencies and non-military accidents afterwards. Medical centers and disaster management units were established by the governments patterned after the military model and based on the war experiences. Such trauma centers started participating and establishing certification programs (e.g. ALSG-Advanced Life Support Group; www.alsg.org) and standards of care. Initial standards of care led to further research and refinement into the delivery of care during transfer within (intra-) and between (inter-) facilities. It is still an ongoing process with air-ambulances (fixed-wings or choppers) being pressed into service where time-critical transfers (like for organ (cardiac)-transplantation) have become standard practice and are being investigated for outcome improvement.

Outcome for adults, especially transport involving trauma and cardiac patients, is significantly improved by emergency transport systems. The same, when asked to respond to pediatric emergency transports have run into problems. Indications for transport of sick children (different from those of sick adults) and the support skills required therein have been the major determinants of the deficiency of transport of a sick child. Transport team members with infrequent exposure to critical sickness in babies and the difficulty in maintaining adequate pediatric skills without frequent application for team members have become reasons for a separate, dedicated pediatric transfer/transport teams with a similar flow of information, political and administrative support and guidelines as for sick adults (Neonatal Emergency Transport (**NET**) and Pediatric Emergency Transport (**PET**) .

STRUCTURE AND LEGISLATION

In established network of pediatric transport services (e.g. in the UK), the guiding principle of the structure of care delivery is that centralization of services at larger dedicated pediatric intensive care improves patient outcome for critical illness. A loco regional efficient **coordinating node** was the focal point of developing and unifying the services for critically ill children. The initial organic, understaffed unit-based and bed-dependent ad-hoc transfer services were improved in terms of structure, training and staff. Progressively, a network of 29 PICUs (www.picsociety.uk) has been reported by 2014. Updates including quality benchmarks and standardized checklists have been developed and published by them.[2] More than 5000 interfacility transfers between these centers, 92% being done by a specialist transport team with a consultant at the helm of affairs—these reports highlight the different models of regional services that have been developed. The defining feature of a coordinated service has come to be single point of telephonic contact activating the conference call between clinicians, a "ready to roll" transport, no anchoring on bed availability and digital recording of the process for review and quality improvement. The various guidelines by societies of pediatric service providers recommend development of local protocols for inter- and intrahospital transport of sick children for diagnostic and therapeutic indications.

For example, Guidelines on transfer of seriously ill children within the hospital should be in use. They should give clear instructions regarding the escort and equipments required for taking babies to specific destinations, e.g. imaging room.

Inter-hospital transfer guidelines: These should cover (a) category of sickness and age of child to be transferred; (b) composition and competencies of the personnel in the escort team; (c) logistic support; (d) drugs, equipment - restraint of children during transfer; and (e) monitoring during transfer. Most hospitals will need to transfer children, for example, for opinions, investigations and treatment. Guidelines should reflect local circumstances and should cover transfer of both stable and unstable children. The advice of the **pediatric critical care operational delivery network** and the Specialist Pediatric Transport Service for the local population may be helpful in developing local guidelines.

The Government of National Capital Territory of Delhi[3] has come up with its legislative framework of requirements for transport ambulances, which has essential equipment for basic life support and advanced life support. It gives details of the equipment and the medications and other logistic supports required including the space and its dimension for registering ambulances in the National Capital Region.

In the private setup of healthcare delivery and transport of sick infants, the categorization of patient transport ambulances into routine transfer (Type B), basic life support (Type C) and advanced life support (Type D) is practiced. However, it remains non-uniform across urban and rural areas of the country.

PEDIATRIC TRANSPORT TEAM

Evidence supports the enhanced safety and quality with specialist transport team(s) with a reduction in the rate of critical incidents, risk adjusted PICU mortality rate, and overall cost of care - actualizing the concept of an outreach for PICU services. The Pediatric Intensive Care Society (PICS) has set up national standards in UK requiring consultant cover for 24 hrs, pediatric specific training and certification, quality assurance of standard pediatric equipment, care of parents and referring facility education. Alternative accreditation standards (Commission on Accreditation of Medical Transport Systems; www.camts.org) are also available for ensuring safety and quality of transport environment. A brief outline about the two types of transport (intra- and interhospital) is discussed here.

Intrahospital Transport

This is usually undertaken for diagnostic evaluation and sometimes for surgical or intervention based therapy. The team, its constitution and knowledge, skill and competence matching is entirely on a case to case basis in resource-limited settings. There is insufficient evidence that a dedicated team improves outcomes significantly compared to even a nurse/nurse practitioner including the bedside care provider in settings where transfers are thought-through and are routine. There are primarily four concerns, which require written intensive care unit policies and procedures: communication, personnel, equipment, and monitoring.

Interhospital Transport

Patient outcomes are dependent on the competence of and equipment available to personnel within each referring and referral unit. When required services overwhelm available resources, a patient must be transferred to an another facility that has the required resources. Obviously, the benefits to the patient should exceed the risks of the transfer. A decision to transfer a patient is the responsibility of the attending physician at the referring institution.[4] In cases of neonatal interfacility transfers, the use of a specialized retrieval team has improved outcomes, in terms of enhanced survival. Significantly, more adverse events occurred when a nonspecialized team transported pediatric patients. These included airway issues, sudden cardiac and/or respiratory events requiring cardiopulmonary resuscitation, hypotension and loss of vascular access. Another study demonstrated a reduction in pediatric mortality rate from 23% to 9% when using specialized transport teams. Having dedicated transport teams especially for high-volume centers with interfacility transfers, improves availability and mobilization as well as response times. Impact of the presence of a physician in the physical transport is not defined yet. There is no scoring tool for the accurate prediction of transport morbidity. One method is to group all transfers based on occurrence of complications during transport. A successful transport team requires good leadership, with team members who demonstrate flexibility, independence, critical thinking, timely judgment and problem solving skills, together with interpersonal and communication skills and appropriate crisis resource management. Team health and safety are also of primary importance, and should be considered when determining the best performance model.[5]

The importance of Inter Professional Education (IPE) and practice is also being increasingly recognized as the most relevant model in terms of safety and quality. It breaks healthcare silos and improves team building. Appreciating discrete roles, responsibilities and intersections of care of a sick child is critical for effective team work and gaining time for critical transfers.

Legal Framework

The dynamic nature of care giving and transfer including physical transport is tested within the framework of the "Bolam test", legally. It says that "If a doctor reaches the standard given by a responsible body of medical opinion, he/she is not negligent". Therefore, it is clear that as long as the reasonable competence in resuscitation skills and inpatient safety matters is maintained, team members would be legally supported. The understanding is that there is no sudden shifts in responsibility for patient care, in the best interest of the child throughout the process. From referral to handover, the child remains the sole responsibility of the referring hospital team. Once the transport team has physically taken over the care of the child, it assumes responsibility of care. Similarly at the point of care at the receiving hospital. The legal responsibility of care of a sick child remains by the patient's bedside and travels with the patient.

APPROACH INCLUDING ACCEPT, REVIEW BASIS[6,7]

A 4-yr old child presents to a primary health center at 8:00 pm with alleged history of drinking the mosquito repellant and vomiting. Her mother informs the ED staff that she had a similar history just a month ago. Her consciousness progressively deteriorates in ED from A to P in AVPU scale The emergency trainee registrar calls the anesthetic trainee registrar who takes control of the airway and ventilation for the child. A CXR shows bilateral lung haziness and drop in SpO_2 *levels on room air as well as supplemental oxygen ventilation. Being a time-critical case, the team in ED decides to activate the ACCEPT approach*:

Assessment

The structured ABCD protocol has now been the safest checklist to be incorporated for assessment even for transport.

Airway: She is intubated by the Emergency Department Physician in view of the progressive neurological deterioration, with a 5.0 mm orotracheal tube taped securely at 13 cm at the lips. A CXR has been done to confirm the tip position.

Breathing: She is on a transport ventilator with $EtCO_2$ at 33 mm Hg.

Circulation: NIBP measures 92/50 mm Hg in the right upper limb in supine position with no signs of compromised perfusion. Two peripheral IV lines have been established.

Drugs/Disability/Diagnostics: Drug infusions are started. Pupils are equal in size and reacting to light when tested.

With respect to time-efficiency, the referring CHC (Community Health Center) supporting the PHC (Primary Health Center)decides to undertake the transfer to the tertiary center. Time-critical transfers, e.g. those requiring surgical procedures and other life-saving complex interventions are usually undertaken by the referring hospital. The team is decided from amongst the referring hospital staff, if one is not already designated and/or present.

Control

Overall control may change hands like baton in a relay race. Leadership is vital to stabilization and safe transfer. Initial stabilization by the ED physician may be followed by pediatric consultant who may subsequently hand over to the anesthetics or transport consultant. Shared or overlapping of care is usual; however, a written/printed checklist at each handover significantly reduces information loss and medical errors.

Communication

Safe transfer of a critically sick child involves multiple individuals working in teams across many sites. Poor quality of communication especially with multiple native languages for the team(s) is usually the reason for the system to fail and the child to suffer. Structured checklists (for communication) may decrease adverse events related to transport. It requires uniform computer interfaces across hospitals (e.g. GPACS for X-ray) so that the team can carry minimum amount of hard data related to the child's condition.

In the above example, the senior anesthetic consultant agrees to transfer the child by road ambulance. The shared care given by the ED physician and the pediatric consultant is formally handed over. The CXR and other images are sent across digitally to the center of care. The patient notes are updated and category (graded as per time-criticality) is escalated to "emergency transfer". Senior consultant second-on call agrees to provide anesthetic cover at the referring hospital.

Evaluation and Preparation

Appropriateness of transfer correlates to the condition of the child and the support at the referring hospital. Senior team members take a call on the time and nature of the transport for the child. Road ambulances are usually preferred for all time-critical transfers. When distances are more than 150 km or time to travel lesser distances may be inordinately long due to absence of a "green-channel" for fast transport, alternatives to road ambulances (air, water, etc.) may be options.

Packaging and Pre-departure Checks

Appropriate preparation and labeling of infusions, size and comfort of pediatric harnesses, transport trolleys and emergency medications, monitoring devices and transport ventilators are some of the specific time-consuming preparations, which determine the smoothness, and safety of transport of a sick child. The usual time consumed for resuscitating and stabilizing the child before transfer must be balanced against the delay in transfer to a better equipped PICU. However, it is clear that hasty transfers often escalate the cost to the patient and the system in terms of the adverse effects of a "quick retrieval".

Transport

A smooth transfer is critical besides time to maintain the physiology of the sick child and reducing the deterioration of resuscitation benefits. Bumpy maneuvering for as quick as possible transfers is to be avoided. Dramatizing the whole process (sirens, lights, screeching turns and repeated accelerations, etc.) only adds "stress (oofff)" to the entire team including the sick(er) infants and premature babies who respond adversely. Ideally, the circumstances of transport must provide a step-up in the level of care than provided by the referring hospital. The parent(s) may or may not accompany the child in the ambulance or by their own means. However, they must be briefed about the entire transfer process before the actual transfer. The receiving center also must be briefed about the clinical status just prior to transfer and an expected time of arrival. The communication may be brief and continued while "en-route" also depending on the condition just prior to transfer. It may be difficult in air ambulances especially a rotor-craft. Contrary to expectations, air retrieval is not superior to road ambulances. Based on at least two decades of experience, the American Academy of Pediatrics and other authorities on the subject have given specific recommendations about the transport (team constitution and functioning, optimizing safe and smooth transport) in transfer of a sick child. Some of them are discussed in the next section.

KEY RECOMMENDATION AND FUTURE[7-10]

An extensive review of 5 years of literature on pediatric critical transport had the following recommendations:

- There is an increased risk for complications with handover and transfers of a sick child.
- Standardized checklists, handover tools, mnemonics for communication(s) must be used.
- The tools (e.g. the ISBAR -Identify Situation Background Assessment Recommendation checklist) for handover do not increase the time for handover.[8,9]
- The tools for handover improve patient outcomes, provider satisfaction, team work and trust.

- The tools for handover reduce technical errors, complications, handoff failures.
- The tools of handover improve workflow.
- Best outcomes are achieved by specialized models who share mental models and trust.
- Specialized teams are associated with decreased mortality.
- Good quality transports DO NOT escalate costs.
- There should be minimum interruptions and distractions during handover.
- An interdisciplinary approach for nursing handover reduces stress for the workforce.
- Quality improvement measurement must be user-friendly.
- Administrators should have the responsibility of time, funding, research into quality improvement metrics.

KEY MESSAGES

- Risk for patient complications (airway compromise, cardiac arrest, loss of IV line, hypothermia, hypoxemia, intracranial hemorrhage) is more with pediatric transport and handovers.
- Standardization of communication using tools and checklists including specialized teams and teamwork is the CRUX for improved outcomes. This is measured in terms of patient outcomes, provider satisfaction and cost.
- Frequent monitoring while transfer and specialized training for specific situations including debriefing for providers improves patient outcomes.

REFERENCES

1. Guidelines for Air and Ground Transportation of Pediatric Patients. American Academy of Pediatrics. Pediatrics. 1986;78: 943.
2. Quality Standards for the Care of Critically Ill Children. Paediatric Intensive Care Society, 5th edition December 2015. Available from: *picsociety.uk/wp-content/uploads/2016/05/PICS_standards_2015.pdf.* Accessed July 24, 2019.
3. Government of Delhi. Registration of Ambulances. Available from: *http://scvriti.delhi.gov.in/wps/wcm/connect/1c884d00 406954a5b44dbc34262e20fd/cat.pdf?MOD=AJPERES&lmod=-288077341.* Accessed August 19th 2019.
4. Warren J, Fromm RE, Orr RA, *et al.* Guidelines for the inter- and intrahospital transport of critically ill patients. Crit Care Med. 2004;32:256-62.
5. Whyte HE, Jefferies AL. Canadian Paediatric Society, Fetus and Newborn Committee. The interfacility transport of critically ill newborns. Paediatr Child Health. 2015;20:265-75.
6. Johnson CM, Gonyea MT. Transport of the critically ill child. Mayo Clin Proc. 1993;68:982-7.
7. Foronda C, Van Graafeil, Quon R, Davidson P. Handover and transport of critically ill children: An integrative review. Int J Nurs Stud. 2016;62:207-25.
8. Thompson JE, Collett LW, Langbart MJ, *et al.* Using the ISBAR handover tool in junior medical officer handover: A study in an Australian tertiary hospital Postgrad Med J. 2011;87:340-4.
9. Müller M, Jürgens J, Redaèlli M, *et al.* Impact of the communication and patient hand-off tool SBAR on patient safety: A systematic review. BMJ Open. 2018;8:e022202.
10. Gilpin D, Hancock S. Referral and transfer of the critically ill child. BJA Education. 2016;16:253-57.

CHAPTER

5

Patient Safety and Medication Errors

Jayashree M, Biraj Parjauli

INTRODUCTION

Intensive care with its advanced technology and faster delivery of care, has brought about a substantial decline in the morbidity and mortality of critical illnesses. Fine tuning of this care, with more emphasis on patient safety and quality is now the need of the hour. Quality improvement in intensive care includes defining goals and standards to be achieved, continuous audit, and learning from data.

BACKGROUND

In the 1960s, quality improvement meant understanding the processes of providing care and improving its quality. Later the focus shifted to the errors in medicine, how to identify and decrease them. Reports from the nineties have shown that medical errors were not only associated with high morbidity and mortality but also high financial burden. Subsequently in the 21st century, landmark reports emphasizing on patient safety initiatives at local and national levels like Institute of Medicine's "To err is human: Building a safer health system"[1] and United Kingdom National Health Service's "An organization with a memory"[2] were published. The exact impact of medical errors in terms of mortality and morbidity, especially in children, is unknown. It is believed to be ranging from 1.81 to 2.96 per 100 discharges[3] but the exact rate in PICU in not known. Children have higher incidence of medical error as compared to adults.[4]

What is a System?

A system is "a set of interdependent human and nonhuman elements interacting to achieve a common aim". It can be a unit or department within a hospital, an entire hospital, or many hospitals. Systems can be simple (linear) or complex, loosely or tightly coupled, and isolated or overlapping with other systems.

In PICU, the system includes the people (patients, healthcare providers, visitors), equipment (monitors, devices, computers), environment (lighting, noise, lack of standardization, staffing) and decision making (complex, multiple data sources, frequent interruptions).

Complex and tightly coupled system have multiple components, interactions and functions. Such systems have very little buffer between actions, and are difficult to change than loosely coupled systems. In tightly coupled systems, one action quickly gives rise to other actions such that it is nearly impossible to recognize failure or intercede and prevent the failure from reaching a patient. Important definitions with respect to patient safety are elaborated in **Table 1**.

Types of Errors

Common medical errors occur when the healthcare provider fails to perform a task perfectly and the system does not have adequate layers to prevent the error from reaching the patient. Active errors occur because of limitations inherent to humans, like the impact of emotions, perceptions, stress, and fatigue on decision-making abilities. Some examples of such errors are listed in **Table 2**.[5]

Medication errors are an important type of medical error that can have serious consequences for patients, families and healthcare systems. It can occur either in or out of the hospital, and accounts for more than 7000 deaths annually.[1] Medication errors are avoidable events that harm or have the potential to harm a patient. These errors can occur at four levels: Prescription, administration,

Table 1: Important definitions with respect to patient safety[5]

Patient safety	Avoidance, prevention and amelioration of adverse events or injuries stemming from the processes of health care	
Adverse event	Unintended event that occurs during medical care not directly related to underlying patient's condition, e.g. adverse drug reaction	
Medical error	Error of commission Failure of planned action to be completed as intended It can be an error in execution or error of judgment Esophageal intubation is an example of the former whereas treating a gram negative organism with a drug that only has gram positive cover is an example of latter	Error of omission Lack of plan or an action
Near miss	Event which has capacity to do harm but does not have adverse consequences due to timely and appropriate identification and correction. E.g. Wrong drug charting identified and corrective measures taken	
Sentinel event	Unanticipated event resulting in death or physical or psychological injury not related to natural course of the disease	

Table 2: Definitions of common errors

Nomenclature	*Definition*
Slips	Observable action that deviates from what was planned
Lapse	Represent a memory failure
Mistake	Knowledge based failure
Active (sharp) error	Occur in a patient care area by frontline provider, effect is immediately apparent
Latent (blunt) error	System based problems and may lead to poor design, incorrect installation, faulty maintenance, etc. These errors are hard to identify and may be hidden within the structure of the system

transcription and dispensing.[6] The severity can be classified into seven levels, ranging from a "potential error without harm" (level 0) to "fatal complications" (level 6).[7] Pediatric population and intensive care are highly prone to medication errors due to their complex settings, large number of medications administered for each patient, and more number of parenteral drugs. In the pediatric age group, errors have been estimated to be 3–37/100 orders during prescription, 5–15/100 orders during dispensing and 72–75/100 orders during administration.[8]

WHY DO ERRORS OCCUR?

The PICU Environment

The physical and psychological environment in a PICU adds to the risk of medical errors. Decision making in PICU is complex and involves interpreting multiple data in a short span of time in an environment that may require multitasking. In PICU, the acuity of illness, constant exposure to death and grieving parents, fatigue, inappropriate staffing, lack of equipment standardization, multiple simultaneous demands, and the use of many interventions associated with narrow therapeutic windows all affect human performance. A study by Grayson and Potter[9] found that errors tend to occur within 30 minutes after sudden changes in patient needs in an environment that is dominated by distractions and interruptions.

***Workload and fatigue*:** Compared to other industries, little is known about human factors and the PICU environment. Recent studies related to increased workload, fatigue, and emotional stress clearly demonstrate the influence of human factors on patient safety.

1. Sleep deprivation has negative impact on performance and is high risk for personal injury, mood disturbances, and stress-related illnesses. Cumulative sleepiness, mood disturbance, and psychomotor vigilance decreases during a week of sleep restricted to 4–5 hours per night.[10]
2. The increased number of patient handovers has become a new source of error due to breach in communication.
3. Nurses play an important role in intensive care settings and the need for adequate rest and appropriate staffing is paramount.[11] Lower patient-to nurse staffing ratios have shown to be associated with a lower risk of adverse events. Appropriate staffing levels, orientation, ongoing education, and rewards for staff nurses is important.

ERROR PREVENTION AND IMPROVING PATIENT SAFETY

System Related Changes

Safety is not the responsibility of a single person, device, or department within a system, but rather the product of the interactions among various components of a system. Complex, tightly coupled systems have been made safer, as demonstrated by successes in aviation and nuclear energy industries.

- "Swiss Cheese Model" described by Reason[12] is a conceptual framework of error prevention in complex systems where the "holes" in the layers represent potential failures points. When multiple holes line up, the downstream effect results in failure. In case of patient care, this translates to occurrence of a medical error.
- Implementation of checklists has been shown to improve outcomes in surgery.
- Standardized procedures using "bundles of care" approach has been shown to improve outcomes, e.g. Prevention bundles for central-line sepsis, ventilator-associated pneumonia and accidental extubation. Patient care should be triaged, as it is difficult to address more than one patient at a time.
- Introduction of computerized physician order entry (CPOE) combined with clinical decision support has led to decrease in medication errors, with respect to calculations, dose modifications and drug contraindications based on organ dysfunction or drug-drug interactions.

Communication: Effective communication is essential to improve safety. The Joint Commission for the Accreditation of Hospitals and Other Organizations (JCAHO) found that poor communication was an important factor in majority of sentinel events. For critically ill infants and children whether in PICU or during transport, communication is fundamental to ensure that patients receive appropriate care be it the handover between nurses or physicians.

A**SBAR** (Situation, Background, Assessment, and Recommendation) is a tool to improve communication between team members and to overcome perceived and real restrictions related to hierarchy. Another communication tool, **"PASS the BATON"**, developed by the Defense Department, provides a structure for transferring patient care from one individual to another. The acronym provides prompts for relaying Patient data, such as name, age, sex, and location. Good communication is ensured only within environments where there are high levels of trust between all members of the team.

Human Factor Engineering

Human factor engineering deals with interactions between humans, the tools they use, and the environment in which they live and work.[1] Industries have used human factors for recognizing where and why systems break down. Investigating aviation accidents demonstrated that take-offs and landings were the times of highest risk during any flight. The concept of the "sterile" cockpit was developed because factors contributing to human error, such as stress were identified as risk factors during crash investigations.

Continuous Quality Improvement

Continuous process of reviewing and improving the practices and procedures of care is known as **Continuous quality improvement (CQI)**.[13] It evaluates structure, process, or outcome, either as independent components of the CQI process or simultaneously.

Staffing for patient acuity levels, the right equipment at the right time, and involvement of an intensivist in the care of critically ill patients are examples of structures influencing quality. Processes refer to how care is delivered, policies and evidence-based medicine guidelines routinely followed. Outcomes summarize the effectiveness of care, including adverse events. Examples are risk-adjusted mortality, hospital-acquired infections, and adverse medication errors.

Studies have shown that CQI leads to improved patient safety and better outcomes. However, lack of formal training in CQI and the progress of the concept catching up has been slow in medical field compared to non-healthcare industries.

QUALITY IMPROVEMENT MEASURES

Critical Incident Reporting: Error Detection

Error reporting system(s), is/are important to improve patient safety in the PICU. Identification of adverse events is the only way to know that issues exist. Types of reporting systems include voluntary reporting, mandatory reporting, concurrent surveillance, automated surveillance, and chart review.[14]

Intensivists should facilitate development of an environment that allows investigation of actual and near-miss events. Key components necessary for supporting an environment in which learning from error occurs are: reporting, just, flexibility and learning.[15] In a "reporting" culture, staff is actively engaged in reporting accidents and near misses. In a "just" culture, safeguards exist that allow the identification of individuals who repeatedly fail to follow policies or who act with malicious intent, while protecting those who report errors and near misses. The willingness and competence to correctly interpret safety data, form correct conclusions, and implement new processes are features of a "learning culture". In a "flexible" culture, individuals must be willing to move between a traditional, hierarchical structure to a horizontal, professional structure, so that individuals with expertise in an area may investigate and design solutions.

When an event occurs or an opportunity to improve safety is prospectively identified, the team is assembled to design a new process. The team should include representation from all areas or service that had a role in the care of the patient. Inclusion of the appropriate personnel helps to ensure that a thorough planning stage occurs.

ERROR ANALYSIS

- *Root cause analysis*[16] is a structured process that retrospectively assists in identifying underlying factors or causes of an adverse event or near-miss. Understanding the contributing factors or causes of a system failure can help develop corrective actions. A cause and effect diagram, called a "**fishbone**" diagram (**Fig. 1**), helps in identifying possible causes of a problem and in sorting ideas into useful categories. The problem or effect is displayed at the head or mouth of the fish. Possible contributing causes are listed on the smaller "bones" under various cause categories.
- Another common error analysis tool is "*Failure Modes and Effects Analysis (FMEA)*" which is prospective unlike the fishbone analysis. The possible failures of a product or services are identified, to determine the frequency and impact of the failure. The information gathered from FMEA provides valuable data for designing a safer process, as failures are anticipated and solutions for preventing patient harm are built into the process.
- Various other work models that provides systematic approach for investigating events and processes include the PDCA cycle (Plan-Do-Check-Act) and the DEPOSE (Design, Equipment, Procedures, Operators, Supplies and materials, and Environment) model.

RESOURCE ALLOCATION

Defining standards and goals of treatment to be offered in the PICU, reasonable allocation of resources, appropriate management of these resources, accountability for the use of the resources, and ongoing feedback to the stakeholders is important for quality care. Both the process of setting standards and goals and resource allocation requires rationing at number of levels, including bedside, institutional and higher levels. Rationing includes the process of making rational, defensible, and ethical decisions as to which intervention to withhold from which

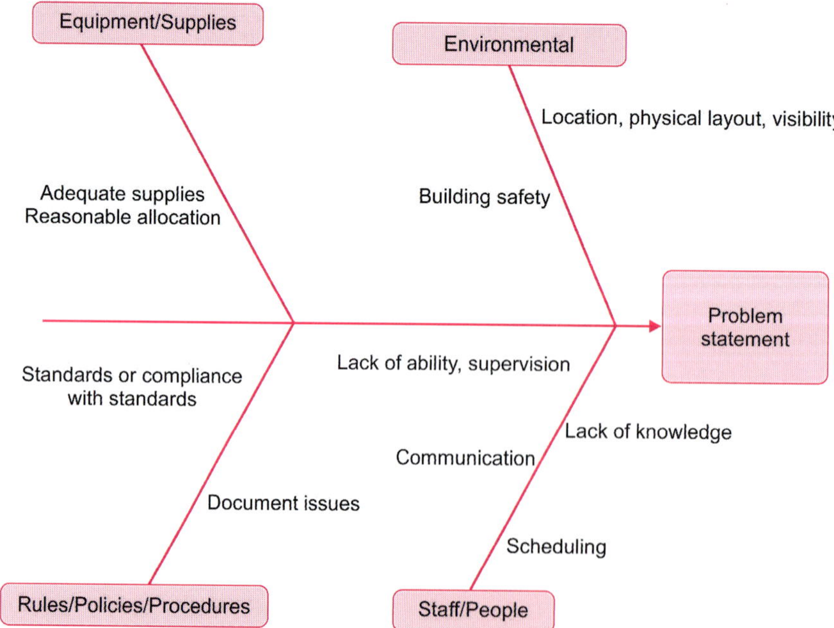

Fig. 1: Fishbone diagram

patients so that resources can be allocated towards other beneficial patients/activities.

Response to an Adverse Event

Recommendations for an appropriate response when an adverse event occurs have been reviewed[17] and include the following:

1. *Managing the patient and his/her family*: Address the problem and ensure patient safety first. The senior member of the team should communicate with the parents about the situation. This communication should happen within 24 hours from the event and depends on the condition of the child and the family. The family should be briefed about the event, condition of the patient and steps taken for prevention of the event.
2. The concerned medical personnel should be given adequate time to recover from the incident. If the primary care provider is unable to cope up, then replacement must be found.
3. Investigating the incident and providing clarity should be immediate and the team should constitute those who have an understanding of the clinical context, and functioning of PICU.
4. All aspects of this process should be appropriately and carefully documented.
5. The events should be reported to the appropriate authorities within the hospital and health system.

KEY MESSAGES

- Reduction in adverse events and errors are important to ensure quality of care delivered to a patient in pediatric intensive care unit.
- It is essential that comprehensive team- and systems-based approaches are employed to improve care and limit errors.
- Ongoing measurement and assessment of systems is an essential component of quality improvement.
- In resource limited settings, areas of concern must be identified and resources diverted to those areas for improving care.

REFERENCES

1. Kohn LT, Corrigan JM, Donaldson MS, editors. To Err is Human: Building a Safer Health System. Washington, D.C.: National Academies Press; 2000.
2. Donaldson L. An organization with a memory: Report of an expert group on learning from adverse events in the NHS. London, England: Stationery Office; 2000.
3. Slonim AD, LaFleur BJ, Ahmed W, *et al.* Hospital-reported medical errors in children. Pediatrics. 2003;111:617-21.
4. National service framework: children, young people and maternity services. Available from: *https://www.gov.uk/government/publications/national-service-framework-children-young-people-and-maternity-services.* Accessed July 24, 2019.
5. Argent AC, Montogomery VL. Quality improvement, patient safety, and medical error. In: David G Nichols, Donald H Shaffner, editors. Rogers' Textbook of Pediatric Intensive Care, 5th edition. Philadelphia: Wolters Kluwer. p. 290-309.
6. ASHP guidelines on preventing medication errors in hospitals. Am J Hosp Pharm. 1993;50:305-14.
7. Hartwig SC, Denger SD, Schneider PJ. Severity-indexed, incident report-based medication error-reporting program. Am J Hosp Pharm. 199;48:2611-6.
8. Alsulami Z, Conroy S, Choonara I. Medication errors in the Middle East countries: A systematic review of the literature. Eur J Clin Pharmacol. 2013;69:995-1008.
9. Grayson D, Boxerman S, Potter P, *et al.* Do transient working conditions trigger medical errors? In: Henrikson KB, Marks ES, Lewin DI, editors. Advances in Patient Safety: From Research to Implementation. Research Findings. Rockville, MD: Agency for Healthcare Research and Quality; 2005 p. 53-64. AHRQ publication 05-0021-1.
10. Dinges DF, Pack F, Williams K, *et al.* Cumulative sleepiness, mood disturbance, and psychomotor vigilance performance decrements during a week of sleep restricted to 4-5 hours per night. Sleep. 1997;20:267-77.
11. Lankshear AJ, Sheldon TA, Maynard A. Nurse staffing and healthcare outcomes: A systematic review of the international research evidence. ANS Adv Nurs Sci. 2005;28:163-74.
12. Reason J. Human error: Models and management. BMJ. 2000; 320:768-70.
13. Counte MA, Meurer S. Issues in the assessment of continuous quality improvement implementation in health care organizations. Int J Qual Health Care. 2001;13:197-207.
14. Aspden P, Corrigan JM, Wolcott J, *et al.*, Institute of Medicine (US) Committee on Data Standards for Patient Safety. Patient Safety: Achieving a New Standard for Care. Washington (DC): National Academies Press (US); 2004. Also available from: *https://www.ncbi.nlm.nih.gov/pubmed/25009854.* Accessed July 24, 2019.
15. Ruchlin HS, Dubbs NL, Callahan MA. The role of leadership in instilling a culture of safety: Lessons from the literature. J Healthc Manag. 2004;49:47-58; discussion 58-9.
16. Phillips J, Simmonds L. Using fishbone analysis to investigate problems. Nurs Times. 2013;109:18-20.
17. Powell SK. When things go wrong: responding to adverse events: A consensus statement of the Harvard hospitals. Lippincotts Case Manag. 2006;11:193-4.

SECTION 2

Initial Stabilization

***Section Editor:** Arvind Bagga*

CHAPTER 6

Emergency Airway Management

Lokesh Guglani

INTRODUCTION

Airway management in infants and children is an important set of skills and practices that can be helpful in the initial and ongoing management of several acute and chronic respiratory disorders. Training and preparedness for acute airway emergencies is important for providers at all levels of healthcare and an ongoing evaluation of competency in these skills through deliberate practice and simulation-based learning can be helpful in improving outcomes. This chapter will focus on the basic principles of airway management in neonates and children in acute care settings.[1-3]

EPIDEMIOLOGY AND ETIOLOGY

Respiratory disorders are a major cause of morbidity and mortality in infants and children across the world.[1] While specific patterns of diseases and their prevalence may differ in different countries or regions, acute and chronic respiratory conditions account for a significant proportion of office and emergency room visits as well as hospitalizations in children. Acute respiratory illnesses comprise the majority of respiratory disease burden in India,[2] and there is now an increasing recognition of rising incidence of several chronic respiratory conditions such as asthma.[3] Prompt recognition of airway and breathing problems can help prioritize care and initiate timely referrals for children needing advanced levels of respiratory support.

PATHOPHYSIOLOGY

It is important to understand the unique features of the pediatric respiratory system and how they could affect the management of various conditions in acute emergencies. Besides anatomic differences, there are several important changes in airway, chest wall and lung physiology that occur with age through infancy and early childhood.

Unique Features of Pediatric Airway

There are significant anatomical differences in the airway anatomy of young children (<2 years of age) when compared to adults. In general, children that are age 8 years and above have airway features similar to those of adults. Between the ages of 2 to 8 years there is a transition in the level of the glottic opening, which is present at the level of first cervical vertebra (C1) in infants. It reaches the C3-C4 level by age 7 years and is present at C5-C6 level in an adult (**Fig. 1B**). The presence of a large tongue relative to the size of the oral cavity in infants can make airway assessment difficult (**Fig. 1A**). The relative size of epiglottis is also much larger in a child (**Fig. 1D**) and this makes it harder to visualize the larynx by using a curved blade inserted up to the vallecula to lift up the epiglottis. This is the reason why a straight blade laryngoscope may be easier to use in children less than 3 years of age to lift the epiglottis from underneath for adequate visualization of the glottic opening. The relatively high and anterior position of the pediatric airway along (**Fig. 1C**) with a large occiput requires placement of shoulder rolls to facilitate neck extension and provide easier access during laryngoscopy. Children may have enlarged tonsils and adenoids and there is a more acute angle between the epiglottis and laryngeal opening, which can make blind

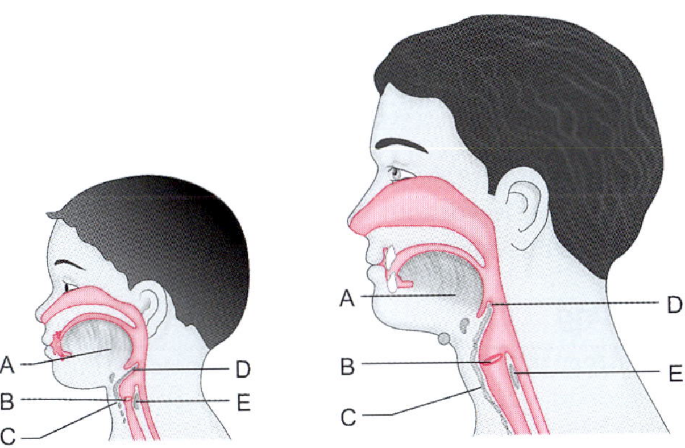

Fig. 1: Differences in pediatric and adult airway anatomy: (A) Tongue is larger in infants relative to the size of oral cavity; (B) Vocal cords are placed at much higher level in infants (C1) as compared to adults (C5–6); (C) Cricothyroid membrane; (D) Epiglottis is much larger in infants and can interfere with visualization of glottic opening during laryngoscopy; (E) Cricoid ring is the narrowest part of the pediatric airway as opposed to the glottic opening in adults

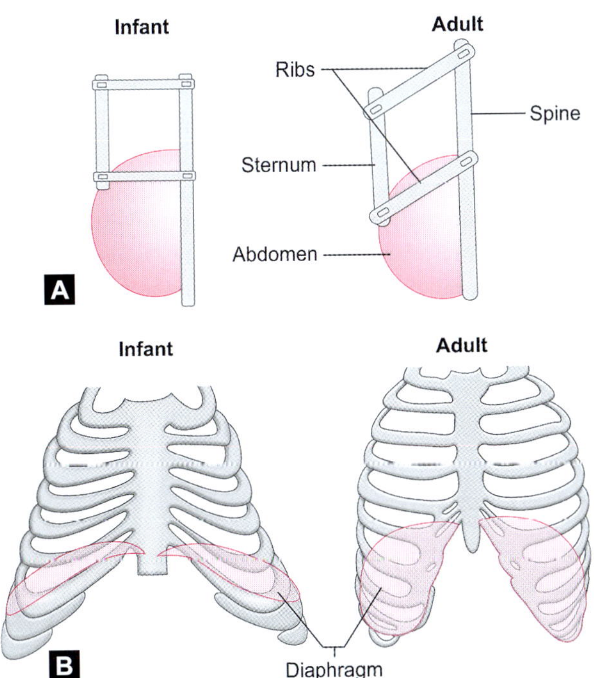

Figs. 2A and B: Comparison of infant and adult chest wall. (A) Comparison of the orientation of the ribs and thoracic cage in infants and adults; (B) Comparison of the insertion of the diaphragm and area of apposition in infants and adults

nasotracheal intubation difficult. The narrowest site of the pediatric airway is the cricoid ring (as opposed to the vocal cord region in adults) (**Fig. 1E**) and therefore endotracheal tube size selection should be based on the patient's age and size. Infants and young children can have a higher vagal response to laryngoscopy or oropharyngeal suctioning and this predisposes them to the development of bradycardia during these procedures.

Infants tend to have a significantly higher basal metabolic rate and have a higher oxygen consumption rate (7 mL/kg/min at birth) as compared to adults (3–4 mL/kg/min). Infants have a higher overall cardiorespiratory demand and lower functional residual capacity (FRC) which makes them susceptible to developing respiratory failure during acute respiratory illnesses. In the first year of life, the chest wall has increased compliance due to horizontally placed ribs (**Fig. 2A**), poorly developed intercostal muscles, and cartilaginous ribs and sternum. This means that the rib cage contributes little during normal tidal breaths as the bucket-handle motion of the rib cage is limited and infants depend more on diaphragmatic activity. The diaphragm inserts into the rib cage in a more horizontal position in infants (**Fig. 2B**) which leads to inward retraction of the lower rib cage leading to subcostal retractions during periods of respiratory distress. The diaphragm and the intercostal muscles act in opposite direction at the level of the costal margin and predominant effect depends on the curvature of the diaphragm. In acute viral illnesses (bronchiolitis) or small airways constriction, the diaphragm is pushed down by hyperinflation of the lungs and this makes its movements less efficient in maintaining tidal volume during inspiration. This also causes additional energy expenditure as more forceful contraction of the diaphragm during inspiration causes the rib cage to be pulled inwards more significantly and this causes further limitation of inspiratory airflow as inward movement of lower rib cage is essentially like an expiratory maneuver. This inward movement of the lower rib cage during inspiration in infants with respiratory distress is called Hoover sign.

The respiratory muscles in infants are mostly comprised of the rapid-twitch, Type II fibers which helps them maintain higher respiratory rates, but during acute illnesses where there is a higher workload imposed on them, they are more likely to fail under this stress and develop respiratory failure relatively quickly. The development of intercostal retractions during periods of respiratory distress is another inefficiency that causes sucking in of the intercostal spaces during inspiration wasting energy that is being expended in generating inspiratory airflow.

To overcome the limitations imposed by their anatomy, infants breathe at higher respiratory rates and maintain their FRC by partially abducting their vocal cords during exhalation to limit expiratory airflow and maintain some degree of diaphragmatic constriction during exhalation as well. During periods of respiratory distress, the lower lung elastic recoil is unable to prevent dynamic collapse of their airways. Any changes in airway diameter lead to a significant increase in resistance of the airways and the lack of collateral ventilation (inter-alveolar pores of Kohn and bronchoalveolar canals of Lambert) does not allow adequate filling of these distal alveoli, making infants more susceptible to atelectasis and ventilation-perfusion mismatch.

CLINICAL FEATURES

Prompt recognition and intervention for acute respiratory symptoms can be provided using a basic standard approach for quick evaluation and decision making. This includes a quick Primary Assessment (a rapid evaluation of respiratory, cardiac and neurologic function including vital signs and pulse oximetry), followed by Secondary Assessment (which includes a more focused medical history and examination).

Primary Assessment

For patients presenting to the clinic or emergency room, a rapid primary assessment using the Airway, Breathing Circulation, Disability, Exposure (ABCDE) approach can help to collect information quickly to determine next steps. This chapter will focus on the airway and breathing evaluation only, and the remaining sections will be covered in subsequent related chapters.

Airway

Airway assessment starts with evaluation of patency of the airway. This can be done by use of visual, auditory and tactile cues as shown below:

- Look—at the movement of chest wall and abdomen.
- Listen—for abnormal breath sounds (audible stridor or wheezes) and auscultation findings.
- Feel—for the air movement at nostrils or in front of mouth.

Based on this evaluation and the overall status of the patient, there can be 3 scenarios:

1. *Clear airway*: The patient has a clear upper airway which is unobstructed.
2. *Maintainable*: Patient has an airway obstruction which can be easily corrected by simple measures (positioning, head-tilt-chin lift, oropharyngeal suctioning).
3. *Not maintainable*: Airway is obstructed, or not maintainable without specific airway interventions (such as intubation).

Breathing

Respiratory effort: If the chest wall shows retractions (intercostal, subcostal or suprasternal) or there is significantly labored breathing, stridor is present, or no breath sounds can be heard despite respiratory effort then airway obstruction is likely to be present.

Respiratory rate and pattern: The next step is to quickly assess the respiratory rate by counting the number of breaths for 10 seconds and then multiplying it by 6. Normal respiratory rates vary by age and are outlined in **Table 1**. An irregular respiratory pattern may be seen with deep gasping breaths followed by apnea or rapid/shallow breathing followed by apnea can be ominous sign of acute respiratory failure and requires immediate intervention. Faster respiratory rates could be due to upper and lower respiratory disorders but can also be seen in non-respiratory conditions such as dehydration, fever, pain, anemia, sepsis and congenital heart disease. A slow respiratory rate can lead to hypoventilation and hypercarbia and can be seen in a variety of conditions outlined in **Table 2**.

Chest expansion and air movement: The degree of chest rise can indicate the adequacy of ventilation and along with auscultation findings to determine symmetry of air entry on both sides can be helpful in determining

Table 1: Normal vital signs by age

Ages	*Heart rate (beats/minute)*	*Respiratory rate (breaths/minute)*	*Blood pressure (mm Hg) systolic/diastolic*
Permature infants	120–170	40–70	55–75/35–45
0–3 months	100–150	35–55	65–85/45–55
3–6 months	90–120	30–45	70–90/50–65
6–12 months	80–120	25–40	80–100/55–65
1–3 years	70–110	20–30	90–105/55–70
3–6 years	65–110	20–25	95–110/60–75
6–12 years	60–95	14–22	100–120/60–75
>12 years	55–85	12–18	110–135/65–85

Table 2: Types of acute respiratory problems and severity

Type	*Common clinical diagnoses*	*Clinical features*	*Severity*
Upper airway obstruction	Croup Epiglottitis Bacterial tracheitis Peritonsillar abscess Airway foreign body Anaphylaxis	Stridor Respiratory distress Retractions Hypoxemia and/or hypercarbia	Respiratory distress Or Respiratory failure
Lower airway obstruction	Bronchiolitis Asthma Lower airway foreign body	Cough Wheezing Respiratory distress Retractions Diminished air entry Rhonchi Hypoxemia and/or hypercarbia	Respiratory distress Or Respiratory failure
Lung parenchymal disease	Pneumonia Aspiration Pulmonary edema Interstitial lung disease	Cough Fever Crackles Hypoxemia and/or hypercarbia	Respiratory distress Or Respiratory failure
Inadequate control of breathing	Trauma Seizures Shock Hypothermia Drug overdose Respiratory muscle fatigue in neuromuscular disorders	Slow breathing rates Gasping breaths Bradycardia Apnea Reduced chest rise Diminished breath sounds Hypercarbia and/or hypoxemia	Respiratory distress Or Respiratory failure

air movement. Diminished air entry on one side may be due to atelectasis, pneumothorax, foreign body or consolidation, while bilateral reduction in air movement may be due to severe bronchospasm or hypoventilation. Limited chest expansion may occur in apnea, central hypoventilation or in patients with neuromuscular weakness.

Lung and airway sounds: Lung and airway sounds can be helpful in diagnosing upper and lower airway pathology. It is important to distinguish upper airway conducted sounds from lower airway sounds. The presence of coarse rhonchi may be due to excessive airway secretions, crackles may represent areas of parenchymal involvement due to infection or fluid (pulmonary edema). Wheezing due to small airways obstruction is generally high pitched and polyphonic in nature and may be heard throughout exhalation or towards the end of exhalation. Sometimes it may also be associated with a prolongation of expiratory phase.

Oxyhemoglobin saturations by pulse oximetry: This is a helpful adjunct to determine the need for oxygen supplementation and to monitor response to interventions. It is important to place the sensor correctly and assess the waveform of the signal before confirming the readings. In the presence of hypothermia, poor peripheral perfusion or abnormal forms of hemoglobin (such as methemoglobin), pulse oximetry can be misleading.

At the end of primary assessment some basic patterns of airway involvement can be determined, and their severity can be established (**Table 2**). This allows for the secondary assessment and diagnostic testing to be focused on these specific conditions.

Secondary Assessment

Secondary assessment includes a focused medical history and a focused physical examination. This can be helpful to narrow down the differential diagnosis and help initiate therapies once airway patency has been established. For hospitalized patients, the occurrence of airway emergencies may be related to the underlying condition and specific evaluations need to be performed rapidly in patients with an advanced airway device. These have been discussed in subsequent sections.

Diagnostic Testing

Diagnostic testing should be performed to confirm the diagnosis and monitor response to interventions. Depending on the healthcare setting, these tests may include chest radiographs, blood gases, laboratory tests for infectious etiologies and blood counts. In acute emergencies, initial stabilization of patient should be prioritized over these diagnostic tests. Once a stable airway has been established then further evaluations can be completed.

TECHNIQUES INVOLVED IN AIRWAY MANAGEMENT

Simple Measures to Maintain an Airway

Positioning: The goal of positioning is to place the child in a position that is comfortable and allows the best alignment for airway patency. In a responsive child, this may be accomplished by elevating the head end of the bed slightly or allowing an older child to sit in a tripod position with neck slightly extended. In an unresponsive child who is not suspected of having cervical spine injury, turning to the side can allow drainage of secretions and prevent the tongue from falling backwards or it may be preferable to perform a head-tilt, chin-lift maneuver (as described below).

Head-tilt, chin-lift maneuver: For children without trauma or suspected cervical spine injury who may be unresponsive, the airway can be maintained in a patent state by placing one hand on patient's forehead and pushing down on it, while the fingers of the other hand are placed under the chin in midline. As the head is tilted back gently with gentle pressure on the forehead, simultaneously the chin is lifted upwards by the other hand **(Fig. 3)**.

Jaw-thrust: For children with suspected cervical cord injury it is important to minimize neck movement while maintaining airway patency. This can be achieved by thrusting the jaw forward in a single motion. The provider should be standing at the head end and rest elbows on the mattress/bed. With forearms lining the sides of the head to minimize sideways motion, place fingertips of each hand under the angle of the jaw. With coordinated forward

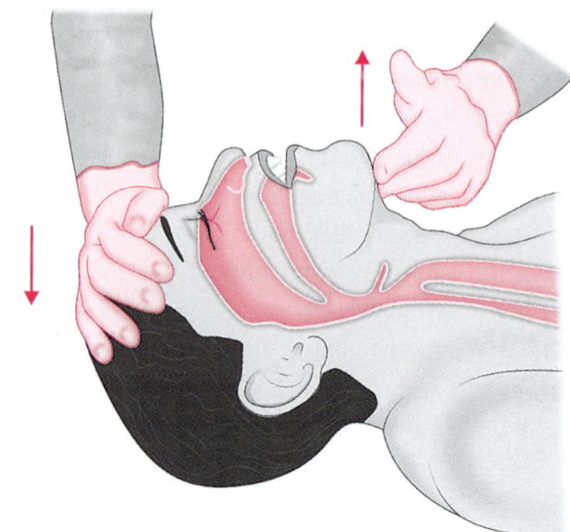

Fig. 3: Head tilt chin lift maneuver

movement of the fingers, lift the jaw upward so that tongue can be moved forward in the mouth thereby opening the airway **(Fig. 4)**.

Suctioning

Suctioning of nasal passages or oropharynx can be very helpful in clearing secretions and maintaining airway patency. Suctioning procedures can cause several complications such as gagging and vomiting, soft tissue injury, agitation, stimulation of vagal nerve in the pharynx leading to bradycardia, or rarely hypoxia if suctioning is performed for a prolonged period of time. It is important to monitor the child's vital signs during suctioning and limit each suction attempt to less than 10 seconds. If there is hypoxia, bradycardia, or clinical worsening, then stop suctioning immediately and give 100% O_2 or positive pressure breaths with bag-mask ventilation if needed until the vital signs become normal.

Techniques for removal of foreign body causing airway obstruction

If there is concern for foreign body obstruction, then immediate interventions should be performed based on age and the responsiveness of the child. For infants, it is important to deliver 5 back slaps and 5 chest thrusts and then re-evaluate the airway. For older children, abdominal thrusts should be performed. If the child becomes unresponsive during this process or presents in an unresponsive state, then it is important to initiate cardiopulmonary resuscitation (CPR).

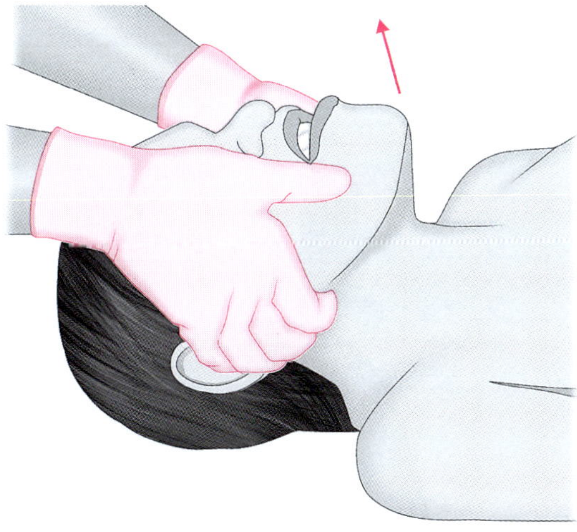

Fig. 4: Jaw thrust maneuver

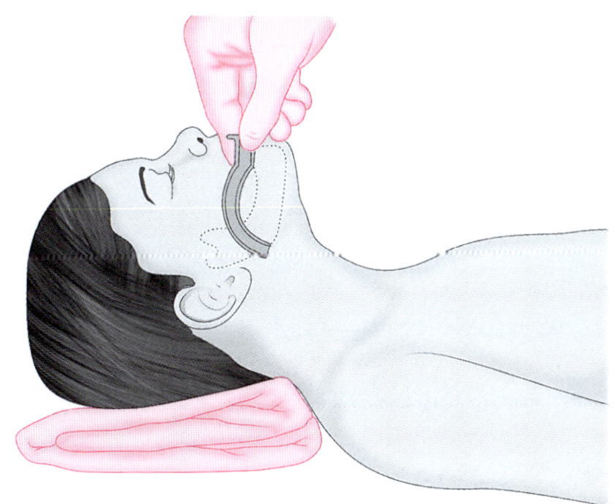

Fig. 5: Determining the appropriate size of oropharyngeal airway

Airway adjuncts

Airway adjuncts such as Guedel airway/oro-pharyngeal airway (OPA) can be helpful in unresponsive patients with adequate spontaneous ventilation when other measures to open the airway have not been successful. Nasopharyngeal airways can be used for conscious patients with soft tissue obstruction of the upper airway. OPA works by preventing the backward collapse of tongue that could potentially cause upper airway obstruction. This device should be used for brief periods during initial stabilization only and should not be used solely as a bite blocker in agitated patients. The device is made of plastic and has an outer flange, a flat bite block region and a curved body. It is hollow to provide easy access for suctioning of pharynx and to permit airflow. Before insertion, it is important to select the appropriate size by placing the device along the side of the patient's face. An appropriately sized device will have the distal curved end ending at the angle of the jaw while the flange is held at the level of the lips (**Fig. 5**). If it is too long, it can induce gagging and bradycardia, while a shorter device may push the base of tongue backwards and worsen upper airway obstruction.

Nasopharyngeal airway (**Fig. 6**) is a flexible nasal tube usually made of rubber that can be inserted via the nose into the nasopharynx to bypass any obstruction caused by tongue and pharyngeal soft tissues. It is less likely to cause gagging and may be better tolerated by conscious patients with acute respiratory distress. It can be particularly helpful in postoperative patients or those with macroglossia or adenotonsillar hypertrophy. To determine the appropriate size of a nasopharyngeal tube, it is important to measure the distance from the patient's nostril to the tragus of the ear. The outer surface of the tube should be lubricated prior to insertion and the bevel of the tube should be pointed towards the nasal septum during insertion to avoid trauma to the nasal mucosa.

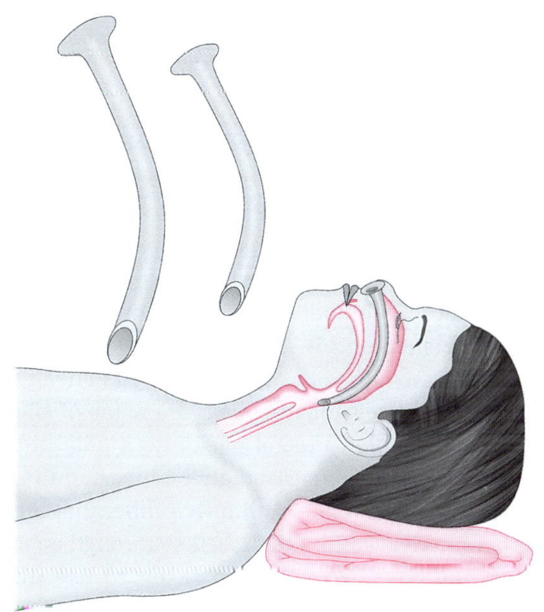

Fig. 6: Nasopharyngeal airway

Bag Mask Ventilation

It is critical to provide bag mask ventilation during emergency airway management to ensure adequate oxygenation. After opening the airways with the head

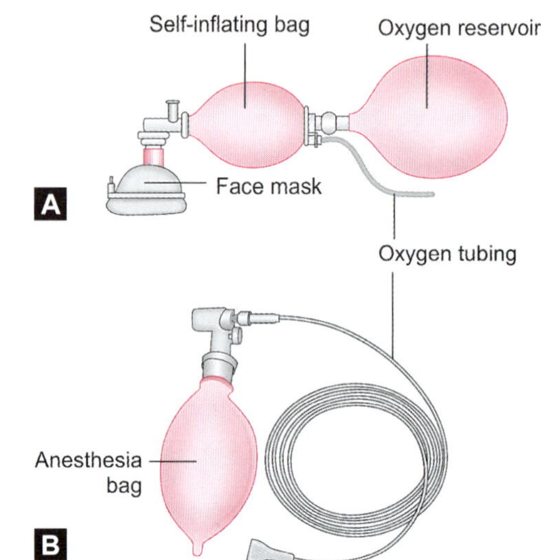

Figs. 7A and B: Two types of bags that are used for bag mask ventilation and their features

tilt-chin lift/jaw thrust maneuvers described above, a ventilation mask is placed over the mouth and nose to provide positive pressure breaths with a self-inflating bag or anesthesia (flow-inflating) bag. This procedure should be practiced and performed by all healthcare providers using simulation methods to ensure adequate technique during acute emergencies.

There are two types of bags that are used in healthcare settings (**Fig. 7**)—self-inflating bags are made of silicone rubber and are able to recoil back into a fully inflated state when pressure is released after squeezing the bag. Anesthesia bags are made of thinner rubber that inflates only when there is continuous gas flow through a circuit. Self-inflating bags are generally easier to use during resuscitation and they have a pop-off valve to minimize barotrauma by limiting peak inspiratory pressures. In situations where there is poor lung compliance or increased airway resistance, higher pressures may be needed to provide adequate ventilation. With anesthesia bags it may be easier to feel the patient effort and lung compliance while bagging and deliver higher FiO_2s as well smaller tidal volumes. For effective bag-mask ventilation, it is important that the mask should fit properly, and this can be determined by ensuring that it covers the patient's mouth and nose but should not cross the chin below or cover the eyes. After identifying the correct size mask, it is important to place the mask on the patient's face to maintain a good seal during positive pressure breaths.

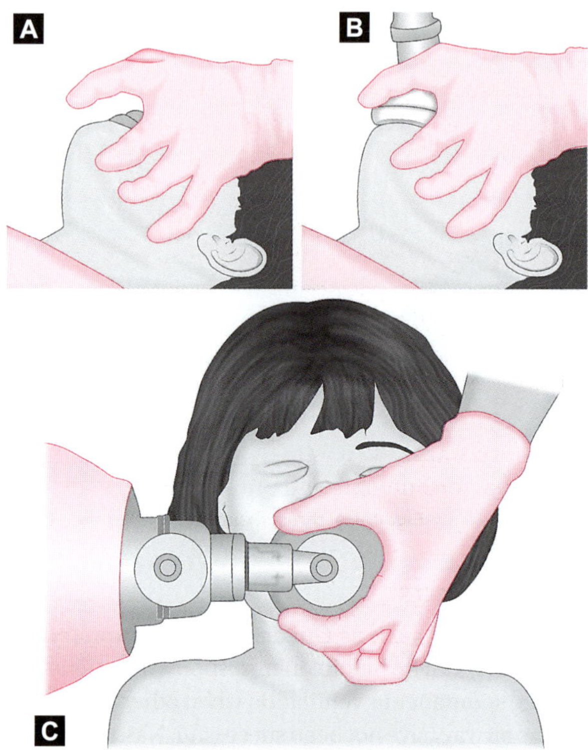

Figs. 8A to C: Bag mask ventilation technique: (A) Placement of non-dominant hand with 3 fingers in the shape of letter E to support the jab; (B) Holding the mask in place with thumb and index finger of the same hand; (C) Placing the index finger and thumb on top of the mask in the shape of the letter C

The E-C Clamp technique (**Fig. 8**) is helpful in ensuring consistent technique during bag-mask ventilation. Starting with the placement of the little finger of the non-dominant hand at the angle of the mandible, the ring and the middle fingers are then placed along the mandible to provide support while forming an E shape (**Fig. 8A**). The index finger and the thumb of the non-dominant hand are used to grasp the mask around the airway opening in a C-shape pattern (**Figs. 8B and C**). The dominant hand is then used to squeeze the self-inflating bag while maintaining a tight seal of the mask around the patient's face. It is important to monitor the degree of chest rise with each breath to ensure adequate volume is being delivered.

Once the airway is positioned properly and a good mask seal is established, then ventilation should be initiated by squeezing the bag steadily over a period of 1 second. Vigorous squeezing of the bag should be avoided to reduce the chances of gastric overinflation. A volume that is just enough to produce a visible chest rise may be adequate to ventilate the patient. The rate of ventilation should be adapted to the clinical situation as outlined in **Table 3**.

Problems can arise during bag mask ventilation if there is an inadequate mask seal, if the size of the mask is not appropriate, if patient position has changed while bagging or if the personnel are inexperienced with optimal bag mask technique. If there is still no chest rise noted during bag-mask ventilation in a child without an advanced airway despite adequate repositioning and maintenance of a good seal with an appropriately sized mask, then it may be due to a foreign body causing complete airway obstruction, significant abdominal distension causing elevation of the diaphragm and poor lung expansion, or bilateral pneumothoraces. Placement of an advanced airway should be considered at this time to secure the airway while other interventions can be performed to establish ventilation. For patients with an advanced airway (such as endotracheal tube or tracheostomy tube), difficulty with bag mask ventilation should prompt an evaluation using the DOPE mnemonic, as shown in **Table 4**. Complications of bag-mask ventilation include: gastric distension, aspiration, hypoventilation and hyperventilation.

Table 3: Rate of ventilation with bag and mask for different clinical situations

Clinical scenario	*Rate of ventilation*
HR ≥ 60 beats per minute with no spontaneous ventilation in a child	12 to 20 per minute (1 breath every 3 to 5 seconds)
HR < 60 beats per minute with no spontaneous ventilation in a child • Single provider • Two providers	2 breaths per 30 chest compressions 2 breaths per 15 chest compressions
Intubated infants and children	8 to 10 breaths per minute without any interruption of chest compressions

Endotracheal Intubation

The process of tracheal tube placement in the upper part of trachea for providing secure access to the airway for ventilation is called endotracheal intubation. This procedure provides respiratory support and oxygenation while minimizing the risk of aspiration of secretions or gastric distension. Elective intubation may be done for surgical procedures or diagnostic tests such as endoscopy, but in emergency situations rapid sequence intubation (RSI) may be necessary. RSI is a series of steps that include preparation, pharmacologic sedation and neuromuscular paralysis to allow easier intubation. RSI is preferable if the patient is not in deeply comatose state or in cardiac arrest, and it is generally safer in patients that may have a full stomach or have varying levels of consciousness. Due to the cessation of spontaneous respiration and the elimination of airway protective reflexes with sedation and paralysis, RSI should be modified for patients with difficult airways.

Endotracheal intubation may be indicated when there is:

- Excessive work of breathing with persistent hypoxemia leading to acute respiratory failure
- Inadequate ventilation due to hypoventilation
- Anatomical or functional airway obstruction

Table 4: Assessment of factors related to inadequate ventilation or desaturations in patients with or without an advanced airway

Factors	*Patients without an advanced airway*	*Patients with an advanced airway (endotracheal tube or tracheostomy tube)*
D—Displacement	Patient positioning is inadequate (no longer in sniffing position) Mask size/position is inadequate Inadequate seal due to mask displacement while bagging	Displacement of the endotracheal tube: • Distally into one of the mainstem bronchi • Esophageal placement Displacement of the tracheostomy tube: • Into a false tract • Improper placement
O—Obstruction	Obstruction of the airway caused by an improperly placed airway adjunct (OPA) Obstruction of the airway caused by foreign body	Obstruction of endotracheal tube by mucous plug Obstruction of tracheostomy tube by mucous plug
P—Pneumothorax	Bilateral pneumothorax will cause no chest rise at all	Can lead to sudden decompensation in patients on mechanical ventilation with an advanced airway
E—Equipment failure	Bag has a leak Mask size is inadequate	Failure of ventilator Disconnection of ventilator tubing Condensed water is collecting in ventilator tubing

- Inability to protect the airway patency (loss of cough or gag reflexes or excessive secretions)
- Need for advancing respiratory support from non-invasive ventilatory support to mechanical ventilation
- Need for controlled ventilation during sedation or anesthesia for surgical or diagnostic procedures
- Need for the patient to be transported to a distant healthcare facility when any of the above factors are present.

Emergency endotracheal intubation differs from rapid sequence intubation (RSI) as it is performed in the setting of cardiorespiratory arrest or during cardiopulmonary resuscitation where there may not be enough time to complete all the steps for sedation and airway access is a priority. The steps involved in performing laryngoscopy and endotracheal tube placement remain the same and will be discussed first. The steps involved in RSI have been outlined in **Table 5**.

Table 5: The seven Ps of rapid sequence intubation

1. Preoxygenation (5 minutes before intubation)
Start preoxygenation as soon as rapid sequence intubation is anticipated. Administer oxygen at the highest concentration available: • *Spontaneously breathing*: 100% FiO_2 (7 L/min oxygen flow) by nonrebreather mask for 3 minutes • *Apneic or inadequate breathing*: Bag-mask ventilation with small tidal breaths using 100% FiO_2 • During induction and paralysis, apneic oxygenation via nasal cannula at flow rate of 1 L/kg/min (maximum flow 15 L/min) may be provided
2. Preparation (4 minutes before intubation)
• Assemble equipment and check for function • Identify conditions that will predict difficult intubation or bag-mask ventilation (e.g. small chin, inability to fully open the mouth, upper airway trauma, or infection) • Identify conditions that will affect choice of medications (e.g. increased intracranial pressure, septic shock, bronchospasm, status epilepticus, or, if succinylcholine use is planned, absolute contraindications for its use as listed below) • Develop contingency plan for failed intubation
3. Pre-intubation optimization (3 minutes before intubation)
• *Atropine*: Although not routinely recommended, many experts suggest atropine as pretreatment for: Children ≤1 year, in shock, <5 years receiving succinylcholine or for older children receiving a second dose of succinylcholine. Dose: 0.02 mg/kg IV without a minimum dose (maximum single dose 0.5 mg; if no IV access, can be given IM) • *Fentanyl*: Optional for increased intracranial pressure in patients with normal or elevated blood pressure. Dose: 1 to 3 µg/kg given over 30 to 60 seconds to avoid respiratory depression and chest wall rigidity. Give 3 minutes before induction agent is administered • *Lidocaine*: Optional for increased intracranial pressure (not recommended for pretreatment in children by some airway experts). Dose: 1 to 2 mg/kg IV (maximum dose 200 mg). Give 2 to 3 minutes before intubation
4. Paralysis with induction
Induction • *Midazolam*: May use in hemodynamically stable patients with status epilepticus. Time to clinical effect is longer, inconsistently induces unconsciousness. May cause hemodynamic instability at doses required for sedation. Dose: 0.2 to 0.3 mg/kg IV (maximum dose 10 mg, onset of effect requires 2 to 3 minutes) • *Propofol*: Causes hypotension. May use in hemodynamically stable patients with status epilepticus. Dose 1 to 1.5 mg/kg IV • *Fentanyl*: Optional for cardiogenic shock or catecholamine-depleted shock (e.g. persistent hypotension despite vasopressor therapy) Limited evidence in children. Give over 30 to 60 seconds to avoid respiratory depression or chest wall rigidity. Dose 1 to 5 µg/kg titrated to effect. Start at lower end of range in hypotensive patients • *Thiopental*: Neuroprotective. Do **not** use with hemodynamic instability. Dose: 3 to 5 mg/kg IV • *Etomidate*: Safe with hemodynamic instability, neuroprotective, transient adrenal cortico-suppression. Do not use routinely in patients with septic shock. Dose: 0.3 mg/kg IV • *Ketamine*: Safe with hemodynamic instability if patient is not catecholamine depleted. Use in patients with bronchospasm and septic shock. Use with caution in hypertensive patients with increased intracranial pressure. Dose: 1 to 2 mg/kg IV (if no IV access, can be given IM dose: 3 to 7 mg/kg) **Paralysis** • *Rocuronium*: Use for children with contraindication for succinylcholine or as primary paralytic if sugammadex is immediately available Dose: 1 mg/kg IV • *Vecuronium*: May be used in children with contraindications to succinylcholine and when rocuronium is not available. Dose: 0.15 to 0.2 mg/kg. Patients may experience prolonged and unpredictable duration of paralysis at this dose • *Succinylcholine*: Do not use with extensive crush injury with rhabdomyolysis, chronic skeletal muscle disease (e.g. Becker muscular dystrophy) or denervating neuromuscular disease (e.g. cerebral palsy with paralysis); 48 to 72 hours after burn, multiple trauma, or denervating injury; patients with history or malignant hyperthermia; or pre-existing hyperkalemia. Dose: Infants and children ≤2 years: 2 mg/kg IV, older children and adolescents: 1 to 1.5 mg/kg IV (if IV access unobtainable, can be given IM, dose: 4 mg/kg)

Contd...

Contd...

5. Protection (30 seconds after induction)
• Put the patient in the "sniffing position" using head-tilt chin lift maneuver if cervical spine injury is not present • Maintain manual cervical spine immobilization during intubation in the trauma patient • Use gentle cricoid pressure to optimize the view of the glottis during direct laryngoscopy
6. Placement of endotracheal tube (45 seconds after induction)
• Perform laryngoscopy • Place endotracheal tube • Confirm tracheal tube placement with end-tidal CO_2 detection and auscultation
7. Post-intubation management (60 seconds after induction)
• Obtain a chest radiograph to confirm the depth of tracheal tube insertion • Provide ongoing sedation (e.g. midazolam), analgesia (e.g. fentanyl 1 µg/kg), and paralysis (if indicated) • If decompensation occurs after successful intubation, use the DOPE mnemonic to find the cause (as listed in **Table 4**)

Laryngoscopy

To perform endotracheal intubation correctly, direct visualization of the airway with a straight line of sight from mouth to larynx is crucial. This can be achieved with direct laryngoscopy using either a curved (Macintosh) or straight (Miller) blade attached to a laryngoscope (**Fig. 9**). Due to the relatively large tongue and acute-angled epiglottis in infants and toddlers, a straight blade may be preferable in children less than 3 years of age as it can be passed posterior to the epiglottis (**Fig. 10A**), with its narrower width allowing easier passage in situations with limited mouth opening. The curved Macintosh blade is wider and has a vertical flange to keep the tongue out of the view (**Fig. 10B**). These blades come in a variety of sizes and can be switched with the same laryngoscope handle. The laryngoscope should be held low on the handle such that the blade's proximal part is at the thenar or hypothenar eminence of the non-dominant hand. It is important to lift the laryngoscope from upward movement at the shoulder joint and to keep the wrists relatively stiff during laryngoscopy. The patient's bed should be elevated to allow the operator to bend their back at the waist and to keep the operator's spine relatively straight during the procedure.

After adequate positioning of the patient's head, the mouth should be opened, and the blade inserted along the right lingual gutter along the inside margin of the molars and keep the tongue to the left. Advance the tip of the blade until the epiglottis is visualized—this is a consistent landmark, as the glottis lies posterior and inferior to it. With a curved blade advanced in the space between the base of tongue and epiglottis, the epiglottis can be lifted out of view to reveal the glottic opening. With a straight blade it has be advanced under the epiglottis to lift it directly. It is important to have familiarity with

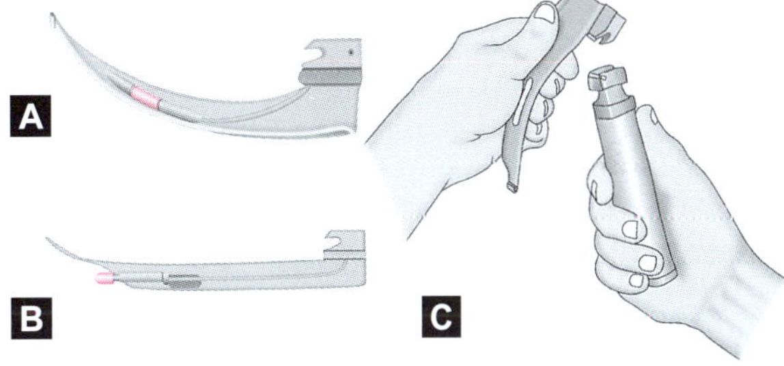

Figs. 9A to C: Laryngoscope and the different types of blades that can be used with it. (A) Curved (Macintosh) blade for laryngoscope; (B) Straight (Miller) blade for laryngoscope; (C) Attaching the laryngoscope blade to the handle

several glottic landmarks as shown in **Figure 11**. If the glottic opening is still not in view as seen in **Figure 11**, then Sellick maneuver (**Fig. 12**) may have to utilized to push the glottic opening into view. This may be especially important for infants whose glottic opening is higher and more anterior and can be done by identifying the cricoid ring beneath the thyroid cartilage and putting pressure on it. The total duration of laryngoscopy should be kept as short as possible and oxyhemoglobin saturations should be closely monitored during the procedure. If there is a delay in completion of intubation, then laryngoscopy should be interrupted, and patient should be given bag mask ventilation to achieve adequate oxygenation before proceeding again with another attempt. Complications of laryngoscopy include: dental or gum injury or bleeding, gagging and vomiting.

Placement of endotracheal tube

After the laryngoscope is in position and glottic opening is adequately visualized, the dominant hand should be

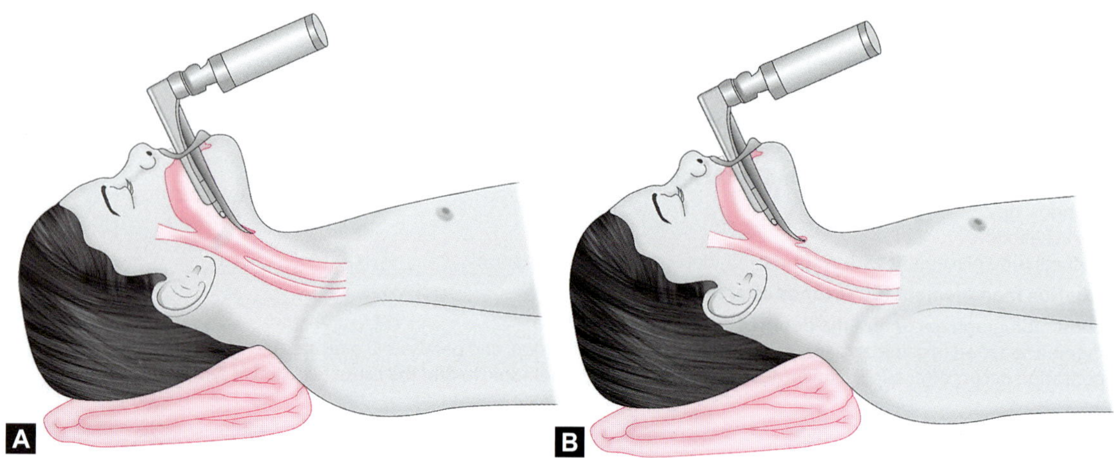

Figs. 10A and B: Laryngoscopy. (A) Laryngoscopy using the straight blade to visualize the glottic opening by lifting the epiglottis; (B) Laryngoscopy using the curved blade to visualize the glottic opening by placing the tip of the blade in the space between the tongue and vallecula

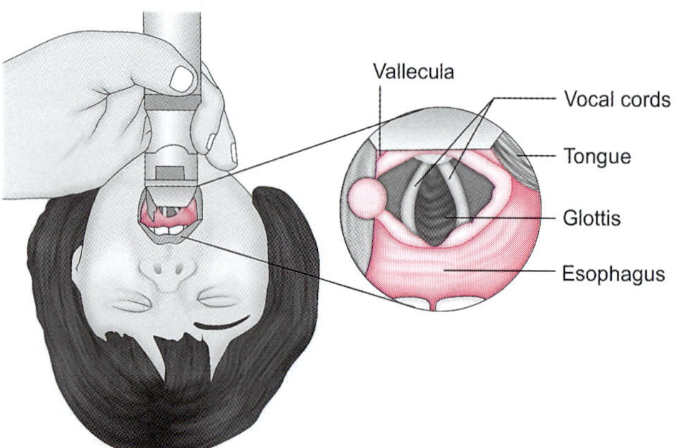

Fig. 11: Glottic landmarks seen on laryngoscopy

used to hold the endotracheal tube and slide it along the laryngoscope blade into the glottic opening. It is important to select the correct endotracheal tube size and lubricate the lower end, especially if using a cuffed endotracheal tube. The size of the endotracheal tube can be determined for children by using the following formula:

Uncuffed endotracheal tube size (mm) = 4 + [Age (in years)/4]
Cuffed endotracheal tube size (mm) = 3.5 + [Age (in years)/4]

It is important to have extra endotracheal tubes 0.5 mm below or above the selected size available at hand during intubation so that if there is significant airway swelling or difficulty in intubation with the selected size, then another size endotracheal tube could be used. For infants less than 1 year of age or less than 4 kg body weight, endotracheal tube size and length can be determined using **Table 6**.

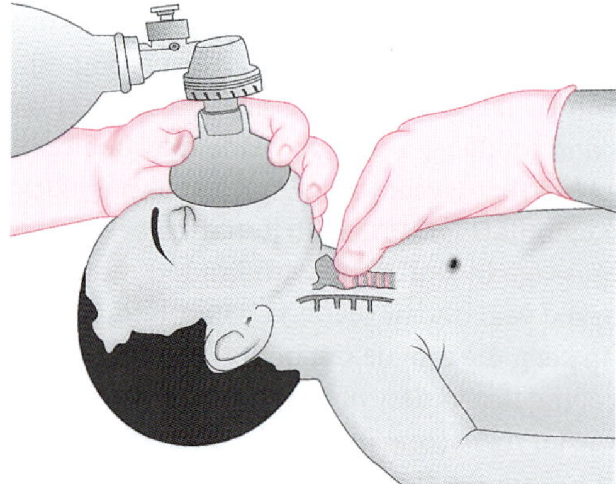

Fig. 12: Sellick maneuver in an infant to push the airway at the level of the cricoid cartilage to allow the glottic opening to be visualized during subsequent laryngoscopy and to prevent aspiration of gastric contents

Table 6: Endotracheal tube sizes and insertion depth (up to lip) for infants based on body weight

Body weight (kg)	*Endotracheal tube size (mm)*	*Depth of insertion of endotracheal tube (measured at lip level in cm)*
<1.0	2.5	5.5
1.0	2.5–3.0	6.0
2.0	3.0	7.0
3.0	3.0	8.5
3.5	3.0–3.5	9.0
4.0	3.5	9.0

A guidewire can be placed inside the endotracheal tube to impart some rigidity to the endotracheal tube.

After endotracheal tube is positioned, this guidewire can be removed while firmly holding the tube at the level of the lip to prevent displacement. The outer end of the endotracheal tube should be immediately connected to a self-inflating bag and few positive pressure breaths should be given to observe chest rise. Simultaneous auscultation of the lungs with bagging can confirm the tracheal position of the distal tip of the endotracheal tube. If there is lack of breath sounds on one side, then the endotracheal tube should be withdrawn by 0.5 to 1 cm and air entry should be checked again. Assessment of exhaled carbon dioxide (CO_2) by colorimetric devices can also be used to confirm tube position. A chest X-ray may also be helpful to assess tube position and lung expansion after endotracheal tube placement. Once the tube position has been confirmed, the marking at the lip should be noted and tape/holding device applied to hold the tube in position. The depth of insertion of the endotracheal tube can be estimated from the child's age or tube size as shown below:

Depth of insertion (cm) for ages >2 years = (Age in years/2) + 12
Or
Depth of insertion (cm) = Tube internal diameter (mm) × 3

Complications of endotracheal intubation include hypoxemia, bradycardia, increased intracranial pressure, soft tissue injury.

Supraglottic Airways

There are several newer devices that can be placed into the upper airway without laryngoscopy and can be used for securing the airway and providing ventilatory support for short periods of time. They can be used as a bridge to advanced airway techniques after achieving some stability. There are now several types of devices available and laryngeal mask airway (LMA) **(Fig. 13)** was the first of these to be introduced in 1981. The second generation LMAs also have a gastric drainage tube included. It is inserted into the mouth with the laryngeal surface directed caudally and the tip of the index finger placed at the cuff-tube junction. The device is advanced over the back of the tongue as far as the length of the operator's index finger will allow. The other hand is used to push it further down into its final seated position. The cuff is then inflated to minimize airleak.

Retroglottic airways such as the Combitube and King laryngeal tube airway have two high-volume, low-pressure balloons where the proximal balloon seals the oropharynx and the distal balloon seals the esophagus. Airflow into the airway is through holes in between these balloons.

Management of Patients with a Tracheostomy

Pediatric patients with a tracheostomy require special attention to a unique set of issues that occur in acute care settings. There is a wide variety of tracheostomy tubes available (**Fig. 14**) and the most common ones used in pediatric patients are either made of silicone (Bivona) or polyvinyl chloride (Shiley). They can have different lengths and inner diameters and these dimensions are usually written on the flange of each tracheostomy tube. The uncuffed tracheostomy (**Fig. 14**) tubes are preferred in pediatric patients (as they are easier to change and can allow vocalization with a Passy-Muir Valve), but cuffed tracheostomy tubes are beneficial in patients who require higher ventilatory settings, who are on night-time support only or those who are at high risk of aspiration. Besides airway humidification, patients with a tracheostomy also require frequent suctioning of the tracheostomy tube to prevent mucus plugging. It is very important to measure out the length of the suction catheter extending from the external connector to the distal tip so that while suctioning, the suction catheter does not extend beyond the distal tip of the tracheostomy tube and cause tracheal injury

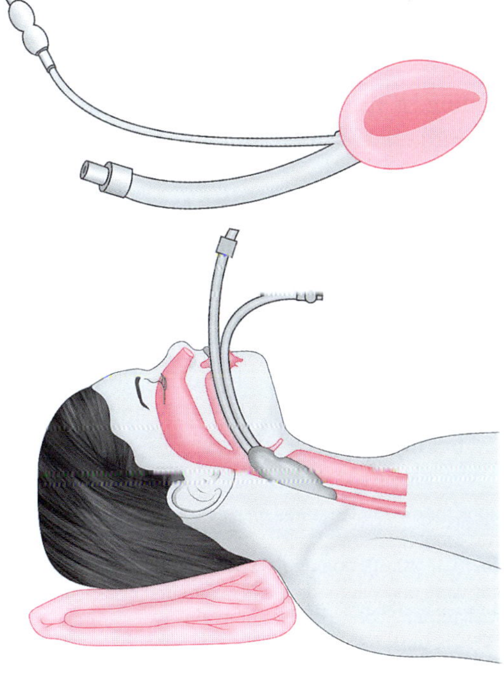

Fig. 13: Laryngeal mask airway in use in a pediatric patient

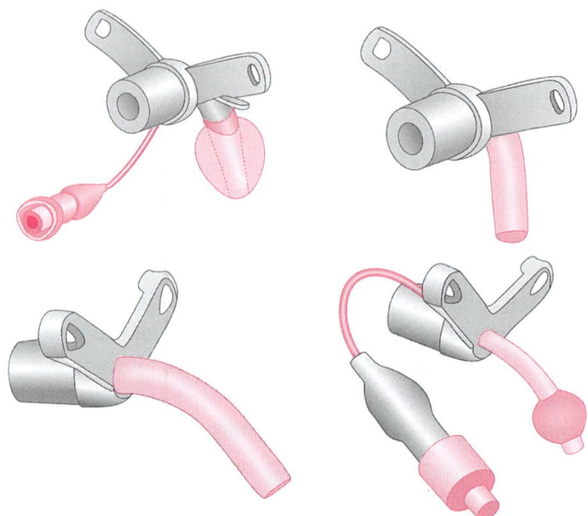

Fig. 14: Different types of tracheostomy tubes

Table 7: Common complications of pediatric patients with a tracheostomy tube
Displacement/accidental decannulation
Obstruction by mucus plugs
Bleeding from tracheostomy tube
Infection (Tracheitis)
Granulation tissue (in the trachea or at the stoma)
False tract/pouch due to improper insertion
Pneumomediastinum
Trachea-innominate fistula

or bleeding. A list of common complications seen in patients with tracheostomy tubes is listed in **Table 7**.

DIFFICULT PEDIATRIC AIRWAY

A difficult pediatric airway occurs when there is difficulty in performing bag-mask ventilation, laryngoscopy or intubation. **Table 8** lists all the congenital and acquired causes of a difficult pediatric airway.

A useful method for the identification of a difficult pediatric airway is called the LEMON approach which is outlined below:

L — Look for external features such as craniofacial anomalies, neck masses
E — Evaluate mouth opening, distance between the thyroid cartilage and the mandible (thyromental distance)
M — Mallampati Scoring of the upper airway
O — Obstruction
N — Neck mobility

Table 8: Causes of difficult pediatric airway

Categories	*Conditions*
Congenital malformations	*Cranial abnormalities*: Macrocephaly, craniosynostosis syndromes *Facial abnormalities*: Apert's syndrome, Goldenhar syndrome *Small oral aperture*: Hallerman Streiff syndrome, Freeman Sheldon syndrome *Small oral cavity*: Treacher Collins syndrome, Pierre Robin sequence *Neck immobility*: Klippel Feil syndrome, mucopolysaccharidoses *Macroglossia*: Down syndrome, Beckwith Wiedemann syndrome *Mass lesions*: Cystic hygromas, hemangiomas, teratomas
Acquired disorders	*Infections*: Epiglottitis, croup, tracheitis, peritonsillar abscess, retropharyngeal abscess Trauma Foreign body Anaphylaxis Extreme obesity Previous airway surgery

If a difficult pediatric airway is anticipated, then it is crucial to plan airway management with experienced personnel and using some of the advanced airway management techniques (such as flexible fibreoptic intubation) outlined in the next section.

ADVANCED AIRWAY MANAGEMENT

Percutaneous Cricothyrotomy

Percutaneous needle cricothyrotomy and transtracheal ventilation can be done in an acute emergency situation where there is "no ventilation, no oxygenation" feasible. This can occur in the setting of complete upper airway obstruction by heavy bleeding in oral cavity, severe maxillofacial trauma, laryngeal foreign body causing complete obstruction or with severe chemical or thermal burns to the upper airway. A needle cricothyrotomy can be subsequently converted to a surgical cricothyroidotomy using the Seldinger technique. An over-the-needle catheter (13 to 16 gauge) is first passed in the midline through the cricothyroid membrane which is present between the inferior margin of the thyroid cartilage and upper margin of cricoid cartilage. Once inside the tracheal lumen, the needle can be withdrawn, and the catheter hub can be connected to an adapter (either a 3 mm endotracheal tube connector or 3 mL Luer lock syringe with plunger removed) for providing ventilation through a ventilator or oxygen source. This technique is feasible in children up to 12 years of age, but in older children and adults surgical cricothyrotomy is associated with less injury. It is important to remember that transtracheal ventilation through a catheter relies on expired air coming out from the mouth and nose. In the setting of complete laryngeal obstruction, the egress of expired air may not be feasible and use of a high pressure oxygen source in this setting can also cause barotrauma **(Fig. 15)**.

Flexible Fiberoptic Intubation

This technique can be utilized in emergency situations and also for elective intubation of patients with a known difficult airway. Familiarity with operation and use of a flexible fiberoptic bronchoscope in pediatric patients is a prerequisite for this technique. The desired size of the endotracheal tube is threaded onto a flexible bronchoscope (generally 3.1 mm size scope) and the bronchoscope along with the tube is advanced either through the mouth or nose of the patient. Once the glottic opening is visualized through the bronchoscope, then the endotracheal tube is pushed along the bronchoscope to advance it into the trachea under direct visualization. This technique generally requires sedation or placement of an oral airway in the patient's mouth so that the patient does not inadvertently bite down on the bronchoscope during the procedure.

Nasotracheal Intubation

Nasotracheal intubation can be performed for anticipated prolonged intubation or for some oral surgical procedures. This requires an extra step of introducing the endotracheal tube through the nasal passages into the pharynx before inserting the laryngoscope. A special instrument called Magill forceps is required to grasp the distal end of the endotracheal tube in the pharynx and advance it under direct laryngoscopic visualization into the glottic opening. The Magill forceps are specially designed such that the bend in their handles keeps them out of the line of sight while they are in use on the right side of the oral cavity. Subsequent steps for endotracheal tube placement confirmation remain the same, but it is important to ensure that the nasal passages have been adequately prepared prior to the procedure to avoid injury to the nasal mucosa.

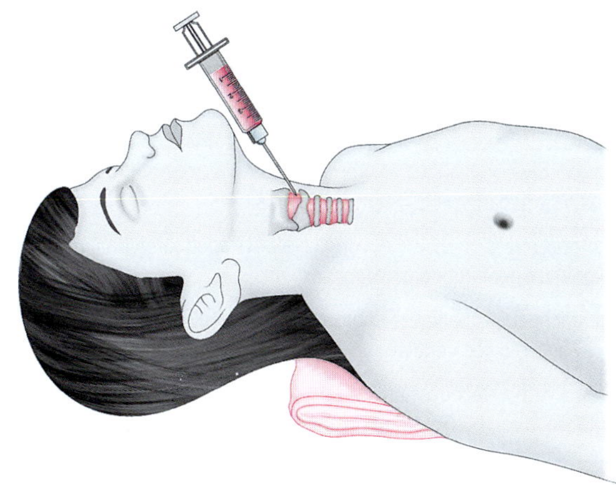

Fig. 15: Percutaneous cricothyrotomy

Single Lung Ventilation

Single lung ventilation is generally done for thoracic, mediastinal, esophageal or video-assisted thoracoscopic surgery (VATS) procedures or during whole lung lavage by placing a double lumen endotracheal tube.

PREVENTION

Prevention of airway problems in hospitalized patients can be achieved by identification of high-risk patients and close monitoring of their vital signs. The disease categories and conditions mentioned in **Table 8** are all associated with greater chances of development of airway related complications. Proper attention to airway humidification can prevent mucus plugging of the airways, especially in intubated patients and in those with a tracheostomy tube. Monitoring of airway secretions for signs of infection (e.g. tracheitis) and instituting daily tracheostomy tube changes for 3 consecutive days in patients with tracheostomy tubes can help reduce the need for repeated airway cultures and antibiotic treatment.

KEY MESSAGES

- Infants and children have significant differences in airway anatomy and chest wall physiology when compared to adults and can develop respiratory failure due to acute illnesses.
- Immediate evaluation of airway and breathing should be performed to determine if a child has a patent airway or not and whether specific interventions are needed to maintain its patency.

- Adequate positioning, use of head-tilt, chin-lift and/or jaw thrust and utilization of airway adjuncts such as oro-/nasopharyngeal airway can improve airway patency.
- Bag mask ventilation should be initiated for children that are unresponsive or cyanotic at presentation while continuing evaluation for airway management.
- Laryngoscopy is an essential skill that allows adequate visualization of the glottic opening during intubation.
- Endotracheal intubation is another essential skill that can secure the airway and provide ventilatory support to critically ill children.
- Patients with a tracheostomy can present with acute emergencies and may require establishment of patency or replacement of tracheostomy tube.
- Use of supraglottic airway devices such as laryngeal mask airway or noninvasive ventilatory support (bilevel positive airway pressure) may be used in initial stages to achieve stabilization.
- Advanced airway management techniques such as percutaneous cricothyrotomy or nasotracheal intubation should be performed in select cases by trained individuals.
- Patients on mechanical ventilatory support can also develop airway complications and it is important to evaluate any acute decompensation for displacement of artificial airway or obstruction; development of pneumothorax or equipment failure.

REFERENCES

1. Zar HJ, Ferkol TW. The global burden of respiratory disease-impact on child health. Pediatr Pulmonol. 2014;49(5):430-4.
2. Selvaraj K, Chinnakali P, Majumdar A, *et al.* Acute respiratory infections among under-5 children in India: A situational analysis. J Nat Sci Biol Med. 2014;5(1):15-20.
3. The burden of chronic respiratory diseases and their heterogeneity across the states of India: The Global Burden of Disease Study 1990-2016. Lancet Glob Health. 2018;6(12):e1363-e1374.

CHAPTER

7

Cardiopulmonary Resuscitation

Javed Ismail, Biraj Parjauli

INTRODUCTION

Cardiopulmonary arrest is defined as cessation of respiration or apnea, unresponsiveness and absent of detectable central pulse. Cardiopulmonary resuscitation (CPR), also called "cardiocerebral resuscitation," is a life-sustaining procedure of delivering oxygen and blood to the vital organs like heart and brain during cardiac arrest and has got a potential to revive an apparently dead child back to life. The main aim of CPR is to provide sufficient myocardial and cerebral blood flow to attain return of spontaneous circulation (ROSC) at a level compatible with survival. If the patients are not rapidly revived from this state, the vital organs (namely brain, heart) sustain an irreversible damage and ultimately die. Majority of arrests in children, in contrast to adults (where arrhythmia is the common cause of cardiac arrest) result from hypoxia due to progression of respiratory failure or shock. Only a small proportion, about 10–15% have sudden cardiac arrest due to arrhythmias.[1] During the cardiac arrest, electrocardiogram may show any of the 4 rhythms; asystole, pulseless electrical activity (PEA), ventricular fibrillation (VF) or ventricular tachycardia (VT) without pulse. Studies have shown a survival of about 11–42% in those undergoing CPR with 8–33% having a intact neurological outcome.[2]

EPIDEMIOLOGY

Pediatric In-Hospital Arrests

Based on registry and administrative data, more than 6000 children in the United States receive in-hospital CPR each year, majority of them in pediatric intensive care units (PICUs). An observational study from north India showed that 6.7% of total admissions required in-hospital CPR and the incidence of CPR in PICU was 15% of all admissions.[3] Among hospitals in the American Heart Association Get With The Guidelines-Resuscitation (GWTG-R) registry, survival to discharge rates improved from ~25% (2000–2005) to >40% (since 2006) with 70%-90% having favorable neurologic outcomes.[4] There has been a trend towards improvement in survival with favorable neurological outcomes for in-hospital CPR if the setting changes from ward to ICU where staff-to-patient ratios, resuscitation experience and expertise are better. Over the last two decades, studies have increasingly used the more rigorous Utstein-style reporting (set of guidelines for uniform reporting of cardiac arrest) for in-hospital pediatric cardiac arrests and CPR.[5]

Pediatric Out-of-Hospital Arrests

Outcomes following pediatric out-of-hospital cardiac arrests (OHCAs) are worse than those following in-hospital arrests due to delay in recognition. OHCAs are not witnessed, and not provided with bystander CPR so the no-flow period is often prolonged and neurologic outcomes are worse. Large-scale population-based studies from North America, Japan, Netherlands, and Finland demonstrate an incidence of 8–10 pediatric out-of-hospital cardiac arrests/100,000 person-years.[6] Infants have a tenfold higher incidence than older children with a high mortality rate, common causes being trauma and Sudden Infant Death Syndrome.

PEDIATRIC CHAIN OF SURVIVAL

The primary goal in sudden cardiac arrest is to achieve a neurologically intact survival and this can be achieved from interlinked intervention termed as "chain of survival" which are carried out together or sequentially (**Fig. 1**). Each step in chain of survival are interlinked and interdependent to the next one.[7] It consists of:

- *Prevention of cardiac arrest*: Avoiding accidental injuries and maintain effective oxygenation and ventilation to prevent asphyxia cardiac arrest.
- *Early effective CPR*: Identify respiratory arrest and provide rescue breathing with or without compression. Identify cardiac arrest and initiate high quality CPR.
- *Rapid activation of emergency response system (ERS)*: Activate ERS for Automated external defibrillator (AED) and CPR.
- *Effective advanced life support*: Stabilization and effective transport to advanced care center.
- *Integrated post ROSC care*: After ROSC, victim's outcome depends on post-resuscitative multiorgan care.

PATHOPHYSIOLOGY

Cardiac arrest is the end result of diverse etiologies culminating into physiological derangements of respiratory, circulatory or neurological systems, which ultimately progress to mechanical cardiac arrest due to progressive hypoxic-ischemic events or metabolic disturbances (**Fig. 2**).

The etiology of cardiac arrest varies in different age groups with cardiorespiratory causes predominate in infant and children whereas arrhythmias are seen in adults. Arrhythmogenic cardiac arrests include ventricular fibrillation or ventricular tachycardia. Some common causes of these arrhythmias are enlisted in **Table 1**.[8] Mechanical ("pump") cardiomyopathic arrests are typically due to inadequate myocardial oxygen delivery from asphyxia, ischemia, metabolic disturbances (e.g. hypocalcemia, hypomagnesemia, severe acidosis), or pharmacologic (e.g. β-blocker, calcium channel blocker, barbiturate) toxicity.

Four Phases of Cardiac Arrest (Table 2)

- Pre-arrest
- No-flow (untreated cardiac arrest)
- Low flow (CPR)
- Post return of spontaneous circulation.

Pre-arrest phase

The pre-arrest phase presents an opportunity to prevent the pulseless cardiopulmonary arrest with vigilant monitoring and thus can reduce mortality and morbidity. Children in their early phase of life-threatening illness maintain their vital parameters with activation of several compensatory mechanisms. If this phase is prolonged, these mechanisms get exhausted and the patient may rapidly progress to cardiac arrest. For identification of patients in early compensatory phase, clinical signs of physiological impairment should be elicited. Recognition

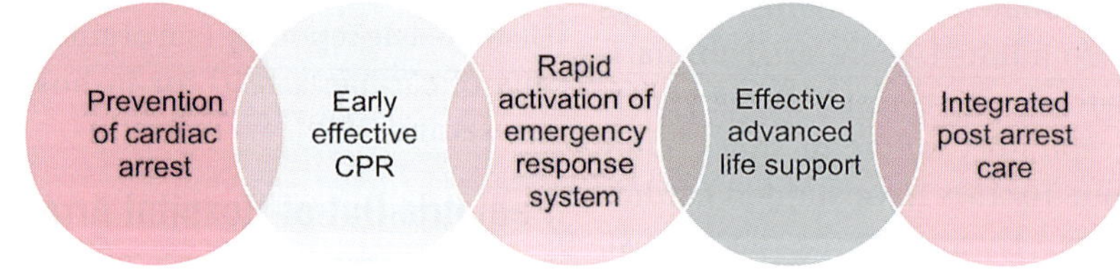

Fig. 1: Pediatric chain of survival[7]

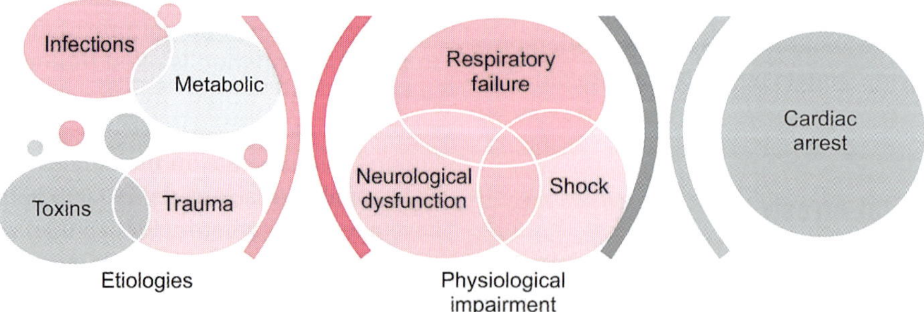

Fig. 2: Pathophysiological pathway of cardiac arrest

Table 1: Causes of sudden cardiac arrest in children

- **Congenital cardiac abnormalities**
  - Associated with myocardial ischemia (e.g. coronary artery anomalies)
  - Genetic channelopathies associated with prolonged QT syndrome
  - Familial cardiomyopathies
  - Mitochondrial diseases
- **Acquired cardiomyopathies**
  - Drugs/toxins (e.g. doxorubicin cardiomyopathy, drug-induced prolonged QT syndrome)
  - Hypoxic-ischemic event with inadequate myocardial oxygen delivery
  - Cardiac surgical injury
  - Commotio cordis
  - Mechanically induced VF
  - Ischemia during CPR
  - Inappropriate unsynchronized cardioversion shock

Table 2: Phases of CPR and effective interventions

Phase	*Effective interventions*
Pre-arrest phase	Early recognition, prompt effective intervention, monitoring to prevent progression to cardiac arrest
No flow/Low flow phase	Early recognition and initiation of *high quality CPR* Identify and treat reversible causes of cardiac arrest Appropriate use of defibrillation, medications
Post-return of spontaneous circulation phase	Prevent secondary cell injury by • Titrating the vasoactive support to optimize the cardiac output and cerebral perfusion • Treating arrhythmias • Avoiding hyperglycemia, hyperthermia, hyperventilation • Mild systemic hypothermia

of patients requiring effective intervention during this phase is assisted using Pediatric early warning scores (PEWS) (**Tables 3 and 4**).[9] Because many pediatric cardiac arrests are due to progressive respiratory failure and shock, the main focus should be early recognition and treatment of these life threatening physiological states and the etiologies causing these. Early recognition, prompt effective intervention, monitoring to prevent progression to cardiac arrest forms the cornerstone of pre-arrest phase.

No-flow and low-flow phase

This phase is characterized by cessation of circulation or absent mechanical cardiac activity. It is recognized by clinical signs of cardiac arrest like unresponsiveness (cessation of blood flow to brain), not breathing or gasping, absent central pulses. The no-flow phase requires an early recognition and prompt initiation of Basic Life Support (BLS) with effective chest compressions to perfuse the coronary and cerebral circulation. ECG rhythms should be evaluated to identify and defibrillate shockable rhythms. Early recognition and initiation of *high quality CPR* forms the cornerstone of this phase. An effective *high quality CPR* generates about 10–25% of the normal coronary blood flow and about 50% of the normal cerebral blood flow.

Post-return of spontaneous circulation

The ischemic hypoxic injury to the cells during the previous phases can trigger the them to follow either of these pathways: apoptosis, mitochondrial hibernation, partial or complete recovery of cellular functions. Thus, the treatment measures during this phase are targeted to reduce the secondary damage caused by reperfusion injury to the recovering cells and to salvage the potential cells. Post-ROSC, the patients are prone for complications like hypotension, arrhythmias, seizures, hyperthermia, brain injury and reperfusion to multiple organs commonly called as post-cardiac arrest syndrome. Hyperoxia, hyperventilation is common and can cause undue adverse effects at cellular level. Management of this phase requires anticipation, identification and treatment of each of these complications by: titrating the vasoactive support to optimize the cardiac output and cerebral perfusion, treating arrhythmias, avoiding hyperglycemia, hyperthermia, hyperventilation, mild systemic hypothermia to minimize reperfusion injury.

Table 3: Pediatric emergency warning score (PEWS)

Score	*Behavior*	*Cardiovascular*	*Respiratory*
0	Playing/appropriate	Pink or Capillary refill time (CRT) 1–2 s	Within normal limits, no retractions
1	Irritable	Pale or CRT – 3 s	RR>10 above normal with accessory muscle use or need of FiO_2 > 30%
2	Irritable	Gray or CRT 4 s or tachycardia HR > 20 beats above normal	RR > 20 above normal with retractions or need of FiO_2 >40%
3	Lethargic/confused or reduced response to pain	Gray, mottled or CRT ≥ 5 s or tachycardia of HR 30 beats above normal or bradycardia	Bradypnea with RR of 5 below normal with retractions and grunting or need for FiO_2 > 50%
+1	If nebulizations are needed every 15 minutes		
+1	If persistent vomiting following surgery		

Table 4: Interpretation of PEWS

PEWS	*Interpretation*
≤2	Low risk, reassess as needed
3–4	Intermediate risk, to inform doctor in charge
≥5	High risk, initiate rapid response team

MANAGEMENT

A high quality early basic life support (BLS) overlapped with Advanced Life Support (ALS) techniques form the basis of management of cardiac arrest. In an out of hospital scenario, first ensure safety of the scene to preclude imminent dangers like electric shocks, fire or road traffic. After ensuring this or in case of in-hospital settings, the care provider rapidly performs a visual assessment of general appearance (looking at tone, alertness, responsiveness) adequacy of breathing (apneic, gasping, respiratory distress or normal respiration) and color (pale, cyanosed, mottling) of the child. **Flowchart 1** shows the algorithm for management of cardiac arrest.

- If there is pulse (heart rate >60/min) and breathing adequately, the child does not require CPR. A systematic primary assessment should be done to identify and grade the severity of physiological impairment if the child is in the pre-arrest state (**Table 5**).
- If the child is unresponsive and apneic/gasping, activate emergency response (call for help) and then rapidly check pulse (brachial in infants, carotids in children; should be done within 10 seconds). If there is no pulse or if the heart rate is <60/min, start CPR (Algorithm). Current recommendations state that chest compressions be initiated by the first responder and the airway, breathing, cardiac rhythms be addressed by the subsequent responders. The sequence is C-A-B (circulation, airway, breathing) for both in-hospital and out of hospital cardiac arrests.
- If there is pulse (with heart rate more than 60/min) and the child is apneic, continue to provide adequate assisted ventilation.

Chest compressions should be initiated as soon as it is recognized that the child is in pulseless arrest. For infants, 2 thumbs over the mid-sternum with hands encircling the chest or 2 fingers over the mid-sternum can be used for providing chest compressions (**Figs. 3A and B**). Whereas, for children >1 year, heel of one hand or two hands placed one above the other can be used with compression delivered over lower half of the sternum (**Fig. 3C**). Care should be taken to avoid injury to the xiphoid or the ribs.

For a single rescuer, the chest compression to ventilation ratio is 30:2 whereas for two rescuers the ratio is 15:2. Ventilation can be provided either by mouth to mouth (out of hospital setting) or bag and mask (in-hospital). It should be delivered at a desired rate of 15–20 breaths/min for children aged ≤8 years; 10–12 breaths/min for >8 years.

A high quality CPR comprises

- Effective chest compressions
  - Push hard (to a depth of at least 1/3rd of anteroposterior diameter of chest or about 4 cm in infants and 5 cm in children). Compression depth should not exceed 6 cm for any age group to avoid chest wall injuries
  - Push fast (compression rate of at least 100/min)
- Allow for complete chest recoil after each compression
- Minimize interruptions between chest compression (compressions should be interrupted only after at least 2 minutes, to check rhythm or to deliver shock. These should not be more than 10 seconds)
- Avoid excessive ventilation.

Flowchart 1: Algorithm for management of cardiac arrest*

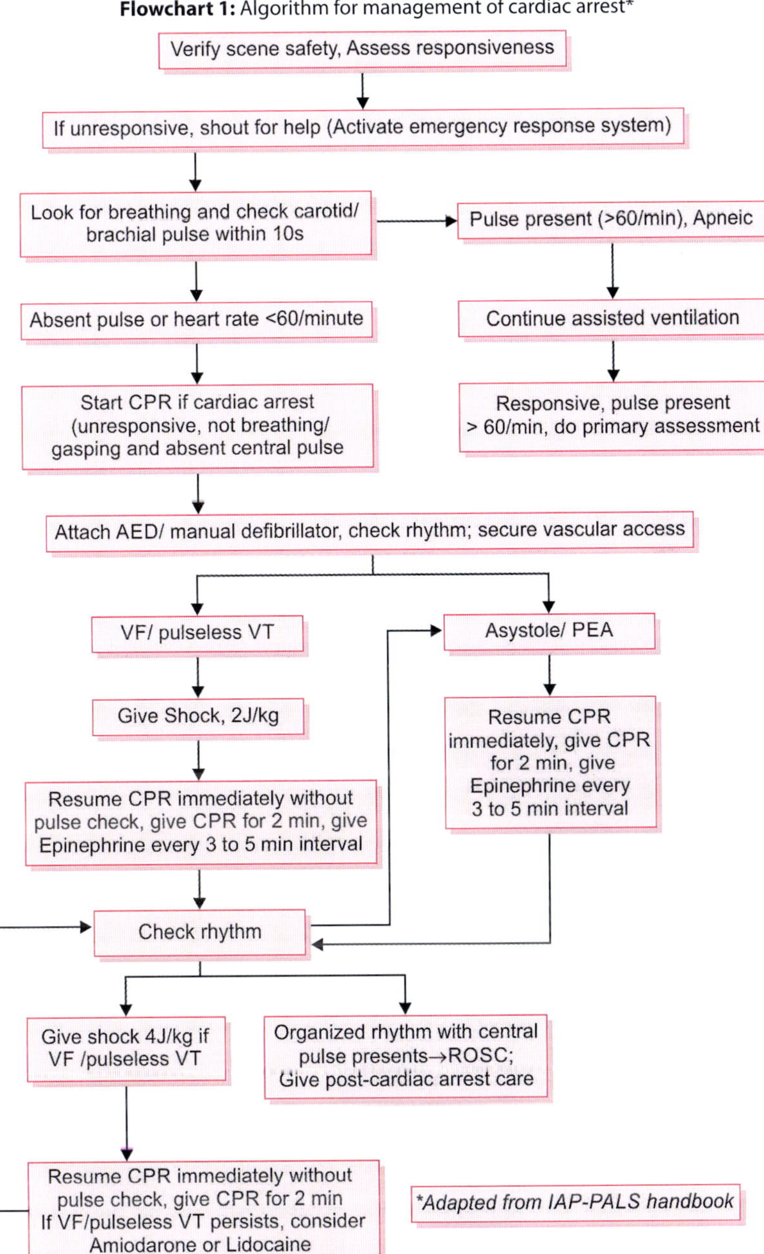

Monitoring during CPR

The ultimate goal of high quality CPR is to achieve a coronary perfusion pressure (arterial pressure minus the right atrial pressure) of > 20 mm Hg during the relaxation phase of CPR or an arterial "diastolic/relaxation" pressure >30 mm Hg. These cut offs have been found to be associated with successful ROSC.[10] In an ideal scenario, an arterial pressure catheter should guide the effectiveness of the chest compressions. Whenever an arterial catheter is not available, end-tidal carbon dioxide ($ETCO_2$) can be used. An $ETCO_2$ of more than 15 mm Hg is associated with higher rate of ROSC.[11]

Often, slow chest compression rates, shallow compressions, prolonged pauses between compressions compromise the quality of CPR. In an out of hospital setting, rescuers should continue *high quality CPR* till

Table 5: Clinical assessment in pre-arrest phase

	Assessment	*Identification*
Airway	Not maintainable, partial or complete obstruction	Open Maintainable Not maintainable
Breathing	Respiratory rate and pattern: Tachypnea, bradypnea, apnea, gasping *Respiratory effort*: Increased with chest retractions, see-saw breathing, jaw breathing, head-bobbing *Chest expansion*: Decreased *Auscultation*: Decreased air entry *SpO_2*: Hypoxia (<94%)	Stable Respiratory distress Respiratory failure
Circulation	*Heart rate and rhythm*: Tachycardia, bradycardia, irregular rhythm *Central, peripheral pulses*: Weak, absent *Capillary refill time*: > 2 seconds *Skin color and temperature*: Cool peripheries, pale, mottled, cyanosed or dusky peripheries	Stable Compensated shock Hypotensive shock
Disability	Altered level of consciousness (low Glasgow Coma Scale), loss of muscle tone, abnormal pupillary size or response, seizures	Stable Cortical dysfunction Brainstem dysfunction
Exposure	Significant bleeding, evidence of trauma, purpura, deformities	

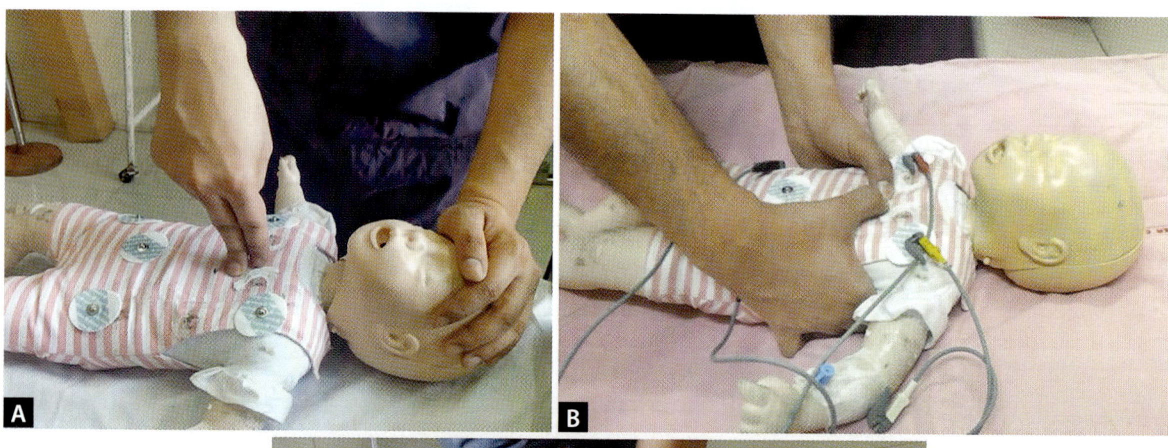

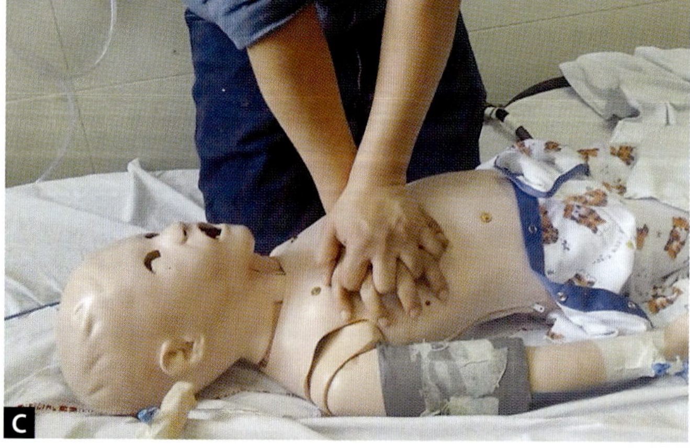

Figs. 3A to C: Position of hand for delivering chest compressions. (A) For infant's and single rescuer; (B) For infants and two rescuers; (C) For children >1 year of age

the emergency response team with automated external defibrillator (AED) arrives or till it is feasible or reasonable as ascertained by the rescuers. In the in-hospital setting, after at least 2 minutes of CPR, an electrocardiogram (ECG) rhythm should guide the further course of action.

The ECG rhythm in a cardiac arrest could be either of the following (**Figs. 4A to D**).

- Asystole
- Pulseless electrical activity (PEA)
- Ventricular fibrillation (VF)
- Ventricular tachycardia (VT) without pulse.

Of these, asystole and PEA are non-shockable rhythms which require continuation of high quality CPR with administration of epinephrine every 2–5 minutes (*see* **Flowchart 1**).

The VF and VT without pulse are shockable rhythms for which in addition to high quality CPR and epinephrine, an emergency defibrillation is essential. Nonshockable rhythms are common in children in contrast to adults. Meanwhile, identify and treat reversible causes of cardiac arrest (6 H's and 5 T's) (**Table 6**).

Table 6: Reversible causes of cardiac arrest (6 H's and 5 T's)

6 H's	*5 T's*
• Hypoxia	• Toxins
• Hydrogen ion (acidosis)	• Tension pneumothorax
• Hypoglycemia	• Tamponade (cardiac)
• Hyper/hypokalemia	• Thrombosis (pulmonary, coronary)
• Hypothermia	• Trauma
• Hypovolemia	

Defibrillation

A defibrillator delivers a high energy electric shock to myocardium in a shockable rhythm (VF or pulseless VT). Various types of defibrillators are available like manual external defibrillator, automated external defibrillator (AED), implantable cardioverter-defibrillator, wearable cardioverter defibrillator and internal defibrillator. Commonly available device in the emergency and ICU settings is the manual external defibrillator whereas in public places like airports, AED is available. Healthcare providers and lay public should be trained accordingly, to use these devices effectively when in need. An AED functions by assessing the heart rhythm and instructs the bystander to deliver the shock if warranted. Whereas in a manual defibrillator, the healthcare provider identifies the rhythm, correlates with the patient's clinical status to decide on defibrillation.

A defibrillator can be used to deliver both synchronized cardioversion and unsynchronized defibrillation depending upon the arrhythmias. As it is switched ON, defibrillator mode is set up by default. The effectiveness of defibrillation depends on current dose, density, paddle size, transthoracic impedance.

The recommended dose of defibrillation is 2 J/kg in the first attempt and 4 J/kg in the subsequent two attempts. A total of 10 J/kg should not be exceeded. Smaller paddle size is recommended only for infants. The paddles can be placed either in an antero-posterior or anterior apex scheme. The anterior-posterior scheme is where one electrode is placed over the left precordium (the lower part of the chest, in front of the heart) and the other electrode is placed on the back between the scapulae. Whereas in the anterior-apex scheme, the anterior electrode is placed on the right, below the clavicle and the apex electrode is applied to the left side of the patient, just below and to the left of the pectoral muscle (**Fig. 5**).

Care should be taken to reduce electrical impedance by applying conducting jelly over the paddles. The provider shall inform loudly to be clear off the patient before delivering shock in order to prevent inadvertent electrical injuries to other care providers. Once the shock is delivered, the chest compressions are resumed immediately without checking the rhythm thereby avoiding interruptions.

Following defibrillation, the rhythm can change to either asystole, pulseless electrical activity or a perfusing

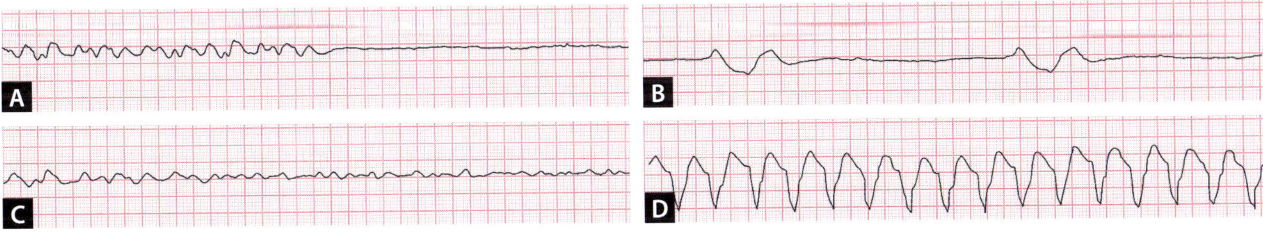

Figs. 4A to D: (A) Asystole; (B) Pulseless electrical activity; (C) Ventricular fibrillation; (D) Pulseless ventricular tachycardia

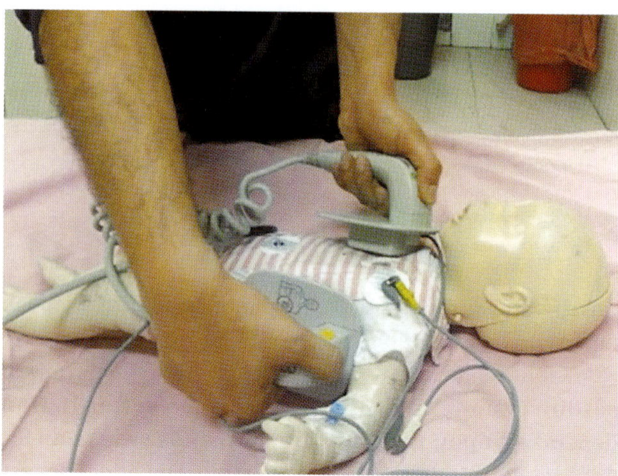

Fig. 5: Position of paddles during defibrillation

rhythm (ROSC). Successful defibrillation requires an adequate current flow for a critical mass of the myocardium to depolarize, resulting in an insufficient remaining muscle mass to continue the arrhythmia. Thus, a sinus rhythm with pulse rate above 60 per minute indicates ROSC, CPR can be stopped and post-arrest care should be continued.

ALS Interventions

Airway and breathing

Respiratory insufficiency resulting in hypoxia being the most common mechanism of pediatric cardiac arrest, providing adequate gas exchange (oxygenation and ventilation) is main aim of assisted ventilation. It is best provided using high quality bag and mask ventilation with supplemental oxygen and a reservoir. Advanced airway placement like endotracheal intubation is not mandatory or emergent. This can be attempted if adequate chest expansion is not achieved with bag and mask ventilation and an airway expert is available. The number of assisted breaths should be limited to 8–10 per minute without interruptions to chest compressions, once advanced airway is in place. Successful placement of endotracheal tube can be confirmed with waveform on capnography connected to the tube. Avoid overventilation (either too rapid or too large breaths) during CPR, as these decrease the cardiac preload to the heart and in turn affects the cardiac output.

Vascular access

Venous access should be established as soon as possible after recognizing cardiac arrest. Veins close to the heart like antecubital vein, veins over the forearm or dorsum of hand are preferred and easier to secure. Great saphenous vein and other lower limb veins or scalp veins can be tried if access is difficult. Intraosseous (IO) access is recommended if venous access could not be established within 90 seconds or 2 failed attempts. Common sites of IO insertion are anteromedial proximal tibia below the epiphyseal plate, just proximal to medial malleolus of tibia, anterior surface of lower end of femur and anterior superior iliac spine. All intravenous medications can be administered through IO access and may require a pressure bag or infusion pump to overcome resistance to flow in the marrow spaces. Fracture of the bone, previous IO insertion attempt in same bone, osteogenesis imperfecta, infection at the insertion site are contraindications to IO insertion. Central venous access can be established if need be, by a trained personnel, after stabilizing the cardiorespiratory status.

Commonly Used Drugs during CPR (Table 7)

Vasopressors: epinephrine and vasopressin

They act by increasing the vascular tone thereby increasing the diastolic blood pressure and blood flow to the heart and brain. In patients with non-shockable rhythm, early administration of adrenaline (within 1 minute of cardiac arrest) has been associated with higher rates of ROSC, survival to hospital discharge and good neurological outcomes. High-dose epinephrine (0.05–0.2 mg/kg) improves myocardial and cerebral blood flow better than standard-dose (0.01–0.02 mg/kg) and thus ROSC.[12] However, high-dose may worsen hemodynamics by increasing myocardial oxygen demand, ventricular ectopy, hypertension, and myocardial necrosis.

Vasopressin causes significant vasoconstriction thereby increasing myocardial and cerebral blood flow, while decreasing splanchnic blood flow during CPR despite presence of acidosis. However, this increased afterload may exacerbate post-cardiac arrest myocardial dysfunction. In randomized, controlled trials of in-hospital and out-of-hospital arrest in adults vasopressin had comparable efficacy to epinephrine.[13,14] Vasopressin has been found to be beneficial in children with prolonged cardiac arrest with failed conventional CPR.[15] Further research is underway regarding the efficacy, safety and long term outcomes of vasopressin in pediatric CPR.

Although vasopressin will not likely replace epinephrine as a first-line agent in pediatric cardiac arrest, preliminary data suggest that its use in conjunction with epinephrine deserves further investigation.[16]

Antiarrhythmic: lidocaine and amiodarone

These medications should be considered after an unsuccessful defibrillation to increase its effectiveness. Epinephrine (with or without vasopressin) is the first drug to be attempted followed by amiodarone or lidocaine. Lidocaine and amiodarone has been shown to improve survival to hospital admission in the setting of out of hospital shock-resistant VF when compared with placebo.[17] There has been no comparative study of antiarrhythmic drugs for pediatric refractory VF, extrapolation from adult studies has led to the recommendation of amiodarone as the preferred antiarrhythmic agent for children.

Post-ROSC Care (Table 8)

During this phase, the patients are prone for complications like hypotension, arrhythmias, seizures, hyperthermia, brain injury and reperfusion to multiple organs commonly called as post-cardiac arrest syndrome. The main aim during this phase is to stabilize and sustain cardiorespiratory function thereby preventing secondary damage to other organ systems. Other goals should be to optimize metabolic derangements and to identify and treat the etiology of cardiac arrest.

Airway should be stabilized with endotracheal tube as indicated. Respiratory support should be adequate to ensure oxygenation (SpO_2 - 94–98% or a PaO_2 > 60 mm Hg) and ventilation (PCO_2 between 35 and 45). Every patient should be presumed to have raised intracranial pressure (ICP) and all the neuroprotective interventions should be instituted accordingly (**Table 8**). There can be multiorgan involvement requiring close monitoring and management and thus, these patients should be monitored preferably in intensive care unit.

Main predictors of outcome of cardiac arrest are, duration of no flow and low flow, quality of CPR, out of hospital arrest and pre-hospital hypothermia. Survival to hospital discharge is equally dependent on the quality of post-arrest care. In long term follow up of these survivors, a comprehensive neurological assessment including vision, hearing, neuroimaging (Magnetic Resonance Imaging) should be done. Supportive care including optimal nutrition, physiotherapy, occupational therapy should be instituted.

TEAM CONCEPT TO PROVIDE EFFECTIVE CPR

To provide a quality CPR, a dynamic team of well-trained professionals is required. A usual team comprises a team leader, well trained team member (at least 4 of them) and effective communication among them. The ideal position and roles of each of the team members is illustrated as below (**Fig. 6 and Table 9**). As the whole team swings into action during a cardiac arrest scenario, the communication and interventions delivered to the patient should be systematic in nature. For an effective communication, the team should follow the 8 core principles of communication (**Table 10**).

Family presence during CPR

The presence of family during CPR has been emphasized by the European Resuscitation Council and American Heart Association. Though it is not mandatory, parents

Table 7: Commonly used drugs during CPR

Drug	*Indication*	*Dose*
Adrenaline	Cardiac arrest	IV or intraosseous – 0.1 mL/kg of 1:10000 dilutions. Repeat every 3 to 5 min Endotracheal – 0.1 mL/kg of 1:1000 dilution
Vasopressin	Cardiac arrest	IV or intraosseous – 0.4 U/kg
Amiodarone	VF or pulseless VT refractory to defibrillation	IV or intraosseous – 5 mg/kg bolus. May be repeated up to 2 times for refractory VF/pVT
Lidocaine	VF or pulseless VT refractory to defibrillation	IV or intraosseous – 1 mg/kg loading dose followed by maintenance: 20 to 50 µg/kg/min infusion Endotracheal – 2 to 3 mg/kg
Magnesium sulfate	Torsades de pointes and hypomagnesemia	IV or intraosseous 25 to 50 mg/kg as infusion (max 2 g)

Table 8: Organ system based management of acute complications during post-ROSC state

Organ system	*Signs and symptoms*	*Interventions*	*Goals of care*
Cardiovascular	Arrhythmias	Antiarrhythmic agents, Correct electrolyte disturbances	Sinus rhythm
	Shock/Hypotension and myocardial dysfunction	Vasoactive infusions, fluid boluses	Therapeutic endpoints of shock 5–50th centile blood pressure
Central nervous system	Seizures	Benzodiazepines, phenytoin	Seizure control
	Cerebral edema, raised intracranial pressure (ICP)	*Anti-raised ICP measures*: • Head of bed elevation • Head in midline • Avoid noxious stimuli • Adequate sedation, analgesia • Normoxia • Normocarbia • Osmotherapy (hypertonic saline) • Prevent fever • Induced hypothermia (32–34°C) for 2 days followed by normothermia for 3 days (36–37.5°C) or strict normothermia (36–37.5°C) for 5 days • Euglycemia	If invasive monitoring available – maintain ICP < 20 cmH_2O; cerebral perfusion pressure of age appropriate cut off; and blood pressure above 50th centile of mean arterial pressures
Respiratory system	Hypoventilation Hypoxia	Provide adequate assisted ventilation and positive pressure to achieve oxygenation Avoid hyperoxia and hyperventilation	$PaCO_2$ – 35–40 mm Hg PaO_2 > 65 mm Hg and SpO_2 – 94–98%
Gastrointestinal tract	Hypoxic liver/ intestinal injury – abdominal distension, ileus	Supportive care, proton pump inhibitors, laboratory monitoring for worsening liver function	Prevent gastrointestinal bleed, avoid secondary injury to liver, intestines
Renal	Oligoanuria, hematuria	Avoid nephrotoxic medications, avoid hypotension, acidosis, monitoring of renal function tests, optimize fluid balance, treat complications like hyperkalemia, volume overload	Adequate urine output
Endocrine	Hypo or hyperglycemia	Avoid hypoglycemia Treat hyperglycemia with blood glucose target less than 180 mg/dL	Euglycemia
	Relative adrenal insufficiency	Treat catecholamine resistant shock with low dose hydrocortisone 2–4 mg/kg/day	Therapeutic end points of shock

or the close family members should be offered to witness the same. If one of the parent choses to witness it, they should be allowed to stand in the corner of the room from where they can view the procedure without interrupting the team. If they choose to decline, the family should be made comfortable in the nearby counseling room. One of the resuscitation team member should be assigned a role to keep the family updated regarding the proceedings. A social worker or a trained nurse can be engaged to communicate the family concerns during CPR.

WHEN TO DISCONTINUE CPR?

The exact time duration to discontinue CPR is variable especially with the advent of E-CPR in developed countries. With high quality CPR, the neurological outcomes were better if ROSC was achieved within 15 minutes and were poor if ROSC is achieved beyond 35 minutes of cardiac arrest. Thus, CPR can be discontinued after an arbitrary duration of 30 minutes of high quality CPR with advanced life support interventions. In patients with severe hypothermia after drowning, or other correctable

Table 9: Roles and responsibilities of team leader and members

Team leader	*Team member*
• Calls for help • Assigns clear roles and responsibilities • Constantly monitors the performance of team members and motivates them • Makes important treatment decisions and delivers a comprehensive patient care • Communicates with the parents • Co-ordinates the team and conducts debriefing	• Should be clear about the role assigned • Should be well trained in performing designated task • Should close the loop of communication after completing the task • Should give constructive inputs • Should be experienced in resuscitation skills • Should be knowledgeable about the cardiac arrest algorithm

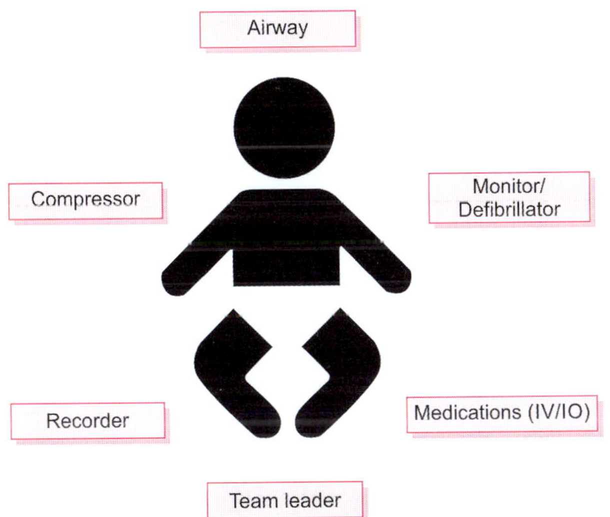

Fig. 6: Ideal position and roles of team members

etiologies like electrolyte disturbance, the resuscitation efforts should be continued beyond this duration till these factors are corrected adequately.

RECENT ADVANCES IN CPR

Extracorporeal Membrane Oxygenation during CPR

Using venoarterial extracorporeal membrane oxygenation (VA-ECMO) during CPR (ECPR) can function as a bridge to recovery to restore effective cardiac output. While high quality CPR is initiated, E-CPR code is activated and a team of cardiothoracic surgeons, ECMO physicians, perfusionists, trained nurses arrive at the scene. Venous cannulation is achieved while chest compressions are continued and ECMO initiated. Post-resuscitation measures like treatment of shock, targeted temperature control, oxygenation, ventilation, anticoagulation can be achieved better with E-CPR. In developed countries, E-CPR is predominantly used in in-hospital cardiac arrest in post-operative cardiac surgical patients and favorable outcome up to 50% have be reported irrespective of duration of CPR. The 2015 American Heart Association guidelines recommend considering ECPR in select cardiac arrest patients in settings with existing protocol, equipment and expertise are available.[18] However, because of the invasive nature, expertise and resources required, its use is limited in Indian settings.

Table 10: Core principles for an effective team communication

- Clear roles and responsibilities
- Clear instructions
- Closed loop communication
- Constructive intervention
- Knowing limitations
- Knowledge sharing
- Mutual respect
- Re-evaluation and summarizing

Active Compression Decompression CPR

This technique involves a device, which is attached to the chest wall over the sternum. It activated, it delivers chest compressions and also actively pulls up to decompress. This decompressing motion results in significant drop in intrathoracic pressure thereby increasing the right ventricular preload and hence the cardiac output during compressions. Such mechanism improves the cerebral blood flow during compressions and also decreases the intracranial pressure by augmenting the venous return away from the brain.

Impedance Threshold Device

This device is connected to the artificial airway of the patient during CPR. It acts by impeding the air flow to the lungs during decompression. This results in further decrease in intrathoracic pressure beyond what is achieved with the active compression decompression CPR. Thereby the beneficial effects of increase in right ventricular preload, cardiac output and cerebral blood flow are also augmented.

KEY MESSAGES

- Recognize respiratory failure and shock as pre-arrest pathophysiological mechanism and act to prevent progression to cardiac arrest.
- Recognize cardiac arrest and start *high quality CPR.*
- Early administration of adrenaline in non-shockable rhythms has good outcome.
- Identify ECG rhythms and deliver shock in case of shockable rhythms (VF, pulseless VT).
- Administer amiodarone or lignocaine in shockable rhythms refractory to defibrillation.
- Administer advanced life support interventions – advanced airway, vascular access.
- Identify and treat reversible causes of cardiac arrest 5 H's and 6 T's.
- For in hospital cardiac arrest, prefer invasive arterial monitoring or capnography to monitor effectiveness of CPR.
- Comprehensive brain protective post ROSC care is the key to secure favorable long term neurological outcomes.
- Practice eight core components of communication to execute an effective team resuscitation.

REFERENCES

1. Jindal A, Jayashree M, Singhi SC. Pediatric cardiopulmonary resuscitation and stabilization. Indian J Pediatr. 2011;78: 1109-17.
2. Torres A, Pickert CB, Firestone J, *et al.* Long-term functional outcome of inpatient pediatric cardiopulmonary resuscitation. Pediatr Emerg Care. 1997;13:369-73.
3. Rathore V, Bansal A, Singhi SC, *et al.* Survival and neurological outcome following in-hospital paediatric cardiopulmonary resuscitation in North India. Paediatr Int Child Health. 2016; 36:141-7.
4. Girotra S, Spertus JA, Li Y, *et al.* Survival trends in pediatric in-hospital cardiac arrests: An analysis from get with the guidelines-resuscitation. Circ Cardiovasc Qual Outcomes. 2013;6(1):42-9.
5. Nadkarni VM, Larkin GL, Peberdy MA, *et al.* First documented rhythm and clinical outcome from in-hospital cardiac arrest among children and adults. JAMA. 2006;295:50-7.
6. Donoghue AJ, Nadkarni V, Berg RA, *et al.* Out-of-hospital pediatric cardiac arrest: An epidemiologic review and assessment of current knowledge. Ann Emerg Med. 2005;46: 512-22.
7. Neumar RW, Shuster M, Callaway CW, *et al.* Part 1: Executive Summary: 2015 American Heart Association Guidelines Update for Cardiopulmonary Resuscitation and Emergency Cardiovascular Care. Circulation. 2015;132:S315-67.
8. Berg RA, Miyasaka K, Rodriguez-Nunez A, et al. Cardiopulmonary resuscitation. In: Nichols DG, Shaffner DH, editors. Rogers' Textbook of Pediatric Intensive Care, 5th edition. Philadelphia: Lippincott Williams & Wilkins; 2015.
9. de Caen AR, Berg MD, Chameides L, *et al.* Part 12: Pediatric Advanced Life Support: 2015 American Heart Association Guidelines Update for Cardiopulmonary Resuscitation and Emergency Cardiovascular Care (Reprint). Pediatrics. 2015;136 Suppl 2:S176-95.
10. Sutton RM, Wolfe H, Nishisaki A, *et al.* Pushing harder, pushing faster, minimizing interruptions... But falling short of 2010 cardiopulmonary resuscitation targets during in-hospital pediatric and adolescent resuscitation. Resuscitation. 2013; 84:1680-4.
11. Sanders AB, Kern KB, Otto CW, *et al.* End-tidal carbon dioxide monitoring during cardiopulmonary resuscitation. A prognostic indicator for survival. JAMA. 1989;262: 1347-51.
12. Jacobs IG, Finn JC, Jelinek GA, et al. Effect of adrenline on surval of out-of-hospital cardiac arrets: A randomised double-blind placebo. Controlled trail. Resuscitation. 2011;82: 1138-43.
13. Wenzel V, Sitter H. A comparison of vasopressin and epinephrine for out-of-hospital cardiopulmonary resuscitation. New Engl J Med. 2004;350:105-13.
14. Stiell IG, Hébert PC, Wells GA, *et al.* Vasopressin versus epinephrine for inhospital cardiac arrest: A randomised controlled trial. Lancet. 2001;358:105-9.
15. Mann K, Berg RA, Nadkarni V. Beneficial effects of vasopressin in prolonged pediatric cardiac arrest: A case series. Resuscitation. 2002;52:149-56.
16. Meert KL, Donaldson A, Nadkarni V, *et al.* Multicenter cohort study of in-hospital pediatric cardiac arrest. Pediatr Crit Care Med. 2009;10:544-53.
17. Paul D, Dan C, Brian S, *et al.* Amiodarone as compared with lidocaine for shock-resistant ventricular fibrillation. New Engl J Med. 2002;346:884-90.
18. Brooks SC, Anderson ML, Bruder E, *et al.* Part 6: Alternative Techniques and Ancillary Devices for Cardiopulmonary Resuscitation: 2015 American Heart Association Guidelines Update for Cardiopulmonary Resuscitation and Emergency Cardiovascular Care. Circulation. 2015;132:S436-43.

CHAPTER

8

Oxygen Therapy

Soonu Udani, Suresh Kumar Angurana

INTRODUCTION

Oxygen is by far the most frequently used intervention in the management of the critically ill child; whether there is respiratory disease or not. There is often, a casual attitude towards the administration of oxygen. We forget that oxygen has well characterized and potentially toxic effects on the lungs and neonatal retina.

Oxygen therapy is the process of increasing the concentration of oxygen in inspired air, to correct or prevent hypoxia. The primary indication is the presence or risk of hypoxemia which may be from a pulmonary or extrapulmonary cause. Many biochemical reactions in the body depend on oxygen utilization. Supply of oxygen to the tissues depends on many factors like ventilation, diffusion across the alveolar-capillary membrane, hemoglobin, cardiac output, and tissue perfusion.

The goal of oxygen therapy is to supply adequate oxygen to the tissues and not just to raise the value in the blood. Reduced oxygen in the blood is hypoxemia, whereas reduced oxygen to the tissues is hypoxia.[1] For oxygen to increase PaO_2, there have to be unit so flow ventilation with normal or near normal perfusion. Any true extra or intrapulmonary right to left shunting will be largely unaffected by an elevation of alveolar oxygen tension (PAO_2).

Oxygen Delivery and Consumption

The quantity of oxygen available to the body in one minute is known as the oxygen delivery. Oxygen delivered (DO_2) = Oxygen carrying capacity of blood (CaO_2) × Cardiac output. Where CaO_2 = (Hb in grams × 1.34 × SpO_2) + (PaO_2 × 0.003), and Cardiac output = Stroke volume × Heart rate.

LIMITATIONS OF OXYGEN THERAPY

The major limitation of oxygen therapy lies in the pulmonary toxicity of increased alveolar oxygen tension. This is clearly related to the duration and level of oxygen administration. An FiO_2 of 0.6 for more than 24 hours is definitely associated with lung damage; whereas 0.4 or less can be given for prolonged periods.

Another feature that limits the usefulness of oxygen therapy in pulmonary disease is the relationship between FiO_2 and the resultant PaO_2 under conditions of varying or increasing intrapulmonary shunting (**Fig. 1**). This is akin to a certain amount of cardiac output by-passing the alveoli without getting oxygen from them. The diseased alveoli do not allow oxygen to diffuse into the capillaries that serve them. The amount of blood not getting oxygenated is expressed as a shunt fraction. Once this is in excess of 30% of the total cardiac output, oxygenation cannot be maintained with less than 0.5 FiO_2. With a greater than 40 percent shunt, oxygen alone will not be enough and some other means of providing oxygen under pressure will be needed (PEEP/CPAP/IPPV).

Oxygen administration for the correction of hypoxia can extend from simple tubes and masks to extraordinary life support systems like ECMO. Oxygen administration to the non-intubated patients only, is elaborated in this chapter.

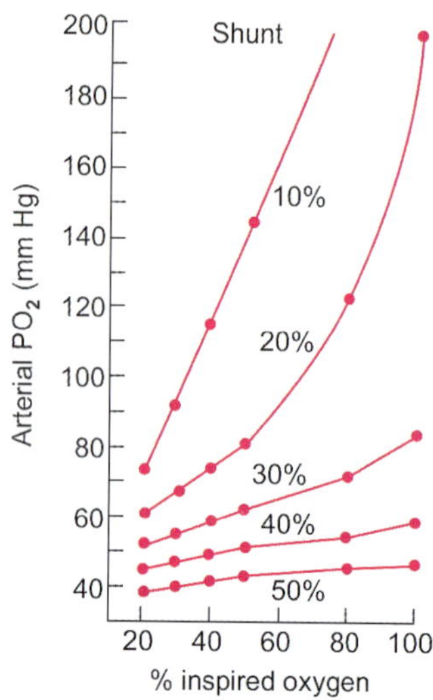

Fig. 1: Shunting: effects of FiO_2 on PaO_2. As the % of shunt rises, increasing the FiO_2 has less and less impact on PaO_2. Under such conditions, reducing the shunt fraction is key to the ability to improve gas exchange and this typically requires PPV and PEEP

USING OXYGEN

Some Basic Principles

- The goal of therapy is to achieve the optimal level of oxygen in the blood at the least possible concentration.
- Clinical assessment of oxygenation includes the five vital signs namely, heart rate, respiratory rate (including level of distress), blood pressure, temperature and SpO_2.
- Patient assessment for distress is more important than any other parameter in deciding further therapy.
- Oxygen should be given without wasting time and thought. Further therapy, amount, duration, can be decided later.
- Usually 0.4–0.6 FiO_2 is adequate in most situations. FiO_2 of 1 is only needed during resuscitation or with severe hypoxemia. However, if needed, it should never be withheld for fear of toxicity.
- SpO_2 monitoring is essential (5th vital sign) and should be kept above 92%. An increasing requirement of oxygen to maintain the same SpO_2 is an ominous sign.
- Children should be nursed in the manner that makes them most comfortable and not by any preconceived notions. Mothers are often the best administrators of oxygen. A frightened and agitated mother will result in a frightened and agitated child so a little time spent in explaining the situation may go a long way in providing comfort. If a child is upset by one method, another should be tried, including a "blow by" flow of gas.

Caution: If a child seems to require O_2, it is mandatory to supply the O_2 first and then determine the cause as quickly as possible. A rise in saturation on institution of therapy should not bring with complacency. If there is an increasing requirement of O_2, this too should be taken seriously and the flow not just dialed up to increase saturations. Very often, this is done to the point where the child's respiratory failure is recognized too late because the O_2 level delivered masked the saturation on the monitor. The indications for further escalation of support are:

- Dropping SpO_2
- Increasing FiO_2
- Fatigue, confusion, agitation, drowsiness (ABG to look for PaO_2, $PaCO_2$, acidosis)
- Poor respiratory effort, obtundation
- Heart rate, BP fluctuations with diaphoresis.

Oxygen Sources and Flow Regulators

Medical gas is provided either from a wall source or a cylinder. A wall source should provide at least 50 psi of pressure at all times. Cylinders operate at 1800–2400 psi. This is too much even to run ventilators. This pressure cannot be delivered directly to the patients and hence, a down regulating valve before a flow meter is required. It is the flow meter and not the valve, that is used to manipulate the flow rate.

Oxygen Delivery Devices

A spontaneously breathing child can be delivered oxygen by a low flow device or high flow device (**Table 1**). **A low flow system** provides FiO_2 that varies with the patient's inspiratory flow rates, e.g. blow-by oxygen, nasal prongs, intranasal catheter, and simple oxygen masks. **A high flow system** provides fixed FiO_2 at flows that meets or exceeds the patient's own inspiratory flow requirements. The patient's own flow requirements depend on the minute ventilation (MV). Normal flow requirements are 3–4 times the MV and MV = tidal Volume (Vt) × respiratory rate (RR). Average Vt is about 6 mL/kg. Therefore a 5 kg child breathing at 60/minute needs about 6–7 L/min of an air oxygen mixture. There are only three real high flow systems; (1) Venturi, (2) Non-rebreathing

Table 1: Low flow and high flow oxygen delivery devices	
Low flow or variable concentration devices	Blow-by oxygen Nasal prongs Intranasal catheter Simple oxygen masks Partial rebreathing mask
High flow or fixed concentration devices	Venturi mask Oxygen hood Oxygen and face tents Non-rebreathing mask High flow nasal cannula Anesthesia circuit

mask, (3) Anesthesia bag and circuit with reservoir. What may be a high flow system for a neonate may result in being a low flow one for an older child.

Nasal cannula

Two soft prongs in the nostrils attached by a long tubing to the oxygen source. The prongs should have some space at the sides for exhalation, as there is only inflow. A single intranasal catheter has little role in any setting. The flow is directed to the nasopharynx, which continues to do the work of humidification and heat exchange. The maximum accepted flow is 2–4 L/min. Irritation and nasal obstruction may occur but these are generally well tolerated. In small premature babies, some inadvertent PEEP may be generated from close fitting prongs like the RAM cannula, and although this device has been used after extubation to provide some pressure, it is inappropriate as a CPAP device and not recommended.[2,3] Neither should these prongs be substituted for the correct CPAP tubings to cut costs, as they are too narrow and offer too much resistance to air flow. The indications for this device are: (1) minimal oxygen requirements less than 30%, (2) weaning off from oxygen, (3) chronic oxygen therapy on low concentrations. This device (**Figs. 2A to C**) offers the single advantage of comfort and conservation of gas.

Simple masks

A mask has perforations, which are exhalation ports. It fits the person's face without much discomfort. As babies vary in size, the most comfortable size must be sought and care must be taken that there are no pressure points or eye damage. Precise FiO_2 is not the aim when using these masks and by their nature, they are used in conditions that are not severe. They provide a maximum of 40% FiO_2 but as this can vary with the flow rate provided with the inspiratory flow rate of the patient a small infant may get considerably more FiO_2 than expected. Hence the importance of checking the concentration provided by using an analyzer.

Partial rebreathing masks

These are simple masks with an additional reservoir that allows the accumulation of oxygen enriched gas for rebreathing. A portion of the exhaled volume from the anatomical dead space is rich in oxygen. This is what enters the reservoir. Up to 60% FiO_2 can be delivered but the pitfalls are similar to those of the simple mask.

Non-rebreathing masks

This works as a high flow system. There is a valve at the entry port that allows only oxygen from the source to enter the reservoir. It prevents room air from being entrained by additional one-way valve at the exhalation port. A well-fitting mask can provide up to 100% FiO_2. When in doubt of the patient's requirements or if the patient is sick, as in the

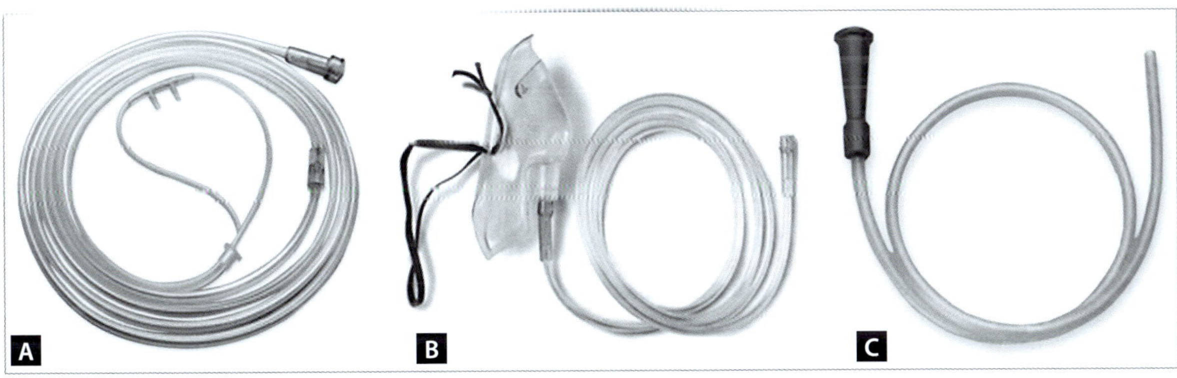

Figs. 2A to C: Low flow oxygen delivery devices: (A) Nasal prongs/cannula; (B) Simple face mask; (C) Intranasal catheter

Table 2: Oxygen percentages with different systems			
Litres/min	*Simple face mask*	*Partial rebreathing*	*Non-rebreathing masks*
5	40%		
6	45–50%	35%	55–60%
8		45–50%	60–80%
10		60%	80–90%
12		60%	90%
15		60%	90–100%

case of shock states, respiratory distress, cardiac failure; this is the mask to choose to institute O_2 therapy as it will provide maximum oxygen and build reserves, even prior to intubation.

The FiO_2 delivered with different systems are summarized in **Table 2**.

Air-entrainment or venturi masks

These are dilutional masks that work on the Bernoulli principle (**Figs. 3A and B**). Oxygen is delivered through a narrow orifice at a high flow. Negative lateral wall pressure is created in the tubing system. There are openings (entrainment ports) near the nozzle that allow room air to be sucked in, diluting the oxygen. Changing the size of the nozzle, the flow rates, as well as ports, allows control of the amount of oxygen (**Table 3**).

The advantages of a Venturi system include: (i) High flow device with guaranteed fixed FiO_2. (ii) Saves oxygen as the high flow comes from the room air. (iii) It can be used to deliver low FiO_2 also. (iv) Helps in deciding whether oxygen requirement is increasing or decreasing. When the FiO_2 requirement is high, the flow rate of O_2 required can be up to 12 L/min and this wastes a lot of O_2. (v) No need for humidification. (vi) Fairly cheap and reliable.

The oxygen concentrations obtained with Venturi devices are depicted in **Table 3**. Each device has will have a table on the package insert as a guide to flow rates required by that particular device. This should be followed.

In children, the problem of fit and comfort is a daily issue. Infants too large for oxyhoods and too small for masks are our usual population. The average infant or even toddler is usually intolerant of a mask and will keep pulling it off. In fact, the infant that remains quiet when the mask is first fitted, is one that may be obtunded from hypoxia or too tired to fight.

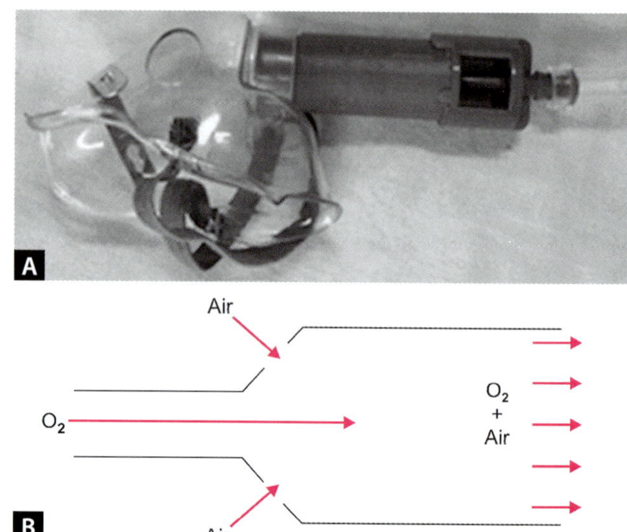

Figs. 3A and B: (A) Air-entrainment or venturi mask; (B) Principle of the air-entrainment or venturi mask

Table 3: Venturi devices and delivery of oxygen		
Liters/min (Oxygen/ Total)	*Oxygen concentration (percent)*	*Air: Oxygen ratio*
2/53	24	25:1
4/45	28	10:1
6/47	31	7:1
8/45	35	5:1
10/33	40	3:1
12/32	50	5:3

The oxyhood

This is small baby's friend. A clear transparent hood that has enough room for the baby's head to fit comfortably and allows free neck and head movement without hurting the baby, is the correct hood size to use (**Figs. 4A and B**). At least 3–4 sizes are available and a unit should keep one of each size. Too big a hood will dilute the oxygen and too small a hood will result in discomfort and result in carbon dioxide accumulation. Adequate flow of humidified oxygen ensures mixing of delivered gases and flushing out of carbon dioxide. Oxygen gradients can vary up to 20% from top to bottom. Continuous flow atleast 6–8 L/min avoids this problem. Cold air will cause heat stress and condense on the baby's head, which will be mistaken for

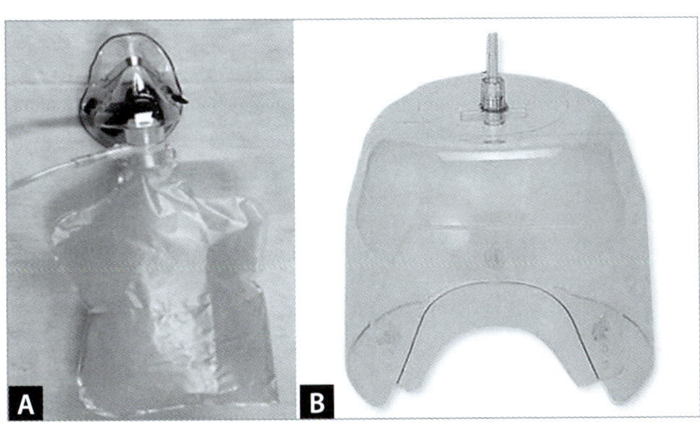

Figs. 4A and B: (A) Non-rebreathing mask; (B) Oxygen hood

perspiration. Adequate flow of at least 6–8 L/min assures that CO_2 does not accumulate and there must be an outlet for this at the top, as CO_2 is lighter than O_2 and will rise to the top.

Face tents and oxygen tents are not used much in India. They do not provide more than about 30% FiO_2 and are cumbersome to use and keep clean and limit access to the child.

Measurement of Delivered Oxygen

An oxygen analyzer or FiO_2 meter is used to measure the concentration of oxygen actually delivered to the patient. The important part of this system is the actual sensor, its quality and accuracy is of paramount importance. It is connected to an instrument that digitally converts the sensed concentration into a reading that is displayed. The sensor has life of about 1000 sensing hours. It is the most expensive part of the machine. It also tells us how wrong our own rough estimates of delivered oxygen can often be. The oxyhood is the ideal place to use it but it can also be held at the mouth/nose within a mask for a quick reading. Calibration with every use is needed.

CONTINUOUS POSITIVE AIRWAY PRESSURE (CPAP)

This is indicated as a possible method for correcting hypoxemia when at the FiO_2 of >60% is not able to maintain PaO_2 of >60 mm Hg. This is the classic criterion but it must be stressed that clinical parameters and the general condition of the patient must also act as the paramount guiding force. CPAP, like background PEEP, it splints and maintains collapsed airways, reduces work of breathing, increases tidal volume, and function residual capacity, reduces oxygen requirement, and improves diaphragmatic activity. CPAP is indicated in bronchial asthma, acute viral bronchiolitis, pulmonary edema, atelectasis, pneumonia, and neuromuscular weakness.

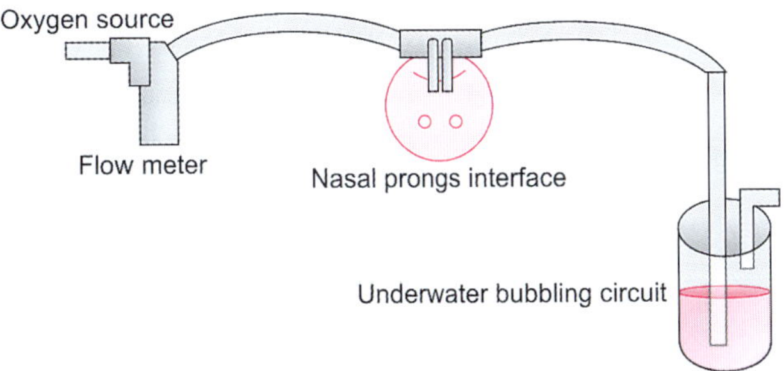

Fig. 5: CPAP circuit using underwater seal[4]

The CPAP can be given using various interfaces like nasal cannula, oro-nasal mask, nasal mask, full face mask, or ET tube. Whatever the method of delivery, it is a versatile tool in the child with early, incipient or even frank respiratory failure. An easy method is to use snugly fitting nasal prongs (the shortest, widest for the snuggest fit with appropriate connection tubing) with a closed mouth. In small neonates <1400 grams this method can also provide noninvasive positive pressure ventilation (**Fig. 5**). A pacifier may help in keeping the mouth closed.

The CPAP systems vary from the unit made underwater seals, bubble CPAP systems with flow drivers readily available but more expensive, to those on ventilators systems. FiO_2 will be inaccurate in locally made systems.[4] Stand-alone CPAP systems with good oxygen blenders may be as expensive as basic ventilators. CPAP can be successfully used in RDS of prematurity, asthma, early ARDS, pneumonia, etc. It could be tried prior to conventional ventilation in any spontaneously breathing patient who does not require emergency ventilation. When using CPAP without intubating the trachea, a proper patient-system interface is important for success.

HEATED HUMIDIFIED HIGH FLOW NASAL CANNULA (HHHFNC)[5]

The HHHFNC is classified as a high flow fixed-performance oxygen delivery system. Flow rate greater than 1 L/min are considered uncomfortable for small babies as the air is cold and dry. HHHFNC uses a large-bore nasal cannula, with a corrugated tubing, proper heated humidification,

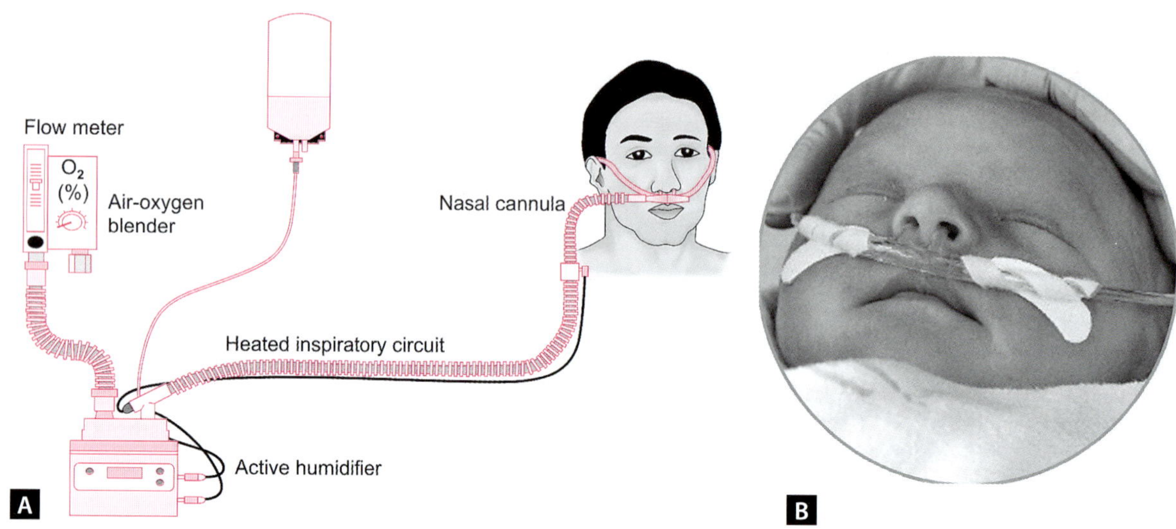

Figs. 6A and B: (A) HHHFNC device with air-oxygen blender, humidifier, flow generator/meter and nasal cannula; (B) Nasal cannula prongs of cannula should cover only 50% of nostril space to allow for good flow and exhalation

and blended oxygen (**Figs. 6A and B**). The flow delivered by this device can vary from 4-70 L/min. The higher flow, above patient's demand flushes the dead space and prevents entrainment of room air. The flow administered is around 2 L/kg/min. The recommended flow rates are <2 L/min for premature or term babies, upto 12 L/min for older infants and toddlers, upto 30 L/min for children, and up to 40 L/min for adults. Some PEEP is expected to be generated, about 4 cm of H_2O, depending upon the flow rate and size of the prongs.

Common indications include acute bronchiolitis,[6,7] pneumonia, congestive cardiac failure, apnea of prematurity, and weaning from mechanical ventilation. It may reduce the need for escalation of respiratory support therapy to CPAP or invasive ventilation by decreasing extrathoracic dead space, increasing pulmonary compliance by providing distending pressure, humidification, and reducing work of breathing.

OTHER ISSUES

Oxygen Concentrator

This device separates oxygen from nitrogen in the air by using adsorption and desorption over a material called zeolite, that adsorbs only the nitrogen. No ventilator or CPAP machine can run on this, as the outlet pressure is only 5 psi. The resultant FiO_2 is about 0.4. This is useful in many situations and is often used in home oxygen therapy. The device costs between Rupees 40,000 and 80,000.

Weaning

This is based on clinical and laboratory parameters. The SpO_2 levels are a boon in this phase and ABGs are usually not needed. Abrupt cessation may precipitate rises in pulmonary pressures in neonates. The flow/concentration should be gradually lowered while monitoring the child. Low flows and concentration can continue without ill effects for a longtime. A high flow system can be replaced by a low flow system, but this doubles the cost.

Hyperbaric Oxygen (HBO)

The goals are to deliver extremely high partial pressure of oxygen >760 torr. This increases the plasma partial pressure of oxygen and the dissociation occurs in the plasma rather than from that bound to hemoglobin.[4] At room air, the PaO_2 is 80–100 torr, at 1 ATA (atomospheric absolute) with 100% FiO_2, it is 500+ torr. At 2ATA in 100% FiO_2 it is 1200+ torr. The indication for HBO are summarized in **Table 4**.[8]

COMPLICATIONS OF OXYGEN THERAPY

- *Hyperoxia*: It is poorly defined. It appears to produce cellular injury through increased production of

Table 4: Indications approved for hyperbaric oxygen

Smoke inhalation	Clostridial myonecrosis
Carbon monoxide poisoning	Osteomyelitis (Refractory)
Cyanide poisoning	Acute traumatic ischemia
Thermal burns	Compromised skin grafts
Anemia due to severe blood loss	Radiation injury
Air embolism	

reactive oxygen species, such as the superoxide anion, the hydroxyl radical, and hydrogen peroxide.[5]

- *Direct lung injury*:[9] The lung injury due to oxygen therapy is akin to injury seen in ARDS and the severity of injury depends on the concentration and duration of oxygen therapy. Breathing at FiO_2 of 100% for even 3 hours leads to chest pain and for longer period to bronchopneumonia. Oxygen toxicity has been observed at a FiO_2 >60%. When the antioxidant stores in the lungs are depleted, oxygen toxicity may develop even at FiO_2 of <60%.
- *Oxidative stress*:[9] The body's antioxidant defense mechanisms (superoxide dismutase, catalase, and glutathione), are either impaired (premature neonates, malnourishment, etc.), or overcome by concentrations of oxygen >50%. The former group is at risk for oxygen toxicity even at lower FiO_2 between 25–50%.
- *Injury*: Catheters, masks and dry and non-humidified gas can cause nasal and oral injuries, thus predisposing to infections.
- *Absorption atelectasis (derecruitment)*: High FiO_2 increases risk of absorption atelectasis by depleting alveolar nitrogen levels. The gases within the alveoli rapidly diffuse into the venous blood leading to collapse.
- *Retinopathy of prematurity (ROP)*: Babies <32 weeks or <1500 g are at higher risk of ROP. ROP can be prevented by keeping the desired PaO_2 <80 mm Hg and SpO_2 between 88–93%. Periodic retinal examination after completion of 32 weeks is mandatory to detect early retinal damage.
- *Fire*: Oxygen supports combustion and hence avoid spark emitting equipments, toys near vicinity.

KEY MESSAGES

- Oxygen is a drug and it should be used judiciously similar to other drugs.
- Oxygen delivery devices are divided into high and low flow devices based on whether or not they meet the flow demand of the patient.
- Oxygen can be decreased by maintaining euthermia, controlling sepsis, optimizing hemoglobin, and cardiac output and work of breathing.
- The FiO_2 used should be as minimal as possible and guided by clinical and laboratory parameters.
- Oxygen should be weaned as soon as possible.

REFERENCES

1. Walsh BK, Smallwood CD. Pediatric oxygen therapy: A review and update. Respir Care. 2017;62:645-61.
2. Myers TR, American Association for Respiratory Care. AARC clinical practice guideline: Selection of an oxygen delivery device for neonatal and pediatric patients: 2002 revision and update. Respir Care. 2002;47:707-16.
3. Vain NE, Prudent LM, Stevens DP, *et al.* Regulation of oxygen concentration delivered to infants via nasal cannulas. Am J Dis Child. 1989;143:1458-60.
4. Jayashree M, Kiran Babu HB, Singhi S, *et al.* Use of nasal bubble CPAP in children with hypoxemic clinical pneumonia-report from a resource limited set-up. J Trop Pediatr. 2016;62: 69-74.
5. Kubicka ZJ, Limauro J, Darnall RA. Heated, humidified high-flow nasal cannula therapy: Yet another way to deliver continuous positive airway pressure? Pediatrics. 2008;121: 82-8.
6. Slain KN, Shein SL, Rotta AT. The use of high-flow nasal cannula in the pediatric emergency department. J Pediatr (Rio J). 2017;93 Suppl 1:36-45.
7. Beggs S, Wong ZH, Kaul S, *et al.* High-flow nasal cannula therapy for infants with bronchiolitis. Cochrane Database Syst Rev. 2014;(1):CD009609.
8. Kindwall EP. Uses of hyperbaric oxygen in the 1990s. C level and Clin J Med. 1992;59:517-20.
9. Fridovich, I. Oxygen toxicity: A radical explanation. J Exp Biol. 1998;201:1203.

CHAPTER

9

Shock

Jayashree M, Reshma Aramanadka

INTRODUCTION

Shock is a dynamic pathophysiologic state of acute circulatory dysfunction, characterized by mismatch between the supply (oxygenation) and metabolic demands of the tissues.[1] This could be due to limitation or maldistribution of blood flow. The ensuing impaired tissue oxygen delivery leads to tissue hypoxia, multiorgan dysfunction and death. Mortality can be averted with early recognition, prompt treatment and intensive monitoring.

PATHOPHYSIOLOGY

Tissue oxygen delivery is a product of cardiac output (CO) and oxygen content of the blood (CaO_2). CO is determined by the preload, myocardial contractility and afterload to cardiac ejection and optimizing one or all the above-mentioned parameters improves cardiac output. CaO_2 on the other hand depends primarily on hemoglobin content and improves with packed red cell transfusion.

Shock results from various causes; whatever be the underlying trigger, the final common pathway is micro-circulatory failure and tissue hypoxia. Broadly, shock is categorized into the following subtypes based on its pathophysiology:

- *Inadequate circulatory blood volume*—hypovolemic shock
- *Abnormality of cardiac function*—cardiogenic shock
- *Inappropriate distribution of circulating blood flow and volume*—distributive shock
- *Obstruction to antegrade flow of blood*—obstructive shock.

Tables 1 and **2** elaborate the various etiologies and underlying pathophysiology of shock respectively. Shock is a dynamic process and the pattern of hemodynamic presentation depends on the severity of insult, degree of compensation, time course and the therapy provided. In the continuum of shock, three severity stages have been recognized—compensated, decompensated and irreversible. In the first phase, when cardiac output falls, the compensatory sympathetic activity increases the heart rate and systemic vascular resistance (peripheries become cold, mottled with weak pulses). The renal and splanchnic vascular resistance also increases, resulting in redistribution of blood flow away from these vascular beds leading to oliguria, vomiting and ileus. It is important to identify shock in the compensated stage as it is more likely to reverse. Signs and symptoms of early shock include tachycardia, tachypnea, prolonged capillary refill time (CRT), cool extremities, mild alteration in sensorium-irritability/lethargy. Blood pressure is maintained for age and sex during this stage. It must be remembered that signs of early shock may be subtle and can be missed. Early septic shock will have bounding pulses and flash CRT.

In the decompensated stage, hypotension (systolic blood pressure < 5th centile for age) sets in. In children between 1 and 10 years age, hypotension is defined as systolic blood pressure (SBP) less than 70 + (child's age in years × 2) mm Hg. Progressive tachypnea and tachycardia are indicators of worsening clinical status. As the shock progresses, microvascular perfusion drops and cellular function deteriorates leading to vital organ dysfunction. Terminal or

Table 1: Etiologies of shock

Hypovolemic shock	Bleeding	• External bleeding—trauma • Internal bleeding—GIT, intracranial
	Plasma loss	• Burns • Capillary leak syndromes—sepsis, scrub typhus, severe dengue
	Fluid and electrolyte loss	• Vomiting, diarrhea • Excessive diuresis—glucosuria in diabetes mellitus, diuretics, diabetes insipidus, cerebral salt wasting
Cardiogenic shock	Arrhythmias – due to any underlying cause	Supraventricular tachycardia, ventricular tachycardia, bradycardia
	Myocardial diseases	*Myocarditis*—viral, bacterial, fungal, protozoal *Metabolic*: a. Hypoglycemia, hypocalcemia, metabolic acidosis b. Fatty acid oxidation disorders, glycogen storage disorders, mitochondrial disorders, hypo/hyperthyroidism *Cardiomyopathies*—dilated, hypertrophic, restrictive *Immunologic disorders*—Kawasaki disease, systemic lupus erythematosus, acute rheumatic fever
	Hypoxic ischemic events	Post-cardiac arrest Cardiopulmonary bypass Prolonged shock Excessive catecholamine release
Distributive shock	Sepsis Anaphylaxis Spinal cord injury	
Obstructive shock	Tension pneumothorax Cardiac tamponade Massive pulmonary embolism Duct dependent heart disease—critical aortic stenosis, hypoplastic left heart	

Table 2: Pathophysiology of different types of shock

Type of shock	*Preload*	*Cardiac contractility*	*Afterload*
Hypovolemic shock	Decreased	Initially normal or increased	Increased
Distributive shock	Normal or decreased	Normal, increased or decreased	Decreased
Cardiogenic shock	Variable	Decreased	Increased
Obstructive shock	Variable	Normal	Increased

irreversible stage ensues when end organ damage has become irreversible. Rapid, focused assessment and identification of the shock in the early compensated stage helps avert the progression to irreversible stage.

Sepsis and Septic Shock

The incidence of pediatric sepsis is highest among infants and decreases with increasing age. The mortality ranges between 6–10% for all age groups. The common infections leading to sepsis include pneumonia, blood stream infections, gastrointestinal and urinary tract infections. The most prevalent organisms are gram positive organisms including streptococci and staphylococci, gram negative bacteria namely *Escherichia coli*, *Klebsiella* and *Pseudomonas*. Clinical manifestations of sepsis have been elaborated in **Table 3**.

Table 3: Physiological/laboratory indicators of severe sepsis

General variables
- Fever (>38.3°C)
- Hypothermia (core temperature <36°C)
- Heart rate >90/min or >2 SD above the normal value for age
- Tachypnea
- Altered mental status
- Significant edema or positive fluid balance (> 20 mL/kg over 24 hr)
- Hyperglycemia (plasma glucose > 140 mg/dL or 7.7 mmol/L) in the absence of diabetes

Inflammatory variables
- Leukocytosis (WBC count > 12,000/cumm)
- Leukopenia (WBC count < 4,000/cumm)
- Normal WBC count with greater than 10% immature forms
- Plasma C-reactive protein > 2 SD above the normal value
- Plasma procalcitonin > 2 SD above the normal value

Hemodynamic variables
- Arterial hypotension (Systolic pressure <90 mm Hg, mean arterial pressure <70 mm Hg, or an systolic pressure decrease >40 mm Hg in adults or <2 SD below normal for age)

Organ dysfunction variables
- Arterial hypoxemia (PaO_2/FiO_2 <300)
- Acute oliguria (urine output <0.5 mL/kg/hr for at least 2 hrs despite adequate fluid resuscitation)
- Creatinine increase > 0.5 mg/dL or 44.2 µmol/L
- Coagulation abnormalities (INR > 1.5, or aPTT> 60 seconds)
- Ileus (absent bowel sounds)
- Thrombocytopenia (platelet count < 10,000/cumm)
- Hyperbilirubinemia (plasma total bilirubin > 4 mg/dL or 70 µmol/L)

Tissue perfusion variables
- Hyperlactatemia (>1 mmol/L)
- Decreased capillary refill or mottling

(SD: Standard deviation); Adapted from Surviving Sepsis Campaign guidelines, 2012.[2]

Pathophysiology

Septic shock follows a trimodal pattern and is multifactorial; hypovolemic, secondary to capillary leak, cardiogenic due to sepsis induced myocardial dysfunction, distributive caused by toxin induced vasodilatation and occasionally obstructive shock. At the microcirculatory level, there is a supply-demand mismatch leading to a state of global ischemia. Anaerobic respiration leads to accumulation of toxic metabolites and lactic acidosis. At the cellular level, energy failure culminates in cell death. Children can present with foci of infection like pneumonia, gastroenteritis and skin/soft tissue abscess or joint infections. Infants with septic shock tend to have non-specific complaints like poor feeding, lethargy and occult sources of infection. Fever is an important symptom of infection in older children whereas infants may have either hyperthermia or hypothermia. Identifying the cause of infection is important to ensure adequate source control.

APPROACH TO MANAGEMENT OF A CHILD WITH SHOCK

Recognition Bundle

The recognition of shock is primarily based on clinical hemodynamic variables.[1] The clinical findings of shock are elaborated in **Table 4**.

Resuscitation Bundle

Airway: Generally, the airway is open and stable in children with septic shock, except when level of consciousness is significantly impaired. The child should be nursed in a position of comfort, with gentle suction to clear the mouth and nose, if necessary.

Table 4: Clinical features of shock

Signs	*Hypovolemic*	*Distributive*	*Cardiogenic*
Airway	Usually open unless consciousness is significantly impaired		
Breathing	Tachypnea	Tachypnea Retractions if there is associated pneumonia/ARDS	Tachypnea; retractions, nasal flaring, grunting
Circulation			
Heart rate	Increased	Increased	Increased
Blood pressure and pulse pressure	Normal blood pressure with narrow pulse pressure or hypotension with narrow pulse pressure	Early warm shock (wide pulse pressure) or later cold shock (narrow pulse pressure) with or without hypotension	Normal or low blood pressure or hypotension with narrow pulse pressure
Pulses	Feeble	Bounding or weak pulses	Weak pulses
Capillary refill	Prolonged	Flash or prolonged	Prolonged
Skin	Cool, pale, mottled	Warm and flushed or pale mottled	Cold, pale, mottled and sweaty
Others	Signs of dehydration	Petechial or purpuric rash (septic shock), angioedema (anaphylactic shock), signs of spinal cord injury (neurogenic shock)	Signs of congestive heart failure (hepatomegaly, raised JVP, gallop), cyanosis, murmur

Source: Adapted from IAP-ALS Handbook 2018- 1st edition

***Breathing*:** All children in shock must be provided with supplemental oxygen, preferably by non-rebreathing mask as it delivers close to 100% FiO_2. If unavailable, start oxygen by nasal prongs, simple oxygen mask or oxygen hood (any oxygen delivery device that is available). Positive pressure ventilation, is required in children with increased work of breathing, impending respiratory failure, ARDS, cardiogenic shock, and shock refractory to fluids and requiring more than one vasoactive agent. This may be either CPAP (indigenous bubble CPAP), non-invasive ventilation or endotracheal intubation and mechanical ventilation, depending on child's condition. Positive pressure ventilation decreases left ventricular transmural pressure, causing decreased afterload, thereby reducing myocardial work. Increased work of breathing demands up to 50% of the cardiac output, which is a huge proportion in children with shock. Mechanical ventilation relieves the work load on respiratory muscles and diverts their blood supply to other vital organs.

***Circulation*:** Optimizing the preload is the first consideration in shock. It is important to both replenish the lost volume and replace the ongoing fluid losses. Obtaining intravenous access (IV) may be difficult in a child in shock. If IV access cannot be secured in 3 attempts or 90 seconds (whichever is lesser), intraosseous access should be obtained.

- *Compensated shock*: 20 mL/kg isotonic crystalloid should be administered over 15–20 minutes, under close monitoring. Fluid boluses may be repeated, after assessing the therapeutic response. Careful monitoring is warranted for fluid overload (as described later).
- *Hypotensive shock*: 20 mL/kg isotonic crystalloid bolus should be administered as rapidly as possible, by push-pull method using a 3-way stop-cock/a pressure bag method. Boluses can be repeated up to 3 times (60 mL/kg), in the absence of clinical improvement, before labeling shock as fluid-refractory.

Choice of Fluid

Traditionally, the resuscitation fluid of choice is isotonic crystalloid—isotonic saline (0.9% NaCl). In view of its high chloride content, and the subsequent hyperchloremic acidosis and renal injury, studies are underway comparing isotonic saline with balanced crystalloids like Ringers' Lactate and Plasmalyte. At present, till evidence conclusively proves otherwise, the choice of fluid is isotonic saline. Studies on colloids like hypo-oncotic albumin in adults (SAFE study) showed earlier resolution of shock with albumin as compared to crystalloids; however, there is not much data in children to support this.[3]

Response to Fluids

Response to fluids needs to be monitored closely with the help of clinical parameters; improvement in tachycardia to normal limits for age, improvement in pulse volume and increase in blood pressure and urine output. At the same time signs of fluid overload, such as appearance of crepitations at the lung bases and increasing liver size and appearance of S3 gallop during the administration of fluid boluses must be carefully watched for. If these occur, further fluid administration should be stopped and vasoactive therapy (described below) should be initiated.

Although monitoring of fluid-responsiveness is done clinically in the ER, if facilities are available, bedside echocardiography for IVC collapsibility or distensibility index may be used to assess the need for further fluid boluses. Passive leg raising test (patient's legs raised to 45 degree for about 1 minute) delivers the blood pooled in the large veins of lower extremities into the systemic circulation. It is akin to administering a fluid bolus, hence also known as an "auto-bolus".[4] Passive leg raising (PLR) test using difference in cardiac index with PLR, or difference in stroke volume with PLR (ΔCI-PLR or ΔSV-PLR) has been shown to have good predictive value for fluid responsiveness. The different indices for fluid responsiveness are shown in **Table 5**. Dynamic variables of fluid responsiveness assessment are more valuable in the clinical monitoring of patient with shock, than the static variables like CVP.

Table 5: Indices for assessment of fluid responsiveness

Static parameters	*Dynamic parameters*
Central venous pressure – not reliable Poor indicator of preload responsiveness	Arterial pressure variation >11–13% • Pulse pressure variation • Systolic pressure variation
Global end diastolic volume index	Stroke volume variation >12%
	IVC distensibility = IVCmax –IVCmin/IVCmin (In mechanically ventilated patients) >18%
	IVC collapsibility = IVCmax –IVCmin/IVCmax (In spontaneously breathing patients) >50%
	Passive leg raising test >10% increase in stroke volume
	Respiratory variation in peak aortic blood flow >12%

Vasoactive Therapy

Shock unresponsive to fluids (after administration of 3 fluid boluses), or associated with signs of fluid overload, require vasoactive support. Vasoactive therapy includes inotropes and vasopressors and are initiated and titrated based on clinical indications.

Cold septic shock

- *Compensated*: The goal in this situation is to enhance myocardial contractility and improve perfusion. Since BP is maintained, low dose epinephrine 0.05 μ/kg/min (inotropic dose) or dopamine at 5–10 μ/kg/min can be started. Dose of epinephrine can be increased to 0.2 μ/kg/min based on response.
- *Hypotensive*: The goal in this situation is to raise BP and hence epinephrine 0.1–0.3 μ/kg/min or dopamine at 10–20 μ/kg/min is preferred. Further titration is based on response.
- In both above cases, milrinone infusion (start at 0.3 μ/kg/min and increase up to 0.75 μ/kg/min) can be added for myocardial dysfunction. In absence of a desired response, norepinephrine (0.05–0.3 μ/kg/min) or vasopressin (start at 0.3 mU/kg/min increased upto 10 mU/kg/min) can be added after ensuring adequate volume.

Warm septic shock

- *Compensated*: The goal in this situation is to raise MAP by vasopressor action and hence, norepinephrine started at 0.05 μ/kg/min, and hiked up to 0.3 μ/kg/min based on response is initial drug of choice. Alternative drugs would be epinephrine at 0.1 μ/kg/min (increased to 0.3 μ/kg/min) or vasopressin at 0.3 mU/kg/min (increased up to 10 mU/kg/min). In patients with co-existent myocardial dysfunction, milrinone infusion at 0.3 μ/kg/min, and increased up to 0.75 μ/kg/min can be added.
- *Hypotensive*: Norepinephrine 0.05 μ/kg/min (increased up to 0.3 μ/kg/min) or vasopressin at 0.3 mU/kg/min (increased up to 10 mU/kg/min) can be added. Epinephrine at 0.1 μ/kg/min (increased up to

0.3 μ/kg/min) can be tried. In patients with co-existent myocardial dysfunction, milrinone infusion at 0.3 μ/kg/min, and increased up to 0.75 μ/kg/min can be added after the BP is stabilized with vasopressors. Ensure adequate volume in all children with non-response.

Early Goal Directed Therapy

Early goal directed therapy (EGDT) is a step-wise targeted approach in the first 6 hours of shock management, demonstrated by Rivers *et al.*, with focus on objective improvements in perfusion and markers of end-organ function.[4] They demonstrated a significant decrease in mortality with a time bound bundle of care, which included early identification of septic shock, early administration of antibiotics, sending relevant body fluid/blood cultures, prioritizing early source control, hemodynamic stabilization by restoring intravascular volume (targeting normal CVP with fluid boluses), myocardial contractility (inotropic agents) and systemic vascular resistance (MAP targeted with vasoactive agents). The oxygen content of arterial blood is increased by blood transfusion based on appropriate hemoglobin targets. Recent randomized controlled trials have failed to replicate the mortality benefits of EGDT possibly related to an overall decreased mortality in septic shock seen over the years. All the three recent trials have emphasized more on individualized physiology based and systems based protocolized management.[5-8]

Adjuvant Therapies

The role of corticosteroids in catecholamine refractory septic shock is a contentious issue. Hydrocortisone (combined glucocorticoid and mineralocorticoid) for septic shock can be given in children at risk for absolute or relative adrenal insufficiency, e.g. on long-term corticosteroid therapy or suspected congenital adrenal hyperplasia.[1] It is given in a dose of 100 mg/m^2 body surface area/day. Blood product transfusion targets in decompensated shock is hemoglobin level of 10 g/dL as against a hemoglobin of 7 g/dL in hemodynamically stable patient.[9] Oxygen consumption can be reduced with invasive or early noninvasive ventilation and adequate sedoanalgesia. Administering appropriate broad-spectrum antibiotics within the first hour of presentation, is a key step during resuscitation bundle of septic shock. Metabolic causes of myocardial dysfunction like hypoglycemia, and hypocalcemia should always be looked for and rectified.

If shock remains refractory to therapy, extracorporeal life support (ECMO) may be necessary and should be considered, if available. The ACCM guidelines for pediatric septic shock management is outlined in **Flowchart 1**.

MONITORING OF SHOCK

Noninvasive Methods

Therapeutic end-points of shock are enumerated in **Table 6**. Bedside clinical monitoring of hemodynamic parameters helps in titrating fluids and vasoactive therapy in most patients. Besides these, many non-invasive monitoring tools are fast becoming point of care in management of shock. Noninvasive measurement of cardiac output, systemic vascular resistance, cardiac index and stroke volume is possible and age-based normative values are available in literature. Bedside ultrasonography with Doppler guided measurement of blood flow over the pulmonary artery or aorta is a reliable noninvasive tool to calculate cardiac output (CO) and systemic vascular resistance (SVR).

Near Infrared Spectroscopy (NIRS) is a noninvasive, continuous bedside method of estimating tissue oxygenation. Optodes can be applied to the renal angle, to measure the renal tissue oxygenation and to the forehead, to assess the cerebral oxygenation. The exact absolute cut-off values for tissue saturation (StO_2) are yet to be established; however, monitoring trends of StO_2 can provide valuable information about the therapeutic response.

Invasive Monitoring

This is required in a small proportion of children who fail to respond well to early aggressive resuscitation.

Table 6: End points of shock

- Warm skin and CRT≤2 seconds (document CRT site and reassess at the same site)
- Good central and peripheral pulses
- Blood pressure targets above 5th centile for age*
- Normal mental status
- Urine output ≥1 mL/kg/hour
- Decreased serum lactate
- $ScVO_2 \geq 70\%$

*ACCM guidelines recommend blood pressure target at 50th centile

Flowchart 1: American College of Critical Care Medicine (ACCM) guidelines for pediatric and neonatal septic shock management

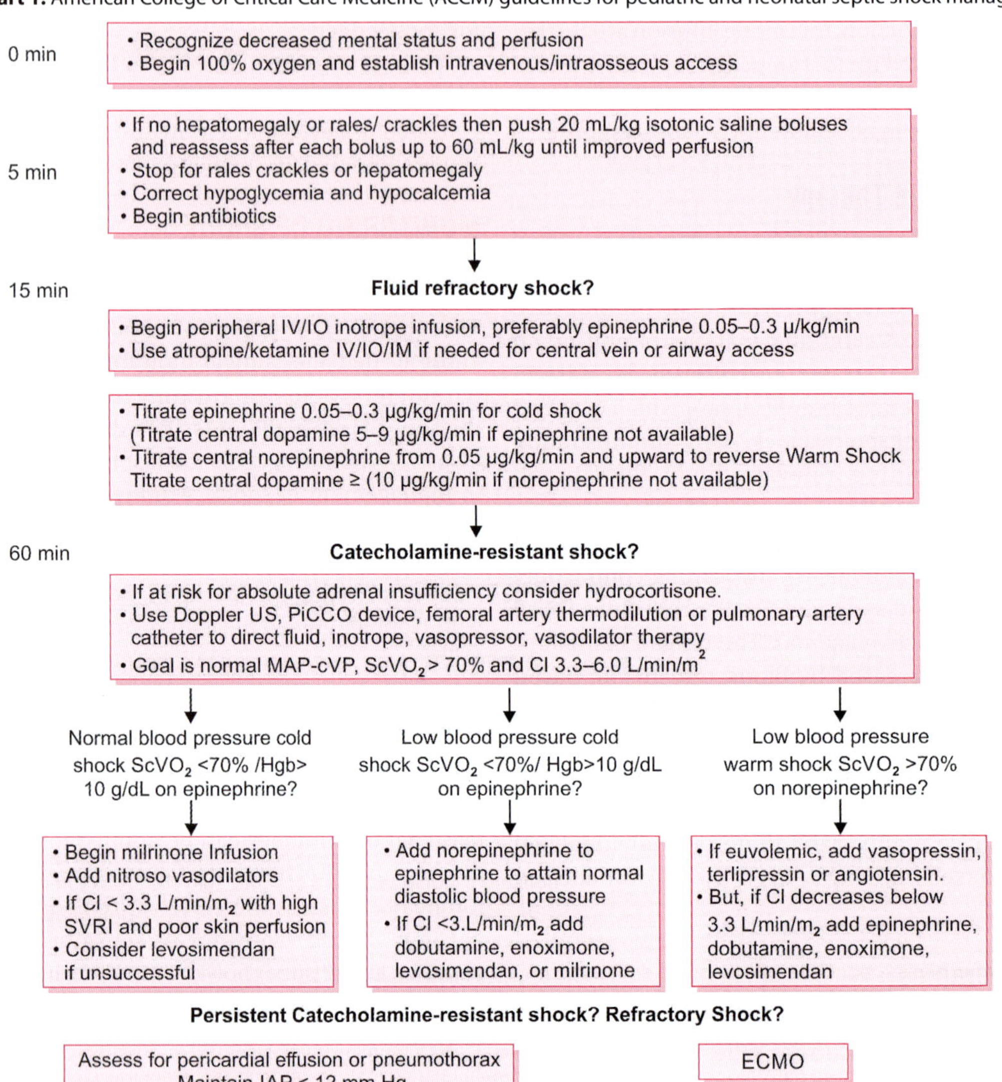

Arterial BP monitoring

Invasive arterial BP monitoring is indicated in children who are on ≥2 vasoactive drugs, severe dengue with shock, in obese children and in patients, where non-invasive BP measurements are likely to be unreliable.[4,10-13] Peripheral arteries like radial, posterior tibial or dorsalis pedis are preferred. With the help of transducers and multi-para-monitors, arterial tracing and arterial blood pressure can be continuously monitored. In situ arterial line also helps in frequent ABG analysis.

Mixed venous oxygen saturation

$ScVO_2$ reflects the balance between oxygen delivery and extraction and is determined by the cardiac output (CO) and oxygen content of blood (CaO_2). It is a surrogate of CO, provided metabolic demand and oxygen content are unchanged. Establishment of internal jugular or subclavian central venous access allows monitoring of $ScVO_2$. Maintaining $ScVO_2$ targets of >70% requires optimization of haemoglobin >10 g/dL and titration of fluids and vasoactive therapy. $ScVO_2$ monitoring can be either continuous or intermittent, depending on the availability.

Arterial lactate levels

The baseline value and serial trend of arterial lactate (lactate clearance) with fluids and vasoactive therapy helps in assessment of severity of oxygen delivery and extraction mismatch. The absolute values of serum lactate > 2 mmol/L (> 3 mmol/L or > 4 mmol/L in some studies,) or a lactate clearance of <10% (<20% in some studies,) at the end of 6 hours, predicts mortality in septic shock.[11-13]

Macrocirculatory versus microcirculatory discordance

In a normal hemodynamic state, there is a concordance between macro and microcirculation. However, in septic shock, this coherence is lost due to endothelial dysfunction, changes in endothelial glycocalyx, adhesion of WBCs and platelets, altered deformability of red blood cells and increase in the diffusion distance for oxygen. Optimizing the macro circulatory parameters therefore does not always translate into adequate microcirculation (tissue perfusion). Areas of poor perfusion aggravate organ dysfunction and mortality correlates with the extent of these microcirculatory abnormalities.[14] Although our understanding of pathogenesis at microcirculatory level has increased enormously, assessment, monitoring and targeted interventions for microcirculation are still under investigation. Surrogates for regional circulation assessment like NIRS, gastric tonometry and sublingual capnography are some of the tools currently available although their clinical application needs more evaluation.

Performance Bundle

Periodic checks should be made to ensure adherence to the recognition and resuscitation bundles.[1]

Specific therapies

Obstructive shock: Tension pneumothorax is urgently drained into underwater seal by needle thoracentesis in 2nd intercostal space. Similarly, an urgent pericardiocentesis is indicated in cardiac tamponade. Duct dependent circulation is treated by Prostaglandin E1 infusion in a dose of 0.01–0.2 μ/kg/min.

Cardiogenic shock: Initial small aliquot of Normal saline/Ringer lactate 5–10 mL/kg over 30–60 min can be tried. Early inotropes (dobutamine/milrinone) to augment cardiac output should be started. In compensated shock either dobutamine at 5 μ/kg/min (increased up to 20 μ/kg/min) or milrinone at 0.3 μ/kg/min (increased up to 0.75 μ/kg/min) can be used. In hypotensive children, epinephrine at 0.05 μ/kg/min (increased upto 0.2 μ/kg/min) or dopamine at 5–10 μ/kg/min should be started to normalize BP. Milrinone or dobutamine can be added after improvement in blood pressure. Positive pressure ventilation by reducing cardiac afterload helps in improving cardiac output.

Anaphylactic shock: Child should be placed in Trendelenburg position and administered 0.01 mg/kg of intramuscular undiluted epinephrine (1:1000). A repeat dose may be required after 10–15 min in severe cases. If hypotension persists, epinephrine as infusion 0.1 to 0.3 μg/kg/min may be started. Fluid bolus may be required to counter shock.

Neurogenic shock is vasodilatory shock and is treated with fluid bolus and vasopressors (norepinephrine/epinephrine).

Targeted De-resuscitation

Once the resuscitation end points are met and there is no further need for fluid boluses and vasoactive infusion doses have stabilized for at least 12–24 hours, targeted de-resuscitation should be initiated in children with features of extravascular/interstitial fluid overload. Since a fluid overload % of >10%, is associated with organ dysfunction, targeted diuresis (diuretic infusions), fluid restriction, or continuous renal replacement therapy may be required to maintain the body homeostasis.

KEY MESSAGES

- Shock is a dynamic state of mismatch between metabolic demands of tissues and supply of the substrates.
- It is multifactorial; common causes being hypovolemic, distributive and cardiogenic
- All these causes progress from compensated to hypotensive shock if untreated leading to anaerobic metabolism, lactic acidosis, end organ dysfunction and MODS.
- A thorough clinical examination coupled with simple, focused laboratory investigations help fine-tune the management.
- High index of suspicion and early recognition of shock along with prompt resuscitative measures is key for good outcome.

REFERENCES

1. Davis AL, Carcillo JA, Aneja RK, *et al.* American College of Critical Care Medicine Clinical Practice Parameters for Hemodynamic Support of Pediatric and Neonatal Septic Shock. Crit Care Med. 2017;45:1061.
2. Dellinger RP, Levy MM, Rhodes A, *et al.* Surviving sepsis campaign: International guidelines for management of severe sepsis and septic shock: 2012. Crit Care Med. 2013;41:580-637.
3. A Comparison of Albumin and Saline for Fluid Resuscitation in the Intensive Care Unit. N Engl J Med. 2004;350:2247-56.
4. Rivers E, Nguyen B, Havstad S, *et al.* Early goal-directed therapy in the treatment of severe sepsis and septic shock. N Engl J Med. 2001;345:1368-77.
5. A Randomized Trial of Protocol-Based Care for Early Septic Shock. N Engl J Med. 2014;370:1683-93.
6. Osborn TM. Severe Sepsis and Septic Shock Trials (ProCESS, ARISE, ProMISe): What is optimal resuscitation? Crit Care Clin. 2017;33:323-44.
7. Goal-Directed Resuscitation for Patients with Early Septic Shock. N Engl J Med. 2014;371:1496-506.
8. Mouncey PR, Osborn TM, Power GS, *et al.* Trial of early, goal-directed resuscitation for septic shock. N Engl J Med. 2015; 372:1301-11.
9. Muszynski JA, Guzzetta NA, Hall MW, *et al.* Recommendations on RBC Transfusions for Critically Ill Children With Nonhemorrhagic Shock From the Pediatric Critical Care Transfusion and Anemia Expertise Initiative. Pediatr Crit Care Med J Soc Crit Care Med World Fed Pediatr Intensive Crit Care Soc. 2018;19(9S Suppl 1):S121-6.
10. NEMJ. Trial of early, Goal-Directed Resuscitation for Septic Shock. Available from: *https://www.nejm.org/doi/full/10.1056/nejmoa1500896*. Accessed July 24, 2019.
11. Jones AE. Lactate clearance for assessing response to resuscitation in severe sepsis. Acad Emerg Med Off J Soc Acad Emerg Med. 2013;20:844-7.
12. Marty P, Roquilly A, Vallée F, *et al.* Lactate clearance for death prediction in severe sepsis or septic shock patients during the first 24 hours in intensive care unit: An observational study. Ann Intensive Care. 2013;12:3:3.
13. Ryoo SM, Lee J, Lee Y-S, *et al.* Lactate level versus lactate clearance for predicting mortality in patients with septic shock defined by sepsis-3. Crit Care Med. 2018;46:e489-95.
14. Cecconi M, De Backer D, Antonelli M, *et al.* Consensus on circulatory shock and hemodynamic monitoring. Task force of the European Society of Intensive Care Medicine. Intensive Care Med. 2014;40:1795-815.

CHAPTER

10

Respiratory Distress and Failure

Praveen Khilnani

INTRODUCTION

Respiratory distress and respiratory failure form a spectrum of illness with respiratory distress being a condition of lesser severity compared to respiratory failure where the compensating mechanism of the body begin to fail leading to cardiopulmonary failure and cardiorespiratory arrest. Respiratory failure is a major cause of morbidity and mortality in children and adults usually preceded by respiratory distress.

EPIDEMIOLOGY

If defined as the necessity for endotracheal intubation and mechanical ventilation, the incidence of acute respiratory failure in Europe is 78–88 cases per 100,000 inhabitants per year.[1,2] Respiratory illnesses contribute to a major proportion of pediatric intensive care unit admissions in India, ranging from 19.7–33.3%.[3-5]

DEFINITION

Respiratory failure is defined as a clinical state in which the respiratory system fails to meet the metabolic demands of the body for oxygenation and removal of carbon dioxide from the pulmonary circulation.

- **Type 1 respiratory failure** is diagnosed when the patient loses the ability to provide sufficient oxygen to the blood leading to hypoxemia, arbitrarily defined as a partial pressure of arterial oxygen (PaO_2) less than 60 mm Hg.
- **Type 2 respiratory failure** occurs when the patient is unable to adequately ventilate which leads to hypercarbia and hypoxemia; partial pressure of arterial carbon dioxide ($PaCO_2$) is greater than 50 mm Hg. Hypercarbia is always associated with hypoxemia, whereas type 1 (hypoxemic) respiratory failure may be associated with a normal or low $PaCO_2$.

Respiratory failure is classified as *acute* when it develops over minutes or days and can be rapidly lethal. *Chronic respiratory failure* develops over a longer period and exists when gas exchange abnormalities persist past one month. It is characterized by certain degree of metabolic compensation with an elevated plasma bicarbonate level to restore the pH close to normal in spite of persistently elevated $PaCO_2$.

PATHOGENESIS AND PATHOPHYSIOLOGY

The frequency of respiratory distress and failure is higher in infants and young children than in adults because of the developmental differences that influence their susceptibility to respiratory failure. The infant, for the first few months of life, is primarily an obligate nose breather. This results in limitation of the ability to convert to oral breathing in those born with choanal atresia or stenosis. A relatively large tongue with relatively undeveloped mandible in an infant has the potential to obstruct the airway particularly if the size of the tongue is further increased, as with a hemangioma or in a child with Down syndrome or hypothyroidism. In contrast to adults, the subglottic region (the cricoid cartilage) being the narrowest part of a child's upper airway, is predisposed to edema from infection (croup) or mechanical trauma (endotracheal intubation or bronchoscopy). In general, airways are small in children below 5 years of age making them more vulnerable to increased airway resistance, due to bronchospasm or mucosal swelling resulting from viral infections of the lower airway. The relative weakness of cartilaginous support in infants compared with that of adults leads to dynamic compression of the trachea in conditions associated with high expiratory flow rates and increased airway resistance.[6]

The smaller alveolar size of the infant not only predisposes to alveolar collapse but also leads to decreased diffusion surface available for gas exchange. Unlike adult lungs, the inability to allow ventilation distal to an obstructed airway by less developed pores of Kohn (interalveolar channels), Lambert channels (bronchiole-alveolar channels) and interbronchiolar channels make the infant and young child at increased risk for atelectasis or emphysematous changes and consequent ventilation/perfusion mismatching.

The pathophysiology of respiratory failure is as follows:

Failure of ventilation: The ventilatory function of the respiratory system is dependent on an intact respiratory pump which consists of feedback mechanism comprising of sensors (chemoreceptors and lung and airway receptors), controllers (cerebrum, brainstem and spinal cord) and effectors (chest wall, muscles of respiration). Failure of the respiratory pump leading to hypoventilation is a common reason for ventilatory failure leading to hypercapnia (**Table 1**).

The increased work of breathing results from abnormal lung mechanics as seen with decreasing pulmonary compliance and/or increasing airway resistance.[7] Pulmonary compliance refers to the volume of gas that can move into the lung for each unit of pressure change. Thus, compliance = V/P where P is the change in pressure required and V is the volume produced. Conditions such as pneumonia, atelectasis, acute respiratory distress syndrome (ARDS), large pleural effusions and tension pneumothorax decrease the pulmonary compliance, whereas tense ascites,[8] obesity and vigorous respiratory muscle contraction lead to a fall in chest wall compliance. As opposed to these, restrictive respiratory disease, iatrogenic reasons such as use of endotracheal tube (even appropriately sized),[9] secretions, post-extubation airway obstruction, bronchiolitis and asthma may be responsible for obstructive causes of increased work of breathing. Lower airway obstructive diseases cause hypercapnia relatively late in the course of the disease because the compensatory hyperventilation results in CO_2 washout.

Significant hypercapnia is always associated with hypoxemia unless the patient receives supplemental oxygen, since increased alveolar carbon dioxide dilutes the available oxygen in the lungs. This is represented by the alveolar air equation:

$$P_AO_2 = PiO_2 - PaCO_2/R$$

where P_AO_2 is the partial pressure of oxygen in the alveoli, P_iO_2 is the partial pressure of inspired oxygen and R is the respiratory quotient.

Table 1: Site of abnormality for failure of ventilation

Central control abnormality	• CNS infections—meningitis, encephalitis • Encephalopathies—hypoxic encephalopathy • Drug overdose—sedatives, anesthetics • Traumatic brain injury—stroke, sleep apnea
Extrathoracic airway obstruction	• Infections—laryngotracheobronchitis, croup, Ludwig angina, retropharyngeal abscess, peritonsillar abscess • Traumatic—post-extubation, burns • Foreign body aspiration • Other causes—hypertrophied tonsils, adenoids • Congenital lesions—craniofacial anomalies, choanal atresia, laryngomalacia, tracheomalacia, subglottic stenosis, web or cyst
Intrathoracic obstruction	• Vascular ring, pulmonary sling, mediastinal mass, bronchogenic cyst, foreign body
Chest wall restriction	• Diaphragm eventration, diaphragmatic hernia, kyphoscoliosis, flail chest, massive ascites
Respiratory muscle paralysis	• Guillain-Barré syndrome, poliomyelitis, post-diphtheric, spinal cord trauma, hypokalemia, hypomagnesemia, hypophosphatemia, muscular dystrophy, spinal muscular atrophy, botulism
Respiratory muscle fatigue	• Severe respiratory distress

Since the lung function is unimpaired in hypoventilation, the difference between the alveolar PO_2 (P_AO_2) and the arterial PO_2 (PaO_2), also known as the alveolar to arterial gradient [$P(A\text{-}a)O_2$] or alveolar-arterial PO_2 difference [A-a DO_2] is relatively small. Thus if the $AaDO_2$ is within normal limits, hypoxemia is entirely due to hypoventilation and not due to problems in pulmonary gas exchange.

Impaired pulmonary perfusion: Impairment of blood flow to alveoli results in increased "dead space" in the lungs. This problem is seen most frequently with pulmonary emboli, a low cardiac output state and obliteration of pulmonary vasculature in certain lung diseases. Pulmonary embolism, although uncommon in pediatric population, may result in a very rapid deterioration of oxygenation without gross impairment of ventilation. It should be suspected in: (i) cases involving abdominal, pelvic or lower extremity trauma, (ii) older and obese children that are immobile, and (iii) children with increased susceptibility to venous thrombosis, such as those with nephrotic syndrome, burns, autoimmune diseases, and protein S, C, or antithrombin-3 deficiency.

Ventilation-perfusion (V/Q) imbalance or mismatch: It is the relative distribution of ventilation and perfusion that is critical to effective oxygenation. Ventilation must take place where perfusion does and perfusion must occur in areas of good ventilation. When considering ventilation and perfusion, there can be four types of alveolar-capillary units. If ventilation and perfusion are normal, the unit is normal. If there is ventilation without perfusion (V/Q = infinity), the unit is considered to be dead space. If there is perfusion without ventilation (V/Q = 0), the unit is considered to be a pure (right-to-left) shunt. If there is neither ventilation nor perfusion, the unit is silent.

Ventilation/perfusion inequality is the most commonly encountered cause of hypoxemia. Commonly seen conditions causing hypoxemia due to V/Q mismatch are pneumonia, pulmonary edema, asthma, bronchiolitis, bronchopulmonary dysplasia and ARDS.

Impaired gas transfer across the alveolar-capillary membrane: Diffusion impairment by itself is never the major cause of respiratory failure primarily because the transfer of oxygen from alveolus to hemoglobin usually requires only a brief time for completion.[10]

Impaired gas transport and uptake by the tissues: Impaired oxygen transport as seen in anemia, carbon monoxide poisoning, cardiogenic shock and failure of tissue oxygen extraction, for example, in cyanide poisoning result in inadequate oxygenation of the tissues, but are not considered under the term respiratory failure.

CLINICAL FEATURES

Clinical Evaluation of a Child with Respiratory Distress and Failure

A five-point quick clinical assessment is invaluable to identify the degree of alteration in the child's respiratory physiological status and to identify any rectifiable life threatening cause of poor gas exchange:

1. *State of consciousness*: Lethargy, confusion, agitation may be signs of hypoxemia and hypercarbia. Decreased level of activity and cry is indicative of impending respiratory failure in an infant with respiratory distress.
2. *Assessment of the presence and probable site of airway obstruction*: One should quickly assess whether the airway is patent or obstructed and if obstructed, the probable site of airway obstruction in child with suspected respiratory failure. Signs such as inspiratory retraction, stridor, wheezing, grunting along with a worried, restless general appearance are suggestive of increasing airway obstruction. Impending collapse due to severe airway obstruction is suggested by the following signs:
   - Markedly decreased respiratory effort, decreased stridor and breath sounds
   - Restless, distracted activity, decreased conscious-ness level, hypotonia
   - Cyanosis or extreme pallor.

   Quick assessment of the site of obstruction is helpful to select appropriate intervention (**Table 1**).
3. *Assessment of breathing and work of breathing*: Assessment of breathing helps to judge the degree of derangement in gas exchange. This is done by assessment of minute ventilation by clinical estimation of tidal volume and respiratory rate.
4. *Cyanosis*: Cyanosis is a fairly late and unreliable sign as it is influenced by skin perfusion and hemoglobin concentration, and subjective error in assessment.

Hypoxemia should be suspected in children with respiratory disease before the appearance of cyanosis.

5. *Heart rate*: Tachycardia, though nonspecific, is an important accompaniment of hypoventilation and hypoxia. The presence of bradycardia in an acutely ill infant or child is suggestive of impending cardiorespiratory arrest due to profound hypoxemia and acidosis. Diminished breath sounds and slow, irregular respiration is indicative of significant hypoventilation.

On the other hand, a markedly increased respiratory rate with nasal flaring, accessory muscle use and marked suprasternal, intercostal and subcostal retractions indicate very significant increase in the work of breathing. Since the state of compensation (**respiratory distress**) may rapidly and unpredictably convert into a decompensated state (**respiratory failure**) in children because of limited ability to compensate, anticipation of respiratory failure and intervention by intubation and mechanical ventilation, is essential.

DIAGNOSIS

Diagnosis is essentially clinical and supported by few investigations.

1. Arterial blood gas analysis can be used to define acute respiratory failure, characterized by a $PaCO_2$ greater than 50 mm Hg and a PaO_2 less than 60 mm Hg.
2. *Complete blood count*: polycythemia suggests chronic hypoxemia.
3. *Electrolyte estimation*: Hypokalemia, hypocalcemia and hypophosphatemia can impair muscle contraction and contribute to acute respiratory failure.
4. *Estimation of hypoxemia*: Most common clinical parameter is to assess oxygen saturation and need for supplemental oxygen.

Calculation of the Alveolar-arterial Oxygen Difference [(A-a) DO_2]

The (A-a) DO_2 is widened when a V/Q mismatch, right-to-left shunt or diffusion defect is the mechanism producing hypoxemia in contrast to hypoventilation as the cause of hypoxemia. Interpretation of values of (A-a) DO_2 should be done with caution at higher oxygen concentrations. The normal (A-a) DO_2 widens with higher fractions of inspired oxygen. This value may reach up to 70 mm Hg when PaO_2 exceeds 350–450 mm Hg and then decreases at a higher PO_2 so inscribing a bell shaped curve. Thus, between the two extremes of inhaled FiO_2 (0.21 and 1.0), the expected (A-a) DO_2 level even in normal subjects is difficult to predict, and there is no reliable reference values for patients with intermediate levels of FiO_2.

PaO_2/FiO_2 ratio is a commonly used indicator of impairment of oxygenation. Normally this ratio is (100/0.21) = 500; values <300 are defined as acute lung injury and <200 as ARDS.

- *Mild* ARDS: PaO_2/FiO_2 between 300 and 200 mm Hg with PEEP or CPAP >5 cm water
- *Moderate* ARDS: PaO_2/FiO_2 between 200 and 100 with PEEP >5 cm water
- *Severe* ARDS: $PaO_2/FiO_2 \leq 100$ mm Hg with PEEP ≥ 5 cm water.

The oxygenation index also takes into account the mean airway pressure as a determinant of oxygenation and is a better indicator of oxygenation in mechanically ventilated patients.

$$\text{Oxygenation index (OI)} = \text{Mean airway pressure (MAP)} \times FiO_2 \times 100/PaO_2.$$

The Pediatric Acute Lung Injury Consensus Conference 2015 suggests the use of oxygen saturation index (OSI).[11]

$$OSI = [FiO_2 \times MAP \times 100]/SpO_2$$

Imaging Studies

Lateral and AP radiographs of the neck can depict a radio-opaque foreign body or a soft tissue structure encroaching the airway lumen. Chest X-rays are useful to evaluate for abnormalities that require immediate intervention (e.g. malpositioned endotracheal tube, pneumothorax). Common findings associated with respiratory failure include focal or diffuse pulmonary disease (e.g. pneumonia, ARDS), bilateral hyperinflation (e.g. asthma), asymmetric lung expansion suggesting bronchial obstruction, pleural effusion and cardiomegaly.

Chest CT can sometimes further define radiodensities due to vascular, pleural, interstitial, or airway lesions. Airway CT scanning, MRI, or angiography can be used to differentiate deep tissue structure, bone lesions and vascular abnormalities from one another. CT angiography may be done to rule out pulmonary embolism if indicated. Fluoroscopy is valuable to evaluate the movement of the diaphragms and dynamic obstructive lesion of both the extra- and intrathoracic airway. Ventilation-perfusion scanning can predict a probability of V/Q mismatch as in pulmonary embolism.

Additional diagnostic procedures may be indicated for confirmation of precise etiologic diagnosis, e.g. bronchoscopy (fiber optic or rigid) may be needed to assess the airway for anatomic abnormalities and foreign body. Bronchoalveolar lavage is done to identify a specific pulmonary pathogen; silver stain and bacterial, viral, fungal and AFB can be sent. Other investigations include thoracentesis, lung biopsy, electromyography nerve conduction velocity. Polysomnography or sleep studies are done is patients with suspected obstructive or central sleep apnea.

MANAGEMENT

Respiratory support for a patient with respiratory failure should be initiated. While supporting the respiratory system and ensuring oxygen delivery, an intervention specifically to correct the underlying conditions may be life saving. Examples of such interventions are: needle aspiration for tension pneumothorax, naloxone for narcotic associated hypoventilation, nebulized beta-agonists and steroids for severe asthma, tracheotomy or cricothyroidotomy for complete or nearly complete airway obstruction and rapid sequence intubation for conditions causing acute respiratory failure.

Airway Management

The first decision is whether a tracheal intubation is needed. While unnecessary or too early intubation may expose the child to hazards of intubation and/or mechanical ventilation, unwarranted delays may result in complications associated with emergency intubation. Upper airway obstruction resulting in markedly compromised air movement, loss of protective airway reflexes such as coughing or gag reflex, and apnea are threat to life. Therefore, establishment of an artificial airway by endotracheal intubation tracheostomy or cricothyrotomy is a priority.

Indications for Admission to the PICU

- Patients too unstable to be managed in ward: Severe respiratory distress, tachypnea and retractions
- Oxygen requirement on the rise >50% to maintain oxyhemoglobin saturation above 90%. Desaturation below 90% on highest flow of oxygen
- Lethargic child
- Arterial blood gas showing hypoxemia, hypercarbia or metabolic acidosis.

High flow nasal cannula (HFNC) and continuous positive airway pressure (CPAP)

The HFNC or CPAP may be indicated if a lung disease results in severe oxygenation abnormalities such that an FiO_2 of more than 0.6 is needed to maintain a PaO_2 of more than 60 mm Hg. Usually HFNC flows 2 mL/kg are used and for CPAP pressure between 3 and 10 cm of water are used. CPAP improves oxygenation by increasing the lung volume, redistribution of fluid from the alveoli and interstitium, increased ventilation in areas of low V/Q by opening up of atelectatic alveolar units and improved respiratory mechanics.

Lung and Respiratory Pump Support

Indications of mechanical ventilation

- Indications are mainly clinical (blood gas though important but not absolutely necessary): PaO_2 <55 mm Hg or $PaCO_2$ >60 despite 100% oxygen therapy.
- Deteriorating respiratory status despite oxygen and nebulization therapy.
- Anxious, sweaty lethargic child with deteriorating mental status.

Positive pressure ventilation

Institution of positive pressure ventilation important advance in the care of children with acute respiratory failure.

DIFFERENTIAL DIAGNOSIS AND SPECIFIC MANAGEMENT

Upper Airway Obstruction

Nasal and pharyngeal causes such as choanal stenosis or atresia will cause cyanosis at rest. Common symptom of upper airway obstruction is stridor in infancy. Important causes of stridor include laryngomalacia vocal cord paralysis, laryngeal web, vascular ring, tracheal stenosis, airway hemangiomas, hypocalcemia and hypoparathyroidism. In older child, infections causing upper airway obstruction (hoarseness, drooling swallowing difficulty, stridor with or without respiratory distress) include: Laryngotracheobronchitis, epiglottitis, diphtheria, tonsillitis/peritonsillar abscess, retropharyngeal abscess, bacterial tracheitis, and tracheobronchomalacia. Other causes of upper airway obstruction should always be looked into such as airway foreign bodies, airway tumors, post intubation stridor, and subglottic stenosis.

Emergency department and management

Oxygen for all patients and no sedation

Is airway maintained? *If stable airway*: Maintain position of comfort. Do not force to examine the airway and do not lay the child forcefully. Accompany child for portable soft tissue anteroposterior and lateral neck X-rays. *If unstable airway*: Secure airway first in best possible location in controlled environment, i.e. operation theater or the PICU with availability of emergency tracheostomy.

Intravenous antibiotics and medications: Ceftriaxone or cefuroxime for tracheitis, peritonsillar abscess and epiglottitis. Adrenaline nebulization and IV methylprednisone or dexamethasone for laryngotracheobronchitis. For angioedema, adrenaline subcutaneously and IV dexamethasone.

Bronchiolitis

Chest radiograph shows hyperinflation as well as perihilar infiltrates but no evidence of lobar consolidation. Treatment is symptomatic until acute phase is over in 24 to 48 hours. Endotracheal intubation and mechanical ventilation is rarely required.

Acute Severe Asthma

Asthma is characterized by inflammation, mucosal exudation and edema as well as reversible lower airway obstruction with bronchospasm, with respiratory distress precipitated by one or combination of viral infection, allergens, exposure to cold environment, exercise induced or induced by use of medication.

Management in emergency department: Oxygen in combination with nebulizer therapy with β-2 agonists intermittent or continuously, and IV steroids is the cornerstone of therapy in the emergency room.

Indications for admission to pediatric intensive care unit: Following conditions may require and possible intubation and mechanical ventilation:

- Altered consciousness, exhaustion
- Respiratory arrest
- Shallow respirations, $PaCO_2$ >50 mm Hg worsening or persistent hypoxia PaO_2 <60 mm Hg, worsening metabolic acidosis
- Patient with pneumothorax.

Acute Respiratory Distress Syndrome (ARDS) and Pneumonia

It is a predominantly alveolar disease with respiratory distress with or without fever affecting oxygenation as well as ventilation.[12]

Emergency department management: Includes quick history and rapid cardiopulmonary assessment: Saturation is assessed by pulse oximetry. Portable chest X-ray is done to confirm alveolar disease, and diffuse infiltrates/consolidation usually with normal sized heart. Complete blood count, blood culture, coagulation profile, electrolytes, urea, creatinine and liver functions are obtained. Intravenous line is secured and fluid bolus is administered if patient is in shock. If hypotension and poor perfusion is present despite fluid therapy, use of inotropes is considered.

Tension Pneumothorax

This is a medical emergency and should be promptly recognized and treated. Severe respiratory distress with shock due to decreased intrathoracic venous return results in acute fall in cardiac output as indicated by hypoxemia, poor perfusion and hypotension. On auscultation, there are absent or reduced breath sounds on the affected side as well as muffled heart sounds and shifted apical impulse. Chest X-ray shows mediastinal shift as well as compression with free air in the pleural cavity depressing the dome of diaphragm. Immediate intervention is often necessary. Thoracentesis with 16 or 18 gauge IV cannula or scalp vein needle may be attempted to relieve tension pneumothorax. Once chest X-ray is obtained the patient will require tube thoracostomy on the affected side in 2nd intercostal space anteriorly in mid-clavicular line or in 4th intercostal space in mid-axillary line.

Neuromuscular Disorders Leading to Respiratory Failure

Central hypoventilation syndrome

Central hypoventilation may be congenital or acquired. The former presents as cyanosis at birth readily responsive to mechanical ventilation with normal chest radiographs but repeated weaning failures. In less severe cases, abnormalities in respirations during sleep such as periodic breathing, apnea or acute life-threatening episodes may occur. This must be differentiated from reversible systemic processes such as sepsis, hypothermia, electrolyte abnormalities, hypocalcemia, hypoglycemia and seizures, CNS infections, intracranial hemorrhage and acute hydrocephalus. The condition needs to be distinguished from obstructive sleep apnea due to hypertrophied tonsils and adenoids, macroglossia, micrognathia, temporomandibular ankylosis, vascular ring and vocal cord paralysis. Therapy is immediate ventilatory support if in acute respiratory failure. Doxapram, theophylline and caffeine have been tried. Tracheostomy with home mechanical ventilatory assistance during sleep is commonly required. Recently noninvasive methods such as use of nasal mask continuous positive airway pressure (nasal CPAP) or noninvasive positive pressure ventilation (NIPPV) have been shown to be effective.

Guillain-Barré syndrome

This condition commonly presents as a post viral immune mediated paralysis affecting skeletal muscles as well as autonomic nervous system leading to ascending muscle weakness and paresthesias. Diaphragmatic and intercostal muscle weakness leads to neuromuscular respiratory failure requiring mechanical ventilation in 20% of children. Frequent assessment of respiratory reserve is imperative, including forced vital capacity below 15 to 20 mL/kg, maximum negative inspiratory pressure <20–30 cm water $PaCO_2$ >50 mm Hg.

Cerebrospinal fluid protein level is usually elevated >45 mg/dL in absence of pleocytosis. EMG shows lower motor neuron disease and nerve conduction velocity is delayed, 2–3 weeks following onset of disease.

Early plasmapheresis within 7 days of onset of disease has been found to be beneficial. Intravenous gamma globulin therapy is more effective, compared to plasmapheresis. Prognosis is satisfactory with recovery in 3–4 weeks, however muscle power and neurological recovery may be incomplete.

Myesthenia gravis

Muscle weakness in myasthenia gravis is attributed to immunological interference with neuromuscular transmission associated with acetylcholine receptor antibodies. While classical or juvenile myasthenia can occur in children as young as 2 years, the illness typically presents in adolescence. Neonatal myasthenia gravis may be associated with severe generalized muscle weakness, with history of similar illness in the mother. Reasons for acute respiratory failure in myasthenia are two-fold: progressive muscle fatigue or excessive treatment with anticholinesterase therapy. Indications for intubation and mechanical ventilation include apnea, hypoventilation, or evidence of severe respiratory muscle fatigue. If muscle weakness is precipitated by viral infection or other systemic stress, treatment with anticholinesterase agents (neostigmine, pyridostigmine) may be life saving. Severe bronchospasm can occur as a side effect of anticholinesterase therapy. Myasthenic patients with muscle weakness due to cholinergic crisis usually show excessive parasympathetic activity such as salivation, lacrimation, diarrhea and bradycardia that can be managed with atropine therapy.

Therapy with prednisone is used as adjunct to anticholinesterase therapy. Thymectomy is useful in juvenile myasthenia and plasmapheresis performed before thymectomy has been found to be useful in adult patents with resistant myasthenia gravis. The prognosis is satisfactory.

Unilateral phrenic nerve paralysis

This condition results from birth trauma to phrenic nerve and usually presents with respiratory distress in infancy. Fluoroscopy shows upward movement of the diaphragm during inspiration. Usually adequate gas exchange can be maintained with CPAP alone or institution of mechanical ventilation, however, long-term management will require surgical plication of affected diaphragm. Other important causes of phrenic nerve injury include direct phrenic nerve injury during open heart surgery and aorto-pulmonary shunt procedures. Transcutaneous phrenic nerve stimulation in the cervical region may be effective.

Tetanus

Clostridium tetani is the usual cause of neonatal tetanus. Widespread immunization has significantly reduced the prevalence of the illness. Tetanolysin and tetanospasmin released at the neuromuscular junction cause severe muscle spasm leading to respiratory failure. Lock jaw or severe masseter spasm is common in 50% to 70% patients. Mental status is normal. Benzodiazepines, muscle relaxants and mechanical ventilation (3-5 weeks) are life saving in addition to antibiotics and proper attention to nutrition and PICU care.

Poliomyelitis

Poliomyelitis is an acute viral infection of the central nervous system that results in widespread muscle paralysis due to involvement of anterior horn cells and secondary respiratory failure. Causative virus can be isolated from fecal and oropharyngeal specimens. Serological confirmation is made by identifying specific antibodies to polio virus. Endotracheal intubation, mechanical ventilation and chest physiotherapy remain the key treatment modalities. Widespread and effective vaccination strategies have resulted in eradication of poliomyelitis from most counties in the world, including India.

KEY MESSAGES

- Respiratory distress and failure is a major cause of morbidity and mortality in children and adults.
- The frequency of acute respiratory failure is higher in infants and young children because of the developmental differences that influence their susceptibility.
- Support of respiratory function of the child in respiratory distress should be initiated instantly, regardless of the primary diagnosis.
- While most etiologies resulting in respiratory failure are treatable, the overall prognosis varies based on the primary condition leading to respiratory failure..

REFERENCES

1. Luhr OR, Antonsen, K, Karlsson M, *et al.* Incidence and mortality after acute respiratory failure and acute respiratory distress syndrome in Sweden, Denmark and Iceland. Am J Respir Crit Care Med. 1999;159:1849-61.
2. Lewandowski K, Metz J, Deutschmann C, *et al.* Incidence, severity, and mortality of acute respiratory failure in Berlin, Germany. Am J Respir Crit Care Med. 1995;151:1121-5.
3. Khilnani P, Devajit S, Singh R, *et al.* Demographic profile and outcome analysis of a tertiary level pediatric intensive care unit. Indian J Pediatr. 2004;71:587-91.
4. Lodha R, Kabra SK, Pandey RM. Acute respiratory distress syndrome: Experience at a tertiary care hospital. Indian Pediatr. 2001;38:1154-59.
5. Yadav RS. Comparative outcome evaluation in children admitted to the pediatric intensive care unit and those admitted to the general pediatric wards. Thesis for M.D. (Pediatrics). Upgraded King George's Medical College: Lucknow; 2002.
6. Wittenborg MH, Gyepes M, Crocker D. Tracheal dynamics in infants with respiratory distress, stridor and collapsing trachea. Radiology. 1967;88:653-57.
7. Guslits BG, Gaston SE, Bryan MH, *et al.* Diaphragmatic work of breathing in premature human infants. J Appl Physiol. 1987;62: 1410-5.
8. Rosado M, Banner MJ. Ascites and its effects upon respiratory muscle loading and work of breathing. Crit Care Med. 1996;24: 538-40.
9. Velarde CA, Short BL, Rivera O, *et al.* Reduced airway resistance and work of breathing during mechanical ventilation with an ultra-thin two-stage polyurethane endotracheal tube. Crit Care Med. 1997;25:276-9.
10. Staub NC. Alveolar-arterial oxygen tension gradient due to diffusion. J Appl Physiol. 1963;18:673-80.
11. The Pediatric Acute Lung Injury Consensus Conference Group. Pediatric Acute Respiratory Distress Syndrome: Consensus recommendations from the pediatric acute lung injury consensus conference. Pediatr Crit Care Med. 2015;16:428-39.
12. Ranieri VM, Rubenfeld GD, Thompson BT, *et al*; ARDS Definition Task Force. Acute respiratory distress syndrome: the Berlin definition. JAMA. 2012;307:2526-33.

CHAPTER

11

Mechanical Ventilation in the Emergency Room

Dinesh Raj

INTRODUCTION

Respiratory failure is a common cause of emergency consultations in the pediatric age group. With the advent of noninvasive ventilation (NIV), many of these patients can be managed without need of invasive ventilation. Some patients may however present with frank respiratory failure where NIV is contraindicated, justifying the need for intubation and mechanical ventilation. Emergency room physicians need to be conversant with basics of respiratory physiology and mechanical ventilation, so as to assist in rapid stabilization of the critically ill child, while he is being shifted to the Pediatric Intensive Care Unit (PICU). Availability of a PICU bed is also a problem and critically ill children may spend significant time in the emergency department.

Though mechanical ventilation is lifesaving in the acute setting, it may lead to complications. It may often be not possible to take enough history while the child is in significant respiratory failure. While important points in history and examination are being elicited quickly, the respiratory management should be done simultaneously. As soon as relevant clinical data is available along with radiological and laboratory investigations, the working diagnosis is appropriately modified.

This chapter will discuss the relevant respiratory physiology of the critically ill child, basics of invasive mechanical ventilation and clinical application of mechanical ventilation in common settings in the emergency room.

Peculiarities of the Pediatric Patient

The respiratory physiology of the child differs from adults. Even in the pediatric age group there are signification variations in the various age group. Starting with around 50 million alveoli at birth in a term infant, the alveoli number gradually increase to upto 300 million by about 5 to 8 years of age, a process called alveolization. Collateral ventilation is often not developed in children till 5 to 6 years of age. Pores of Kahn (interalveolar communications) develop in the first few years of age, whereas Lambert channels (bronchoalveolar communications) develop by 5 to 6 years of age. Absence of collateral ventilation increase the risk of atelectasis in children.[1]

Compliance is defined by volume change per unit pressure change ($C = \Delta V/\Delta P$). Children have more compliant chest walls compared to adults. Because of this increased compliance, children have to work harder to breathe a certain tidal volume compared to adults. Compliance can change in different disease processes. Furthermore, it can change during the disease process in a patient, either recovering or worsening. At extremes of inflation and deflation, the compliance decreases (**Fig. 1**). Alveolar filling is dependent on lung compliance, hence decrease in lung compliance leads to reduced tidal volume. This would lead to increased respiratory rate and work of breathing to maintain minute ventilation.

Static compliance is the lung compliance measured at zero airflow (as during an inspiratory pause) and dynamic compliance is measured during airflow through the lungs. Dynamic compliance reflects lung and chest wall stiffness, besides airway resistance. In a stiff lung (e.g. pulmonary edema, consolidation), both are low. If only the dynamic compliance has decreased, it suggests that the airway might be obstructed, e.g. ET tube obstruction or bronchospasm.[2]

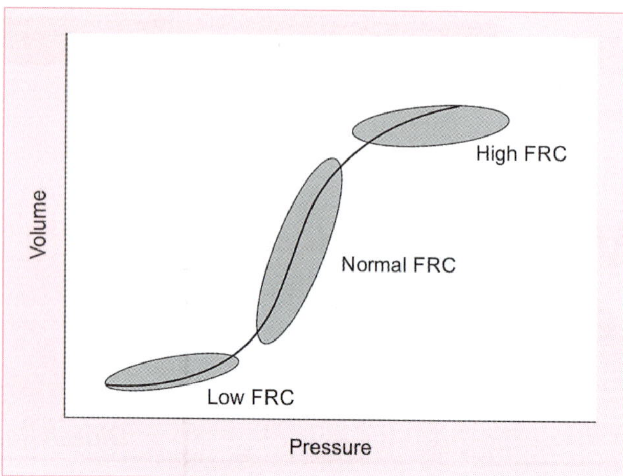

Fig. 1: Pressure-volume curve—compliance curve (FRC: Functional residual capacity)

As resistance is inversely proportional to the fourth power of radius airway resistance is increased in children because of smaller sized airways. This increases further in the airway diseases. Even a small reduction in airway size due to edema or mucus may markedly increase respiratory resistance. The peripheral airway resistance in young children is significantly higher than adults, leading to increased likelihood of lower airway obstructive symptoms.

Oxygenation

Oxygenation is primarily determined by partial pressure of oxygen in alveoli (PAO_2) which is given by the alveolar gas equation

$$PAO_2 = PiO_2 - PACO_2$$

where PiO_2 is the partial pressure of inspired oxygen and $PACO_2$ is partial pressure of carbon dioxide (CO_2) in the alveoli. PiO_2 can be calculated by multiplying fraction of inspired oxygen (FiO_2) to the atmospheric pressure [barometric pressure (Pb) minus water vapor pressure (Pw)]. Moreover, $PACO_2$ is equal to the partial pressure of arterial carbon dioxide ($PaCO_2$) divided by respiratory quotient (RQ). The alveolar gas equation after putting these variables is:

$$PAO_2 = FiO_2\,(Pb\text{-}Pw) - PaCO_2/RQ$$

If we put physiological variables in this equation, PAO_2 comes to around 100 to 120 mm Hg at sea level in room air. This equation suggests that PAO_2 (or oxygenation) may be affected by change in FiO_2, altitude and depth/rate of respiration.[1]

Partial pressure of arterial oxygen (PaO_2) is usually around 10 mm Hg less than PAO_2 which is maintained by the diffusion barrier of the alveolar-capillary membrane and ventilation-perfusion matching. This gradient can be affected in various respiratory diseases by reducing lung volumes, atelectasis and V-Q mismatch. Atelectatic lung may get perfused but not ventilated leading to intrapulmonary shunting.

Alveolar Ventilation

$PaCO_2$ is inversely related to alveolar ventilation which is given by:

$$\text{Alveolar ventilation} = RR\,(Vt - Vd)$$

where, RR is respiratory rate, Vt is tidal volume, and Vd is dead space. In normal lungs, dead space includes only the large conducting airways which do not take part in gas exchange (anatomic dead space), but in diseased lungs atelectatic alveoli which are perfused but not ventilated also contribute to dead space (alveolar dead space).

Hypoxemia

Based on the above, causes of hypoxemia are: (i) hypoventilation; (ii) ventilation-perfusion mismatch, (iii) diffusion abnormalities, (iv) high altitude, and (v) true shunt related to congenital heart disease.

Indications for Mechanical Ventilation

Almost all indications of mechanical ventilation can be grouped under conditions which threaten spontaneous respiration or conditions where spontaneous respiration is not sufficient for adequate gas exchange (**Table 1**).

VENTILATOR VARIABLES

Inspiration is controlled in mechanical ventilation, whereas expiration is passive. The four variables which can be controlled during inspiration are pressure, volume, flow and time. The manner in which each of these variables is controlled decides the mode of ventilation. Phase variables are parameters which control the various phases of the respiratory cycle. Trigger variable controls the initiation of inspiration, limit variable maintains inspiration, and cycle variable switches from inspiration to expiration.[2]

Initiation of the inspiration is determined by triggering. Mandatory breaths initiated by the machine are time-triggered as set by the operator. Ventilator can also assist

Table 1: Indications for mechanical ventilation in children

- Any condition causing hypoxemia and/or hypercarbia [pneumonia, acute severe asthma, acute lung injury (infections, inhalational injuries), respiratory distress syndrome, pulmonary edema, heart diseases; e.g. like myocarditis, congenital heart disease]
- Increased work of breathing (septic shock, pneumonia, bronchiolitis, heart diseases)
- Decreased respiratory drive (head trauma, poisonings, apnea, altered mentation)
- Neuromuscular diseases (Guillain-Barré syndrome, spinal muscular atrophy)
- Reduction of raised intracranial pressure
- Issues related to chest wall, diaphragm and pleura (flail chest, congenital diaphragmatic hernia, pneumothorax, massive pleural effusion)
- Elective ventilation for surgeries, invasive procedures; postoperative state

Table 2: Description of ventilator terminology

Variable	*Definition*	*Comments*
Peak inspiratory pressure (PIP)	Maximum pressure during inspiration	Needed to inflate alveoli and oxygenation High PIP may lead to barotrauma
Positive end expiratory pressure (PEEP)	Pressure maintained in airways at the end of exhalation to keep alveoli open	Improves FRC, oxygenation, and avoiding atelectotrauma (due to reopening and closing of alveoli) High PEEP can lead to overdistension, reduced venous return and tidal volume
Respiratory cycle	One respiratory cycle includes inspiration and expiration	
Inspiratory time (Ti)	The duration of inspiration	
Expiratory time (Te)	The duration of expiration	
I:E ratio	The ratio of inspiratory time and expiratory time	Normally, I:E ratio is kept at 1:1.5 to 1:2 Inverse ratio ventilation may be needed in ARDS to improve oxygenation
Tidal volume (TV)	Volume delivered in each breath	Needed for oxygenation and CO_2 removal
Rise time	Defines the beginning of a breath, either fast or slow depending on the flow rate	A square waveform, with a faster rise, is needed for patients who are air hungry Ramp waveform leads to slower rise providing laminar flow and better gas distribution
Mean airway pressure (MAP)	The average airway pressure during one complete respiratory cycle.	$MAP = \frac{K(Ti \times PIP) + (Te \times PEEP)}{Ti + Te}$ K = constant based on the shape of waveform
Plateau pressure (PPlat)	The pressure at equilibrium applied to small airways and alveoli during inspiration	PIP is slightly above Pplat in normal lungs. With increasing TV and worsening compliance, both PIP and Pplat increase proportionately Increased airway resistance due to any cause leads to increase in PIP with no change in Pplat
Fraction of inspired oxygen (FiO_2)	Fraction of inspired oxygen	Ranges from 0.2 to 1 To avoid oxygen toxicity, it is desired to keep FiO_2 below 0.6

the breaths initiated by the child by sensing change in pressure or change in flow in the circuit. Based on whether the trigger set if flow or pressure, the ventilator detects a reduction in flow or a drop in pressure in the circuit and initiates inspiration.[2]

Limit variable maintains inspiration and is not allowed to exceed a preset level. Pressure, volume or flow may be used as a limit variable.[2] Cycle variable determines the transition from inspiration to expiration. The commonly used cycle variable is time. But pressure, volume or flow can also be used as cycle variable. Using flow as a cycle variable facilitates synchronization of expiration.[2]

VENTILATION CONTROLLERS

In mechanical ventilation, inspiration is controlled but expiration is passive. The four variables which can be controlled during inspiration are pressure, volume, flow and time. The mode of ventilation is decided by the manner in which each of these is controlled. The ventilator terminology is described in **Table 2**.

Pressure Control Ventilation

In this mode, a constant pressure is maintained during inspiration which is irrespective of the compliance and

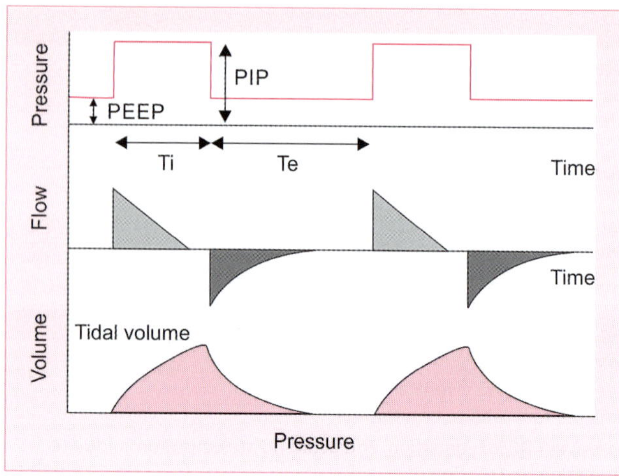

Fig. 2: Scalar waveforms for pressure-controlled ventilation

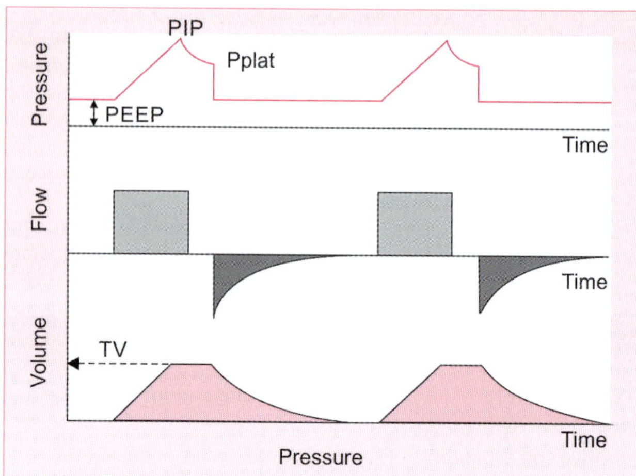

Fig. 3: Scalar waveforms for volume-controlled ventilation

resistance; volume and flow are dependent variables in this setting (**Fig. 2**). The tidal volume will therefore vary with changes in compliance and resistance. The flow utilized in pressure control ventilation has a decelerating pattern, i.e. high flow during the beginning of inspiration followed by gradual decline. Expiration ensues once inspiratory time is completed. In most of the current ventilators, expiration ensues once flow decreases to a certain predetermined fraction (usually 25%) of the initial flow (flow cycling).

This mode is preferred in children with an uncuffed tube with a leak around the tube. This mode is useful in neonates where flow sensor is at the ventilator end instead of endotracheal tube end, as measurement at the ventilator end may not be representative of patient's respiratory physiology due to the long ventilator circuit. Disadvantages include diseases with rapidly changing lung mechanics (e.g. neonate with respiratory distress syndrome after surfactant administration) leading to variable tidal volumes.

Volume Control Ventilation

In this mode, a preset volume is delivered with each breath using a constant flow pattern. This mode should be called flow control as ventilators measure flow and calculate volume from flow measurement. The flow and volume remain constant with variable pressure (**Fig. 3**). Though earlier avoided in neonates and infants, with accurate measurement of volumes at the patient end and accumulating evidence, this is now the preferred mode even in small babies. Disadvantages include tubal leaks leading to variable tidal volume delivery. A comparison of volume and pressure control is given in **Table 3**.

Type of Breaths

Breaths in a ventilated patient can be either mandatory, assisted or spontaneous. Mandatory breaths are initiated and terminated by the ventilator, i.e. inspiratory cycling is determined by the machine. Triggered or assisted breaths are initiated by the patient. In spontaneous breaths, both cycling (inspiratory and expiratory) and limit, are determined by the patient. In supported breaths, inspiratory and expiratory cycling is determined by the patient, but supported by the ventilator to a preset limit.

VENTILATOR MODES

Intermittent Mandatory Ventilation (IMV)

The IMV is a ventilation mode in which the machine delivers control (mandatory) breaths irrespective of patient efforts. As machine frequency is preset and independent of the patient's own efforts, breath stacking may occur leading to asynchrony. In this mode, patient often has to be put on sedation or neuromuscular blockade. The control could be either volume control or pressure control. IMV has now been replaced by more sophisticated modes which allow synchronization and other benefits.

Synchronized Intermittent Mechanical Ventilation (SIMV)

The SIMV is a ventilation mode, which gives either assisted breaths (patient-triggered) or time-triggered

Table 3: Comparison of volume control and pressure control ventilation

	Volume control	*Pressure control*
Tidal volume	Set	Variable
Airway pressure	Variable	Set
Inspiratory flow	Constant	Decelerating
Minute ventilation	Set	Variable
Advantages	Less risk of volutrauma Automatic weaning as compliance improves	Less risk of barotraumas Initial high flow (decelerating flow) better for stiff lungs
Disadvantages	Risk of barotrauma in stiff lungs with unmonitored peak pressures Flow starvation in air hungry patients due to constant flow	Variable tidal volume Volutrauma can result if peak inspiratory pressure not decreased with improvement in compliance

machine breaths. This mode allows both mandatory breaths and spontaneous breaths. The control could be either pressure or volume control. Just prior to time-triggered breath, there is a synchronization window, during which if the patient triggers a breath, it is assisted. If no effort is observed from the patient, the machine delivers the time-triggered breath (mandatory period). In between mandatory breaths (spontaneous period), patient is free to take spontaneous breaths which are limited by the patient. The spontaneous period begins after termination of mandatory period.[1]

Synchronization prevents breath stacking (i.e. mandatory breath over and above spontaneous breath). SIMV has the advantages of maintenance of spontaneous respiratory activity, lowering MAP, decreasing respiratory muscle atrophy and facilitating weaning. The patients need not be put on excessive sedation and neuromuscular blockade. Disadvantages include rapid weaning leading to muscle fatigue. However, this can be offset by adding pressure support to SIMV. SIMV is indicated in actively breathing patient to provide partial ventilatory support.

Assist Control Mechanical Ventilation (ACMV)

The ACMV is a ventilation mode in which patient determines the respiratory rate and minute ventilation. It is used in patients with a spontaneous and stable respiratory drive. The ventilator delivers a breath of a preset tidal volume in response to patient's trigger (assist. If the patient triggers less than the set frequency, the machine delivers time-triggered mandatory breaths (control). The patient is not allowed to breathe spontaneously.

Advantages include decreased work of breathing, and ability to control the minute ventilation by the patient. However, it can lead to respiratory alkalosis in an anxious child due to excessive triggering, as all breathing efforts detected will trigger the ventilator to deliver the breath.

Pressure Support Ventilation (PSV)

The PSV mode allows supporting of spontaneous breaths with pressure. The child triggers the breath and controls the cycling to expiration by change in flow. These breaths are supported to a preset pressure support level, and are terminated when the inspiratory flow demand falls below a certain threshold. Advantages of PCV include promotion of spontaneous breathing leading to reduction in work of breathing and better patient comfort. This mode is often used as an adjunct to SIMV. Gradual reduction in pressure support can be used as a weaning modality. For obvious reasons it can be used in a spontaneously breathing patient only.

Pressure-regulated Volume Control (PRVC)

The PRVC is a dual control or hybrid mode of mechanical ventilation.[3] A preset tidal volume is delivered at the lowest possible pressure by alterations in inspiratory flow rate and inspiratory time. This mode provides the best of pressure and volume control. In volume control, the flow being constant, so change in airway resistance leads to change in peak pressure to deliver the desired volume. However, in PRVC, with an increase in airway resistance, the inspiratory flow decreases to prevent peak pressure from rising, but the inspiratory time increases to deliver the set tidal volume. PRVC thus controls both volume as well as pressure in a way. The advantages of PRVC include delivering a constant TV while minimizing peak pressure. PRVC can be utilized in patients with fluctuating lung mechanics.

Airway Pressure Release Ventilation (APRV)

The APRV mode of ventilation provides continuous prolonged higher levels of positive airway pressure with intermittent releases in airway pressure. The prolonged "inspiratory time" leads to higher MAP and oxygenation, justifying its utility in ARDS. The intermittent release of pressure leads to volume delivery and removal of carbon dioxide. The use of prolonged high airway pressures helps in recruitment leading to ventilator cycle operating well above the lower inflection point. APRV mode allows spontaneous breathing throughout the cycle leading to decreased use of sedation and patient comfort. Spontaneous breathing adds to the minute ventilation and also leads to redistributing aeration of the dependent lung. The main indication of APRV is ARDS with poor compliance.[4]

High-Frequency Ventilation (HFV)

The HFV mode employs supraphysiologic frequencies along with small tidal volume even below the anatomical dead space. HFV utilizes open lung strategy with high MAP and low tidal volume, leading to lower peak pressure and avoidance of lung injury.[5] The most common mode of HFV used in neonates and in children is high frequency oscillatory ventilation (HFOV). HFOV employs an oscillatory diaphragm which generates an oscillatory waveform or a rapidly altering gas flow which provides active inspiration and expiration. With the back and forth motion of the diaphragm, air is pushed into the lungs and actively withdrawn. This waveform can be produced by a variety of methods in various machines including piston pump oscillator, electromagnetic flow generator and linear motor generators.

The mechanism for gas exchange in HFV is complex and quite different from conventional ventilation. As the tidal volume utilized in HFOV is even smaller than anatomical dead space, the mechanism for gas exchange is not alveolar filling and emptying as seen in conventional ventilation.

Evidence is accumulating on successful use of HFOV predominantly in neonates but also in children.[5] Neonatal data suggests improvement in oxygenation and long term outcomes. As of now, HFOV is used as a rescue mode in patients who fail conventional lung protective ventilation primarily due to poor oxygenation. HFOV has been used with success in acute lung injury and persistent pulmonary hypertension of the newborn. Use in obstructive airway diseases should be cautious as HFOV may lead to intrinsic PEEP and air-trapping, and even active expiration of this modality may not be very effective in these conditions. Other disadvantages include increased need of sedation and neuromuscular blockade to improve patient comfort and avoid spontaneous breathing. Never modes of ventilator include neutrally adjusted ventilatory assist.[6]

VENTILATOR SETTINGS

The goal of mechanical ventilation is to provide adequate gas exchange with minimal lung injury. The ventilator setting should be optimized to achieve this goal. Definition of acceptable gas exchange is not same for every situation. For example, in a setting of acute lung injury with poor compliance, slightly lower oxygenation and higher PCO_2 (permissive hypercapnia) may be accepted to avoid lung injury. In some conditions, permissive hypercapnia may be deleterious (intracranial hypertension, for example). The settings of mechanical ventilation should, therefore, be tailored to each clinical scenario in terms of target oxygenation and PCO_2, based on the pathophysiology of the underlying disease. Initial settings for pressure and volume controlled mode are given in **Table 4**.

Table 4: Initial settings for pressure and volume control mode

Settings	*Pressure-controlled mode*	*Volume-controlled mode*
Rate	Age-related	Age-related
PEEP	3–5 cm H_2O (lower for obstructive diseases)	3–5 cm H_2O (lower for obstructive diseases)
Volume	—	6–10 mL/kg
PIP	Titrate to chest rise	—
Ti	Usually I:E ratio 1:2; can increase Te in case of obstructive diseases	Usually I:E ratio 1:2; can increase Te in case of obstructive diseases
FiO_2	Target adequate oxygenation	Target adequate oxygenation

(FiO_2: fraction of inspired oxygen; PEEP: positive end-expiratory pressure; PIP: peak inspiratory pressure; Ti: inspiratory time; Te: expiratory time)

Healthy Lungs

Ventilation of children with healthy lungs is usually not difficult but may lead to ventilator associated complications. For healthy lungs, no specific mode is recommended. The ventilation settings are essentially physiological. A PCO_2 tidal volume of 6–8 mL/kg is appropriate. If PCV is chosen, a pressure level can be guided by adequate chest rise and optimal saturation is acceptable; pressures usually 8–10 cm H_2O above PEEP. A physiological PEEP of 3–4 cm H_2O is appropriate. Inspiratory time is 0.4 sec for newborns and infancy, 0.6 sec for toddlers and preschool children, and 0.8–1 sec for older children and adolescents.

Severe Asthma

Asthma is an obstructive airway disease which is characterized by increased airway resistance due to bronchospasm, mucosal edema and airway secretions. Mechanical ventilation of a child with severe asthma is difficult as the obstruction to airflow is predominantly during expiration, and expiration is passive in mechanical ventilation. This leads to increased risk of airtrapping and air leaks complicating ventilation. Therefore, non invasive ventilation should be given a try and invasive mechanical ventilation be avoided as much as possible.

There is some evidence that volume controlled ventilation is better tolerated than PCV, as tidal volume may vary with fluctuating airway resistance and bronchospasm the latter. PRVC appears an attractive mode in this scenario where tidal volume can be delivered with minimum pressures. Plateau pressures need to be carefully monitored in VCV, and limited to less than 30 cm H_2O. The ventilation strategy is low rates, low or zero PEEP with prolonged expiratory time.[7] The targets of oxygenation and carbon dioxide elimination need to be considered carefully to prevent ventilator induced damage and maintaining just appropriate gas exchange. Permissive hypercapnia is encouraged while accepting pH as low as 7.2. Sedation and neuromuscular blockade need to be used to minimize air leaks. Dynamic hyperinflation (or auto PEEP) should be closely monitored by real time flow time curves and total PEEP H_2O measured by the ventilator. If total PEEP is above set PEEP, auto PEEP is said to be present.

Ketamine and fentanyl are the preferred drugs for sedation and morphine is contraindicated. One should be wary of expected complications including pneumothorax and pneumomediastinum during ventilation by way of careful monitoring. In a patient with deteriorating cardiopulmonary function because of air trapping, disconnecting the patient from the ventilator for a brief while may lead to dissipation of air trapping.

Acute Lung Injury (ALI)/Acute Respiratory Distress Syndrome (ARDS)

The ALI/ARDS is characterized with decreased lung compliance leading to respiratory failure. Although diffuse infiltrates (whiteout in some cases) are evident on chest radiographs, the pattern of involvement is heterogeneous with predominant involvement of dependent regions and sparing of nondependent regions. As there are areas of atelectasis and consolidation interspersed with normal lung parenchyma, the ventilation is difficult and prone to ventilator-induced lung injury (VILI). Alveoli in the dependent areas or consolidated part of lung have a closing volume near end-expiration leading to alveolar collapse. These alveoli need to be reopened during inspiration. The repeated opening and closing lead to alveolar damage (atelectrauma). The strategy in ALI is to recruit lungs, keeping the alveoli patent and avoiding overdistension of healthy areas of the lung at the same time. This can be done using optimal PEEP which is needed to keep lung open and preventing atelectrauma.[8,9]

As a general principle, one should use the lowest possible tidal volume with appropriate PEEP to avoid atelectasis and maintain adequate gas exchange. Start with a PEEP of 6–8 cm H_2O and increase in increments of 1–2 cm H_2O till adequate oxygenation (saturation of 90–92%) is attained along with improvement in lung mechanics. The fraction of inspired O_2 (FiO_2) is kept at 60% or below to prevent oxygen toxicity. If FiO_2 above 60% is needed, despite high PEEP, other measure including prone positioning need to be utilized. Low tidal volume (4–6 mL/kg) with low Pplat (<28–30 cm H_2O) are used to prevent volutrauma and barotraumas. These lung protective strategies can cause hypercapnia which is acceptable provided the pH is above 7.2 (permissive hypercapnia).

The recent Pediatric Acute Lung Injury Consensus Conference described the recommendations for mechanical ventilation management of pediatric patients with ARDS. There was strong consensus that severe ARDS may need PEEP greater than 15 cm H_2O, but it should be carefully monitored with markers of oxygen delivery, respiratory compliance and hemodynamics. Hemodynamics should be optimized by adequate intravascular volume and vasopressor support.

Air Leak

While ventilating a child with air leak, the aim should be to reduce MAP as much as possible. FiO_2 can be increased to attain optimum oxygenation. Higher rates may be tried as alveoli have much shorter time constant than the interstitial air. If reduction in MAP is not tolerated, high frequency oscillatory ventilation (HFOV) may be attempted.

Weaning and Extubation

Weaning is the transition of assisted breathing to spontaneous breathing. The process includes reduction of ventilatory support while evaluating spontaneous breathing. At the end of weaning, patient should be able to breathe spontaneously to maintain adequate gas exchange, following which the patient can be extubated.[2]

While prolonged mechanical ventilation is definitely harmful, premature extubation has risks of reintubation and other complications. A careful assessment needs to be done while taking a decision for extubation (**Table 5**). ALI/ARDS may have to be weaned slowly once the stormy phase is over. Critically ill children with fluid overload often have decreased lung compliance affecting oxygenation and may prolong/delay weaning. Risk factors for extubation failure in children include young age, severity of lung disease, duration of mechanical ventilation, high oxygenation index (above 5) and intravenous sedation.

Various weaning techniques have been described in literature.[2] Gradual reduction of ventilatory support (SIMV) is the commonly used technique of weaning as SIMV permits spontaneous breaths between machine breaths. The ventilator rate, PEEP and/or the level of pressure or volume support is reduced gradually while monitoring the oxygen saturation and blood gases. The rapidity with which the rates can be lowered depends on the cardiopulmonary function of the patient.

Spontaneous breathing trials (SBT) have also been used to facilitate weaning. They are usually tried either alone or with low levels of pressure support (5–7 cm H_2O) or with CPAP for around half-an-hour. Most patients who fail an SBT usually do so within 20–30 minutes. Pressure support ventilation either alone or in combination with SIMV is sometimes used to facilitate weaning. PSV is started at around 5–10 cm H_2O and titrated upward to achieve a desired spontaneous tidal volume (10–15 mL/kg) and desired frequency of 25/min or less. If patient tolerates this well, then pressure support can be gradually reduced. Automatic tube compensation available in some ventilators can also be used to facilitate weaning.

Weaning failure should be distinguished from extubation failure. Weaning failure refers to inability to maintain adequate gas exchange while settings are being reduced. Whereas, extubation failure refers to the need for reintubation after successful extubation. However, successful weaning does not necessarily guarantee successful extubation.

Table 5: Prerequisites for weaning

- Cause of respiratory failure is passive or has improved substantially
- Absence of acidosis
- Adequate oxygenation: maintains arterial oxygen saturation and partial pressure of arterial oxygen above 90% and 60 mm Hg, respectively on fraction of inspired $O_2 < 0.4$
- Hemodynamic stability
- Absence of anemia
- Adequate mental status (presence of good respiratory drive and protective reflexes)

COMPLICATIONS OF MECHANICAL VENTILATION

Mechanical ventilation is life saving but it is associated with numerous deleterious effects,[10] as shown on **Table 6**.

Ventilator-induced Lung Injury (VILI)

Lung damage caused or exacerbated by positive pressure ventilation is designated as VILI. The pathophysiologic mechanisms of VILI are complex including biophysical disruption of cellular membranes and alveolar spaces due to mechanical forces (alveolar overdistension) and aberrant cellular response leading to inflammation. Degree of lung inflation (volutrauma and overdistension) is a key determinant of lung injury. Repeated opening and causing (recruitment-derecruitment) of alveoli also leads to VILI (atelectrauma), when ventilating at lower lung volumes. High inspired oxygen (FiO_2 above 0.6) also contributes to lung injury due to oxidant stress. The key strategies to reduce VILI include: Judicious use of oxygen, optimal PEEP, limiting Pplat to less than 30 cm H_2O), and avoidance of overdistension.

Table 6: Complications and adverse physiological effects of mechanical ventilation

Respiratory effects	• Upper airway injury – secondary to traumatic intubation • Laryngeal edema and ulceration • Subglottic stenosis • Nasal/perioral tissue damage • Air leaks – pulmonary interstitial emphysema, pneumomediastinum, pneumothorax, pneumopericardium, subcutaneous emphysema • Ventilator associated pneumonia • Atelectasis • Disuse atrophy of diaphragm • Pulmonary arterial hypertension
Central nervous system effects	PEEP may increase intracranial pressure and decrease cerebral perfusion pressure
Cardiovascular effects	• Reduced venous return, stroke volume and cardiac output • Hypotension • Pulmonary vasoconstriction
Renal effects	Reduction in renal water and sodium excretion; oliguria
Hepatic effects	Reduced portal venous flow; hepatic dysfunction
Miscellaneous	Oxygen toxicity

Ventilator-associated Pneumonia (VAP)

Pneumonia diagnosed in patients ventilated for 48 hours or more with signs of a new lower respiratory infection is known as VAP. VAP occurs in 3–20% of all mechanically ventilated children, and risk of VAP increases at around 1% per day of ongoing ventilation. VAP pathophysiology includes colonization of upper respiratory tract, microaspiration of oropharyngeal secretions and contaminated equipment or aerosolized medications. Prolonged duration of ventilation, use of neuromuscular blockade, severe underlying disease and supine positioning also increase the risk of VAP. Preventive strategies include head end elevation by 30°, avoidance of gastric distension by nasogastric tubes, frequent oropharyngeal suctioning, oral hygiene with antiseptics, in-line suctioning, and changing ventilator circuits only when visibly soiled or malfunctioning.[2]

Air Leaks

Excessive transpulmonary pressure and overdistension may cause the respiratory epithelium to rupture during positive pressure ventilation leading to air entering the lung parenchyma or the pleural space. Air tracking proximally along the bronchovascular bundle leads to pulmonary interstitial emphysema (PIE), and followed by pneumomediastinum and pneumopericardium. Pneumothorax may occur if air reaches the pleural cavity. Tension pneumothorax must be kept in mind when a child on mechanical ventilation deteriorates suddenly. If pneumothorax is suspected in a child with cardiorespiratory compromise, immediate needle decompression must be attempted, followed by a chest drain insertion. If even after 48 hours of putting the chest drain the lung does not reexpand or air continues to bubble through the drain, a bronchopleural fistula is the likely possibility. Lung protective strategies limiting plateau pressure and TV reduce the chances of air leak.

Auto-PEEP

Auto-PEEP (also called occult PEEP, intrinsic PEEP, or inadvertent PEEP dynamic hyperinflation) is caused by incomplete exhalation leading to air-trapping or hyperinflation. The most frequent underlying cause is severe airflow limitation due to obstructive diseases (e.g. asthma). However, many other scenarios lead to auto-PEEP without airflow limitation, including inverse ratio ventilation (too short inspiratory time), blocked endotracheal tube and high tidal volume. Auto PEEP can be measured by applying end-expiratory pause for 0.5–1.5 seconds, while the patient is not exerting significant respiratory effort. Careful observation of the ventilator graphics can help identifying the presence of auto PEEP. The persistence of expiratory flow even at the end of expiration indicates presence of auto PEEP.

Auto-PEEP leads to increased work of breathing, worsening gas exchange, deterioration in hemodynamic status (reduction in venous return and cardiac output) and barotrauma.

KEY MESSAGES

- Respiratory failure is a common cause of emergency consultations in the pediatric age group.
- Absence of collateral ventilation makes children at increased risk of atelectasis.
- Phase variables are parameters which control the various phases of the respiratory cycle, including triggering which controls the initiation of inspiration, limit variable maintains inspiration, and cycle variable switches from inspiration to expiration.
- With accurate measurement of volumes at the patient end and accumulating evidence, volume controlled mode is now the preferred mode even in small babies.
- Apart from conventional SIMV mode, increasing evidence is accumulating on newer modes including PRVC, APRV, NAVA and other volume targeted modes.
- APRV mode of ventilation provides continuous prolonged higher levels of positive airway pressure with intermittent releases in airway pressure and allows spontaneous breathing.
- HFOV is increasingly being used as a recue mode in neonates and children with hypoxemia and poor compliance.
- Mechanical ventilation of a child with acute severe asthma is challenging and volume control mode with low rates, low PEEP and prolonged expiratory time is preferred.
- The strategy of mechanical ventilation in ALI/ARDS is to recruit lungs, keeping the alveoli patent and avoiding overdistension of healthy areas of the lung at the same time using optimal PEEP.
- Mechanical ventilation, though life-saving, is associated with lots of complications, which need to be considered and managed appropriately.

REFERENCES

1. Kornecki A, Kavanagh BP. Mechanical ventilation. In: Wheeler DS, Wong HR, Shanley TP, editors. The Respiratory Tract in Pediatric Critical Illness and Injury. London: Springer; 2009. p. 67-80.
2. Raj D, Lodha R. Mechanical ventilation. In: Gupta P, Menon PSN, Ramji S, Lodha R, editors. PG Textbook of Pediatrics, 2nd edition. New Delhi: Jaypee Brothers Medical Publishers; 2018. p. 317-26.
3. The ABCs of ventilator modes. Available from: *https://getinge.training/DesktopModules/Documents/ViewDocument.aspx?AddToLog=1&DocumentID=1903*. Accessed August 27, 2019.
4. Lalgudi Ganesan S. Airway pressure release ventilation in children. Curr Opin Crit Care. 2019;25:63-70.
5. Hupp SR, Turner DA, Rehder KJ. Is there still a role for high-frequency oscillatory ventilation in neonates, children and adults? Expert Rev Respir Med. 2015;9:603-18.
6. Beck J, Emeriaud G, Liu Y, *et al.* Neurally-adjusted ventilatory assist (NAVA) in children: a systematic review. Minerva Anestesiol. 2016;82:874-83.
7. Pardue Jones B, Fleming GM, Otillio JK, *et al.* Pediatric acute asthma exacerbations: Evaluation and management from emergency department to intensive care unit. J Asthma. 2016; 53:607-17.
8. Kneyber MCJ, de Luca D, Calderini E, *et al.* section Respiratory Failure of the European Society for Paediatric and Neonatal Intensive Care. Recommendations for mechanical ventilation of critically ill children from the Pediatric Mechanical Ventilation Consensus Conference (PEMVECC). Intensive Care Med. 2017;43:1764-80.
9. Pediatric Acute Lung Injury Consensus Conference Group. Pediatric acute respiratory distress syndrome: consensus recommendations from the Pediatric Acute Lung Injury Consensus Conference. Pediatr Crit Care Med. 2015;16:428-39.
10. Principi T, Fraser DD, Morrison GC, *et al.* Complications of mechanical ventilation in the pediatric population. Pediatr Pulmonol. 2011;46:452-7.

CHAPTER

12

Anaphylaxis

Sandeep Kumar Kanwal

INTRODUCTION

An international multidisciplinary symposium defines anaphylaxis as "a serious, generalized or systemic, allergic or hypersensitivity reaction that can be life-threatening or fatal.[1] Clinical diagnostic criteria (**Table 1**) and management guidelines have also been defined.[2]

EPIDEMIOLOGY AND ETIOLOGY

The incidence of anaphylaxis is reported to be 1.5–7.9/1,00,000 person years in Europe[3]; whereas in North America, patients with anaphylaxis comprise approximately 0.1% to 0.4% of total emergency visits at all age groups.[4] The frequency of hospital admissions for anaphylaxis in children less than 18 years has more than doubled from the year 2000 to 2009.[5] The triggering cause for an anaphylactic reaction is identified in less than one-third children. Food is the most commonly associated trigger, followed by *Hymenoptera* (bee/wasp) stings, preservatives in food and drugs and medications.[6] Foods such as peanuts, tree nuts, fish, milk, eggs, soya and shellfish (e.g. shrimp, lobster, crab, scallops and oysters) are implicated as trigger in 35–50% of anaphylaxis in children.[7] Environmental allergens such as pollens, molds, and dust mites are an infrequent cause. Other triggers include infection, opiates, radiocontrast dye and exercise, which mediate anaphylaxis via a different pathway.

PATHOPHYSIOLOGY

Only limited data are available on immunologic mechanisms of anaphylaxis from human subjects because of

Table 1: Clinical criteria for diagnosing anaphylaxis

Anaphylaxis is highly likely when any one of the following three criteria are fulfilled:
1. Acute onset of an illness (minutes to several hours) with *involvement of the skin*, mucosal tissue or both (e.g. generalized hives, pruritus or flushing, or swollen lips-tongue-uvula) and *at least one* of the following: a. Respiratory compromise (e.g. dyspnea, wheeze-bronchospasm, stridor, reduced PEF or hypoxemia) b. Reduced BP or associated symptoms of end-organ dysfunction (e.g. hypotonia collapse, syncope or incontinence)
2. *Two or more of the following* that occur rapidly after exposure to a likely allergen for that patient (minutes to several hours): a. Involvement of the skin-mucosal tissue (e.g. generalized hives, itch-flush or swollen lips tongue-uvula) b. Respiratory compromise (e.g. dyspnea, wheeze-bronchospasm, stridor, reduced PEF or hypoxemia) c. Reduced BP or associated symptoms of end-organ dysfunction (e.g. hypotonia, syncope or incontinence) d. Persistent gastrointestinal symptoms (e.g. crampy abdominal pain or vomiting)
3. Reduced BP after exposure to a known allergen for that patient (minutes to hours) a. Infants and children: low systolic BP (age specific)* or greater than 30% decrease in systolic BP from normal.
* Low systolic blood pressure for children is defined for 1 month–1 year: < 70 mm Hg; for 1 to 10 years less than (70 mm Hg + [2 × age]); for 11 to 17 years: < 90 mm Hg

ethical concerns due to life-threatening nature of anaphylaxis. The term **anaphylaxis** generally refers to IgE-mediated reactions, whereas **anaphylactoid reaction** generally refers to non-immune mediated reactions that can occur even without previous exposure to a triggering agent. Both conditions are clinically indistinguishable. The pathophysiologic model of anaphylaxis may be both active systemic anaphylaxis which is the induction of antibodies involved in anaphylaxis through antigen sensitization of naive hosts or passive anaphylaxis, which is an adoptive transfer of IgE or IgG antibodies that leads to anaphylaxis on subsequent challenge with antigens recognized by such antibodies.

IgE-dependent Anaphylaxis

IgE antibodies have been regarded as a key risk factor for the development of allergy, anaphylaxis or both. Normally in healthy humans, concentration of IgE antibody is the lowest in circulation (50–200 ng/mL, compared to IgG ~10 mg/mL). But they are at much higher levels in patients with allergic diseases. It is proposed that on initial exposure to antigen, the B cells in the peripheral lymphoid tissues differentiate into IgE-producing cells via the activity of CD4- helper T cells (Th2 cells). IgE then binds to the high-affinity epsilon receptor I (FcεRI) on the surfaces of tissue-resident mast cells and basophils, and to lesser extent on neutrophils, eosinophils, monocytes, dendritic cells and platelets.[8] On re-exposure to a bivalent or multivalent allergen, cross-linking of FcεRI-bound IgE leads to the activation of mast cells and basophils and immediate release of preformed mediators, such as histamine and various proteases, as well as *de novo* synthesis of many inflammatory mediators, such as leukotrienes (LT), prostaglandins, and cytokines (**Table 2**).

Histamine

Histamine is an important mediator of anaphylaxis, although its effect is less potent than the LT.[9] Intravenous administration of histamine in volunteers can reproduce many of the signs and symptoms including cutaneous flushing, headache, airway obstruction, and transient hemodynamic changes like hypotension, tachycardia, and increased left ventricular output. Some systemic effects of histamine (airway obstruction, tachycardia) are mediated by H1 receptor, while others (cutaneous flushing, headaches) are mediated by both H1 and H2 receptors. H1 antihistamines are commonly used as adjunctive treatment for acute anaphylaxis and anaphylactoid reactions.

Platelet activation factor

Platelet activation factor is a potent phospholipid-derived mediator implicated in platelet aggregation with an

Table 2: Mediators of anaphylaxis

	System involved	*Clinical features*	*Primary mediator*	*Other mediators*
1.	Upper respiratory system	Rhinorrhea Sneezing Angioedema Stridor	Histamine	
2.	Lower respiratory system	Cough Wheeze Dyspnea	Histamine	Cys LT
3.	Cardiovascular system	Tachycardia Syncope Vasodilatation Capillary leak Hypotension Cardiac arrest	Histamine	PAF Cys LT
4.	Skin	Flushing Urticaria Angioedema Hives	Histamine	Anaphylatoxins PAF Cys LT
5.	Gastrointestinal system	Nausea Vomiting Diarrhea Abdominal pain	Histamine	

(PAF: platelet factor; CysLT: cytokines leukotrienes activation)

important role in a variety of immune and inflammatory responses.[10] The factor can be released by a variety of human cells, including purified lung mast cells and blood basophils after *ex vivo* stimulation with anti-IgE antibodies. Circulating factor levels increase and acetyl hydrolase activity decreases in proportion to the severity of anaphylaxis.

Cytokines leukotriene (CysLT)

A third class of potential mediators of anaphylaxis was originally termed slow-reacting substance of anaphylaxis and consists of 3 bioactive cytokines leukotriene (cysLT): LTB4, LTC4 and LTD4. CysLT are synthesized from arachidonic acid by a variety of cells, including mast cells, basophils and macrophages. Intradermal injection of LTB4, LTC4 and LTD4 induces a wheal-and-flare reaction and aerosol administration of LTC4 and LTD4 in healthy subjects induces bronchoconstriction.[9]

Following triggering agents are usually associated with IgE-mediated anaphylaxis:

- Foods and additives like walnuts, peanuts, shellfish, fish, milk, egg, spices
- Insect stings and bites (Hymenoptera venom, horse flies, ants)
- Medications (e.g. beta-lactam antibiotics, NSAIDs)
- Anesthetic drugs (e.g. suxamethonium, atracurium, rocuronium, sugammadex)
- Contrast media (iodinated, technetium, fluorescein)
- Occupational allergens (natural rubber latex, hair dye).

IgE-independent and Non-immune Mediated Anaphylaxis

Role of IgG and FcgRs

The role of IgG-mediated anaphylaxis is unclear in humans.[11] However, human IgG receptors (FcgRs) are capable of activating macrophages and neutrophils to secrete platelet-activating factor, which activates mast cells causing immune complex mediated anaphylaxis. This mechanism has been implicated in reactions to protamine, dextran and infliximab.

Role of complement

Activation of the complement cascade occurs in response to many stimuli and leads to generation of the small polypeptides C3a, C4a, and C5a, also named anaphylatoxins, which are potent inflammatory mediators, and might be involved in anaphylaxis.[12]

Direct activation of mast cells

Opioids, alcohol and physical factors (e.g. cold, heat, exercise, sunlight) are believed to induce anaphylaxis via direct activation of mast cells by unknown mechanism.

Other mechanisms

Medications like NSAIDS and, over-sulfated chondroitin sulfate can cause rare anaphylactic reactions or isolated angioedema due to the excessive production and/or accumulation of bradykinin.

CLINICAL FEATURES

Anaphylaxis may present with mild symptoms that resolve spontaneously due to the endogenous production of compensatory mediators (e.g. adrenaline, angiotensin II) or it may be severe and may progress within minutes to respiratory or cardiovascular compromise and death. Mild to moderate reactions present as swelling of lips, face, eyes, urticarial rash, tingling in mouth, abdominal pain and vomiting. Cutaneous manifestations are common occurring in 90% of individuals but absence of skin manifestations does not exclude the diagnosis. Severe signs and symptoms are difficult or noisy breathing, progressive swelling of tongue and tightness in throat, difficulty in talking and/or hoarse voice, wheeze or persistent cough, dizziness, vomiting and/or abdominal pain. Tachycardia, hypotension to severe cardiovascular collapse is noted in rapid and up to 45% cases. Severe cardiovascular symptoms sometimes develops without skin or respiratory symptoms.[13]

Anaphylaxis can be further classified on the basis of progression as follows:

Uniphasic anaphylaxis: It is the most common type accounting for 80–90% of all episodes. The uniphasic response peaks within 30 to 60 minutes after exposure to allergens and resolves either spontaneously or with treatment in 30–60 minutes.

Biphasic anaphylaxis: This has an estimated incidence of 20–25% of all anaphylactic reactions. These reactions are characterized by an initial response, followed by an asymptomatic period of 1-hr or more and subsequent recurrence of symptoms without re-exposure to the antigen. These reactions can happen in all age groups.

Protracted anaphylaxis: These anaphylactic reactions last hours, days or even weeks without resolving completely.

Fatal or near fatal anaphylactic reactions: There are many anaphylaxis deaths reported each year although this may be an underestimation. According to a case series, fatal food anaphylactic reactions caused collapse and respiratory arrest typically within 30–35 minutes, insect stings after 10–15 minutes and intravenous medication within 5 minutes. Death generally is not reported more than 6 hours after contact with a trigger.[14] Patients at risk of severe and fatal anaphylaxis include adolescents, those with peanut and tree nut allergy, pre-existing respiratory or cardiovascular disease, asthma, delayed administration of epinephrine, history of previous biphasic anaphylactic reactions and mast cell disease.[7]

APPROACH TO DIAGNOSIS

Use of Clinical Diagnostic Criteria

Signs and symptoms of anaphylaxis are usually rapid in onset and can progress in severity over minutes to hours. The diagnosis of anaphylaxis is clinical and is based on the history and physical examination. Typically, at least two organ systems get involved, although only one organ system might be initially involved. Due to the broad spectrum of clinical features, the National Institutes of Allergy and Infectious Disease, Food Allergy and Anaphylaxis Network (NIAID/FAAN) USA has provided diagnostic criteria (**Table 1**), which were adopted in 2005.[2] These criteria have 97% sensitivity, 82% specificity, 98% negative predictive value and 69% positive predictive value for diagnosis of anathylasis.[15] These criteria are useful but do not substitute for clinical findings. It is important for physicians to recognize the variable clinical presentation and progression of anaphylaxis. Recognition of milder anaphylaxis is critical not only to prevent progression to a more serious outcome but in preventing recurrent episodes in future.

Serum Tryptase Level

Tryptase is the most abundant serine protease of mast cells with both mature and immature forms; basophils have lower levels of tryptase.[10] The immature form is released constitutively by unstimulated mast cells, whereas the mature form is released on mast cell activation, such as in anaphylaxis. Serum tryptase determination seems to hold promise in the diagnosis or monitoring of mast cell disorders, including anaphylaxis, mastocytosis, myeloproliferative conditions and in prediction of severity risk in some allergic conditions.[16] Elevated levels can be detected 3–6 hours after the anaphylaxis reaction and normalize in 12–14 hours.[17] An elevated acute serum tryptase level (% change >141% above base level, or absolute tryptase level of >15.7 µg/L) has been reported to be highly predictive of IgE-mediated anaphylaxis.[5]

At present serum tryptase levels are neither easily nor rapidly available. These levels are not elevated in most patients with food induced anaphylaxis. However, if diagnosis of anaphylaxis is uncertain, a high serum tryptase level aids the clinical diagnosis. Serial monitoring of tryptase levels at the time of presentation, 1–2 hr later and following resolution of symptoms may improve its sensitivity.[18]

Differential Diagnosis

There are some medical conditions that imitate anaphylaxis closely:

Acute disorders: Acute asthma, acute generalized urticaria, acute angioedema, cardiovascular events (myocardial infarction, pulmonary edema).

Flush syndromes: Carcinoid syndrome, hyperthyroidism, red man syndrome (vancomycin), pheochromocytoma.

Excess histamine production: Mastocytosis, basophilic leukemia.

Shock: Hypovolemic, cardiogenic, septic, distributive (e.g. spinal cord injury).

MANAGEMENT

Symptoms of anaphylaxis have the potential to progress rapidly and become life threatening so, immediate triage of patients is required with thorough assessment of airway, breathing and circulation. The management of a patient who presents with symptoms of anaphylaxis within few minutes after exposure to a suspected trigger might be different from one exposed few hours previously. Sometimes anaphylaxis can be self-limited and patient presents when symptoms have nearly resolved and may no longer require epinephrine for acute management. At a same time, a patient who presents with acute symptoms of anaphylaxis should immediately receive epinephrine even if the initial symptoms are not life threatening, because anaphylaxis can progress rapidly from mild symptoms to severe life-threatening symptoms.

During the triage of anaphylaxis, patient should be placed in a supine position to counteract any circulatory collapse. However, patients in respiratory distress alone can be placed in a more upright position while they are monitored carefully for any circulatory collapse. Oxygen should be administered to patients exhibiting respiratory or cardiovascular symptoms or with decreased oxygen saturation.

The first line of treatment in anaphylaxis is epinephrine. Its physiologic effects include vasoconstriction, cardiac chronotropic and inotropic effects, bronchodilatation. Epinephrine suppresses the release of histamine and other mediators from mast cells and basophils, leading to increased cardiac output, increased peripheral vascular tone, decreased mucosal edema and airway resistance. The recommended dose of epinephrine is 0.01 mg/kg (maximum dose, 0.5 mg) of 1:1000 concentration administered intramuscularly (IM) every 5 to 15 minutes as necessary to control symptoms. **Table 3** lists the age, weight and the approximate dosage in ready to use charts for the emergency room. Auto-injector syringes are also available for use in settings outside the hospital, in a vulnerable child particularly at home or school use.

The 5-minute interval between two doses of epinephrine injections can be reduced, as determined by the clinical state. Pharmacokinetic studies in children and adult reported that epinephrine administered IM into the anterolateral thigh resulted in a higher and rapid peak plasma concentration as compared to subcutaneous or IM administration in the arm.[19,20] In the setting of anaphylaxis, there is no absolute contraindication for administration of epinephrine. Nevertheless, a significant proportion of patients do not receive epinephrine for this indication, adversely affecting severe outcomes.[21]

Patient with hypotensive require rapid infusion of normal saline 20 mL/kg IV by a wide bore IV access. Further fluid resuscitation may be required to manage distributive shock, counteract significant plasma leak and complement parenteral epinephrine therapy. Fluid therapy should be adjusted to achieve goals of shock therapy and to prevent volume overload. In hypotensive patient or patient requiring multiple IM doses of epinephrine, the use of epinephrine infusion at 0.1 µg/kg/minute may be considered.[22] If IV access is not readily available, epinephrine may be given by intraosseous route. Bolus administration of IV epinephrine is associated with an increased risk of cardiac arrhythmias, and should therefore be avoided.

Norepinephrine, vasopressin, and other pressors have been used with success in patients in anaphylaxis with refractory hypotension.[23]

Monitoring, preferably continuous hemodynamic, is essential for patients of anaphylaxis and patient should be managed in PICU. This should include pulse oximetry, blood pressure, continuous pulse rate and electrocardiographic monitoring. They should be used to monitor response to therapy and direct subsequent intervention. Airway management, including intubation is required if there is any suggestion of severe airway edema (e.g. hoarseness or stridor) or associated respiratory or cardiopulmonary compromise. Once the patient is intubated, post-intubation management should continue with ventilator management.

Many clinical manifestations of anaphylaxis, including vasodilatation, vascular permeability, bronchospasm, and increased airway secretions are mediated by histamine. While therapy with antihistamines in anaphylaxis is believed to be justified based on efficacy in other allergic diseases (allergic rhinitis and allergic conjunctivitis), there is no direct evidence of effectiveness of these medications in anaphylaxis.[24] The use of antihistaminic drugs and steroids are second-line adjunct treatment and should never be considered as an alternative to epinephrine.[25]

Bronchospasm is a part of symptomatology of anaphylaxis and can persist despite initial treatment with epinephrine. Inhaled β-agonist should be administered

Table 3: Epinephrine dosage chart in emergency department

Age (years)	*Weight (kg)*	*Volume 1:1000 adrenaline*	*Auto-injector**
<1 yr 1–2 yr 2–3 yr	5–10 10 10–15	0.05–0.1 mL 0.1 mL 0.15 mL	
4–6 yr 7–10 yr	20 30	0.2 mL 0.3 mL	>15–30 kg 0.15 mg device
10–12 yr >12 yr and adults*	40 >50	0.4 mL 0.5 mL	≥30 kg 0.3 mg device

*In settings other than hospital or clinical establishment, auto-injector devices (EAI) may be used depending upon availability.

if bronchospasm has not responded to epinephrine, and there is no reason to believe that the treatment of bronchospasm during anaphylaxis is different than treatment of bronchospasm in patients who are not in anaphylaxis.

Various case reports have reported favorable results following treatment with glucagon infusion, when standard therapy has failed treatment of refractory anaphylaxis in patients on β-blockers.[26] The recommended dose of glucagon in children is 20–30 μg/kg (maximum 1 mg) administered intravenously over 5 minutes and followed by an infusion of 5–15 μg/min titrated to clinical response. Airway protection is important because emesis and possible aspiration is a possible side effect of glucagon. Use of methylene blue in refractory anaphylaxis with hypotension has been advocated in some case reports. Methylene blue, a selective nitric oxide cyclic GMP inhibitor, prevents nitric oxide induced vasodilation and reverse the course of anaphylaxis refractory to epinephrine, oxygen, and IV fluid resuscitation.[5,27]

A patient is admitted to the hospital based on severity of symptoms, response to initial treatment, past history of allergies or anaphylactic reaction, coexistent medical conditions, patient education status and access to medical care. If the patient is not admitted, observation for 4–8 hours should be strongly considered in all patients diagnosed with mild anaphylaxis. Biphasic reactions occur in patients who develop anaphylaxis and involve organ systems not affected in the initial reaction due to waning serum epinephrine levels. Corticosteroids have not shown to prevent biphasic reactions. The time of observation should be individualized based on the same criteria used to determine the need for admission.[28]

Flowchart 1 represents the diagrammatic view of the emergency management of patient with anaphylaxis. A written protocol for detection and management of anaphylaxis is highly recommended.[29]

OUTCOME

Anaphylaxis is one of the most urgent medical emergencies in which rapid diagnosis and prompt and appropriate treatment can mean the difference between life and death. The overall prognosis of anaphylaxis is good if managed appropriately during acute phase, and patients receive an epinephrine injection before arrival in the emergency. Failure to recognize the severity of anaphylaxis and delayed injection of epinephrine, defined as that given following 1-hr of management, is associated with poor outcome.

PREVENTION

Resolution of an acute episode of anaphylaxis does not mean end of the management. A child who is either at risk of anaphylaxis or had an episode of anaphylaxis previously requires prevention and management of recurrences. Patients leaving healthcare facility post discharge are prescribed to carry at least two *epinephrine autoinjectors (EAI)* or epinephrine ampoules or epinephrine prefilled syringes (EPFS) to manage such episodes in community. The EAIs are preferred and available in two strengths. Children weighing 15–30 kg receive a 0.15-mg dose of epinephrine from the auto-injector; those ≥30 kg and adults receive a 0.3-mg dose of epinephrine. Each EAI contains a single dose of epinephrine for single use and should be used to administer intramuscularly into the anterolateral aspect of the thigh, through clothing if necessary. With severe persistent anaphylaxis, repeat injections with an additional epinephrine injection, may be necessary. Studies show that up to 30% of patients who develop anaphylaxis will require more than 1 dose of epinephrine.[30] If two sequential doses of epinephrine are administered, the third should be administered under direct medical supervision. Older children and their caregivers also should be given structured training in anaphylaxis and in administering these devices. Currently EAI are expensive, needs to be stored in temperature range of 20–25°C and are current not available in India. Epinephrine in ampoules (1:1000, 1 mg/mL) are the only available epinephrine in India, and is less expensive with a shelf-life of 6–12 months.

Anaphylaxis emergency action plan card or identification bracelets need to be issued by a proper medical specialist to the child at the time of discharge.

The causative agent of anaphylaxis is frequently unknown at the time of discharge from the ED or at the time of admission to the hospital. Therefore, follow-up with an allergist-immunologist for assessment of sensitization to allergen and long-term risk reduction by avoidance and/or immune modulation is recommended.[5] Assessment of sensitization to relevant allergens is done by measurement of allergen-specific serum IgE levels or allergen sensitization detection skin test or medically supervised provocation tests few weeks post episode of anaphylaxis and discharge from hospital.

Flowchart 1: Emergency management of patient with anaphylaxis[29]

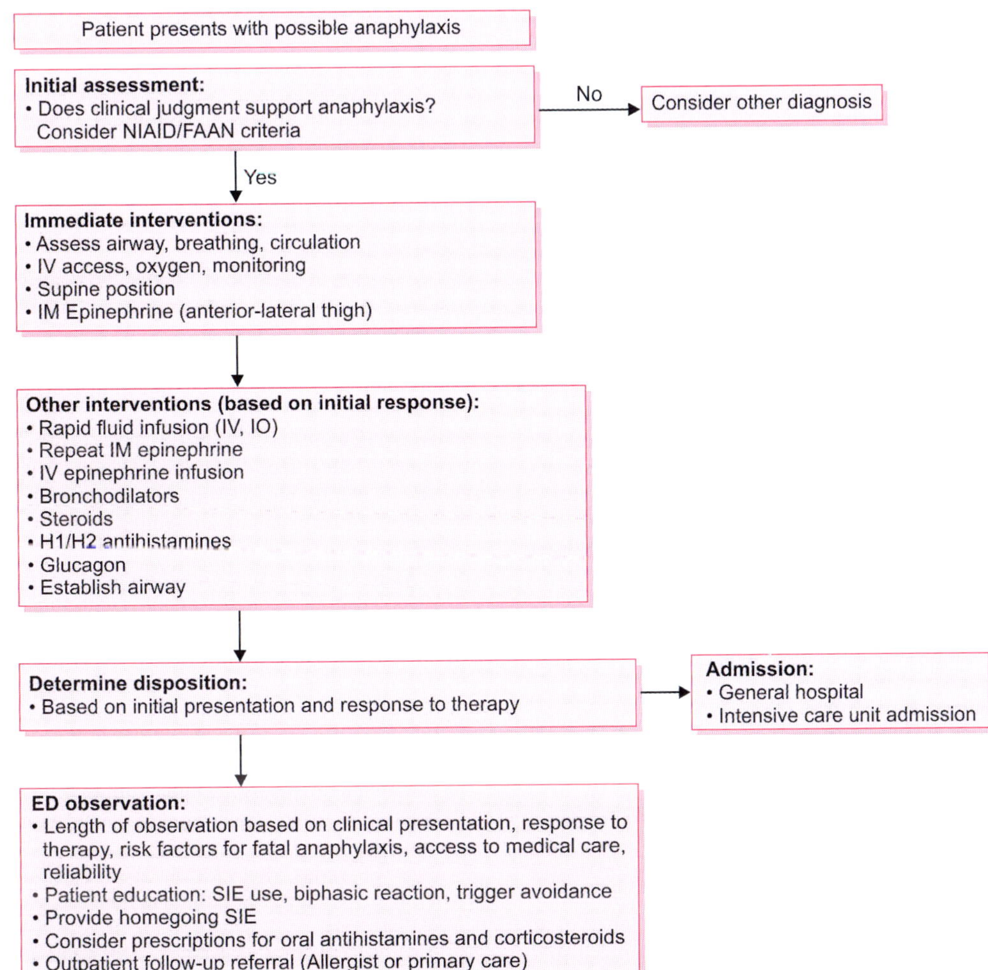

Long-term risk reduction/immunomodulation is recommended for food-triggered anaphylaxis by strict avoidance of relevant food(s), subcutaneous venom immunotherapy for stinging insect-triggered anaphylaxis, avoidance of relevant medications and use of safe substitutes for medication-triggered anaphylaxis. Glucocorticoid and non-sedating H1-antihistamine prophylaxis is recommended for 2–3 months infants with for idiopathic recurrent anaphylaxis.[18]

Omalizumab, an anti-IgE monoclonal antibody which is at present is used to control symptoms and prevent exacerbations in severe chronic asthmatics not controlled on steroids[31] and chronic idiopathic urticaria.[32] Recently, the drug has been used to prevent recurrent anaphylaxis in a women[33] and exercise induced anaphylaxis.[34]

KEY MESSAGES

- Food such as peanuts, tree nuts, fish, milk, eggs, soya and shellfish (e.g. shrimp, lobster, crab, scallops and oysters) are implicated as trigger in 35–50% of anaphylaxis in children.
- Epinephrine (adrenaline) is the medication of first choice in anaphylaxis. Early injection of epinephrine (within 1 hour) in anaphylaxis is associated with favorable outcome.
- Use of antihistaminic drugs as well as steroids is second-line adjunct treatment and should never be considered as an alternative to epinephrine.

- Self-carrying of epinephrine auto-injectors (EAI) or epinephrine ampoules or epinephrine prefilled syringes (EPFS) are highly recommended to manage such episodes in community or outside the hospital settings.
- Anaphylaxis emergency action plan card or identification bracelets or wallet cards are highly recommended. Training of older children, their caregivers like siblings, parents and school teachers are in emergency management of anaphylaxis and giving injection epinephrine to a vulnerable child are recommended.

REFERENCES

1. Simons FE, Ardusso LR, Bilo MB, *et al.* International consensus on (ICON) anaphylaxis. World Allergy Organ J. 2014;7:9.
2. Sampson HA, Muñoz-Furlong A, Campbell RL. Second Symposium on the Definition and Management of Anaphylaxis: Summary Report - Second National Institute of Allergy and Infectious Disease/Food Allergy and Anaphylaxis Network Symposium. J Allergy Clin Immunol. 2006;117: 391-7.
3. Panesar SS, Javed S, desilva D, *et al.* Epidemiology of anaphylaxis in Europe: A systematic review. Allergy. 2013;68:1353-61.
4. Brown SGA, Mullins RJ, Gold MS. Anaphylaxis: Diagnosis and management. Med J Aust. 2006;185:283-9.
5. Simons FER, Ebisawa M, Borges MS, *et al.* 2015 update of the evidence base: World Allergy Organization anaphylaxis guidelines. World Allergy Organ J. 2015;8:1-16.
6. Greenberger P, Rotskoff BD, Lifschvitz B. Fatal anaphylaxis: post-mortem findings and associated comorbid diseases. Ann Allergy Asthma Immunol. 2007;98:252-7.
7. CDC. Voluntary guidelines for managing food allergies in schools and early care and education programs. Available from: *https://www.cdc.gov/healthyschools/foodallergies/index.htm.* Accessed March 03, 2019.
8. Kraft S, Kinet JP. New developments in Fc epsilon RI regulation, function and inhibition. Nat Rev Immunol. 2007;7: 365-78.
9. Weiss JW, Drazen JM, Coles N, *et al.* Bronchoconstrictor effects of leukotriene C in humans. Science. 1982;216:196-8.
10. Reber LL, Hernandez JD, Galli SJ. The pathophysiology of anaphylaxis. J Allergy Clin Immunol. 2017;140:335-48.
11. Finkelman FD, Khodoun MV, Strait R. Human IgE-independent systemic anaphylaxis. J Allergy Clin Immunol. 2016;137:1674-80.
12. Wuepper KD, Bokisch VA, Muller-Eberhard HJ, *et al.* Cutaneous responses to human C3 anaphylatoxin in man. Clin Exp Immunol. 1972;11:13-20.
13. Chapman J, Lalkhen AG. Anaphylaxis. Anaesth Intensive Care Med. 2017;18:16-21.
14. Liew WK, Williamson E, Tang ML. Anaphylaxis fatalities and admissions in Australia. J Allergy Clin Immunol. 2009;123: 434-42.
15. Campbell RL, Hagan JB, Manivannan V, *et al.* Evaluation of National Institute of Allergy and Infection Disease/Food Allergy & Anaphylaxis Network criteria for the diagnosis of anaphylaxis in emergency department patients. J Allergy Clin Immunol. 2012;129:748-52.
16. Vitte J. Human mast cell tryptase in biology and medicine. Mol Immunol. 2015;63:18-24.
17. Komarow HD, Hu Z, Brittain E, *et al.* Serum tryptase levels in atopic and nonatopic children. J Allergy Clin Immunol. 2009;124:845-8.
18. Simons FER, Ardusso LRF, Bilo MB, *et.al.* 2012 update: World Allergy Organization Guidelines for the assessment and management of anaphylaxis. Curr Opin Allergy Clin Immunol. 2012;12:389-99.
19. Simons FE, Roberts JR, Gu X, *et al.* Epinephrine absorption in children with a history of anaphylaxis. J Allergy Clin Immunol. 1998;101:33-7.
20. Simons FE, Gu X, Simons KJ. Epinephrine absorption in adults: intramuscular subcutaneous injection. J Allergy Clin Immunol. 2001;108:871-6.
21. Humphrey RS. Lessons for management of anaphylaxis from a study of fatal reactions. Clin Exp Allergy. 2000;30:1144-50.
22. Soar J, Humphrey R, Cant A, *et.al.* Emergency treatment of anaphylactic reactions guidelines for health care providers. Resuscitation. 2008;77:157-69.
23. Schummer C, Wirsing M, Schummer W. The pivotal role of vasopressin in refractory anaphylactic shock. Anesth Analg. 2008;107:620-4.
24. Sheikh A, Ten Brock V, Brown SG, *et al.* H1 Antihistamine in the treatment of anaphylaxis. Cochrane Database Syst Rev. 2007; 62:830-7.
25. Campbell RL, Li James TC, Nicklas RA, *et al.* Emergency department diagnosis and treatment of anaphylaxis: A practice parameter. Ann Allergy Asthma Immunol. 2014;113:599-608.
26. Pollack CV. Utility of glucagon in the emergency department. J Emerg Med. 1993;11:195-205.
27. Bauer CS, Vadas P, Kelly KJ. Methylene blue for the treatment of refractory anaphylaxis without hypotension. Am J Emerg Med. 2013;31:264.
28. Brady WJ, Luber S, Carter CT, *et al.* Multiphasic anaphylaxis: an uncommon event in the emergency department. Acad Emerg Med. 1997;4:193-7.
29. Campbell RL, Li James TC, Nicklas RA, *et al.* Emergency department diagnosis and treatment of anaphylaxis: A practice parameter. Ann Allergy Asthma Immunol. 2014;113:599-608.
30. Jarvinen KM, Sicherer SH, Sampson HA, *et al.* Use of multiple doses of epinephrine in food-induced anaphylaxis in children. J Allergy Clin Immunol. 2008;122:133-8.
31. Lommatzsch M, Korn S, Buhl R, *et al.* Against all odds: Anti-IgE for intrinsic asthma? Thorax. 2013;69:94-6.
32. Maurer M, Rosén K, Hsieh HJ, *et al.* Omalizumab for the treatment of chronic idiopathic or spontaneous urticaria. N Engl J Med. 2013;368:924-35.
33. Gomez G. Current strategies to inhibit high affinity FcεRI-mediated signaling for the treatment of allergic disease. Front Immunol. 2019;10:175.
34. Peterson RM, Christopher A. Long-term omalizumab use in the treatment of exercise-induced anaphylaxis. Allergy Rhinol. 2017;8:170-2.

CHAPTER

13

Fluid and Electrolyte Disturbances

Krishna Mohan Gulla, Rakesh Lodha, Arvind Bagga

The extraordinarily complicated functions of the human body depend on the preservation of a narrow range of volume and composition of the body fluids. Even slight variations can have dramatic manifestations and consequences. On the other hand, there is an immense capability to maintain homeostasis, i.e. the dynamic equilibrium between the intake of water, inorganic substances and organic molecules, their distribution between body compartments, and their excretion. Before considering the conditions that affect this delicate balance, it is important to discuss the principles of fluids and electrolyte balance in our body. In children, the influence of growth on physiology is striking in terms of: (a) the body composition of fluids and electrolytes, (b) metabolic turnover, and (c) the progressive maturation of organ systems (e.g. the kidneys) with time.

PHYSIOLOGY

Body Water and Its Distribution

Water is the largest component of the human body. Total body water (TBW) in healthy, term neonates at birth is 75–80% of the body weight; this gradually declines to 60–65% by 1 year of age. In adolescent boys, TBW is 60% of body weight, while in adolescent girls, it is about 55% of the body weight.[1]

The TBW is divided into two main compartments: the fluid inside the cells (intracellular fluid, ICF) and the fluid outside (extracellular fluid, ECF). The ICF remains relatively constant at 40% of the body weight, while ECF as a proportion of body weight reduces with age (**Table 1**). The

Table 1: Changes in body water (% body weight) with age

Age	*Total body water*	*Extracellular fluid*	*Intracellular fluid*
Neonate			
Preterm	80–85	50–60	25–30
Term	75–80	40–45	35
1-year-old	65	25	40–45
Adolescent			
Boy	60	20	40–45
Girl	55	15–20	40

ECF is further divided into the intravascular (or plasma) volume and the interstitial fluid by the capillary membrane. In addition, ECF also includes the transcellular fluid, i.e. cerebrospinal fluid, intraocular fluid, synovial fluid, and pleural and peritoneal fluids.

The composition of ICF is important, as it is the site of all metabolic activity. The ECF regulates the ICF and composition, since both ECF and ICF are under osmotic equilibrium.

Electrolyte Composition of Body Fluids

The electrolyte composition of these compartments is different. The major cation in plasma is sodium (Na^+), with smaller contributions from calcium (Ca^{2+}), potassium (K^+) and magnesium (Mg^{2+}); chloride (Cl^-), bicarbonate (HCO^-) and proteins are the major anions. In addition, there are a number of anions that are present, but are not routinely estimated; these undetermined anions constitute the anion gap.

Sodium is the focus of homeostatic mechanisms concerned with maintenance of intravascular volume. If osmolality is maintained, then the water movement tends to follow the Na^+ movement across various compartments. Therefore, total body Na^+ and TBW generally parallel one another. By contrast, the dominant cation in ICF is K^+, with small amounts of Na^+ and Mg^{2+}. Most of the anions are organic phosphates, proteins, organic acids and sulfate.

It is important to understand three important concepts in fluid and electrolyte therapy namely, cell membrane permeability, osmolality/effective osmolarity (tonicity) and electro neutrality. Cell membrane permeability refers to the ability of the membrane to allow certain substances such as water and urea to pass freely, while charged ions such as Na^+ cannot freely cross the membrane and are trapped on one side.

Osmolarity is defined as the number of osmotically active particles in 1 liter water in a solution (mOsm/L). Osmolality, on the other hand, refers to the number of osmotically active particles per kilogram water (mOsm/kg). The number of dissolved particles in a solution determines its osmolality and osmolarity. For instance, one molecule of sodium chloride will dissociate into two ions: Na^+ and Cl^-. One mOsm sodium chloride thus yields a two mOsm solution.

Plasma osmolality can be estimated by the following formula:

Osmolality (mOsm/kg)

2Na + Glucose (mg/dL)/18 + BUN (mg/dL)/2.8

Tonicity/effective osmolarity can be defined as net vector of force on cells relative to a semipermeable membrane when in solution. Isotonic fluids do not cause osmotic shifts and size of cells do not change. In case of hypotonic fluids, cell expands as the free water is high in the extracellular environment and crosses the semipermeable membrane easily. Whereas, in case of hypertonic fluids, free water shifts out of the cells, causing cell shrinkage. Osmolality is distinct from tonicity in that tonicity relates to both the effect on a cell of a fluid (dependent on the selective permeability of the membrane) and the osmolality of the fluid. For example, urea affects serum osmolality but not tonicity because urea moves freely across cell membranes with no effect on tonicity. Tonicity of IVF is primarily affected by the sodium. Though, dextrose affects the osmolarity of IVFs, it is not a significant contributor to the tonicity unless uncontrolled hyperglycemia such as uncontrolled diabetes mellitus. Hence, dextrose in maintenance fluid, in clinical practice, is not believed to affect tonicity of fluids. As already discussed, effective osmolality (tonicity) is defines as two times serum Na^+ plus glucose (mg/dL)/18. As is evident, the concentration of Na^+ is the major determinant of plasma osmolality. The normal plasma osmolality ranges from 280–295 mOsm/kg and changes of as little as 1% elicit regulatory mechanisms. Finally, the principle of electro neutrality implies that the total electrical charge of cations equals that of the anions. In conditions where there is loss of bicarbonate anions (e.g. in diarrhea or renal tubular acidosis), chloride is retained leading to a hyperchloremic metabolic acidosis.

Regulation of the Water Balance

The TBW and plasma osmolality are maintained in a narrow range by regulating the intake and loss of water. Water is available to the body by oral intake, oxidation of fats and carbohydrates, and from release of water during tissue catabolism. The intake of water is governed by the thirst mechanism (controlled by the hypothalamic osmoreceptors that are sensitive to change in plasma osmolality and blood volume). Intravascular volume preservation takes precedence over osmolality. Thus, thirst may occur even when the body water is hypo-osmotic.[2]

The amount equivalent to the intake is lost by the way of insensible water losses (lungs, skin), urine and losses through the gastrointestinal tract. Under normal circumstances, there is no significant control over the extrarenal fluid losses. The renal excretion of water and solutes is under the control of antidiuretic hormone (ADH, the release of which is controlled by changes in plasma osmolality and volume) and natriuretic peptides. Hypovolemia is a stronger stimulus for release of ADH than hyperosmolarity. The renin-angiotensin-aldosterone axis contributes to the regulation of Na^+, and thereby, water excretion. In older children and adults, ADH is a more important regulatory mechanism than thirst as water intake is commonly influenced by social and cultural factors rather than physiological needs.

Changes in plasma osmolality, which are determined mainly by plasma Na^+ concentrations, are sensed by the hypothalamic osmoreceptors. These receptors influence water intake by regulating thirst, and water excretion by regulating the release of ADH. Thus, osmoregulation is primarily achieved by changes in water balance without any significant changes in Na^+ handling.

On the other hand, volume regulation aims to maintain tissue perfusion. Various sensors located in the carotid sinus, afferent arterioles, and atria detect changes in the effective circulating volume. Urinary Na^+ excretion is modified to achieve changes in the volume by renin-angiotensin-aldosterone system, sympathetic nervous system, atrial natriuretic peptide and ADH. Thus, the osmoregulatory and volume regulatory pathways are essentially independent except for the overlap involving ADH.

Normal Requirements of Fluids and Electrolytes

Physiology based fluid replacement can be divided into four distinct phases. Phase I: Bolus IVFs are required to rebuild tissue perfusion and to avoid or decrease end-organ injury. Phase II: IVFs are shifted from boluses to maintenance fluids which is a critical window to maintain balance between fluid intake and losses. Phase III: Fluids to achieve balance between requirements and losses. Phase IV: IVF administration is stopped and body's intrinsic fluid regulation takes over. Fluid administration during these 4 phases of fluid therapy needs to be carefully titrated based on the physiology of each patient.

Normal requirement of water was calculated by Holliday and Segar based on the energy expenditure of healthy children, with 1 mL of fluid provided for each kilocalorie expended, or 1500 mL/m^2 per day. The insensible water loss (by evaporation from skin and lungs) is about 40–60 mL per 100 cal metabolized. The renal water loss varies from 50 70 mL and the stool water loss is 5–10 mL per 100 Cal. On the other hand, the water produced during oxidation of carbohydrates, proteins and fats is about 12–17 mL and tissue catabolism contributes 3 mL per 100 Cal. The net requirement of water is thus 100–110 mL for 100 Cal metabolized. The approximate requirements for Na^+ are 3 mEq/100 Cal, K^+ about 2 mEq/100 Cal and Cl^- 2 mEq/100 Cal that are utilized. **Table 2** shows the maintenance requirements for fluids based on body weight.[3] However, the resting energy expenditure in healthy children is different from those children with acute illness or after surgery. Using more reliable calorimetric methods, average basal metabolic rate of ill children varies from 50 to 60 kcal/kg/day, which is much lower than the historical practice.

Table 2: Fluid requirements in relation to body weight

Body weight	*Fluid requirement*	
Up to 10 kg	100 mL/kg	
11–20 kg	1000 mL plus	50 mL/kg above 10 kg
>20 kg	1500 mL plus	20 mL/kg above 20 kg

The following issues should be considered while calculating the requirements for maintenance fluids and electrolytes: (i) Is insensible water loss normal? (ii) Is the urine output as expected? (iii) Are there any abnormal losses? (iv) Is there an altered metabolic rate? (v) Is Na^+ and K^+ homeostasis normal?

Apart from the above, type of fluid which is to be infused also to be determined. Children have been administered hypotonic maintenance IV fluids for years which is based on theoretical calculations from 1950s.[4,5] Hypotonic fluid administration lead to increased incidence of acute hospital acquired hyponatremia resulting in hyponatremic encephalopathy at times.[6,7] Due to hyponatremia caused by use of hypotonic fluids, use of 0.2% saline was decreased along with increase in use of isotonic/near isotonic fluids (0.45% and 0.9% saline) in clinical practice.[8] However, concerns regarding safety of these isotonic maintenance fluids was questioned due to side effects such as hypernatremia, hypertension, fluid overload, and metabolic acidosis. Recent clinical practice guideline by American Academy of Pediatrics recommends the use of isotonic fluids in children from 1 month to 18 years of age with appropriate potassium and glucose to mitigate the risk of hyponatremia (strong recommendation).[9] But, use of isotonic fluids in children with neurosurgical disorders, cardiac disease, renal failure, malignancy, diabetes insipidus, severe burns is not well studied and the fluid composition needs to individualized based on serum electrolytes in these clinical scenarios. Commonly used maintenance fluids and their composition are shown in **Table 3**. Oral fluid therapy is preferred provided the child is hemodynamically stable and is able to accept and retain fluids given orally.

For acutely expanding the intravascular volume, intravenous fluid solutions that can be used safely, include normal (0.9%) saline and Ringer's lactate. These crystalloid solutions are limited by the short retention time of their solutes. When isotonic sodium-containing solutions are given intravenously, only 15–30% of administered salt

Table 3: Composition of commonly used intravenous fluids

Fluid	Glucose (g/dL)	Sodium (mEq/L)	Chloride (mEq/L)	Potassium (mEq/L)	Calcium (mg/L)	Magnesium (mEq/L)	Buffer (mEq/L)	Effective osmolarity (Tonicity) (mOsm/L)
Isolyte -P	5	23	29	20		3	23 Acetate 3 phosphate	75
$D_5$0.2% NaCl	5	34	34	0	0	0	0	78
D_5 0.45% NaCl	5	77	77	0	0	0	0	154
D_5 0.9% NaCl	5	154	154	0	0	0	0	308
Ringer lactate	0	130	109	4	3	0	28 Lactate	273
Plasmalyte	0	140	98	5	0	3	27 Acetate 23 Gluconate	294

Table 4: Work-up of a child with suspected fluid and electrolyte disturbance

Serum electrolytes	Provide information about Na^+, K^+, Cl^- and anion gap
Blood urea, creatinine	Blood creatinine is a useful indicator of renal dysfunction. Raised blood urea may reflect intravascular volume depletion
Urine examination	Specific gravity is related to the hydration status and presence of abnormal solute, e.g. glucose. Urinary electrolytes and specific gravity are useful in assessing patients with renal dysfunction
Plasma and urine osmolality	Osmolal gap (difference between measured and calculated plasma osmolality) >10 mOsm/kg suggests presence of additional substances, e.g. mannitol. Plasma osmolality shows whether or not a patient is in an isotonic state. Urine osmolality helps in evaluation of the concentrating capacity of kidneys
Serum protein and albumin	Total protein and albumin levels determine the intravascular oncotic pressure. Reduced in liver disease, nephrotic syndrome and malnutrition
Blood gases	Provides information on blood pH, oxygen and carbon dioxide tension and bicarbonate

and water remains in the intravascular space while the remainder contributes to the interstitial fluid.[10] Hypertonic solutions, such as 3% saline, permit greater expansion of circulating blood volume with lower fluid load and less edema. Infusion of colloids such as albumin or blood products, which have some oncotic pressure by virtue of their protein content, has a longer lasting effect. This issue is addressed in detail in another chapter.

Fluid and Electrolyte Disturbances

Of various fluid and electrolyte disturbances, diarrheal dehydration is the commonest. This is discussed elsewhere.

Regular clinical evaluation and relevant investigations are important for monitoring a child receiving parenteral fluid therapy. Investigations that are useful in working up a child with suspected fluid or electrolytes disturbance are listed in **Table 4**. Clinical evaluation of the hydration status and peripheral perfusion should be performed every 8–12 hours, and more frequently in an unstable child. Urine output charting should be done every 6–8 hours. In some patients, particularly those with low urine output, urine specific gravity may aid in fluid management. Serum electrolytes should be estimated every 24–48 hours and more frequently, if there is dyselectrolytemia. Blood urea and creatinine levels should be measured every other day.

DISORDERS OF SODIUM HOMEOSTASIS

The concentration of Na^+, the main cation of ECF, determines the intravascular and interstitial volumes. The dietary intake of salt varies with food habits. Normal Na^+ losses in feces and sweat are small and kidney is the chief regulator of Na^+ excretion.

The ECF concentration of Na^+ is maintained around 135–145 mEq/L and the ICF concentration 10 mEq/L. The latter is achieved by active efflux of Na^+ from the cells mediated by magnesium dependent Na^+-K^+- ATPase system. Changes in Na^+ concentration of serum are followed by parallel changes in its concentration in ECF and interstitial fluid. The Na^+ concentration of transcellular fluids (gastrointestinal secretions, cerebrospinal fluid, pleural, peritoneal and synovial fluid) is highly variable, as these fluids do not have a simple diffusion relationship with plasma.

Retention or loss of Na^+ is usually accompanied by a proportionate change in water handling, leading to expansion or shrinkage of ECF volume, but with little changes in serum Na^+ concentration. In disease states, inappropriate retention or loss of water or Na^+, or a combination of both may lead to hypo- or hypernatremia. Alterations in levels of serum Na^+ that arise slowly or are chronic in nature tend to be better tolerated clinically than acute alterations. Chronic or slow changes allow for maximal counter-regulation that involves loss or gain of organic osmolytes (idiogenic osmoles) and fewer clinical sequelae. On the other hand, profound acute alterations are often accompanied by neurologic complications.

Hyponatremia

Hyponatremia, serum Na^+ level below 130 mEq/L is a common abnormality detected in children hospitalized after the newborn period.[11] Mild hyponatremia is defined as serum sodium between 130–135 mEq/L, moderate hyponatremia is 125–129 mEq/L and profound hyponatremia is below 125 mEq/L. Hyponatraemia considered to be acute when it is documented to exist in less than 48 hrs duration. Whereas, chronic hyponatremia is considered when it lasts more than 48 hrs.[12] In a majority of the cases, hyponatremia is mild and asymptomatic and does not require treatment. However, in occasional situations, especially when the serum Na^+ rapidly falls to very low levels, neurological symptoms and even irreversible brain damage may occur.

Causes

Important conditions that lead to hyponatremia are listed in **Table 5**. Hyponatremic dehydration is the most common condition, resulting from replacement of acute diarrheal fluid losses with plain water or very hypotonic solutions. Nephrotic syndrome, congestive cardiac failure and syndrome of inappropriate ADH secretion are the other important causes. Hyponatremia also is frequently observed in acute or chronic renal failure, when excessive fluids have been given.[13]

In the absence of accumulation of abnormal solutes, hyponatremia is associated with low serum osmolality. Occasionally, hyponatremia results from shift of water from cells due to solutes restricted to the ECF (e.g. mannitol); the osmolality is increased in these cases. Similarly, hyperglycemia, by causing water to move out of cells, leads to hyponatremia. An increase of blood glucose by 100 mg/dL reduces the serum Na^+ concentration by 1.6 mEq/L. Excessive loss of K^+ may also cause hyponatremia as Na^+ shifts into the cells in exchange for K^+.

Pseudohyponatremia

Falsely low levels of serum Na^+ may be obtained if it contains very high concentrations of lipids. The true Na^+ value can be measured by separating the lipids and measuring Na^+ in plasma water. Measurement of plasma osmolality is of help since the osmolality depends upon the number of solutes in plasma water and is not affected by hyperlipidemia. An accurate osmo-meter is used to measure plasma osmolality. If the measured osmolality exceeds the calculated osmolality (see above) by 10 mOsm/kg, either pseudo-hyponatremia is present or the plasma contains some unmeasured substance (e.g. mannitol, ethanol or acetone).

Pathophysiology of neurological complications

The intrinsic characteristics of the blood brain barrier cause the brain to respond to osmolal gradients as if it were a single cell. Most solutes, including Na^+, take several hours to equilibrate across the blood brain barrier. Because of the free movement of water, brain responds to hypo-osmolality by swelling and to hyperosmolality

Table 5: Causes of hyponatremia

Circulating volume	*Urinary <20 mEq/L*	*Na^+ >20 mEq/L*
Decreased	Gastroenteritis chronic diuretic therapy Burns	Adrenal insufficiency Salt wasting states
Normal or increased	Congestive heart failure Cirrhosis liver Nephrotic syndrome	Renal tubular acidosis Obstructive uropathy Diuretic phase of ATN Renal failure SIADH Compulsive water drinking Excessive fluid therapy

(ATN: acute tubular necrosis; SIADH: syndrome of inappropriate ADH secretion)

by shrinking. The brain when compared to the other organs is more likely to experience a change in its total size in response to an acute change in plasma osmolality.

Since skull is a rigid structure, increasing cerebral edema may lead to severe intracranial hypertension and brainstem herniation. In infants with open fontanelles and unfused sutures, there is relative protection from a rapid increase in intracranial pressure. Children are more prone to neurological damage due to hyponatremia since (i) the ratio of the brain to skull size is such that less room exists for expansion of the pediatric brain in skull than in adults, and (ii) the relative amount of cerebrospinal fluid is lower in children than in adults. Adults thus have more space for brain to expand than do children.

The pathological findings in severe hyponatremia include cerebral edema, and demyelinating lesions in the basal ganglia, periventricular white matter and cerebral cortex. Central pontine myelinolysis is characterized by demyelination within the central portion of basal pons with sparing of axis cylinders and neurons. Clinical manifestations of pontine myelinolysis include spastic quadriplegia, pseudobulbar paralysis and behavioral changes without focal abnormalities. The lesions can be detected on CT and MRI scanning. There is considerable controversy on whether this condition occurs as a consequence of hyponatremia or its treatment, since it has been associated with both.[14]

In chronic hyponatremia brain water tends to gradually decrease. Initially there is extrusion of Na^+ from the cells. Subsequently, there may be extrusion of idiogenic osmoles (e.g. taurine). Symptomatic hyponatremia usually occurs relatively acutely in a previously well patient or when serum Na^+ rapidly falls further in a patient with chronic hyponatremia.

Clinical features

Symptoms are related to the severity as well as the rapidity of development of hyponatremia. A very gradual fall in serum Na^+ level may not cause any abnormality even at levels below 110 mEq/L. Apathy, anorexia, nausea, vomiting, agitation, headache, altered sensorium, convulsions and coma are the usual manifestations. With the development of cerebral edema and a rise in intracranial pressure, brainstem herniation may occur causing respiratory depression and apnea. Moderately severe hyponatremia is defined by nausea without vomiting, confusion, headache and severe hyponatremia is characterized by seizures, coma, abnormal and deep somnolence, cardiorespiratory arrest.

Evaluation

A careful clinical evaluation of the state of ECF volume is important. Serum and urinary electrolytes and osmolality should be measured. Nonhypotonic hyponatremia is to be excluded **(Table 6)**.

The rapidity of development of hyponatremia, whether acute or chronic, should be determined. Symptoms ascribed to low serum Na^+ should be noted and the state of hydration assessed. Hypovolemia is indicated by thirst, dry mucous membranes, decreased skin turgor and hypotension. The urinary Na^+ concentration is low, unless adrenal insufficiency or renal salt wasting has led to hyponatremia. The most common cause of normovolemic hyponatremia is the syndrome of inappropriate ADH secretion. Approach to hyponatremia is shown in **Flowchart 1**.

Treatment

In a patient with hyponatremic dehydration, the foremost aim is to restore the circulatory adequacy with 20–40 mL/kg of normal saline or Ringer's lactate. In patients with symptomatic hyponatremia (presence of lethargy, altered sensorium, seizures) serum Na^+ level should be rapidly increased by intravenous infusion of 3% saline (514 mEq Na^+/L), 5–6 mL/kg body weight over 10–15 minutes.[15] A rapid increase in the serum Na^+ level by 4–5 mEq/L usually causes relief of symptoms. If clinical improvement does not occur, an additional 3–4 mL/kg may be administered. The amount of Na^+ needed to raise the serum Na^+ by a given amount can be calculated by the formula.

$$\text{mEq } Na^+ \text{ required} = [\text{desired—actual serum } Na^+] \times 0.6 \times \text{body weight (kg)}$$

Table 6: Causes of non-hypotonic hyponatremia

Setting	*Serum osmolarity*	*Examples*
Presence of "effective" osmoles that raise serum osmolality and can cause hyponatremia	Isotonic or hypertonic	Glucose, Mannitol
Presence of "ineffective" osmoles that raise serum osmolality but do not cause hyponatremia	Isotonic or hyperosmolar	Urea, Alcohols, Ethylene-glycol
Presence of endogenous solutes that cause pseudohyponatremia (laboratory artifact)	Isotonic	Triglycerides, Cholesterol intravenous immunoglobulins

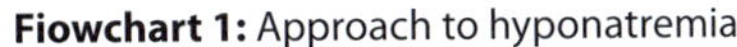

Fiowchart 1: Approach to hyponatremia

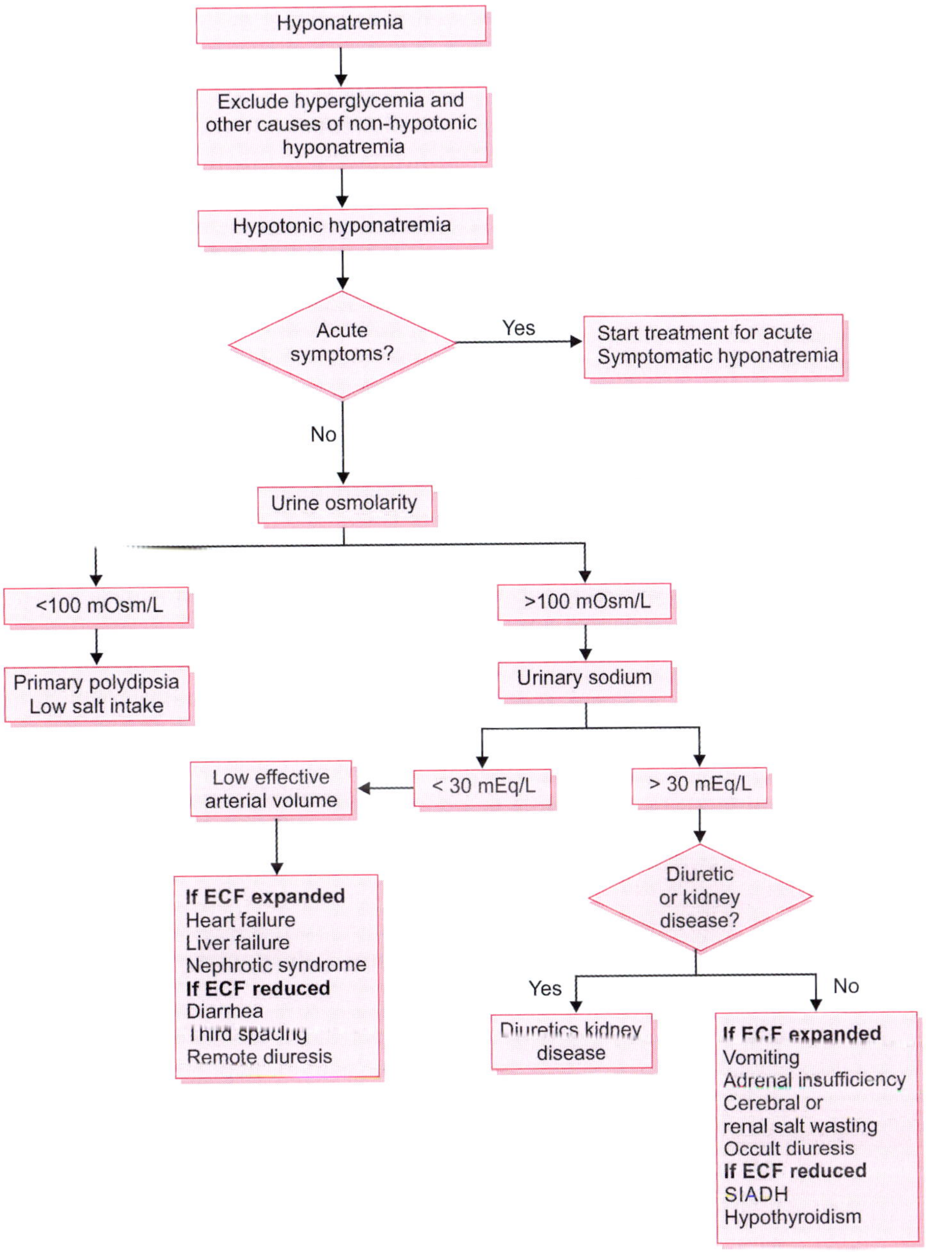

Further increase in serum Na^+ should be at a rate of 0.5 mEq/L per hour. The increase in plasma Na^+ concentration should not exceed 10–12 mEq/L in the first 24 hours. If neurological symptoms persist the possibility of some CNS pathology (hemorrhage, infections) should be considered.

$$\text{Change in serum } [Na^+] = \frac{\text{Infusate } [Na^+] - \text{Serum } [Na^+]}{\text{Total body water} + 1}$$

Current evidence suggests that it is safe to raise the plasma Na^+ concentration in asymptomatic patients by 10–12 mEq/L on the first day and 18 mEq/L over the first two days.[16]

Water intake should be restricted in patients with an expanded ECF volume (e.g. cardiac or renal failure) or those who have received excessive fluids. In some patients, administration of diuretics is required. Some hyponatremic patients with congestive heart failure may benefit from a combination of a loop diuretic and an ACE inhibitor.[17]

Syndrome of Inappropriate Secretion of Antidiuretic Hormone (SIADH)

The SIADH is an important cause of hyponatremia in hospitalized patients.

Clinical features

The SIADH is characterized by hyponatremia and hyposmolality, oliguria, modest expansion of body fluid volume and mild urinary Na^+ wasting. The urine osmolality is inappropriately high. The blood pressure and renal function are normal and a cardiac or endocrine disorder is absent. There is no/mild edema. There may be no abnormal clinical findings and hyponatremia is often detected incidentally. Occasionally the serum Na^+ levels are very low (below 120 mEq/L) and lead to sensorial disturbances and seizures.

Causes

Intracranial infections and pulmonary diseases are the common causes of SIADH (**Table 7**). Hyponatremia in the postsurgical period might be due to SIADH caused by administration of anesthetic agents.

Table 7: Important causes of syndrome of inappropriate ADH secretion

Neurologic disorders	
Tuberculous meningitis	Pyogenic meningitis
Brain abscess	Tumor
Head injury	Subarachnoid hemorrhage
Guillain-Barre syndrome	Status epilepticus
Drugs	
Cyclophosphamide	Vincristine
Barbiturates	Carbamazepine
Chlorpropamide	Indomethacin
Pulmonary disorders	
Tuberculosis	Pneumonia
Chronic obstructive disease	Positive pressure ventilation
Acute respiratory failure	
Miscellaneous	
Hodgkin's disease	Postoperative patient
Malignancies	

Diagnosis

The Essential criteria for diagnosis of SIADH are: Low plasma Na^+(<135 mEq/L) and effective osmolality (<275 mOsm/kg), Urine osmolarity >100 mOsm/kg, clinical euvolemia, urinary sodium >30 mEq/L with normal salt intake, absence of adrenal, thyroid, pituitary or renal insufficiency, no recent use of diuretics. Supplementary criteria are serum uric acid <4 mg/dL, serum urea <21.6 mg/dL, failure to correct hyponatraemia after 0.9% saline infusion, fractional sodium excretion >0.5%, fractional urea excretion >55%, fractional uric acid excretion >12%, correction of hyponatraemia through fluid restriction.[12]

Treatment

The treatment of SIADH consists of restriction of water intake, which will gradually lead to a rise in the serum Na^+ level. However, if neurological abnormalities are present, 3% saline should be slowly infused to partly correct hyponatremia. Intravenous furosemide in a dose of 1–2 mg/kg will cause excretion of free water and increased levels of serum Na^+. Drugs like lithium or demeclocycline that inhibit ADH effect on the kidney are not recommended in children. Urinary Na^+ and K^+ losses should be measured and replaced.

Cerebral Salt Wasting

The syndrome of cerebral salt wasting (CSWS) is characterized by the development of excessive natriuresis and subsequent hyponatremic dehydration in patients with intracranial diseases.[18] Differentiation of this condition from the syndrome of inappropriate secretion of ADH is important (**Table 8**).

Table 8 : Differentiation between SIADH and CSWS

Feature	*SIADH*	*CSWS*
Serum urea	Normal-low	Normal-high
Serum uric acid	Low	Normal-high
Urine volume	Normal-low	High
Urine sodium	>30 mEq/L	>>30 mEq/L
Blood pressure	Normal	Normal—orthostatic hypotension

The syndrome of cerebral salt wasting occurs in the setting of an acute disease involving the central nervous system, e.g. head injury, brain tumor, intracranial surgery, intracerebral hemorrhage and tuberculous meningitis. The exact mechanism underlying renal salt wasting is unclear. It is hypothesized that urinary Na^+ loss results from an exaggerated renal pressure-natriuresis response caused by increased activity of the sympathetic nervous system and dopamine release. Another hypothesis involves the presence of circulating natriuretic factors in patients with cerebral salt wasting. The clinical features are those of hyponatremia. The urine is dilute and its flow rate high (unlike urine that is concentrated and with reduced flow in patients with SIADH). Urine sodium concentrations are typically >40 mEq/L. However, urinary sodium excretion (product of urine sodium concentration and urine volume) is high in patients with cerebral salt wasting and normal in SIADH. This results in a negative sodium balance in the former. Serum uric acid concentrations are low in patients with SIADH but normal in cerebral salt wasting.[19]

The management of CSWS comprises correction of volume depletion and hyponatremia, and replacement of ongoing urinary fluid and electrolyte losses using intravenous fluids. Once the patient is stabilized, enteral salt supplementation can be considered. Fludrocortisone, which enhances sodium reabsorption in the renal tubule resulting in expanded extracellular fluid volume, may be beneficial in some cases.[20]

Adrenal Insufficiency

Hyponatremia is a common complication of adrenal insufficiency, chiefly attributed to cortisol deficiency, diarrhea, vomiting and renal losses (due to lack of aldosterone). Cortisol deficiency results in an increased release of ADH, reduced water excretion and hyponatremia. Replacement of cortisol improves water excretion and increases plasma Na^+.[21] A mineralocorticoid, such as fludrocortisone, may be required to correct the urinary Na^+ losses and hyperkalemia that are commonly seen. Administration of fludrocortisone alone does not normalize renal water excretion and is not required in conditions that have normal aldosterone.

Hypernatremia

Hypernatremia, defined as serum Na^+ level above 150 mEq/L, represents net water deficit in relation to Na^+ stores, which can result from a net water loss or hypertonic Na^+ gain. Majority of patients with hypernatremia have net water loss; this may occur in absence of Na^+ loss (pure water loss) or in its presence (hypotonic fluid loss). Hypertonic Na^+ gain is usually due to therapeutic interventions or its accidental administration (**Table 9**).

Table 9: Causes of hypernatremia

Water loss
Increased insensible losses
Increased sweating, respiratory infections, burns
Gastrointestinal loss
Osmotic diarrhea, infectious diarrhea
Renal loss
Diabetes insipidus (central/nephrogenic), osmotic diuresis
Hypothalamic disorders
Primary hypodipsia
Sodium excess
Administration of hypertonic saline or sodium bicarbonate
Salt poisoning
Improperly prepared oral rehydration solution

The condition is mainly encountered in children with diarrhea and dehydration. It is more common in children who have been given oral or parenteral fluids having a high Na^+ content. It is more common in summer months when insensible losses are increased. Other causes of hypernatremia include substitution of salt for sugar in preparation of formula feeds and accidental ingestion of salt. Excessive intake of Na^+ leads to increase in body Na^+ and extracellular fluid volume.

Hypernatremia results in a movement of organic acids and free H^+ ions into the extracellular fluid, leading to acidosis. Hyperglycemia may occur due to inappropriately low levels of insulin. Hyperosmolality of the ECF causes a shift of water from the cells, which in the case of brain, leads to distension of cerebral vessels. These may rupture causing intracerebral, subdural or subarachnoid hemorrhage. Idiogenic osmoles are generated in the cells in patients with sustained and severe hypernatremia.[22] This is a protective phenomenon, which reduces the efflux of water, thereby preventing the consequences of hypernatremia.

Clinical features

In hypernatremic dehydration, extracellular fluid volume is relatively well preserved and features of hypovolemia and clinical shock are less prominent. Compared to older children and adults, infants and young children are at increased risk for hypernatremic hypovolemia due to their higher ratio of surface area to volume, resulting in greater insensible water losses from the skin and their inability to communicate and independently access for fluid intake. Children with about 10% loss of body weight have reduced skin turgor and a characteristic doughy feel. Hypernatremia usually manifests with nonspecific symptoms such as include irritability, restlessness, weakness, vomiting, muscular twitching, fever, and, in infants, high-pitched cry and tachypnea. Severe symptoms are seen with acute rise of sodium above 160 mEq/L which include altered mental status, lethargy, coma, and seizures. In the most severe cases, such as salt poisoning, the rapid rise in sodium leads to acute brain shrinkage, resulting in vascular rupture with cerebral and subarachnoid hemorrhage, demyelination, and irreversible neurologic injury.[2] Seizures may be present before the institution of fluid therapy or develop subsequently.

Evaluation

A detailed history of fluid loss in the form of gastrointestinal losses, polyuria, oral intake along with clinical signs of dehydration, neurological examination, midline defects etc. are to be noted. Measurement of urinary osmolality and urinary Na^+, serum urea and creatinine are useful in determining the etiology. Patients showing hypernatremia with urine osmolality less than 800 mOsm/kg usually have at least a partial defect in ADH release or action. In diabetes insipidus, urinary osmolality is usually less than 300 mOsm/kg. Desmopressin administration increases urine osmolality only if there is impaired endogenous secretion. Patients with nephrogenic diabetes insipidus or osmotic diuresis do not show increased urine osmolality following desmopressin administration.

Provided kidney functions are normal, fractional excretion of (FENa) may be useful, as FENa >2% suggestive of excessive salt intake and FENa <1% is suggestive of hypernatremia secondary to dehydration. Urinary Na^+ is usually below 25 mEq/L when hypernatremia is due to water loss but well above 100 mEq/L if there is Na^+ overload.[23] If diabetes insipidus is suspected, a water deprivation test should be carried out.[24]

Treatment

The management of hypernatremia requires correction of the underlying cause and the prevailing hypertonicity. Patients showing features of severe dehydration or shock are managed with parenteral administration of normal saline or Ringer's lactate.

Prior to treating a child with hypernatremia, few questions need to be addressed. 1. What is the volume status? 2. Need for fluid resuscitation to restore intravascular volume and tissue perfusion? 3. What is the water deficit? 4. What is the rate of hypernatremia correction? 5. How to address ongoing fluid loss? 6. What is the underlying cause of hypernatremia?

Ongoing monitoring of child's volume status with frequent clinical examinations and laboratory evaluation, including frequent measurement of sodium levels. Based on the clinical status and laboratory parameters, initial fluid prescription may be revised.

In any child with significant fluid loss, priority should be directed towards fluid resuscitation irrespective of sodium level. In patients with moderate to severe dehydration, initiate fluid resuscitation with isotonic fluid (0.9% saline, Ringer lactate)at the rate of 10–20 mL/kg.

Calculate the free water deficit: After restoration of effective circulatory volume, or in cases where there is no need for fluid resuscitation, calculate free water to correct the hypernatremia. Free water deficit = 0.6 × weight × ([current plasma Na/140] – 1); Example: 10 kg infant with a plasma sodium of 160, the free water deficit is: (0.6 L/kg) × (10 kg) × ([160/140] – 1) = 0.65 liters or 650 mL.

Rate of correction: For children with chronic hypernatremia (plasma sodium ≥150 mEq/L for greater than 24 hours) or those with acute severe hypernatremia (plasma sodium >160 mEq/L), rate of correction should not exceed a fall of sodium greater than 0.5 mEq/L per hour (i.e. 10 to 12 mEq/L per day).

Ongoing losses and maintenance needs: Children do have ongoing normal maintenance needs and may also have excess free water losses not accounted for by calculations for maintenance fluids (e.g. continuing diarrhea or persistent fever), and should receive replacement of these ongoing losses to prevent further electrolyte derangement. Since ongoing losses can fluctuate over time, it can be challenging to try to estimate them for inclusion in a fluid and electrolyte prescription

Treatment of specific etiologies: Initial evaluation and management of hypernatremia should occur simultaneously. Although most young children develop hypernatremia related to acute illness or inability to take in fluid, in cases where an underlying condition is identified, such as nephrogenic or central diabetes insipidus, treatment should be directed towards treating the cause. (e.g. administration of desmopressin in addition to providing free water replacement).

Example: A 10 kg child is estimated to have a 10% dehydration (approximately 1 litre) and a serum sodium concentration of 156 mEq/L. The following calculations can be made:

Total fluid deficit: 10% of 10 kg = 1000 mL; Free water deficit: 6 L [(156/140 mEq/L)–1] = 686 mL; Isotonic loss: Total fluid deficit - Water deficit = 314 mL.

During resuscitation, 20 mL/kg bolus of normal saline (200 mL) was given. Subsequent fluid regimen includes replacement of the free water deficit (686 mL) and remaining isotonic loss (314–200 = 114 mL), maintenance of usual daily sodium and fluid needs (1000 mL/day of N/2 saline), and any excess ongoing loss of fluid and electrolyte. The water deficit should be replaced over at least 36 hours so that the sodium is lowered at a rate below 0.5 mEq/L per hour. This is often accomplished by replacing two-thirds of the free water deficit over the first 24 hours and the remainder over the next 12 or more hours. Over the first 24 hours, fluid includes: Free water deficit (two-thirds of total water deficit) = 460 mL; Remaining isotonic deficit = 114 mL of water and 17 mEq of sodium; Maintenance needs = 1000 mL of water and 30 mEq of sodium. In this case, administration of one-quarter isotonic saline at 65 mL/hour would provide adequate replacement of maintenance needs and remaining isotonic deficit, and would provide free water at a rate lower than the maximum threshold rate of 0.5 mEq/L per hour. Enteral fluids can also be used to replace free water deficits and provide maintenance needs. In case seizures occur during rehydration, and serum Na^+ level has been lowered too rapidly, 3–5 mL/kg of 3% saline may be slowly injected. In most cases, hypernatremic dehydration can be treated with oral rehydration solution. Twice the clinically estimated deficit is administered either using the standard WHO oral rehydration solution, or the standard WHO solution and water in a ratio of 2:1 over 12–24 hours. Correction of hypernatremic dehydration with oral fluids is as effective as parenteral therapy but with considerably lower risk of complications.[25] Hypocalcemia is an occasional complication during treatment of hypernatremia and should be treated with administration of calcium gluconate. Severe acute hypernatremia (as in salt poisoning) should be treated with urgent dialysis (see further).

Hypernatremia in Diabetes Insipidus

Increasing the oral intake of water is usually sufficient in hemodynamically stable children. Administration of intravenous fluids containing 5% dextrose causes glucosuria and further loss of free water should be avoided. If there is peripheral circulatory failure, immediate measures are taken to expand the intravascular volume with isotonic solution. Thereafter, administration of fluids as calculated above along with administration of desmopressin is recommended.

An appropriate dose of vasopressin or desmopressin is the cornerstone of management of central diabetes insipidus. Intranasal desmopressin may be used in conscious patients. In unconscious patients, intravenous vasopressin infusion is started at 0.5 mU/kg/hour and titrated upward to achieve the desired effect.[26]

Salt Poisoning/Severe Hypernatremia (Plasma Na^+ >180 mEq/L)

In cases of salt poisoning, peritoneal dialysis is performed using a 8–10% dextrose solution without electrolytes.[27] Three cycles one hour apart are usually sufficient. Simultaneously fluids calculated as above should be administered. In patients with hypernatremia that has developed rapidly over a period of hours, rapid correction improves the prognosis without increasing the risk of cerebral edema. Severe hypernatremia due to causes other than salt poisoning, particularly if present for some time should be corrected gradually using commercially available peritoneal dialysis fluid (1.7–3%).

DISORDERS OF POTASSIUM HOMEOSTASIS

Potassium (K^+) is the chief cation of intracellular space. Of the total body K^+, over 90% is in the intracellular compartment, mostly in the muscle; the intracellular concentration is about 150 mEq/L of cell water. Its plasma concentration is closely maintained between 3.8–5.0 mEq/L (higher in newborn and preterm infants) and depends upon total body K^+ as well as its distribution between intracellular and extracellular compartments. The ECF K^+ modulates the electrical potential across cell membranes.

The high concentration of K^+ inside the cells is due to active influx of the ion mediated by the enzyme Na^+-K^+-ATPase. This enzyme is present in all cell membranes and pumps in two molecules of K^+ in exchange for 3 molecules of Na^+. K^+ efflux from the cells is stimulated by exercise, decrease in extracellular pH and increase in plasma osmolality. Its movement into the cells is increased by a rise in extracellular pH and by insulin, epinephrine, thyroxin and growth hormone. Insulin increases Na^+-K^+-ATPase activity and stimulates K^+ uptake within minutes. Beta-adrenergic agonists, such as salbutamol and terbutaline stimulate movement of K^+ into the cells.

K^+ is chiefly excreted by the kidney. Fecal losses are small, but may increase with high K^+ intake or when renal function is impaired. K^+ loss in sweating is normally negligible. Renal excretion of K^+ is slow with only 50% of an ingested load excreted in the first 4 hours. The major adaptation to a K^+ load is a shift of K^+ into the intracellular pool.

An intake of 2 mEq/kg/day of K^+ is adequate. Dairy products, foods from animal sources, some green vegetables and fruits are rich in K^+.

Hypokalemia

Important causes of hypokalemia (plasma K^+ below 3.5 mEq/L) are listed in **Table 10**. Common conditions such as protein energy malnutrition, chronic diarrhea, malabsorption and excessive diuretic use can easily be diagnosed. Diarrheal stools may contain as much as 15 mEq/L of K^+, while gastric juice contains about 10 mEq/L. In hypokalemia due to gastrointestinal or other non-renal conditions (e.g. excessive sweating, severe burns), the urinary K^+ concentration is below 10–20 mEq/L. The hypokalemia that occurs with vomiting or nasogastric suction is not caused by extrarenal losses from the gastrointestinal tract alone but is also consequence of renal loss that occurs secondary to metabolic alkalosis and secondary hyperaldosteronism.

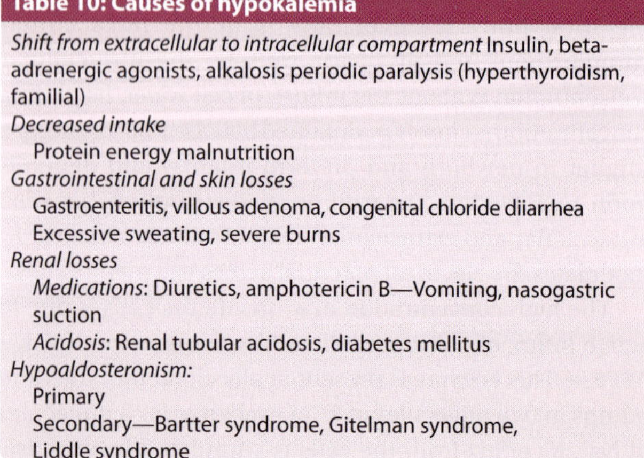

Table 10: Causes of hypokalemia

Shift from extracellular to intracellular compartment Insulin, beta-adrenergic agonists, alkalosis periodic paralysis (hyperthyroidism, familial)
Decreased intake
  Protein energy malnutrition
Gastrointestinal and skin losses
  Gastroenteritis, villous adenoma, congenital chloride diiarrhea
  Excessive sweating, severe burns
Renal losses
  Medications: Diuretics, amphotericin B—Vomiting, nasogastric suction
  Acidosis: Renal tubular acidosis, diabetes mellitus
Hypoaldosteronism:
  Primary
  Secondary—Bartter syndrome, Gitelman syndrome, Liddle syndrome

Important tubular disorders associated with excessive K^+ losses in urine (spot urinary K^+ >30 mEq/L) include Fanconi syndrome, distal renal tubular acidosis and Bartter syndrome. Excessive use of diuretics, mineralocorticoid excess and situations when large amounts of Na^+ are presented at the distal Na-K exchange sites lead to increased urinary K^+ losses and hypokalemia. Occasionally hypokalemia may result from a shift of K^+ from the extracellular to intracellular compartment, as in hypokalemic periodic paralysis. Treatment with β2-agonists such as salbutamol and terbutaline, in usual doses may occasionally cause hypokalemia.

Clinical and laboratory features

Mild to severe muscle weakness is characteristic. It is initially noted in limbs before involving trunk and respiratory muscles. In infants, paralytic ileus and gastric dilation are common. Cardiac arrhythmia and eventually cardiac arrest may occur. ECG shows depression of ST segment, low voltage T waves and appearance of U waves; premature ventricular contractions are common and rarely complete AV block may occur (**Fig. 1**). Hyponatremia and alkalosis aggravate ECG abnormalities. Chronic hypokalemia leads to impairment of urinary concentrating capacity and urinary acidification. Tubular glutamine synthesis and ammonia formation is increased resulting in alkaline urine with a high ammonium content. The levels of plasma K^+ by and large reflect the severity of its deficiency; levels below 2 mEq/L indicate a massive loss of intracellular K^+. Severe hypokalemia can cause paralysis and rhabdomyolysis.

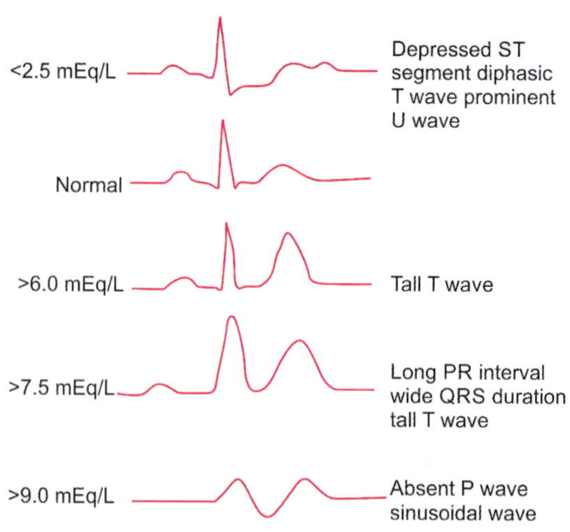

Fig. 1: ECG changes in potassium disturbances

Urinary K^+ excretion is helpful in evaluation of a patient with hypokalemia. If urinary K^+ is below 15 mEq/L, then extrarenal loss is likely. On the other hand, increased urinary K^+ in the presence of normal urinary output implies renal wasting.

Treatment

If severe muscle weakness, paralytic ileus or ECG abnormalities are present, K^+ is infused intravenously in an amount not exceeding 0.5–0.75 mEq/kg body weight in the first hour. In severe hypokalemia that does not respond to the above, infusion rates of 1 mEq/kg body weight per hour may be used for short periods under cardiac monitoring. The concentration of K^+ in the intravenous fluid should not exceed 40 mEq/L in a peripheral and 60 mEq/L in a central vein. In some situations, much higher concentrations of K^+ in the intravenous fluid may be used provided there is facility for continuous cardiac monitoring.[28] Potassium should be infused using an infusion pump, using a large vein for the infusion, e.g. femoral vein. Some authors recommend against use of a CVP line whose tip is in the heart for administration of high concentrations as the local increase in the K^+ concentration may have a deleterious effect on the cardiac conduction. K^+ is given in saline without glucose, since the latter may cause of shift of K^+ into the cells and aggravate hypokalemia. Continuous ECG monitoring and frequent estimations of serum K^+ levels are done to detect hyperkalemia.

Oral supplementation of K^+ may suffice if hypokalemia is relatively asymptomatic. Potassium chloride syrup (10%) contains 20 mEq K^+/15 mL solution. If hypokalemia is associated with metabolic alkalosis administration of chloride along with K^+ is crucial. In the presence of metabolic acidosis, K^+ should be administered as its acetate or citrate salt.

Patients showing lack of response to K^+ replacement may benefit with magnesium supplementation (magnesium sulfate 50%, 0.2 mL/kg twice daily for 3 days).[29]

Hyperkalemia

Hyperkalemia (serum K^+ level >5.5 mEq/L) is a relatively common emergency in children with renal disorders. The blood sample for K^+ measurement should be carefully obtained. Use of tourniquet, repeated clenching and opening of fist, and hemolysis (pushing blood sample through a fine needle) may cause a false rise in the level of serum K^+. Severe thrombocytosis and leukocytosis may also cause an increase in serum level of K^+ during clot retraction.

Causes

Important causes of hyperkalemia are listed in **Table 11**. Excessive intake of K^+ may lead to hyperkalemia if renal function is impaired, e.g. in the neonate or in the presence of renal disease. In such situations infusion of stored blood and drug formulations with high K^+ content may result in hyperkalemia. Acute renal failure is a common cause of hyperkalemia. In chronic renal failure, serum K^+ levels are kept within the normal range because of an adaptive increase in aldosterone secretion that causes increased K^+ excretion from the remaining normal nephrons and colonic mucosa. These are overcome toward the terminal phase of chronic renal failure, when hyperkalemia is observed.

True hyperkalemia can occur from K^+ shift from the intracellular to extracellular space, as seen with acidosis and lack of insulin. Several adrenal disorders (salt losing type of congenital adrenal hyperplasia, Addison disease and hypoaldosteronism) are characterized by hyperkalemia. Administration of certain drugs such as β-adrenergic blockers and angiotensin converting enzyme inhibitors leads to K^+ retention. High serum levels of K^+ (7–9 mEq/L) may be observed in very low birth weight infants.

Clinical and laboratory features

Muscular weakness, paresthesia, flaccid paralysis and cardiac arrhythmia are the chief manifestations.

Table 11: Important causes of hyperkalemia
Renal
Renal failure • Type IV renal tubular acidosis • Renal immaturity in very low birth weight babies
Endocrine
• Salt-losing congenital adrenal hyperplasia Addison disease • Pseudohypoaldosteronism type I and II • Spironolactone, amiloride, triamterene, cotrimoxazole ACE inhibitor therapy
Increased K^+ load
• Drugs (potassium chloride, penicillin) • Repeated blood transfusions • Rhabdomyolysis, hemolysis, large tissue bleeds • Hypercatabolic states (burns, surgery) • Tumor lysis syndrome
Shift of K^+ from cells
• Metabolic acidosis • Hyperkalemic periodic paralysis • Insulin deficiency • β-blocker drugs

Mild elevation in serum K^+ level (6.0–6.5 mEq/L) is associated with symmetrical peaking and increase in amplitude of T waves. At higher levels of serum K^+ there is widening of QRS complex and prolongation of PR interval. At serum K^+ levels of 7–8 mEq/L there is broadening and ultimately disappearance of P waves and further widening of QRS complexes results in a sine wave pattern. Arrhythmias include sinus bradycardia, atrioventricular block, idioventricular rhythm and asystole. A rapid rise in serum K^+ may cause ventricular asystole, tachycardia and fibrillation. Acidosis, hyponatremia and hypocalcemia increase the cardiac effects of hyperkalemia.

The transtubular K^+ gradient (TTKG) is a measure of net K^+ secretion by the distal nephron. The TTKG accounts for changes in urine osmolality that occur with water reabsorption in the collecting duct. It is expressed as:

$$\text{TTKG} = \frac{\text{Urine } K^+ \times \text{serum osmolality}}{\text{Serum } K^+ \times \text{urine osmolality}}$$

A value below 5–7 in the setting of hyperkalemia implies impaired distal tubular secretion of K^+ (aldosterone deficiency or resistance), whereas a value >10 suggests increased K^+ load and normal distal nephron handling of K^+.

Treatment

The urgency of treatment of hyperkalemia depends upon its severity, best assessed by ECG abnormalities. These are largely related to serum K^+ levels, but wrong techniques in blood sampling and laboratory error occasionally create confusion. Serum K^+ levels below 6.0 mEq/L usually do not produce ECG changes, while higher levels cause peaking of T waves. When QRS widening or arrhythmias are present severe hyperkalemia must be inferred and immediate treatment initiated.

Measures to treat hyperkalemia are listed in **Table 12**. Infusion of 10% calcium gluconate has an instantaneous but brief effect. Calcium gluconate antagonizes the toxic effect of hyperkalemia by raising the depolarization threshold for myocytes. It should be administered very slowly with ECG monitoring. The dose may be repeated if ECG abnormalities persist. Infusion of sodium bicarbonate and insulin-glucose should follow the administration of calcium gluconate. Glucose-insulin infusion may lower plasma K^+ concentration by 0.5–1.5 mEq/L, an effect that begins within 1 hour and may last for several hours.[30]

β2-agonists, administered parenterally or by nebulization, are effective in lowering blood levels of K^+. The dosage of salbutamol that is required for this effect is higher than used for bronchodilation.[31,32]

Measures to reduce total body K^+ should be instituted. If the patient has normal renal function and is volume depleted, saline infusion (2–4 mL/kg/hr) will increase the distal delivery of Na^+ and enhance K^+ excretion. Loop diuretics (furosemide 1 mg/kg) may be administered if there is volume overload. If there is poor renal function, K^+ clearance should be promoted either by enhancing its gut excretion (with K^+ binding resins), or by dialysis. Hyperkalemia in acute renal failure is usually associated with acidosis and other complications. Dialysis should be promptly instituted in such cases. Hyperkalemia is usually corrected after 4–6 hours of peritoneal dialysis.

Chronic hyperkalemia

In chronic renal failure, preventive measures should be taken. Dietary K^+ should be restricted, and K^+ retaining drugs such as β-blockers, ACE inhibitors and spironolactone avoided. Dehydration should be promptly treated. K^+ exchange resins [polystyrene sulfonate (Kayexalate) 1 g/kg/dose orally or rectally every 6 hours] decrease serum K^+ by 0.5–0.7 mEq/L over 6–8 hours. The drug is administered with enough fluids and sorbitol or lactulose to prevent constipation.

Table 12: Treatment of acute hyperkalemia

Drug	*Dose*	*Onset of action*	*Duration of action*	*Remarks*
Calcium gluconate (10%)	0.5–1 mL/kg IV	1–3 minutes	30 minutes	Give slowly under ECG control; bradycardia may occur
Sodium bicarbonate (7.5%)	1–2 mEq/kg IV	10–30 minutes	2 hours	Effect unpredictable; monitor ECG
Insulin and glucose	0.1–0.2 U/kg insulin with 0.5–1 g/kg glucose	20–30 minutes	2–4 hours	Risk of hypoglycemia
Salbutamol inhalation	0.15 mg/kg nebulization	30 minutes	4–6 hours	Tremor, hypokalemia, tachycardia
Polystyrene sulfonate	1 g/kg/dose	4 hours	6–8 hours	Bowel obstruction may occur with sorbitol and each g/kg of sorbitol reduces serum levels by 0.5–0.7 mEq/L

DISORDERS OF CALCIUM HOMEOSTASIS

Calcium is a cation available in extracellular fluid. Molecular weight of calcium is 40 g/mol and its valency is +2. Normal total serum calcium concentration is 8.5–10.2 mg/dL whereas ionic concentration of calcium is 4–5.2 mg/dL.

Hypocalcemia

Hypocalcemia is defined as serum calcium level less than 8.5 mg/L. Hypocalcemia causes several physiological changes in three major organs, i.e. bone, kidney and intestines to bring back the plasma calcium level to the normal levels. Hence, hypocalcemia activates calcium-sensing receptors in parathyroid and renal tubules. Action on parathyroid results in increased biosynthesis and secretion of parathyroid hormone (PTH) which acts in three different ways. (1) Increased calcium absorption and decreased phosphate absorption at renal tubular level. (2) Stimulation of osteoclasts in bone to cause its resorption to maintain serum calcium levels. (3) Stimulation of 1α-hydroxylase enzyme in the proximal renal tubule to increase 1,25-dihydroxyvitamin which in turn augments intestinal calcium absorption.[33] Common causes of hypocalcemia are listed in **Table 13**.

Symptoms and signs

The symptoms of hypocalcemia are related to disturbances in nerve and muscle conduction as hypocalcemia causes neuromuscular excitability. Paraesthesia, muscle cramps, seizures, tetany are common manifestation of hypocalcemia. Uncommon symptoms are stridor secondary to laryngeal spasm and apnea in infants. On examination, chvostek and trousseau signs can be elicited in hypocalcemia. ECG reveals prolonged QT interval. Chvostek and Trousseau signs can be elicited in hypocalcemia. Chvostek sign is gentle tapping 0.5–1.0 cm below the zygomatic process and anterior to ear lobe. A positive chvostek sign defined as twitching of ipsilateral corner of the mouth. Trousseau's sign is elicited by inflating BP cuff over the systolic pressure for 3 minutes which results flexion of wrist and metacarpophalangeal joints along with extension of the interphalangeal joints and adduction of fingers.[34]

Table 13: Etiology of hypocalcemia[33]

Vitamin D deficiency
• Impaired vitamin D metabolism • Impaired renal function
PTH related problem • Reduced PTH secretion • Impaired PTH function • Vitamin D disorder
Calcium-sensing receptor (CaSR) problem • Gain-of-function mutations in the gene encoding the CaSR • Activating antibodies to the CaSR

Investigations

Total serum calcium level including ionized calcium levels is desired. If ionic calcium levels are available, look at the albumin levels to measure corrected calcium levels as approximately 50% total calcium is bound to serum albumin. One of the commonly used methods to correct serum calcium: add 0.8 mg/dL of calcium for decrease in every 1 g/L serum albumin (considering 4 g/L as normal albumin level).[35] Example: For total serum calcium level of 7.5 mg/dL with serum albumin level of 2 g/L, corrected calcium would be 7.5 + [0.8(4–2)] = 9.1 mg/dL. Basic investigations which are to be ordered in case of hypocalcemia are listed in **Table 14**. Classification of hypocalcemia based on PTH levels is shown in **Table 15**.

Treatment

Management of hypocalcemia in emergency depends on severity of symptoms and underlying etiology of

Table 14: Basic investigations in hypocalcemia

Serum calcium, phosphate, alkaline phosphatase
Serum vitamin D, parathyroid hormone (PTH), X-ray wrist or knee
Serum albumin, creatinine and magnesium
Urine calcium/creatinine ratio

Table 15: Classification of hypocalcemia based on PTH levels[33]

Undetectable or low PTH levels • Hypoparathyroidism • Hypomagnesemia
Normal PTH levels • Abnormality of the calcium-sensing receptor
Elevated PTH levels • Pseudohypoparathyroidism • Vitamin D deficiency • Impaired vitamin D metabolism • Chronic renal failure • Osteopetrosis

Table 16: Symptoms and signs of hypercalcemia[38]

System	*Mild (10.5–11.9 mg/dL)*	*Moderate (12.0–13.9 mg/dL)*	*Severe (>14 mg/dL)*
Neuropsychiatric	Anxiety, depression	Cognitive dysfunction	Lethargy, confusion, stupor, coma
Gastrointestinal	Anorexia, nausea, constipation	Anorexia, nausea, constipation	Pancreatitis
Renal	Polyuria	Dehydration	Renal insufficiency, dehydration
Cardiac	Shortened QT interval	Shortened QT interval	Arrhythmia, ventricular tachycardia
Musculoskeletal	None	Weakness	Weakness

hypocalcemia. Intravenous calcium is required in case of seizures, laryngospasm, tetany, cardiovascular compromise such as septic shock. Commonly available intravenous calcium preparation is 10% calcium gluconate (1 mL contains 9.3 mg of elemental calcium). Intravenous dose of 0.5–1 mL/kg (maximum of 2 mL/kg) calcium gluconate diluted with normal saline or 5% dextrose (1:10 dilution) over 20 minutes i.e, not more than 5 mg of elemental calcium/min.[33] Intravenous calcium should be always infused under cardiac monitoring. Observe periodically for extravasation of intravenous calcium gluconate which may cause necrosis and subsequent scarring of the skin and subcutaneous tissues. Once the acute severe symptoms are subsided, discontinue intravenous supplementation and initiate oral calcium supplementation if feasible. For those children who do not need urgent correction of serum calcium, oral calcium supplementation can be administered upto maximum of 400 mg/kg/day. Once, acute symptomatic hypocalcemia is resolved, investigate for underlying etiology of hypocalcemia and manage accordingly.

Table 17: Etiology of hypercalcemia

PTH mediated causes
- Adenoma/hyperplasia of parathyroid gland
- Familial hypocalciuric hypercalcemia
- Multiple endocrine neoplasia syndromes (type 1, 2A)

Autosomal dominant hypocalciuric hypercalcemia

Malignancy
- Leukemia and lymphomas
- Rhabdomyosarcoma
- Renal carcinoma

Hypervitaminosis D
- Iatrogenic
- Excessive milk intake
- Granulomatous conditions such as sarcoidosis, tuberculosis or fungal infections

Hypervitaminosis A

Endocrine causes
- Thyrotoxicosis
- Hypoadrenalism
- Pheochromocytomas

Syndromic causes
- Williams syndrome, Murk Jansen syndrome

Miscellaneous
- Acute/Chronic renal failure
- Thiazide diuretics or lithium
- Milk-alkali syndrome
- Subcutaneous fat necrosis
- Prolonged immobilization

Hypercalcemia

Hypercalcemia is uncommon in children compared to hypocalcemia. Hypercalcemia is defined as serum calcium more than 10.2 mg/dL and symptoms usually appear when levels exceed 12 mg/dL.[36]

Symptoms and signs

Symptoms of hypercalcemia can be summarized as "groans, bones, stones and psychic moans". Common symptoms are polyuria, polydipsia, poor weight gain and failure to thrive, easy fatigability, irritability, confusion, anorexia, nausea, pain abdomen, vomiting and constipation. Severe hypercalcemia inhibits neuromuscular and myocardial depolarization causing arrhythmias and neuromuscular weakness. Severe acute abdominal pain could be a clue to suspect pancreatitis. Serum levels more than 14 mg/dL may result in encephalopathy. Bone related symptoms include bone pain, fractures, subperiosteal and endosteal bone resorption. Cardiovascular effects include prolonged PR interval, short QT interval, widened QRS complex, and bradycardia[37] (**Table 16**).

Etiology

Most common etiology of hypercalcemia is hyperparathyroidism. Various causes of hypercalcemia are listed in **Table 17**.

Table 18: Management of hypercalcemia[39]

Increasing calcium elimination	Twice maintenance fluid (isotonic fluid) Loop diuretics (I.V furosemide 1–2 mg/kg/day) in case of renal or cardiac disease only Hemodialysis (low calcium dialysate)
Reducing bone resorption	Bisphosphonates *Pamidronate*: 0.5–1.0 mg/kg as an infusion over 4–6 hours *Calcitonin*: 4 units/kg I.M/S.C q 12 hrly
Reducing calcium absorption (granulomatous conditions)	Steroids (1–2 mg/kg/day; 20–40 mg/day)

Treatment[39]

Treatment is required for symptomatic hypercalcemia and asymptomatic hypercalcemia with serum calcium more than 15 mg/dL. Management is shown in **Table 18**.

DISORDERS OF MAGNESIUM

Magnesium (Mg) is fourth most abundant cation and second most abundant intracellular cation in the human body. Less than 1% of total body Mg is present extracellular compartment. Mg acts as a co-factor for more than three hundred enzymatic reactions and required for bone stability, muscular relaxation, neurotransmission, etc. Serum Mg concentration is 1.5-1.9 mEq/L and 65% is ionized, 27% is protein bound and 8% is bound to citrate, phosphate and bicarbonate (8%). Common causes of magnesium deficiency are: malabsorption, sepsis, protein-energy malnutrition, hypoalbuminemia, hypothermia, prolonged gastrointestinal aspiration, blood transfusion, catecholamine excess, drugs such as loop diuretics, amphotericin B, aminoglycosides, cisplatin, calcineurin inhibitors, proton pump inhibitors, Bartter's syndrome, Gitelman syndrome and postoperative state.[40,41] Hypomagnesemia is defined as Mg level <1.4 mEq/L and hypermagnesemia is defined as >2 mEq/L. Hypermagnesemia is uncommon and hence is further not discussed.

Symptoms of Hypomagnesemia

Mg is essential for secretion of PTH and its activation and hence it exacerbates hypocalcemia. Hypomagnesemia is usually asymptomatic and may present with symptoms of hypocalcemia, tetany, cardiac arrhythmia, decreased bone stability, reduced seizure threshold, renal stones. Clinical and biochemical manifestations of hypocalcemia are shown in **Table 19**.

Table 19: Biochemical and clinical manifestations of hypomagnesemia

Biochemical Hypokalemia, renal potassium wasting, hypocalcemia, Impaired PTH secretion and resistance to vitamin D
Neuromuscular Tetany, carpo-pedal spasm, seizures, vertigo, ataxia, nystagmus, muscle weakness, tremor, fasciculation
Cardiovascular VT, SVT, AF, prolonged PR and QT interval, wide QRS, tall T waves, ST depression Vasospasm, hypertension

Table 20: Treatment of hypomagnesemia

Hypomagnesemia *Neonate*: 25–50 mg/kg/dose every 8–12 hours for 2–3 doses *Child*: 25–50 mg/kg/dose every 4–6 hours for 3–4 doses (maximum 2 g/dose)
Seizures *Child*: 20–100 mg/kg/dose every 4–6 hours (maximum 2 g/dose, however in severe cases doses as high as 200 mg/kg dose have been used)
Oral therapy (MgO) *Child*: 10–20 mg/kg per dose up to 4 times a day

Treatment of Hypomagnesemia[42]

Usual rate of Intravenous administration of magnesium is over 2-4 hours and not to exceed 125 mg/kg/min. recommended concentration of magnesium for infusion in peripheral line is 60 mg/mL and for central venous line is 200 mg/mL. Treatment of hypomagnesemia is shown in **Table 20**.

KEY MESSAGES

- Unlike adults, total body water (TBW) in healthy children decreases gradually from infancy to adolescence and ideal body weight is to be used especially in obese children while prescribing maintenance fluids.
- Fluid prescription to critically ill children based on Holliday and Segar formula may result in fluid overload and hence, fluid volume to be infused should be based on clinical scenario.
- Always consider lab error, false positive and false negative conditions while interpreting serum electrolyte values, especially when the clinical scenario does not match.

- Clinical symptoms and chronicity of electrolyte disturbance is to be taken into account while treating electrolyte imbalance (especially sodium).
- Urine sodium estimation is of paramount importance to identify etiology of sodium disturbances.
- Renal replacement therapy may be needed at times in refractory hypernatremia.
- Protein energy malnutrition, diarrheal losses and renal losses are the most common causes of hypokalemia and for asymptomatic hypokalemia, oral potassium supplementation is usually sufficient.
- Sodium bicarbonate, Insulin/Dextrose, Salbutamol nebulization are used for reducing serum potassium in very short duration, while polystyrene sulfonate should not be used as a sole agent to reduce serum potassium in case of hyperkalemia.
- Always consider serum albumin while interpreting serum calcium levels, and hypomagnesemia should be thought of in refractory hypocalcemia.
- Observe for extravasation of intravenous calcium gluconate which may cause necrosis and subsequent scarring of the skin and subcutaneous tissues.
- Treat severe electrolyte disturbances (K, Ca, Mg) always under continuous ECG monitoring.

REFERENCES

1. Friis-Hansen B. Body water compartments in children: Changes during growth and related changes in body composition. Pediatrics. 1961;28:169-81.
2. Finberg L. Water metabolism and regulation. In: Finberg L, Kravath RE, Hellerstein S, editors. Water and Electrolytes in Pediatrics: Physiology, Pathology, and Treatment, 2nd edition. Philadelphia: WB Saunders; 1993. p. 17-21.
3. Holliday MA, Segar WE. The maintenance need for water in parenteral fluid therapy. Pediatrics. 1957;19:823-32.
4. Freeman MA, Ayus JC, Moritz ML. Maintenance intravenous fluid prescribing practices among paediatric residents. Acta Paediatr. 2012;101(10):e465-68.
5. Lee JM, Jung Y, Lee SE, *et al.* Intravenous fluid prescription practices among pediatric residents in Korea. Korean J Pediatr. 2013;56:282-85.
6. Hoorn EJ, Geary D, Robb M, *et al.* Acute hyponatremia related to intravenous fluid administration in hospitalized children: An observational study. Pediatrics. 2004;113:1279-84.
7. Choong K, Arora S, Cheng J, *et al.* Hypotonic versus isotonic maintenance fluids after surgery for children: A randomized controlled trial. Pediatrics. 2011;128:857-66.
8. Drysdale SB, Coulson T, Cronin N, *et al.* The impact of the National Patient Safety Agency intravenous fluid alert on iatrogenic hyponatraemia in children. Eur J Pediatr. 2010; 169(7):813-7.
9. Feld LG, Neuspiel DR, Foster BA, *et al.* Clinical practice guideline: Maintenance intravenous fluids in children. Pediatrics. 2018;142:e 20183083.
10. Lamke LO, Liljedahl SO. Plasma volume changes after infusion of various plasma expanders. Resuscitation. 1976;5:93-102.
11. Singhi S, Prasad SVSS, Chugh KS. Hyponatremia in sick children: A marker of serious illness. Indian Pediatr. 1994;31:19
12. Spasovski G, Vanholder R, Allolio B, *et al.* Clinical practice guideline on diagnosis and treatment of hyponatraemia. Intensive Care Med. 2014;40(3):320-31.
13. Gruskin AB, Sarnaik A. Hyponatremia: Pathophysiology and treatment, a pediatric perspective. Pediatr Nephrol. 1992;6: 280-6.
14. Ayus JC, Krothapalli RK, Arieff AI. Changing concepts in treatment of severe symptomatic hyponatremia: Rapid correction and possible relation to central pontine myelinosis. Am J Med. 1985;78:897-902.
15. Sarnaik AP, Meert K, Hackbarth R, *et al.* Management of hyponatremic seizures in children with hypertonic saline: A safe and effective strategy. Crit Care Med. 1991;19:758-62.
16. Sterns RH, Cappuccio JD, Silver SM, *et al.* Neurologic sequelae after treatment of severe hyponatremia: A multicenteric perspective. J Am Soc Nephrol. 1994;4:1522-30.
17. Packer M, Medina N, Yushak M. Correction of dilutional hyponatremia in severe chronic heart failure by converting enzyme inhibition. Ann Intern Med. 1984;100:782-9.
18. Harrigan MR. Cerebral salt wasting syndrome: A review. Neurosurgery. 1996;38:152-60.
19. Maesaka JK, Gupta S, Fishbane S. Cerebral salt-wasting syndrome: Does it exist? Nephron. 1999;82:100-9.
20. Sakarcan A, Bocchini J. The role of fludrocortisone in a child with cerebral salt wasting. Pediatr Nephrol. 1998;12:769-71.
21. Raff H. Glucocorticoid inhibition of neurohypophyseal vasopressin secretion. Am J Physiol. 1987;252:R635.
22. Lee JH, Arcinue E, Ross BD. Organic osmolytes in the brain of an infant with hypernatremia. N Engl J Med. 1994;331:439-42.
23. Meadow R. Non-accidental salt poisoning. Arch Dis Child. 1993;68:448-52.
24. Srivastava RN, Bagga A. Pediatric Nephrology, 3rd edition. New Delhi: Jaypee Brothers Medical Publishers; 2001. p. 20.
25. Guzman C, Pizarro D, Castillo B, *et al.* Hypernatremic diarrheal dehydration treated with oral glucose-electrolyte solution containing 90 or 75 mEq/L of sodium. J Pediatr Gastroenterol Nutr. 1988;7:694-8.
26. Ralston C, Butt W. Continuous vasopressin replacement in diabetes insipidus. Arch Dis Child. 1990;65: 896-7.
27. el-Dahr S, Gomez RA, Campbell FG, *et al.* Rapid correction of acute salt poisoning by peritoneal dialysis. Pediatr Nephrol. 1987;1:602-4.
28. Kruse JA, Carlson RW. Rapid correction of hypokalemia using concentrated intravenous potassium chloride infusions. Arch Intern Med. 1990;150:613-7.
29. Whang R, Flink EB, Dyckner T, *et al.* Magnesium depletion as a cause of refractory potassium depletion. Arch Intern Med. 1985;145:1686-9.
30. Salem MM, Rosa RM, Batlle DC. Extrarenal potassium tolerance in chronic renal failure: Implications for the treatment of acute hyperkalemia. Am J Kidney Dis. 1991;18:421-40.
31. Greenberg A. Hyperkalemia: Treatment options. Semin Nephrol. 1998;18:46-57.

32. Mandelberg A, Krupnik Z, Houri S, *et al.* Salbutamol metered dose inhaler with spacer for hyperkalemia: How fast? How safe? Chest. 1999;115:617-22.
33. Allgrove J, Shaw NJ. Calcium and Bone Disorders in Children and Adolescents, 2nd, revised edition, volume 28. Endocr Dev. Basel, Karger; 2015. p. 84-100.
34. Schaaf M, Payne CA. Effect of diphenylhydantoin and phenobarbital on overt and latent tetany. N Engl J Med. 1966; 274:1228-33.
35. Parent X, Spielmann C, Hanser AM. "Corrected" calcium: Calcium status underestimation in non-hypoalbuminemic patients and in hypercalcemic patients. Ann Biol Clin (Paris). 2009;67(4):411-8.
36. Allgrove J, Shaw NJ. Calcium and Bone Disorders in Children and Adolescents, 2nd, revised edition, volume 28. Endocr Dev. Basel, Karger; 2015. p. 101-18.
37. Naganathan S, Gossman WG. Hypercalcemia. StatPearls; 2019. Available from: *http://www.ncbi.nlm.nih.gov/books/NBK430714*. [Accessed August 27, 2019].
38. Malangone S, Campen C. Hypercalcemia of malignancy. J Adv Pract Oncol. 2015;6(6):588.
39. Carrick AI, Costner HB. Rapid fire: Hypercalcemia. Emerg Med Clin North Am. 2018;36(3):549-55.
40. Singhi SC, Singh J, Prasad R. Hypo- and hypermagnesemia in an Indian Pediatric Intensive Care Unit. J Trop Pediatr. 2003; 49(2):99-103.
41. Haque A, Saleem AF. On admission hypomagnesemia in critically ill children: Risk factors and outcome. Indian J Pediatr. 2009;76(12):1227-30.
42. Kaplinsky C, Alon US. Magnesium homeostasis and hypomagnesemia in children with malignancy. Pediatr Blood Cancer. 2013;60(5):734-40.

CHAPTER

14

Acid-Base Disturbance

Samriti Gupta, Rakesh Lodha, Arvind Bagga

PHYSIOLOGY

Acid-base homeostasis influences the functioning of all body proteins, including enzymes thereby critically affecting tissue and organ performance. According to the Bronsted and Lowry definition, an acid is a donor of hydrogen ion (or proton) and base is an acceptor or hydrogen ion.[1,2] The pH of the body must be maintained within a narrow range of 7.35 to 7.45. Most body systems function optimally at a pH of near 7.4. Deviations of systemic pH in either direction can have adverse consequences and, when severe, can be life-threatening. Yet it is the nature of the condition responsible for severe acidemia or alkalemia that largely determines the patient's status and prognosis.

As the pH changes, enzymes may cease to function, nerve and muscle activity weakens, and finally all metabolic activity becomes deranged.[3] The composition of the cell depends upon the pH for two reasons: (i) as the pH changes so will the degree of ionization and, hence, the concentration of ionized substances; (ii) if the degree of ionization changes greatly, a substance may cease to be ionized and move out of the cell. In practice we neither measure nor directly treat the pH inside the cell. It is much closer to neutral (pH 6.8 at 37°C) than the extracellular fluid, but it varies from one part of the cell to another.

The extracellular fluid provides nutrition and oxygenation to the cell and determines its temperature, and alkalinity. The normal pH (7.4) represents a hydrogen ion (H^+) concentration of 40 nmol/L.[4] This is about one quarter its concentration inside the cell, 160 nmol/L. This four-fold concentration gradient favors H^+ elimination from the cell, but is counter-balanced by the intracellular potential of –60 mV (which tends to retain the ion within the cell). Regulation of the H^+ concentration at these low levels is essential for normal functioning of cells because of the high reactivity of H^+, particularly with the proteins.[3] H^+, because of its small size, is more strongly attracted to negatively charged portions of molecules and is more tightly bound than Na^+ or K^+.

Under normal circumstance, the H^+ concentration varies little from the normal value of approximately 40 nmol/L.[4] This maintenance of H^+ concentration in a very narrow range occurs even though acids and bases are continually being added to the extracellular fluid. The process of H^+ regulation involves: chemical buffering, control of the partial pressure of CO_2 in the blood by alterations in the rate of alveolar ventilation and control of the plasma bicarbonate (HCO_3^-) concentration by changes in the renal H^+ excretion.

Buffers are the substances that maintain the pH in the normal range even when the acid or base is added to the body. The pH at which an acid or base is in half of the dissociated form is called dissociation constant and is depicted as pK. Weak acids and bases have pK close to 7.4 and accept or donate the H^+ easily and hence they are best buffers.

The intracellular buffers include proteins, organic and inorganic phosphates, and hemoglobin within the erythrocytes. Bone also acts as an important buffering site.[5] Hemoglobin has a property that enables it to maintain pH within the capillaries. When combined with O_2, hemoglobin tends to release H^+ that have attached to the imidazole chain (it becomes a stronger acid). When hemoglobin is exposed to acid and lower O_2 concentrations in the capillaries, it gives up the O_2. It then becomes a weaker acid, taking up the extra H^+. This change maintains the pH in the capillaries despite the higher CO_2 concentration. An opposite change occurs when hemoglobin is exposed to the higher O_2 concentration in the lung. As it takes up oxygen, it becomes more acidic (more prone to release the H^+). The H^+ reacts with HCO_3^- to form carbonic acid, which in turn is converted to CO_2 and released into the alveoli. Hemoglobin is therefore not only an O_2 transporting molecule, but is also an acid-transporting system.

Other buffers exist in the human system of which the carbonic acid-bicarbonate buffer is the clinically most relevant. The carbonic acid-bicarbonate system is a classic chemical buffer. The body eliminates chemicals from either end of the chemical reaction to maintain the pH. In the case of bicarbonate in this buffer, the chemical reaction is:

$$H^+ + HCO_3^- \leftrightarrow H_2CO_3 \leftrightarrow H_2O + CO_2$$

This buffering system is very effective because of the ability to convert carbonic acid to carbon dioxide (through the enzyme carbonic anhydrase) which is then removed from the body through respiration. Changes in carbonic acid concentration occur rapidly (seconds) in response to hypo- or hyperventilation. On the other hand, changes in bicarbonate require hours or days through the relatively slow process of elimination by the kidney. The ratio of bicarbonate to carbonic acid determines the pH of the blood. Normally this ratio is about 20:1. This relationship is described in the Henderson-Hasselbalch equation:

$$pH = pK + \log(HCO_3^-/H_2CO_3)$$

(pK, the dissociation constant of the buffer is 6.10 at body temperature. The change in pK with temperature is the reason pH determinations must be adjusted for patients with abnormal temperatures).

As carbon dioxide is directly proportional to the carbonic acid (H_2CO_3), and can be directly measured, it will be substituted into the above equation.[6]

$$PaCO_2 = 33 \times H_2CO_3 \text{ or } H_2CO_3 = 0.03 \times PaCO_2$$

By substituting,

$$pH = pK + \log[HCO_3^-/(PaCO_2 \times 0.03)]$$

Thus by measuring serum pH and $PaCO_2$, the serum bicarbonate can be calculated as in most blood gas measurements:

$$\log(HCO_3^-) = pH + \log(PaCO_2) - 7.604$$

ACID ELIMINATION AND COMPENSATION

The body's own regulators of acid-base balance are the lungs and the kidneys, which are responsible for excreting the respiratory and metabolic acids respectively. The power of the lungs to excrete large quantities of carbon dioxide enables them to compensate rapidly. Unless the respiratory system is diseased or depressed, metabolic disturbances promptly stimulate partial respiratory compensation.

The elimination of acid is achieved by H^+ secretion ($Na^+ - H^+$ exchange in the proximal tubule and thick ascending limb of Henle; and active H^+ ATPase pump in the collecting tubules). The hydrogen ions are produced in the body from dietary protein metabolism, partial metabolism of fats and carbohydrates and excretion of bicarbonate in stool which is more significant in children with diarrhea. The daily acid load is not excreted as free H^+ ions; the secreted H^+ ions are excreted by binding either to filtered buffers such as HPO_2^-, or to NH_3 to form NH^+. The rate of NH_3 production can be varied according to the physiologic needs. The excretion of daily acid load also requires almost complete resorption of filtered HCO_3^-, as HCO_3^- loss in the urine is equivalent to addition of H^+ ions to the body.

There is a sequential response to H+ load in an attempt to restore the acid-base balance. Extracellular buffering of the excess H^+ by HCO_3^- occurs almost immediately. Respiratory compensation begins within several minutes. The hyperventilation leads to decrease in PCO_2 and increase of pH towards normal. In about 2–4 hours, the intracellular buffers, primarily proteins and organic phosphates, and bone provide further buffering. These responses prevent wide swings is the arterial pH until acid base homeostasis can be restored by the renal excretion of H^+. The corrective renal response begins early and is usually complete within 5 6 days. If there is metabolic alkalosis, the corrective renal action is more rapid, as the excess HCO_3^- is rapidly excreted in the urine.[7]

On the other hand, alterations in pH induced by changes in PCO_2 elicit a different response. There is no extracellular buffering since HCO_3^- cannot effectively

Table 1: Expected compensatory response to acid-base disorder

Abnormality	*Primary change*	*Expected compensatory response*
Metabolic acidosis	↓ HCO_3^-	Expected $PaCO_2$ = 1.5 [measured HCO_3] + 8 ± 2 mm Hg (Winter's formula)[8] or $PaCO_2$ decreases by 1–1.5 mm Hg for each 1 mEq/L fall in HCO_3^-
Metabolic alkalosis	↑ HCO_3^-	Expected $PaCO_2$ = 0.7 [measured HCO_3^- – 24] + 40 ± 2 mm Hg[9] or $PaCO_2$ increases by 0.25–1 mm Hg for each 1 mEq/L rise in HCO_3^-
Acute respiratory acidosis	↑ $PaCO_2$	↑ HCO_3^- by 1 mEq/L for each 10 mm Hg rise in $PaCO_2$
Chronic respiratory acidosis	↑ $PaCO_2$	↑ HCO_3^- by 4 mEq/L for each 10 mm Hg rise in $PaCO_2$
Acute respiratory alkalosis	↓ $PaCO_2$	↓ HCO_3^- by 1–3 mEq/L for each 10 mm Hg fall in $PaCO_2$
Chronic respiratory alkalosis	↓ $PaCO_2$	↓ HCO_3^- by 2–5 mEq/L for each 10 mm Hg fall in $PaCO_2$

buffer CO_2. There is no compensatory change in alveolar ventilation, since the abnormality in gas exchange is the primary problem. The intracellular buffering is the initial response occurring in 10-30 minutes. The intracellular buffers increase plasma HCO_3^- concentration by only 1 mEq/L for each 10 mm Hg rise in PCO_2. The renal compensation, by excretion of H^+ ions, begins within several hours, but takes a few days to complete.[5] In respiratory alkalosis, there is reduction of plasma HCO_3^- because of intracellular buffering and decrease in net acid excretion.

These changes discussed above are compensatory but not corrective. Acid-base homeostasis cannot be restored unless the primary problem is taken care of. **Table 1** shows the expected compensatory response.

ACID-BASE DISORDERS

Acidemia is defined as a decrease in the blood pH or an increase in H^+ concentration and alkalemia as an elevation in the blood pH. On the other hand, acidosis and alkalosis refer to processes that tend to lower and raise the pH, respectively. Usually, an acidotic process leads to acidemia and alkalotic process to alkalemia. However, in the mixed acid base disturbances, the final pH depends on the balance between the different disorders present.

Acidemia and alkalemia indicate the pH abnormality; acidosis and alkalosis indicate the pathologic process that is taking place.

Evaluation of acid-base status begins with the pH. If the pH is greater than 7.44, the patient is alkalemic and pH less than 7.36, the patient is acidemic. If the HCO_3^- is shifted in the direction of the pH, it may be the primary culprit. CO_2 is likely to be the primary culprit if it is shifted opposite to the pH. The pH is abnormal in majority of the patients with acid-base disturbance except in few circumstances where the pH will be maintained in normal range despite the acid base disturbance which includes, mixed metabolic acidosis and respiratory alkalosis in which the change in hydrogen ion concentration occur in the opposite direction in equal magnitude and the simple chronic respiratory alkalosis that can have adequate metabolic compensation.

After identifying the abnormal parameter (CO_2 or HCO_3^-), the other value is assessed. If that other value is abnormal, but in a direction that would move the pH back towards normal, then compensation is present.

Diagnosis of mixed acid-base disorders can be made if one takes into account the expected compensatory responses **(Table 1)** and deviations from these.

Metabolic Acidosis

Metabolic acidosis is characterized by low arterial blood pH, reduced plasma HCO_3^- and compensatory hyperventilation. Low plasma HCO_3^- alone is not diagnostic of metabolic acidosis since it may also result from the renal compensation to chronic respiratory alkalosis. These can be differentiated by measurement of the arterial pH. However, the plasma HCO_3^- of 10 mEq/L or less is indicative of metabolic acidosis, as the renal compensation to chronic hypocapnia does not lead to such low levels of plasma HCO_3^-.

Etiology

Metabolic acidosis results from either an inability of the kidney to excrete the dietary H^+ load or an increase in the generation of H^+ or the loss of HCO_3^-. Decreased H^+ excretion usually produces a slowly developing acidemia, while an acute increase in the H^+ load can overwhelm renal excretory capacity, leading to the rapid onset of significant metabolic acidosis. Rapid expansion of the extracellular fluid with a bicarbonate free solution may reduce bicarbonate concentration of extracellular fluid and cause acidosis. Loss of bicarbonate in gastrointestinal tract (diarrhea) and failure of its renal reabsorption (renal tubular acidosis) are common causes. The bicarbonate is replaced by chloride and serum chloride is elevated. Increased production of nonvolatile acids in the body such as phosphate, sulfate or organic acids (as in starvation, diabetes mellitus or renal failure) titrate bicarbonate and leads to metabolic acidosis. The blood chloride levels, in these cases, are normal. Several inborn errors of metabolism and poisonings are also important causes of metabolic acidosis. **Table 2** shows the important causes of metabolic acidosis.

Clinical features

The clinical manifestations of the underlying disorder causing metabolic acidosis are more prominent. The clinical manifestations of the metabolic acidosis depend on the severity of the acidosis and the respiratory function. Mild metabolic acidosis with appropriate respiratory compensation is clinically manifested by rapid and deep breathing (Kussmaul respiration). Fall in serum pH below 7.2 is associated with myocardial dysfunction with impaired contractility and when arterial blood pH falls below 7.1 there is increased risk of fatal ventricular arrhythmias and attenuate response to catecholamines.[10]

Table 2: Causes of metabolic acidosis

High anion gap
- Lactic acidosis
- Ketoacidosis: diabetes, starvation
- Renal failure
- Toxins, medications: salicylates, ethylene glycol, methanol, paraldehyde
- Inborn errors of metabolism
- Liver failure

Normal/low anion gap acidosis
- Gastrointestinal losses of bicarbonate
- Diarrhea
  - External intestinal drainage
  - Ureterosigmoidostomy, small bowel loops
  - Drugs causing diarrhea
- Renal tubular acidosis
- Acetazolamide
- Hypoaldosteronism
- Ammonium chloride loading
- Excessive administration of high chloride containing intravenous fluids such as normal saline

This myocardial dysfunction occur more so in children with underlying cardiac disease or when there is associated electrolyte abnormality is present. The decrease in ventricular function may have a role in persistence of shock-induced lactic acidosis. In newborn period the metabolic acidosis causes pulmonary vasoconstriction which aggravates persistent pulmonary hypertension.

Neurological symptoms, varying from lethargy to coma have been described in metabolic acidosis. However, these abnormalities are more common in respiratory acidosis. Chronic acidemia, as with renal failure and renal tubular acidosis, can result in skeletal problems due to release of calcium ions and phosphate during bone buffering of the excess H^+ ions. This also manifests in impaired growth. Other metabolic impairment that may occur with metabolic acidosis are hyperkalemia, insulin resistance, increased protein catabolism and reduced ATP synthesis that are seen more commonly with long-standing metabolic acidosis. In infants and young children, there may be non-specific symptoms as anorexia, vomiting, weight loss, muscles weakness and listlessness.[11] Failure to thrive and recurrent episodes of respiratory distress are also common in infants with longstanding metabolic acidosis.

Laboratory findings

The blood pH and HCO_3^- as well as PCO_2 levels are decreased. For every 1 mEq/L fall in blood HCO_3^-, the PCO_2 decreases by 1-1.5 mm Hg as a compensatory response; failure of that to occur indicates a respiratory contribution to acidosis. After confirming the presence of metabolic acidosis, calculation of the serum anion gap is a useful step in determining the underlying cause. The anion gap is equal to the difference between concentrations of the major cations (Na^+) and the major measured anions (Cl^- and HCO_3^-). The normal value of the anion gap is 12 ± 2 mEq/L. The normal value for anion gap should be revised downward by 2.5 mEq/L for every 1 g/dL decline in the plasma albumin concentration.[12] **Table 2** lists the causes of metabolic acidosis according to the anion gap.

The plasma anion gap is useful in various clinical settings. In the first setting, the presence or absence of increased anion gap is useful for determining the cause of metabolic acidosis. Thus, metabolic acidosis with an increased anion gap is usually attributable to disorders associated with the accumulation of either endogenous organic acids (lactic acidosis, ketoacidosis, renal failure) or exogenous organic acids (methanol, ethylene glycol, salicylate). The magnitude of the increase in the anion gap is important. With an anion gap of >25 mEq/L, an organic acidosis is nearly always present.[13] However, mild increases in the anion gap may be relatively insensitive for detecting the presence of mild-to-moderate organic acidoses, such as the lactic acidosis encountered in critically ill patients. In even classic cases considered to be characterized by the presence of an increased anion gap metabolic acidosis, such as diabetic ketoacidosis, an increase in anion gap often cannot be demonstrated due to other acid-base disturbances and variations in fluid status.

The second setting in which the anion gap may be useful is when ascertaining if a mixed acid-base disturbance is present through the calculation of the ratio of the change in the anion gap and the change in the serum bicarbonate termed as delta-delta gap.[14] This calculation is based on the assumption that each milliequivalent of acid added to the body will reduce the serum bicarbonate by an equivalent amount. The normal value is between 1 and 2. Therefore, when the change in the anion gap is larger than the change in the serum bicarbonate, this implies an additional source of base (metabolic alkalosis). When the change in the anion gap is less than the change in the serum bicarbonate, this implies an additional source of acid (non-anion gap metabolic acidosis).

Measurement of urinary pH cannot reliably differentiate acidosis of renal origin from that of extrarenal origin. A useful method to distinguish extrarenal from renal causes of metabolic acidosis is to measure urinary ammonium excretion. Extrarenal causes of metabolic acidosis are associated with an appropriate increase in urine acid excretion, primarily shown by high levels of urinary ammonium. In contrast, the net acid excretion and urinary ammonium levels are low in metabolic acidosis of renal origin. Measurement of urinary ammonium excretion is, however, cumber- some and not a commonly available test in most laboratories. One can, however, indirectly assess the amount of urinary ammonium by calculating the urine anion gap.[15]

Urinary anion gap

$$(UAG) = (UNa^{+} + UK^{+}) - UCl^{-}$$

Under normal conditions the urinary anion gap is positive, with values between 20–50 mEq/L. A negative value suggests presence of increased renal excretion of an unmeasured cation (other than Na^{+} or K^{+}). One such cation is ammonium. Metabolic acidosis of extrarenal origin is associated with an increase in urinary ammonium, and a negative urinary anion gap. If the metabolic acidosis is of renal origin like in renal tubular acidosis, urinary ammonium excretion is low and the urinary anion gap is positive. However, the urinary anion gap becomes unreliable when polyuria is present, when the urine pH exceeds 6.5, or when urinary ammonium is excreted with an anion other than chloride (e.g. keto acids, acetylsalicylic acid, D-lactic acid, and large quantities of penicillin).[16] The usefulness of the urinary anion gap is questionable when the urinary sodium level is less than 20 mmol per liter as urinary acidification depends upon adequate delivery of sodium to the distal collecting tubule.[17] In such cases, the urinary osmolal gap is generally more reliable.

The urinary osmolal gap determines the difference between measured and calculated urinary osmolality. The urinary osmolality is calculated as follows:

$$(2 \times [Na^{+}] + 2 \times [K^{+}]) + (\text{urine urea nitrogen in millimoles/L}) + (\text{urine glucose in millimoles/L}).$$

A urinary osmolal gap below 40 mmol per liter in normal anion-gap acidosis indicates impairment in excretion of urinary ammonium. The urinary osmolal gap reflects the level of ammonium in most of the cases, except in the presence of large quantities of a nondissociated acid, such as β-hydroxybutyric acid in ketoacidosis. The urinary osmolal gap is better correlated with the urinary ammonium value as compared to the urinary anion gap.[18]

Blood urea, creatinine, blood glucose, electrolytes and urinalysis are done to look for the cause of metabolic acidosis. The serum potassium level is most important as it is elevated abnormally and can cause fatal cardiac arrhythmia. If there is hypokalemia with metabolic acidosis, the differential diagnoses are narrowed which include, the diarrhea, renal tubular acidosis (proximal and distal) and use of diuretic acetazolamide.

Treatment

While in most conditions, correction of the acidemia can be achieved by the administration of $NaHCO_3$, it is more important to correct the underlying disorder. The initial therapeutic goal in patients with severe acidemia is to raise the systemic pH to above 7.1–7.2, a level at which arrhythmias become less likely. At this pH, the cardiac contractility and responsiveness to catecholamines is likely to be restored. Rapid administration of sodium bicarbonate is important only in patients with severe metabolic acidosis; this should be done only if ventilation is adequate. Exogenous sodium bicarbonate is usually not required if the initial arterial pH is greater than 7.20, the child is asymptomatic and the underlying process can be controlled.

The amount of HCO_3^- required to correct the acidemia can be estimated by the formula:

$$HCO_3^- \text{ required} = 0.6 \times \text{body weight} \times HCO_3^- \text{ deficit/L}$$

Another formula for requirement of bicarbonate infusion is:

$$HCO_3^- (mEq) \text{ deficit} = [HCO_3^- \text{ desired} - HCO_3^- \text{ actual}] \times \text{weight (kg)} \times 0.3 \text{ where } HCO_3^- \text{ desired} = 15 \text{ mEq/L.}$$

Desired bicarbonate level of 15 is usually taken with distribution volume of 30% to tide over the critical situation and also to avoid potential side effects.

The intravenous bicarbonate solution should be isosmolar (about 1.5%), diluted with equal volume of distilled water and preferably be administered through a central venous line. Half of the calculated dose is administered in 1–4 hours. Further requirement will depend upon clinical assessment and repeat measurement. The added HCO_3^- produces a large increase in the plasma HCO_3^- concentration within a few minutes. Thereafter, the change is attenuated as the exogenous HCO_3^- equilibrates with the intracellular and bone buffers. Therefore, measurement of pH shortly after administration of HCO_3^- may overestimate the final effect of the treatment. Sodium bicarbonate may be given as a bolus at a dose of 1 mEq/kg in emergency situation.

The infused volume and amount of sodium provided simultaneously must be considered. Alternative approach is to add sodium bicarbonate or sodium acetate with simultaneous removal of equal amount of sodium chloride from patient's intravenous fluids.

Alkali therapy is usually not required in lactic acidosis or ketoacidosis where the metabolism of the organic anions will regenerate HCO_3^-. Similarly, citrate salts of sodium or potassium may be preferable in the chronic treatment of renal tubular acidosis.

Metabolic acidosis due to diarrheal losses should be corrected by expansion of extracellular fluid with Ringer's lactate solution. Correction of the underlying disorder is the primary therapy in lactic acidosis. For example, reversal of circulatory failure will reduce the output of lactate and allow metabolism of lactate to HCO^-_3. The role of sodium bicarbonate therapy in lactic acidosis is controversial.[19] Theoretically, the benefits of increase in arterial blood pH include improvement in tissue perfusion, by correction of vasodilatation and improvement in cardiac contractility. However, the potential adverse effects are volume overload, hypernatremia, hypocalcemia, hypokalemia, metabolic alkalosis and paradoxical intracellular acidosis. Current evidence does not support routine use of sodium bicarbonate in treatment of lactic acidosis.[20] However, a small amount of sodium bicarbonate may be administered to patients with severe metabolic acidosis to raise the pH to 7.10.

In diabetic ketoacidosis, insulin is the mainstay of therapy. However, sodium bicarbonate therapy may be beneficial if there is marked acidemia (pH < 6.9). It may also be useful in patients with relatively normal anion gap because of excretion of ketoacids in the urine; as in this condition, the quantity of sodium bicarbonate generated from metabolism of organic anions is likely to be low.

In renal failure, exogenous alkali therapy is not used routinely. Usually in most patients, the arterial pH is maintained close to 7.3 because of respiratory compensation. Attempts to increase pH in presence of hypocalcemia can precipitate tetany. There is also a risk of volume expansion. Sodium bicarbonate therapy is indicated if the plasma HCO_3^- is less than 12 mEq/L, the patients are symptomatic or there is persistent hyperkalemia. In children, alkali therapy is used more frequently, as acidemia interferes with growth. In renal failure, the alkali of choice is sodium bicarbonate. Citrate may increase aluminum absorption in children receiving aluminum hydroxide.[21]

The aim of correction of acidosis in renal tubular acidosis is to allow normal growth, to minimize nephrocalcinosis, renal calculus formation and to prevent osteopenia due to calcium loss from the bone, and to diminish excessive urinary K^+ losses.[11] Patients may be treated with sodium bicarbonate or citrate salts.

Sodium bicarbonate administration is helpful in poisoning due to salicylates, tricyclic antidepressant, ethylene glycol and methanol as they help in eliminating the poisonous agent through renal route. Long term sodium bicarbonate therapy may be necessary in cases of inborn error of metabolism.

Tromethamine (Tris-buffer or Tham) causes neutralization of acids without releasing CO_2 and hence is an option in mixed metabolic and respiratory acidosis. It can be used in conditions where $NaHCO_3$ cannot be administrated because of risk of hypernatremia.[22] However, this preparation is not currently available in India.

Dialysis, either peritoneal or hemodialysis, may be an option in treatment of severe metabolic acidosis due to renal failure or methanol or ethylene glycol poisoning.

Metabolic Alkalosis

Metabolic alkalosis is characterized by an increase in the arterial pH, an increase in the plasma HCO_3^- concentration and compensatory hypoventilation. The kidney normally responds to an increase in HCO_3^- by rapidly excreting the excess alkali. Sustained metabolic alkalosis thus occurs when some additional factor disrupts the renal regulation of body alkali stores. Metabolic alkalosis commonly occur secondary to vomiting in children.

Etiology

Most of the conditions leading to metabolic alkalosis are characterized by enhanced renal reabsorption of bicarbonate due to depletion of volume, chloride or potassium[23] (**Table 3**). Removal of gastric secretions leads to metabolic alkalosis. Since there is no stimulus for pancreatic HCO_3^- secretion; this results in increase in plasma HCO_3^-.[24] Persistent vomiting is also associated with increased renal H^+ loss. In conditions with mineralocorticoid excess, aldosterone promotes H^+ secretion by stimulating the distal H^+-ATPase pump. In addition, hypokalemia, due to increased K^+ losses plays an important role in metabolic alkalosis by causing volume contraction and increase in urinary H^+ loss.

The causes of metabolic alkalosis can be divided into chloride responsive and chloride resistant.

Often alkalosis is seen in patients in whom chronic respiratory acidosis is corrected rapidly. The compensatory response to respiratory acidosis is increase in urinary H^+ secretion and increase in plasma HCO_3^-. If such a patient is mechanically ventilated and CO_2 brought down rapidly, the plasma HCO_3^- still remains high and leads to metabolic alkalosis.

Table 3: Causes of metabolic alkalosis

Chloride responsive alkalosis (Urine Cl^- < 25 mEq/L)
- Vomiting or gastric drainage
- Diuretics
- After correcting prolonged hypercapnia
- Low chloride intake
- Chloride losing diarrhea
- Cystic fibrosis

Chloride-resistant alkalosis (Urine Cl^- > 40 mEq/L)

High blood pressure:
- Cushing syndrome
- Primary hyperaldosteronism
- Renovascular disease
- Renin-secreting tumor
- Congenital adrenal insufficiency

Normal/Low blood pressure:
- Bartter syndrome
- Gitelman syndrome
- Severe hypokalemia
- Excessive bicarbonate therapy
- Milk alkali syndrome

The causes of chloride responsive metabolic alkalosis are vomiting or nasogastric suction, diuretics, low chloride intake and post-hypercapnia. These conditions can be reversed by administration of sodium chloride and water, by intravenous or oral route. These act by (1) reversing the depletion of volume and Cl^- thereby removing stimulus for renal Na^+ retention, and allowing sodium bicarbonate excretion in the urine; and (ii) by increasing distal Cl^- delivery, which promotes HCO^- secretion.

The chloride resistant causes are the ones where K depletion, not hypovolemia, is responsible for alkalosis. These include edematous states, mineralocorticoid excess, severe hypokalemia and renal failure. In edematous states, frequent use of diuretics is responsible for metabolic alkalosis. Even though volume depletion contributes to the pathogenesis, saline administration is not indicated as it will increase the edema and the risk of pulmonary edema.

Hypokalemia is frequently observed in patients with metabolic alkalosis. This is because (i) many conditions cause both H^+ and K^+ loss; (ii) hypokalemia causes migration of K^+ out of the cells and H^+ into the cells; and (iii) hypokalemia increases urinary acid excretion and HCO_3^- reabsorption.

Clinical features

The clinical features of metabolic alkalosis depend on the underlying cause. Mild metabolic alkalosis is well tolerated with no clinically significant adverse effects. The most serious effects of moderate metabolic alkalosis (HCO_3^- >40 mEq/L) occur due to associated hypokalemia and hypocalcemia. Chloride responsive metabolic alkalosis is associated with volume depleted and can have the manifestations of hypovolemia while chloride unresponsive metabolic alkalosis may have features of hypertension. With more severe metabolic alkalosis, hypoxemia can develop as a result of the hypoventilation. Patients may present with seizures, tetany and altered sensorium.

Diagnosis

The finding of serum HCO_3^- > 28–30 mEq/L in association with hypokalemia is diagnostic of metabolic alkalosis.

Elevated plasma bicarbonate, hypercapnia, and hypoxemia may be seen in respiratory acidosis also, but this can be differentiated easily by the pH. However, a combination of respiratory acidosis and metabolic alkalosis may be difficult to interpret.

The etiology of metabolic alkalosis usually can be elicited from history. Measurement of urinary chloride is helpful in differentiating chloride responsive (Cl^- < 25 mEq/L) from chloride resistant (Cl^- > 40 mEq/L) forms. Primary hyperaldosteronism is characterized by a combination of hypertension and metabolic alkalosis. Measurement of plasma renin and aldosterone levels is useful in differentiating syndromes of mineralocorticoid excess from those with apparent mineralocorticoid excess. In a normotensive or hypotensive child with chloride resistant metabolic alkalosis, the diagnosis of Bartter or Gitelman syndrome is highly probable.

Therapy

The aim of therapy is to correct the volume, Cl^- and K^+ deficits. Efforts should be directed at correction of underlying disease. Oral or intravenous administration of sodium chloride and water is indicated in chloride responsive causes of metabolic alkalosis. With the exception of hypotension or shock or severe metabolic derangement, gradual correction is preferable to avoid complications of volume overload. The efficacy of such treatment can be assessed bedside by monitoring the urine pH. Urine pH, which is often below 5.5 before therapy, increases to beyond 7.0 once volume and chloride are replaced.

The administration of saline is usually ineffective in chloride resistant causes of metabolic alkalosis and can worsen hypertension. In patients with edematous states, withholding diuretics is the corrective therapy. Acetazolamide may be used to treat both edema and alkalosis, where withholding diuretics alone does not help.[25] Correction of severe hypokalemia (as in states of mineralocorticoid excess) leads to correction of alkalosis.

Respiratory Acidosis

Respiratory acidosis is characterized by a reduced arterial blood pH, an elevated PCO_2 and an increase in plasma HCO_3^- concentration.

Etiology

Hypercapnia and respiratory acidosis are almost always due to a reduction in alveolar ventilation and not due to increase in CO_2 production (**Table 4**). Hypoventilation, as seen in patients with reduced respiratory drive or neuromuscular dysfunction, leads to a generalized fall in the alveolar ventilation. On the other hand, CO_2 retention in intrinsic pulmonary disease occurs primarily due to an imbalance between ventilation and perfusion.

If the ventilation is not improved, the cell buffers and increase in renal H^+ secretion minimize the decrease in pH. However, the latter occurs over several days and the protection of the extracellular pH in acute respiratory acidosis is much less efficient than that seen in chronic respiratory acidosis.

The common causes of acute respiratory acidosis include severe pneumonia, asthma, pulmonary edema, acute exacerbation of existing pulmonary disease and suppression of the respiratory center following drug toxicity or administration of excessive oxygen to a patient with chronic hypercapnia.

Important causes of chronic respiratory acidosis in children are chronic lung disease, cystic fibrosis, extensive bronchiectasis and neuromuscular defects. Upper airway diseases cause hypoventilation secondary to decreased

Table 4: Causes of respiratory acidosis

Acute
Normal (A-a) O_2 difference
• Central respiratory center depression
– Cerebral disease (encephalitis or trauma)
– Drugs (narcotics, barbiturates, or benzodiazepines)
High (A-a) O_2 difference
• Acute airway obstruction
– Acute exacerbation of asthma
– Obstructive sleep apnea
• Pneumonia
• Acute respiratory distress syndrome
• Pulmonary edema
• Pneumothorax
Chronic
Normal (A-a) O_2 difference
• Neuromuscular disease -Myasthenia gravis, Guillain-Barré syndrome, muscular dystrophy, amyotrophic lateral sclerosis
• Chest wall deformities-Kyphoscoliosis
• Extreme obesity
High (A-a) O_2 difference
• Chronic obstructive pulmonary disease

(A-a) O_2 difference: alveolo-arterial oxygen gradient

air entry into lungs. Children with mild or moderate lung diseases cause respiratory alkalosis due to hyperventilation which occurs as a result of mild hypoxia or stimulation of lung mechanoreceptors. Severe lung diseases will have respiratory acidosis either due to hypoventilation secondary to airway obstruction or respiratory muscle fatigue or due to severe ventilation: perfusion mismatch.

Clinical features

The clinical features of respiratory acidosis depend on the underlying cause. In children with respiratory acidosis due to hypoventilation due to central nervous system depression or respiratory muscle fatigue and respiratory failure will have bradypnea, hypoxia and altered sensorium while respiratory acidosis due to pulmonary or airway obstruction will have tachycardia, tachypnea, respiratory difficulty and features of hypoxia. Severe acute respiratory acidosis may lead to symptoms of restlessness, anxiety, headache, blurred vision and excessive sweating.[26] Excessive CO_2 retention may lead to CO_2 narcosis as manifested by tremors, asterixis, delirium and excessive sleep. There may be features of raised intracranial pressure. Severe acidosis may also lead to significant vasodilatation and hypotension. With fall in arterial pH, the impairment in cardiac function, altered response to catecholamine and cardiac arrhythmia can also occur similar to metabolic acidosis. Rise in serum potassium can also occur in children with respiratory acidosis but less prominent compared to metabolic acidosis.

Diagnosis

The presence of acidemia and elevated PCO_2 is diagnostic of respiratory acidosis. In order to determine whether it is acute or chronic, an accurate history and good examination are essential. Children with altered sensorium may have severe central nervous system disease, drug intoxication or carbon dioxide narcosis. Tachypnea, respiratory distress, wheezing, crepitations and stridor may be present in pulmonary or airway diseases.

It is always important to remember the expected compensations in acute and chronic respiratory acidosis to determine presence of mixed metabolic and respiratory abnormalities.

Calculation of alveolo-arterial oxygen gradient [(A-a) DO_2] can assist in determining the etiology. It is usually increased in patients with intrinsic pulmonary disease. A normal gradient usually excludes pulmonary disease and indicates central alveolar hypoventilation or abnormalities of chest wall or muscles of breathing.

Treatment

Patients with acute respiratory acidosis often have both hypercapnia and hypoxemia. While the hypoxemia can usually be corrected by increasing the FiO_2, correction of hypercapnia requires increase in alveolar ventilation. This can be achieved by reversing the underlying condition or by mechanical ventilation. Mechanical ventilation in respiratory acidosis is indicated in following conditions: PCO_2 >75 mm Hg, CNS depression, hypoxia refractory to supplemental oxygen, or increased work of breathing with impending respiratory failure. While the primary aim of therapy is to restore normal alveolar ventilation, some authors recommend infusion of small doses of $NaHCO_3$ to correct the pH, particularly in status asthmaticus.[27] This is done primarily to minimize the ventilatory settings in order to prevent barotrauma and air leaks, while accepting higher PCO_2 values. However, there are risks of volume overload, hypernatremia, and persistence or worsening of tissue acidosis.

Usually, the conditions leading to chronic respiratory failure are not entirely correctable. Hence, the goal of therapy is to maintain adequate oxygenation and if possible improve alveolar ventilation. Because of the efficient renal compensation, the pH is usually maintained. In children with cor pulmonale, use of diuretics may be helpful in raising the pH further. Attempts should be made to correct reversible components, e.g. appropriate use of bronchodilators, treatment of infections. Sedatives and excessive O_2 supplementation should be avoided as they act as respiratory depressants. Low flow O_2 therapy is useful in reversing hypoxemia and improving blood flow. Mechanical ventilation is usually limited to condition with an acute exacerbation. In this setting, the goal of therapy is restoration of the baseline $PaCO_2$ of the patient if known rather than targeting for normal $PaCO_2$ or attaining $PaCO_2$ of 60 mm Hg is acceptable if the baseline $PaCO_2$ is not known. PCO_2 should be lowered gradually, as a rapid decline can lead to alkalemia.

The current therapeutic approach in mechanical ventilation is use of lung protective strategy which includes low tidal volumes of 5–8 mL/kg of ideal body weight and plateau pressure below 30 cm of H_2O in order to prevent ventilator-induced lung injury by avoiding volutrauma along with permissive hypercapnia in which a pH goal above 7.25 should be maintained for maintaining adequate cellular and myocardial function irrespective of pCO_2 levels.[28] Sedation with or without neuromuscular paralysis is usually required to overcome patient discomfort commonly associated with lung protective strategies. Noninvasive ventilation is another option for respiratory acidosis in selected patients with normal sensorium. Other measures to decrease production of CO_2 include reducing the dietary carbohydrate load, treatment of fever and sedation to reduce anxiety in patients.

Respiratory Alkalosis

Respiratory alkalosis is characterized by elevated arterial blood pH, a low PCO_2 and a reduction in plasma HCO_3^- concentration.

Etiology

A decrease in PCO_2 will occur when the alveolar ventilation is increased beyond the level needed to eliminate the load of CO_2 produced. Primary hyperventilation leading to respiratory alkalosis can result from hypoxemia, anemia and pulmonary disease (**Table 5**). Pain, anxiety, stimulation of mechano-receptors within the respiratory systems, and direct stimulation of respiratory center by various conditions and chemicals can also cause hyperventilation.

Clinical features and diagnosis

The clinical features are due to the ability of alkalosis to impair cerebral function and to increase cell membrane excitability. Profound respiratory alkalosis can reduce cerebral blood flow. The symptoms include altered consciousness, paresthesiae, cramps and carpopedal spasms. In critically ill patients, supraventricular and ventricular arrhythmias may also occur. The diagnosis can be confirmed by the arterial blood gas result. Based on the clinical setting, history and examination, the underlying condition can be diagnosed.

Treatment

Hyperventilation is done in some patients with raised intracranial tension. Correction of alkalemia is not required and the management should be directed at the diagnosis and correction of the underlying disorder. In severely symptomatic patients, rebreathing into a reservoir (to increase PCO_2 in inspired air) may partially increase PCO_2 and relieve the symptoms. Iatrogenic respiratory alkalosis is to be corrected by adjusting mechanical ventilator settings. For hyperventilation secondary to anxiety, child should be reassured; benzodiazepines may be useful.

Table 6 lists terminologies used in blood gas analysis reports. **Flowcharts 1** and **2** demonstrate the diagnostic approach to acidosis and alkalosis respectively.

Table 5: Causes of respiratory alkalosis

Acute
Normal (A-a) O_2 difference Fever, Pain, anxiety, severe anemia, stroke, meningitis, trauma, salicylate toxicity
High (A-a) O_2 difference Pneumonia, aspiration, pulmonary edema, pulmonary embolism, sepsis, congestive heart failure
Chronic
Normal (A-a) O_2 difference Pregnancy, hyperthyroidism, hepatic failure
High (A-a) O_2 difference Liver failure with aspiration pneumonia

Table 6: Terminology used in blood gas analysis reports

Term	*Explanation*	*Normal values*
pH	Negative logarithm of H^+ ion concentration	7.35–7.45
PCO_2	Partial pressure of CO_2 in blood	36–44 mm Hg
PO_2	Partial pressure of O_2 in blood	80–100 mm Hg
Base excess (BE)	Actual base excess in variance from (above or below) total buffer base	–2 to +2 mEq/L
Buffer base (BB)	Buffer base represents the buffering capacity	48–50 mEq/L
HCO_3^-	Actual plasma bicarbonate concentration (derived from blood pH, PCO_2)	22–26 mEq/L
Standard HCO_3^- (SBC)	Plasma bicarbonate value at PCO_2 40 mm Hg and temperature 37°C	22–26 mEq/L

Contd...

Contd...

Term	*Explanation*	*Normal values*
TCO_2	Total CO_2 is the sum of HCO_3^- and the amount of CO_2 dissolved in plasma (for each mm Hg PCO_2, 0.03 mL CO_2 is dissolved in 100 mL plasma)	23–27 mmol/L
Standard pH	pH adjusted for PCO_2 of 40 mm Hg and a temperature of 37°C. This represents pH purely due to metabolic status	7.35–7.45
O_2 content	Sum of O_2 bound to hemoglobin and oxygen dissolved in plasma (For each gram of saturated hemoglobin, 1.34 mL O_2 is bound to it, and for each mm Hg PO_2 0.003 mL O_2 is dissolved in 100 mL plasma)	

Flowchart 1: Diagnostic approach to acidosis[29]

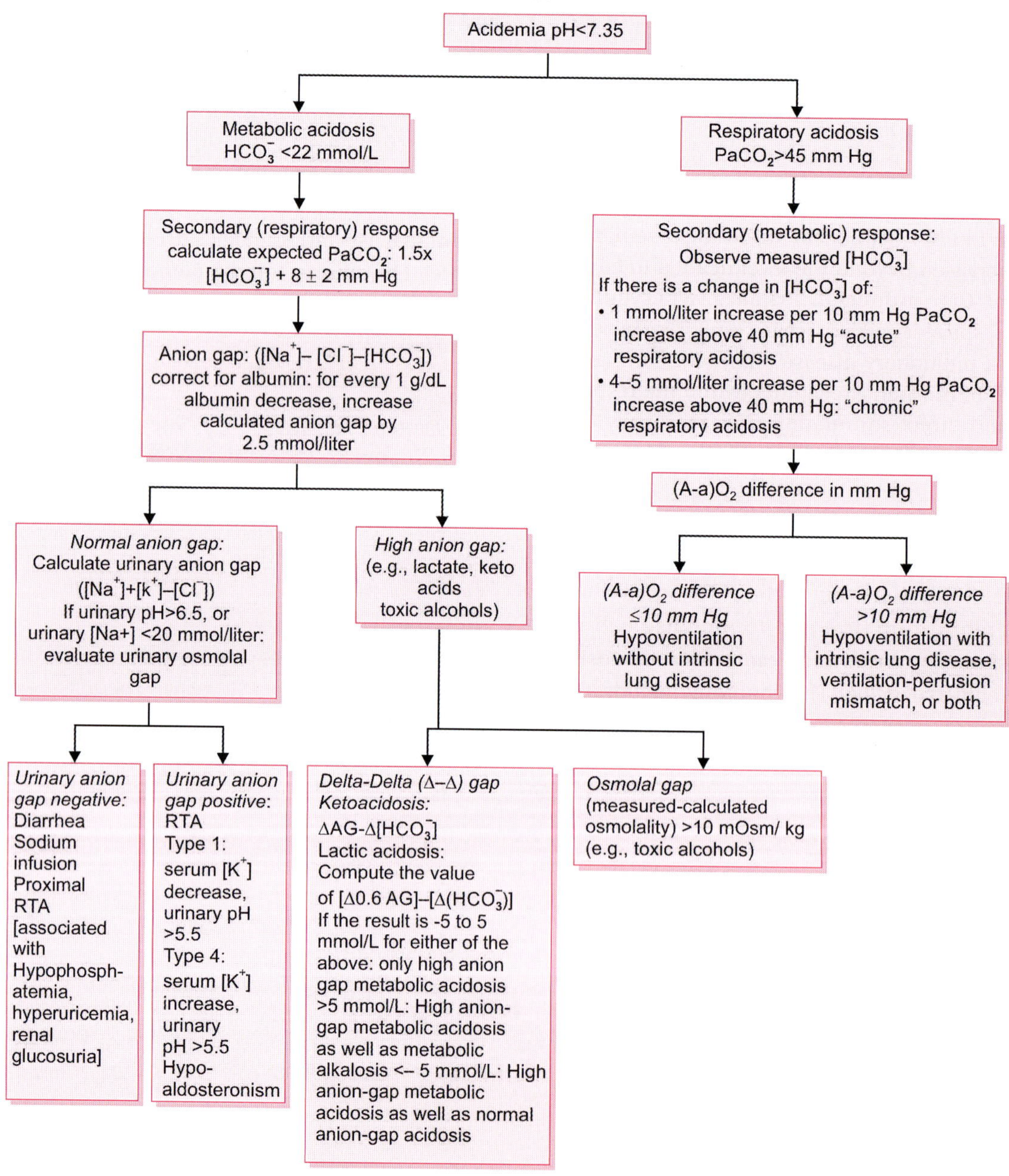

Flowchart 2: Diagnostic approach to alkalosis[29]

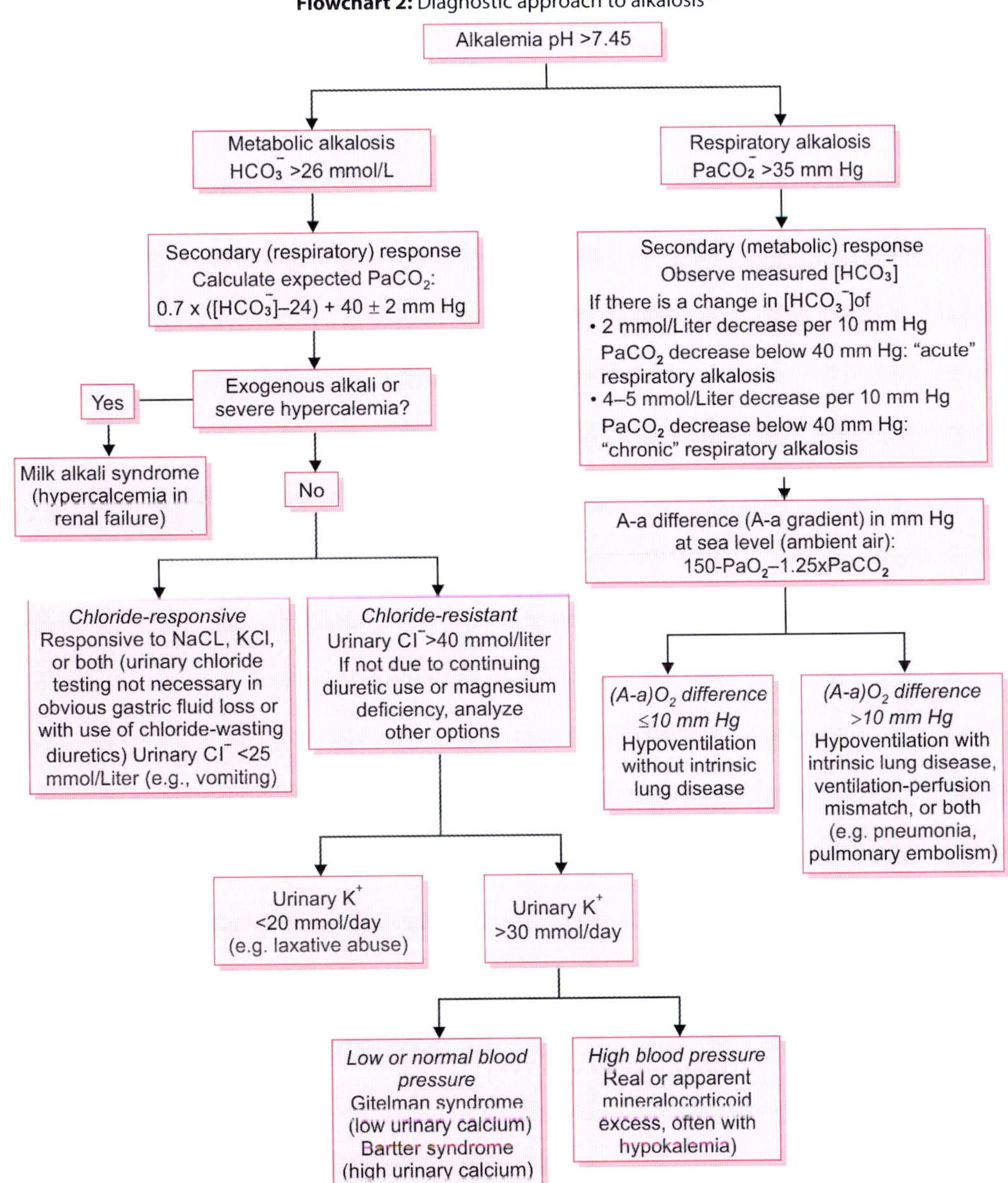

KEY MESSAGES

- Identification of acid base disorders requires a stepwise methodological approach for arterial blood gas analysis and basic pathophysiological mechanisms.
- Interpretation of arterial blood gas should always be done in consideration with the clinical status of the patient.
- Knowledge of expected compensatory responses helps in detection of mixed acid base disorders.
- Delta gap, osmolal gap and urinary anion gap are useful concepts for differentiating different causes of metabolic acidosis.
- Underlying cause should be addressed for the treatment of metabolic acidosis.
- Bolus of sodium bicarbonate should be avoided in management of metabolic acidosis unless pH is <7 which increases the risk of myocardial depression.
- Respiratory acidosis (permissive hypercapnia) in mechanically ventilated patient may not always require intervention unless pH <7.2 in order to avoid ventilator induced lung injury.

REFERENCES

1. Relman AS. What are "acids" and "bases"? Am J Med. 1954; 17:435.
2. Madias NE, Cohen JJ. Acid-base chemistry and buffering. In Cohen JJ, Kassier JP, editors. Acid/Base. Boston: Little, Brown; 1982.
3. Relman AS. Metabolic consequences of acid-base disorders. Kidney Int. 1972;1:347-59.
4. Kurtz I, Maher T, Hulter HN, *et al.* Effect of diet on plasma acid-base composition in normal humans. Kidney Int. 1983;24: 670-80.
5. Lemann J, Lennon EJ. Role of diet, gastrointestinal tract and bone in acid-base homeostasis. Kidney Int. 1972;1:275-9.
6. Rose BD, Post TW. Acid-base physiology. In: Rose BD, Post TW, editors. Clinical Physiology of Acid-Base and Electrolyte Disorders, 5th edition. New York: McGraw Hill; 2001. p. 299-324.
7. Rose BD, Post TW. Regulation of acid-base balance. In: Rose BD, Post TW, editors. Clinical Physiology of Acid-Base and Electrolyte Disorders, 5th edition. New York: McGraw Hill; 2001. p. 325-71.
8. Albert MS, Dell RB, Winters RW. Quantitative displacement of acid-base equilibrium in metabolic acidosis. Ann Intern Med. 1967;66:312-22.
9. Javaheri S, Kazemi H. Metabolic alkalosis and hypoventilation in humans. Am Rev Respir Dis. 1987;136:1011-6.
10. Mitchell JH, Wildenthal K, Johnson RL Jr. The effect of acid-base disturbance on cardiovascular and pulmonary function. Kidney Int. 1972;1:375-89.
11. McSherry E. Renal tubular acidosis in childhood. Kidney Int. 1981;20:799-809.
12. Gabow PA. Disorder associated with an altered anion gap. Kidney Int. 1981;27:472-83.
13. Rose BD, Post TW. Metabolic acidosis. In: Rose BD, Post TW, editors. Clinical Physiology of Acid-Base and Electrolyte Disorders, 5th edition. New York: McGraw Hill; 2001. p. 578-646.
14. Reilly RF, Anderson RJ. Interpreting the anion gap. Crit Care Med. 1998;26:1771-2.
15. Battle DC, Hizon M, Cohen E, *et al.* The use of the urinary anion gap in the diagnosis of hyperchloremic metabolic acidosis. N Engl J Med. 1988;318:594-9.
16. Katzir Z, Dinour D, Reznik-Wolf H, *et al.* Familial pure proximal renal tubular acidosis — a clinical and genetic study. Nephrol Dial Transplant. 2008;23:1211-5.
17. Finkel KW, Dubose TF. Metabolic acidosis. In: Dubose T Jr, Hamm L, editors. Acid Base and Electrolyte Disorders: A Companion to Brenner & Rector's The Kidney. Philadelphia: Saunders; 2002. p. 55-66.
18. Reddy P, Mooradian AD. Clinical utility of anion gap in deciphering acid-base disorders. Int J Clin Pract. 2009;63: 1516-25.
19. Adrogue HJ, Madias NE. Management of life-threatening acid base disorders. N Engl J Med. 1998;338:26-34.
20. Stacpoole PW. Lactic acidosis: The case against bicarbonate therapy. Ann Intern Med. 1986;105:276-8.
21. Walker JA, Sherman RA, Cody RP. The effect of oral bases on enteral aluminum absorption. Arch Intern Med. 1990;150: 2037-39.
22. Kallet RH, Jasmer RM, Luce JM, *et al.* The treatment of acidosis in acute lung injury with tris-hydroxymethyl aminomethane (THAM). Am J Respir Crit Care Med. 2000;161:1149-53.
23. Palmer BF, Alpern RJ. Metabolic alkalosis. J Am Soc Nephrol. 1997;8:1462-9.
24. Kassirer JP, Schwartz WB. The response of normal man to reflective deletion of hydrochloric acid; Factors in the generic of persistent gastric of persistent gastric alkalosis. Am J Med. 1996;40:10-8.
25. Preisig PA, Toto RD, Alpern RJ. Carbonic anhydrase inhibitors. Renal Physiol. 1987;10:136-59.
26. Kelburn KH. Neurologic management of respiratory failure. Arch Inter Med. 1965;116:409-15.
27. Menitove SM, Goldring RM. Combined ventilator and bicarbonate strategy in the management of asthmatics. Am J Med. 1983;74:898-901.
28. Pediatric Acute Respiratory Distress Syndrome: Consensus Recommendations From the Pediatric Acute Lung Injury Consensus Conference. Pediatr Crit Care Med 2015;16(5):428-39.
29. Berend K, de Vries APJ, Gans ROB. Physiological approach to assessment of acid-base disturbances. N Engl J Med. 2014; 371:1434-45.

CHAPTER

15

Blood Component Therapy

Pooja Dewan, Neha Rastogi

Transfusion of blood and blood products is often a life-saving procedure, however, it is not without risks and complications. Since, blood and blood products are derived from human donors, there is an inherent risk of infectious disease transmission despite of meticulous screening. Additionally, several non-infectious complications may also result from blood transfusion. Hence, their judicious use is crucial for their usefulness. In this chapter, we will discuss various blood components, blood group antigens, blood transfusion practices for different blood products and adverse reactions to blood products transfusions.

BLOOD COMPONENTS AND THEIR PREPARATION

Whole blood, 350 or 450 mL, is collected in bags with anticoagulant namely citrate-phosphate-dextrose with adenine (CPDA) followed by the separation into its components by centrifugation. This process needs to be completed within 8 hours of collection. The process of separation of collected blood into its various components is referred to as "fractionation of blood".

Centrifugation of one unit of whole blood will yield different components based on their size and relative density. The components in increasing order of relative density are plasma, white blood cells or buffy coat (BC), platelets, and red blood cells. "**Apheresis**" involves collection of one or more than one component from a donor while the rest of blood components are returned to the donor.

Preparation of packed red blood cell (PRBC) component and fresh frozen plasma (FFP) involves a single-step heavy spin centrifugation (5000 G for 10–15 min). However, preparing platelet concentrates, PRBC concentrates and FFP is by two-step centrifugation (light spin 1500 G for 5 min followed by heavy spin). The components can be separated using an extractor.

Plasma is fresh-frozen at -30°C within 6 hours of collection and stored for further use. The rapid freezing prevents the degradation of the clotting factors and helps maintain their viability. Following the process of thawing of frozen plasma before transfusion, the clotting agents get reactivated, albeit a minor reduction in Factor V and Factor VIII does occur. Thawing is usually done in a water bath over 30–45 minutes before use. FFP can be stored at –18°C for up to 12 months. Once thawed, it must be used as soon as possible, or can be used up to 5 days if stored at 1–6°C.

If FFP is thawed slowly at 1–6°C and thereafter centrifuged at an RPM of 5000 for 6 minutes, and the supernatant (cryo-poor plasma) is removed; the insoluble precipitate left behind is dispensed in 10–15 mL of plasma and refrozen at –18°C and is referred to as cryoprecipitate. This is rich in clotting factors, Factor VIII, fibrinogen, von Willebrand factor and Factor XIII. Cryoprecipitate can be stored at –18°C for up to 12 months.

Plasma can be fractionated into several component protein fractions, which also need to be purified before use. Several units of plasma from different donors must be pooled together to yield therapeutic protein preparations. Processing of pooled plasma involves mixing with ethanol and varying temperatures, pH and ionic strength concentrations to precipitate different groups of proteins like fibrinogen, albumin and immunoglobulins.

Since blood components are derived from donors and hence they are foreign to the patient, their transfusion is liable to produce adverse reactions like mild allergic manifestations, hemolytic reactions and even transfusion transmitted infections (TTIs). To minimize these adverse events, blood products are modified by techniques like leukoreduction, irradiation, saline washing and pathogen inactivation procedures.

BLOOD PRODUCTS

Blood can be fractioned to yield either the basic components (RBC concentrates, Platelet concentrates, Plasma), or undergo additional processing to yield special components like washed/filtered/irradiated basic components, plasma protein fractions like albumin, clotting factors, etc. or their combinations. We will discuss each of these in the following sections.

Red Cell Components

Whole blood: The uncentrifuged blood suspended in CPDA constitutes the whole blood. It includes RBCs, platelets, and leukocytes suspended in plasma containing plasma proteins and clotting factors. It is usually stored at 4°C for 28–35 days. It has a hematocrit of about 35–40%. The current indications for transfusion of whole blood are limited. These include: acute blood loss (>30% blood loss within 24 hours), exchange transfusion and in emergency situations where appropriate fraction is unavailable. Exchange transfusion may be indicated in certain poisonings, some infections like severe septicemia or malaria, and in neonates for hyperbilirubinemia. While performing exchange transfusion, whole blood used must not be older than 4–5 days. Transfusion of whole blood may be associated with complications due to white blood cells or platelets. These include febrile non-hemolytic transfusion reactions, alloimmunization, graft versus host disease and transmission of infections and pyrogens. These are discussed in detail later in the chapter.

Packed red blood cell (PRBC) concentrate: Red cell concentrate is extracted from whole blood by centrifugation and separation of plasma, such that the red cell concentrate has a hematocrit of about 60%. Before, we elaborate on processing of PRBCs let us understand the grouping of blood based on the presence of red cell antigens.

Blood Grouping

Red blood cells express multiple antigens on its surface. Additionally, blood in every individual has innate antibodies against certain antigens on the RBCs. Based on this, an individual may be characterized to have a blood group or type. These antigens and antibodies are inherited from parents and generally the blood group of an individual remains the same for life. Rarely, the blood group of an individual can change due to special conditions like receiving bone marrow transplant from person with different blood group, or in certain autoimmune conditions.

Currently, about 36 human blood group systems and 346 RBC antigens are recognized. The major antigen systems are ABO and Rh blood grouping systems. *For safe blood transfusion services, we need to find at least ABO and Rh compatible donors.*

The RBC antigens are clinically important in their immune-mediated destruction.[1] Antibodies present in the recipient blood against these antigens in the donor blood are responsible for immune destruction of RBCs in allogeneic blood transfusions, fetomaternal blood group incompatibility, immune hemolytic anemia, and tissue/organ transplantation.

ABO blood group system

This system involves the presence of two antigens (antigen A and antigen B) on RBCs and two antibodies (antibody A and antibody B) in serum. ABO antigens are detectable on the fetal RBCs of 5- to 6-week-old embryos, but they are fully developed by 2 to 4 years of age.[1] The genes for the A and B blood group antigens are co-dominant so a person can have AB blood group. Antibodies against A and B antigens are known as isohemagglutinins and they are naturally occurring. They develop as a result of environmental stimulants, such as bacterial cell walls, that carry similar antigens.

Depending upon the combination of antigen and antibodies, either of the 4 major blood types are possible (**Table 1**). Blood transfusion should always be ABO compatible because ABO incompatibility is the most common cause of fatal hemolytic transfusion reactions.

Table 1: ABO blood group

Antigen	Antibody	Blood group (Phenotype)	Genotype
Antigen A	Antibody B	A	AA or AI
Antigen B	Antibody A	B	BB or BI
Antigen A and antigen B	None	AB	AB
None	Antibody A and antibody B	O	II

Table 2: Choice of donor ABO group for blood products administration to children

Recipient blood group	Choice	Choice of red blood cells	Choice of platelet	Choice of fresh frozen plasma
A	First choice	A	A	A
	Second choice	O*	O*	AB
B	First choice	B	B	B
	Second choice	O*	O*	AB
AB	First choice	AB	AB	AB
	Second choice	A or B or O	A or B or O	–
O	First choice	O	O	O
	Second choice	–	A or B or AB	A or B or AB

*O blood component must have low titers of anti A and anti-B
Rh compatibility is not so much of an issue with platelet and FFP transfusion.

Routine testing of blood group consists of testing the red cells with anti-A and anti-B (cell or forward type) and testing the serum or plasma with A and B red cells (serum or reverse type).[2]

Rhesus (Rh) blood typing

The Rh blood grouping involves about 50 antigens; most importantly D antigen, and is the second most significant blood group system in humans. The terms "Rh positive" and "Rh negative" refer to the presence or absence of the red cell antigen D.[2] Now, other Rh antigens are also being recognized (C, E, c, e).[1] These five principal antigens (D, C, E, c, e) and their corresponding antibodies are responsible for most of clinically relevant issues involving the Rh system.[2] In contrast to individuals with blood groups A and B who have inherent antibody B and antibody A respectively, persons whose RBCs lack the D antigen do not have natural anti-D antibodies. Exposure to red cells possessing the D antigen through transfusion or pregnancy, leads to anti-D formation. The D antigen has greater immunogenicity than other red cell antigens; it is estimated that 30% to 85% of D-persons who receive a D+ transfusion will develop anti-D.[2]

Minor blood group systems

Other RBC antigen systems are Kell system, Lewis system, MNS system, Duffy system. These are more relevant in multi-transfused individuals who may develop antibodies to these groups and may require to be matched for minor blood groups in addition to ABO and Rh groups (extended phenotyping).

Matching of blood groups before transfusion

The ABO and Rh compatible RBC transfusion is mandatory. Platelets express on their surface antigens of the ABO system while they do not express any antigens of the Rh system. For platelet and FFP transfusions, ABO and Rh compatibility should be ensured, whenever possible. Both products contain enough red cell stroma to stimulate Rh immunization. **Table 2** shows choice of ABO group for blood product administration.[3]

Special Processing of Packed Red Blood Cells

Leukodepletion

Removal of leukocytes from various blood products has been shown to minimize febrile non-hemolytic transfusion reactions, HLA alloimmunization, platelet refractoriness in multi-transfused patients and prevention of transmission of leukotropic viruses.[4] Current guidelines mandate that WBC count of transfused PRBCs should be $< 5 \times 10^6$ per unit. This can mitigate the risk for CMV transmission especially for infants <1.5 kg, immunodeficient patients and stem cell recipients.

Methods for leukodepletion:[5]

- *Manual buffy coat removal*: This is a crude method which can reduce WBC content by 80%. However, it also leads to loss of 20% of RBCs.
- *Filtration*: Filtration using special filter with diameter <40 μ removes 90% to 99.99% WBCs. The older generation of leukodepleting filters (first and second generation) were capable of removing 90–95% of leukocytes. In contrast, the current generation of leukofilters (third and fourth) have excellent leukoreduction efficiency (99.99%). Leukofiltration of blood components can be done either at the time of blood collection in the blood bank, post-collection within the blood bank (before storage), or at bedside (post-storage).
- *Pre-storage filtration* of whole blood or packed RBCs is the preferred method for leukodepletion. It not only eliminates the leukocytes but also eliminates cytokine generation due to leukocytes during storage thereby reducing non-hemolytic febrile reactions. Pre-storage leukofiltration can also reduce the risk of leukotropic virus transmission.
- Bedside filtration refers to the packed red cell unit, which is filtered at the bedside, at the time of transfusion.[5] **Table 3** illustrates the WBC content of various fractions used for transfusion.

Table 3: White blood cell (WBC) content of blood products

Blood component	*WBC content (cells/unit)*
Whole blood	$2–3 \times 10^9$
Filtered (leukocyte reduced) RBC concentrate	$<1 \times 10^6$
RBC concentrate - resuspended buffy coat free	$1–5 \times 10^8$
Plasma	2×10^7
Platelet concentrate	0.5×10^8

Washed red blood cells

Washed RBCs (and also platelets) are prepared using 0.8% sodium chloride which helps to reduce plasma proteins, potassium, free hemoglobin and antibodies.[4] Washing is not effective for leukoreduction. Instead, washing should be used in conjunction with filtration.[5] Indications for use of washed red blood cell include:

- Ig A deficient individuals
- History of anaphylactic reaction to blood components
- Extracorporeal membrane oxygenation (ECMO) or cardiopulmonary bypass patients when fresh red blood cells are unavailable
- Paroxysmal nocturnal hemoglobinuria
- Intrauterine transfusion (fetal transfusion)
- Anemia with hyperkalemia and impaired kidney.

Irradiation

Transfusion-associated graft versus host disease (TA-GVHD) is a rare complication after transfusion of cellular products.[1] Patients who are the most susceptible include premature neonates, some patients with congenital immunodeficiency syndromes, patients on chemotherapy, and patients receiving immunosuppressive drugs for hematopoietic stem cell transplantation (HSCT) and solid organ transplantation.[1]

It is preferable to irradiate all red cell and platelet components (with the exception of frozen red cells and fresh frozen plasma) for:[3]

- Intrauterine transfusion (IUT)
- Exchange transfusion (ET) of red cells or Top-up transfusion after IUT
- When the donation is from a first- or second-degree relative or a human leukocyte antigen (HLA)-selected donor
- When the child has proven or suspected immunodeficiency
- HSCT recipients
- Preterm neonates.

Irradiation dose is minimum of 25 Gy. Red cells may be irradiated at any time up to 14 days after collection, and thereafter stored for a further 14 days from irradiation. All granulocytes should be irradiated for patients of any age and transfused as soon as possible after.[3] It is possible that on rare occasions, even some of the immunocompetent recipients may develop transfusion associated graft versus host disease (TA-GVHD), hence some blood banks routinely irradiate all cellular blood products.[1]

Cryopreservation

Frozen red cell concentrate, or cryopreserved PRBC: Red cells are treated with a cryoprotective solution and frozen. It can be stored for 10 years, if storage temperature is maintained below –65°C.

Peripheral blood hematopoietic stem cells are also cryopreserved for autologous or allogeneic transplants if required to be stored beyond 3 days.

Red Blood Cell Component Transfusion

Packed RBC components should be transfused through a standard blood giving set with a screen filter (170–200 μ). The primary indication for transfusion of RBCs is to restore or maintain oxygen-carrying capacity to meet tissue demands.[7] In critically ill patients, strategy for RBC transfusion can be liberal or restrictive. A liberal transfusion policy is the one in which PRBC transfusions are given to patients when their Hb level is below 10 g/dL and a restrictive transfusion policy involves giving PRBC transfusion to patients when their Hb level is below 7 g/dL. Neonates fare better with a liberal transfusion strategy but in pediatric age group and in critically ill patients, a restrictive strategy is better.[1]

Indications and threshold for transfusions might vary with age and underlying disorders (**Table 4**).[4] About 10–15 mL/kg of PRBCs are transfused at 3–5 mL/kg/h and the transfusion should be completed within 3–5 hours. RBC compatibility testing must be performed before RBC transfusion.[4]

Artificial blood/blood substitute

Artificial blood is being developed to carry out oxygen carrying functions of blood. These are usually perfluorocarbon based oxygen carriers. Most of these products are in the clinical trial phase and yet to be marketed. Theoretically, these could be useful in avoiding the risks of disease transmission, cover shortage of blood and be offered in groups who have religious beliefs to avoid blood transfusion like the *Jehova witnesses*.

Platelet Component

Separation of a unit of platelet (Random donor platelet, RDP) from a unit of whole blood is a two-step process involving a soft spin to separate RBCs and WBCs from a platelet rich plasma which is further subjected to a heavy spin to separate platelet concentrate from plasma. Each unit of RDP usually has at least 5.5×10^{10} platelets. In order to reach the therapeutic dose, usually platelets are pooled from more than one donor. A single donor platelet (SDP) involves apheresis of platelets from one donor to reach at least 3×10^{11} platelets per unit (equivalent to 6 RDPs/bag). While RDP is cost effective, SDP offers the advantage of greater dose of platelet, better protection from alloimmunization and lesser risk for infection. Use of leukocyte filters can reduce risk for febrile reactions.

Table 4: Indications for red cell transfusion
Premature infant
Stable, growing, hemoglobin (Hb) <7 g/dL
Respiratory distress syndrome: not requiring oxygen therapy, (Hb) <10 g/dL; with oxygen requirement, (Hb) <12 g/dL
Mildly symptomatic anemia (apnea, tachycardia, poor wight gain), (Hb) <10 g/dL
Severely symptomatic (e.g. worsening apnea, hypotension, acidosis, heart disease), (Hb) <12 g/dL.
Term infant <4 months of age
Symptomatic anemia (apnea, tachycardia, poor weight gain), Hb <7 g/dL
Perioperative anemia, Hb <10 g/dL
Hypoxia or on extracorporeal membrane oxygenation Hb <12 g/dL
Cyanotic heart disease, Hb <13 g/dL
Acute blood loss >10% blood volume, not responsive to other forms of therapy
> 4 months of age
Acute blood loss >15% of blood volume, or anticipation thereof, or hypovolemia not responsive to other forms of therapy
Postoperatively with signs of anemia (e.g. apnea) Hb <10 g/dL
Severe cardiopulmonary disease, Hb <12 g/dL
Patients receiving chemotherapy or irradiation, or patients with chronic anemia not responsive to medical therapy, Hb <7 g/dL (symptomatic patients may be transfused at a higher hemoglobin level)
Chronic hemolytic anemia like thalassemia, complications of sickle cell disease, Hb <9 g/dL

Platelet units are stored at room temperature between 20 and 24°C and kept horizontally on an agitator to maintain viability with a shelf life of 5 days; after which risk of bacterial overgrowth is very high.[6]

The usual dose of platelet is 10–15 mL/kg for children. It is transfused rapidly over 30 minutes.[6] One unit of RDP is expected to raise the platelet count by 50,000/μL to 100,000/μL in a neonate weighing 3 kg and about 30,000/μL to 50,000/μL in a child weighing 10 kg. Transfused platelets have a life of only 3–4 days and may need to be transfused repeatedly.

Preferably, ABO compatible and RhD compatible platelets should be used because non-identical transfusion is associated with poorer response, but in case of emergency non group specific platelets can also be used. Transfusion of Rh positive platelets units to Rh negative patient may be done except in females of childbearing age.

Platelet refractoriness is defined when platelet counts do not rise above a threshold value despite repeated transfusions, and when there is poor increment, even after two ABO-compatible transfusions (stored less than 72 h).[6] To compare the effectiveness of platelet transfusion, the best ratio to use is the corrected count increment (CCI).[1] Platelet refractoriness is defined as CCI <5,000 at 1 hour.

CCI = (platelet increment per μL) × (body surface area in m^2)/number of platelets transfused ($\times 10^{11}$).

For example, a platelet increment of 50,000/μL in a child with BSA of 0.6 m^2 after a single donor platelet would represent a CCI of (50,000 × 0.6/3) = 25,000.

Platelet transfusion thresholds in neonates:[4,6]

- Stable neonate: <20,000/μL
- Unstable or sick neonate: <30,000–50,000/μL
- Active bleeding or invasive procedure: <50,000/μL.

Platelet transfusion thresholds in older children

- Non-infected, clinically stable (without any additional risk factors like sepsis, coagulopathy, bleeding, use of antibiotics, etc.): <10,000/μL
- Neonates with sepsis, coagulopathy, bleeding, etc.: > 10, 000/μL
- In immune thrombocytopenic purpura (ITP) platelet transfusion is not indicated except in life-threatening bleeding
- In thrombotic thrombocytopenia (TTP) and heparin induced thrombocytopenia (HIT) platelet transfusion is relatively contraindicated as this may precipitate thrombotic episodes
- For procedures like lumbar puncture, epidural anesthesia, upper gastrointestinal endoscopy, transbronchial biopsy, laparotomy: The platelets should be >50,000/μL
- For surgeries involving the eyes and brain: The platelets should be >100,000/μL.

Platelet cryopreservation: Cryopreservation of platelets is mainly used for autologous transfusions for a few selected patients who are refractory to allogeneic platelets.

Plasma and Its Fractions

Plasma is frozen at –18°C or colder within 6 hours of donation to get fresh frozen plasma (FFP). FFP should not be used for volume expansion or for single factor deficiency when that factor concentrate is available.

Indications for FFP transfusion include:

- Liver disease with increased prothrombin time (PT) and partial thromboplastin time (PTT) with clinical bleeding
- Large quantities of PRBC transfusion to counter dilutional coagulopathies
- Disseminated intravascular coagulation with active bleeding
- Rapid reversal of warfarin effect
- Protein C, protein S, anti-thrombin III deficiencies, or other single-factor deficiency where no product is available and patient is bleeding
- Since FFP contains all clotting factors it is sometimes used in patients with clotting factor deficiencies. One mL of fresh frozen plasma contains 1 unit of factor activity.

Dose of FFP: A dose of 12–15 mL/kg of FFP should be administered at a rate of 10–20 mL/kg/h. Once thawed, FFP should be used within 24 hours.

Other plasma fractions include Factor VIII concentrate, Factor IX concentrate, prothrombin concentrate, intravenous immunoglobulin (IVIG) preparations (Normal IVIG, Specific IVIG, RhD immunoglobulin) and cryoprecipitate.

Cryoprecipitate concentrate

Cryoprecipitate is prepared by thawing FFP at 4°C and then removing the supernatant (cryo-depleted plasma) from the cryoprecipitable proteins following centrifugation at 1–6°C.[7] Cryoprecipitate contain concentrated Factor VIII:C, von Willebrand factor, fibrinogen, Factor

XIII and fibrinogen. Thus, cryoprecipitate contains almost exclusively procoagulants and, unlike FFP, does not contain appreciable quantities of physiologic anticoagulants such as protein C, proteins S, and others. Therefore, cryoprecipitate alone may not be the optimal replacement strategy in patients with disease processes that deplete both procoagulants and anticoagulants such as disseminated intravascular coagulation or severe hepatic failure.[7] Cryoprecipitate is used mainly for congenital or acquired hypofibrinogenemia but can also be used for von Willebrand disease or hemophilia A if Factor VIII concentrate is not available. A bag of cryoprecipitate made from one unit of FFP (200–250 mL) contains 70–80 units of factor VIII in a volume of 30–40 mL.

Cryo-depleted plasma

The main use of cryo-depleted plasma is for the treatment of thrombotic thrombocytopenic purpura (TTP).

Plasma-derived clotting factor concentrates

These are intermediate and high purity plasma derived clotting factor concentrates (pdCFC) mainly Factor VIII and Factor IX concentrates available in lyophilized forms and are used in hemophilia patients. Hemostatic level of Factor VIII is 25–30 U/dL and Factor IX is 15–30 IU/dL. The dose of factor to be used depends upon the type of bleed and indication (prophylactic or therapeutic) (**Table 5**). Each unit of Factor VIII per kilogram of body weight infused intravenously is expected to increase the plasma Factor VIII level by 2 IU/dL if the patient does not have any inhibitors to the Factor VIII. Likewise, each unit of Factor IX concentrate per kilogram of body weight infused intravenously is expected to increase the plasma Factor IX level by 1 IU/dL. The use of pdCFC is associated with risk of transmission of viral infections especially HIV and hepatitis C and hence are being replaced by recombinant factors.[8]

Prothrombin complex concentrates

Factor IX concentrates that also contain Factors II, VII, IX, and X, also known as prothrombin complex concentrates (PCCs). To prevent activation of these factors, most PCC contain heparin. Indications for use include urgent reversal of over-anticoagulation with warfarin, and

Table 5: Dosage of Factor VIII/ Factor IX replacement therapy in bleeding in hemophilia A and B

	Factor VIII (U/kg)	*Factor IX (U/kg)*
Hemarthrosis	20–30	30
Superficial muscle bleeding Deep muscle bleeding (initial 1–2 days) Deep muscle bleeding (3–5 days)	20–30 40–50 15–30	20–30 30–40 15–30
Dental extraction	20	30
Epistaxis	20	30
Intracranial bleeding	40–50 (initial); 20–30 (maintenance)	30
Major trauma	15–25	30–50
Gross hematurtia	25	20
Gastrointestinal bleeding	40–50 (initial); 20–30 (maintenance)	20–40 (initial); 15 (maintenance)
Head and neck bleeding	40–50 (initial); 20–30 (maintenance)	30–40 (initial); 20 (maintenance)
Major surgery Preoperative Postoperative (day 1–3) Postoperative (day 4–6) Postoperative (day 7–14)	 40–50 30–40 20–30 15–25	 30–40 20–30 15–25 10–20
Minor surgery Preoperative Postoperative	 25–40 15–40	 25–40 15–40

congenital deficiency of any of the vitamin K-dependent coagulation factors. Its adverse effects include risk for thromboembolic complications, anaphylactic reactions and heparin-induced thrombocytopenia.

Human Albumin

Human albumin is derived from human plasma by cold ethanol fractionation and chromatographic purification. It is available commercially as 5% or 20% concentration. Albumin solution is used in treating hypovolemic conditions where use of colloids is indicated, treatment of fluid loss where electrolyte or fluid load is contraindicated, and in certain hypoalbuminemic states. Adverse effects to use of albumin include anaphylaxis, renal toxicity, cardiac failure, pulmonary edema, and hypotension due to sepsis due to contamination. Risk for transmission of viral infections also exists. Albumin use should be avoided in children with hypertension, cardiac failure, bleeding diathesis, esophageal varices, azotemia, severe anemia and pulmonary edema.

Granulocyte Infusion

Granulocyte transfusion should be ABO compatible and is collected by leukapheresis. Leukapharesis involves separation of anticoagulated blood into components by a suitable apheresis machine. The granulocytes so separated are suspended in a portion of the plasma before infusing in the recipient or storage, while the remaining elements are returned to the donor. A minimum dose of $2–3 \times 10^{10}$ neutrophils should be given to adults. The indications for granulocyte infusion include life-threatening severe neutropenia (absolute neutrophil count, ANC<0.5 × 10^9/L) with severe bacterial or fungal sepsis in patients with cancer, bone marrow failure conditions like aplastic anemia or congenital neutropenia. The half-life of the neutrophil is approximately 7 hours. Granulocyte infusion should always be irradiated.

ADVERSE REACTIONS TO BLOOD PRODUCT TRANSFUSIONS

The adverse reactions can be infectious or non-infectious. Additionally, these could be categorized as immediate, early or delayed. Non-infectious complications of blood transfusions four broad categories of transfusion reactions: (i) acute immunologic, (ii) acute non-immunologic, (iii) delayed immunologic, and (iv) delayed non-immunologic complications.

Non-infectious Complications

Acute (<24 hrs) immunologic complications

Acute hemolytic reactions: These reactions occur due to immune destruction of transfused RBCs by the antibodies present in the recipient. As less as 10 mL of transfused blood can cause acute hemolysis characterized by the abrupt onset of fever, chills, lower back pain, dyspnea, hemoglobinuria, oliguria, and shock. These unusual reactions most commonly arise from errors in patient identification or blood typing and compatibility testing.[5] As soon as acute hemolytic reaction is suspected, the transfusion should be stopped immediately and intravenous fluids should be administered to maintain intravascular volume. Verify the patient identity and check donor blood group. Send the recipient blood sample for direct Coomb's test, renal function test, serum haptoglobulin, and serum bilirubin.

Febrile non-hemolytic transfusion reactions (FNHTR): The fever here occurs due to the preformed cytokines from the donor WBCs or the recipient antibodies reacting with donor WBC antigens. Depending upon the fraction used, the content of WBCs in the component transfused can vary (**Table 3**). Leukoreduction, especially pre-storage leukoreduction, and premedication with paracetamol can minimize FNHTR.[5] Always, try to exclude other causes of fever following transfusion like acute hemolysis or bacterial contamination.

Allergic reactions: These usually include urticaria, pruritus and flushing. Those with severe manifestations can develop stridor, bronchospasm, or hypotension, especially in patients with IgA deficiency and anti-IgA antibodies.[5] These reactions are caused due to antibodies to donor plasma proteins and are mediated by IgE.[7] Use of antihistamines or corticosteroids before transfusion might help in preventing them. Recurrent allergic reactions can be minimized by use of washed PRBCs. Patients with IgA deficiency and severe allergic reactions may even require blood from IgA-deficient donors.[5]

Transfusion related acute lung injury (TRALI): It is a potentially life-threatening reaction that is usually caused by specific anti-neutrophil or anti-HLA antibodies. Clinical picture is of "noncardiogenic pulmonary edema".[7] Signs and symptoms include dyspnea, hypoxemia, hypotension, fever, and a chest X-ray showing bilateral infiltrates with pulmonary edema during or within six hours of transfusion. Oxygen therapy, steroids and diuretics, and assisted ventilation can be used in such situations.[5]

Acute (<24 hours) non-immunologic complications

Transfusion-associated circulatory overload: It may occur when the rate of transfusion is very fast or in the presence of underlying cardiac dysfunction. Patient may develop dyspnea, orthopnea, cough, tachycardia, hypertension, and headache. Chest radiograph will reveal the classical findings of pulmonary edema.[7] Treatment includes upright posture, oxygen, diuretics and cardiac support, as required.

Non-immune hemolysis: It is a rare complication caused by physical or chemical destruction of blood (heating, freezing, hemolytic drug, or solution added to blood). Signs and symptoms include hemoglobinuria and hemoglobinemia. Management includes identification and removal of the cause.

Air embolism: It is a rare complication due to air infusion via intravenous line. Patient develops sudden shortness of breath, acute cyanosis, pain, cough, hypotension, cardiac arrhythmia. The minimum volume of air embolism that is potentially fatal for an adult is approximately 100 mL.[2] If air embolism is suspected, the patient should be placed on the left side with the head down, to displace the air bubble from the pulmonic valve.

Hypocalcemia: Rapid citrate infusion as in case of massive transfusion of citrated blood, and apheresis procedures causes hypocalcemia. Signs and symptoms include paresthesia, tetany, and arrhythmias. Investigations show low ionized calcium and prolonged Q-T interval on electrocardiogram.[2]

Hypothermia: It can happen after rapid infusion of cold blood especially in smaller babies.

Bacterial contamination: These can range from mild pyrexial reactions to septic shock. Diagnosis is established by blood culture of both the blood component and the recipient.[4]

Hyperkalemia: This can be avoided by using fresh blood (<7 days old).

Delayed (>24 hours) immunologic complications

Delayed transfusion reactions usually occur 5–14 days after transfusion and are characterized by unexpected levels of anemia, as well as malaise and jaundice.[5] They are caused by anamnestic immune response to red cell antigens.[2]

Alloimmunization against RBC or HLA antigens: It is an immune response to foreign antigens on RBCs, or WBCs and platelets (HLA). Management includes avoiding unnecessary transfusions and using leukodepleted blood products.

Transfusion-associated graft versus host disease (TA-GVHD): It is a rare but often fatal complication of transfusion caused by the viable lymphocytes in the transfused units which engraft in recipient and mount attack on host tissues.[5] Immunosuppressed patients are at an increased risk, but TA-GVHD may also occur in immunocompetent recipients when they receive blood from a haploidentical donor such as a family member. TA-GVHD usually occurs within 1–4 weeks of transfusion and is characterized by fever, rash, liver dysfunction, diarrhea and pancytopenia due to bone marrow failure. It can be prevented by avoiding blood from a family member, or use of irradiated PRBCs.[5]

Post-transfusion purpura: This rare event is caused by the recipient platelet antibodies (apparent alloantibody, usually anti-HPA-1) destroy autologous platelets. Patients presents with thrombocytopenic purpura, bleeding, 8–10 days after transfusion.[2] Diagnostic testing includes platelet antibody screen and identification. Treatment includes IVIG, HPA-1-negative platelets and plasmapheresis.

Delayed (>24 hours) non-immunologic complications

Iron overload: Every PRBC unit contains approximately 200 mg of iron. Chronically transfused patients, especially those with hemoglobinopathies, have progressive and continuous accumulation of iron and no physiologic means of excreting it thus leading to iron overload.[2]

Infectious Complications of Transfusion (Transfusion Transmitted Diseases)

The commonly used screening tests in most blood banks are based on the detection of viral antibodies in donor blood (exception: Hepatitis B). However, there is always some risk of TTI if a donation was made during the window period (before a detectable antibody response). Use of antigen testing and nucleic acid testing (NAT) can help circumvent these issues to some extent.[4] Various common transfusion transmitted diseases are HIV, Hepatitis B, Hepatitis C, West Nile virus, Parvovirus B19, Human T-cell lymphotrophic virus 1 (HTLV-1), Cytomegalovirus, Plasmodium (Malaria).

KEY MESSAGES

- Centrifugation of one unit of whole blood will yield the following blood components in increasing order of relative density: plasma, white blood cells or buffy coat (BC), platelets, and red blood cells.
- Plasma when frozen at –30°C within 6 hours of collection yields fresh frozen plasma (FFP) which is rich in all clotting factors. Once thawed, fresh frozen plasma must be used within 24 hours.
- Cryoprecipitate is rich in clotting factors: factor VIII, fibrinogen, von Willebrand factor and Factor XIII, and can be stored at –18°C for up to 12 months.
- Leukodepletion of blood minimizes febrile non-hemolytic transfusion reactions, HLA alloimmunization, platelet refractoriness in multi-transfused patients and prevention of transmission of leukotropic viruses.
- Irradiated blood prevents transfusion-associated graft versus host disease (TA-GVHD) and is especially useful in organ/tissue transplant recipients.
- Platelet units are stored at room temperature between 20 and 24°C and kept horizontally on an agitator to maintain viability with a shelf life of 5 days.
- One unit of random donor platelet is expected to raise the platelet count by 50,000/µL to 100,000/µL in a neonate weighing 3 kg and about 30,000/µL to 50,000/µL in a child weighing 10 kg.

REFERENCES

1. Sloan SR. Transfusion medicine. In: Orkin SH, Nathan DG, Ginsburg D, Look AT, Fisher DE, Lux SE, editors. Nathan and Oski's Hematology of Infancy and Childhood, 7th edition. Pennsylvania: Elsevier; 2008. p. 1127-1164.e10.
2. Brecher ME. Technical Manual, 15th edition. United States: AABB; 2005.
3. Gibson BE, Todd A, Roberts I, *et al.* British Committee for Standards in Haematology Transfusion Task Force: Writing group. Transfusion guidelines for neonates and older children. Br J Haematol. 2004;124:433-53.
4. Dewan P. Hematology. In: Gupta P, editor. Textbook of Pediatrics, 2nd edition. Delhi: CBS Publishers; 2018.
5. Cappellini MD, Cohen A, Eleftheriou A, *et al.* Guidelines for the Clinical Management of Thalassemia, 2nd edition. Nicosia, Cyprus. Thalassemia International Federation; 2008.
6. Kickhs TS. Principles of platelet transfusion therapy. In: Hoffman R, Benz EJ, editors. Hematology: Basic Principles and Practice, 4th edition. Pennsylvania: Elsevier; 2005. p. 2433-40.
7. Klumpp TR, Seigal DL. In: Kahn, Marc J, Gregory, Stephanie A, editors. ASH-SAP: American Society of Hematology Self-assessment Program, 3rd edition. Washington, DC: American Society of Hematology; 2007. p. 409-44.
8. World Federation of Hemophilia. Guidelines for the management of hemophilia. Available from: <*https://www1.wfh.org/publication/files/pdf-1472.pdf*. Accessed July 2>4, 2019.

CHAPTER

16

Sedation, Analgesia and Anesthesia

Anil Sachdev, Bharat Mehra

INTRODUCTION

The treatment and reduction of pain is a basic human right for all, regardless of age.[1] Unfortunately, children frequently receive no treatment or inadequate treatment for pain and painful procedures, with newborn and critically ill children being especially vulnerable. This is because of the conventional "wisdom" that children neither respond to nor remember painful experiences to the same degree that adults do, which is simply untrue. In fact, all of the nerve pathways essential for the transmission and perception of pain are present and functioning by 24 weeks of gestation.[2]

Painful diagnostic or therapeutic procedures are often necessary during emergency care of children who already have painful and frightening injuries and illnesses.[3] There are many reasons why effective anxiolysis, analgesia and sedation are not commonplace in the emergency department. The explanations for less use of analgesia or sedation include lack of consensus about optimal safe effective methods, medications, patient monitoring, lack of physician familiarity with local anesthetic techniques and dosing, insufficient time to carry out sedation and belief that children have only short-term memory of pain.

NEUROPHYSIOLOGY OF PAIN

The International Association for the Study of Pain (IASP) defines pain as "an unpleasant sensory and emotional experience associated with actual or potential tissue damage, or described in terms of such damage." The American Pain Society defines pain as "the result of a dynamic integration of biological processes, psychological factors and social/cultural context considered within a developmental trajectory.[4] This type of pain includes persistent (ongoing) and recurrent (episodic) pain with possible fluctuations in severity, quality, regularity, and predictability.

The basic mechanism of pain perception has four components, transduction, transmission, perception and modulation.[5] Noxious mechanical, thermal or chemical stimuli excite afferent nerve fibers that transmit information about the potential injurious stimuli from the periphery to the dorsal horn of the spinal cord. The pain impulse is transmitted via A-delta (large, myelinated) and C (small, unmyelinated) fibers. The tissue injury causes release of inflammatory mediators (e.g. bradykinin, prostaglandins, cytokines, catecholamines, substance P) that senitize the A and C fibers and recruit other neurons resulting in hyperalgesia. This nociceptive sensory input reaches the second order neurons in spinothalamic, spinoreticular and spino-mesoencephalic tracts and is then widely distributed throughout the brain. As there is no single pain center, the perception and modulation occur within a distributive neuromatrix.

Pain can occur in single or multiple body regions and can involve single or multiple organ systems. According to the above definitions, tissue damage does not need to be present in order for the child to experience pain. Therefore, as a profession, we no longer refer to pain as "real" or "psychosomatic." Pain is now categorized as "structural pain," "pain associated with tissue damage," or "functional pain," "pathological pain not associated with ongoing tissue damage". Patients undergoing the same surgical procedure may respond in a completely different manner, depending on their age, gender, previous pain experiences, and coping skills.

Pain perception is a highly subjective experience. Any procedure by its very nature causes pain, and the stress of being in an unfamiliar environment and awakening to changes in physical functioning can compound this sensation. The clinician has a unique challenge when attempting to predict pain intensity and duration. Failure to assess the patient's pain symptoms and behaviors, as well as to act on them, can result in unrelieved pain and suffering. Infants and young children may not be able to conceptualize or articulate either the intensity and/or the quality of their pain. Therefore, reliable tools for analyzing pain behaviors are necessary. Lack of pain assessment may result from multiple misunderstandings or misconceptions regarding pain in children.[6]

PRINCIPLES OF SEDATION AND ANALGESIA

Before deciding the choice of drugs and its posology for sedating a child, it is first essential to clearly identify the goals of sedation, i.e. whether the child requires "only sedation" or "sedation with analgesia". Not all procedures demand both, and commonly there is a greater need for one or the other. Simultaneosly, physician needs to address the current physiologic condition of the patient and the clinical scenario.

Lets understand the common terminologies used while describing sedation:

- *Minimal sedation (anxiolysis)*: A drug-induced relief of apprehension with minimal effect on sensorium. Although cognitive function and coordination might be impaired, ventilatory and cardiovascular functions are unaffected.
- *Moderate sedation (formerly conscious sedation)*: A drug-induced depression of consciousness in which patients can respond to external stimuli. Reflex withdrawal from a painful stimulus is not considered a purposeful response. Airway reflexes, spontaneous ventilation, and cardiovascular function are maintained.
- *Dissociative sedation*: A trance-like cataleptic state induced by the dissociative drug ketamine in which a patient feels no pain, and has no memory of unpleasant events, but can cooperate with commands and suggestions. Eyes are open with distorted perception of sight and sound and produce feelings of detachment – dissociation – from the environment and self.
- *Deep sedation*: A drug-induced depression of consciousness during which patients cannot be easily aroused but respond purposefully following repeated or painful stimulation. The patient may not be able to maintain airway reflexes or spontaneous ventilation, but cardiovascular function is preserved.
- *General anesthesia*: A drug-induced loss of consciousness during which patients are not arousable, even by painful stimulation.

Thus, different levels of sedation are, rather, a continuum, and a child may pass from a state of light sedation to deep sedation with unexpected ease and rapidity depending upon the drug and its dose used. Moreover, individual patient response to medications can vary and are unpredictable, i.e. a dose of medication that causes light sedation in one child may produce deep sedation and an impaired reflexive ability to protect the airway in another child. The drugs chosen and the underlying clinical condition of the patient may make this transition more or less likely. Physicians must always be prepared for the possibility that the patient may pass into a greater depth of sedation than initially anticipated, and should have emergency apparatus available in case problems arise.

PRE-EVALUATION

Before subjecting the patient to sedation, every patient must have a medical evaluation to determine what underlying clinical conditions, if any, will affect the choice of the sedative drug and its posology.[7,8] The major issues that must be addressed relate to four general areas:

1. Ability to maintain patent airway and adequate ventilation,
2. Cardiovascular status (including hydration and adequacy of intravascular filling),
3. Factors affecting drug metabolism and disposition, and
4. Nothing-by-mouth (NPO) status and risk for aspiration.

ASSESSMENT TOOLS

Pain Assessment Tools

Although assessing pain is a simple task, it is one that is infrequently performed. Clinicians continue to estimate the presence or absence and amount of pain that a child is experiencing based on their own perceptions. This subjective data can result in inaccurate documentation of pain scores and failure to implement appropriate pain management practices. There are a myriad of pediatric pain tools available that demonstrate good reliability and validity, are user friendly, and time efficient. The neonatal pain, agitation, and sedation scale (NPASS) is used for premature infants up to 44 weeks post conception.[9] The FLACC is a behavioral pain assessment tool that evaluates the infant/toddler's facial expression, leg movement, activity, cry, and ability to be consoled.[10] The Wong-Baker FACES pain rating scale is used for developmentally appropriate 3 year olds and older and is probably the most widely known and well received of all pain tools used for young children who can conceptualize that an event can have an escalation in intensity.[11]

Sedation Scores

Although pain assessment is the first step in evaluating pain, a sedation level assessment is equally important and should be done to assist the clinician in analyzing whether or not pain medications need to be withheld or titrated down. When a child is receiving opioids, a sedation assessment should be performed with every pain assessment, including the post-intervention assessment. The most commonly used procedural sedation assessment tool is the University of Michigan Sedation Scale.[12] The COMFORT scale is another commonly used PICU pain and sedation tool that utilizes both behaviors and physiologic parameters.[13] Other scoring systems, such as the Sedation-Agitation Scale, also eliminate the use of physiologic parameters and visually assess the level of the patient's comfort, grading it from 1 (nonarousable) to 7 (dangerous agitation such as pulling at the endotracheal tube).[14] A commonly used sedation scale in the adult ICU population is the Ramsay sedation score.

MONITORING

The potential risks of sedation include airway obstruction, hypoventilation, apnea, and cardiopulmonary impairment. All patients receiving sedatives must have basic monitoring of SpO_2 (using pulse oximetry) and cardiovascular status by monitoring heart and blood pressure. Visual inspection of chest wall movements and capnography using sidestream $EtCO_2$ (end-tidal CO_2) monitoring help in assessing the adequacy of ventilation.

Table 1: Fasting guidelines

Age	*Solids, liquids and non-clear liquids, including milk (hours)*	*Clear liquids (hours)*
> 36 months	6–8	2–3
6 to 36 months	6	2–3
<6 months	4–6	2

Paramount to the safe conduct of sedation is the presence of an independent monitoring clinician whose roles are to monitor the patient and attend to the airway, administer drugs, and record clinical data and events.[15] Thus, physician performing the procedure should be different from the physician administering the sedative drugs.

Fasting Guidelines for Conscious or Deep Sedation

Fasting guidelines are the same as for any anesthetic regardless of how "light" the sedative technique be (**Table 1**).[16]

Is an Intravenous Catheter Necessary?

Needle phobia is universal among children. Previously healthy children who present for painful procedures will not have pre-existing IV access. It would be difficult to manage a child during a painful procedure without IV access. Intravenous access is important for any emergency drugs to be administered, for fluid administration, if there is any hypotension and to administer sedative or analgesics intravenously. If eutectic mixture of local anesthetic (EMLA) is available it can be applied an hour before the procedure for better success of IV access.

Is Sedative or Analgesic Best for Children Undergoing Painful Procedures?

Choice of the sedative or anesthetic agent depends on pediatrician's preferences and comfort, and the answers to the following question; (i) Is the procedure painful? e.g. lumbar puncture, bone marrow aspiration, (ii) What is the duration of the procedure?; (iii) Does the child need to be motionless (EEG, CT scan, MRI); and (iv) Is the child outpatient or inpatient?

The character of an ideal sedative or analgesic are depicted in **Table 2**. General recommendations for that use are shown in **Table 3**.

Table 2: Characteristics of an ideal sedative

- Rapid onset
- Predictable duration
- No active metabolites
- Rapid recovery
- Multiple routes of delivery
- Easy to titrate
- Minimal cardiopulmonary effects
- Not altered by renal or hepatic disease
- No drug interactions
- Wide therapeutic index

Table 3: General recommendations for sedation and analgesia

- Assess the child and beware of "full stomach" in emergency situation
- NPO guidelines
- Obtain consent
- Establish venous access
- Check airway and resuscitative equipment including suction apparatus
- Monitor heart rate and oxygen saturation
- All the medications to be diluted and labeled and injected at a very slow rate. After administration of each drug flush the line
- After injecting one drug before injecting another drug, wait at least for 15 to 20 seconds. Watch the respiration
- In the midazolam + fentanyl combination, inject midazolam first
- Atropine/glycopyrrolate, then midazolam and finally ketamine
- Document before and after sedation
- Pediatrician should be trained in pediatric advanced life support

Table 4: Routes and dosages

Route	Dose (mg/kg)	Onset (minutes)	Duration of action
Midazolam			
Oral	0.5–0.7	15–20	45–90 min
Per rectum	0.25–0.5	10–30	60–90 min
Intranasal	0.2–0.5	5–15	45–60 min
Intramuscular	0.05–0.15	10–20	60–120 min
Intravenous	0.05–0.15	2–3	30–60 min
Morphine			
Subcutaneous	0.1–0.15	10	4–5 hr
Intramuscular	0.1–0.15	10	4–5 hr
Intravenous	0.1–0.15	2–5	4 hr
Ketamine			
Oral	6–10	10–30	1–2 hr
Intramuscular	3–5	2–10	60–90 min
Intravenous	1–2	0.5–1	10–30 min
Dexmedetomidine			
Buccal	1 µg/kg	15–30	
Intranasal	1–3 µg/kg	8–10	
Intravenous	0.5–2 µg/kg	2–3	
Etomidate			
Intravenous	0.2–0.4	5–30 secs	

SPECIFIC DRUGS

Benzodiazepines

Benzodiazepines are sedatives, anxiolytic, anticonvulsant but *not analgesic*. The biggest advantage of these drugs is their *amnesic* property. Of all the drugs, benzodiazepines have best anterograde and retrograde amnesia. Of the benzodiazepines, midazolam is a preferred agent for sedation in the emergency room because it is water soluble, has shorter duration and quicker onset of action than diazepam and lorazepam. Because of pain during intravenous, erratic absorption intramuscular injection and long duration of action, diazepam is not a suitable sedative in the emergency department.

Midazolam has minimal hemodynamic effects and is metabolized by liver and excreted by the kidneys. Intravenous flumazenil can reverse midazolam sedation at a dose of 0.01 mg/kg/dose up to a maximum of 0.04 mg/kg. The recommended dosage of midazolam for various routes is given in **Table 4**.

When a combination of midazolam and narcotic is contemplated the dosage of narcotic and midazolam must be individualized and administered by titration rather than by fixed dosage schedule.

Triclofos Sodium

Triclofos sodium has been used for rendering children immobile during painless procedures to keep the child motionless, like ophthalmological examinations, echocardiogram, EEG, CT scan and MRI scan. Despite the safe records and absence of respiratory depression in sedated children, it is advisable to have continuous pulse oximetry monitoring during the procedure. A combination of triclofos and paracetamol can be used if a mild analgesic effect also is required. The dose is 50 to 100 mg/kg and the onset of action is in 30 to 40 minutes and duration of action is 90 to 120 minutes.

Pethidine/Promethazine/Chlorpromazine

The combination of pethidine (2 mg/kg), promethazine (1 mg/kg), and chlorpromazine (1 mg/kg) called "lytic cocktail" has been used for many years for sedation in children especially for cardiac catheterization. Due to availability of better drugs and significant episodes of hypotension, apnea, prolonged recovery and dystonic reactions, the above combination is no longer recommended.

Morphine

Morphine is the gold standard narcotic agent by which other narcotic analgesics are compared. Although a very good analgesic, its main disadvantages are histamine release (not suitable for reactive airway disease children), long duration of action and possible hypotension especially in hypovolemic children. Its metabolite morphine-6-glucuronide is also a potent narcotic. Morphine causes much more nausea and vomiting than other opiates. Though, it is an excellent analgesic for postoperative analgesia, it is not an ideal agent for emergency room procedures due to its longer duration of action. The recommended dosage for various routes is given in **Table 4**.

Fentanyl

Fentanyl[17] is a potent synthetic opiate agonist and is 100 times more potent than morphine. Its faster onset of action, short duration and potent analgesic effect make this drug narcotic of choice for wide variety of painful procedures in the emergency room. It should be given in a dose of 1–3 µg/kg. Fentanyl has an onset of action within 2–3 min and the duration of action is 45–60 min. If fentanyl is given fast, it might cause respiratory depression and apnea. Fentanyl causes mild decrease in the heart rate and peculiar effect to chest wall rigidity, which may impair ventilation. Naloxone will reverse the adverse effects of fentanyl. The combination of fentanyl and midazolam is very good for severe painful procedures but one should be cautious of respiratory depression or even arrest due to its synergistic effect. The newer drugs, ultrashort acting alfentanil and sufentanil, have not entered the Indian market yet.

Ketamine

Ketamine[18] was introduced as an intravenous anesthetic agent. It produces dissociative anesthesia, profound analgesia and sedation while maintaining spontaneous respiratory effort. Though it was introduced as an anesthetic agent it is being used widely for many procedure related pains by the non-anesthesiologist because its potent analgesic effect occurs even when the laryngeal and pharyngeal reflexes are preserved. Because of its bronchodilatory effect, it is a very good analgesic agent for asthmatic children. It increases heart rate and blood pressure. The unpleasant hallucinations seen often in adult occur less frequently in children. Since ketamine increases salivation, it is mandatory to administer antisialogogue (glycopyrrolate or atropine) before injecting ketamine. No reversal agent for ketamine exists. Ketamine should never be taken lightly and resuscitation equipment and drugs should be ready when it is administered. The recommended dosage for various routes is given in **Table 5**. Premedication with atropine or glycopyrrolate (causes less tachycardia) 0.01 to 0.02 mg/kg IV or IM.

Propofol

Propofol, which was used initially as a general anesthetic, due to its short half-life, is now widely used for short-term sedation. The recommended dosage is 1–4 mg/kg intravenously; the onset of action is within 60 sec and the duration of action lasts for 10–15 min. Though long-term (> 48 h) sedation with propofol may cause severe metabolic acidosis, it is being recommended for procedures like CT scan, MRI, intercostal drainage insertion and central venous line placements.

Its main advantage is immediate and smooth recovery. Propofol, a lipid emulsion, is very painful during IV injection. The pain can be alleviated by prior administration of 0.5 mg/kg of lignocaine or mixing it with propofol solution itself. If propofol is to be given in a small doses it is advisable to dilute with 5% dextrose. This agent is associated with some drawbacks like apnea, hypotension, and airway obstruction. So, it is mandatory that a pediatrician should be well trained in airway management.

Table 5: Dosage of some local anesthetics

Drug	*Dose (mg/kg)*	*Onset (min)*	*Duration (min)*
Lignocaine (plain)	4	3–6	60–90
Lignocaine (adrenaline)	7	5–10	90–120
Bupivacaine	2.5	10–15	180–240

Dexmedetomidine

Dexmedetomidine[19] (Dexmed) is a highly selective central α2-adrenergic agonist that provides anxiolysis and cooperative sedation without respiratory depression. It does not have analgesic effect. It has an opioid sparing effect and is rapidly gaining acceptance as a medication of choice in short procedures done in both ICU and emergency room. It induces normal sleep pattern, in contrast to benzodiazepines, thus patients are easily arousable and it does not cause respiratory depression. Respiratory and EEG patterns during Dexmed sedation shows that it preserves epileptiform activity in children with seizure disorders, facilitating localization and identification of seizure foci during EEG studies. In combination with ketamine, its use has extended to painful procedures such as lumbar puncture, bone marrow biopsy, burn dressing changes, chest tube insertion, and femoral cut-down for tunneled central venous catheter placement.

Dexmed causes dose dependent decrease in heart rate and cardiac output. However, literature supports that concurrent hemodynamic collapse or need for pharmacological resuscitation does not occur. Thus, clinician should be well versed with hemodynamic responses while administering dexmedetomidine. Caution should be exercised when administering anticholinergics to treat isolated Dexmed-associated bradycardia in children, because IV glycopyrrolate has been shown to elicit immediate, significant hypertension.

Etomidate

Etomidate[20] is a non-barbiturate hypnotic agent with an ultrashort onset of action (5–30 seconds). Because of its rapid onset of action and rapid recovery, minimal hemodynamics and respiratory effects with few residual effects, it is gaining rapid popularity for sedation during brief non-painful procedures, especially for children who require ongoing clinical assessment of consciousness (e.g. patients with head injury). It reduces ICP and maintains hemodynamic stability, thus a good choice for sedating patients in whom cardiovascular status is uncertain or compromised (e.g. multiple system trauma patients).[21]

There are side effects that sometimes discourage its use. Nausea and vomiting occurs due to activation of nausea center, pain on injection (caused by propylene glycol which is used a preservative), superficial thrombophlebitis 48–72 hours after injection and myoclonus. Pain during IV administration that can be reduced by IV pretreatment with 0.5 mg/kg of systemic *lidocaine* that is injected into the vein one minute prior to etomidate with a tourniquet applied. Pain is also lessened by injecting into an antecubital rather than a hand vein. Etomidate also causes a dose-dependent, temporary and reversible inhibition of steroid synthesis. However, adrenal suppression from single doses of etomidate has not been associated with any negative outcomes in healthy children undergoing procedural sedation.

Non-narcotic Analgesics

Weak analgesics like paracetamol and nonsteroidal anti-inflammatory drugs are the most commonly used drugs in general pediatric practice and sometimes in postoperative analgesia. Though, they are very useful in mild pain, they are not suitable for the procedure related pain in the emergency room.

Local Anesthetics

Local anesthetic[22] agents are sodium channel blockers preventing depolarization of the nerve. To act at the sodium channel, local anesthetics must first enter the cell in non-ionized form and then act inside the cell. Local anesthetics are weak bases, so at physiological pH they exist primarily in the ionized state. In certain local conditions like infection and inflammation, a state of relative tissue acidosis exists and the local anesthetic is not effective. Adding epinephrine to the local anesthetics causes vasoconstriction, decreases rate of absorption and thereby prolongs the duration of the block and reduces the toxicity. Epinephrine containing local anesthetics should never be used in areas supplied by end arteries such as finger, toes, penis and the tip of the nose.

The two drugs, which are commonly used are lignocaine and bupivacaine. Lignocaine has quicker onset and shorter duration of action and bupivacaine has slower onset and longer duration of action. Toxicity includes tinnitus, anaphylaxis, convulsions, cardiac arrhythmias and cardiovascular collapse. The arrhythmias are more common with bupivacaine than lignocaine and it is difficult to treat these drug-induced rhythm disturbances.

The general guidelines for using local anesthetic agents include:

- Use smallest possible needle (24 or 25G) to raise the wheal. First inject subcutaneously and then raise the intradermal wheal to prevent pain.
- All resuscitative equipment and drugs should be ready to manage possible overdosage and toxicity.
- It is always safer to have intravenous line in place.
- To prevent intravascular injection, always aspirate before injecting the local anesthetic.

Infiltration of local anesthesia as an adjunct to sedative drugs is very useful in the following situations: (i) Lumbar puncture; (ii) Suturing small lacerated wounds; (iii) Central venous line placement; (iv) Arterial line placement; (v) Intercostal drainage tube insertion (vi) Bone marrow aspiration and biopsy; and (vii) Liver and kidney biopsy.

Eutectic mixture of local anesthetics

The EMLA is a eutectic mixture of local anesthetic cream, which is a mixture of lignocaine, and prilocaine in water based cream, which provides analgesia even in intact skin. It should be applied at least 60 minutes before the procedure. There are some reports of methemoglobinemia after its application in children less than 6 months of age due to the presence of prilocaine. Its main usage is for intravenous placement but it can be used for lumbar puncture and circumcision.

The dosage of some local anesthetics is given in **Table 5**.

Digital Nerve Block

Of all the regional nerve blocks, the most useful block to be learnt by the pediatrician is digital nerve block. The paired digital nerves enter the digits medially and laterally. Inject 1 to 2 mL of local anesthetic in the web space on either side of the finger or the toe. The usual approach is to enter from the dorsal surface where it is less painful. Epinephrine containing local anesthetic should never be used. It is very useful for suturing finger injuries, removal of warts and foreign body removal.

Synergism

If two drugs of different mechanisms of action are combined, one may potentiate the other one and reduce the dose requirement of each of them for optimal usage. But at the same time, it may carry the increased risk of respiratory depression.

Example 1: *Midazolam and fentanyl*[17]

Combining sedative and analgesic will be very effective for many procedures like lumbar puncture, wound suturing, closed fracture reduction and immobilization. The main advantage of midazolam is amnesia with mild muscle relaxation. Both the drugs should be diluted and injected slowly and titrated to the desired effect without exceeding the upper dose limit of each drug for that particular child. When these combinations are given, it is mandatory to monitor the patient by pulse oximetry. The pediatrician administering these combinations must be skilled in airway management and resuscitation.

Example 2: *Atropine or glycopyrrolate (0.02 mg/kg), midazolam (0.05 mg/kg), ketamine (0.5 to 1 mg/kg); all intravenous.*

It is a statifactory combination for painful procedures like wound suturing and fracture reduction. This cocktail effect is not reversible and airway reflexes may not be maintained.

Example 3: *Dexmedetomidine (0.25 μg/kg) and ketamine (0.5 to 1 mg/kg), all slow intravenous.*[23]

This combination provides sedation, analgesia, amnesia, and hemodynamic stability for painful procedural procedures.

Example 4: *Ketamine (0.5 to 1 mg/kg) and propofol (0.5 mg/kg).*[24] *The opposing effects become complimentary and minimize overall adverse events*

Advantages of combo over ketamine alone are:

- Shorter recovery time;
- Result in smaller doses of each medication needed than either alone;
- Decreased incidence of nausea and vomiting;
- Lower incidence of emergence reactions; and
- Fewer adverse respiratory events.

KEY MESSAGES

- In choosing a technique for sedating an infant or child, it is first essential to identify clearly the goals of the sedation plan and to differentiate between sedation and analgesia. Not all procedures or clinical situations demand both, and there is commonly a greater need for one or the other.
- The most commonly used procedural sedation assessment tool is the University of Michigan Sedation Scale. The COMFORT scale is another commonly used PICU pain and sedation tool.

- Choice of the sedative or anesthetic agent depends on pediatrician's preferences and comfort, and the answers to the following question; (i) Is the procedure painful? e.g. lumbar puncture, bone marrow aspiration; (ii) What is the duration of the procedure?; (iii) Does the child need to be motionless (EEG, CT scan, MRI); and (iv) Is the child outpatient or inpatient?
- Drugs used for sedation and analgesia in children include midazolam, triclofos, fentanyl, ketamine, propofol, dexmedetomidine, etc.

REFERENCES

1. Schechter NL, Berde CB, Yaster M, editors. Pain in Infants, Children, and Adolescents. Baltimore: Williams and Wilkins; 1993.
2. Lee SJ, Ralston HJ, Drey EA, *et al.* Fetal pain: A systematic multi-disciplinary review of the evidence. JAMA. 2005;294: 947-54.
3. Anand KJ, Craig KD. New perspectives on the definition of pain. Pain. 1996;67(1):3-6; discussion 209-11.
4. Bursch B, Collier C, Joseph M, *et al.* Policy statement on pediatric chronic pain. APS Bulletin. 2000;10.
5. Fitzgerald M. Development biology of inflammatory pain. Br J Anaesth. 1995;75:177-85.
6. Rodriguez E, Jordan R. Contemporary trends in pediatric sedation and analgesia. Emerg Med Clin North Am. 2002;20: 199-222.
7. Goad RN, Webster D. Sedation, analgesia, and anesthesia issues in the pediatric patient. Clin Pediatr Med Surg. 1997;14: 131-48.
8. Joint Commission on Accreditation of Healthcare Organizations. Comprehensive Accreditation Manual for Hospitals. Oakbrook Terrace, IL: Joint Commission on Accreditation of Healthcare Organizations; 2005.
9. Puchalski M, Hummel P. The reality of neonatal pain. Adv Neonatal Care. 2002;2:233-44; quiz 245-7.
10. Merkel S, Voepel-Lewis T, Malviya S. Pain assessment in infants and young children: The FLACC scale. Am J Nurs. 2002;102:55-8.
11. Wong DL, Baker CM. Pain in children: Comparison of assessment scales. Pediatr Nurs. 1988;14:9-17.
12. Malviya S, Voepel-Lewis T, Tait AR, *et al.* Depth of sedation in children undergoing computed tomography: Validity and reliability of the University of Michigan Sedation Scale (UMSS). Br J Anaesth. 2002;88:241-5.
13. Ambuel B, Hamlett KW, Marx CM, *et al.* Assessing distress in pediatric intensive care environments: The COMFORT scale. J Pediatr Psychol. 1992;17:95-109.
14. Simmons LE, Riker RR, Prato BS, *et al.* Assessing sedation during intensive care unit mechanical ventilation with the Bispectral Index and the Sedation-Agitation Scale. Crit Care Med. 1999;27:1499-504.
15. Committee on Drugs Section on Anesthesiology. Guidelines for the monitoring and management of pediatric patients during and after sedation for diagnostic and therapeutic procedures. Pediatrics. 1992;89:1110-5.
16. Cote CJ. Sedation protocols: Why so many variations? Pediatrics. 1994;94:281-3.
17. Johnson KL, Erickson JP, Holley FO, *et al.* Fentanyl pharmacokinetics in the pediatric population. Anesthesiology. 1984;61:441-5.
18. Rauch DA. Use of ketamine in a pain management protocol for repetitive procedures. Pediatrics. 1998;102:404-5.
19. Mahmoud M, Mason KP. Dexmedetomidine: Review, update, and future considerations of paediatric perioperative and periprocedural applications and limitations. Br J Anaesth. 2015;115:171-82.
20. Amidate® prescribing information. Drugs.com, January 2009. Available from: *www.drugs.com/pro/amidate.html.* Accessed August 31, 2019.
21. Bramwell KJ, Haizlip J, Pribble C, *et al.* The effect of etomidate on intracranial pressure and systemic blood pressure in pediatric patients with severe traumatic brain injury. Pediatr Emerg Care. 2006;22:90-3.
22. Smith GA, Starugbaugh SD, Harbeck-Weber C, *et al.* Comparison of topical anesthetics with lidocaine infiltration during laceration repair in children. Clin Pediatr (Phila). 1997; 36:17-23.
23. Tobias JD. Dexmedetomidine and ketamine: An effective alternative for procedural sedation? Pediatr Crit Care Med. 2012;13:423-7.
24. Shah A, Mosdossy G, McLeod S, *et al.* A blinded, randomized controlled trial to evaluate ketamine/propofol versus ketamine alone for procedural sedation in children. Ann Emerg Med. 2011;57(5):425-33.e2.

CHAPTER 17

Acute Asthma

Joseph L Mathew

INTRODUCTION

Bronchial asthma is a complex disease with genetic, as well as environmental factors contributing to the etiopathogenesis, clinical manifestations, therapeutic response, clinical course and prognosis. The traditional model considering asthma as a single inflammatory disease characterized by the classic triad of airway (hyper) reactivity, mucosal edema and bronchoconstriction is now giving way to better understanding of the heterogeneous nature of the condition.[1] In fact, it is now believed that there can be fixed as well as reversible limitations to airflow in the broad entity labeled "asthma". Emphasis is being placed on understanding the factors involved in the causation of "asthma" in an individual child and development of personalized therapy protocols.

Irrespective of the background mechanism, asthma is characterized by recurrent, episodic, reversible exacerbations that contribute to significant morbidity for individual children as well as the society at large. The Global Initiative for Asthma (GINA) 2018 guidelines,[2] define "asthma exacerbation" as a progressive increase in symptoms or change from baseline status. This can manifest as shortness of breath, increased cough, wheezing, or chest tightness (in older children/adolescents). This type of change from baseline status is easier to determine in a child with a "known" diagnosis of asthma. However, children can also present for the first time, with an acute episode. In current practice, the term "acute severe asthma" is the preferred term to denote exacerbations. This term is also easier for parents/families to understand. Alternate terminologies include acute episode, flare-up, attack, acute attack, etc.[2] Formerly, the term "status asthmaticus" was used to convey the same concept, although it was sometimes used to signify an episode unresponsive to standard initial treatment. Some authors insist that the term "acute attack" should be used as it better emphasizes the seriousness of the condition, and potential for adverse outcome.[3] In addition, there is now evidence that uncontrolled asthma in children has the potential to restrict lung growth in the long-term.[4]

Management of childhood asthma in general, and acute severe asthma in particular, has been the subject of intense clinical research. In fact, almost every aspect of management has been extensively studied through well-designed randomized controlled trials and systematic reviews. However, there is considerable diversity amongst the various trials (comprising the body of current evidence) in terms of methodological quality, age of children included, definitions of acute asthma, healthcare setting where the trial was conducted, severity grading systems, restrictions to inclusion in the trial, etc. Further, the reported outcomes are also very diverse and include patient centric (hard) outcomes such as treatment success/failure, hospitalization rate, length of hospital stay, changes in clinical parameters documented objectively, occurrence of complications, need for advanced management, etc.; as well as a host of surrogate outcomes such as markers of oxygenation, patient symptoms, clinical signs, respiratory rate, and indirect markers of well-being. More recent studies include economic assessments as well. Since mortality is not very common with appropriate management of acute asthma in clinical trial settings, this is not usually included as an outcome. The diversity in studies on acute asthma management, sometimes makes it difficult to directly compare studies against each other and/or pool the data together for an informed decision. Nevertheless, several clinical practice guidelines have been developed by professional societies and agencies to provide optimal management in a cost-effective manner.[2,5-8] While some of the elements of management are common across the various guidelines, some elements are entirely context specific and cannot be easily extrapolated. This chapter summarizes the current evidence for the management of acute severe asthma in children, focusing on the Indian setting.

EPIDEMIOLOGY AND ETIOLOGY

Some years back, the World Health Organization (WHO) calculated that almost 250 million people suffer from asthma all over the world. In many developed countries, it is the most frequent chronic condition affecting children, and accounts for a very large number of emergency visits and hospital admissions.[8] In the United Kingdom alone, over one million children suffer from asthma; this translates to a prevalence of almost 10% in the pediatric age group.[6] Asthma is often reported as the most common chronic disease of childhood.[40]

The ISAAC phase three study suggested that in India, about 6% children in the age group 6–7 years, as well as in the age group 13–14 years have asthma.[9] However, the precise burden of childhood acute asthma is difficult to calculate on a nation-wide basis. In referral hospitals, it constitutes a significant part of pediatric emergency visits. In the Pediatric Emergency at PGIMER Chandigarh, acute asthma was observed to be the third most frequent cause of visits to the emergency.[10,11] A publication from the All India Institute of Medical Sciences, New Delhi reported that acute asthma comprised about 4% of all pediatric emergency room visits, and overall less than 1% children with acute asthma required intensive care.[12]

Acute asthma often occurs in children with pre-existing asthma who have been appropriately diagnosed and are taking regular controller medication. In such situations, there is usually an identifiable trigger for the worsening (i.e. acute episode). This could be a viral upper respiratory infection, or exposure to known environmental triggers, or a decline in treatment adherence in terms of dose, frequency, or regularity. Personal experience suggests that diminished treatment adherence and/or incorrect technique of controller inhalation therapy are very frequent causes of acute exacerbations. Exposure to aero-allergens, air pollution, and tobacco smoke can also trigger acute episodes. Some medications, strenuous physical exertion and often emotional stress are well known triggers of acute episodes. Less commonly, uncontrolled comorbidities and/or complications such as Allergic Bronchopulmonary Aspergillosis (ABPA) may be the triggering factors. However, it should be remembered that acute exacerbations may be the first manifestation of bronchial asthma in some children. In such situations, no obvious trigger may be evident.

PATHOPHYSIOLOGY

Asthma is characterized by the classic triad of airway inflammation, mucosal edema and airway (hyper) reactivity. Acute asthma is characterized by episodic worsening of these three pathophysiologic components, usually in response to a known or unknown trigger. This leads to obstruction in the distal small airways by mucus secretions, airway edema and bronchospasm. The resultant reduction in airway caliber leads to higher airway resistance, thereby reducing expiratory airflow; there is more inflow than outflow with each breath leading to hyperinflation of the lungs. This in turn creates mechanical disadvantages to normal respiration, decreasing the forced vital capacity and expiratory volume. Ventilation-perfusion mismatches then follow (due to increasingly aerated alveoli but no corresponding increase in perfusion) along with increased intra-pulmonary shunting.[13] Pulmonary vascular resistance increases along with decreased systemic blood pressure due to higher left ventricular afterload (on account of deeper negative intrathoracic pressure).[10] Thus, acute severe asthma can be complicated and present with several clinical signs reflecting compromised cardiovascular status.

CLINICAL FEATURES

The diagnosis of acute severe asthma in children is based almost entirely on clinical grounds. Unlike adults and adolescents where documentation of airflow limitation using spirometry or peak expiratory flow

(PEF) measurement is part of the standard management protocol,[2] these are often not feasible in children. Clinical evaluation of symptoms and signs are generally sufficient to guide the diagnosis and management. In children with pre-existing asthma, symptoms suggesting an acute severe episode include increased cough, wheezing, chest tightness, and shortness of breath. However, the degree of wheezing may not directly correlate with disease severity.[12] Other symptoms include inability to lie down (in older children), difficulty in speaking complete sentences, sweating, etc.

In children younger than 5 years, reduced exercise tolerance (or limitation in physical activity), and/or decreased feeding may be additional symptoms. A combination of increased daytime cough, daytime wheezing, and need for reliever medication at night may predict an imminent acute exacerbation.[2] Young children often have exacerbations in association with upper respiratory tract infection (cold), hence the above symptoms/signs in the presence of a viral upper respiratory infection are consistent with acute asthma. Clinical signs include tachypnea, increased work of breathing, generalized polyphonic wheeze (i.e. variable pitch/tone in different parts of the lung), and use of accessory muscles of respiration. Transcutaneous measurement of oxygen saturation helps to determine hypoxia.

In children who present one or more of the above symptoms and signs, for the first time (i.e. without a pre-existing diagnosis of asthma), it may be difficult to make a clinical diagnosis of acute asthma with certainty, as some other clinical conditions can present similarly. These are highlighted in the section on Differential Diagnosis.

Although clinical symptoms/signs are sufficient for diagnosing acute asthma, it should be recognized that symptoms do not always correlate with objective measures of airway obstruction. Even clinical scoring systems often do not relate to lung function tests.[14,15] This is why many guidelines in developed countries emphasize objective measurements of airflow and/or lung function.

Clinical signs that can help to identify cases of acute asthma associated with high(er) mortality are referred as "red flag signs". These are well described in the GINA 2018 guidelines.[2] The situations relevant to Indian children include the following:

- Previous episode(s) requiring endotracheal intubation and mechanical ventilation.
- Previous episode(s) requiring hospital admission or Emergency room management within the preceding 12 months.
- Inappropriate treatment of current asthma.
- Excessive usage of rescue/reliever medication.
- Absence of a written asthma management plan.

Respiratory failure may be associated with central cyanosis, pulsus paradoxus >20 mm Hg, paradoxical breathing, silent chest and low oxygen saturation not ameliorated by oxygen.

Complications

Acute severe asthma can result in respiratory failure, cardiovascular compromise, and cardiac failure if not managed appropriately. In can be associated with other life-threatening complications including air-leaks manifesting as pneumothorax, pneumo-mediastinum, and subcutaneous emphysema. Obstruction of airways can lead to atelectasis further compromising gas exchange. All complications of hypoxemia can become evident. Rarely, children can present with the syndrome of inappropriate antidiuretic hormone (SIADH) manifesting as signs of fluid overload and oliguria.

DIFFERENTIAL DIAGNOSES

Although there are only a limited number of clinical conditions mimicking the features of acute asthma in a child with pre-existing physician diagnosed asthma, it may not be easy to distinguish these alternate diagnoses in a child presenting for the first time. Further, younger children and infants may have diagnoses other than asthma, even if they have had wheezing episodes previously and loosely been labeled as asthma.

The first episode of clinical features mimicking acute asthma may be seen in infants/toddlers with acute bronchiolitis (caused by RSV and other viruses). Such children have wheezing as the most prominent symptom and sign, although cough, runny nose, and fever may be present.

Foreign body inhalation is generally associated with localized signs in a child with a history of sudden onset coughing or choking while feeding or playing with toys. However, unwitnessed foreign body aspiration may be difficult to pinpoint especially in young infants/children wherein localization of wheeze is sometimes difficult. In such situations, the presence of an older sibling in the habit of trying to feed the infant may give a clue. The classic radiographic feature of localized hyperinflation can clinch the diagnosis. Rarely, the foreign body may lodge in the trachea or glottis, producing stridor that may be mistaken as wheeze. There are also instances of vegetable foreign bodies splitting and lodging in the airways on both sides, creating bilateral wheeze. In such cases, the absence of localizing signs and absent antecedent history makes it difficult to distinguish acute asthma from foreign body aspiration.

Aspiration syndromes in young infants can mimic asthma symptoms in terms of recurrent, episodic wheeze sometimes necessitating hospitalization. A history of respiratory symptoms during feeding suggests a direct communication between the airway and esophagus, as in a tracheoesophageal fistula. The usual history in gastro-esophageal reflux disease is regurgitation of feed, and/or respiratory symptoms several minutes after completing feeding.

Congenital heart disease can sometimes present with recurrent episodic wheezing. The mechanism is either congestive heart failure, or enlarged vessels compressing the airways. Generally, a history suggesting congenital heart disease and/or physical examination of the cardiovascular system reveals the diagnosis. However, dilated cardiomyopathy with resultant cardiac failure is one condition that can present without a murmur. Astute clinical judgment with radiographic evidence of a wide cardiac shadow can provide a clue.

Vascular malformations can present with wheezing related to airway compression/narrowing. Aberrant right subclavian artery passing behind the airway has sometimes been missed until imaging studies are done. Similarly, other vascular anomalies including airway hemangiomas, pulmonary artery sling, etc. may cause mild wheezing that intensifies with episodes of infection.

Congenital airway and pulmonary anomalies usually present with symptoms starting early in life. Upper airway anomalies resulting in obstruction of the airway generally produces stridor that can be misinterpreted as wheezing by the family and/or primary physician. Similarly, airway collapse in laryngomalacia and trachea/bronchomalacia produces stridor that can be mistaken as wheeze. Pulmonary adenomatoid malformation, bronchogenic cysts, esophageal duplication cysts, sequestered lobe, mediastinal masses, etc. can sometimes be mistaken as asthma.

It should be remembered that pulmonary infections can pour secretions into the airways creating wheezing. In such cases, crackles are present with auscultable wheeze. Moreover, acute asthma can be associated with crackles even without the presence of infection. In an acute setting wherein clinical examination reveals both crackles and wheeze, other clues may be required viz wet-sounding cough, presence of fever, systemic toxicity, expectoration of sputum, etc. Clinical conditions associated with bronchiectasis (cystic fibrosis, primary ciliary dyskinesia, primary or secondary immune deficiency, idiopathic bronchiectasis, etc.) can present with acute exacerbations associated with wheezing.

MANAGEMENT

Management of acute severe asthma in the hospital.

Step 1: Stabilization

As in all pediatric emergencies, the first step is to stabilize the child through a rapid assessment of vital signs, and focus on the A, B, C components of emergency care. The Airway (A) should be checked for patency and ensured that it is open; Breathing (B) is assessed and supported if required, and Circulation (C) is assessed by confirmation of peripheral pulse volume, capillary refill time, etc. If any of the components of ABC is/are impaired, the child qualifies for immediate resuscitation. Other clinical clues demanding immediate attention including endotracheal intubation include altered sensorium (drowsy, lethargic, unresponsive), bradycardia, silent chest, and low oxygen saturation.

Step 2: Focused History

This should be directed to identifying the timing of acute episode, possible trigger cause(s), compliance to previously prescribed therapy, status of devices, and any home-based management provided. Other relevant history to be sought include presence of features of a viral (or other) respiratory infection.

Step 3: Clinical Examination

Assess the vital signs (consciousness, heart rate, peripheral pulse, respiratory rate, blood pressure, and oxygen saturation). Thereafter, assess the severity of the acute episode by evaluating the ability to complete sentences,

Table 1: PRAM scoring system

	0	1	2	3
Oxygen saturation*	≥ 95%	92–94%	<92%	
Suprasternal retraction (visual assessment)	Absent		Present	
Scalene muscle contraction (palpatory assessment)	Absent		Present	
Air entry**	Normal	Decreased at the base	Decreased at the apex and base	Minimal or absent
Wheezing**	Absent	Only during expiration	Present during inspiration (± expiration)	Audible without stethoscope or silent chest

*In gen*eral, a score ranging from 0 to 3 represents mild exacerbation, 4–7 represents moderate exacerbation and 8–12 is considered severe.

* Oxygen saturation should be checked when the child is breathing room air. For serial assessments, the oxygen should be turned off for approximately 1 minute. In case saturation falls <92%, a score of 2 is given and the oxygen can be turned on immediately. However, some guidelines do not recommend turning off supplemental oxygen for measurement of saturation.[8]

** Air entry and wheezing are described for lung fields. The Right anterior lung field represents the Right upper and middle lobes, the Right posterior lung field represents the Right upper and lower lobes, the Left anterior lung field and the Left posterior lung field both represent the Left upper and lower lobes. In case different lung fields have different scores, the field with the greatest score is taken into consideration.

Adapted from References 16 and 17.

use of accessory muscles, and presence of wheeze on auscultation.

Clinical scoring systems can be used to judge the severity of acute episodes as well as guide the intensity of treatment. Currently, the Pediatric Respiratory Assessment Measure (PRAM) Score is considered a validated, reliable and applicable system.[16,17] It is a twelve-point clinical scoring system that evaluates scalene muscle contraction, suprasternal retractions, wheezing, air entry, and oxygen saturation. It has been validated for children in the age group 1–17 years. The scoring can be done by any medical personnel in the Emergency Unit including physicians, nurses and other members of the team. **Table 1** shows the scoring criteria.

The GINA guidelines[2] proposed a somewhat different system of severity categorization. Mild to moderate exacerbation in an older child is characterized by one who is alert, not agitated, and able to talk in phrases. Although respiratory rate is higher than normal, accessory muscle use is not evident. Oxygen saturation in room air is above 90% and PEF is usually >50% of the predicted value or personal best. Children younger than 5 years with mild exacerbation may be breathless, agitated, and have heart rate less than 180 per minute. Oxygen saturation is >92%.

In contrast, an older child who is sitting hunched forward, agitated, unable to speak more than words, and with evident usage of accessory muscles, would be categorized as severe exacerbation. Such children may have oxygen saturation less than 90% and PEF <50% of the predicted value or personal best.

Those children in a drowsy or confused state and/or a silent chest are categorized as having life threatening exacerbation. The last two categories need immediate management in an institution. The corresponding criteria in pre-school children are inability to speak, refusal of feed, confusion/drowsiness, heart rate >200/min in children <3 years, and >180/min in those 3–5 years, significant chest retractions, and oxygen saturation <92%.[2]

In comparison to these guidelines, the British Thoracic Society (BTS) and Scottish Inter-Collegiate Guideline Network (SIGN) guideline define acute severe asthma in children older than one year of age by inability to speak complete sentences in a single breath (or inability to feed in infants), tachycardia (defined as heart rate >125/ minute in children older than 5 years, and >140/minute in those younger than 5 years), tachypnea (defined as respiratory rate >30/minute in children older than 5 years and >40/ minute in those younger than 5 years), oxygen saturation <92%, peak expiratory flow between 33% and 50%.[3] In this guideline, a life-threatening episode is identified by features such as silent chest, cyanosis, hypotension, exhaustion, confusion, oxygen saturation <92% and peak expiratory flow <33%. However, it is unclear whether physicians following these guidelines are expected to attempt objective measures of lung function in acutely sick children.

Placing too much reliance on absolute cut-off values for tachycardia or tachypnea may not be prudent because these are affected by a variety of factors. There is also no consensus on what the exact cut-off values should be. For example, the Italian guidelines.[8] use heart rate upper limit of 100/min in children between 2 and 8 years, and 120/min in children 1–2 years.

Investigations such as spirometry are not routinely feasible in children with acute exacerbation. Similarly, arterial blood gas analysis is not recommended in most situations. This may be required in children who fail to improve as expected or show clinical signs of worsening. Likewise chest radiography is not routinely recommended in acute asthma, unless the history or physical examination suggest alternate diagnoses (such as foreign body inhalation, pneumonia, etc.) or a complication such as pneumothorax. One guideline developed for children in Italy,[8] incorporated arterial blood gas $PaCO_2$ values in the classification of severity. Suggested cut-off values in mild, moderate and severe acute episodes were <38, 38–42, and >42 mm Hg, respectively.

Investigations

Laboratory investigations are generally not required for confirmation of the diagnosis in acute asthma. However, sometimes a chest radiograph may be required to rule out other clinical conditions that mimic acute asthma. The most common is suspected foreign body aspiration wherein the classical signs of localized airway obstruction are difficult to discern. In such situations, a posteroanterior (if possible) or supine chest radiograph (if standing/sitting is not possible) may be obtained. Since community acquired pneumonia does not routinely warrant chest radiography, there is no need to obtain one in children with acute asthma suspected of having underlying pneumonia. If a congenital airway malformation is suspected on clinical grounds, sometimes a chest radiograph may help to strengthen the diagnosis. In the event of a suspected complication such as pneumothorax suspected clinically, a chest radiograph may be helpful in planning the site of intercostal tube insertion.

Computed tomography (CT) of the chest is not advisable in children presenting with acute asthma.

Blood gas analysis is also not routinely required in children with acute asthma. It should be reserved for children who fail to respond to standard therapy in the expected timeframe, or show unusual/unexpected clinical course, or secondary worsening. It is very useful to guide escalation of management in pediatric intensive care units (PICU). Once a child is in the PICU, there is no need of "routine" blood gas analysis to assess the clinical status.

Some centers managing adult (and sometimes pediatric) acute asthma in developed countries emphasize the value of measuring Fractional Exhaled Nitric Oxide (FeNO) which is a marker of airway eosinophilic inflammation. This is not routinely available in our country.

Other laboratory investigations may be planned based on clinical need.

Step 4: Pharmacologic Management

This revolves around the three-pronged strategy of providing oxygen, short acting beta-2 agonist (SABA) reliever medication and systemic steroid therapy.

Short-acting beta-2 agoinsts

In exacerbations with PRAM score less than 8 (i.e. mild to moderate severity), SABA can be delivered using MDI with spacer.[18] This was shown in a Cochrane review with multiple trials in adults as well as children.[18] In children, the duration of stay in the emergency was shorter with spacer. Heart rate was also lower among children using spacers, and the incidence of tremors was also reduced. Metered dose inhaler with spacer can be used in children of all ages, although an additional face mask may be added in younger children and infants. An overview of systematic reviews exploring treatment of acute asthma in children identified 7 reviews related to efficacy of SABA.[19] The overall conclusion was that SABA inhaled through a metered dose inhaler and spacer was superior to nebulizer, reducing the need for hospitalization, duration of emergency room stay and improving clinical score. The overall safety profile was also better with spacers.

An older Cochrane review suggested that even home-made spacers can be as efficacious as commercial spacers.[20] More recent trials have also confirmed the same.[21] However, "home-made" is a somewhat loose term and hence all such "spacers" may not be efficacious. A dosage of 400 to 1000 μg salbutamol is recommended every 20 minutes during the first hour in older children. A slightly lower dose ranging from 200 to 600 μg may be used in younger children and infants. If there is adequate clinical response, subsequent doses may range from 400–1000 µg every 3–4 hours to as much as 600–1000 µg every hour in older children, and 200–600 µg in younger children. In older children who do not have severe exacerbation, SABA can be delivered by dry powder inhalers (DPI) also.[2] However, DPI require patients to breathe in with an effort which is usually possible in children older than 5 years. If this is not possible, then DPI should not be used.

Although nebulized SABA is not required for children with mild to moderate exacerbations, it is generally preferred in severe asthma as the body of evidence for MDI in this situation is limited. Also, in children in mild-moderate exacerbations, who are not being treated with MDIs, it may not be feasible to administer SABA with MDI in an emergency setting; in such situations, nebulization is often used. Nebulization has the advantage of delivering uninterrupted humidified oxygen if a central supply oxygen is used to create the aerosol. However, this benefit is lost when air-driven nebulizer machines are used; in fact such machines can make children more hypoxemic.[13] Further, the inner parts of the nebulizer are not cleaned creating the theoretical risk of contamination, and spread of infection. It is unclear whether nebulized salbutamol is more efficacious when delivered intermittently or continuously. The GINA guidelines recommended that initially continuous delivery may be used, followed by intermittent delivery.[2]

In older children with PRAM >8, continuous nebulization with salbutamol in the dosage 0.5 mg/kg may be used children, whereas the usual nebulizer dose in mild to moderate exacerbation is 0.15 mg/kg delivered intermittently. In those younger than 5 years, the GINA guidelines recommend that salbutamol may be administered by nebulizer in the dose of 2.5 mg per dose diluted with 3 mL normal saline. However, dosage per kg body weight can be used in this situation also. Nebulized route is especially useful in young children whose oxygen saturation is low, as it ensures that oxygen can be provided even during inhalation of SABA. In those whose saturation is not low, metered dose inhaler and spacer with or without a mask can be used. The dose range is 200–600 µg salbutamol depending on the severity.

While the therapeutic benefits of inhaled SABA are undeniable in acute asthma, it should be remembered that some portion will always be absorbed into the systemic circulation. SABA can end up reversing the vasoconstriction (in response to alveolar hypoxia) and potentially worsen ventilation-perfusion mismatch.[13]

Oxygen therapy

Oxygen should be provided to children with all severity levels targeting a saturation of 94–98% in children 6–11 years old, although 93–95% is an acceptable target in adolescents.[2,5] Low flow oxygen may be provided using a tightly fitting face mask or nasal cannula. In general, all guidelines recommend that oxygen should be humidified.[8]

Steroids

Systemic corticosteroid therapy: It may be delivered as oral prednisolone in the dosage 1–2 mg/kg up to a maximum of 40 mg. The upper limit is 30 mg per day for children 2–5 years old and 20 mg per day for infants <2 years old.[2] The daily upper limits in the BTS/SIGN guideline are 10 mg for children less than 2 years old, 20 mg for children 2–5 years old, and 30–40 mg in older children.[5] This guideline has an additional provision that if a child is taking oral steroids as maintenance therapy (very rare in the Indian context), the upper limit may be 60 mg per day.

Alternate steroid medications are one or two doses of oral dexamethasone (0.15–0.3 mg/kg/day) or intravenous hydrocortisone (in the dose of 10 mg/kg) followed by 5 mg/kg/dose every 6 hourly (upper limit 100 mg/dose). Systemic steroid therapy enhances clinical resolution and prevents relapses. Ideally systemic steroids should be administered within the first hour itself, although some experts delay it until the end of the first hour of treatment with SABA.[2] Oral administration is as efficacious as intravenous administration, and liquid preparations can be used in children. However, it should be remembered that oral corticosteroids (OCS) require about 4 hours for a discernible improvement in symptoms. Intramuscular route has been used in some settings but this is less preferred in children. The usual duration of systemic steroids is 3–5 days. This can then be omitted without tapering of dose. There is emerging evidence that oral dexamethasone for 1–2 days may be as effective as other steroid preparations. An updated meta-analysis confirmed comparable efficacy, although frequency of vomiting was decreased with dexamethasone.[22] Nevertheless, some physicians do not prefer dexamethasone on account of metabolic effects beyond 2 days of treatment.

Inhaled corticosteroid therapy

There is evidence that high dose ICS administered within the first hour can reduce the need for hospital admission. In fact, one of the pioneering studies demonstrating efficacy was conducted in PGIMER, Chandigarh itself.[23] Usually, three doses of Budesonide 800 µg are administered at 20 minute intervals within the first hour. Some studies have attempted comparison of ICS versus systemic steroids, and shown clinically similar benefits. An older Cochrane review identified 13 trials in children and reported that those receiving ICS had decreased hospitalization, and some improvement in peak expiratory flow as well as FEV_1. The authors suggested that ICS therapy is beneficial in patients who are not treated with systemic corticosteroids.[24] A more recent systematic review with 8 pediatric trials found no difference between ICS and systemic steroids for hospitalization.[25] One placebo-controlled, double-blinded, double-dummy design RCT compared 2000 µg/day nebulized fluticasone propionate versus 1 mg/kg/day oral methylprednisolone in children with moderate acute asthma. Objective changes in symptom scores and peak expiratory flow appeared similar in both the groups. The authors concluded equivalent efficacy of inhaled fluticasone with oral methylprednisolone.[26] An Indian trial with a double dummy design among children 5–12 years of age, compared 800 µg inhaled budesonide (three doses at 20 minute intervals) versus single dose of 2 mg/kg oral prednisolone. The clinical outcomes were similar in both groups, although in the group receiving budesonide had more patients who could be discharged by 2 hours.[27] Despite these pieces of individual and collective evidence, most guidelines have not recommended switching to ICS.[8] Further, addition of ICS to systemic steroids has not been shown to have added advantage in children with moderate severity of acute asthma, although there was some benefit in children with severe exacerbations.[28]

Anticholinergics

Ipratropium bromide is also used in the initial management of moderate to severe exacerbations. The onset of bronchodilator effect is slower with ipratropium (compared to SABA), but the combination can be synergistic as the mechanisms of action are different. Thus, some studies in moderate to severe exacerbations have shown beneficial effects when SABA and ipratropium were administered together in the emergency department, compared to SABA alone. A Cochrane review with 20 trials including almost 2700 children confirmed that the requirement of hospitalization was reduced.[29] Although there was no reduction in the length of hospitalization in those admitted for treatment.[30] Pulmonary function tests were better and the risk of tremor was lower with the combination.[29] The usual dose range is 250 µg delivered via nebulizer (GINA), although the recent Italian guidelines recommended nebulization with 125–250 µg per dose in preschool children and 250–500 µg per dose in older children.[8] However, continuous nebulization with ipratropium is not advised.

A Cochrane review comparing inhaled anticholinergic alone versus SABA as well as anticholinergic plus SABA in children over two years old identified six trials. Treatment failure rate was higher with anticholinergic alone versus SABA, as well as anticholinergic alone versus the combination.[31]

ICS-LABA combinations

There is insufficient evidence for the efficacy of ICS-LABA combinations in children for the management of acute severe asthma in the hospital setting.

Magnesium sulfate

A 2016 Cochrane review with 5 trials showed that intravenous magnesium reduced hospitalization in children with moderate to severe acute exacerbations.[32] A more recent systematic review with 6 randomized and quasi-randomized trials in children, reported that intravenous magnesium improved pulmonary function as well as reduced hospitalization.[33] This was reiterated in a detailed exploration of current evidence relevant to the Indian context as well.[34] Intravenous magnesium sulfate has been observed to be efficacious in children who do not respond well to the initial treatment, and is preferable to starting other medications such as aminophylline/terbutaline.[35] Thus, it is generally used after the first hour of management. The usual dose is 50 mg/kg and this can be repeated 4 times at 6 hourly intervals.

Some investigators reported beneficial effects of inhaled magnesium in trials where salbutamol was nebulized using magnesium sulfate rather than normal saline as the vehicle, however the evidence base is weak.[8] In a large Cochrane review examining the efficacy of inhaled magnesium sulfate, there were 12 trials with children.[36] Addition of inhaled magnesium to inhaled SABA and ipratropium showed inconsistent benefit. Although initial hospitalization appeared to be reduced, there was no impact on step-up care and re-admission. Addition of magnesium sulfate to SABA also failed to show a consistent benefit with the combination. A recent systematic review with 4 trials also did not find significant benefits on pulmonary function or hospitalization.[33] More recently, a well-designed trial has been initiated across seven centers in Canada to explore the potential place of nebulized magnesium in treatment of childhood acute asthma.[37]

A limited number of studies undertaking direct comparison between inhaled magnesium and inhaled SABA were mostly in favor of SABA. Nevertheless, the BTS/SIGN guideline provided a weak recommendation to add 150 mg magnesium sulfate to every dose of nebulized salbutamol and ipratropium within the first hour of management itself.[5]

Intravenous salbutamol is recommended as a second-line treatment in unresponsive children older than 5 years in the BTS/SIGN guideline[5] and Italian guideline.[8] The dose is 15 µg/kg. This is probably based on an older Cochrane review comparing intravenous SABA versus intravenous aminophylline that included only two pediatric trials and found insufficient evidence to favor one over the other.[38] However, intravenous preparation of the drug is not available in India.

A Cochrane review evaluating the addition of intravenous SABA to inhaled SABA identified two trials in a small number of children. One trial reported shorter recovery time with the combination, and earlier discharge from the emergency. However, the other trial conducted in an ICU setting did not find similar benefits.[39]

Aminophylline, terbutaline and theophylline

The GINA guidelines[2] strongly recommend against the use of these medications on account of inferior efficacy (compared to SABA) and safety issues. However, these continue to be used in pediatric intensive care units in India when a child has not responded to the initial management. Intravenous terbutaline is given in a loading dose of 10 µg/kg followed by infusion of 0.1–10 µg/kg/min. The infusion rate may require titration at 20 minute intervals to achieve the required clinical response. The dose for aminophylline is 5 mg/kg loading dose infused over 20 minutes followed by a continuous infusion at 0.5–1.0 mg/kg/hr. Both drugs have a low safety profile; hence, careful clinical and/or ECG monitoring is required. It is not advisable to attempt using these medications outside an intensive care unit. There is little to choose between aminophylline and terbutaline,[35] although some intensivists prefer aminophylline.[40] However, a detailed systematic review of 14 trials observed that the dose of intravenous aminophylline in children did not correlate well with clinical outcomes such as resolution of symptoms, length of hospital stay or need for mechanical ventilation.[41]

Intravenous theophylline is sometimes considered as a second line treatment for acute asthma in children. The target serum theophylline level is believed to range from 10 to 20 mg/L. A systematic review examining the clinical outcomes of children receiving theophylline who achieved serum levels in this range (versus those who did not) failed to discern any differences in symptom duration, length of hospital stay, requirement of mechanical ventilation or pulmonary function parameters.[42] Interestingly, serum level >20 mg/L was not associated with greater incidence of adverse events.

Leukotriene receptor antagonists (LTRA)

These are not generally recommended in acute severe asthma,[8] although some physicians have tried this in younger children/infants. A Cochrane review including three trials in children did not find any significant difference in hospitalization rate or objective lung function parameters with oral LTRA.[43] A recent placebo controlled, blinded RCT examined montelukast (in addition to standard pharmacotherapy) in children 2–5 years of age with acute asthma. However, there were no significant differences with respect to FEV_1 or peak expiratory flow at any time point during the course of treatment.[44]

Heliox

A 2014 systematic review of heliox driven nebulization with SABA identified only 3 pediatric trials. Overall, it was associated with better lung function parameters, especially in those with severe exacerbation.[45] Thus, the current guidelines do not recommend the routine use of heliox in the management of acute asthma, unless it is severe and not responding to the usual therapeutic regimens.[8] It is not readily available in the Indian setting.

Heated, humidified, high flow nasal cannula (HHHFNC) oxygen therapy

This was shown to be useful in one study (compared to conventional delivery of oxygen by face mask) in terms of better symptom score and resolution of hypoxemia within the initial two hours of treatment.[46] In another retrospective study, HHHFNC was compared to NIV with respect to treatment failure. Although NIV was superior in terms of efficacy, length of stay in the PICU was similar.[47]

Noninvasive ventilation (NIV)

Small scale studies suggest that NIV could relieve symptoms in acute asthma, but the evidence is limited in terms of quantity and quality to offer definite recommendations for clinical practice. Details of noninvasive and invasive mechanical ventilation strategies are outside the scope of this chapter.

Antibiotics

In a Cochrane review examining antibiotics for acute asthma in adults and children, three trials included children less than 18 years of age. However, the overall evidence was limited in terms of quantity and quality to offer confident conclusions in favor of antibiotics.[48] Although some experts advocate antibiotics, these are not generally recommended.[2]

General supportive measures include provision of a calm environment, maintenance of hydration, maintaining normothermia, and attention to electrolyte levels, especially as salbutamol can result in hypokalemia.

Generally, acute asthma is managed taking into consideration the age of the child, clinical severity, and response to the initial treatment. **Table 2** provides a broad summary of the management protocol. However, individual adjustments may be made depending on the clinical need. Escalation of therapy and management options in intensive care units is beyond the scope of this chapter.

Clinical monitoring

It is ideal to monitor children with an acute severe episode frequently, generally hourly. Periodic monitoring of heart rate, pulse, blood pressure, accessory muscle use, respiratory rate, auscultatory findings and oxygen saturation form the backbone of clinical monitoring. The PRAM score is useful for objective determination of response and hourly monitoring can be continued till the PRAM is less than 4. If objective measures of airflow or lung function are feasible, these can be recorded along with clinical monitoring. However, there are considerable challenges in using these routinely for children.

Clinical monitoring should also include detection of medication side effects. SABA therapy is associated with tachycardia and tremors. In addition, the risk of hypokalemia should be remembered. Anticholinergic medications may be associated with dryness of mouth.

Step 5: Hospital Admission and Transfer to Intensive Care Unit

The criteria for hospitalization of children with acute severe asthma may vary from institution to institution. Clinical criteria include markers of deterioration or non-response. Objective criteria include FEV_1 less than 60% of predicted or personal best.

The specific criteria to transfer children to pediatric ICU may depend on the individual unit, but in general, those who respond poorly to initial treatment, require continuous salbutamol inhalation, have severe hypoxia, impending or established respiratory failure, etc., are suitable candidates.[40] Some authors use the term "critical asthma" for children with acute asthma requiring intensive care or a need for treatment escalation.[40]

Step 6: Discharge

Criteria for discharge from hospital include relief of symptoms, and oxygen saturation >94% while breathing room air. At discharge, pharmacologic prescription should include reliever medication as needed, and controller medication in a dose higher than the previous dose. In children whose first episode necessitated hospitalization, controller medication should be initiated. In addition, oral prednisolone may be continued for 3–5 days. A Cochrane review comparing single dose intramuscular dexamethasone versus oral prednisone (for a few days) at discharge identified a comparable risk for relapse and no significant differences in the adverse event profile between the arms.[49] Although single dose intramuscular dexamethasone was not superior to a short course of oral prednisone for preventing relapse, it may be an option in children where compliance to prescribed therapy may be a concern. Another Cochrane review could not conclude

Table 2: Outline of clinical management of acute asthma

	Mild acute asthma	*Moderate acute asthma*	*Severe acute asthma or Life-threatening acute asthma*
PRAM score	<3	4–7	8–12
Initial management after stabilization	Oxygen if required Inhaled SABA* 3 doses at 20 minute intervals	Oxygen if required Inhaled SABA* 3 doses at 20 minute intervals Consider addition of ICS 3 doses at 20 minute intervals Consider addition of Ipratropium 3 doses at 20 minute intervals	Continuous oxygen Continuous inhaled SABA** + Ipratropium 3 doses at 20 minute intervals + Systemic steroid Consider addition of ICS 3 doses at 20 minute intervals
At the end of 1st hour	If PRAM improved, use inhaled SABA as required Observe for 1 hour and consider discharge on inhaled ICS and SABA as required If PRAM is >3, step up therapy to moderate severity protocol	If PRAM <4, use inhaled SABA as required Observe for 1 hour and plan discharge	If PRAM >8 or clinical worsening is evident, continue above + add intravenous magnesium sulfate If PRAM 4-7, continue treatment as for moderate severity If PRAM <3, observe hourly
At the end of 2nd hour		If PRAM is 0–3, discharge on OCS (for 3–5 days), ICS and inhaled SABA as required If PRAM is 4–7, re-start moderate severity protocol If PRAM >8, step up to severe exacerbation protocol	If PRAM >8 or clinical worsening is evident, continue above treatment and consider transfer to ICU Step-up treatment to include IV aminophylline, OR consider noninvasive ventilation OR intubation and mechanical ventilation In the ICU, ketamine may be considered 4 doses of IV magnesium sulfate and hydrocortisone at 6 hourly intervals to continue
			Continue above therapy till child is stable for 6–12 hours Step down therapy decreasing dose and/or frequency of administration, starting with the medications added last Consider transfer to ward once child has improved and is stable for at least 6–12 hours Plan discharge when the child is receiving inhaled salbutamol not more than every 8 hours At discharge, the child should be prescribed OCS for 5 days, ICS and inhaled SABA as required

*Ideally delivered by metered dose inhaler with spacer (and additional mask in young children/infants).
**Delivered by nebulizer driven by oxygen.

whether shorter or lower-dose oral corticosteroid regimens were significantly different from longer or higher-dose regimens, in terms of efficacy or safety.[50]

Children may require a temporary step-up in the therapy protocol for a few weeks, although this decision is not universal and must be individualized. The precise duration for this is also unclear. The GINA guidelines[2] recommend a duration as short as 1–2 weeks to as long as 12 weeks depending on the possible cause(s) of exacerbation.

At the time of discharge, a formal action plan for management should be provided as a written document. This is despite the fact that there is weak evidence to support this as a systematic review of three trials in adults did not observe reduction in relapse rate.[51] The action plan should ideally include the treatment protocol, home-based self-monitoring using peak flow measurement (where possible) and a clear plan for identification and management of worsening. Instructions of avoidance of common triggers, and emphasis on adherence to treatment should be mentioned.

Children discharged from hospital after an acute exacerbation should be followed up soon after discharge,

Table 3: Advice at discharge
• Inhaled corticosteroids (ICS): Initiate ICS if the child is not already receiving ICS. If the child is already on ICS, increase dosage for 2–4 weeks. • Oral corticosteroids (OCS): Prednisolone @ 1–2 mg/kg/day (maximum dose 40 mg/day) for 3–5 days. Alternatively, dexamethasone for a total of 1–2 days • SABA: Use 100–200 µg salbutamol as and when required. If it is required too frequently, the child should be seen by a physician • Avoidance of triggers • Emphasis on treatment adherence • Education on correct inhalation technique, and maintenance of inhalation devices • Offer a written management plan for home-based actions • Schedule a follow-up: Outpatient visit 1–2 weeks after discharge

generally within 1 week. **Table 3** summarizes the advice at discharge.

HOME-BASED MANAGEMENT OF ACUTE ASTHMA

Ideally, all children with asthma should be provided a written, action plan detailing the steps to recognition, and immediate management of acute episodes. While providing written plans, careful consideration should be given to issues like patient/family understanding, motivation for appropriate management, access to care, and other socio-cultural issues that can create added risk to individual children.

Reliever medication (short-acting beta 2 agonist) inhalation should be initiated using multiple doses delivered by metered dose inhaler (MDI) and spacer with or without a mask. In children, this translates to 200 µg salbutamol, with the provision of repeating thrice at 20 minute intervals, if required. However, if there is insufficient relief, the child should be seen by a physician rather than continuing with this. In general, usage of >600 µg salbutamol should prompt seeking professional advice. However, the BTS/SIGN guideline recommends seeking medical attention if symptoms remain uncontrolled despite 1000 µg salbutamol.[5]

Inhaled corticosteroid: Some experts advise doubling the dose of the current preventer ICS for a brief period of 5-7 days to tide over the acute episode. However, the data to support this is limited and more evidence is required for using this routinely. Further, the beneficial effect is limited if there is delay in initiating this measure. In younger children, this may not be advisable.

Combination of ICS with long acting bronchodilator: Formoterol is a rapid onset LABA and combination with ICS in a single inhaler has been shown to effectively prevent acute exacerbations when initiated at the early stages of worsening control. The maximum permissible daily dosage of formoterol is 72 µg.

Oral corticosteroids: If the symptoms are not relieved with inhalation of SABA and/or increased dose of preventer ICS, oral prednisolone (1-2 mg/kg/day) can also be initiated at home. However, parents should review the response and take the child to a physician for further care. Such treatment is not generally recommended at home for children younger than 5 years.

Obviously, home-based management as described above should not be implemented too frequently, and parents should be cautioned to seek medical care if the child does not improve within 1-2 days. In addition, any alarming symptoms should be brought to the attention immediately. Further, the family should visit their physician within 1-2 weeks for review of status and management. In such situations, physicians should confirm that the inhalation technique and inhalation devices are appropriate. Effort must also be made to identify possible cause(s) of the acute episode.

PREVENTION OF ACUTE SEVERE EPISODES

Discussion with children/family members about the mechanisms and possible causes of acute exacerbations can help to empower families to introduce lifestyle changes that can help prevent acute exacerbations. Some of these lifestyle changes include avoidance of obvious triggers such as dust, smoke, tobacco smoke, cold wind, etc. In case there are documented exacerbations with other specific triggers such as cosmetics, specific food items, processed food, etc., then families should be advised to exercise caution with this. Some triggers may not be entirely avoidable including pollution, cold weather, etc. Physical exercise and some forms of breathing exercises may help to enhance asthma control, although their role in preventing exacerbations is unclear. Overweight children and adolescents should be encouraged to lose weight. Stress is a significant trigger for acute episodes; hence, children may require temporary step up of medication and closer monitoring during periods of anticipated stress such as school examinations. In children with asthma associated with particular seasons or events such wheat harvesting/threshing, it is prudent to cover the season with appropriate inhaler therapy. Children who have exercise induced symptoms should be encouraged to continue physical activity with the support of reliever medication if required. Home based peak expiratory flow monitoring and maintaining an asthma symptom diary can help families detect imminent acute episodes even if the child is not feeling unwell.

KEY MESSAGES

- Acute severe asthma represents an acute deterioration in asthma control in children who have been previously diagnosed to have bronchial asthma. However, it can be the first clinical manifestation of asthma in some children.
- Acute asthma is diagnosed clinically in children based on signs of airflow limitation and/or consequent hypoxemia. There is no need of investigations to make a diagnosis.
- The Pediatric Respiratory Assessment Measure (PRAM) Score is a validated, almost entirely clinical scoring system that can help to categorize the severity of acute asthma, and for serial evaluation during treatment.
- The mainstay of therapy in acute asthma is a three-pronged approach of using oxygen, inhaled short acting beta-2 agonists, and systemic steroids.
- For most children with mild to moderate severity acute asthma, SABA can be delivered using a metered dose inhaler and spacer; a mask may be added for young children/infants. Nebulization may be reserved for children with severe episodes, and/or those with hypoxia requiring oxygen.
- Children who do not respond in the expected manner despite appropriate doses of these medications delivered through appropriate devices, require stepping up therapy. This includes intravenous magnesium sulfate, continuous nebulization with SABA, and sometimes additional medications such as systemic aminophylline or terbutaline or salbutamol.
- Mild acute asthma can be managed at home if families are provided a clear, written, action plan of steps to be taken for immediate management and subsequent visit in case of insufficient relief.

REFERENCES

1. Spycher BD, Silverman M, Kuehni CE. Phenotypes of childhood asthma: Are they real? Clin Exper Allergy. 2010;40:1130-41.
2. Global Initiative for Asthma. Global strategy for asthma management and prevention, 2018. Available from: *www.ginasthma.org*. Accessed July 24, 2019.
3. Gupta A, Bhat G, Pianosi P. What is new in the management of childhood asthma? Indian J Pediatr. 2018;85:773-81.
4. McGeachie MJ, Yates KP, ZhouX. Patterns of growth and decline in lung function in persistent childhood asthma. N Engl J Med 2016;374:1842-52.
5. British Thoracic Society, Scottish Intercollegiate Guidelines Network. 2016. British guideline on the management of asthma. Available from: *https://www.brit-thoracic.org.uk/quality-improvement/guidelines/asthma/*. Accessed July 24, 2019.
6. National Institute of Health and Clinical Excellence. Asthma: diagnosis and monitoring of asthma in adults, children and young people. NICE NG 80, Methods, evidence and recommendations, November 2017. Available from: *https://www.nice.org.uk/guidance/ng80/evidence/full-guideline-asthma-diagnosis-andmonitoring-pdf-4656178047*. Accessed July 24, 2019.
7. National Asthma Council Australia. Australian asthma handbook. Available from: *http://www.asthmahandbook.org.au*. Accessed January 20, 2019.
8. Indinnimeo L, Chiappini E, Miraglia Del Giudice M; Italian Panel for the management of acute asthma attack in children. Guideline on management of the acute asthma attack in children by Italian Society of Pediatrics. Ital J Pediatr. 2018;44:6.
9. Asher MI, Montefort S, Björkstén B, *et al.* Worldwide time trends in the prevalence of symptoms of asthma, allergic rhinoconjunctivitis, and eczema in childhood: ISAAC Phases One and Three repeat multicountry cross-sectional surveys. Lancet. 2006;368:733-43.
10. Grover S, Jindal A, Bansal A, *et al.* Acute bronchial asthma. Indian J Pediatr. 2011;78:1388-95.
11. Singhi S, Jain V, Gupta G. Pediatric emergencies at a tertiary care hospital in India. J Trop Pediatr. 2003;49:207-11.
12. Saharan S, Lodha R, Kabra SK. Management of status asthmaticus in children. Indian J Pediatr. 2010;77:1417-23.
13. Bush A, Griffiths C. Improving treatment of asthma attacks in children. BMJ. 2017;359:j5763.
14. Bekhof J, Reimink R, Brand PL. Systematic review: Insufficient validation of clinical scores for the assessment of acute dyspnoea in wheezing children. Pediatr Respir Rev. 2014;15:98-112.
15. Eggink H, Brand P, Reimink R, *et al.* Clinical scores for dyspnoea severity in children: A prospective validation study. PLoS One. 2016;11:e0157724.
16. Ducharme FM, Chalut D, Plotnick L, *et al.* The Pediatric Respiratory Assessment Measure: A valid clinical score for assessing acute asthma severity from toddlers to teenagers. J Pediatr. 2008;154:476-80.
17. PRAM (Pediatric Respiratory Assessment Measure) Score Assessment for Asthma. Available from: *https://www.childhealthbc.ca/sites/default/files/BCCH%20PRAM%20score%20for%20assessment%20for%20Asthma%20(2).pdf*. Accessed July 24, 2019.
18. Cates CJ, Welsh EJ, Rowe BH. Holding chambers (spacers) versus nebulizers for beta-agonist treatment of acute asthma. Cochrane Database Syst Rev. 2013;9:CD000052.

19. Castro-Rodriguez JA, J Rodrigo G, E Rodríguez-Martínez C. Principal findings of systematic reviews of acute asthma treatment in childhood. J Asthma. 2015;52:1038-45.
20. Rodriguez-Martinez CE, Sossa M, Lozano JM. Commercial versus home-made spacers in delivering bronchodilator therapy for acute therapy in children. Cochrane Database Syst Rev. 2008;2:CD005536.
21. Leelathipkul L, Tanticharoenwiwat P, Ithiawatchakul J, *et al.* MDI with DIY spacer versus nebulizer for bronchodilator therapy in children admitted with asthmatic attack. J Med Assoc Thai. 2016;99 Suppl 4:S265-74.
22. Mathew JL. Oral Dexamethasone versus oral prednisolone in acute asthma: A new randomized controlled trial and updated meta-analysis: Evidence-based medicine viewpoint. Indian Pediatr. 2018;55:155-9.
23. Devidayal SS, Kumar L, Jayshree M. Efficacy of nebulized budesonide compared to oral prednisolone in acute bronchial asthma. Acta Pediatr. 1999;88:835-40.
24. Edmonds ML, Milan SJ, Camargo CA Jr, *et al.* Early use of inhaled corticosteroids in the emergency department treatment of acute asthma. Cochrane Database Syst Rev. 2012; 12:CD002308.
25. Beckhaus AA, Riutort MC, Castro-Rodriguez JA. Inhaled versus systemic corticosteroids for acute asthma in children. A systematic review. Pediatr Pulmonol. 2014;49:326-34.
26. Demirca BP, Cagan H, Kiykim A, *et al.* Nebulized fluticasone propionate, a viable alternative to systemic route in the management of childhood moderate asthma attack: A double-blind, double-dummy study. Respir Med. 2015;109: 1120-5.
27. Arulparithi CS, Babu TA, Ravichandran C, *et al.* Efficacy of nebulised budesonide versus oral prednisolone in acute severe asthma. Indian J Pediatr. 2015;82:328-32.
28. Alangari AA, Malhis N, Mubasher M, *et al.* Budesonide nebulization added to systemic prednisolone in the treatment of acute asthma in children: A double-blind, randomized, controlled trial. Chest. 2014;145:772-8.
29. Griffiths B, Ducharme FM. Combined inhaled anticholinergics and short acting beta2-agonists for initial treatment of acute asthma in children. Cochrane Database Syst Rev. 2013; 8:CD000060.
30. Vézina K, Chauhan BF, Ducharme FM. Inhaled anticholinergics and short-acting beta(2)-agonists versus short-acting beta2-agonists alone for children with acute asthma in hospital. Cochrane Database Syst Rev. 2014;7:CD010283.
31. Teoh L, Cates CJ, Hurwitz M, *et al.* Anticholinergic therapy for acute asthma in children. Cochrane Database Syst Rev. 2012;4:CD003797.
32. Griffiths B, Kew KM. Intravenous magnesium sulfate for treating children with acute asthma in the emergency department. Cochrane Database Syst Rev. 2016;4:CD011050.
33. Su Z, Li R, Gai Z. Intravenous and nebulized magnesium sulfate for treating acute asthma in children: A systematic review and meta-analysis. Pediatr Emerg Care. 2018;34:390-5.
34. Mathew JL. Systematic review on efficacy of magnesium (intravenous or nebulized) for acute asthma episodes in children: Evidence-based medicine viewpoint. Indian Pediatr. 2017;54:133-6.
35. Singhi S, Grover S, Bansal A, *et al.* Randomised comparison of intravenous magnesium sulphate, terbutaline and aminophylline for children with acute severe asthma. Acta Paediatr. 2014;103:1301-6.
36. Knightly R, Milan SJ, Hughes R, *et al.* Inhaled magnesium sulfate in the treatment of acute asthma. Cochrane Database Syst Rev. 2017;11:CD003898.
37. Schuh S, Sweeney J, Freedman SB, *et al.* Magnesium nebulization utilization in management of pediatric asthma (MagNUM PA) trial: Study protocol for a randomized controlled trial. Trials. 2016;17:261.
38. Travers AH, Jones AP, Camargo CA Jr, *et al.* Intravenous beta(2)-agonists versus intravenous aminophylline for acute asthma. Cochrane Database Syst Rev. 2012;12:CD010256.
39. Travers AH, Milan SJ, Jones AP, *et al.* Addition of intravenous beta(2)-agonists to inhaled beta(2)-agonists for acute asthma. Cochrane Database Syst Rev. 2012;12:CD010179.
40. Shein SL, Speicher RH, Filho JO, *et al.* Contemporary treatment of children with critical and near-fatal asthma. Rev Bras Ter Intensiva. 2016;28:167-78.
41. Cooney L, Sinha I, Hawcutt D. Aminophylline dosage in asthma exacerbations in children: A systematic review. PLoS One. 2016;11:e0159965.
42. Cooney L, Hawcutt D, Sinha I. The evidence for intravenous theophylline levels between 10-20 mg/L in children suffering an acute exacerbation of asthma: A systematic review. PLoS One. 2016;11:e0153877.
43. Watts K, Chavasse RJ. Leukotriene receptor antagonists in addition to usual care for acute asthma in adults and children. Cochrane Database Syst Rev. 2012;5:CD006100.
44. Wang X, Zhou J, Zhao X, *et al.* Montelukast treatment of acute asthma exacerbations in children aged 2 to 5 years: A randomized, double-blind, placebo-controlled trial. Pediatr Emerg Care. 2018;34:160-4.
45. Rodrigo GJ, Castro-Rodriguez JA. Heliox-driven β2-agonists nebulization for children and adults with acute asthma: A systematic review with meta-analysis. Ann Allergy Asthma Immunol. 2014;112:29-34.
46. Ballestero Y, De Pedro J, Portillo N, *et al.* Pilot clinical trial of high-flow oxygen therapy in children with asthma in the emergency service. J Pediatr. 2018;194:204-10.e3.
47. Pilar J, Alapont V, Lopez-Fernandez YM, *et al.* High-flow nasal cannula therapy versus non-invasive ventilation in children with severe acute asthma exacerbation: An observational cohort study. Med Intensiva. 2017;41:418-24.
48. Normansell R, Sayer B, Waterson S, *et al.* Antibiotics for exacerbations of asthma. Cochrane Database Syst Rev. 2018;6:CD002741.
49. Kirkland SW, Cross E, Campbell S, *et al.* Intramuscular versus oral corticosteroids to reduce relapses following discharge from the emergency department for acute asthma. Cochrane Database Syst Rev. 2018;6:CD012629.
50. Normansell R, Kew KM, Mansour G. Different oral corticosteroid regimens for acute asthma. Cochrane Database Syst Rev. 2016;5:CD011801.
51. Villa-Roel C, Voaklander B, Ospina MB, *et al.* Effectiveness of written action plans for acute asthma: A systematic review. J Asthma. 2018;55:188-95.

CHAPTER

18

Stridor and Foreign Body Inhalation

Kana Ram Jat

INTRODUCTION

Stridor is a high-pitched inspiratory sound generated by turbulence in airflow through a partly occluded airway. Always remember that stridor is not a disease, but a manifestation of one of the many diseases, and evaluate the child systematically to identify the underlying diagnosis. It is very pertinent in emergency department to identify acute life-threatening condition for stridor or upper airway obstruction to initiate timely and appropriate management.[1] Foreign body (FB) aspiration may be one of the such acute life-threatening conditions. The chapter discusses about etiology, approach to diagnosis, and management of stridor and FB aspiration in children.

STRIDOR

Epidemiology and Etiology

Stridor is not uncommon in children and it results from infectious and non-infectious causes (**Table 1**). Croup is most common cause of acute stridor and laryngomalacia is most common cause of chronic stridor in children. In this chapter, we are focusing on the common conditions.

Laryngotracheobronchitis (LTB)/Croup

Croup occurs mostly in children between 6 months to 36 months of age and more common in boys than girls with ratio of 1.5. The croup is caused by viruses with parainfluenza (1 and 3) and influenza being most common agents. Most cases of croup are mild to moderate and about 8% require hospitalization and less than 1% requiring admission in Pediatric Intensive Care Unit (PICU).[1]

Bacterial tracheitis

It is a bacterial infection of trachea and caused by *Staphylococcus aureus* (most common), *Streptococcus pneumoniae, Haemophilus influenzae* b (Hib), *Moraxella catarrhalis*, and group A streptococci.

Epiglottitis

The occurrence of epiglottitis has decreased markedly after introduction of Hib vaccine. It is caused by *Haemophilus parainfluenzae*, non-typeable *Haemophilus influenzae, Staphylococcus aureus, Streptococcus pneumoniae*, and group A streptococci. The mean age of presentation is also changed from school age to adolescent age group.

Pathogenesis/Pathophysiology

As children have smaller airway, they are more likely to develop stridor after airway obstruction. Further, children have large tongue and large epiglottis compared to oral cavity making them more susceptible for early development of stridor. As per Poiseuille's law, resistance in airway is proportional to 4th power of its radius when air flow is laminar and the resistance is proportional to 5th power of its radius when airflow is turbulent. This is the explanation that some children do not have stridor at rest, but stridor become evident when child cries or is agitated because airflow becomes turbulent on crying/getting agitated.

Table 1: Causes of stridor in children

Acute		*Chronic*	
Infectious	**Non-infectious**	**Mass lesions/growths**	**Non-neoplastic**
Laryngotracheobronchitis (croup)	Anaphylaxis	Airway hemangioma	Choanal atresia/stenosis
Bacterial tracheitis	Foreign body aspiration	Airway papilloma	Laryngomalacia
Epiglottitis	Hypocalcemia-laryngeal spasm	Cystic hygroma	Laryngeal cleft, laryngeal web
Infectious mononucleosis	Burn injury to airway	Compression from outside	Sub-glottic stenosis-congenital, post-intubation
Diphtheria	Vocal cord palsy after cardiac surgery	Malignancy-lymphoma	Tracheomalacia
Retropharyngeal abscess		Lymphadenopathy	Tracheal stenosis-complete tracheal ring
Ludwig angina		Mediastinal tumors	Vascular ring
Peritonsillar abscess			Foregut duplication cysts-bronchogenic cyst, neuro-enteric cyst
			Syndromes associated with micrognathia and macroglossia, e.g. Pierre Robin
			Vocal cord paralysis-hydrocephalus, Arnold-Chiari malformation

Clinical Features

Laryngotracheobronchitis (LTB)/Croup

Croup typically presents after 2–3 days of upper respiratory tract infection (mild fever, cough, cold) like illness and it is characterized by presence of barking cough, inspiratory stridor, and hoarseness of voice. Symptoms usually start in the second half of night. Croup can be classified as mild, moderate, and severe. Children with mild croup appear comfortable with mild or no chest retractions and have stridor only on exertion like coughing or crying. In moderate croup, there is stridor at rest, child is fussy, and has chest wall retractions. In severe croup, stridor is associated with lethargy or restlessness, cyanosis, and child may be exhausted.

Bacterial tracheitis

It starts with upper respiratory tract infection like croup, but instead of improvement in symptoms over time, there is acute worsening of fever and child appears acutely ill. Compared to epiglottitis (see below), children with bacterial tracheitis often have cough and there is no drooling of saliva.

Epiglottitis

Epiglottitis is characterized by acute onset of high-grade fever and within hours of fever onset there is drooling of saliva, difficulty in swallowing and child prefers to sit in tripod position. The cough is usually absent or mild in epiglottitis.

Vocal cord paralysis

Vocal cord paralysis may be unilateral or bilateral. There is mainly change in voice with unilateral vocal cord paralysis and bilateral vocal cord paralysis often results in stridor.

Approach to Diagnosis

First step to approach a child with stridor is to confirm the sound as stridor and to differentiate it from other respiratory sounds. Stridor is high-pitched inspiratory sound; wheezing is low-pitched expiratory sound; snoring (sound during sleep) and stertor (sound during awake state) sounds originate from obstruction in nasopharynx or nose.[2] Next step is history and examination as good detailed history and examination is sufficient to make diagnosis in most of the cases of stridor in children.

History

Age of onset of stridor is a very important clue for diagnosis. Croup is common in children between 6 months to 36 months of age; bacterial tracheitis between 3 to 8 years of age; foreign body aspiration between 1 to 3 years of age; retropharyngeal abscess is common around 5 years of age and peritonsillar abscess in adolescents; and laryngomalacia usually presents in 2nd week of life and improves by 2 years of age.[3,4] Acute onset stridor, barking cough, hoarseness of voice, and respiratory distress after 2–3 days of viral prodrome in children between 6 month and 3 years of age is almost diagnostic of croup.

Rapidity of onset of stridor is another clue for diagnosis. Croup, bacterial tracheitis, and epiglottitis start acutely; but epiglottitis has most sudden onset amongst these. Retropharyngeal abscess, laryngomalacia, tracheal anomalies, and vocal cord problems have gradual onset stridor. Associated symptoms and precipitating factors can also provide a clue for diagnosis. Croup is typically worst at night and is preceded by upper respiratory tract infection (URTI). Bacterial tracheitis and epiglottitis are associated with fever and children are sick looking. Laryngomalacia is worsened by feeding and is better in prone position. Birth trauma may suggest vocal cord palsy, and history of intubation and ventilation in past will suggest sub-glottic stenosis. If a child with suspected croup does not respond to usual therapy, bacterial tracheitis should be considered.

Examination

First look at child may give a clue for possible diagnosis. Children with epiglottitis often sit in tripod or sniffing position. A child with retropharyngeal abscess often keeps neck hyperextended, and a child with peritonsillar abscess had trismus and has problem in swallowing and speaking. Both inspiratory and expiratory noisy breathing is suggestive of compression of airway from within or from outside, such as seen with hemangioma, laryngeal web, vascular ring, mediastinal masses. Presence of hoarseness of voice will indicate anaphylaxis or croup. Associated urticaria and past history of allergy/anaphylaxis will suggest anaphylaxis. A child with vocal cord involvement may have a weak cry. Abnormal facies may suggest upper airway obstruction by large tongue or by retrognathia. Asymmetrical air entry may suggest a foreign body beyond carina. A child with hypotonia (like Down syndrome) may have tracheomalacia, bronchomalacia, or tracheal stenosis.

Investigations

In most of the cases of stridor, good history and examination is sufficient to make a diagnosis and blood and radiological investigations are not required. Imaging is only required if there is doubt in diagnosis or the condition does not respond to appropriate therapy as expected. Though croup is a clinical diagnosis, an X-ray of neck will reveal classic "steeple sign" due to narrowing of subglottic area, but many children with croup may have a normal X-ray. The lateral X-ray in epiglottitis will reveal classic "thumb sign" due to edematous epiglottis, though it may not be required if there is classic history. In bacterial tracheitis, lateral X-ray of neck may show "candle dripping sign" due to irregular wall of trachea. Direct laryngoscopy may be considered in case of epiglottitis (but only after securing airway), burn injury to larynx and in case of laryngomalacia. Fiberoptic laryngoscopy is diagnostic for vocal cord dysfunction, but now even ultrasound has good sensitivity for diagnosis vocal cord dysfunction.

CT and MRI are usually not required unless a surgery is planned like for a large retropharyngeal abscess.

Flexible bronchoscopy may be required for diagnosis of bacterial tracheitis, subglottic stenosis, airway hemangioma and papilloma, and foreign body aspiration.

Differentiating features of various causes of stridor is summarized in **Table 2**.

Management of Stridor

General management in emergency department

First step is to define severity of respiratory difficulty to determine need for immediate intervention to keep the airway patent. Altered consciousness or marked agitation, hypoxia on oxygen and fatigue will indicate severe airway obstruction and need appropriate quick intervention. Altered consciousness in absence of hypoxia may be due to hypercarbia and should be assessed by arterial blood gas.

Agitation and crying will induce turbulent airflow and may worsen airway patency, therefore, child should be kept calm as far as possible by avoiding unnecessary intravenous cannulation, by giving oxygen via non-threatening manner (like blow-by method in mother's lap), and avoiding unnecessary examination of oral cavity. Child should be allowed to sit in their position of comfort that may be tripod position as it will minimize airway obstruction.[1] Avoid sedation as it may worsen airway obstruction.

The emergency team should be ready for all measures to support airway in case of worsening such as keeping ENT and anesthesiology team on standby, informing operation theater staff for possible need, keeping appropriate size

Table 2: Differentiating features of various common causes of stridor in children

Condition	*Clinical features*	*Investigations*	*Treatment*
Croup	Sudden onset of stridor, associated with barking cough and hoarseness of voice (usually in second half of night), after 2–3 days of viral prodrome	In a typical case, no investigation required	Corticosteroids ± nebulized adrenaline (in moderate to severe cases)
Bacterial tracheitis	Child is acutely sick after 2–5 days of viral prodrome in form of high grade fever, toxic look, and may have severe respiratory distress that respond poorly to croup management If intubation needed, trachea will reveal thick secretions	X-ray of neck may reveal irregular tracheal border	(IV) ceftriaxone with cloxacillin or vancomycin antibiotics, airway management
Epiglottitis	There is sudden onset high grade fever, difficulty in swallowing with drooling of saliva, and child prefers typical sniffing position (sitting with hands' support with neck extension). There is no barky cough	Usually not require If done, thumb sign in X-ray neck	Intravenous ceftriaxone, airway management
Retro/para-pharyngeal abscess	May have stridor, difficulty in swallowing with drooling, respiratory difficulty, stiffness of neck, and lymph node enlargement on one side of neck. Torticollis and restricted neck movements may be present	Lateral X-ray neck may reveal bulging soft tissue in the posterior pharynx	IV antibiotics with or without surgical drainage
Foreign-body in trachea or esophagus	Sudden onset stridor without preceding fever or barking cough History of foreign body aspiration may not be always there	Chest X-ray, flexible bronchoscopy	Removal by rigid bronchoscopy
Anaphylaxis	Rapid onset airway obstruction with or without dysphagia, urticarial rash, swelling of face and tongue after a drug or other allergen There may be history of similar episodes in past or a known allergy	In a typical case, no investigation required	IM adrenaline, IV steroids, H1 and H2 antihistaminics
Vocal cord paralysis	Biphasic stridor. Cry may be weak and feeble in unilateral vocal cord paralysis, paralysis of both vocal cord may cause severe respiratory distress with good quality of voice	Flexible laryngoscopy/ bronchoscopy	Speech therapy, wait and watch or airway management
Diphtheria	Gradual onset low grade fever, cervical lymphadenopathy followed, stridor, and/or dysphagia History of partial vaccination may be there On examination, typical grayish membrane is seen	Special stain for diphtheria	Anti-diphtheric toxin and antibiotic (penicillin)

of endotracheal tube (keep smaller than age-appropriate size also) and tracheostomy tube. If sedation is required for a procedure, agents causing laryngospasm such as ketamine should be avoided.

Management of croup (LTB)

Corticosteroids are first line of treatment for croup of any severity and it should be used for all severity. There is no difference in efficacy of oral versus intramuscular steroids and oral route should be preferred if child is accepting orally.[5] Further, three doses of dexamethasone [0.6 mg/kg (max 12 mg), 0.3 mg/kg, and 0.15 mg/kg (max 3 mg)] are found to be equally effective for croup, therefore lower dose of 0.15 to 0.3 mg/kg should be used.[6,7] Recently, single dose of high dose (2 mg) of inhaled budesonide has been reported to have equal efficacy. Similarly, oral dexamethasone and oral prednisolone (1 mg/kg) are found to have similar efficacy. At present, there is no additional benefit of adding two routes (such as inhaled budesonide plus oral or intramuscular dexamethasone) of corticosteroids for croup.[8,9] Still, there is lack of evidence for single versus multiple doses of steroids for croup. To summarize, steroids in croup may be used as intramuscular, oral or nebulized as per convenience of treating physician, severity of croup, oral tolerability of child, or even as per parents' choice.

Addition of nebulized adrenaline is indicated for moderate and severe croup. The nebulized adrenaline had quicker action within 30 minutes, but effects lasts for about 2 hours only.[10] Both l-adrenaline (dose is 5 mL of 1 mg/mL solution) and racemic adrenaline (dose is 0.5 mL of 2.25% strength in 4 mL saline) are equally efficacious for croup and either can be used depending on availability.[11] Child with croup receiving nebulized adrenaline should be observed for 2–4 hours for rebound worsening in ED before sending home.

There is no role of antibiotics (as croup is caused by viruses), oral decongestants, bronchodilators, cough remedies, mucolytics, and steam inhalation in croup; rather they may harm child such as burn by steam inhalation. A child with croup can be discharged from ED once there is no stridor at rest after observing for 2–4 hours without any therapy, no respiratory distress, no requirement of oxygen, and child is accepting orally.

Epiglottitis

Epiglottitis is an emergency and keeping airway patent is a priority. Almost all cases of epiglottitis require airway support. ENT specialist and anesthetist should be informed immediately for possible need for tracheostomy or cricothyrotomy. The intubation (endotracheal tube size should be 0.5 to 1 mm less than the age appropriate size) is preferred in operation theater with backup arrangement for emergency tracheostomy. As epiglottitis is caused by bacteria, all children with epiglottitis should be started on injection ceftriaxone 100 mg/kg/day in two divided doses. Duration of antibiotic is usually for 10 days. There is no role of steroids, adrenaline nebulization and bronchodilators for epiglottitis.

Bacterial tracheitis

It is caused by bacteria and may cause serious airway obstruction. Treatment of bacterial tracheitis includes broad-spectrum antibiotics in form of ceftriaxone plus cloxacillin or vancomycin if methicillin resistant *Staphylococcus aureus* (MRSA) is suspected. Antibiotics are given intravenously initially and can be shifted orally once child is afebrile and accepting orally to complete a total duration of 10–14 days.[12] Meticulous airway management is required including endotracheal intubation in few cases. If intubated, a smaller tube should be used because of inflamed trachea and good suctioning is needed to keep airway clear from secretions.

Diphtheria

If untreated, diphtheria may cause severe airway obstruction and extra-respiratory complications. Mainstay of treatment is diphtheria antitoxin (DAT) and intravenous penicillin (erythromycin if child is allergic to penicillin). Dose of DAT is single dose of 20,000–1,00,000 units depending on severity of disease, and extent of membrane; higher doses in severe cases and extensive membrane. DAT should be used after a test dose; if there is reaction, desensitization should be done. Dose of aqueous penicillin G is 1–1.5 lakh units/kg/day every 6 hourly intravenously (IV) and dose of erythromycin is 40–50 mg/kg/day every 6 hourly oral or IV. The total duration of antibiotic therapy is 14 days. If pseudomembrane is causing severe obstruction, child may require intubation or tracheostomy.

Anaphylaxis

Anaphylaxis is a life-threatening condition and intramuscular injection of adrenaline in dose of 0.01 mg/kg (0.01 mL/kg of adrenaline with 1 mg/mL solution, maximum dose 0.3 mg) is first-line treatment. In case of autoinjector of adrenaline, the dose is 0.15 mg for children below 25 kg and 0.3 mg for children above 25 kg. If there is poor response to first dose of adrenaline, second dose may be used. Other drugs used for anaphylaxis include corticosteroids, H_1 and H_2 blockers. If there is poor perfusion, a normal saline bolus should be used.

Vocal cord dysfunction

Most children with bilateral vocal cord paralysis will require tracheostomy. If presenting to emergency with acute worsening, frequent shallow breathing, pursed-lip breathing, and breathing with a straw may help in opening the airway. Bilateral vocal cord paralysis may recover in 2 months to 5 years after diagnosis, so regular follow-up is required.[13] For unilateral vocal cord paralysis, speech therapy may be useful for strengthening closure of glottis and improving feeding and vocalization.

Laryngomalacia

Laryngomalacia improves with time, so conservative therapy in form of feeding in upright position, thickening of food, and use of proton pump inhibitors (if there is associated gastroesophageal reflex) is only that is required in most of the cases. Severe cases of laryngomalacia causing repeated LRTI despite conservative therapy may require surgery in form of supraglottoplasty.[14]

Airway hemangiomas

Propranolol is first line of management for airway hemangiomas and there is dramatic improvement after starting propranolol.[15] Dose regimen of propranolol for hemangioma include: start with 1 mg/kg/day in three divided doses for 1 week; monitor for side effects such as bradycardia, hypotension, and hypoglycemia; if dose is tolerated after 1 week, increase to 2 mg/kg/day in three divided doses and continue same dose throughout the therapy.[15] The duration of propranolol therapy is not well studied; it should be continued till hemangioma is subsided completely and usual duration of therapy is 3–12 months. It should be tapered off before stopping over 1–3 weeks to prevent rebound tachycardia.

FOREIGN BODY ASPIRATION

Foreign body (FB) aspiration is a life-threatening condition occurring most commonly between 1–3 years of age.[16] It is more common in boys compared to girls. The most common site of FB lodgment is right main bronchus.[17] Among 70 cases of FB aspiration in a study from India, 42 (60%) were due to peanuts, 13 (18.6%) pulses and seeds, and 4 (5.7%) were due to almonds.[17]

Diagnosis

If there is sudden onset of symptoms and parents noticed foreign body inhalation, diagnosis is straightforward and the child is referred directly for foreign body removal after initial stabilization. But, in many cases, there is no history of FB aspiration. FB aspiration should be suspected when there are sudden onset respiratory symptoms along with unilateral findings (wheeze or decreased air entry) on chest examination.

Frontal chest X-ray or lateral film will identify radio-opaque FB and will also localize foreign body in trachea or esophagus; foreign body in esophagus will be flat in antero-posterior X-ray and vertical in lateral X-ray. Chest X-ray may be helpful even in radio-lucent FB as it may be show unilateral lung collapse (complete airway obstruction) or unilateral hyperinflation (ball valve mechanism) (**Fig. 1A**). Sometimes, chest X-ray in inspiration and expiration may help in identifying FB aspiration. If still diagnosis is not clear, flexible bronchoscopy is diagnostic for FB aspiration (**Fig. 1B**).

Management

If there is severe (complete) airway obstruction by foreign body aspiration, BLS (Basic Life Support) maneuvers like alternate back blow and chest thrust for infants, and Heimlich maneuver (abdominal thrust) for older children should be started immediately and continued till either foreign body is removed or victim become unresponsive; in the later situation, cardiopulmonary resuscitation should be started and advance airway and removal of foreign body by rigid bronchoscopy should be planned. If there is partial obstruction with stridor and maintained airway, child should be kept calm to prevent conversion of partial to complete obstruction and should be referred to center where facility for foreign body removal is available. If foreign body is above vocal cords, it may be removed with Magill forceps. FB in lower airways is removed by rigid bronchoscopy under general anesthesia. A few centers

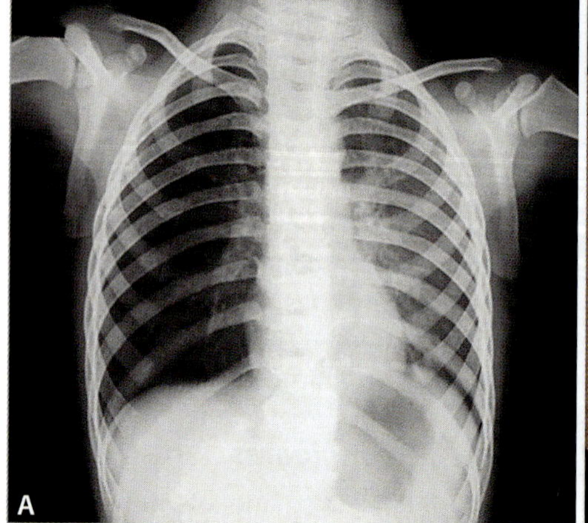

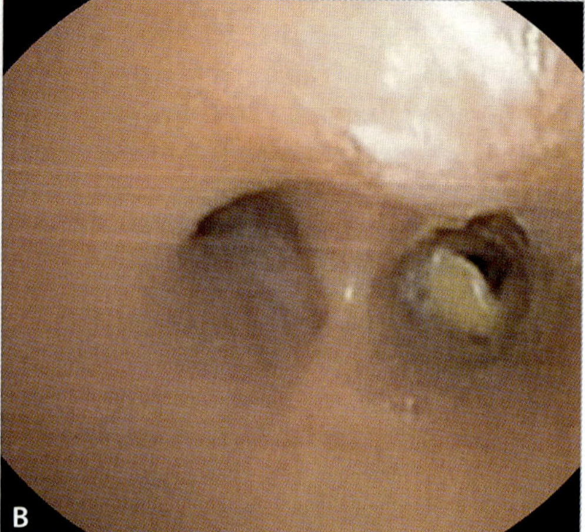

Figs. 1A and B: A 2.5-year-old boy with 2 months history of sudden onset persistent cough, no history of FB aspiration: (A) Chest X-ray showing hyperinflation on right side; (B) Flexible bronchoscopy revealed peanut in right main bronchus

remove FB in children with a flexible bronchoscopy,[18] but it should be considered by an experienced and trained person only with backup of rigid bronchoscopy. During removal of FB or sometimes spontaneously, FB may be dislodged in trachea causing severe hypoxia and may need immediate intervention in form of Heimlich maneuver or needle cricothyroidotomy or tracheostomy.[19]

KEY MESSAGES

- Children had wide range of etiologies for stridor, both infectious (croup is the most common) and non-infectious.
- To maintain airway patency is the first priority in all cases of stridor in children either by simple measures like positioning or by advanced airway such as intubation or tracheostomy.
- Oral corticosteroids are first line therapy for croup and both oral or intramuscular route and lower doses are equally effective.
- Antibiotics are not required for all cases of stridor; they are needed for bacterial tracheitis, epiglottitis, diphtheria, retropharyngeal abscess, and peri-tonsillar abscess.
- Vocal cord dysfunction is frequently mis-diagnosed as poorly-controlled asthma, therefore, a high index of suspicion is needed for diagnosis.
- Laryngomalacia improves overtime itself and conservative management is sufficient in most of the cases.
- Sudden onset of symptoms and unilateral chest findings suggest FB aspiration.

REFERENCES

1. Marchese A, Langhan ML. Management of airway obstruction and stridor in pediatric patients. Pediatr Emerg Med Pract. 2017;14:1-24.
2. Boudewyns A, Claes J, Van de Heyning P. Clinical practice: An approach to stridor in infants and children. Eur J Pediatr. 2010;169:135-41.
3. Bjornson CL, Johnson DW. Croup in children. Can Med Assoc J. 2013;185:1317-23.
4. Passàli D, Lauriello M, Bellussi L, *et al.* Foreign body inhalation in children: An update. Acta Otorhinolaryngol Ital. 2010;30:27-32.
5. Leung AKC, Kellner JD, Johnson DW. Viral croup: A current perspective. J Pediatr Health Care. 2004;18:297-301.
6. Geelhoed GC, Macdonald WBG. Oral dexamethasone in the treatment of croup: 0.15 mg/kg versus 0.3 mg/kg versus 0.6 mg/kg. Pediatr Pulmonol. 1995;20:362-8.
7. Chub-Uppakarn S, Sangsupawanich P. A randomized comparison of dexamethasone 0.15 mg/kg versus 0.6 mg/kg for the treatment of moderate to severe croup. Int J Pediatr Otorhinolaryngol. 2007;71:273-7.
8. Geelhoed GC. Budesonide offers no advantage when added to oral dexamethasone in the treatment of croup. Pediatr Emerg Care. 2005;21:359-62.
9. Petrocheilou A, Tanou K, Kalampouka E, *et al.* Viral croup: Diagnosis and a treatment algorithm. Pediatr Pulmonol. 2014; 49:421-9.
10. Eghbali A, Sabbagh A, Bagheri B, *et al.* Efficacy of nebulized L-epinephrine for treatment of croup: A randomized, double-blind study. Fundam Clin Pharmacol. 2016;30:70-5.
11. Bjornson C, Russell K, Vandermeer B, *et al.* Nebulized epinephrine for croup in children. Cochrane Database Syst Rev. 2013;(10):CD006619.
12. Al-Mutairi B, Kirk V. Bacterial tracheitis in children: Approach to diagnosis and treatment. Paediatr Child Health. 2004;9:25-30.
13. Kothur K, Singh M, Dayal D, *et al.* Bilateral idiopathic vocal cord palsy. Pediatr Emerg Care. 2007;23:171-2.
14. Faria J, Behar P. Medical and surgical management of congenital laryngomalacia: A case-control study. Otolaryngol Head Neck Surg. 2014;151:845-51.
15. Darrow DH, Greene AK, Mancini AJ, *et al.* Diagnosis and management of infantile hemangioma. Pediatrics. 2015; 136: e1060-104.
16. Shivakumar AM, Naik AS, Prashanth KB, *et al.* Tracheobronchial foreign bodies. Indian J Pediatr. 2003;70:793-7.
17. Sehgal A, Singh V, Chandra J, *et al.* Foreign body aspiration. Indian Pediatr. 2002;39:1006-10.
18. Kim K, Lee HJ, Yang EA, *et al.* Foreign body removal by flexible bronchoscopy using retrieval basket in children. Ann Thorac Med. 2018;13:82-5.
19. Maraynes M, Agoritsas K. Inhaled foreign bodies in pediatric patients: Proven management techniques in the emergency department. Pediatr Emerg Med Pract. 2015;12:1-14; quiz 15.

CHAPTER

19

Lower Respiratory Tract Infections

Mehak Bansal, Dhiren Gupta

INTRODUCTION

Acute respiratory infections are one of the most common childhood illnesses, with most of the children experiencing about four to six episodes of acute respiratory infections (ARI) per year.[1] Infections above the glottis, from nostrils to vocal cords are classified as upper respiratory tract infections (URTI), such as acute rhinitis, acute sinusitis, pharyngitis, tonsillitis and otitis media. Whereas, infections below the glottis including the larynx below the vocal cords trachea, bronchi, bronchioles and alveoli are considered as lower respiratory tract infections (LRTI), such as bronchiolitis, bronchitis and pneumonia.

EPIDEMIOLOGY AND ETIOLOGY

Globally, LRTIs are responsible for around 12% of the deaths in children under 5 years of age, with India accounting for the highest overall number of deaths due to LRTI in under 5-year olds.[2] Around one third of these LRTI deaths are attributed to two bacteria—*Pneumococcus* (55.8%) and *H. influenzae* Type b (8.3%). However, respiratory syncytial virus (RSV) and influenza virus together account for 6.6% of under 5 mortality due to LRTI.[3] Among the viruses, RSV is the most notorious virus that causes a very high rate of hospitalizations (around 3.2 million) and in-hospital deaths (about 59,000) in children younger than 5 years; 45% of these hospitalizations and deaths occur in infants less than 6 months of age.[3] The severity of RSV LRTI is higher in very preterm babies and rate of hospitalization among them is three times higher as compared to term babies.[4] Developing countries have a much higher incidence of LRTIs and a higher mortality rate as opposed to developed nations owing to factors like malnutrition, overcrowding, indoor air pollution and lack of immunization.

CLINICAL FEATURES

- Cough, fever, tachypnea, difficulty in breathing, wheeze or crackles on auscultation are the key features of LRTI, while cough, fever, coryza, ear pain or throat pain are the symptoms associated with URTIs.
- The severity of the disease can be assessed by sensorium of the child, refusal to feeds, head bobbing, nasal flaring, use of accessary muscles of respiration and cyanosis.
- Tachypnea, which is the pathognomonic feature of LRTIs is absent in upper respiratory tract infections.
- It is very crucial to look for increased work of breathing along with tachypnea while assessing the child, as tachypnea alone can be present in other conditions like severe metabolic acidosis and diabetic ketoacidosis. In these conditions, tachypnea is present without any increased work of breathing.
- The presence of adventitious sounds along with tachypnea points towards the site of infection. For example, tachypnea with stridor is present in upper airway obstruction (croup or laryngotracheobronchitis), tachypnea with audible wheeze suggests lower airway obstruction (asthma) and tachypnea with grunting points towards lung parenchymal disease (pneumonia).

BRONCHIOLITIS

It is the most common lower respiratory tract infection in infants with peak incidence in the first 6 months of life. American Academy of Pediatrics has defined bronchiolitis as a clinical syndrome which is preceded by upper respiratory prodrome and subsequently followed by inflammation of lower respiratory tract, resulting in increased respiratory distress and wheezing in children <2 years.[5]

Epidemiology

About one-third of the children develop bronchiolitis during the first year of their life, and 2–3% of these infants require hospitalization.[5,6] Bronchiolitis leads to significant morbidity and huge costs to healthcare system.

Etiology

Respiratory syncytial virus (RSV) is the most common causative agent of bronchiolitis, followed by Rhinovirus. Majority of the children are infected with RSV by their 2nd birthday, and up to 40% of them develop LRTI.[7,8] Infection with RSV does not confer lifelong immunity and children experience reinfections even till adulthood. Influenza A and B, parainfluenza type 1–3, adenovirus, human metapneumovirus, coronavirus, human bocavirus and enterovirus are the other virus implicated in bronchiolitis.[9,10] Co-infection with two or more viruses can also occur and is detected in 10–30% of the admitted children.[11] Bacterial superinfections rarely occur.

Pathogenesis

Viral infection is first acquired by the inoculation of upper respiratory tract. After approximately 2–5 days, the virus infects mainly the bronchioles and alveoli. This results in inflammation of bronchial epithelial cells and alveolar pneumocytes, which triggers an innate immune response by secreting chemokines, cytokines and interleukins. This immune response results in cellular recruitment and infiltration of the peribronchial tissue with CD4 and CD8 T lymphocytes, Natural Killer cells, granulocytes. Consequently, partial or complete obstruction of the airways occurs, owing to increased mucus production, sloughing of necrotic epithelium and fibrin deposits, causing air trapping and overinflation. The obstruction becomes even more severe during expiration due to positive intrathoracic pressure, causing wheeze. Since the resistance of airways is inversely proportional to the fourth power of the radius, any obstruction causes severe restriction of the airflow during both phases of respiration in children in severe cases. Furthermore, in case of complete obstruction, there is air trapping distal to the obstructed airways, causing a ball-valve mechanism and leading to adsorption atelectasis, ventilation-perfusion (V/Q) mismatch and hypoxemia. Severe obstruction leads to hypercapnia eventually.

Risk Factors

Children with the following risk factors have a greater chance of progressing to severe disease and are associated with greater morbidity and mortality due to bronchiolitis (**Table 1**).

Clinical Features

- A detailed birth history, past medical history, history of atopy or any allergies, social history and family history should be taken to assess for any above-mentioned risk factors.
- Ask for history of initial upper respiratory prodrome-mild cough and coryza symptoms lasting for 1–3 days followed by tachypnea and increased work of breathing in case of bronchiolitis.
- On physical examination look for cough, tachypnea, increased work of breathing, use of accessory muscles, intercostal, subcostal and suprasternal recessions, tracheal tugging and nasal flaring.
- Wheeze or crackles on auscultation.
- Look for hydration status, as child can have dehydration and signs of poor perfusion due to vomiting or refusal of feeds.
- Apnea can be present especially in preterm babies and infants.

Table 1: Risk factors of bronchiolitis
1. Infants < 12 weeks old
2. Prematurity (<37 weeks)
3. Chronic lung disease (CLD) (cystic fibrosis, bronchopulmonary dysplasia, congenital lung anomaly)
4. Hemodynamically significant congenial heart disease (pulmonary hypertension)
5. Immunodeficiency disorders
6. Neurological disorders
7. Environmental factors such as overcrowding, passive smoking and indoor air pollution and winter season

- Pulse oximetry is a significant part of clinical examination to identify hypoxemia, which is not sometimes evident on physical examination.

Severe bronchiolitis

Following are signs and symptoms of severe bronchiolitis:

- Lethargic or signs of exhaustion
- Apnea
- Severe respiratory distress with RR >70/min or presence of nasal flaring, subcostal, intercostal, suprasternal recessions, tracheal tugging, head bobbing, grunting
- Central cyanosis
- Dehydration and poor peripheral perfusion
- Silent chest on auscultation
- Respiratory failure - Hypoxemia or hypercapnia
- Persistently low oxygen saturation of <92% on room air on pulse oximetry.

Course of Bronchiolitis

The initial coryza symptoms are followed by lower respiratory tract symptoms and signs on second or third day of illness. These LRTI symptoms peak on 5–7 days, following which they gradually resolve. Child may require hospitalization during peak period of bronchiolitis and usually recovers after 3–4 days of hospitalization, but the cough and wheeze may persist for 2–3 weeks. The symptoms may persist even longer in children with risk factors and comorbid conditions.

Diagnosis

Bronchiolitis is a clinical diagnosis; diagnostic tests are not routinely indicated as they are not very informative and can result in unnecessary hospitalizations and administration of inappropriate therapy. Differential diagnoses are listed in **Table 2**.

Table 2: Differential diagnosis of bronchiolitis

Pulmonary causes	*Non-pulmonary causes*
Asthma	Congenital heart disease
Foreign body aspiration	Congestive heart failure
Aspiration pneumonia	Vascular rings
Virus induced wheeze	Mediastinal mass
Pneumonia	
Anomalies of airways	
Chronic lung disease	

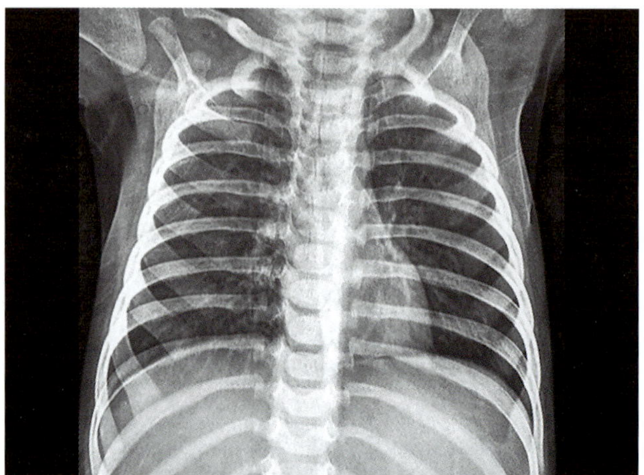

Fig. 1: Chest X-ray of 9 months old with bronchiolitis. Notice bilateral hyperinflated lung fields

1. *Chest X-ray*: It shows hyperinflation of lung fields and patchy atelectasis in bronchiolitis (**Fig. 1**). However, these findings can mimic the findings of consolidation and infiltrates in pneumonia or can be misinterpreted, leading to inappropriate treatment with antibiotics. Hence, Chest X-ray should be done only in case of severe disease, to rule out complications and in case where the patient is not improving, to rule out any other diagnosis. Also, X-rays do not correlate well with the severity of disease.[12]
2. *Rapid antigen detection to detect viruses using immunofluorescence and polymerase chain reaction (PCR) assays of respiratory or nasopharyngeal secretions*: RSV can be detected in 60–75% cases of RSV bronchiolitis using PCR assay of nasopharyngeal secretions.[13,14] Even co-infection with two or more viruses can be identified. These tests are not useful in the outpatients, but in inpatients identifying the virus using PCR technique helps in cohorting of the admitted patients, helps in decision making to discontinue antibiotics, give anti-influenza treatment and anti-influenza prophylaxis to high-risk contacts. The major disadvantage of PCR is that sometimes it detects prolonged viral shedding from previous illness which may not be relevant in the current clinical situation. Few rapid diagnostic tests are also available; however their sensitivity is lower than that of PCR.
3. *Complete blood counts, acute phase reactants and cultures*: They may be abnormal in secondary bacterial

infections or systemic bacterial infection in children less than 2 months of age or in children with strong suspicion of bacterial infection. These tests are not routinely recommended.

4. *Blood gas*: Analysis will be useful to ascertain hypercarbia and hypoxemia in sick babies that might require or are admitted in intensive care unit.
5. *Electrolytes*: In children requiring admission to intensive care unit, electrolytes should be monitored, especially sodium.

Management of Bronchiolitis

Outpatient management

Mild cases of bronchiolitis are managed conservatively as an outpatient, no specific therapy is required, just conservative management along with reassurance to the mother. However, the pediatricians should keep in mind that a close observation is required as the children can deteriorate on the 3–5th day of illness and might require hospitalization.

Admission criteria of bronchiolitis

1. Apnea
2. Oxygen Saturation on Pulse oximetry (SpO_2) <92% in room air
3. Presence of moderate to severe respiratory distress and use of accessory muscles of respiration
4. Inadequate fluid intake or presence of signs of dehydration or inadequate perfusion
5. Lethargy or signs of exhaustion
6. Presence of history of risk factors like, prematurity, CLD, congenital heart disease, immunological disorders, neurological disorders.

Respiratory and other support

1. *Oxygen*: Humidified oxygen is the mainstay of therapy. It should be given to children with saturation <90% in order to maintain a target saturation of >90%.[5] Oxygen can be given via nasal cannula, non-rebreathing mask or head box in infants.
2. *Noninvasive respiratory support*: High flow nasal cannula (HFNC) is device that can deliver high flow humidified oxygen which is better tolerated by children than any other high flow oxygen device and also provides 3–5 cm H_2O of PEEP that splints the atelectatic airways open. HFNC has been shown to reduce the need for ventilation.[15,16] Nasal CPAP support (PEEP 5–6 mm Hg) can be tried in case of worsening distress with close monitoring. The children that develop recurrent apnea, rising oxygen requirements, severe respiratory distress with signs of exhaustion have to be intubated and ventilated.
3. *Mechanical ventilation*: Endotracheal intubation and ventilation is indicated in cases of bronchiolitis with severe respiratory distress or impending respiratory failure, lack of clinical improvement or worsening respiratory distress on noninvasive respiratory support (CPAP or HFNC), FiO_2 requirement >60% in order to maintain saturations >90%, persistent or recurrent apnea, deterioration of sensorium or seizure. Low tidal volume ventilation with permissive hypercapnia and early weaning is important while ventilating children of bronchiolitis.
4. *Regular suctioning*: It helps the patient clear out the secretions to alleviate distress.
5. *Chest physiotherapy*: It is not regularly required and has not shown to reduce the hospital stay.
6. *Hydration*: Dehydration occurs due to increased insensible water losses owing to high work of breathing or due to refusal to feeds and vomiting. Therefore, frequent feeding should be promoted to maintain hydration. Some infants with tachypnea and increased work of breathing have a risk of aspiration of feeds, so in such cases, nasogastric feeds (NG) are advocated. Dehydrated children with refusal to feeds or vomiting will require fluid bolus to optimize the intravascular volume, followed by maintenance IV fluids to optimize hydration status and maintain electrolyte balance. In case of severe respiratory distress and possible intubation, children should be made nil by mouth and are started on maintenance IV fluids. In case of severe bronchiolitis, 2/3rds of isotonic (5% dextrose with 0.9% saline) maintenance fluids are preferred to prevent fluid overload and hyponatremia.

Adjunct therapies

1. *3% hypertonic saline nebulization*: Hypertonic saline is thought to improve mucociliary clearance of airways and hydration of the airway surface liquid. A Cochrane review has shown that 3% saline nebulization can reduce the length of stay in cases where hospital stay

is >3 days.[17,18] Four mL of 3% saline is nebulized over 5–10 min.

2. *Nebulized beta-adrenergic agonists*: Since smooth muscle constriction is not a mechanism of bronchiolitis, bronchodilation with beta agonists (salbutamol) is not beneficial. Studies have shown that beta agonists do not affect resolution of the disease or reduce the rates of hospitalization or length of hospital stay.[19,20] Hence, they are not recommended in bronchiolitis. However, they are widely used as it is very difficult to differentiate bronchiolitis from virus induced wheeze. Only in case of a child with wheeze, a trial of salbutamol can be given, and continued if a clinical response is documented. Salbutamol is administered in dose of 0.15 mg/kg (minimum 2.5 mg; maximum 5 mg) administered over 10–15 minutes or 4–6 puffs of metered dose inhaler using spacer and face mask.
3. *Epinephrine nebulization*: Epinephrine causes vasoconstriction and is thought to reduce mucosal swelling. However, studies suggest that it should be used a rescue therapy in severe disease instead of routine use as it has not been found to be beneficial in reducing length of stay.[21]
4. *Oral and nebulized corticosteroids*: Corticosteroids have anti-inflammatory properties and can reduce airway edema and infiltration of airways, but there is no evidence to support the use of inhaled or oral steroids in bronchiolitis.[22] Steroids along with bronchodilators are also not indicated.
5. *Antibiotics*: Bronchiolitis is a viral disease and antibiotics are not advised unless there is a strong suspicion or evidence to support concomitant bacterial infection.
6. *Antivirals*: Ribavirin has limited benefit and thus, not recommended.[23]
7. *Heliox*: Helium and oxygen mixture can improve respiratory scores and work of breathing in children with severe bronchiolitis as it reduces airway turbulence. However, its use is cumbersome and is of limited benefit.
8. *Dornase, surfactant, anticholinergics*: These agents have no role in bronchiolitis.

Complications

1. *Apnea*: RSV infection is known to cause apnea, especially in infants less than 2 months old and premature babies. A child can also present with apnea without any other signs suggestive of bronchiolitis.
2. *Respiratory failure*: Hypoxemia and hypercarbia in bronchiolitis is caused by mucous plugging, atelectasis, which impair gaseous exchange. Such children require ventilatory support and monitoring in intensive care unit.
3. *Secondary bacterial infection*: Bacterial infections can complicate a few cases of bronchiolitis and subsequently result in bacterial pneumonia.

Prognosis

Mortality due to bronchiolitis is about 1–2% and is attributable to apnea and respiratory failure. Mortality is more in developing nations and in infants with high-risk factors. The incidence of asthma and wheezing in children in the 1st decade of life is more in children with history of bronchiolitis.

Prevention

Good hand hygiene, minimizing exposure to tobacco smoke, breastfeeding and reducing contact with adults with respiratory infections reduces the risk of bronchiolitis.

Palivizumab: It is a human monoclonal antibody directed against RSV F protein and may administered to children with history of prematurity <32 weeks, bronchopulmonary dysplasia and hemodynamically significant CHD in the first year of their life.[5] It reduces mortality in these high-risk groups due to RSV infection.

COMMUNITY-ACQUIRED PNEUMONIA

Introduction

Community-acquired pneumonia (CAP) is characterized by the inflammation of the lung parenchyma in a previously healthy child by as a result on an infection acquired from the community.[24] Hospital-acquired pneumonia (HAP) is the clinical spectrum of pneumonia that develops 48 hours after admission to a hospital. Pneumonia is the second leading cause of under 5 mortality (16%, 0.92 million deaths), after preterm birth complications in 2015.[2,25]

Etiology (Table 3)

Bacterial agents

Streptococcus pneumoniae is the most common bacteria and responsible of causing 30–40% of total cases of

Table 3: Classification of etiological agents according to age group

	Common etiological agents	*Less common etiological agents*
Less than 3 weeks	***Bacteria*** *Escherichia coli* *Streptococcus pyogenes* Other gram-negative bacteria	***Bacteria*** *Streptococcus pneumoniae* *Haemophilus influenzae* type b ***Viruses*** Cytomegalovirus Herpes simplex virus
3 weeks to 3 months	***Viruses*** RSV Influenza A and B Parainfluenza Rhinovirus Adenovirus Enterovirus ***Bacteria*** *Streptococcus pneumoniae* *Haemophilus influenzae* type b *Chlamydia trachomatis*	***Bacteria*** *Bordetella pertussis* *Staphylococcus aureus* *Moraxella catarrhalis* ***Viruses*** Cytomegalovirus
4 months to 5 years	***Viruses*** RSV Influenza A and B Parainfluenza Rhinovirus Adenovirus Human metapneumovirus Enterovirus ***Bacteria*** *Streptococcus pneumoniae* *Haemophilus influenzae* type b *Mycoplasma pneumoniae* *Chlamydia pneumoniae*	***Bacteria*** *Staphylococcus aureus* Group A *Streptococcus* ***Viruses*** Varicella Zoster virus
5 years to adolescence	***Bacteria*** *Mycoplasma pneumoniae* *Chlamydia pneumoniae* *Streptococcus pneumoniae* ***Viruses*** Influenza A and B Adenovirus	***Bacteria*** *Staphylococcus aureus* Group A *Streptococcus* ***Viruses*** RSV Rhinovirus Parainfluenza virus Human metapneumovirus Enterovirus

community-acquired pneumonia.[26,27] Less frequent bacterial pathogens are Group A *Streptococcus* and *Staphylococcus aureus* and *H. influenzae* type b (Hib). Group A *Streptococcus* and *Staphylococcus aureus*, especially methicillin resistant *Staphylococcus aureus* (MRSA) are associated with more severe disease and complications like empyema. *Staphylococcus* can complicate influenza in children. *Mycoplasma pneumoniae* and *Chlamydia pneumoniae* are more frequent causes of pneumonia among school-age children (>5 years of age) and cause atypical pneumonia. Pneumonia caused by gram negative bacteria, such as, *Klebsiella pneumoniae* and *Pseudomonas aeruginosa* and fungal agents like *Aspergillus fumigatus*, *Histoplasma* and *Coccidioides* are uncommon, and are mainly present in children with immunodeficiency disorders (HIV) or in patients with HAP. With the introduction of conjugate pneumococcal vaccines, the incidence of pneumococcal pneumonia has decreased in certain regions, which are well covered with the vaccine.[28]

Viral agents

Viruses account for 30–67% of the cases of childhood pneumonia and the viral pneumonias are more predominant in children less than 1 year of age.[29,30] RSV contributes to 30% of the cases of viral pneumonia. Rhinovirus, influenza and parainfluenza virus, adenovirus, human metapneumovirus and enteroviruses are the other viruses isolated from children with pneumonia. Mixed viral and bacterial infections are present in 30–50% of the cases of CAP in children.[31]

Noninfectious causes

Pneumonia can also occur due to noninfectious causes like aspiration (gastric contents, foreign bodies), drug or radiation induced pneumonitis and hypersensitivity reactions.

Pathogenesis

The lungs protect themselves using various defense mechanisms like coughing, mucociliary clearance, innate immunity (macrophages, granulocytes and complement cascade) and adaptive immunity (T-cells and B-cells). In viral pneumonias, the viruses cause damage to the respiratory epithelium, resulting in airway edema, deposition of cellular debris and obstruction of airways. Obstruction of airways leads to hypoxemia, V/Q mismatch and hypercarbia. In bacterial pneumonias, the bacteria travel to the lower airways through the upper airways or via hematogenous route. They initiate inflammatory response and damage the endothelial and epithelial cells. In *Streptococcus pneumoniae*, local edema, inflammatory cells and microorganisms together result in formation of lobar pneumonia and consolidation. Group A *Streptococcus* causes diffuse interstitial pneumonia. It causes necrotizing hemorrhage and edema of tracheobronchial mucosa. *Staphylococcus aureus* pneumonia is characterized by extensive areas of hemorrhagic necrosis and cavitation of the lung parenchyma, resulting in empyema, pneumatoceles or bronchopulmonary fistulae.

Risk factors for severe disease

1. Children younger than 5 years
2. History of prematurity
3. History of immunodeficiency disorders
4. History of chronic lung disease (bronchopulmonary dysplasia)
5. History of congenital heart disease
6. History of cystic fibrosis
7. History of neurological disabilities
8. Malnourished
9. History of gastrointestinal disorders (gastroesophageal reflux disease)
10. Environmental factors such as winter season, indoor pollution, tobacco smoke exposure and overcrowding.

Clinical Features

- History of fever, tachypnea **(Table 4)**, dyspnea and difficulty in breathing. Cough is usually present. Older children may present with tachypnea, fever and chest pain.
- History of gastrointestinal symptoms, such as vomiting, diarrhea and abdominal distention can be present sometimes in a child with pneumonia.
- Physical examination—fever, tachypnea, tachycardia, increased work of breathing, use of accessary muscles of respiration, subcostal, intercostal, suprasternal recessions, nasal flaring, grunting.
- Tachypnea is the most important sign and has a high negative predictive value (97.4%).[32] It has a good predictor of radiologically defined pneumonia and hypoxemia. However, severely malnourished children may not have tachypnea.
- On auscultation, crackles or rales or bronchial breathing may be identified. Decreased air entry in lung fields on auscultation and dull note on percussion can be present in pleural effusion or empyema.
- Presence of lethargy, cyanosis, severe respiratory distress with subcostal, intercostal, suprasternal recessions, nasal flaring, grunting suggest severe pneumonia. SpO_2 <90% on pulse oximetry indicates hypoxemia.
- In bacterial pneumonias children look toxic and unwell.
- In viral pneumonias, the upper respiratory symptoms are followed by respiratory distress, increased work of breathing and wheeze. The toxic appearance is absent.

Table 4: The WHO age-based definition of tachypnea[24]
1. Respiratory rate (RR) > 60/min if age <2 months old
2. RR > 50/ min in 2–12 months old
3. RR > 40/ min in >12 months to 5 years

- Atypical pneumonia caused by *Mycoplasma* presents with atypical symptoms—cough, chest pain, headache, generalized malaise, arthralgia, sore throat and wheeze.

Atypical pneumonias are more commonly associated with wheeze.

Pulse oximetry: Monitoring oxygen saturation of blood using pulse oximetry is important part of respiratory assessment and detects hypoxemia before cyanosis is evident.

Differential diagnosis

1. Bronchiolitis
2. Aspiration pneumonia
3. Gastroesophageal reflux disease
4. Sepsis
5. Foreign body aspiration
6. Bronchiectasis
7. Congestive heart failure.

Complications of Pneumonia

Pleural effusion and empyema

Parapneumonic effusion (fluid collection in pleural space in association with underlying pneumonia) and empyema (pus collection in pleural space are caused due to immune response to the pathogenic organism, resulting in pleural inflammation, increased vascular permeability and migration of inflammatory cells in pleural space. This results in parapneumonic fluid or pus collection in pleural space. Later on, deposition of fibrin causes formation of septations and loculations. Persistence of fever beyond 7 days or inadequate response to antimicrobial therapy after 48 hours should raise the suspicion of empyema. *Streptococcus pneumoniae*, *Streptococcus pyogenes* and MRSA are the common organisms associated with parapneumonic effusions and empyema. X-ray chest anteroposterior and lateral views and ultrasound lung aid in the diagnosis and lung ultrasound also helps in quantifying the amount of fluid in the pleural space. Treatment includes antibiotics, antifibrinolytics (urokinase), and drainage of the fluid or pus via chest drain. Small effusions can be conservatively managed. However, large effusions require drainage by thoracostomy or surgical removal via Video Assisted Thoracoscopic Surgery (VATS) or decortication if treatment with chest drainage and urokinase fail.

Necrotizing pneumonias

It is a serious complication of pneumonia and is caused by necrosis and liquefaction of the lung parenchyma. *Streptococcus pneumoniae* (type 3 and serogroup 19), Group A *Streptococcus* and *Staphylococcus aureus* are the causative agents of necrotizing pneumonia. The symptoms of necrotizing pneumonia are quite severe, and child appears toxic. Presence of radiolucent area on X-ray and computed tomography (CT chest) confirms the diagnosis. Treatment is the same as complicated pneumonia.

Lung abscess

It is an accumulation of pus in lung parenchyma. The predisposing factors for lung abscesses are congenital cysts, bronchiectasis and immunodeficiency disorders. Diagnosis is confirmed by thick walled cavity in the lung parenchyma with air-fluid level on X-ray or CT chest. Prolonged antibiotic course along with USG or CT-guided drainage of pus is required. Surgical intervention may be required in few cases.

Pneumatoceles

They are thin-walled air-filled cysts in the lung parenchyma. It is a pathognomonic feature of *Staphylococcus aureus*, and its rupture can lead to pneumothorax.

Hematological spread of the bacteria can result in septicemia.

Diagnosis

1. *White cell count*: A high white cell count with neutrophil predominance suggests bacterial infection. Leukopenia with lymphocytosis suggests a viral pathology.
2. *Urea, creatinine and electrolytes*: They should be monitored in hospitalized cases of pneumonia to look for renal dysfunction and electrolyte imbalance.
3. *Acute phase reactants*: CRP and procalcitonin are high in bacterial infections, but significant overlap with viral infections occur especially adenoviruses and enteroviruses. Hence, they should not be used in isolation to predict bacterial infections.
4. *Blood culture*: They are positive in only in less than 10% cases of CAP. Blood culture specimen should be collected for child requiring hospitalization.
5. *Sputum and respiratory secretions culture and sensitivity*: Obtaining sputum in children is quite

tricky as children are not able to produce sputum. Bronchoalveolar lavage is required to obtain lower respiratory tract secretions.

6. *Pleural fluid culture and sensitivity*: Pleural fluid obtained in case of pleural effusion can be sent for cytology, pneumococcal antigen, PCR and culture. Pleural fluid cultures have poor yield.
7. *Pneumococcal antigen testing in blood and urine*: It has a good negative predictive value.
8. *Rapid diagnostic tests (RDT) for viral antigens using PCR assays and immunofluorescence techniques using nasopharyngeal secretions*: RDTs for viruses have very good sensitivity and specificity in detecting viral infections like influenza. However, a positive test does not rule out a bacterial infection.
9. *Paired serology and PCR assay for mycoplasma and chlamydia infection*: Acute and convalescent serology is the diagnostic test to detect *Mycoplasma pneumoniae*, whereas PCR assays can also be used.
10. *Chest X-rays*: Chest radiographs are suggested in moderate to severe cases of pneumonia that require hospitalization. It also helps to assess the complications of pneumonia-empyema, pneumothorax and pleural effusion. However, chest radiograph cannot differentiate between viral and bacterial etiology. Consolidation (**Fig. 2**), pneumatoceles, pleural effusion or empyema and cavitation on chest X-Ray point towards bacterial pneumonia. *Mycoplasma pneumoniae* has diffuse bilateral infiltrates on chest X-ray. Presence of hyperinflation and bilateral interstitial infiltrates on chest X-ray suggest viral pneumonia (**Fig. 3**).
11. *Lung ultrasound* is helpful in diagnosing consolidation, pleural effusion and empyema. It is noninvasive and avoids exposure to radiation associated with chest X-rays.

Management of Pneumonia

Outpatient management

Children with mild symptoms of pneumonia can be managed at home with antipyretics for fever management and oral fluids to prevent dehydration. The parents must be explained about the danger signs of pneumonia, and to visit the pediatrician if the child shows signs and symptoms of deterioration.

Criteria of hospitalization in pneumonia

1. Apnea or grunting
2. SpO_2 <92% in room air or cyanosis
3. Lethargy, poor feeding or dehydration
4. RR>70/min for infants and RR>50/min for older children
5. Tachycardia, poor perfusion, prolonged capillary refill time
6. Comorbidities like chronic lung disease, congenital heart disease, neuromuscular disorders, immunodeficiency disorders

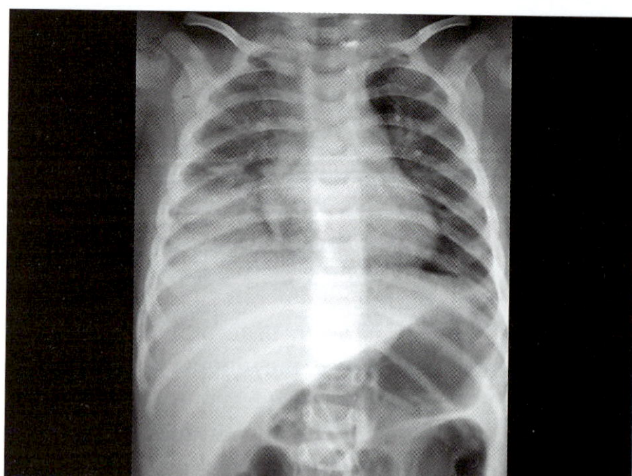

Fig. 2: Chest X-ray of a 3-year-old child with community acquired pneumonia-right middle and lower lobe pneumonia due to *Streptococcus pneumoniae*

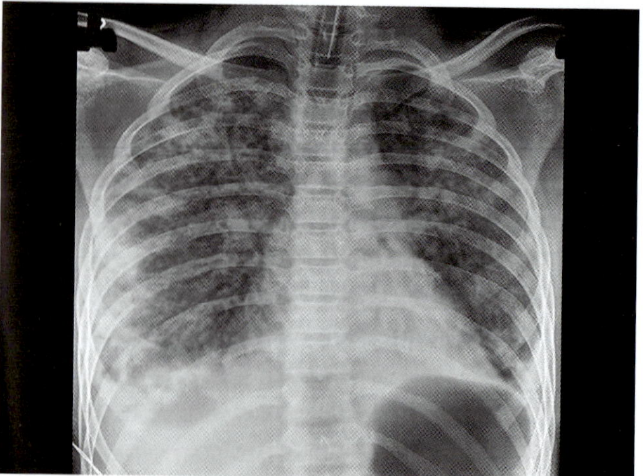

Fig. 3: A 6-year-old with influenza A pneumonia with bilateral patchy infiltrates

7. Complications of pneumonia—Pleural effusion or empyema
8. Failure of outpatient treatment, social issues (like parents not confident).

Criteria for admitting to intensive care unit

1. SpO_2 <92% on FiO_2 >60%
2. Hemodynamic instability
3. Signs of respiratory failure or severe respiratory distress with signs of exhaustion
4. Recurrent apnea or intermittent shallow respirations.

General management

1. *Oxygen*: Oxygen should be given via nasal cannula, non-rebreathing mask or head box if the oxygen saturation (SpO_2) is less than 92%, in order to maintain SpO_2 > 92%. High flow nasal cannula can also be used to deliver heated humidified high flow oxygen in children with moderate distress. Severe cases of pneumonia may require intubation and ventilatory support.
2. *Feeds*: Fluid resuscitation with isotonic fluids may be required in case of dehydration. Thereafter, nasogastric feeds should be started in case of respiratory distress to prevent aspiration. Restricted IV fluids can be started if child is not tolerating any feeds. Electrolytes should be monitored in children with IV fluids to look for electrolyte imbalance due to SIADH.
3. *Antipyretics*: Paracetamol, oral or intravenous, should be given for fever and discomfort.
4. *Suctioning and chest physiotherapy*: Gentle suction of secretions may be required. Chest physiotherapy has not been found to be beneficial in children with pneumonia.
5. *Antimicrobial therapy:*
   - Antimicrobial therapy should be based on the age of the child, the severity of the disease and the resistance pattern of local pathogens.
   - Infants less than 3 months of age usually are managed as in-patients.
   - Antibiotics are usually not required for children in the preschool age group with mild symptoms suggestive of viral infection, as viruses are responsible for most of the illnesses in this age group. Antibiotics should be commenced on clinical suspicion of bacterial infection or if investigations are supporting a bacterial disease.
   - In all children with high suspicion of bacterial infection or moderate to severe pneumonia, antibiotics should be started empirically to treat and prevent complications of bacterial pneumonia, as it is difficult to distinguish between viral and bacterial pneumonia.
   - Use of oral antibiotics is safe and effective and is the preferred route.
   - Parenteral route should be used in case of vomiting and inability to tolerate oral fluids or if the child is having signs of septicemia or complicated pneumonia.
   - Change antibiotics from intravenous to parenteral route as soon as the child shows clinical improvement, is afebrile and is accepting oral feeds.

Antibiotic Therapy[27,33,34]

Outpatient treatment (Table 5)

- Amoxicillin is antimicrobial of choice in children as it acts against most of the bacteria prevalent in children, especially streptococci. The emergence of penicillin resistant streptococci in certain regions, a higher dose of amoxicillin is advocated in such areas (90 mg/kg/day); this is not applicable to India.
- Co-amoxiclav (amoxicillin and clavulanic acid), second or third generation cephalosporins (cefuroxime, cefaclor) are effective alternatives.
- Macrolides (azithromycin and clarithromycin) are advised as second line agents in case of no response to first line therapy.
- If *Mycoplasma* or *Chlamydia pneumonia* is suspected macrolides should be used as first line agent.

Table 5: Antimicrobial therapy for CAP—outpatient

Age group	*First line*	*Second line*
3 months – 5 years	Amoxicillin	Co-amoxiclav or cefuroxime or Amoxicillin plus cloxacillin (if *Staphylococcus* suspected)
>5 years	Amoxicillin Or Azithromycin (10 mg/kg/day once daily) (suspected atypical pneumonia)	Co-amoxiclav Or Azithromycin

- If the child is allergic to penicillin group, then cephalosporins or macrolides can be used.
- If the child is suspected to have moderate to severe pneumonia due to influenza virus, prompt treatment with antiviral agent—oseltamivir should be started. The treatment should not be delayed awaiting laboratory confirmation.
- Children suspected with mild staphylococcal infection require cefuroxime or co-amoxiclav or a combination of amoxicillin and cloxacillin.

Inpatient therapy (Table 6)

- Infants less than 3 months with pneumonia should be admitted and treated with IV ceftriaxone/cefotaxime with or without aminoglycoside. Co-amoxiclav can be used alternatively with aminoglycoside.
- Intravenous antibiotics that can be used to treat severe pneumonia are broad-spectrum antibiotics like ampicillin, amoxicillin, co-amoxiclav, ceftriaxone, cefuroxime or cefotaxime.
- Macrolides should be given if atypical pneumonia is suspected, or as an add on therapy in severe disease.
- If clinical and radiological features are suggestive of pneumonia due to *Staphylococcus aureus*, use anti-staphylococcal antibiotics **(Table 7)**. If MRSA is suspected, start clindamycin or vancomycin. Linezolid is an effective alternative and can be given orally or intravenously.

Duration of antibiotics

Antibiotics should be given for 7–10 days. Shorter courses (3–5 days) can also be given for mild cases, especially on OPD basis. Macrolides are given for 5 days. In case of complicated staphylococcal pneumonia (empyema) antibiotics are indicated for longer duration (3–4 weeks).

Table 6: Antimicrobial therapy for CAP—inpatient

Age group	*Parenteral antibiotic therapy*
0–3 months	Co-amoxiclav (30 mg/kg/dose 12 hourly) + amikacin (15 mg/kg/day Once daily) /gentamicin (7 mg/kg/day Once daily) Or Ceftriaxone (50–100 mg/kg/day once or twice daily) + amikacin /gentamicin Or Cefotaxime (150 mg/kg/day 8 hourly) + amikacin /gentamicin
3 months to 5 years	Amoxicillin (50 mg/kg/dose twice daily) Or Co-amoxyclav (30 mg/kg/dose 8 hourly) Or Ceftriaxone (50–100 mg/kg/day once or twice daily) Or Cefotaxime (150 mg/kg/day 8 hourly) Or Azithromycin (if atypical pneumonia is suspected) (10 mg/kg/day once daily) *Azithromycin can be added to amoxicillin, cefotaxime and ceftriaxone as add on therapy in case of severe infections*

Table 7: Treatment of suspected staphylococcal pneumonia or complicated pneumonia

Methicillin sensitive *Staphylococcus aureus* (MSSA)	Cefuroxime (30 mg/kg/day iv 8 hourly) Or Co-amoxyclav (30 mg/kg/dose 8 hourly) Or Ceftriaxone (100 mg/kg/day once or twice daily) with + cloxacillin Or Cefazolin
Methicillin resistant *Staphylococcus aureus* (MRSA)	Ceftriaxone/Cefotaxime with clindamycin (10 mg/kg/dose 6 hourly) Or Ceftriaxone/Cefotaxime with vancomycin (15 mg/kg/dose 6 hourly) (septic patients with hemodynamic instability)

Table 8: Treatment of influenza with oseltamivir

Age group	*Treatment dose x 5 days*	*Chemoprophylaxis dose × 10 days*
<3 months	3 mg/kg/dose twice daily	Not recommended
>3 months	3 mg/kg/dose twice daily	3 mg/kg/dose once daily
>1 year	Weight 15 kg 30 mg twice daily 16–23 kg 45 mg twice daily 24–40 Kg 60 mg twice daily >40 kg 75 mg twice daily	30 mg once daily 45 mg once daily 60 mg once daily 75 mg once daily

Table 9: Treatment of hospital-acquired pneumonia

Gentamicin 7.5 mg/kg per day once daily or Amikacin 15 mg/kg/ once daily
Plus
Piperacillin-tazobactam 90 mg/kg/dose 6 hourly
Or
Meropenem 60 mg/kg/day in 8 hourly
Or
Ceftazidime 100–150 mg/kg /day 8 hourly
Vancomycin 15 mg/kg/dose 6 hourly to be given in suspected or confirmed MRSA pneumonia

Influenza Pneumonia

Treatment[35]

Infants and children with confirmed or suspected infection due to influenza virus require treatment (**Table 8**) in the following situations:

- Children less than 5 years old
- They require hospitalization
- Rapidly progressive, severe or complicated disease
- Presence of risk factors such as chronic lung disease, immunodeficiency disorders, neurodegenerative or neurodevelopmental disorders, liver, renal, endocrine and metabolic disorders.

Chemoprophylaxis

It is given to the high-risk cases who come in contact with an individual who is in the infective phase of influenza and if they have come in contact with the infectious person in the last 48 hours.

Hospital-acquired Pneumonia

The antibiotics in HAP should be directed towards nosocomial organisms like *Klebsiella pneumoniae*, *Pseudomonas aeruginosa*, *Acinetobacter* (gram negative organisms), and MRSA (gram positive organisms). So, empirical treatment comprises of a combination of an antibiotic cover for gram negative and gram positive organisms (**Table 9**).

KEY MESSAGES

- Bronchiolitis is clinical syndrome in children less than 2 years of age characterized by upper respiratory symptoms followed tachypnea and/or wheezing.
- Bronchiolitis is primarily caused by respiratory syncytial virus.
- Risk factors for severe diseases and/or complications include gestational age less than 37 weeks, ago less than 12 weeks, chronic pulmonary disease, congenital and anatomic defects of the airways, congenital heart disease, immunodeficiency and neurologic disease.
- Bronchiolitis is diagnosed clinically. Chest radiographs and laboratory tests are not routinely indicated.
- Anticipatory guidance, adequate clinical monitoring and supportive management are essential. Bronchodilators may have a role in some patients.
- Children with pneumonia usually present with fever, tachypnea, productive cough, and chest pain. In pneumonia caused by atypical pathogens, a more gradual onset associated with low grade fever or no fever, headache, non-productive cough and malaise may be present.
- Chest X-rays are not routinely in patients being treated on OPD basis with a strong clinical suspicion of pneumonia.
- In previously healthy children with suspected bacterial pneumonia being treated on OPD basis, amoxicillin is the first line antibiotic in a dose of 50 mg/kg/day, given in two or three divided doses.
- Children with severe or very severe pneumonia (as per WHO definitions) should be hospitalized for management.
- Children with severe and life-threatening bacterial pneumonia should be started on parenteral antibiotics and offered supportive therapy.

REFERENCES

1. World Health Organization. (1995). The Management of acute respiratory infections in children: practical guidelines for outpatient care. Geneva: World Health Organization. Available from: *http://www.who.int/iris/handle/10665/41803*. Accessed August 16, 2019.
2. GBD 2015 LRI Collaborators. Estimates of the global, regional, and national morbidity, mortality, and aetiologies of lower

respiratory tract infections in 195 countries: A systematic analysis for the Global Burden of Disease Study 2015. Lancet Infect Dis. 2017;17:1133-61.

3. Shi T, McAllister DA, O'Brien KL, *et al.* Global, regional, and national disease burden estimates of acute lower respiratory infections due to respiratory syncytial virus in young children in 2015: A systematic review and modelling study. Lancet. 2017;390:946-58.
4. Hall CB, Weinberg GA, Blumkin AK, *et al.* Respiratory syncytial virus-associated hospitalizations among children less than 24 months of age. Pediatrics. 2013;132:341-8.
5. Ralston SL, Lieberthal AS, Meissner HC, *et al.* Clinical practice guideline: The diagnosis, management, and prevention of bronchiolitis. *Pediatrics*. 2014;134:1474-502.
6. Zorc JJ, Hall CB. Bronchiolitis: Recent evidence on diagnosis and management. Pediatrics. 2010;125:342-9.
7. Meissner HC. Selected populations at increased risk from respiratory syncytial virus infection. Pediatr Infect Dis J. 2003; 22:S40-4.
8. Hacımustafaoğlu M, Celebi S, Bozdemir SE, *et al.* RSV frequency in children below 2 years hospitalized for lower respiratory tract infections. Turk J Pediatr. 2013;55:130-9.
9. Miller EK, Gebretsadik T, Carroll KN, *et al.* Viral etiologies of infant bronchiolitis, croup and upper respiratory illness during 4 consecutive years. Pediatr Infect Dis J. 2013;32:950-5.
10. Meissner HC. Viral bronchiolitis in children. N Engl J Med. 2016;374:62-72.
11. Paranhos-Baccalà G, Komurian-Pradel F, Richard N, *et al.* Mixed respiratory virus infections. J Clin Virol. 2008;43:407-10.
12. Friedman JN, Rieder MJ, Walton JM. Canadian Paediatric Society, Acute Care Committee, Drug Therapy and Hazardous Substances Committee. Bronchiolitis: Recommendations for diagnosis, monitoring and management of children one to 24 months of age. Paediatr Child Health. 2014;19:485-91.
13. Mansbach JM, Piedra PA, Teach SJ, *et al.* MARC-30 Investigators. Prospective multicenter study of viral etiology and hospital length of stay in children with severe bronchiolitis. Arch Pediatr Adolesc Med. 2012;166:700-6.
14. Mansbach JM, McAdam AJ, Clark S, *et al.* Prospective multicenter study of the viral etiology of bronchiolitis in the emergency department. Acad Emerg Med. 2008;15:111-8.
15. McKiernan C, Chua LC, Visintainer PF, *et al.* High-flow nasal cannulae therapy in infants with bronchiolitis. J Pediatr. 2010;156:634-8.
16. Hilliard TN, Archer N, Laura H, *et al.* Pilot study of vapotherm oxygen delivery in moderately severe bronchiolitis. Arch Dis Child. 2012;97:182-3.
17. Zhang L, Mendoza-Sassi RA, Wainwright C, *et al.* Nebulized hypertonic saline solution for acute bronchiolitis in infants. Cochrane Database Syst Rev. 2008;(4):CD006458.
18. Gupta HV, Gupta VV, Kaur G, *et al.* Effectiveness of 3% hypertonic saline nebulization in acute bronchiolitis among Indian children: A quasi-experimental study. Persp Clin Res. 2016;7:88-93.
19. Gadomski AM, Brower M. Bronchodilators for bronchiolitis. Cochrane Database Syst Rev. 2010;8:CD001266.
20. Hartling L, Fernandes RM, Bialy L, *et al.* Steroids and bronchodilators for acute bronchiolitis in the first two years of life: Systematic review and meta-analysis. BMJ. 2011;342: d1714.
21. Skjerven HO, Hunderi JO, Brugmann-Pieper SK, *et al.* Racemic adrenaline and inhalation strategies in acute bronchiolitis. N Engl J Med. 2013;368:2286-93.
22. Fernandes RM, Bialy LM, Vandermeer B, *et al.* Glucocorticoids for acute viral bronchiolitis in infants and young children. Cochrane Database Syst Rev. 2010;CD004878.
23. American Academy of Pediatrics, Subcommittee on Diagnosis and Management of Bronchiolitis. Diagnosis and management of bronchiolitis. Pediatrics. 2006;118:1774-93.
24. British Thoracic Society Standards of Care Committee. British Thoracic Society guidelines for the management of community acquired pneumonia in children: update 2011. Thorax. 2011; 356:1-23.
25. Liu L, Oza S, Hogan D, *et al.* Global, regional, and national causes of under-5 mortality in 2000-15: An updated systematic analysis with implications for the Sustainable Development Goals. Lancet. 2016;388:3027-35.
26. Thomson A, Harris M. Community-acquired pneumonia in children: what's new? Thorax. 2011;356:927-8.
27. Bowen SJ, Thomson AH. British Thoracic Society Paediatric Pneumonia Audit: A review of 3 years of data. Thorax. 2013;356: 682-3.
28. Black SB, Shinefield HR, Ling S, *et al.* Effectiveness of heptavalent pneumococcal conjugate vaccine in children younger than five years of age for prevention of pneumonia. Pediatr Infect Dis J. 2002;21:810-15.
29. Michelow IC, Olsen K, Lozano J, *et al.* Epidemiology and clinical characteristics of community-acquired pneumonia in hospitalized children. Pediatrics. 2004;113:701e7.
30. Cilla G, Onate E, Perez-Yarza EG, *et al.* Viruses in community-acquired pneumonia in children aged less than 3 years old: High rate of viral coinfection. J Med Virol. 2008;80:1843e9.
31. Stuckey-Schrock K, Hayes BL, George CM. Community-acquired pneumonia in children. Am Fam Physician. 2012; 86(7):661-7.
32. Taylor JA, Del Beccaro M, Done S, *et al.* Establishing clinically relevant standards for tachypnea in febrile children younger than 2 years. Arch Pediatr Adolesc Med. 1995;149:283-7.
33. Bradley JS, Byington CL, Shah SS, *et al.* Executive summary: The management of community-acquired pneumonia in infants and children older than 3 months of age: Clinical Practice Guidelines by the Pediatric Infectious Diseases Society and the Infectious Diseases Society of America. Clin Infect Dis. 2011;53: 617-30.
34. Haq IJ, Battersby AC, Eastham K, *et al.* Community-acquired pneumonia in children. BMJ. 2017;356:j686.
35. CDC. Recommendations for Use of Antiviral Medications for the Management of Influenza in Children and Adolescent for the 2009-2010 Season—Pediatric Supplement for Healthcare Providers. Available from *https://www.cdc.gov/h1n1flu/recommendations_pediatric_supplement.htm*. Accessed August 16, 2019.

CHAPTER

20

Emergencies in Chronic Respiratory Disorders

Sankaran Krishnan, Daniel Krich

INTRODUCTION

Respiratory illnesses contribute to major morbidity and mortality in children. In India, the level of disability adjusted life years (DALYs) secondary to chronic respiratory diseases has increased from 4.6% to 6.4% in the past 25 years (1990–2016). As of 2016, India had 32% of the global DALYs.[1] Acute lower respiratory infections are among the top three causes of childhood death.[2] Those who survive may be predisposed to sequelae of chronic respiratory conditions, with intermittent exacerbations. In this chapter, we will discuss management approaches to chronic respiratory conditions including asthma, bronchopulmonary dysplasia, cystic fibrosis, primary ciliary dyskinesia, hypoventilation syndromes, neuromuscular disease, interstitial lung diseases, and related disorders.

ASTHMA

Asthma is a multifactorial disease affecting both children and adults. It is one of the most common chronic diseases in children,[3] affecting 14% of children globally,[2] and in some regions of India as high as 18%.[4] It is characterized as a chronic inflammatory disorder of the airways, by variable and recurring symptoms (cough or wheeze), airflow obstruction, bronchial hyper-responsiveness, and an underlying inflammation. The reversibility of airway flow obstruction can be spontaneous or with treatment.[3] However, the ability to fully reverse airflow obstruction through lung function testing following bronchodilator may be incomplete in some individuals, classified as "fixed obstruction".[5]

The pathogenesis of asthma is multifactorial, consisting of both genetic and environmental factors.[6] Those exposed to tobacco smoke or those with parents with tobacco smoke exposure have an increased risk of developing asthma.[7] Individuals with parental history of asthma, or personal atopic features (eczema) carry an increased risk.[8]

Complications of uncontrolled asthma can lead to serious morbidity and/or mortality. Children with asthma may be missing out on peer activities, exercise, and education with prolonged illnesses including those with or without hospitalizations.[9] Caregivers of children with asthma report burdens upon their financial resources. For adults, an individual with asthma can lose up to 17 working days/year.[10] The yearly cost of asthma in India as of recent estimates in 2015 may be as high as 139 billion INR. This does not include the mortality secondary to asthma, which in 2015 was attributable for 82,000 deaths.[11-13]

Risk factors for severe asthma exacerbations[14,15] *(from GINA guidelines, 2016, Box 4-1)*

- Any history of near-fatal asthma requiring intubation and ventilation
- Hospitalization or emergency care for asthma in last 12 months
- Not currently using ICS, or poor adherence with ICS
- Currently using or recently stopped using OCS (indicating the severity of recent events)
- Over-use of short-acting beta agonists (SABAs), especially if more than 1 canister/month
- Lack of a written asthma action plan
- History of psychiatric disease or psychosocial problems
- Confirmed food allergy in a patient with asthma.

Flowchart 1: Management of acute asthma

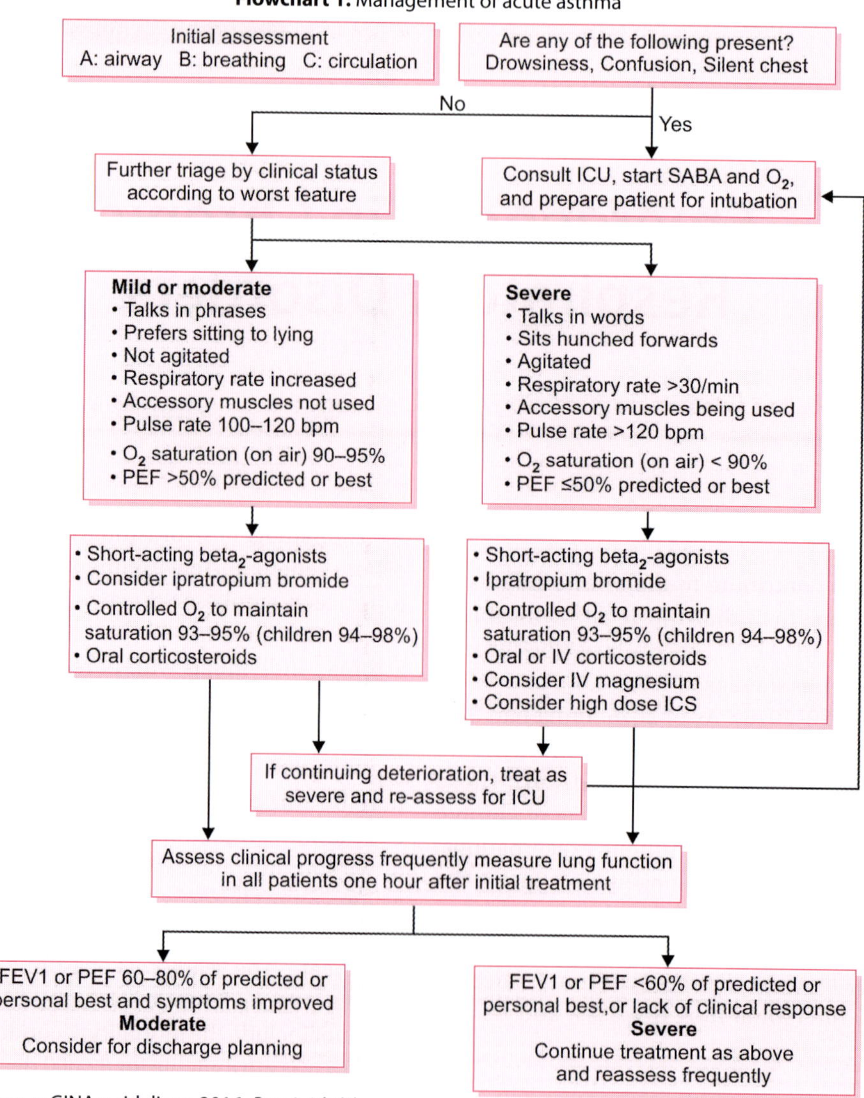

*Source***:** GINA guidelines, 2016, *Box 4-4 (1/4)*

Management of Acute Asthma[14]

(From the GINA guidelines, 2016, *Box 4-4 (1/4)* See **Flowchart 1**. Also, see chapter on management of acute asthma for details on pharmacotherapy. If presenting with a severe asthma exacerbation that is not responsive to standard pharmacotherapy and oxygen, noninvasive ventilation or invasive ventilation may be necessary. Approximately 2–4% of patients presenting in status asthmaticus will require mechanical ventilation.[16] Noninvasive ventilation has added benefits of aerosolized delivery of medications.[17-19] Invasive ventilation may present additional irritants for bronchospasm, dynamic hyperinflation, necessitate sedation medications, and may worsen gas exchange.

Physiologic Changes in Status Asthmaticus

- Dynamic hyperinflation
- Progressive increased lung volumes stretching pulmonary vasculature,
- Increased pulmonary vascular resistance
- Increased right ventricular afterload further exacerbated with pulmonary vasoconstriction, secondary to hypoxia and acidosis

- Increased left ventricular afterload, decreased cardiac output, secondary to high negative pulmonary pressures during inspiration
- Exaggerated decrease in systolic blood pressure during inspiration. A decrease in SBP >10 mm Hg during inspiration is termed pulsus paradoxus
- Negative intra-pleural pressure generated favors trans-capillary fluid edema to the alveolar space.

Dynamic hyperinflation occurs with increasing hyperinflation in obstructive lung disease, with incomplete exhalation of tidal volume. With each successive delivered breath, further hyperinflation occurs. More time is needed in the exhalation phase in order to exhale the appropriate tidal breath. Measuring Plateau airway pressure (Pplat-represents average end-alveolar inspiratory pressures) and auto-PEEP (Peak end expiratory pressure) can yield information regarding dynamics hyperinflation, occurring during volume cycled ventilation.[16-19]

Mechanical Ventilation Strategies in ICU for Asthma

- Noninvasive ventilation,[18,19] with or without backup rate. Appropriate pressures selected for IPAP and EPAP to ensure adequate chest expansion and improvement in blood gases.
    - Small dose of benzodiazepines or propofol with or without a low-dose ketamine infusion or dexmedetomidine may facilitate the tolerance for NPPV.
- Invasive ventilation strategies[19,20]
    - Permissive hypercapnia
    - Lung protective strategies, allowing for sufficient exhalation to minimize the amount of dynamic hyperinflation
    - Ventilator mode
        - Pressure-limited ventilation
        - Pressure regulated volume control,
            - Results in a lower peak airway pressure and a higher mean airway pressure than a volume control mode
            - Positive end-expiratory pressure should surpass the lower inflection point of alveolar collapse duration exhalation (as observed on the Pressure-Volume Curve).

Suggested target range for ventilator parameters[15-19]

- Plateau pressures (Pplat)—upper limit of 30 cm H_2O.
    - Higher pressures may result in barotrauma/air-leak syndromes or hypotension
- PEEP (auto-PEEP)—ranging between 10 and 15 cm H_2O
- Minute ventilation—avoid too high or low
- Adequate flow rate
- Square wave form
- Decreased I:E ratio with increased expiratory phase
- Permissive hypercapnia to limit dynamic hyperinflation.

Options for sedation while intubated[15-19]

- *Ketamine*: 0.5–1 mg/kg/minute for initial general anesthesia, titrate as needed. Note: ketamine is also a bronchodilator, combine with midazolam to decrease "emergent behaviors" when terminated, can increase pulmonary artery pressures.
- *Propofol*: 25–75 µg/kg/minute; initiate at 15 µg/kg/minute with increments of 5 µg/kg/minute every 5 minutes until sedated or a max dose of 50 µg/kg/min.
- *Fentanyl*: 1–3 µg/kg fentanyl over 1–2 min as needed or infusion at 0.05–3 µg/kg/hour, titrate as needed.
- *Midazolam*: 1–2 µg/kg/min IV; Start: 0.05–0.2 mg/kg IV and titrate; Note: use ideal body weight (IBW) in obese patients; titrate to effect; taper dose gradually if long-term use. Alternate: 0.05–0.15 mg/kg IV q1–2h as needed.

BRONCHOPULMONARY DYSPLASIA

Bronchopulmonary dysplasia (BPD) is a chronic lung disease most commonly found in preterm infants who required mechanical ventilation (invasive or non-invasive) with prolonged needs of oxygen. First described by Northway in 1967, it was reported in infants who had received respiratory support via mechanical ventilation and elevated levels of oxygen concentration. The degrees of BPD were based on chest radiography findings, thought to be associated with barotrauma and oxygen toxicity, termed "Hyaline Membrane Disease".[20] With advances in medicine including surfactant replacement, as well as gentler modes of ventilation (including non-invasive ventilation) and more carefully targeted oxygen saturations (with carefully titrated oxygen concentration), current BPD, or "new BPD" has associations with arrested lung development, with less lung fibrosis.[21]

Epidemiology

The incidence of BPD in premature infants born less than 28 weeks gestation has remained stable around 40%.[21] The definition of BPD encompasses both oxygen requirements as well as duration of oxygen needs **(Table 1)**.

The pathophysiology and degree of BPD is related inversely to the gestational age at birth. The arrest of lung development, and thereby the stage of lung development attained by the infant, coincides with normal embryologic growth. Factors that can affect development include infection (chorioamnionitis), intrauterine growth retardation (IUGR), antenatal steroids, as well as ventilation and fluid overload.

Pathophysiology

Barotrauma alone induces injury, with overdistention of alveoli, as evidence by BPD found in those with mechanical ventilation.[21,22] Oxygen toxicity is associated with promotion of free radicals and oxidative stress, leading to release of cytokines including tumor necrosis factor alpha (TNFα), IL-8, IL-1β and IL-6, as well as neutrophils with damaging molecules such as neutrophil elastase and oxidative burst. Nutrition as well plays a role in optimizing lung growth, and minimizing fluid overload, which would cause edema in the developing alveoli and induce injury.[22]

Treatment

Therapies aimed at prevention of BPD have incorporated each of the above etiologic concerns. Gentle ventilation with permissive hypercapnia and noninvasive ventilation have been accepted methods of managing premature infants to minimize barotrauma to the developing alveoli.[23,24] Based on large multicenter trials [Surfactant, Positive Pressure and Oxygenation Randomization Trial (SUPPORT)[25] and Benefits of Oxygen Saturation Trials (BOOST II)],[26] oxygen saturations of 93–96% have been targeted. Antenatal steroids are used before delivery to improve surfactant quality (aside from surfactant administration), though postnatal steroids remain controversial with the potential risk of cerebral palsy, and overall neurodevelopmental effects on the growing infant.[27] Caffeine, which has central modulatory effects in minimizing apnea of prematurity, has been a long standing accepted therapy in minimizing BPD.[24, 27]

Some infants with BPD have "wet lungs" and benefit from diuretics, as evidenced by improved oxygenation following trials of furosemide and chronic diuretics. The doses of diuretics are for chlorothiazide (20–40 mg/kg/day, divided BID) and spironolactone (1–3 mg/kg/day). Infants treated with these medications may need periodic evaluation of electrolytes, particular sodium and potassium. These infants may benefit from chronic diuretics, weaned as the infant grows.[28]

Management of BPD following early infancy includes modalities as mentioned above (**Flowchart 2**). There is a large prevalence of asthma in BPD infants, with reports ranging from 25% to 50%. These infants respond to bronchodilators and are often treated with standard asthma therapies.[28] In prevention of BPD exacerbations, appropriate hand hygiene as well as avoidance of tobacco exposure remain extremely important.[22-24,28]

Palivizumab is a monoclonal antibody against RSV (Synagis) which is given to the following: premature infants born <29 weeks gestational age (in first year of life), those with hemodynamically significant CHD, and those premature infants, in second year of life, if on chronic corticosteroid therapy.[29] Despite best management, some of these infants will continue to have a "fixed obstruction" to their airways, and may have significant exercise limitations when older.[30] The greatest preventative strategies for BPD remains adequate prenatal care and avoiding premature birth.[22-28]

Table 1: Bronchopulmonary dysplasia classification

Gestational age	*<32 weeks*	*≥32 weeks*
Time point of assessment (Treatment with oxygen >21% for at least 28 day **plus)**	36 weeks PMA or discharge to home, whichever comes first	>28 days but <56 days postnatal age or discharge to home, whichever comes first
Mild BPD	Breathing room air at 36 weeks PMA or discharge, whichever comes first	Breathing room air by 56 days postnatal age or discharge, whichever comes first
Moderate BPD	Need for <30% oxygen at 36 weeks PMA or discharge, whichever comes first	Need for <30% oxygen at 56 days postnatal age or discharge, whichever comes first
Severe BPD	Need for ≥30% oxygen and/or positive pressure, (PPV or NCPAP) at 36 weeks PMA or discharge, whichever comes first	Need for ≥30% oxygen and/or positive pressure (PPV or NCPAP) at 56 days postnatal age or discharge, whichever comes first

Adapted from Davidson and Berkelhamer.[23]

Flowchart 2: Management pathway for bronchopulmonary dysplasia exacerbation

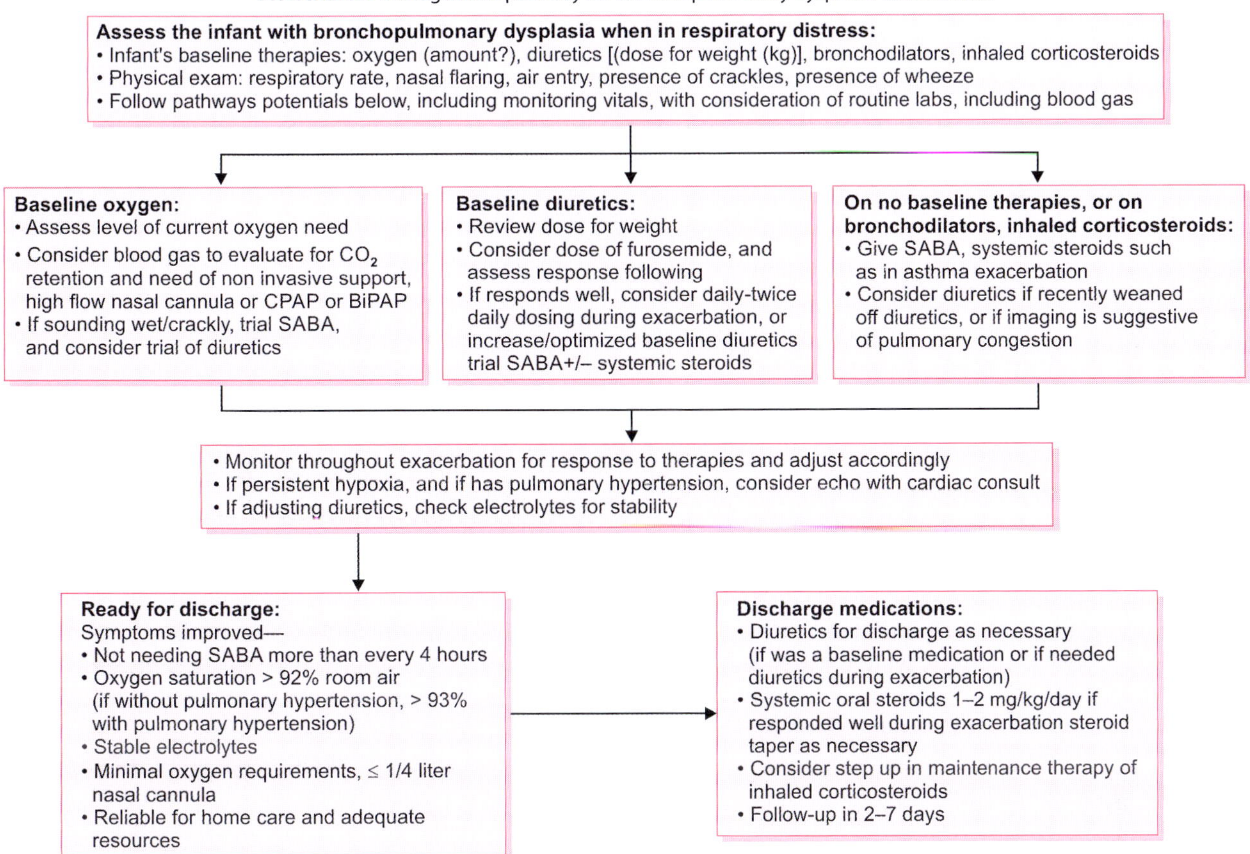

Adapted from: Bhandari A and Panitch H[28]

CYSTIC FIBROSIS

Etiopathogenesis

Cystic fibrosis (CF) is an autosomal recessive inherited disorder associated with lung infections and malnutrition amongst other organ dysfunction.[31,32] It is caused by a mutation in the CFTR (Cystic fibrosis transmembrane conductance regulator) gene located on chromosome 7. CFTR is a chloride channel found in multiple sites of the body. It allows for chloride movement with water passively following the chloride. Its function is well known throughout the lungs, gastrointestinal tract, and sexual organs. Its dysfunction in the lungs leads to thickened mucus in the airways, decreased airway clearance, promoting a bacteria rich region (with entrapped base enzymes for bacterial nutrients), cyclical inflammation and infection. This further promotes bronchiectasis, and decreased lung function. In the gastrointestinal tract, it promotes pancreatic exocrine dysfunction, leading to fat malabsorption, as well as potentially diabetes.[31,32] In the sexual organs, it interferes with basic egg and sperm motility in their respective ducts, leading to fertility issues.[31,32]

Epidemiology

There are approximately 2000 known mutations associated with CF. There are 6 classes of mutations determined by the production, configuration, cell membrane insertion/functionality, and lastly, degradation of the protein. Based on the combinations of class mutations, there is a wide variation in manifestations of the dysfunction, ranging from severe lung disease and pancreatic malabsorption with potential needs for lung transplant, to mild asthma type patterns and possible pancreatitis. The prevalence of CF in the Indian population is approximately 1/10,000 to 1/40,000.[32,33] Homozygous F508del comprises approximately 19–56% of the CF diagnosis, with other heterogeneous mutation combinations for remainder of the CF population.[32,33]

Treatment

The long-term care of individuals with CF requires a multidisciplinary approach. In CF lungs, as mentioned above, the airway surface layer is altered with thickened mucus, leading to poor airway clearance, colonization/chronic infection with bacteria, potential long-term bronchiectasis, and decline in lung function. Optimizing airway clearance through mechanical devices such as chest vest therapy, mucolytics (such as hypertonic nebulizer saline, dornase alpha) are used to maintain optimal lung function.[34-40] Routine screening of lung bacteria though throat culture (in those unable to produce sputum), induced sputum, or if necessary bronchoscopy (though no longer routine), guides choice of antibiotics in pulmonary exacerbations (see further), and may guide potential attempts at bacterial eradication when colonized with *Pseudomonas aeruginosa*, which is associated with lung function decline.[34-40]

Exacerbations in CF include pulmonary exacerbations, hemoptysis, acute pneumothorax, and distal intestinal obstructive syndrome (DIOS).

Pulmonary exacerbations

Pulmonary exacerbations are common in CF, though incidence rates are difficult to assess with no consensus on exact criteria for an exacerbation.[40,41] Most experts agree that an exacerbation is associated with increased cough or sputum, weight loss, or decline in lung function. Evaluation includes sputum to assess for alterations in colonized bacteria. Airway clearance is increased, and oral antibiotics are prescribed, typically a 10–14-day regimen. If not improving, then intravenous (IV) antibiotics are initiated, with standard use of two intravenous antibiotics, for durations of 10–21 days, based on clinical response. Selection of antibiotics is based on most recent bacterial culture results, while awaiting results from current testing. Though combination antibiotic therapy has not been validated in the treatment of CF lung infections, the standard of care has been to use combination antibiotics as treatment of *P. aeruginosa*, typically including an aminoglycoside.[41] Once-daily dosing of aminoglycosides is preferable to 3-times daily dosing.[42] Monitoring for improvement includes quality/quantity of sputum, cough, weight gain, and improved FEV_1 (if able to be performed) obtained via spirometry.[34-40] The North American CF Foundation guidelines recommends continuing chronic therapies for maintenance of lung health, including inhaled antibiotics and/or azithromycin, during treatment of an acute exacerbation of pulmonary disease.[41] Routine use of corticosteroids in the treatment of an acute exacerbation is not recommended, though may reduce inflammation in select cases.

Hemoptysis (Flowchart 3)

Mild to moderate hemoptysis defined as scant blood streaks (<5 mL) or small amounts of blood in sputum, can be present with an exacerbation, and airway clearance should be continued as well as antibiotics as in a general pulmonary exacerbation.[41] Any nonsteroidal anti-inflammatories should be temporarily stopped. Persistent or massive hemoptysis, defined as 240 mL in a 24-h period or recurrent bleeding 100 mL/d over several days, predominantly occurs in older patients with more advanced disease. It is an acute emergency, with possible airway obstruction from the blood itself, or with hypotension from volume loss.

Management is two-fold, controlling for the acute hemoptysis, and assessing for collateral bronchial arteries in bronchiectatic regions (tortuous arteries adjacent to bronchi). Management of the acute bleed includes stopping aerosolized hypertonic saline. Tranexamic acid at 4-hourly dosing, recommended at a level of 10 mg/kg IV and 30–40 mg/kg orally, is an option in massive hemoptysis.[42] If this is inadequate to control the bleeding, then bronchial artery embolization can be used (though embolization of potential future bleeding arteries remains controversial).[41,42] If still failing to control for the bleed, a last resort may include lung wedge resection. During these hemoptysis episodes, noninvasive pressure support should not be withheld.[41]

Acute spontaneous pneumothorax

Acute spontaneous pneumothorax **(Flowchart 4)** in cystic fibrosis is treated with standard care as indicated for any spontaneous pneumothorax, including expectant observation, and thoracostomy tube placement if indicated.[41] Positive pressure or percussive airway clearance devices may be withheld during the acute period.[41] If a persistent leak occurs, the management is more controversial. Surgical pleurodesis has been

Flowchart 3: Management of hemoptysis in cystic fibrosis

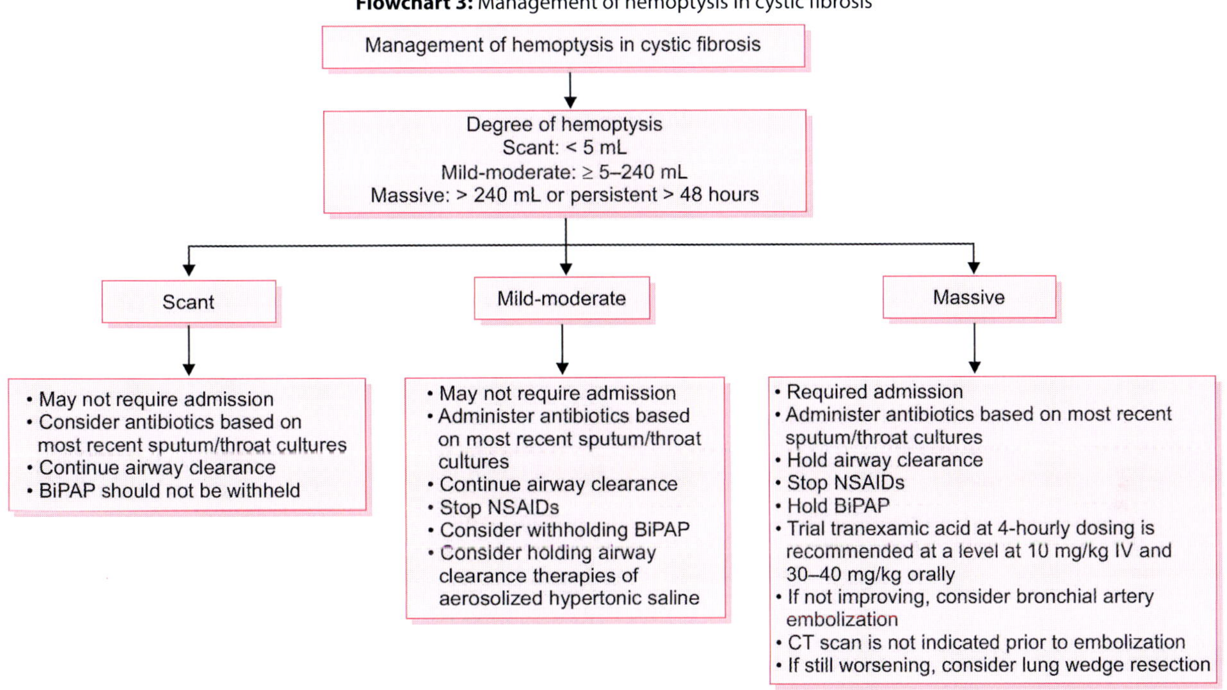

Adapted from Flume et al.[41]

performed, though can complicate long-term management for potential lung transplant if ECMO should be needed.[41] Alternatively, an autologous blood patch can be performed, with some case reports demonstrating good results.[41,43]

Pneumothorax occurs in cystic fibrosis due to the underlying obstruction and may not represent lung function decline with particular aims at prevention. Hemoptysis episodes however do occur primarily in worsening disease, with indication of ongoing lung function decline. Prevention aims at preserving lung function through optimized airway clearance, adherence to therapies and routine visits with a CF specialist to adjust therapies as necessary.[41]

Distal intestinal obstructive syndrome

The DIOS is a gastrointestinal emergency in CF, the result of the accumulation of viscid fecal material within the bowel, which combines with mucus produced in the CF intestine.[44] This material adheres to the intestinal wall, commonly in the terminal ileum and cecum, making it fixed in position and difficult to remove. This can lead to partial or complete obstruction. It affects between 10% to 22% of individuals with CF. One study found that children with CF had complete DIOS at a rate of 5 to 12 episodes per 1000 patients per year, with the figures for incomplete DIOS being higher. The incidence increases through adulthood, with an average rate of 35.5 episodes per 1000 patient years. Recurrence risks can be as high as 77%.[44,45]

Comorbidities for DIOS include meconium ileus, dehydration, poor adherence to pancreatic enzyme replacement, liver disease, diabetes mellitus, and *Pseudomonas aeruginosa* infection. Differential diagnoses for DIOS include the following: constipation (usually involves the colon), meconium ileus (found at birth, DIOS occurs later), intestinal obstruction secondary to adhesions from prior abdominal surgery, appendicitis; appendicular abscess, mucocele of the appendix, intussusception, and fibrosing colonopathy (associated with overuse of enzymes).

Management[44-46]

Diagnosis is based on abdominal radiography; stool-filled bowel loops are noted. Medical interventions include polyethylene glycol (2 g/kg/day, maximum 80–100 g/day, or as a ready to use iso-osmotic PEG solution, at a dose of 20–40 mL/kg/h up to a maximum of 1 L/h over 8 hours. Titrate dosing based on response based on clinical evaluation and abdominal X-rays as indicated); and oral diatrizoate (50 mL in 200 mL of water or juice for children

Flowchart 4: Management of spontaneous pneumothorax in cystic fibrosis

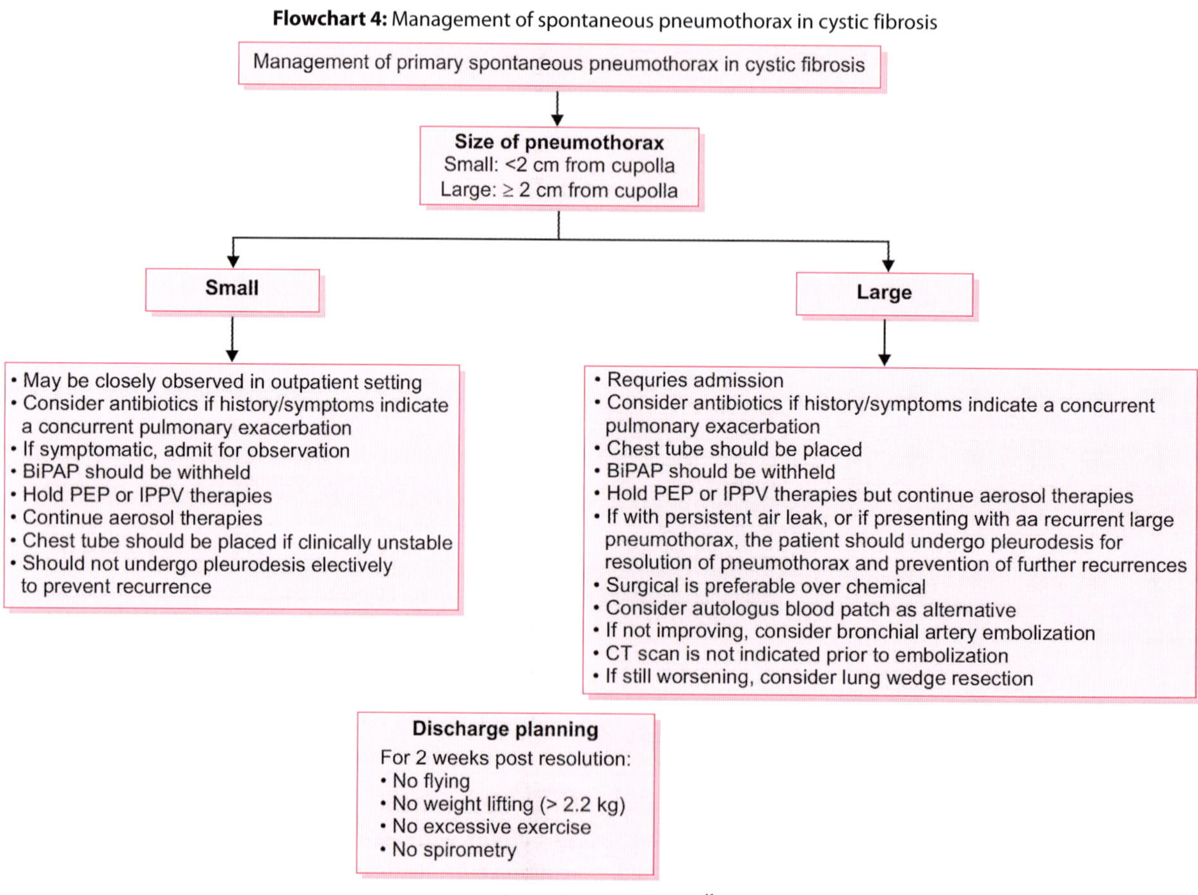

Adapted from Flume et al.[41]

<6 years; and 100 mL diluted in 400 mL for older patients on day 1, and half doses on subsequent days). Stimulant laxatives, senna, and oral N-acetylcysteine have also been used. Rarely surgical evacuation may be indicated. Newer intestinal chloride channel openers including lubiprostone have been tried,[46] especially in recalcitrant cases.

NEUROMUSCULAR DISORDERS AND HYPOVENTILATION

Neuromuscular disorders (NMDs) affect approximately on average 1–10/100,000 children. These include heterogeneous disease states of muscle, nerve, or neuromuscular junction **(Table 2)**. In most neuromuscular disorders there is involvement of the respiratory system.[47] The respiratory muscles, i.e. diaphragm or accessory muscles, may be affected leading to decreased vital capacity, atelectasis, and possible respiratory insufficiency.[48] Children with NMD have increased compliance of the rib cage similar to that of neonates, predisposing them to atelectasis with the lung tissue recoil unopposed.[49] In addition, children with NMD often have accompanying scoliosis, leading to restrictive lung defects, further compromising ventilation.[50]

Depending on the severity of muscular weakness, these individuals can present with varying respiratory comorbidities. These include restrictive lung defects as mentioned above. In addition, there is an overall decreased vital capacity associated with ineffective cough and poor airway clearance of their secretions, with further morbidity during periods of respiratory illness.[51] In general, a healthy individual should be able to generate a cough peak flow of > 360 L/min. Those with diminishing cough peak flows are indicative of inadequate cough, and those with vital capacity < 40% predicted, signals need for nocturnal non-invasive ventilation **(Table 3)**.

Individuals with NMD should be screened for sleep disordered breathing, including obstructive sleep apnea and nocturnal hypoventilation.[52-54] In NMD, with weakened musculature and altered respiratory compliance, the respiratory load is disproportionate to the respiratory muscles, with an increased respiratory load 2–3 times that of a healthy individual.[52-54] With the imbalance, the central respiratory drive will be increased, but with progressive weakness, alveolar hypoventilation will occur during sleep, as well as during illness, leading to increased risk for respiratory failure.

Management of Respiratory Failure in Children with NMD (Flowchart 5)

Respiratory infections in these children present as emergencies with necessity of increased airway clearance, either through chest physiotherapy, or if with an ineffective cough, through cough augmenting devices.[53-55] Augmentation of noninvasive ventilation is often required.[48,56,57] For the child with NMD presenting in respiratory distress, one needs to have suspicion for respiratory muscle fatigue, acute aspiration pneumonia and possible impending respiratory failure as they are weak at baseline.[58,59] Asthma in present in up to 26% of children with NMD, and a trial of bronchodilators with possible steroids is warranted.[55] Laboratory tests should include blood gases to assess for degree of hypoventilation and/or possible respiratory failure. There is a higher prevalence of pneumonias in children with NMD which may be attributed to their poor airway clearance.[59] Scoliosis, often associated in children with NMD, makes standard physical exam findings less reliable in assessing for pneumonia.[58,59] Chest radiography should be considered in patients presenting with respiratory symptoms. In addition, to community acquired pneumonia, aspiration pneumonias are more prevalent in children with NMD, secondary to dysphagia.[55,58,59] Airway clearance is of critical importance, and there are many devices available to augment their chest physiotherapy.[55,58] If found to be in acute distress, or if found to be having respiratory compromise based on labs, ventilatory support should be initiated. For those already using noninvasive ventilatory support, increased use or increased settings for pressure/volume may be needed. Caution is needed in over-correcting hypercapnea in those with chronic respiratory failure. Rather than attempting to fully correct their CO_2 levels on blood gasses or end tidal CO_2, attempts should be made to return them to their baseline levels.[57,58] Prevention of respiratory morbidity and mortality in individuals with neuromuscular disorders is aimed at optimizing airway clearance and baseline ventilation.[48,55-59]

Table 2: Neuromuscular disorders in children

Type of disorder	*Disorders*
Muscle	
Muscular dystrophy	Duchenne, Beckers
Myotonic dystrophy type I	Congenital or childhood myotonic dystrophy
Congenital myopathy	Nemaline myopathy, core myopathy, centronuclear myopathy, myosin storage myopathy
Metabolic myopathies	Metabolic myopathies, fatty acid oxidation defects, glycogen storage disease (Pompe's)
Neuromuscular Junction	
Myasthenia gravis	Juvenile, transient neonatal
Nerve fibers	
Hereditary motor and sensory neuropathies	HMSN type I and II
Anterior horn cell	
Spinal muscular atrophy	SMA type I, II, III
Acquired, central nervous system	Cerebral palsy, traumatic brain injury

Adapted from Yang and Finkel[68]

Table 3: Cough strength and indications for cough augmenting devices

Cough peak flow (liters/minute)	*Adequacy of cough*
>360	Normal
>270	Adequate cough
160–270	Adequate cough when well; when ill, may benefit from cough assist
< 160	Cough assist needed at baseline

Adapted from Finder et al.[69]

AIRWAY CLEARANCE

Airway clearance forms the mainstay in the management of respiratory distress across many chronic respiratory disorders. Following is a description of airway clearance techniques that are currently available and commonly used.

Airway Clearance Techniques

Mucus is swept from distal to proximal airways. In the small airways, a thin mucus gel layer is produced by columnar secretory (Clara) cells and in large airways by surface secretory cells and glands. The mucus ascends the trachea and is propelled by ciliary epithelium in the posterior commissure of the larynx. It then enters the pharynx and is swallowed. For those with impaired mucociliary clearance, there is increased risk for morbidity of potential sequelae.[60] Airway clearance methods are detailed in **Table 4**. Postural (gravity-assisted) drainage is shown in **Figure 1**.

High frequency chest wall oscillation[62-64] *(VEST) therapy*

- *Principle*: Several small cups are built into the VEST, which oscillate at high frequencies (5 Hz and above). These oscillations induce cough when the frequency

Flowchart 5: Management of respiratory failure in children with neuromuscular disease

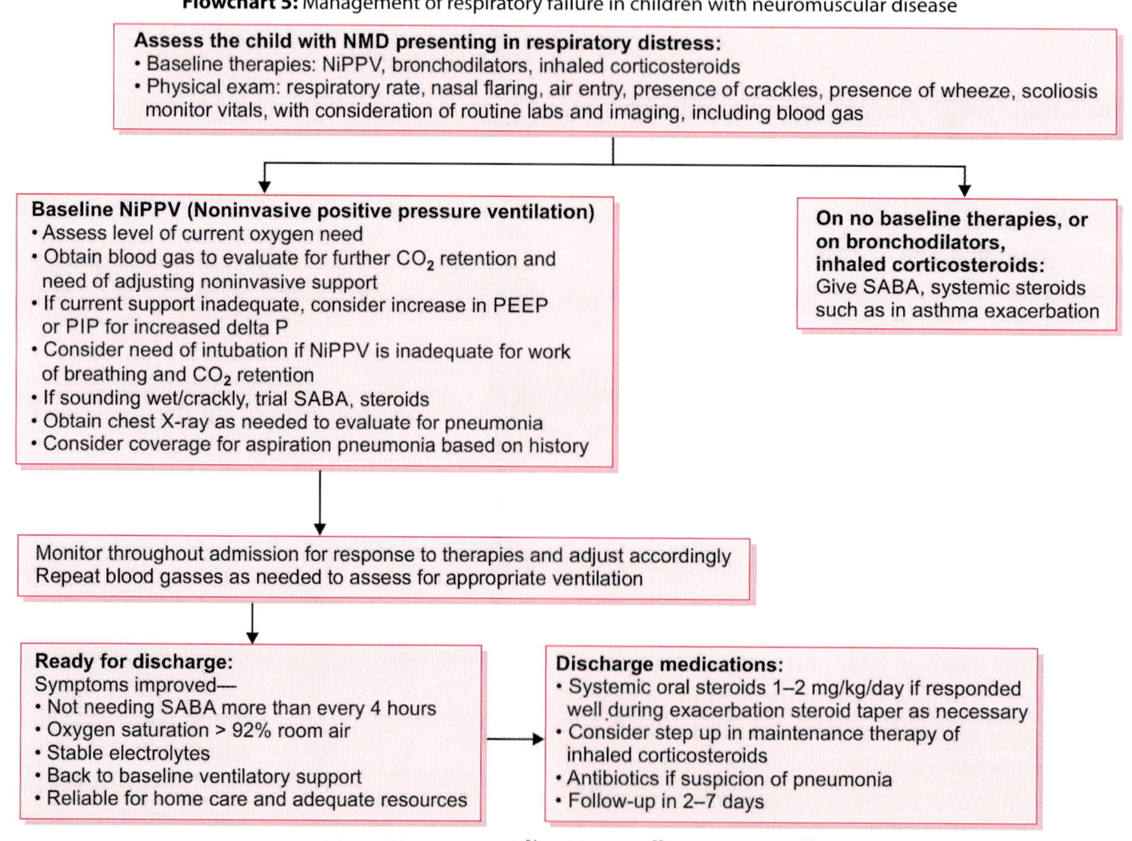

Adapted from: Kao et al.,[54] *Seddon et al.*[55] *and Racca et al.*[58]

Table 4: Airway clearance techniques in children

Technique	*Age range*	*Advantages*	*Disadvantages*
Gravity assisted (postural) drainage	All ages	Suitable for infants and small children who are not yet old enough to cooperate with more active techniques Option for those unable to use or too fatigued to use independent techniques	Discomfort, time consuming, symptoms of gastroesophageal reflux or breathlessness, specific contraindications or precautions
Percussion and vibrations	All ages	Suitable for infants and small children who are not yet old enough to cooperate with more active techniques Option for those unable to use or too fatigued to use independent techniques	Passive, require assistant, discomfort, inconvenient, socially limiting
Assisted autogenic drainage	Infants	Minimal equipment required	Requires assistance, difficult technique to master and for caregivers to learn
Active cycle breathing technique	Toddler to adolescent	Independent, flexible, requires no equipment, can be combined with other techniques	

Contd...

Contd...

Technique	*Age range*	*Advantages*	*Disadvantages*
Autogenic drainage	Toddler to adolescent	Independent technique, nil equipment required	Effect and feedback required to master the technique including sensitivity to auditory and vibratory cues of secretions
PEP with mask	Toddler to adolescent	Independent technique, can be combined with other ACTs, beneficial for those with unstable or compliant airways	
PEP with mouthpiece	Toddler to adolescent	As above Easy for younger children to use Can be used in conjunction with hypertonic saline nebulizer	
High frequency chest wall oscillation	Toddler to adolescent	Independent technique	Time consuming Heavy device, not easily portable Cost

Adapted from Lee et al.[61]

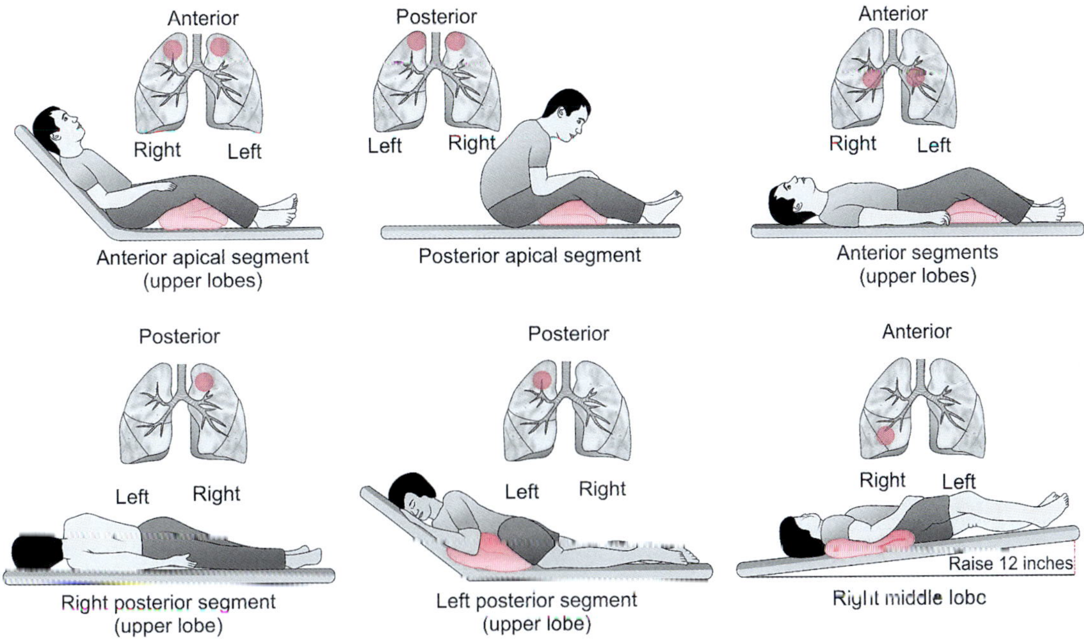

Fig. 1: Postural drainage in children
Adapted from: Sutton et al.[70]

hits a critical point (resonant frequency of the airways). Standard regimen consists of therapy 2–4 times per day of 20 minutes each at a frequency of 10 Hz for 6 min; then 12 Hz for 6 min; then 15 Hz for 6 min (**Fig. 2**).

- *Pressure*: Start with 3 and decrease/increase to patient tolerance/comfort. Pressure should be set at the highest level that is comfortable for the patient.

Metaneb

It is a newer lung expansion/airway clearance device and combines 3 therapies in one device (**Figs. 3 and 4**): lung expansion (CPEP); airway clearance (CHFO); and medication delivery: bronchodilators can be done in-line. Maximizes treatment efficacy and minimizes clinician time.[64,65]

Cough assist:[66,67] This is device to assist airway clearance; and uses positive pressure during inspiration and facilitates expiration using negative pressure. Typical settings are given here:

- *Control setting*: Automatic
  - *Inspiration*: Time 1.5 seconds, Pressure +20 to + 40 cmH_2O

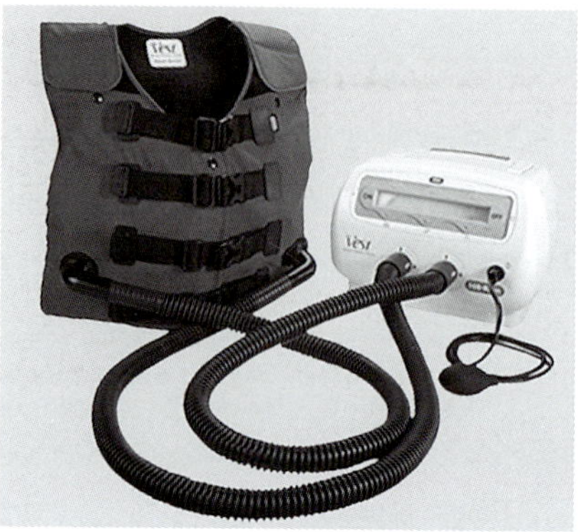

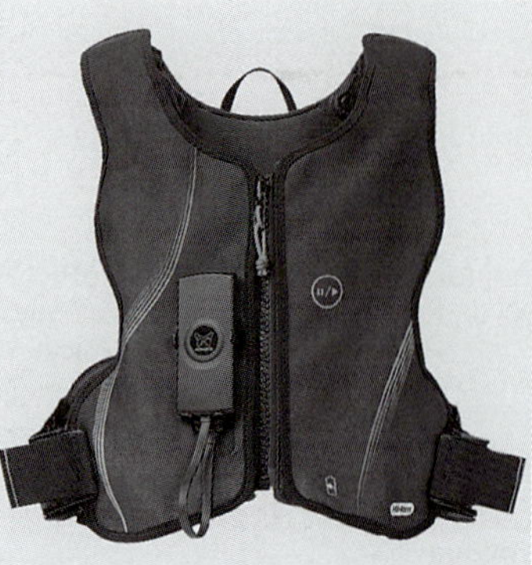

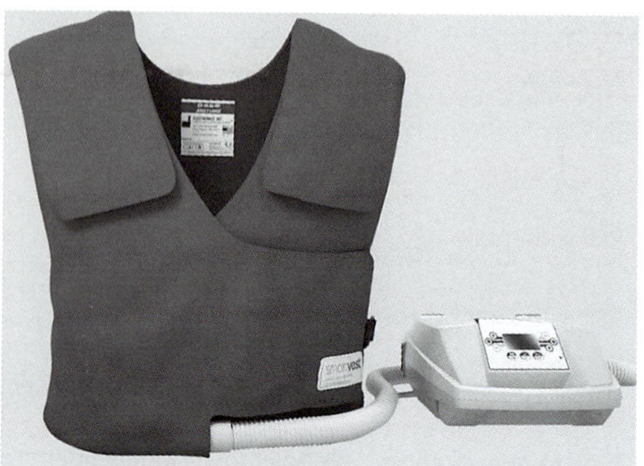

Fig. 2: Different types of VEST therapy devices (Images from manufacturers' websites)

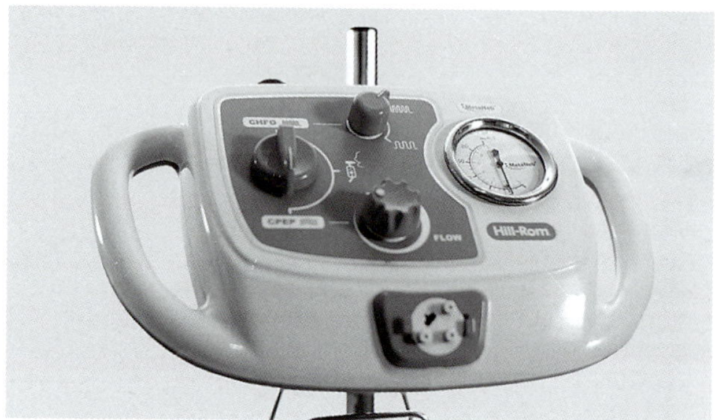

Fig. 3: Metaneb device (image from manufacturers website)

- *Expiration*: Time 1.5 seconds, Pressure –20 to –40 cmH_2O
- *Pause*: Time 2 seconds
- *Flow*: Full (if discomfort, can change to reduced).

- *Sequence*:
  - Inhale + exhale + pause = Cough cycle
  - Perform 4 to 6 cycles (sequence)
  - Allow 20 to 30 seconds for rest period between sequences
  - 3 to 6 sequences = Full treatment
  - Always end with manual inspiration to allow for re-recruitment of atelectatic/de-recruited lung.

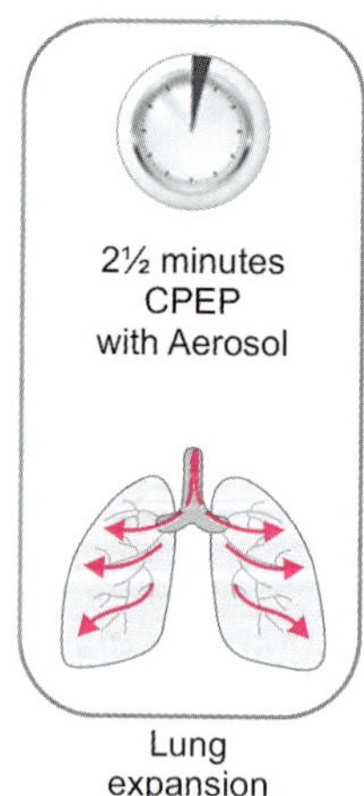
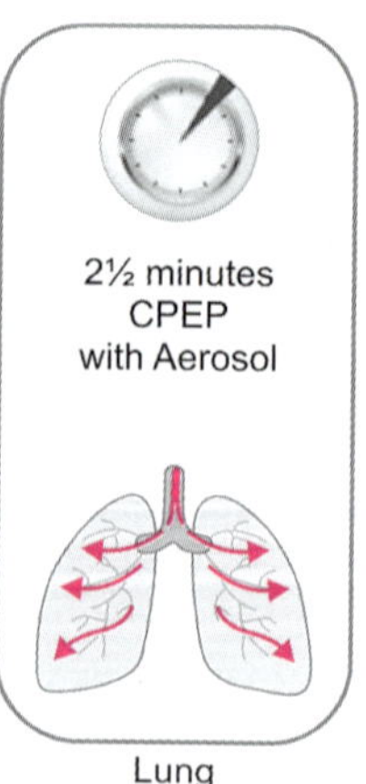
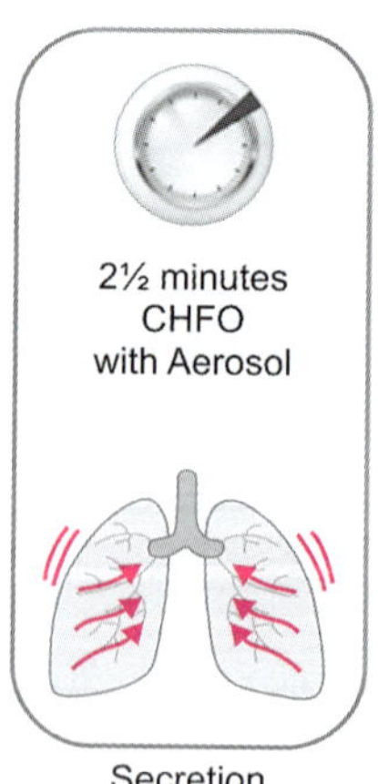

Fig. 4: Use of Metaneb device (Images from https://respiratorycare.hill-rom.com/en/patients/products/the-metaneb-system/)

KEY MESSAGES

- Respiratory illnesses contribute to major morbidity and mortality in children.
- Chronic respiratory disorders comprise a wide spectrum of illnesses, each with their specific complications and emergencies, though some overlap exists between them.
- Prompt recognition and early intervention, using a guidelines-based protocolized approach can minimize morbidity and/or mortality in emergencies.
- Children with neuromuscular disorders are particularly vulnerable for respiratory emergencies and have poorer outcomes.
- Optimal airway clearance is a cornerstone of respiratory care in both acute and long-term care settings in many respiratory disorders.

- Close follow-up and routine care is crucial for prevention and management of complications. .

REFERENCES

1. Salvi S, Kumar GA, Dhaliwal RS, *et al.* The burden of chronic respiratory diseases and their heterogeneity across the states of India: the Global Burden of Disease Study 1990-2016. India State-Level Disease Burden Initiative CRD Collaborators. Lancet Glob Health. 2018;6:e1363-e74.
2. WHO. The Global Impact of Respiratory Disease. Available from: *https://www.who.int/gard/publications/The_Global_Impact_of_Respiratory_Disease.pdf.* Accessed August 17, 2019.
3. National Asthma Education and Prevention Program. Expert Panel Report 3 (EPR-3): Guidelines for the Diagnosis and Management of Asthma-Summary Report 2007. J Allergy Clin Immunol. 2007;120(5 Suppl):S94-138.
4. Mukesh Kumar Gupta, Jyoti Patodia, Pawan Chaudhary, *et al.* The rising trend of asthma prevalence in urban school children of Jaipur: A questionnaire based study. Indian J Asthma Allergy Immunol. 2018;32:10-4.
5. Calhoun WJ, Haselkorn T, Miller DP, *et al.* Asthma exacerbations and lung function in patients with severe or difficult-to-treat asthma. J Allergy Clin Immunol. 2015;136:1125-7.
6. Mukherjee AB1, Zhang Z. Allergic asthma: influence of genetic and environmental factors. J Biol Chem. 2011;286:32883-9.
7. Miller ME, Levin L, Bernstein JA. Characterization of a population of monozygotic twins with asthma. J Asthma. 2005; 42:325-30.
8. Michelle Fox Huffaker, Wanda Phipatanakul. Utility of the Asthma Predictive Index in predicting childhood asthma and identifying disease-modifying interventions. Ann Allergy Asthma Immunol. 2014;112:188-90.
9. Van den Bemt L, Kooijman S, Linssen V, *et al.* How does asthma influence the daily life of children? Results of focus group interviews. Lisette van den Bem. Health Qual Life Outcomes. 2010;8:5.
10. Patel MR1, Brown RW, Clark NM. Perceived parent financial burden and asthma outcomes in low-income, Urban Children. J Urban Health. 2013;90:329-42.
11. Aneeshkumar S, Singh RB. Economic burden of asthma among patients visiting a private hospital in South India. Lung India. 2018;35:312-5.
12. Koul PA, Dhar R. Economic burden of asthma in India. Lung India. 2018;35:281-3.
13. Kumar P, Ram U. Patterns, factors associated and morbidity burden of asthma in India. PLoS One. 2017;12:e0185938 .
14. Reddel HK, Bateman ED, Becker A, *et al.* A summary of the new GINA strategy: a roadmap to asthma control. Eur Respir J. 2015;46:622-39.
15. Ramratnam SK, Bacharier LB, Guilbert T. Severe asthma in children. J Allergy Clin Immunol Pract. 2017;5:889-98.
16. Leatherman J. Mechanical ventilation for severe asthma. Chest. 2015;147:1671-80.
17. Ortiz-Alvarez O, Mikrogianakis A; Canadian Paediatric Society, Acute Care Committee. Managing the paediatric patient with an acute asthma exacerbation. Paediatr Child Health. 2012;17:251-62.
18. Bond KR, Horsley CA, Williams AB. Non-invasive ventilation use in status asthmaticus: 16 years of experience in a tertiary intensive care. Emerg Med Australas. 2018;30:187-92.
19. Mortamet G, Emeriaud G, Jouvet P, *et al.* Non-invasive ventilation in children: Do we need more evidence? Arch Pediatr. 2017;24:58-65.
20. Northway WH Jr, Rosan RC, Porter DY. Pulmonary disease following respirator therapy of hyaline-membrane disease. Bronchopulmonary dysplasia. N Engl J Med. 1967;276:357-68.
21. Mosca F, Colnaghi M, Fumagalli M. BPD: Old and new problems. J Matern Fetal Neonatal Med. 2011;24 Suppl 1:80-2.
22. Jobe AH, Bancalari E. Bronchopulmonary dysplasia. Am J Respir Crit Care Med. 2001;163:1723-9.
23. Davidson LM, Berkelhamer SK. Bronchopulmonary dysplasia: Chronic lung disease of infancy and long-term pulmonary outcomes. J Clin Med. 2017;6(1):4.
24. Higgins RD, Jobe AH, Koso-Thomas M, *et al.* Bronchopulmonary dysplasia: Executive summary of a workshop. J Pediatr. 2018; 197:300-8.
25. Carlo WA, Finer NN, Walsh MC, *et al.*; SUPPORT Study Group of the Eunice Kennedy Shriver NICHD Neonatal Research Network. Target ranges of oxygen saturation in extremely preterm infants. N Engl J Med. 2010;362:1959-69.
26. Khadawardi E, Al Hazzani F. Oxygen Saturation and Outcomes in Preterm Infants. The BOOST II United Kingdom, Australia, and New Zealand Collaborative Groups. J Clin Neonatol. 2013;2:73-5.
27. Schmidt B1, Roberts RS, Davis P, *et al*; Caffeine for Apnea of Prematurity Trial Group. Caffeine therapy for apnea of prematurity. N Engl J Med. 2006;354:2112-21.
28. Bhandari A, Panitch H. An update on the post-NICU discharge management of bronchopulmonary dysplasia. Semin Perinatol. 2018;42:471-7.
29. Committee on Infectious Diseases. From the American Academy of Pediatrics: Policy statements--Modified recommendations for use of palivizumab for prevention of respiratory syncytial virus infections. Pediatrics. 2009;124:1694-701.
30. Caskey S, Gough A, Rowan S, *et al.* Structural and functional lung impairment in adult survivors of bronchopulmonary dysplasia. Ann Am Thorac Soc. 2016;13:1262-70.
31. Farrell PM, White TB, Ren CL, *et al.* Diagnosis of cystic fibrosis: Consensus guidelines from the cystic fibrosis foundation. J Pediatr. 2017;181S:S4-S15.
32. Kabra SK, Kabra M, Lodha R, *et al.* Cystic fibrosis in India. Pediatr Pulmonol. 2007;42:1087-94.
33. Ashavaid TF, Raghavan R, Dhairyawan P, *et al.* Cystic fibrosis in India: A systematic review. J Assoc Physicians India. 2012; 60:39-41.
34. Flume PA, Robinson KA, O'Sullivan BP, *et al.* Clinical Practice Guidelines for Pulmonary Therapies Committee. Cystic fibrosis pulmonary guidelines: Airway clearance therapies. Respir Care. 2009;54:522-37.
35. Flume PA, Mogayzel PJ Jr, Robinson KA, *et al.*; Clinical Practice Guidelines for Pulmonary Therapies Committee. Cystic fibrosis pulmonary guidelines: Treatment of pulmonary exacerbations. Am J Respir Crit Care Med. 2009;180:802-8.
36. Mogayzel PJ Jr, Naureckas ET, Robinson KA, *et al.* Pulmonary Clinical Practice Guidelines Committee. Cystic fibrosis

pulmonary guidelines: Chronic medications for maintenance of lung health. Am J Respir Crit Care Med. 2013;187:680-9.
37. Borowitz D, Robinson KA, Rosenfeld M, *et al.* Cystic Fibrosis Foundation evidence-based guidelines for management of infants with cystic fibrosis. J Pediatr. 2009;155(6 Suppl):S73-S93.
38. Lahiri T, Hempstead SE, Brady C, *et al.* Clinical practice guidelines from the cystic fibrosis foundation for preschoolers with cystic fibrosis. Pediatrics. 2016;137(4):pii:e20151784.
39. Yankaskas JR, Marshall BC, Sufian B, *et al.* Cystic fibrosis adult care: Consensus conference report. Chest. 2004;125 (1 Suppl):1S-39S.
40. Stallings VA, Stark LJ, Robinson KA, *et al.*; Clinical Practice Guidelines on Growth and Nutrition Subcommittee; Ad Hoc Working Group. Evidence-based practice recommendations for nutrition-related management of children and adults with cystic fibrosis and pancreatic insufficiency: Results of a systematic review. J Am Diet Assoc. 2008;108:832-9.
41. Flume PA, Mogayzel PJ Jr, Robinson KA, *et al.*; Clinical Practice Guidelines for Pulmonary Therapies Committee; Cystic Fibrosis Foundation Pulmonary Therapies Committee Cystic Fibrosis. Pulmonary Guidelines: Pulmonary Complications: Hemoptysis and Pneumothorax. Am J Respir Crit Care Med. 2010;182:298-306.
42. Hurley M, Bhatt J, Smyth A. Treatment of massive haemoptysis in cystic fibrosis with tranexamic acid. J R Soc Med. 2011;104 Suppl 1:S49-52.
43. Kioumis IP, Zarogoulidis K, Huang H, *et al.* Pneumothorax in cystic fibrosis. J Thorac Dis. 2014; 6(Suppl 4):S480-S7.
44. Colombo C, Ellemunter H, Houwen R, *et al.*; ECFS. Guidelines for the diagnosis and management of distal intestinal obstruction syndrome in cystic fibrosis patients. J Cyst Fibros. 2011;10 Suppl 2:S24-8.
45. Green J, Carroll W, Gilchrist FJ. Interventions for treating distal intestinal obstruction syndrome (DIOS) in cystic fibrosis. Cochrane Database Syst Rev. 2018;8:CD012798.
46. O'Brien CE, Anderson PJ, Stowe CD. Lubiprostone for constipation in adults with cystic fibrosis: A pilot study. Ann Pharmacother. 2011;45:1061-6.
47. Deenen JC, Horlings CG, Verschuuren JJ, *et al.* The epidemiology of neuromuscular disorders: A comprehensive overview of the literature. J Neuromuscul Dis. 2015;2:73-85.
48. Mellies U, Ragette R, Dohna Schwake C, *et al.* Long-term noninvasive ventilation in children and adolescents with neuromuscular disorders. Eur Respir J. 2003;22:631-6.
49. Papastamelos C, Panitch HB, Allen JL. Chest wall compliance in infants and children with neuromuscular disease. Am J Respir Crit Care Med. 1996;154(4 Pt 1):1045-8.
50. Inal-Ince D1, Savci S, Arikan H, *et al.* Effects of scoliosis on respiratory muscle strength in patients with neuromuscular disorders. Spine J. 2009;9:981-6.
51. Kravitz RM. Airway clearance in Duchenne muscular dystrophy. Pediatrics. 2009;123:S231-S5.
52. Fauroux B, Khirani S. Neuromuscular disease and respiratory physiology in children: putting lung function into perspective. Respirology. 2014;19:782-91.
53. Rose L, McKim D, Leasa D, *et al.* Patterns of healthcare utilisation for respiratory complications of adults with neuromuscular disease: A population study. Eur Respir J. 2018;52(3):pii:1800754.
54. Kao WT, Tseng YH, Jong YJ, *et al.* Emergency room visits and admission rates of children with neuromuscular disorders: A 10-year experience in a medical center in Taiwan. Pediatr Neonatol. 2019;60(4):405-10.
55. Seddon PC, Khan Y. Respiratory problems in children with neurological impairment. Arch Dis Child. 2003;88:75-8.
56. Castro Codesal ML, Featherstone R, Martinez Carrasco C, *et al.* Long-term non-invasive ventilation therapies in children: A scoping review protocol. BMJ Open. 2015;5:e008697.
57. Hess DR. Noninvasive ventilation for neuromuscular disease. Clin Chest Med. 2018;39:437-47.
58. Racca F, Del Sorbo L, Mongini T, *et al.* Respiratory management of acute respiratory failure in neuromuscular diseases. Minerva Anestesiol. 2010;76:51-62.
59. Hirsch AW, Monuteaux MC, Fruchtman G, *et al.* Characteristics of children hospitalized with aspiration pneumonia. Hosp Pediatr. 2016;6:659-66.
60. Fahy JV, Dickey BF. Airway mucus function and dysfunction. N Engl J Med. 2010;363:2233-47.
61. Lee AL, Button BM, Tannenbaum EL. Airway-Clearance techniques in children and adolescents with chronic suppurative lung disease and bronchiectasis. Front Pediatr. 2017;5:2.
62. Kempainen RR, Milla C, Dunitz J, *et al.* Comparison of settings used for high-frequency chest-wall compression in cystic fibrosis. Respir Care. 2010;55:695-701.
63. Varekojis SM, Douce FH, Flucke RL, *et al.* A comparison of the therapeutic effectiveness of and preference for postural drainage and percussion, intrapulmonary percussive ventilation, and high-frequency chest wall compression in hospitalized cystic fibrosis patients. Respir Care. 2003;48:24-8.
64. Morrison L, Innes S. Oscillating devices for airway clearance in people with cystic fibrosis. Cochrane Database Syst Rev. 2017;5:CD006842.
65. Bidiwala A, Volpe L, Halaby C, *et al.* A comparison of high frequency chest wall oscillation and intrapulmonary percussive ventilation for airway clearance in pediatric patients with tracheostomy. Postgrad Med. 2017;129:276-82.
66. Auger C, Hernando V, Galmiche H. Use of Mechanical insufflation-exsufflation devices for airway clearance in subjects with neuromuscular disease. Respir Care. 2017;62:236-45.
67. Sheers N, Howard ME, Berlowitz DJ. Respiratory adjuncts to NIV in neuromuscular disease. Respirology. 2019;24(6):512-520.
68. Yang ML, Finkel RS. Overview of paediatric neuromuscular disorders and related pulmonary issues: Diagnostic and therapeutic considerations. Paediatr Respir Rev. 2010;11:9-17.
69. Finder JD, Birnkrant D, Carl J, *et al.* Respiratory care of the patient with Duchenne muscular dystrophy: ATS consensus statement. Am J Respir Crit Care Med. 2004;170:456-65.
70. Sutton PP, Parker RA, Webber BA, *et al.* Assessment of the forced expiration technique, postural drainage and directed coughing in chest physiotherapy. Eur J Respir Dis. 1983;64:62-8.

CHAPTER

21

Heart Failure

Vivek Chaturvedi, Anita Saxena

INTRODUCTION

Heart failure is a pathophysiological state in which an abnormality of cardiac structure or function is responsible for the failure of the heart to pump blood at a rate commensurate with the requirements of the metabolizing tissues, or does so only at elevated filling pressures.[1,2] The current American College of Cardiology (ACC)/American Heart Association (AHA) guidelines defines heart failure as a "complex clinical syndrome" that can result from any structural or functional cardiac disorder that impairs the ability of the ventricle to fill with or eject blood.[3] Heart failure can have multiple manifestations which determine the terminology used as well as the intended management. New onset severe heart failure, acute heart failure, and decompensated chronic heart failure can all have an emergency presentation, signifying the relative fast development of symptoms rather than severity per se. Our current understanding of heart failure is that of not just a case of cardiac dysfunction but that of a multiorgan syndrome which explains the myriad pathophysiological and clinical features that accompany it.

The pathophysiology and etiologies for heart failure in children are very different from those in adults. Common causes of adult heart failure including ischemia, hypertension and valvular inflammation are less common in children. Infants and children develop heart failure more commonly due to volume overload secondary to shunt lesions, and obstructive lesions of the heart. Less common causes include homeostatic abnormalities and cardiomyocyte dysfunction secondary to myocarditis/cardiomyopathies. Palliated congenital heart disease (CHD) leading to heart failure is increasingly being recognized.

With the aim of keeping this chapter focused on clinical aspects and management of heart failure, the pathophysiology of heart failure shall not be discussed in detail. Briefly, the manifestations of heart failure arise due to mismatch of the circulatory load and the ability of heart, or its components, to pump it in an adequate fashion. These can be accompanied or followed by compensatory changes in the regional perfusions and renal, muscular and endocrine physiology (notable among changes in virtually every organ). The outcome of this, manifesting as symptoms, is excess extracellular volume in lungs and periphery (over a longer duration) and decreased perfusion of vital organs like kidneys and brain as well as the muscles. The time course of development of these changes is variable (and different in younger children), hence the presentation especially during an emergency may vary.

CAUSES OF HEART FAILURE IN INFANTS AND CHILDREN

The prominent causes of heart failure or ventricular dysfunction in children are provided in **Table 1**. **Table 2** enumerates the likely causes of heart failure by age at presentation. This is important, as the symptoms and signs of heart failure can be confusing or fairly nonspecific in children. It is notable that all these causes can present initially in an emergency as acute heart failure, while

Table 1: Causes of heart failure in children by underlying pathology

Cause	*Comment*
Volume overload (relative or absolute)	CHD with increased pulmonary blood flow (VSD, PDA, AVSD, TGA, Truncus, TAPVC, etc.)[1] AV fistula or malformations, anemia, thyrotoxicosis[3]
Obstructive lesions/atretic valves or great vessels	AS, PS, MV atresia or stenosis, coarctation of aorta, aortic interruption[2]
Regurgitant lesions (MR/TR)	Congenital (e.g. as part of AVSD, Ebstein's), acquired (e.g. RF/RHD), postoperative[1]
Myocyte dysfunction • Primary • Inflammatory • Hemodynamic • Abnormal rate/rhythms • Abnormal morphology • Ischemic • Postoperative	 Inborn errors of metabolism, muscular dystrophies, DCM, drug-induced, hemoglobinopathies[3] Myocarditis, Chagas, HIV[1] Obstructive or regurgitant lesions, HT[2] Tachycardiomyopathy, bradycardia, AV dyssynchrony[3] Single ventricle physiology[2] ALCAPA, CAD (including premature IHD)[3] Post-bypass, SV surgeries, post-TGA repair[2]
Abnormal homeostasis	Hypothermia, hypoxia, hypocalcemia, hypoglycemia, sepsis[3] *[Peculiar to neonatal period]*

Table 2: Common causes of heart failure by age at presentation

Day 1 of life/fetal		*1 to 2 months*	
Asphyxia Systemic AV fistula Myocarditis	Metabolic Arrhythmias Ebstein anomaly	VSD AVSD Transposition and malposition complexes ALCAPA	PDA Aorto-pulmonary window Unobstructed TAPVC
1st week of life (after day 1)		*2 to 6 months*	
Critical AS/PS HLHS Adrenal insufficiency TGA with IVS	Obstructed TAPVC Coarctation Hypertension	Causes at 1–2 months Coarctation Aortic stenosis	
2nd week of life		*Older children*	
Large VSD AV septal defect Unobstructed TAPVC	Large PDA Persistent truncus arteriosus	CHD with complications Rheumatic heart disease Cardiomyopathies Palliated CHD/postoperative Corrected transposition great arteries (TGA) PS, TR Tachycardiomyopathy	

volume overload lesions, rheumatic heart disease, and myocyte dysfunction (intrinsic or postoperative) can also have a chronic course with recurrent decompensation. In general, the younger the age, more likely is an acute presentation of heart failure.

Heart failure presenting on the first day of life is commonly due to metabolic abnormalities. Structural diseases that cause heart failure in neonates usually do not manifest on the first day of life. The cardiac causes of heart failure on day one of life are same as those for heart failure in fetus, like Ebstein anomaly, supraventricular tachycardia, complete heart block, etc. About 90% of all cases of heart failure in children occur before the end of first year of life with CHD as the dominant cause. In the first week of life, obstructive and duct-dependent lesions can present with acute heart failure or circulatory shock. Development of heart failure due to left-to right shunts usually follows the fall in pulmonary vascular resistance at 4–6 weeks, though large VSD, PDA, AVSD and aortopulmonary window can cause heart failure by the second week of life, especially if associated with coarctation of the aorta. Isolated ASD are mostly asymptomatic in children and if an infant is diagnosed to have ASD and is in failure, the likely diagnosis is TAPVC.

The myocardium per se is normal in most CHD and the heart failure, if not presenting in the first year, is unlikely to develop for the next 10 years unless complicated by infective endocarditis, anemia, infections or arrhythmias. Thus, older children (usually beyond 2 years) are likely to have other causes for heart failure like acute rheumatic fever with carditis, decompensated chronic rheumatic heart disease, myocarditis, cardiomyopathies and palliated CHD (post-Senning operation for transposition of great arteries or Fontan group of surgeries for univentricular hearts).

EPIDEMIOLOGY OF HEART FAILURE

In Germany, a hospital-based study at University Children's Hospital at Essen studied the epidemiology of heart failure between 1989 and 1998.[4] Heart failure occurred in 40% of all admissions for CHD and one- third of all admissions for all heart disease (congenital and acquired, n = 1755); if postoperative congestive heart failure was excluded, heart failure accounted for a quarter of all CHD admissions. Incidence of heart failure was 289/1000 heart disease patients and 20.1/ 1000 of all pediatric admissions. In 70%, it occurred in the first year of life. Overall mortality in children with heart failure was 14%, more than double when compared to mortality in all heart disease patients. One large database from US found out that the heart failure in children (<18 years of age) was complicated by more frequent procedures, longer stay, but similar mortality as adults (7.5%).[5] The cause was predominantly congenital heart disease in infants (<1 year of age) at 83% while it was present in only 34% in children older than 1 year of age.

In developed countries, the annual incidence of CHD is about 8 per 1000 (0.8%) of live births, of which one-third to on-half are severe enough to warrant attention. Of these, about half result in heart failure, often as an emergency; thus, due to CHD, the incidence of heart failure is about 0.1–0.2% of all live births.[6]

Ninety percent of all cardiomyopathies in children are of the dilated variety, others being hypertrophic and restrictive type. The reported population incidence of idiopathic dilated cardiomyopathy (DCM) in children is 0.6/100, 000 children[7] with recent studies showing 5 year rates of death or transplantation of 46%.[8] More than 50% present within the first year of life. Children with myocarditis as a cause of DCM have a favorable prognosis, with 50–80% showing resolution within 2 years of presentation. The population-based studies on childhood cardiomyopathies systematically excluded cardiomyopathies secondary to cancer drug therapy. At least in the past, anthracycline toxicity has accounted for 50% of admissions due to congestive cardiomyopathy in Boston Children's Hospital.[6]

Prevalence of heart failure in palliated or operated CHD cases is unknown. It has been estimated that 10–20% of operated cases with Mustard/Senning surgery for transposition of vessels and those with Fontan-type of operation have symptoms of heart failure and a significant proportion develop recurrent decompensation.

Rheumatic fever/rheumatic heart disease is an important cause of heart failure in children in developing countries like India. While the incidence and prevalence of RF/RHD are well documented, there are no data on presentation with heart failure in this group, though a significant majority of acute rheumatic carditis and established juvenile mitral stenosis will present with acute heart failure.

CLINICAL FEATURES

The clinical features of heart failure in children vary according to the cause and the age of the child. The presentation of heart failure in fetus is that of hydrops fetalis and fetal wastage, while in newborns acute heart failure can often have prominent non-cardiac findings.

An important point to remember is that raised jugular venous pressure, peripheral edema, effusions and chest crepitations (commonly used to diagnose heart failure in adults) are not seen in neonates and are unlikely in young children as signs of acute or decompensated heart failure. Chest crepitations in fact suggest the possibility of underlying chest infection, which so often accompanies heart failure in children especially in high pulmonary flow situations.

Common clinical features of heart failure in children are given in **Table 3**. Certain features deserve mention:

- The clinical features of heart failure in a newborn can be fairly nonspecific; sometimes the clinical picture resembles that of septicemia. Thus, a high index of suspicion is required.
- Cardiogenic shock as a presentation is more likely in neonates with left ventricular outflow tract obstruction like hypoplastic left heart, interrupted

Table 3: Clinical features of heart failure by age and associated findings

	Newborn/Neonates	
Tachypnea Hepatomegaly Feeding difficulties Subcostal recession Shock	Tachycardia Cardiomegaly Excessive sweating Cyanosis and wheeze Third heart sound	Bounding pulses in AV malformations, PDA Asymmetric upper and lower limb blood pressure in aortic arch anomalies Central cyanosis in TGA, TAPVC, Truncus, TA with no PS Differential cyanosis in PPHN and R-L shunt through patent ductus Wide split second sound with cyanosis in TAPVC, Ebstein's and AVSD Multiple heart sounds in Ebstein's anomaly Ejection systolic murmur in AS/PS Syndromic anomalies (Down's, Noonan syndromes) HLHS, Coarctation of aorta, Interrupted aortic arch, critical AS, tachyarrhythmias, myocarditis
	Infants	
Poor feeding Excessive sweating Slow weight gain	Lethargy Tachypnea, tachycardia Hepatomegaly Third heart sound	Precordial bulge, signs of pulmonary artery hypertension and less impressive systolic murmurs suggest larger L-R shunts Cyanosis in TAPVC, TGA with VSD, AVSD, Truncus Findings of CHF and cyanosis in suspected ASD suggest TAPVC Later onset of heart failure in infancy can be due to certain forms of TAPVC and ALCAPA
	Older children	
Poor weight gain Cardiomegaly Peripheral edema Fatigue Raised JVP	Effort intolerance, orthopnea Gallop rhythm, murmurs Basilar crepitations Hepatomegaly	Diastolic murmur in a child with known VSD suggests associated AR Pericardial rub in appropriate settings suggests acute RF Hypertension and unequal pulses or bruits suggest Takayasu arteritis

aortic arch, severe coarctation of aorta and critical aortic stenosis.

- Unequal upper and lower limb pulses, peripheral bruits or raised/asymmetric blood pressure indicating aortic obstruction (including nonspecific aorto-arteritis, Takayasu arteritis) should always be looked for in a child with unexplained heart failure at any age.
- An interrupted aortic arch or coarctation of aorta in neonates can have normal femoral pulsations in presence of patent ductus arteriosus (PDA); when the ductus closes, these babies may present with acute shock.
- Coarctation of the aorta usually does not cause heart failure after one year of age, when sufficient collaterals have developed.
- Central cyanosis, even if mild, associated with heart failure and soft or no murmurs in a newborn, should always be taken seriously (seen in transposition of great arteries, pulmonary atresia, obstructed total anomalous pulmonary venous connection, etc.).
- An ASD or VSD does not cause heart failure in first 2 weeks of life; their presence with heart failure should prompt evaluation for associated TAPVC or coarctation of aorta respectively.
- A premature newborn with significant respiratory distress and a systolic murmur should be evaluated for patent ductus arteriosus causing heart failure.
- Heart rates above 220/min are unusual in a neonate even with heart failure and should always be investigated to rule out tachyarrhythmias as a cause of heart failure.
- Several children with CHD or cardiomyopathies have associated chromosomal anomalies or extra-cardiac manifestations, which provide clues for diagnosis.
- Older children with TOF physiology can have heart failure due to complicated course (anemia, infective endocarditis, bicuspid aortic valve with aortic regurgitation) or over shunting from aorto-pulmonary shunts.

Unlike adults, children (especially neonates) presenting in emergency with heart failure often have specific causes that need immediate diagnosis and specific treatments beyond those for relief of symptoms and volume overload. Thus, prompt management can often have salutary impact on amelioration of heart failure in children.

INVESTIGATIONS

The cornerstones for rapid clinical diagnosis of heart failure in children are chest radiograph and an electrocardiogram, once immediate therapy including resuscitation, if required, has been administered. Prompt evaluation of arterial blood gases, oxygen saturation, metabolites, plasma glucose and temperature are as important in newborns, who often have non-cardiac causes for heart failure.

Chest Radiograph

This should be done in all patients with suspected heart failure; an echocardiogram is not a substitute for radiograph. It enables diagnosis of cardiomegaly, quantification of pulmonary blood flow, presence of associated chest infection, pleural effusion, etc., as well as being pathognomonic in certain disease states. A cardiothoracic ratio of >60% in neonates and >55% in older children suggest cardiomegaly though expiratory films should be interpreted with caution. A large thymus can also give false impression of cardiomegaly in neonates and infants (**Fig. 1**). Cardiomegaly with increased pulmonary blood flow (pulmonary plethora), prominent main and branch pulmonary arteries, left atrial enlargement, etc. are signs of significantly increased pulmonary blood flow (a finding not appreciable on echocardiogram!) which could cause heart failure (**Fig. 2**). Typical radiographs strongly suggestive of certain diagnosis include those with transposition of great arteries (egg-on-side, **Fig. 3**), obstructed TAPVC (snowstorm appearance, **Fig. 4**), unobstructed TAPVC (figure of 8 appearance in older children, **Fig. 5**), Truncus arteriosus (waterfall appearance of hila, **Fig. 6**), Ebstein anomaly (globular cardiomegaly with decreased pulmonary flow), constrictive pericarditis (calcification in RV/AV groove), juvenile mitral stenosis (left atrial appendage enlargement), etc. It must be remembered however that such typical X-rays are seen in a minority of cases.

Electrocardiogram

An electrocardiogram is very useful in heart failure for elucidation of cardiac diagnosis. It shows biventricular hypertrophy with volume overload of the left ventricle in the most common cause of heart failure in the infant, i.e. a large VSD. Tachycardiomyopathy, a potentially reversible cause of heart failure, due to incessant supraventricular tachycardias (like ectopic atrial tachycardia) can only be picked up by ECG (**Fig. 7**). Similarly, bradyarrhythmias due to congenital complete heart block are detected on ECG (**Fig. 8**). Certain patterns on ECG are virtually diagnostic of specific cardiac pathologies.

The ALCAPA can present with pathognomonic pathologic q waves in anterolateral leads (**Fig. 9**). A superior or northwest axis with biventricular hypertrophy suggests

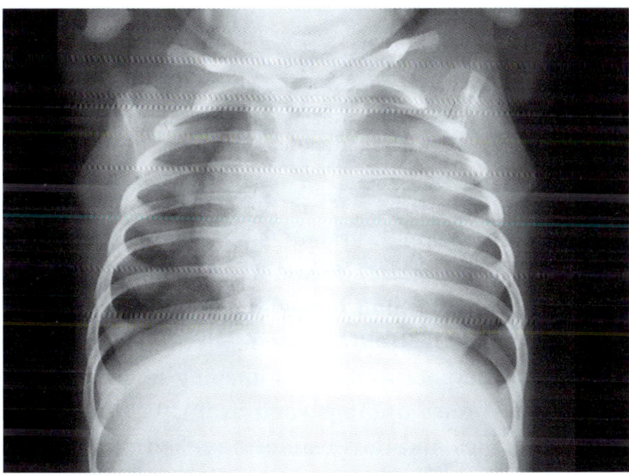

Fig. 1: X-ray chest of a normal neonate with a large thymus

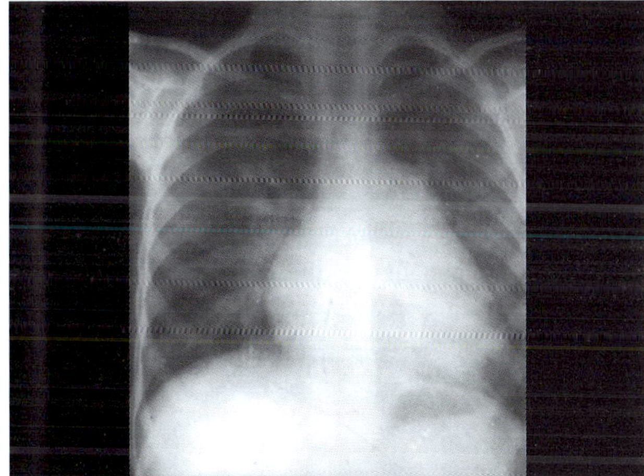

Fig. 2: Chest radiograph showing cardiomegaly, prominent pulmonary artery segment and increased pulmonary blood flow in a case of large VSD

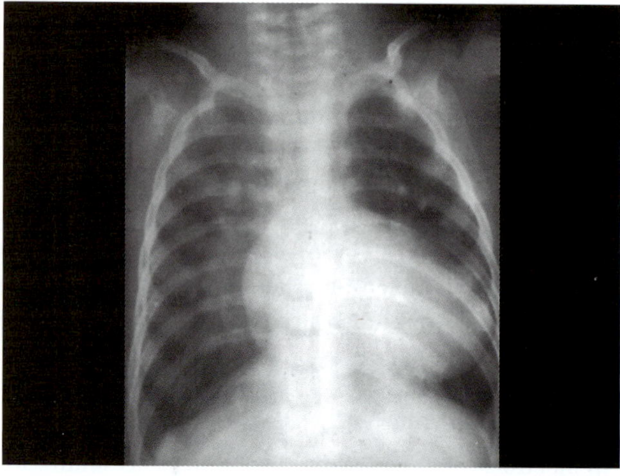

Fig. 3: Chest radiograph of a newborn with transposition of great arteries (egg-on-side)

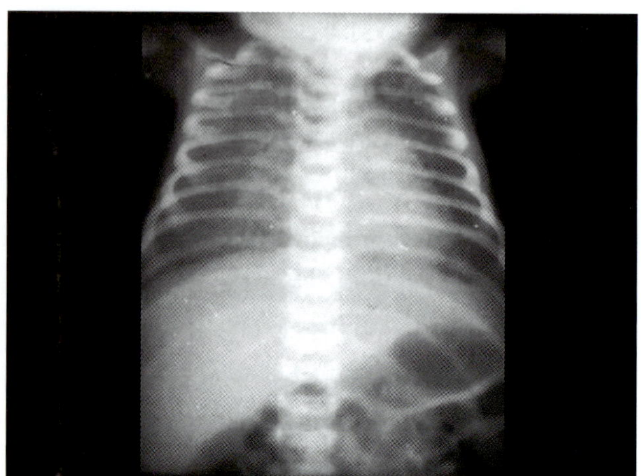

Fig. 4: Chest radiograph of a newborn with obstructed TAPVC showing the 'snow-storm' appearance

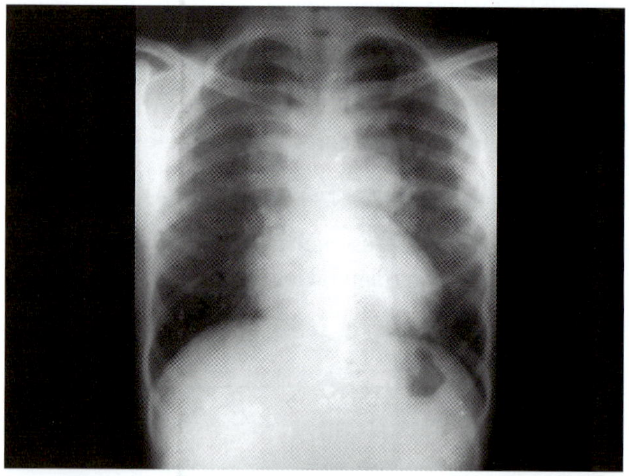

Fig. 5: Chest radiograph in an older child with unobstructed TAPVC showing the typical 'figure of 8' appearance of the mediastinum

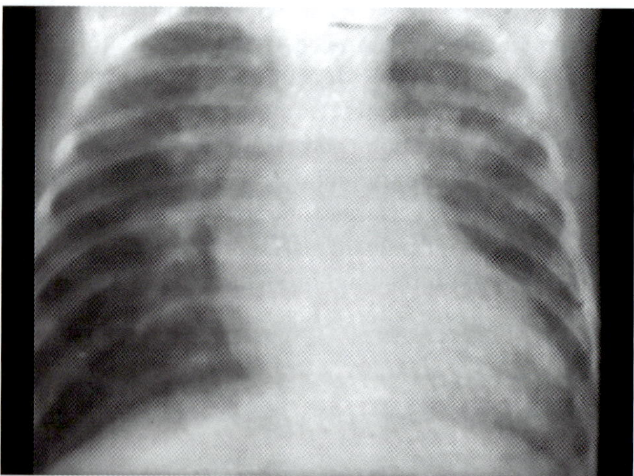

Fig. 6: Chest radiograph in an infant with persistent truncus arteriosus

atrioventrcular septal defect as a cause of heart failure (**Fig. 10**). In a neonate with unexplained heart failure, a prolonged QTc interval with terminal T wave inversion are suggestive of hypocalcemia as the cause of left ventricular dysfunction (**Fig. 11**).

Echocardiogram

An echocardiogram is invaluable in the diagnosis of heart failure. It confirms the presence of structural heart disease and great vessel anomalies and aids in the acute and long-term management strategy. While an echocardiogram is essential for diagnosis of heart disease in heart failure, it should always be interpreted in an integrated fashion with clinical, radiographic and ECG findings. Owing to its dependence on operator skills and inherent problems of imaging small children, an echo can miss findings such as TAPVC and aortic arch anomalies and thus cannot be relied upon as the only screening tool. However, an echocardiogram by a skilled physician is adequate for diagnosis and initial management of practically all diseases causing heart failure.

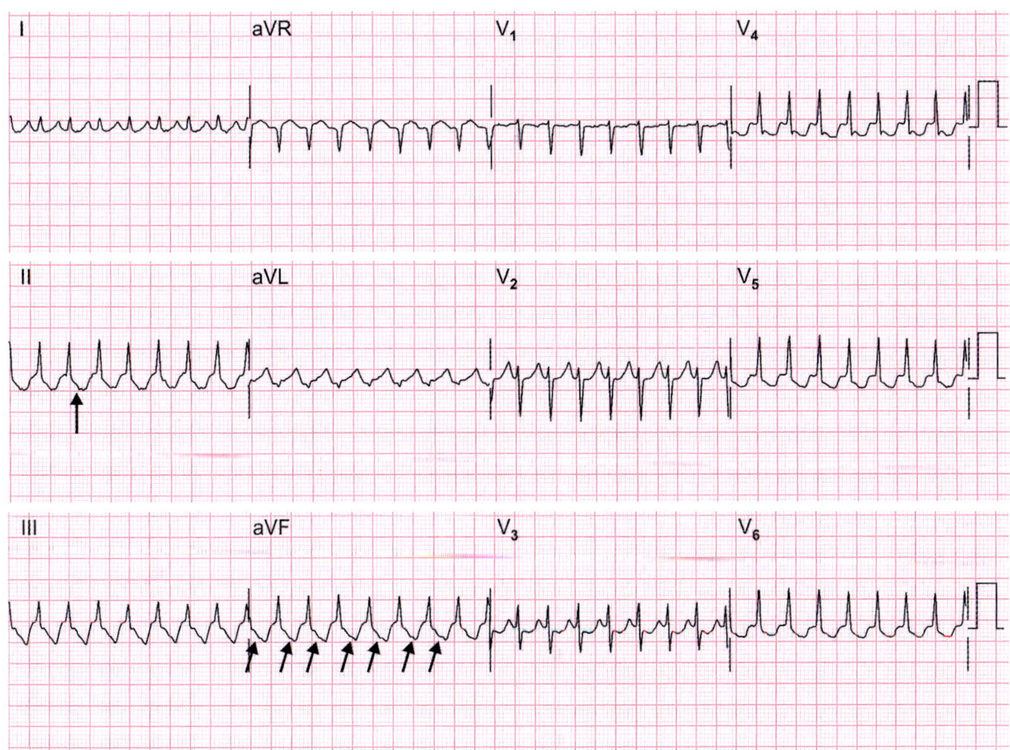

Fig. 7: Electrocardiogram of a child presenting with heart failure due to atrioventricular re-entrant tachycardia at the rate of 200 beats per minute. Arrows point to P waves. Note that RP interval is shorter than PR interval

Other Investigations

B-type natriuretic peptide (BNP)

BNP, a cardiac natriuretic hormone secreted in escalating fashion in ventricular dysfunction and progressive heart failure, is increasingly used in acute settings for differentiation of heart failure from pulmonary causes of respiratory distress. Elevated natriuretic peptide levels might be associated with worst outcome in heart failure.[9] Plasma BNP elevation is a reliable test however for recognizing ventricular dysfunction in children with a variety of CHD.[10] The use of serial BNP or NT-ProBNP measurements in children with heart failure to guide therapeutic intervention or to monitor heart failure status is promising.

Other tests

Hemoglobin is important in diagnosis of heart failure in children; while protracted values around 5 g/dL can cause heart failure even with a normal heart, hemoglobin of 7–8 g/dL can cause decompensation in cases with underlying heart disease. *Electrolytes* like serum calcium, phosphorus and blood glucose should be routinely measured in all children with heart failure, especially neonates, where these abnormalities are an uncommon but reversible cause of ventricular dysfunction. Similarly, screening for hypoxia and sepsis also constitute evaluation of heart failure in a newborn. *ASO* (anti-streptolysin O) and *CRP* (C-reactive protein) are invaluable in work up for diagnosis of suspected primary attack of rheumatic fever or its recurrence in cases with rheumatic heart disease. Metabolic and genetic testing may be considered in primary cardiomyopathy as recent reports suggest a genetic cause for over 50% of patients with dilated cardiomyopathy. [11]

Staging the Severity of Heart Failure

While several systems exist for grading severity of heart failure in adults, including universally known New York Heart Association Class, it is difficult to grade heart failure or apply these classifications in children especially infants. A common system followed is that advocated by Ross[12]

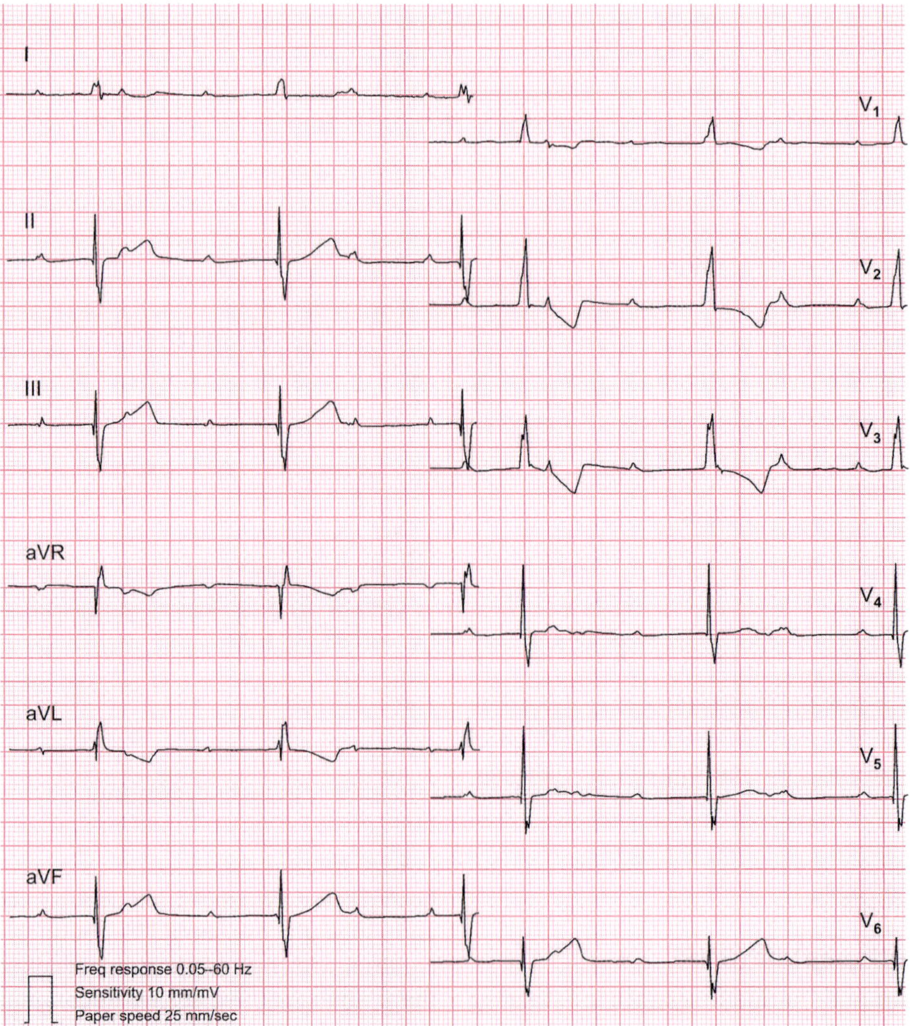

Fig. 8: Holter trace of an infant with bradycardia (ventricular rate of 40 beats per minute) due to congenital complete heart block. Note that there is no relationship between P waves and QRS complexes

for classification of heart failure (**Table 4**) and scoring its severity.

MANAGEMENT OF HEART FAILURE

General Measures

The management of heart failure in emergency settings in children depends on the age of presentation and the suspected pathology. Foremost, cardiopulmonary resuscitation should be instituted, if required, followed by general measures like oxygen inhalation, head end elevation (in relatively stable and older children) and correction of metabolic abnormalities, hypothermia, hypoglycemia and dehydration. It should be remembered that in children with evidence of peripheral shock or who are moving too much, pulse oximetry as a guide to oxygenation status may be unreliable. Furthermore in several lesions it is undesirable to aim for, and maintain, oxygen saturation of 90–100%. These include duct dependent lesions like left ventricular outflow obstruction (hypoplastic left heart syndrome, severe coarctation, interrupted arch) where high oxygen saturation can cause over circulation in pulmonary bed (with worsening of congestion) and may close the ductus. Similarly, in

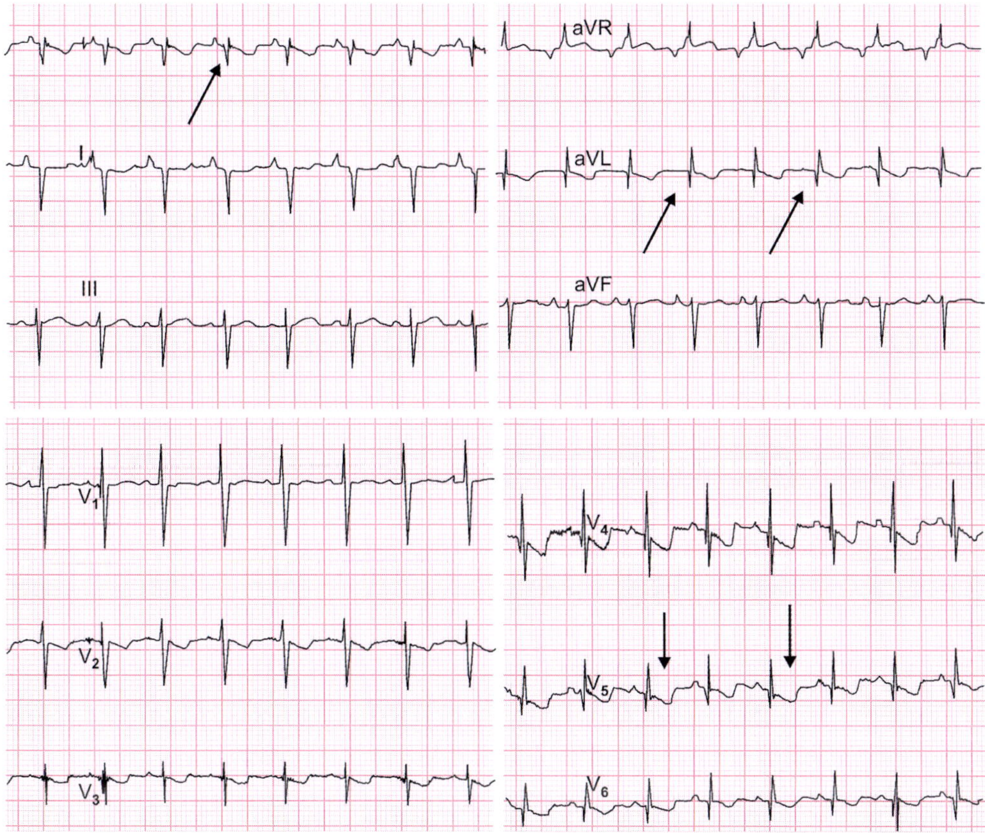

Fig. 9: Electrocardiogram of a child with ALCAPA showing presence of pathologic Q waves and ST–T changes (arrows) in lateral leads

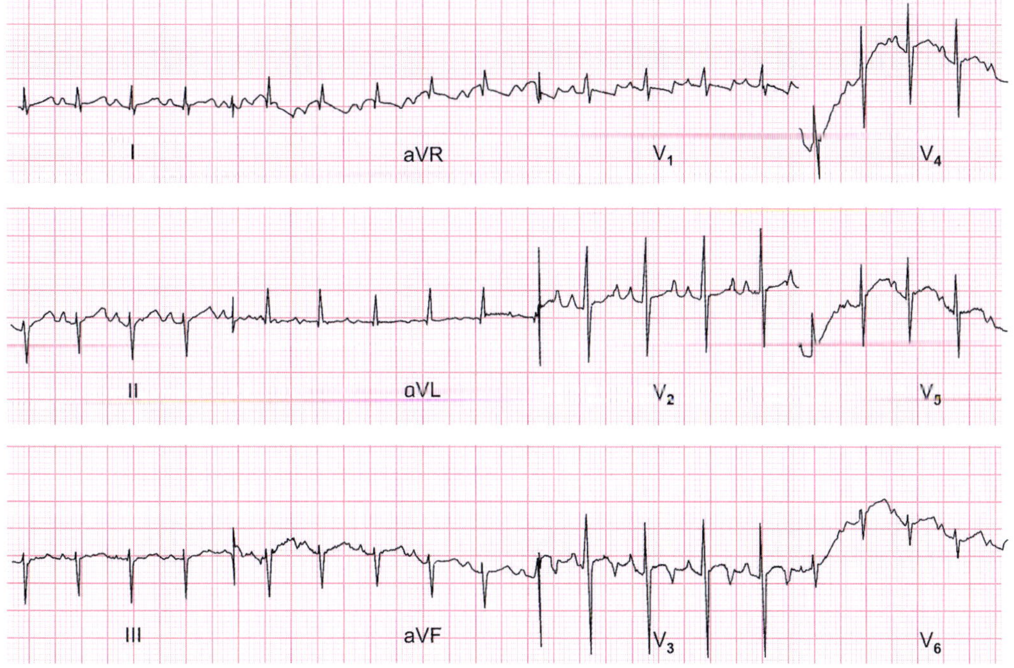

Fig. 10: Electrocardiogram of a child with atrioventricular septal defect showing left axis deviation and right ventricular hypertrophy

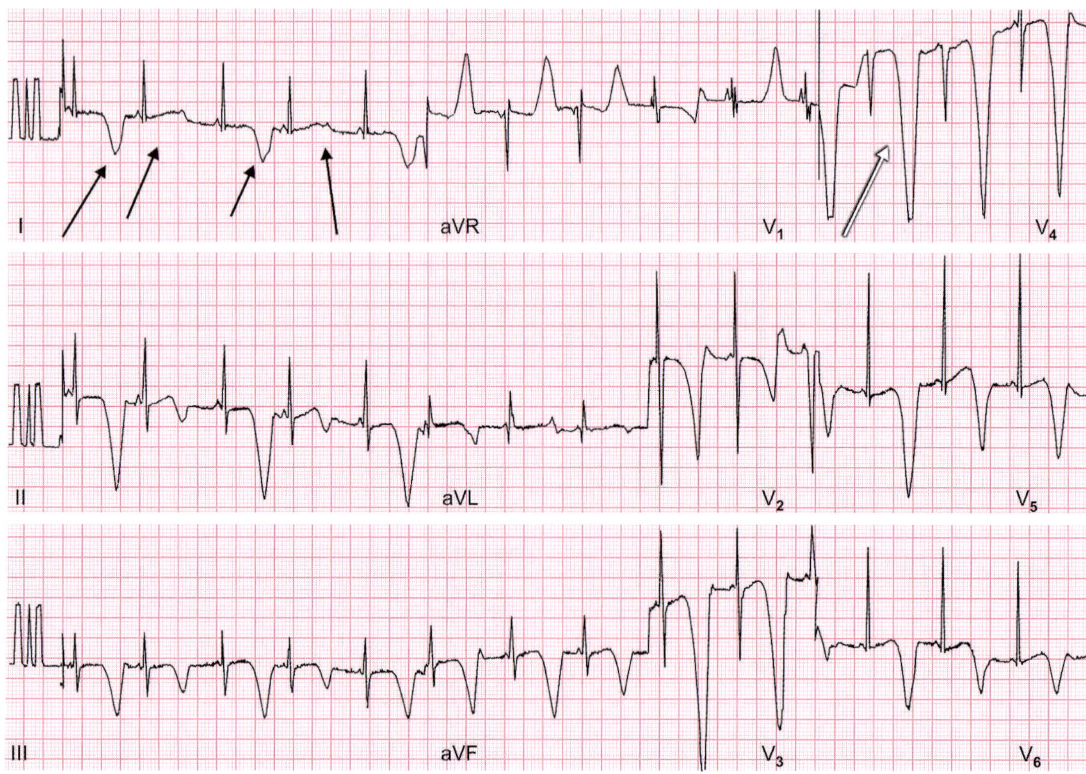

Fig. 11: Electrocardiogram from a child with hypocalcemia showing long QTc interval and bizarre, inverted T waves (white arrow)

Table 4: Ross classification of heart failure in infants

Class I	No limitations or symptoms
Class II	Mild tachypnea or diaphoresis during feeding in infants
	Dyspnea on exertion in older children. No growth failure
Class III	Marked tachypnea or diaphoresis during feeds or exertion Prolonged feeding times Growth failure
Class IV	Symptoms at rest with tachypnea, retractions, grunting or diaphoresis

children with obligatory admixture and high pulmonary flow like transposition or TAPVC physiology, it is wiser to aim for an O_2 saturation of 75–80% and PaO_2 of 50–60.

If there is severe tachypnea, oral feeding should be withheld, as there is risk of aspiration. The fluid and caloric intake should be adequate as the requirement is increased during heart failure. Intravenous fluid is generally restricted to 65–80 mL/kg/day in newborns. It must be ensured that adequate calories are provided in restricted amount of fluids. Some sick neonates may have reduced intravascular volume at the time of admission to emergency room. They should be given fluid boluses of 5 mL/kg normal saline over 20 to 30 minutes till they improve.

Treatment of Precipitating Causes

An attempt should also be made to address any possible precipitating cause for the acute or decompensated heart failure. These may be extracardiac like infection (especially chest infection), anemia, coexistent renal failure or due to arrhythmias (commonly seen with diuretic/digoxin/inotrope therapy), acute rheumatic fever (decompensating chronic RHD), infective endocarditis, myocardial depression due to drugs and others.

Therapy for Acute Heart Failure

Acute therapy for heart failure consists of diuretics, inotropes and vasodilator agents besides specific measures targeted at the underlying pathology (like prostaglandin infusion for ductus dependent CHD in newborns).

Table 5: Treatment for acute heart failure	
Supportive measures	
Avoid hypothermia and hypoglycemia, check for hypocalcemia	
Maintenance of adequate oxygenation	Monitoring of blood gases if perfusion is poor. Ventilate, if required, with modest PEEP to achieve PaO_2 of 50–60 mm Hg and SaO_2 of 75–85% to avoid pulmonary congestion
Adequate hydration	Stop oral feeds if severe tachypnea
Intravenous access	IV and CVP lines (umbilical vein cannula)
Intravenous inotropes for shock	Isoproterenol 0.5–2 µg/kg/min
	Dopamine 5–20 µg/kg/min
	Dobutamine 5–20 µg/kg/min
	Avoid digoxin or use cautiously
Milrinone	Load with 25–50 µg/kg/min. Maintain at 0.25–1 µg/kg/min
Levosimendan	Load with 12 µg/kg over 10 minutes followed by 0.1 µg/kg/min infusion
Diuretics	Furosemide 2–4 mg/kg PO/IV 3–4 times a day
	Spironolactone: neonates 1–3 mg/kg/d PO in 1–2 divided doses, Children 1.5–3.5 mg/kg/d in 1–2 divided doses
	Torsemide: 0.4 mg/kg/day PO (1 mg of furosemide = 0.2 mg of torsemide)
Vasodilators	Captopril 0.1–1 mg/kg/day PO q 8 hrly
	Sodium nitroprusside 0.5–4 µg/kg/min
	IV nitroglycerin 0.05–20 µg/kg/min IV infusion
	Careful monitoring of blood pressure necessary
Prostaglandin (PGE1) infusion for ductus-dependent lesions	Start at 0.1 µg/kg/min (uptil 0.4 µg/kg/min if no response), taper to lowest dose possible (0.005 µg/kg/min); monitor for apnea, keep minimum required dose

Table 6: Drugs used to treat chronic heart failure	
Digoxin	10 µg/kg/day (in two divided doses for children <5 years)
Furosemide	1–4 mg/kg/day (1-2 doses)
Spironolactone	2–4 mg/kg/day (2 doses)
Torsemide	0.2 mg/kg/day (single dose)
Captopril	Neonates: (0.4–1.6 mg/kg/day) in 3 divided doses; Infants and children: 0.5–4 mg/kg/day in 3 divided doses
Enalapril	0.1–0.5 mg/kg/day (2 doses) avoid in neonates
Losartan	0.5 mg/kg/day once daily
Metoprolol	0.1–0.2 mg/kg/dose (2 doses) and increase to 1 mg/kg/dose or maximally tolerated dose over weeks or months
Carvedilol	0.05 mg/kg/dose (twice daily) and increase to 0.4–0.5 mg/kg/dose or maximally tolerated dose

The doses of commonly used drugs in acute and chronic settings are given in **Tables 5 and 6** respectively. In sick children, it is preferable to start the parenteral drugs on continuous cardiac monitoring because of their direct or indirect arrhythmogenic potential. Furthermore, evaluation of heart rate is very useful in assessing response to therapy.

Diuretics

- Intravenous furosemide is usually given in acute heart failure for diuresis and relief of pulmonary congestion and reducing preload. It should be used with caution in newborns who are prone to hypovolemia. There is some evidence to show that continuous infusion of furosemide may be better than intermittent bolus doses. Aggressive monitoring of electrolytes especially potassium is required while using parenteral diuretics. Hypokalemia in these settings can be fatal due to arrhythmias, especially with concomitant use of digoxin.

- Spironolactone is usually given orally in older children along with furosemide. It has potassium preserving action and also has been shown to confer mortality benefit in advanced heart failure in adults.
- Torsemide is a relatively newer diuretic that has action similar to furosemide with better bioavailability and longer action. It is more potent and has some potassium sparing action.[13]
- Metolazone is a potent thiazide type diuretic that has been used in refractory cases of heart failure or volume overload at a dose of 0.2–0.4 mg/kg/day. It also helps in cases with diuretic resistance, but requires close electrolyte monitoring.

Inotropes

While digoxin is used in less sick children as an inotrope, intravenous sympathomimetics are used in acute settings. These include dopamine, dobutamine, and epinephrine. They require close monitoring however because of their arrhythmogenic potential. Dobutamine is a good initial choice to support failing heart because it has less proarrhythmic properties but should not be used alone in cases with hypotension. In cases with failure and hypotension, dopamine initially should be used and dobutamine may be added later. Levosimendan is a relatively new calcium-sensitizing agent being used in infants and children with severe heart failure, mostly as a rescue drug.[14]

Milrinone is also a good choice in children in acute heart failure settings because it reduces afterload while increasing the contractility. This drug is also a pulmonary vasodilator and is useful when heart failure occurs in the setting of pulmonary hypertension. None of these drugs has however been shown to have mortality benefit in adults or children.

Vasodilators

These agents decrease afterload and thus are an important part of acute heart failure therapy due to failing myocardium or volume overload conditions. However, they should not be used in obstructive conditions like aortic stenosis, mitral stenosis, and coarctation of the aorta. Commonly used vasodilators are ACE inhibitors, sodium nitroprusside (both drugs dilate systemic venous and arterial systems) and nitroglycerin (predominantly venous dilator). All these agents require careful monitoring of blood pressure while administration and should be used with caution in presence of renal dysfunction. Use of sodium nitroprusside should always be accompanied by invasive pressure monitoring. Among ACE inhibitors, captopril is favored in children owing to shorter period of action but still should be used carefully in neonates.

Mechanical devices

Ventricular assist devices, intra-aortic balloon counter-pulsation and extracorporeal membrane oxygenators have also been used in acute heart failure to temporarily unload the failing myocardium. However, they are expensive and only available in select tertiary referral centers and are used mostly in postoperative settings.

Newer agents

Several new agents have been used in acute or decompensated heart failure; their role however is still investigational, in adults and in children. These include natriuretic peptides (e.g. nesiritide), vasopressin antagonists (e.g. tolvaptan), renin inhibitors (e.g. aliskiren), endothelin antagonists (e.g. sitaxentan), etc. Nesiritide is used in decompensated heart failure but is not widely available and its incremental benefit over standard regimen is not clear. Several other classes of drugs including anti-inflammatory molecules and vasopeptidase inhibitors have either not been found useful or have unacceptable side effects.

Management of CHF in children, whether acute or long-term, is complex because of frequent presence of structural heart disease (on which medical treatment has little effect) and variable presentation and spontaneous resolution of some diseases. Most of this evidence base has been generated in adults in whom randomized trials usually happen earlier. Conducting such trials in children has been difficult on account of ethical issues and logistical problems. These dilemmas are exemplified by the recently published randomized controlled trial for carvedilol in children[15] with heart failure, where beta-blockade did not improve outcomes over those with placebo. While smaller uncontrolled studies earlier had shown significant benefit with carvedilol, the neutral results of this trial were presumably due to inadequate sample size (due to high rate of spontaneous improvement in placebo group) and heterogeneous effect of drug on type of systemic ventricle (benefit seen in systemic left ventricle only).

Specific Therapy for Various Etiologies

Specific management of heart failure in children can be divided into following categories:

CHD presenting with acute shock

In neonatal period, several causes of heart failure can present with acute circulatory collapse or progress to shock if not recognized early. These can be as follows:

- ***A closing ductus*** where antegrade systemic flow is compromised (e.g. tight coarctation of aorta, interruption of aortic arch, critical AS, hypoplastic left heart syndrome), and TGA with intact septum and restrictive inter-atrial communication. These disorders require maintenance of duct patency with prostaglandin infusion till the time more definitive treatment can be employed. This consists of percutaneous procedures for critical AS (valvuloplasty), TGA (balloon atrial septostomy) as well as surgical procedures. In cases where surgery for coarctation of aorta is not possible due to severe comorbid conditions, a balloon dilatation is performed, although the restenosis rates are likely to be higher.
- Conditions like mitral atresia (requiring emergency atrial septostomy) and obstructed TAPVC (requires emergency surgery) can cause severe elevations in pulmonary venous pressure.
- Non-cardiac cause of neonatal heart failure, tachyarrhythmias and neonatal myocarditis can also rapidly progress to shock if not managed early.
- Lesions like AS, PS and coarctation of aorta, if associated with corresponding ventricular dysfunction or heart failure should undergo urgent relief of obstruction, irrespective of magnitude of gradient at baseline.

As these children are generally sick, they should be transferred to tertiary centers with expertise in their care, after initial resuscitation and prostaglandin infusion (if required). They require intensive monitoring because of frequent comorbidities and likely requirement of ventilation (due to pulmonary edema, chest infections or due to apnea as an adverse effect of prostaglandin therapy).

Prostaglandins in congenital heart disease: Prostaglandins are arachidonic acid metabolites, of which PGE_1 is used as an infusion in duct dependent lesions. An increase in O_2 tension after birth reduces the dilatory effect of endogenous PGE_1 produced by fetal ductus (a physiological mechanism for ductal closure). Thus, congenital lesions that require ductal patency for further survival can be fatal if ductal flow is not established in time. These include lesions that require ductal flow for severely restricted pulmonary blood flow (e.g. pulmonary atresia), for restricted systemic flow (examples given above) and for admixture lesions like TGA.[16] The timing of the infusion is crucial because it does not open an anatomically closed ductus (usually 7–10 days after birth). It is given as a continuous infusion through an infusion pump (dosage, **Table 5**) intravenously with initial requirement for higher dosage. Once the desired response is achieved, the minimum rate required for sustaining the desired response should be used as a maintenance dose. It should also be remembered that this infusion is only a "bridge therapy" prior to a definitive management. Reasons for poor response include closed ductus, low birth weight (2 kg), older age (> 96 hours), high arterial pO_2 and hypoplastic pulmonary vasculature. Babies on prostaglandin infusion require intensive level of monitoring because of high incidence of adverse effects. Up to 12% children develop apnea (which is dose-dependent but more in low weight and cyanotic children), which may require artificial ventilation, while other significant side effects are bradycardia, hypotension, lethargy, jerks and increased rates of infection. Prostaglandin E_1 should be avoided in obstructed TAPVC where it may actually aggravate the heart failure.

CHD awaiting surgery

Short-term medical therapy is needed for stabilization and alleviation of symptoms till surgery is done. The exceptions may be some patients with VSD and PDA in premature babies, which may close spontaneously. These children present with heart failure and frequently have comorbidities like sepsis or chest infection. They tolerate repeated bouts of heart failure and chest infection (which enters into a vicious cycle with heart failure) poorly and should undergo surgery or nonsurgical catheter intervention promptly after stabilization of medical condition.[17] These conditions include:

- Large VSD/PDA/AVSD/Persistent truncus arteriosus with uncontrolled CHF or history of life-threatening infection

- Severe AS or coarctation of aorta
- TGA with intact ventricular septum
- Unobstructed TAPVC.

A special group is that of intractable or severe heart failure due to non-closing ductus in premature babies. These children require a trial of prostaglandin antagonists like indomethacin or ibuprofen. However, it should be remembered that these drugs, beyond their recommended duration, have no effect on patency of the ductus and it is futile to merely observe these sick babies while expecting the PDA to close with prolonged drug administration. These babies should be promptly sent for surgical ductal ligation, which often dramatically improves their status.

CHD requiring long-term medical therapy

Several causes of heart failure in children require prolonged medical therapy because of tendency for spontaneous resolution or a cure for the condition in long-term or due to the fact that the surgical treatment is problematic. These babies often have recurrent episodes of heart failure, mostly exacerbated by chest infection:

- Ventricular septal defect is one of the commonest causes for heart failure after the neonatal period, in infancy. About 10% of non-restrictive VSD die in 1st year of life, primarily due to heart failure. However, up to 30–40% of small or moderate sized defects close spontaneously (mostly by 3–5 years of age) and 25% decrease in size.[18] A minority of VSD with large L-R flow can also close spontaneously.[19] Thus, at least some VSD presenting in infancy with less than severe heart failure can be judiciously followed on medical therapy and watched for spontaneous closure. Similarly, small PDA in term babies until 3 months of age, and those in premature babies not in heart failure (with or without the use of indomethacin) may be observed for spontaneous closure.
- Myocarditis in children is a potentially reversible cause of heart failure provided the acute phase is cared for with the best available medical care (ventricular assist devices, if necessary). Similarly, some uncommon causes of cardiomyopathies (e.g. carnitine deficiency) can be treated effectively with supplementation.
- Some conditions like congenital mitral stenosis are problematic to manage in infancy and it is prudent to defer surgery till later if the child is growing normally.

Long-term therapy

This group of conditions causing heart failure where there is established myocardial dysfunction. This can be due to cardiomyopathies (primary and secondary), decompensated systemic ventricle (single ventricle physiology, corrected transposition), valvular diseases where surgery is not an option, and following palliative surgeries. This group displays the whole spectrum from asymptomatic ventricular dysfunction to decompensated heart failure and requires long-term medical therapy. Treatment options and a step-wise guide for managing chronic heart failure are suggested in **Tables 7 and 8**.

Management of Acute and Chronic Heart Failure

- Treatment of heart failure in children, like in adults, should consist of treatment of the cause, precipitating factors (like anemia, infective endocarditis, infections, acute rheumatic fever, non-compliance with drug or diet, arrhythmias) and treatment of the congested state.
- Digoxin has a very narrow safety window in children and adults alike. It can be used in emergency settings in mild cases but should be avoided in premature babies, those with renal compromised state and cases with acute myocarditis. Electrolytes (K^+, Ca^{++}, Mg^{++})

Table 7: Treatment options for chronic heart failure

Established	*Investigational*
Pharmacotherapy	
• ACE Inhibitors	• Angiotensin receptor blocker
• Beta-blockers	• Nesiritide
• Digoxin	
• Diuretics	
• Aldosterone antagonists	
• Anticoagulants (with severe ventricular dysfunction)	
Cardiac transplantation	
Surgery	
Definite (for structural disease)	Ventricular remodeling
Ventricular assist devices	Cardiac resynchronization therapy
Extracorporeal membrane oxygenation	
Intermittent inotrope infusion	Stem cell therapy

Table 8: Stepwise guide to management of heart failure

Step 1	In acute decompensation: bed rest, propped up position, humidified oxygen. Sodium and, if required, volume restriction
Step 2	Start diuretics. Digoxin may be used in select cases (e.g. tachyarrhythmias) Assess reversible causes and precipitating causes Assess the need for surgery or interventional procedure in case of structural heart disease
Step 3	Add ACE inhibitor. In case of ACEI induced cough, switch to losartan (angiotensin receptor blocker). Switch to nitrates if above therapy not tolerated
Step 4	Add carvedilol in compensated heart failure especially in cases with tachycardia
Step 5	Once or twice weekly dobutamine therapy
Step 6	Cardiac transplantation • Ventricular assist device as bridge therapy

should be carefully monitored to avoid potentiation of toxicity and development of arrhythmias (which are more often bradyarrhythmias in children).

- Generally, initial total digitalization is not performed. One can start directly with oral maintenance dose at 10 µg/kg/day (The available digoxin elixir has 50 µg/mL, hence the dose is 0.1 mL/kg twice daily).
- Continuous infusion of diuretics is recommended in cases of acute decompensated heart failure. Monitoring and supplementation of K^+ is necessary at higher doses, as deficiency is associated with increased risk of arrhythmia.
- During early infancy supplementation with potassium is usually not required up to 2 mg/kg of dose or equivalent. In cases requiring higher doses of furosemide and in older children, usually a combination of furosemide of loop diuretic and spironolactone (or other potassium sparing diuretics) is used. In cases requiring chronic therapy, development of diuretic resistance is quite common. Addition of low dose dopamine may help in this situation by increasing renal blood flow.
- ACE inhibitors should be avoided in heart failure caused by lesions having pressure overload physiology, e.g. in aortic stenosis, as they might interfere with compensatory hypertrophy. The incidence of ACE inhibitor induced cough is much less in children as compared to adults.
- Beta blockers should not be administered in acute decompensated heart failure. They should be started once child is stable, at low dose initially, and slow up-titrations (once every two weeks through 4 levels according to pediatric carvedilol study group trial[15]) should be done as this determines the occurrence and degree of side effects. In case up-titration is not tolerated, lower doses should be continued rather than discontinuing the drug. In the carvedilol trial, overall about 20% children had worsening of heart failure in both carvedilol and placebo population, of which 11% each withdrew from the study.
- Persistently high heart rates (>180/min in older children) with absence of normal variability during sleep or exercise should always be investigated to rule out tachycardiomyopathy as the cause of heart failure.

Myocarditis/Cardiomyopathy

The management of acute myocarditis and cardiomyopathy is a challenge.[8] Several small studies have been conducted with immunoglobulin and immunosuppressive therapy in children with acute myocarditis. Intravenous immunoglobulins may be used in infants with a short history of heart failure, especially if heart failure is preceded by a viral infection. However, robust trials are few, with the outcome that there is still no consensus on use of these therapies.[20,21] Of note, studies in myocarditis indicate a high prevalence of resolution of cardiomyopathy in 2 years to the tune of 50–80%.[22] Children with fulminant myocarditis with a high chance of recovery, do well when put on extracorporeal membrane oxygenation (ECMO) and ventricular assist devices.[23,24] These findings suggest that a diagnosis of myocarditis is a positive prognostic factor in children with heart failure even if requiring mechanical support.

Cardiac Transplantation

Heart transplantation has been used for treatment of end-stage heart disease in children for nearly 4 decades with first infant transplant done in late 1960s. More than 600 pediatric cardiac transplantations are done annually, mostly in developed countries, representing about 10% of total cardiac transplantations. Majority of the transplantations are carried out for end-stage heart disease due to cardiomyopathies. Other causes include congenital heart diseases like hypoplastic heart syndrome and other complex CHD, single ventricle, palliated heart disease, etc. One year survival has approached 90% and estimated 10 year survival is more than 80% according to a recent publication.[25] However, given the fact that the surgery is done in few centers globally and the available donor hearts have remained static over last many years to few hundreds, it is clear that heart transplantation can be a solution for a minority only.

Cardiac Resynchronization Therapy

Cardiac resynchronization therapy is a new treatment option for individuals with symptomatic and severe systolic dysfunction with ventricular dyssynchrony, and consists of pacing the right atrium, right ventricle and the left ventricle (through coronary sinus). It has shown significant mortality and morbidity benefit in adults[26] and is now being used in pediatric patients as well. While there are no large trials in children, available data suggest improvement in functional class and left ventricular function indices in those with systemic left ventricle morphology and in those who have received prior right ventricular pacing.[27]

Pulmonary Artery Banding

Reversible pulmonary artery banding in left ventricular dilated cardiomyopathy with preserved right ventricular function has been tried in 12 infants and toddlers with promising results.[28] The mechanism of improvement in left ventricular function is related to ventricular interaction.

KEY MESSAGES

- Heart failure in children is often a transient state secondary to congenital heart defects.
- Most common causes include large left to right shunts such as a large ventricular septal defect or patent ductus arteriosus. Causes of heart failure vary according to the age at presentation. Some of the cyanotic congenital heart defects can cause heart failure very early in life.
- The conventional clinical features of heart failure (raised jugular venous pressure, pedal edema and basal crepitations in lungs) are often absent in infants and small children.
- Echocardiography is the best tool for establishing the structural diagnosis. However, the importance of X-ray chest and ECG cannot be overemphasized.
- Conventional therapy of heart failure includes use of diuretics and vasodilators. Digoxin has a limited role. Long-term medical therapy is required in a minority of patients as heart failure secondary to congenital heart disease is amenable to definite treatment with surgery or non-surgical interventions.

Note: Parts of this chapter are reproduced with permission from Indian Journal of Pediatrics, Feb 2009;76(2);198-205, for published article "Heart Failure in Children: Clinical Aspect and Management" authored by Dr Anita Saxena and Dr Vivek Chaturvedi.

LIST OF ABBREVIATIONS

ACEI	Angiotensin converting enzyme inhibitors
ALCAPA	Anomalous left coronary artery from pulmonary artery
AR	Aortic regurgitation
ARB	Angiotensin receptor blocker
AS	Aortic stenosis
ASD	Atrial septal defect
AV	Arteriovenous
AVSD	Atrioventricular septal defect
CAD	Coronary artery disease
CCP	Chronic constrictive pericarditis
CHD	Congenital heart disease
COA	Coarctation of aorta
CTGA	Corrected transposition of great arteries
DCM	Dilated cardiomyopathy
HIV	Human immunodeficiency virus
HLHS	Hypoplastic left heart syndrome
HT	Hypertension
ICD	Intracardiac defibrillator
IHD	Ischemic heart disease
IVS	Intact ventricular septum
JVP	Jugular venous pressure
MR	Mitral regurgitation
MV	Mitral valve
NSAA	Nonspecific aorto-arteritis
PAH	Pulmonary arterial hypertension
PDA	Patent ductus arteriosus
PPHN	Persistent pulmonary hypertension of the newborn
PS	Pulmonary stenosis
RCMP	Restrictive cardiomyopathy
RF	Rheumatic fever
RHD	Rheumatic heart disease
SV	Single ventricle
TA	Tricuspid atresia
TAPVC	Total anomalous pulmonary venous connection

TGA	Transposition of great arteries
TOF	Tetralogy of Fallot
TR	Tricuspid regurgitation
VSD	Ventricular septal defect

REFERENCES

1. Dickstein K, Cohen Solal A, Filippatos G, *et al*. ESC guidelines for the diagnosis and treatment of acute and chronic heart failure 2008: The task force for the diagnosis and treatment of acute and chronic heart failure 2008 of the European Society of Cardiology. Developed in collaboration with the Heart Failure Association of the ESC (HFA) and endorsed by the European Society of Intensive Care Medicine (ESICM). Eur J Heart Fail. 2008;10:933-89.
2. Braunwald E, Grossman W. Clinical aspects of heart failure. In: Braunwald E, editor. Heart Disease: A Textbook of Cardiovascular Medicine, 4th edition. Philadelphia: Saunders; 1992. p. 444-63.
3. Hunt SA, Baker DW, Chin MH, *et al*. ACC/AHA Guidelines for the Evaluation and Management of Chronic Heart Failure in the Adult: Executive Summary, A Report of the American College of Cardiology/ American Heart Association Task Force on Practice Guidelines. Circulation. 2001;104:2996-3007.
4. Sommers C, Nagel BH, Neudorf U, *et al*. Congestive heart failure in childhood. An epidemiologic study. Herz. 2005;30: 652-62.
5. Webster G, Zhang J, Rosenthal D. Comparison of the epidemiology and co-morbidities of heart failure in the pediatric and adult populations: a retrospective cross-sectional study. BMC Cardiovasc Disord. 2006;6:23.
6. Kay JD, Colan SD, Graham TP. Congestive heart failure in pediatric patients. Am Heart J. 2001;42:923-8.
7. Lipshultz SE, Sleeper LA, Towbin JA, *et al*. The incidence of pediatric cardiomyopathy in two regions of the United States. N Engl J Med. 2003;348:1647-55.
8. Towbin JA, Lowe AM, Colan SD, *et al*. Incidence, causes, and outcomes of dilated cardiomyopathy in children. JAMA. 2006;296:1867-76.
9. Deshpande SR. B-type natriuretic peptide at presentation of dilated cardiomyopathy in children predicts outcome. Congenit Heart Dis. 2011;6:539-40.
10. Law YM, Keller BB, Feingold BM, *et al*. Usefulness of plasma B-type natriuretic peptide to identify ventricular dysfunction in pediatric and adult patients with congenital heart disease. Am J Cardiol. 2005;95:474-8.
11. Kindel SJ, Miller EM, Gupta R, *et al*. Pediatric cardiomyopathy: Importance of genetic and metabolic evaluation. J Card Fail. 2012;18:396-403.
12. Ross RD, Bollinger RO, Pinsky WW. Grading the severity of congestive heart failure in infants. Pediatr Cardiol. 1992;13: 72-5.
13. Senzaki H, Kamiyama M, Masutani S, *et al*. Efficacy and safety of torsemide in children with heart failure. Arch Dis Childhood. 2008;93:768-71.
14. Namachivayam P, Crossland DS, Butt WW, *et al*. Early experience with Levosimendan in children with ventricular dysfunction. Pediatr Crit Care Med. 2006;7:445-8.
15. Shaddy RE, Boucek MM, Hsu DT, *et al*. Carvedilol for children and adolescents with heart failure: a randomized controlled trial. JAMA. 2007;298:1171-9.
16. Saxena A, Sharma M, Kothari SS, *et al*. Prostaglandin E1 in infants with congenital heart disease: Indian experience. Indian Pediatrics. 1998;35:1063-9.
17. Saxena A; for 'Working Group on Management of Congenital Heart Diseases in India'. Consensus on timing of intervention for common congenital heart disease. Indian Pediatr. 2008;45: 117-26.
18. Keith JD, Rose V, Collins G, *et al*. Ventricular septal defect: incidence, morbidity, and mortality in various age groups. Br Heart J. 1971;33:81.
19. Saxena A, Tandon R, Shrivastava S. Clinical course of isolated ventricular septal defect: An Indian experience. Indian J Paediatr. 1993;60:777-82.
20. Robinson JL, Hartling L, Crumley E, *et al*. A systematic review of intravenous gamma globulin for therapy of acute myocarditis. BMC Cardiovasc Disord. 2005;5:12.
21. Hia CP, Yip WC, Tai BC, *et al*. Immunosuppressive therapy in acute myocarditis: An 18 year systematic review. Arch Dis Child. 2004;89:580-4.
22. Canter CE, Shaddy RE, Bernstein D, *et al*. Indications for heart transplantation in pediatric heart disease: A Scientific Statement from the American Heart Association Council on Cardiovascular Disease in the Young; the Councils on Clinical Cardiology, Cardiovascular Nursing, and Cardiovascular Surgery and Anesthesia; and the Quality of Care and Outcomes Research Interdisciplinary Working Group. Circulation. 2007;115;658-76.
23. Duncan BW, Bohn DJ, Atz AM, *et al*. Mechanical circulatory support for the treatment of children with acute fulminant myocarditis. J Thorac Cardiovasc Surg. 2001;122:440-8.
24. Stiller B, Dahnert I, Weng YG, *et al*. Children may survive severe myocarditis with prolonged use of biventricular assist devices. Heart. 1999;82:237-40.
25. Dipchand AI. Current state of pediatric cardiac transplantation. Ann Cardiothorac Surg. 2018;7:31-55.
26. Cleland JG, Daubert JC, Erdmann E, *et al*. Cardiac Resynchronization-Heart Failure (CARE-HF) Study Investigators. The effect of cardiac resynchronization on morbidity and mortality in heart failure. N Engl J Med. 2005;352: 1539-49.
27. Janousek J, Gebauer RA, Abdul-Khaliq H, *et al*.; for the Working Group for Cardiac Dysrhythmias and Electrophysiology of the Association for European Paediatric Cardiology. Cardiac resynchronisation therapy in paediatric and congenital heart disease: differential effects in various anatomical and functional substrates. Heart. 2009;95:1165-71.
28. Schranz D, Rupp S, Müller M, *et al*. Pulmonary artery banding in infants and young children with left ventricular dilated cardiomyopathy: A novel therapeutic strategy before heart transplantation. J Heart Lung Transplant. 2013;32:475-81.

CHAPTER

22

Cardiac Arrhythmias

Utkarsh Kohli, Srikant Das

INTRODUCTION

Primary heart rhythm problems are common in otherwise healthy children and are often difficult to recognize, especially in younger children, due to nonspecific symptoms. In the United States, arrhythmias account for 13.9 per 100,000 emergency department (ED) visits and 55.1 per 100,000 pediatric ED visits in children under 18 years of age.[1] The most common arrhythmias in children presenting to ED include sinus tachycardia (50%); supraventricular tachycardia (SVT) (13%); nonspecific arrhythmia (10.6%); bradycardia (6%) and atrial fibrillation (AFib) (4.6%).[1] Junctional or ventricular arrhythmias, though rare, are more likely to be associated with hemodynamic perturbations and carry more morbidity and mortality. Patients admitted to pediatric cardiac intensive care unit (CICU) have a high incidence of arrhythmias (29%); ventricular tachycardia non-sustained (VT) (18.0% of admissions) being the most common.[2]

EPIDEMIOLOGY AND ETIOLOGY

Premature atrial (PACs) and ventricular contractions (PVCs) are common in otherwise healthy children. PACs were documented in 51% and PVCs in up to 27% of healthy children over a 24-hour period in an ECG surveillance study.[3] Among supraventricular rhythms, sinus tachycardia is by far the commonest. Supraventricular arrhythmias include supraventricular tachycardia (SVT) with an estimated prevalence of between 1/250 and 1/1000,[4] ectopic atrial tachycardia (EAT) with an estimated prevalence of 0.34% to 0.46%,[5] atrial flutter (AF) and atrial fibrillation (AFib). Junctional ectopic tachycardia (JET) is common after operative repair in patients with congenital heart disease (incidence 1–15.4%)[6,7] but is extremely rare in otherwise healthy children. A congenital form (onset <6 months of age) of JET has however been described.[8] Ventricular tachycardia (VT), is distinctly uncommon in children with structurally normal hearts (0.3 to 0.8/10,000)[9] but is relatively more common in children with underlying structural or hemodynamic abnormalities. Primary or idiopathic ventricular fibrillation is extremely rare in pediatric patients (**Table 1**).

Bradyarrhythmias such as sinus bradycardia, first-degree and Mobitz type 1 second-degree heart block are frequently encountered in pediatric patients. Advanced heart blocks, which include Mobitz type 2 second-degree and third-degree (complete) heart block, are rarely seen in children with structurally normal hearts, but are more common in children with cardiac structural abnormalities, particularly after operative repair.

Three broad mechanisms underlie the pathogenesis of pediatric tachyarrhythmias—enhanced automaticity, reentry, and triggered activity (early [phase 3 of action potential] and delayed after depolarization [phase 4 of action potential], both of which require normal action potential for their initiation).

PREMATURE ATRIAL CONTRACTIONS

Premature atrial contractions (PACs) are usually clinically silent in children. They are often picked up on auscultation as "irregular heart rate" or "skipped beats" during well

Table 1: Acute and long-term management of arrhythmogenic channelopathies

Condition	*Recommended treatment during acute VT*	*Long-term treatment*
Long QT syndrome	Torsades de pointes • **Pulseless:** Defibrillation (2–4 up to 10 J/kg) • **With a pulse:** Stop all QTc prolonging drugs, normalize electrolytes, IV magnesium sulfate, lidocaine, pacing (90–100 bpm for older children and adults), intravenous β-blocker (esmolol) (avoid in pause or bradycardia dependent Torsades), isoproterenol (drug or bradycardia induced LQTS, congenital LQTS 2), stellate ganglion block, thoracic epidural anesthesia, ECMO, heart transplant. Avoid QTc prolonging drugs such as amiodarone, procainamide and sotalol	• β -blocker (Nadolol or Propranolol, others are not as effective) • Mexiletine (LQTS type 2 and 3) • Ranolazine, flecainide, phenytoin and propranolol (LQTS type 3) • Avoid QTc prolonging drugs • Good nutrition and hydration during illness • Restriction from intense or competitive exercise • ICD and sympathectomy if drug refractory
Catecholaminergic polymorphic ventricular tachycardia (CPVT)	• **Pulseless:** Defibrillation (2–4 up to 10 J/kg), magnesium administration (20–50 mg/kg), intravenous β-blocker therapy (esmolol 500 µg/kg bolus followed by a drip of 50–300 µg/kg per minute), and amiodarone (5 mg/kg, may be repeated twice up to 15 mg/kg, maximum dose 300 mg) • **With a pulse:** Sedation, paralysis, avoid sympathomimetics and inotropes, intravenous beta-blocker (esmolol), flecainide, stellate ganglion block, thoracic epidural anesthesia, ECMO, heart transplant	• Nadolol • Flecainide • ICD and sympathectomy
Brugada syndrome	• **Pulseless:** Defibrillation (2–4 up to 10 J/kg), magnesium administration (20–50 mg/kg), amiodarone (5 mg/kg, may be repeated twice up to 15 mg/kg, maximum dose 300 mg) • **With a pulse:** Isoproterenol, deep sedation, catheter ablation of inciting PVCs, RF modification of the substrate • Avoid sodium channel blockers such as procainamide or flecainide	• Promptly treat fever • Avoid drugs that can precipitate Brugada syndrome. (https://www.brugadadrugs.org/) • ICD implantation in symptomatic or high risk patients • Quinidine • Substrate modification
Short QT syndrome	• **Pulseless:** Defibrillation (2–4 up to 10 J/kg), amiodarone (5 mg/kg, may be repeated twice up to 15 mg/kg, maximum dose 300 mg) • **With a pulse:** Due to rarity of the disease, optimal therapy is not known	• ICD implantation in symptomatic and asymptomatic patients with a strong family history of SCD • Sotalol • Quinidine
Abnormal early repolarization	• **Pulseless:** Defibrillation (2–4 up to 10 J/kg), magnesium administration (20–50 mg/kg), amiodarone (5 mg/kg, may be repeated twice up to 15 mg/kg, maximum dose 300 mg) • **With a pulse:** Isporoterenol, quinidine and bepridil	• ICD in symptomatic patients • Quinidine • Experimental agents: Phosphodiesterase III inhibitors (milrinone) and bepridil
Idiopathic ventricular fibrillation	Defibrillation (2–4 up to 10 J/kg), isoproterenol	• ICD implantation • Quinidine

child visits by healthcare providers. PACs, which fail to conduct to the ventricles (blocked PACs), can sometimes present as pseudo-bradycardia in neonates (**Fig. 1**).

The ECG criteria for diagnosis of PACs include the documentation of premature P waves with abnormal P-wave axis or morphology. The AV conduction may be normal, aberrant (bundle branch block) or blocked (**Figs. 1 to 3**).[10] The likely mechanism of genesis of PACs is enhanced automaticity. PACs with aberrant conduction can sometimes be confused with PVCs (**Fig. 3**). To differentiate, search for P wave before the preceding aberrant QRS complex.

The PAC burden typically decreases during the first year of life and no treatment is usually warranted.[10] In fetal life, PACs have been associated with a small risk (<1%) of fetal tachycardia, although a higher risk has been suggested for atrial bigeminy and couplets.

PREMATURE VENTRICULAR CONTRACTIONS

Premature ventricular contractions (PVCs) are highly prevalent in neonates (20%) and older children (30%) with a slight decrease in prevalence during middle childhood (10%).[9] The likely mechanism of genesis of PVCs is enhanced automaticity.

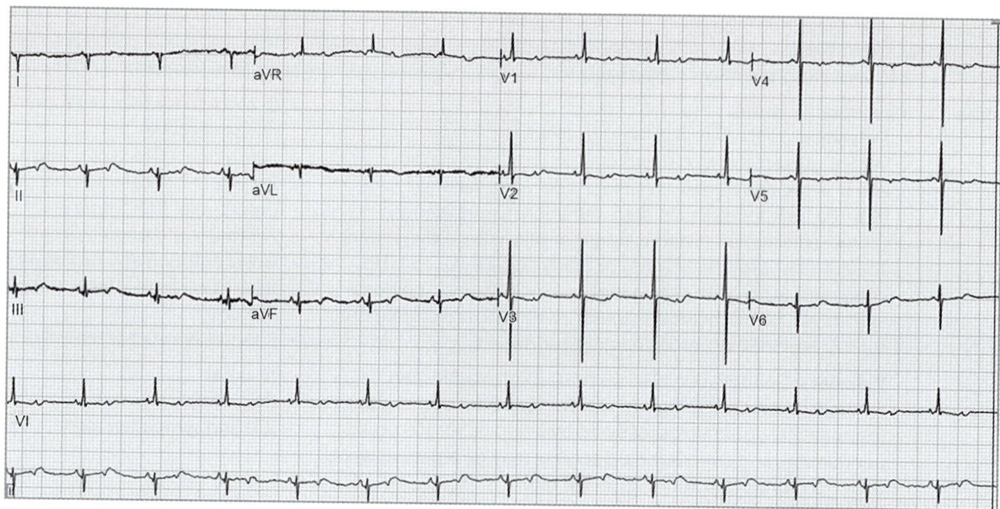

Fig. 1: Pseudo-bradycardia in a neonate with blocked PACs (P waves are best seen in leads V1 and V2)

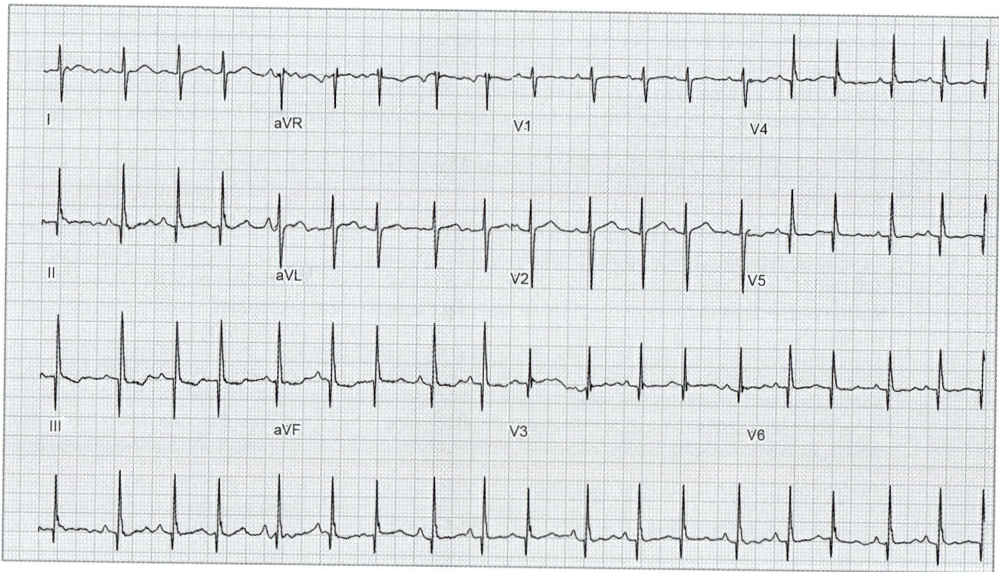

Fig. 2: Normally conducted PACs are seen in a trigeminal pattern. The QRS morphology following the PAC is similar to the QRS seen during sinus rhythm

Like PACs, PVCs are usually clinically silent in children. They are often picked up on auscultation as "irregular heart rate" or "skipped beats" during encounters with healthcare providers. Rarely, the child may complain of "skipped or hard heartbeat". The ECG diagnosis is based on a premature QRS complex that is not preceded by a P wave. Moreover, the QRS morphology of the PVC differs from normally conducted ventricular beats.[10]

Isolated monomorphic (all with similar morphology) PVCs which suppress with exercise are typically benign and do not require any treatment unless the PVC burden is high. Work-up for a child with frequent PVCs (>10% of the total rhythm) should include a 24-hour Holter monitor to quantify the PVC burden and also to screen for runs of non-sustained or sustained VT. In addition, cardiac imaging (echocardiogram) and exercise stress testing should

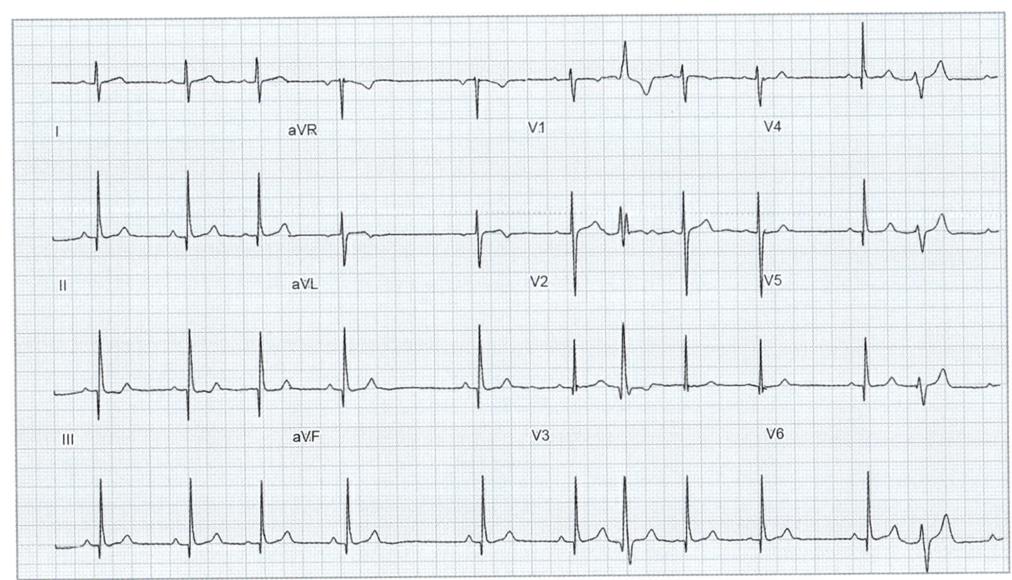

Fig. 3: Aberrantly conducted PACs (the 7th beat from the start of the strip). Note a small P wave before the aberrant beat which is best seen in lead V2. The last beat on this strip is a PVC

be performed to evaluate the left ventricular size and function and to demonstrate suppression with exercise, respectively. Children with frequent PVCs should be followed annually with cardiac imaging (echocardiogram, cardiac MRI) as a high PVC burden has been shown to be associated with a decrease in the left ventricular function (PVC-induced cardiomyopathy).[11] Therapeutic options for PVC-induced cardiomyopathy include medical therapy with drugs such as β-blockers, flecainide, mexiletine, sotalol or amiodarone or catheter ablation which has an acute success rate of between 60–80%.[11] In our experience, children with frequent PVCs are best managed by a pediatric cardiac electrophysiologist. PVCs with a short (<300 msec) coupling interval (interval from preceding R wave to the PVC R wave) can lead to ventricular fibrillation due to R-on-T phenomenon (**Fig. 4**). These PVCs are therefore considered high-risk and a more aggressive approach towards these PVCs is recommended.

Polymorphic PVCs (**Fig. 5**) are also considered high-risk and should prompt a workup to evaluate for underlying structural or electrical cardiac abnormalities. Lastly, PVCs, which appear on exercise (**Figs. 6 and 7**), particularly polymorphic PVCs, are also considered high-risk as they are often associated with structural cardiac disorders such as arrhythmogenic right ventricular cardiomyopathy (ARVC), hypertrophic cardiomyopathy (HCM) or channelopathies such as catecholaminergic polymorphic ventricular tachycardia (CPVT).

SUPRAVENTRICULAR TACHYCARDIAS

Atrioventricular Reentry Tachycardia (AVRT) or Atrioventricular Nodal Reentry Tachycardia (AVNRT)

Paroxysmal supraventricular reentry tachycardia (SVT) (**Fig. 8**) is the most common arrhythmia in children (82%) with an estimated incidence which ranges from 1 in 250 to 1 in 1000, with a peak during the neonatal and prepubescent ages.[12] The mechanism of the arrhythmia is reentry via an accessory pathway which is invariably located along the tricuspid or mitral valvular fibrous ring (atrioventricular groove) or within the atrioventricular (AV) node.

Pathophysiology

The SVT due to an accessory pathway, which is located along the tricuspid or mitral valvular fibrous ring (atrioventricular groove), is defined as **AV reentry tachycardia (AVRT)** and is the most common form of tachycardia in pediatric patients. AVRT has 2 peaks of incidence: the first year of life and then between 8 and 12 years. Accessory pathways, when they are capable of anterograde conduction, show ventricular pre-excitation on ECG,

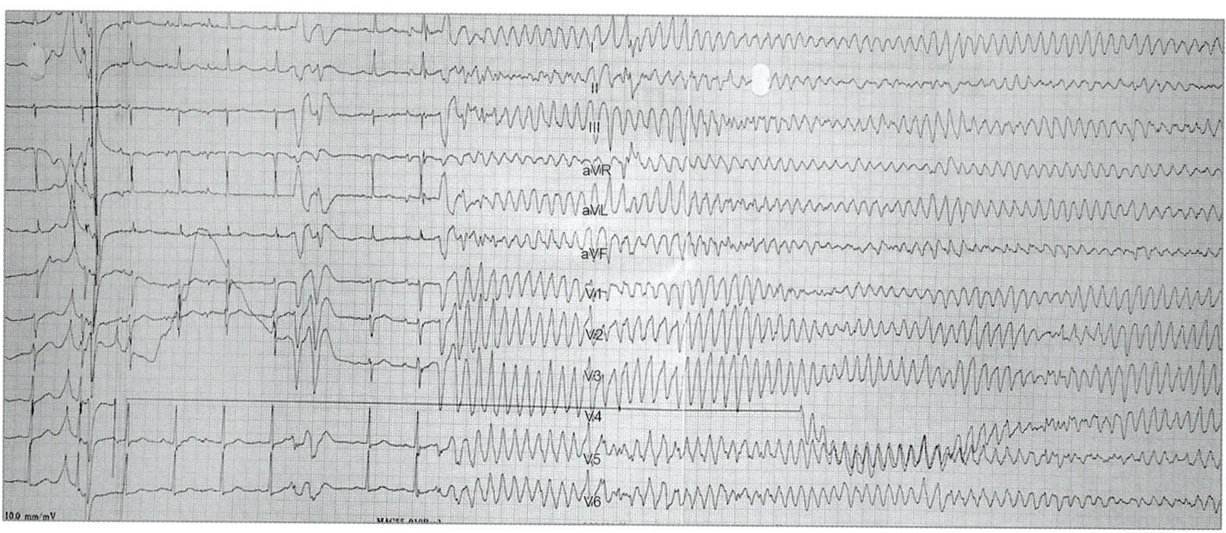

Fig. 4: PVC-triggered ventricular fibrillation. A short-coupled PVC initiates ventricular fibrillation in this patient (*Courtesy:* Drs Hemal Nayak and Roderick Tung, The University of Chicago Pritzker School of Medicine)

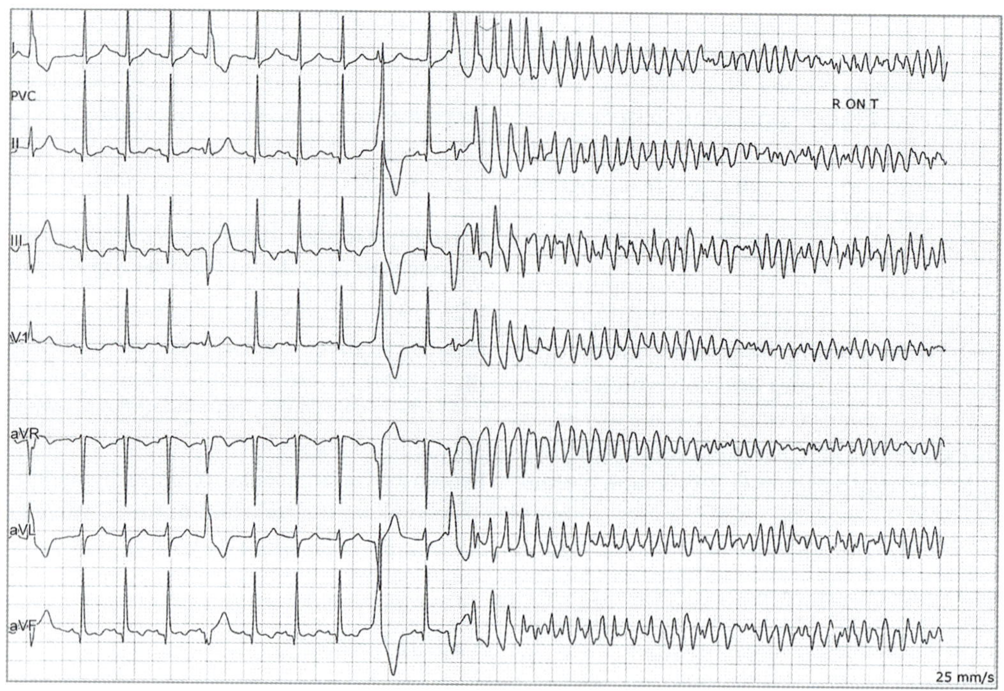

Fig. 5: Polymorphic PVCs and VT following unroofing of the anomalous right coronary artery in a 13-year-old girl (*Courtesy:* Dr Chenni Sriram, Children's Hospital of Michigan, Wayne State University School of Medicine)

which when associated with symptoms is called Wolff–Parkinson–White syndrome (**Fig. 9**).[12] A vast majority of children with this arrhythmia have a structurally normal heart; however, association with Ebstein anomaly,[13] mitral valve prolapse,[14,15] criss-cross hearts,[16] and congenitally corrected transposition of the great arteries[17,18] has been reported. In neonates, SVT can be frequent because it is initiated by PACs, or by the rapid acceleration of sinus

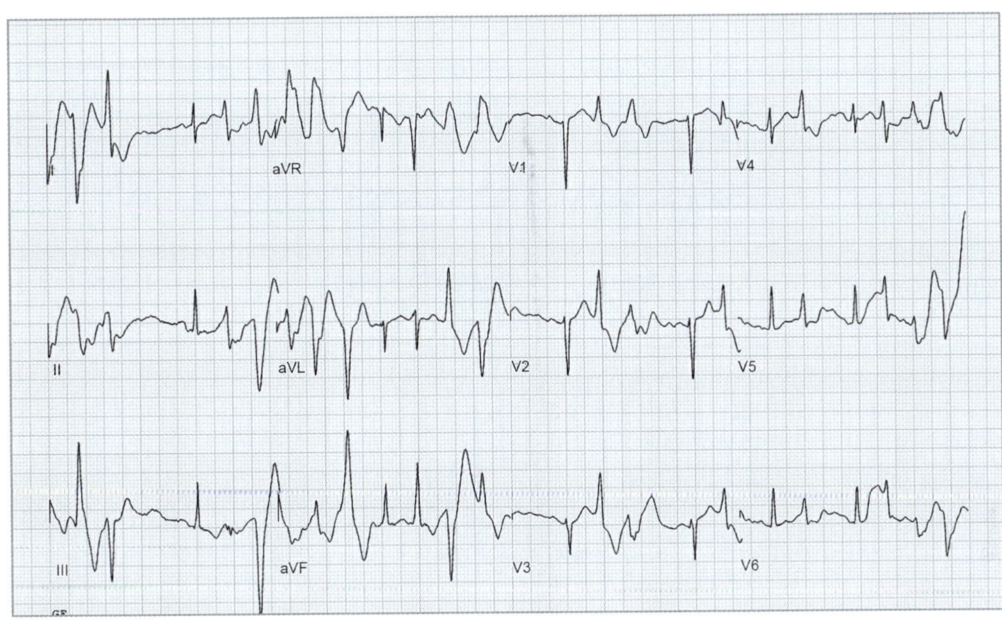

Fig. 6: Polymorphic PVCs and non-sustained VT are seen in a patient with CPVT during exercise stress testing

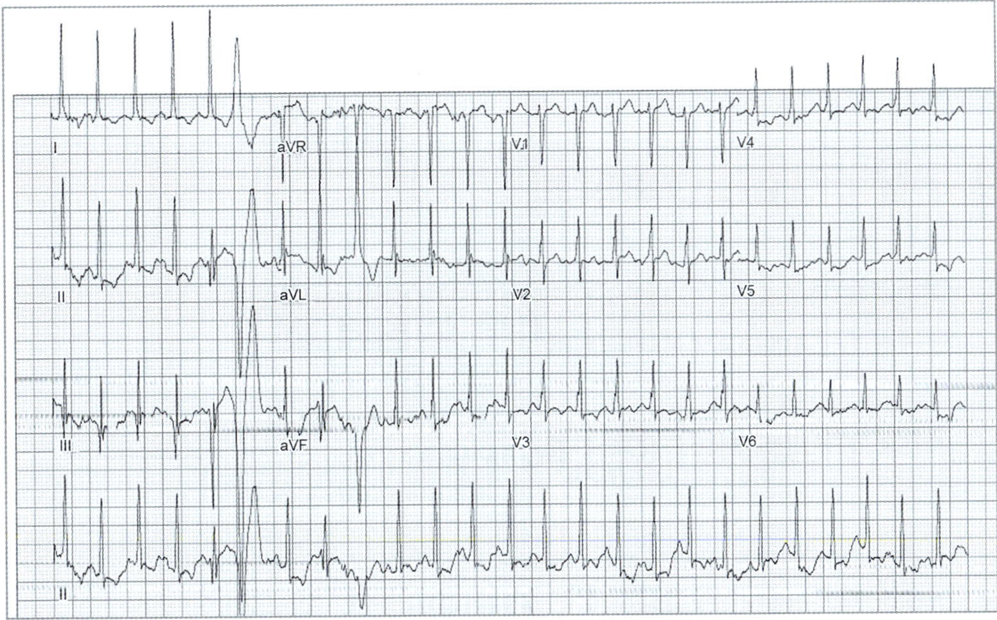

Fig. 7: A PVC is seen during exercise stress testing (heart rate 150 bpm) in patient with hypertrophic cardiomyopathy

rhythm during feeding or crying. After the first year of life, the frequency of recurrences tends to decrease because of a decrease in the number of PACs and a better sympathovagal balance. Transesophageal pacing shows disappearance of the reentry circuit in 50% of infants at 1 year of age.[12,29]

A paroxysmal SVT owing to a reentry in the AV node is defined as **AV nodal reentry tachycardia (AVNRT)** which is rather rare in infants; however, an increase in prevalence is noted through the childhood years with a peak in young adulthood. AVNRT is caused by a reentry through 2 different pathways within the AV node, most commonly,

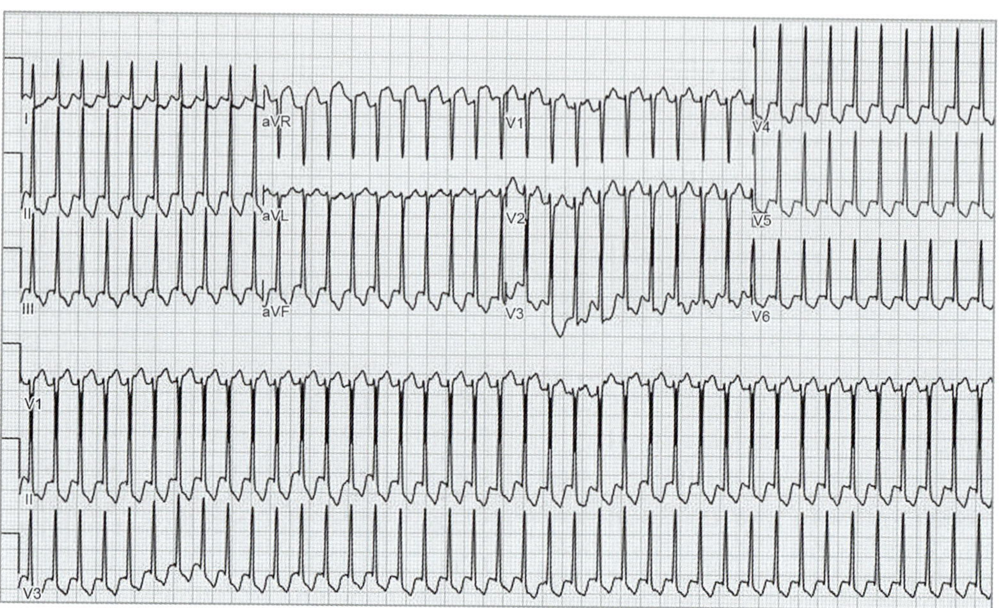

Fig. 8: This 12-lead ECG shows SVT. AVNRT was induced during electrophysiology study in this 16-year-old girl

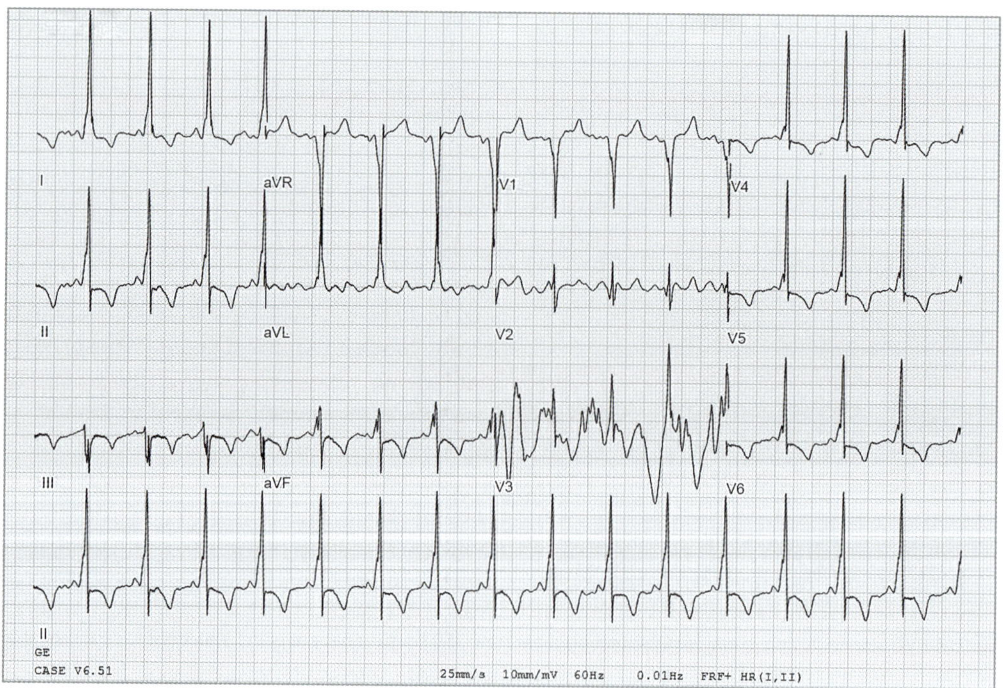

Fig. 9: Pre-excitation through a likely mid-septal pathway is seen in a 12-year-old asymptomatic boy. The echocardiogram showed normal biventricular function

the slow pathway and the fast pathway. However, only 30% to 40% of children with AVNRT show dual AV nodal conduction during electrophysiology study. Interestingly, AVNRT with 2:1 transient AV conduction block is present in 17% of children during electrophysiology study, a much greater proportion than seen in adults (9%).

Clinical features

Clinical manifestations of AVNRT are variable and females are usually more symptomatic than males. AVNRT overall is a benign tachyarrhythmia and effective ablation techniques exist for its treatment (cryoablation or radiofrequency (RF) ablation with 3-dimensional mapping). Preschool children often describe palpitations as precordial pain, heaviness or discomfort; when the SVT is fast and not hemodynamically tolerated, weakness, dizziness, and syncope may occur. The heart rate during reentry tachyarrhythmias can vary from 180 to 340 bpm.[12]

Diagnosis

The ECG during tachycardia sometimes shows a retrograde P wave immediately following the QRS (short RP tachycardia). The retrograde P wave can be difficult to identify in patients with AVNRT (**Fig. 8**). The QRS morphology is typically regular and narrow complex unless there is a rate-related bundle branch block. A delta wave is seen if there is anterograde pathway conduction during sinus rhythm (Wolff-Parkinson-White syndrome) (**Fig. 9**).[10]

In neonates with heart rates greater than 200 bpm, sinus tachycardia can be confused with SVT due to difficulty in identifying P waves. Certain narrow QRS VTs such as intrafascicular VT can also be confused with SVT. The QRS axis in intrafascicular VT is often superior whereas the QRS vector in SVTs is typically inferiorly directed.

Treatment

- For a patient who is *hemodynamically unstable*, PALS protocol should be initiated without delay and synchronized cardioversion is recommended (0.5–1.0 J/kg of energy is recommended for first cardioversion and 2.0 J/kg for the following cardioversions). It is reasonable to administer adenosine to terminate the tachycardia while preparation is being made for cardioversion, this however should not delay the cardioversion.
- *For a hemodynamically stable patient*, vagal maneuvers such as ice-to-face (neonates and infants), Valsalva maneuver, handstands and head down position can be tried. Carotid sinus massage and pressure on the eyeballs are not recommended due to associated complications. Success rates of vagal maneuvers have varied from 19.4% to 54.3%, as reported in different studies.[19]

If the SVT does not terminate in response to vagal maneuvers, a rapid intravenous bolus of adenosine should be administered from an intravenous cannula which should be placed as close to the heart as possible. The adenosine bolus should always be chased by a rapid saline flush (10 mL neonates, 20 mL in older children and young adults). Adenosine can be repeated up to 3 times (0.1 mg/kg for the first dose, maximum dose 6 mg; subsequent doses 0.2 mg/kg, maximum of 12 mg). In patients with pre-excitation, ventricular fibrillation can be precipitated during adenosine administration. Therefore, it is recommended to have a defibrillator on standby while adenosine is being administered. It is also important to record the effect of adenosine on cardiac rhythm and conduction on a 12-lead ECG (rhythm strip) as response to adenosine can help in determining the precise etiology of the tachyarrhythmia.

If adenosine is unsuccessful, our practice is to initiate therapy with esmolol (intravenous β-blocker) in infants and younger children. Older children can be administered a dose of an oral β-blocker such as atenolol or nadolol. Detailed dosages and adverse effects of all antiarrhythmic drugs are provided in *Annexure* 2. These children will often require admission and observation. Class 1A or 1C class drugs such as (flecainide 1.5–2 mg/kg in 3–5 minutes or propafenone 1.5 mg/kg in 3–5 minutes) can be considered if there is no or inadequate response to a β-blocker. Amiodarone can be used in refractory patients or in patients with a reduced ejection fraction (5 mg/kg in 20 minutes followed by infusion of 10–15 mg/kg in 24 hours). Given the long half-life of oral β-blockers and antiarrhythmic drugs, it can take a few days to achieve therapeutic serum concentrations. Intermittent adenosine boluses, which are sometimes only transiently effective, can meanwhile be tried to prevent tachycardia-induced cardiomyopathy.

In cases of severe heart failure or cardiogenic shock and non-response to synchronized external electric cardioversion (0.5–1.5 J/kg), transesophageal atrial overdrive pacing can be tried. This modality however is associated with complications such as esophageal perforation and burns particularly if a high output is used for a prolonged period of time to capture the atrium.

Prophylaxis

In all forms of paroxysmal SVTs, antiarrhythmic prophylaxis should be started after acute management to avoid recurrence. Our preference is to start infants and young children on oral propranolol unless pre-excitation is present on resting electrocardiogram in which case flecainide is preferred. The therapy is initiated in the inpatient unit with careful monitoring of pre-feed blood sugars and blood pressure for at least 48 hrs. Approximately two-thirds of newborns are likely to outgrow SVT by 1 year of age (33% of them will eventually relapse later in childhood),[20] therefore, if the child has no recurrence, we do not weight adjust propranolol after 8–9 months of age and let the child outgrow the dose. The therapy is discontinued at one year of age. The parents are taught heart rate monitoring with a stethoscope, which is done twice a day by them at home until the child is old enough to vocalize the symptoms. Heart rate is typically greater than 200 bpm during SVT in infants and young children, which is the threshold for them to come to ED or to contact the treating physician. Digoxin has been shown to have an efficacy, which is equivalent to propranolol for treatment of SVT.[21] However, it is contraindicated in patients with pre-excitation. Calcium channel blockers are contraindicated in children less than 1 year of age due to a risk of myocardial depression.

Refractory SVT

For refractory SVT, flecainide (2–7 mg/kg/d in 3 divided doses), propafenone (10–15 mg/kg/d in 3 divided doses), amiodarone (loading dose of 10–20 mg/kg/d in 1–2 divided doses for 7–10 days; maintenance dose of 3–7 mg/kg/d in 1–2 divided doses), or sotalol (2–8 mg/kg/d in 2–3 divided doses) can be tried as either stand-alone medications or used in conjunction with β-blockers (propranolol 1–3 mg/kg/d in 3–4 divided doses, nadolol 0.5 to 1 mg/kg/d in 1–2 divided doses, metoprolol 2–2.5 mg/kg/d in 2 divided doses). Transcatheter RF or cryoablation can be used emergently for drug refractory SVT. Elective catheter ablation is indicated if there is poor response to drug therapy, if there are intolerable side effects or if the child is unwilling to take the medications. The risk of complications is lower when the child weighs more than 20 to 25 kg (beyond 7–8 years).[12]

Prolonged incessant SVT can be associated with tachycardia-induced cardiomyopathy, which presents as poor feeding, lethargy, color change and decreased activity in neonates and young children. Therefore, our practice is to instruct the families to watch for the above-mentioned symptoms and signs of low cardiac output and to report to the nearest ED if the child is symptomatic or if the SVT does not terminate within 45 to 60 minutes of detection. The recommendations are similar for older children in whom the clinical presentation is often quite different. Older children can present with syncope or dizziness during an acute episode, particularly if the SVT rate is >250 bpm. Incessant SVT can lead to tachycardia-induced cardiomyopathy, which presents with symptoms of heart failure such as exercise intolerance, fatigue, and shortness of breath in older children.

Patients with ventricular pre-excitation can present with heart failure due to ventricular dys-synchrony-induced cardiomyopathy. The cardiac function and symptoms rapidly improve after ablation of the pathway in these patients. This presentation however is extremely rare.[22] Patients with pre-excitation are predisposed to atrial fibrillation (AFib). Rapid conduction of AFib via the accessory pathway to the ventricles can precipitate ventricular fibrillation, which in turn can lead to sudden death (**Fig. 10**). The risk is higher in patients who are symptomatic or have underlying structural or hemodynamic cardiac abnormalities. Exercise stress test is helpful in risk stratifying these patients. The presence of single-beat loss of pre-excitation during exercise stress testing indicates a low-risk pathway which is not associated with an added risk of sudden death (**Figs. 11A to C**); however, the sensitivity and negative predicted value of exercise stress testing have been found to be low.[23] Persistence of pre-excitation through the exercise stress test indicates (**Fig. 12**) a possible high-risk pathway and therefore an electrophysiology study is indicated in these patients to for risk stratification.

Conclusion

To conclude, acute onset SVT is associated with a low mortality. However, incessant SVT can present with heart failure which rapidly responds to rate and rhythm control. Ventricular pre-excitation is associated with a small risk of sudden cardiac death in the asymptomatic. The risk is higher in those with symptoms or underlying structural or hemodynamic cardiac abnormalities. Fortunately, the risk is modifiable as the accessory pathways are readily amenable to catheter ablation. Overall, the prognosis of patients with appropriately managed SVT is excellent.

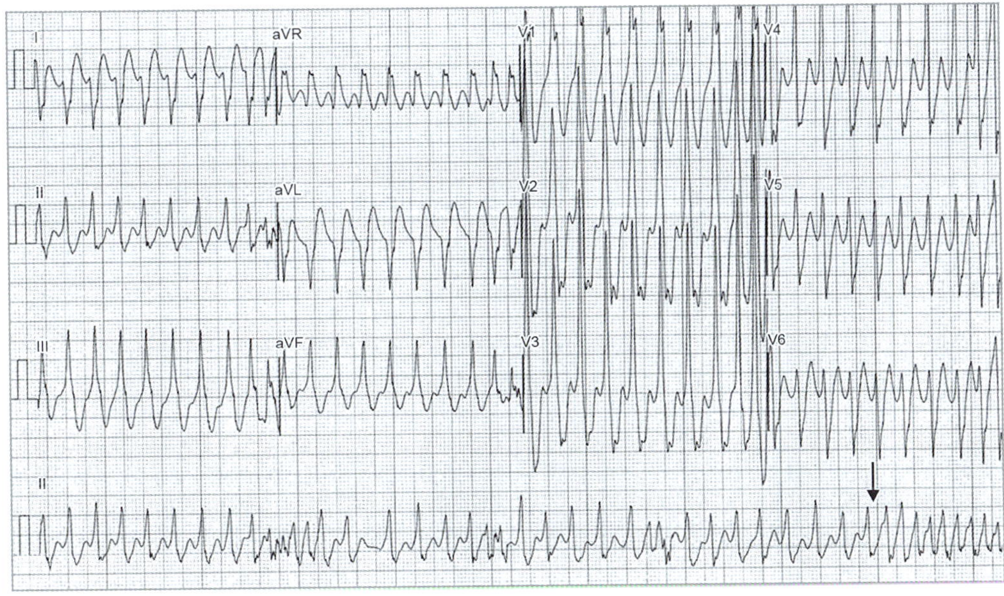

Fig. 10: Ventricular fibrillation in patient with pre-excited atrial fibrillation (with permission from the authors)

Permanent Junctional Reciprocating Tachycardia

The PJRT constitutes approximately 4% of all pediatric SVTs. It is due to the presence of an accessory pathway (usually on the right side of the heart in the posteroseptal region) which is capable of decremental retrograde conduction. PJRT is incessant in approximately half the patients, often leading to tachycardia-induced cardiomyopathy, which presents with symptoms of heart failure. Left ventricular dysfunction at presentation has been reported in approximately 18–30% patients with PJRT.

Diagnosis

The ECG tracings of PJRT are characterized by negative P waves in the inferior leads (II, III and aVF) and a long RP interval (long RP tachycardia) (**Figs. 13 and 14**).[12] Usually, PJRT onset is caused by an increase in sinus rate rather than a PAC. This tachycardia needs to be differentiated from other long RP tachycardias such as sinus tachycardia (upright P waves in leads II, III, and aVF), atypical AVNRT (slow-slow reentry) and ectopic atrial tachycardia (EAT). Response to adenosine can help in differentiating EAT from PJRT; only 10% of EATs terminate in response to adenosine whereas PJRT terminates with a retrograde P wave which does not conduct through the AV node.

Treatment

The PJRT is highly resistant to drug therapy in approximately 30–50% the patients. For this reason, often the only treatment option in patients with PJRT is transcatheter ablation which has been reported to have an acute success rate of 90% with a recurrence rate of 10–20% on long-term follow-up. Spontaneous resolution of PJRT has also been reported in approximately 12% of the patients. For these reasons, medical therapy is preferred as the first-line option in infancy and early childhood, whereas in older and symptomatic patients catheter ablation is a safe and effective option. A combination of amiodarone and a β-blocker has been shown to be clinically beneficial in 100% of the patients.

Ectopic Atrial Tachycardia

Ectopic atrial tachycardia (EAT) is due to increased automaticity of myocardial cells in a non-sinus atrial focus and is uncommon in pediatric patients (14% of all SVTs). The ectopic foci are frequently localized to the right side (~60%) (the right atrial appendage and crista terminalis, 25% each). Other common locations include the pulmonary veins (9%), the left atrial appendage (11%) or the left atrium (11%). A focus can, however, exist at any place in the right or the left atrium. EAT is detected as an incidental finding in the absence of other presenting symptoms or signs in approximately 40% of the children.

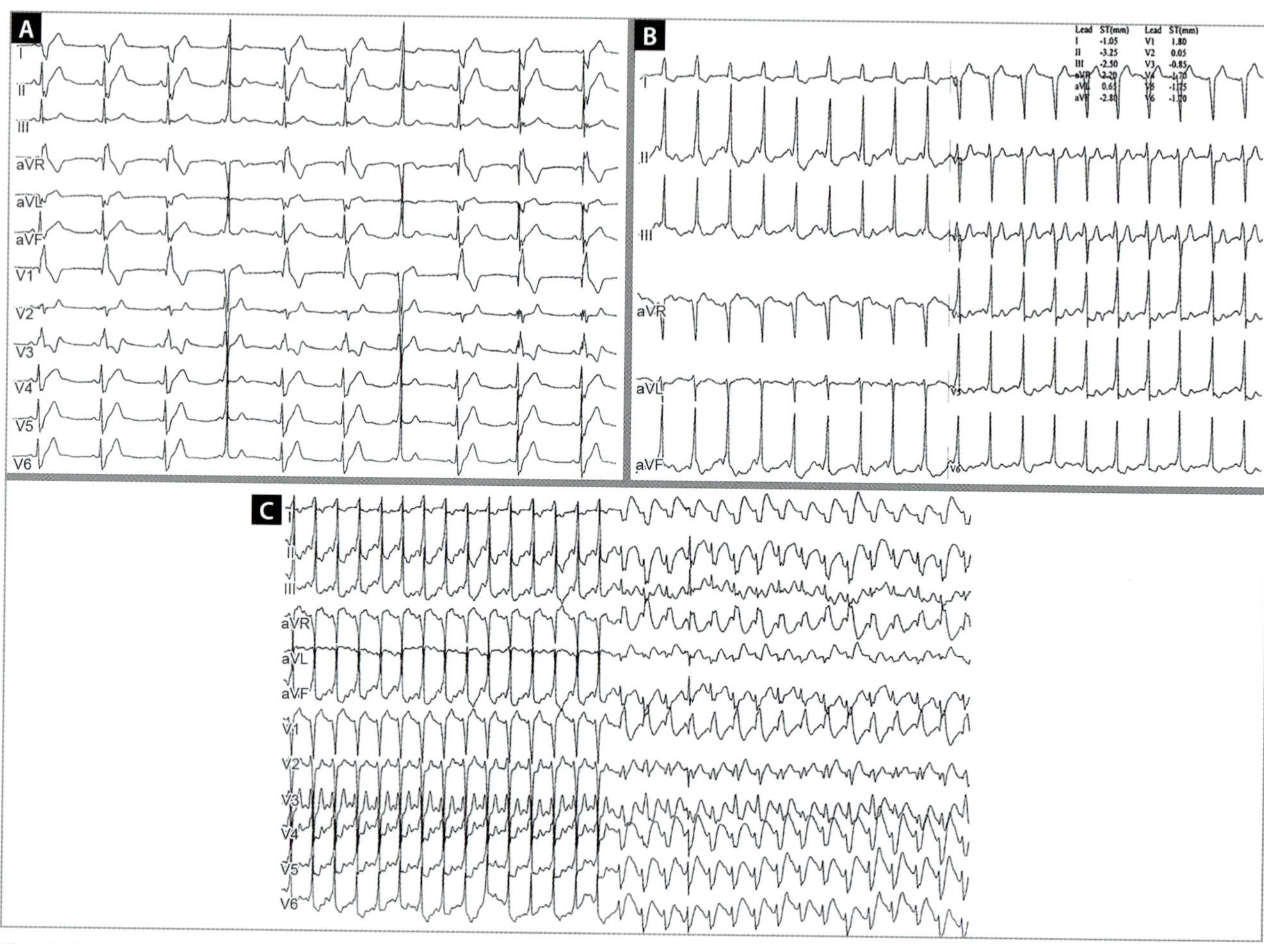

Figs. 11A to C: Single-beat loss of pre-excitation is seen during exercise stress testing. Baseline ECG shows right bundle branch block (RBBB) and intermittent pre-excitation (A). 1:1 pre-excitation is noted at a heart rate of 114 bpm (B). Abrupt loss of pre-excitation and RBBB pattern is noted at a heart rate of 180 bpm (C)
(*Courtesy*: Dr Chenni Sriram, Children's Hospital of Michigan, Wayne State University School of Medicine)

Diagnosis

For symptomatic children, common presenting symptoms include palpitations, heart failure due to tachycardia-induced cardiomyopathy, and syncope. Of note, approximately 40% of the children are hospitalized at the time of diagnosis. ECG during EAT reveals P waves which are different from the sinus P wave and the RP interval is typically long (**Figs. 15 and 16**). Atrial rate during EAT is influenced by variation in autonomic tone and usually ranges between 130 and 300 bpm. First- and second-degree AV blocks can also be present (**Figs. 17 and 18**). Also, in contrast to pathway mediated SVT which is fairly regular, beat-to-beat variation is common with EAT. In addition, warm-up or cool-down is often noted at the start and termination of EAT. Common differentials include other long RP tachycardias such as sinus tachycardia, PJRT and atypical AVNRT.

Treatment

In hemodynamically stable patients, first line drugs include β-blockers (propranolol, nadolol and metoprolol); class IC antiarrhythmic drugs can be used (flecainide & propafenone) as an alternative. In patients with reduced ejection fraction or resistance to other antiarrhythmic drugs, amiodarone is recommended. The overall response to medical therapy in patients with EAT is approximately 70%.

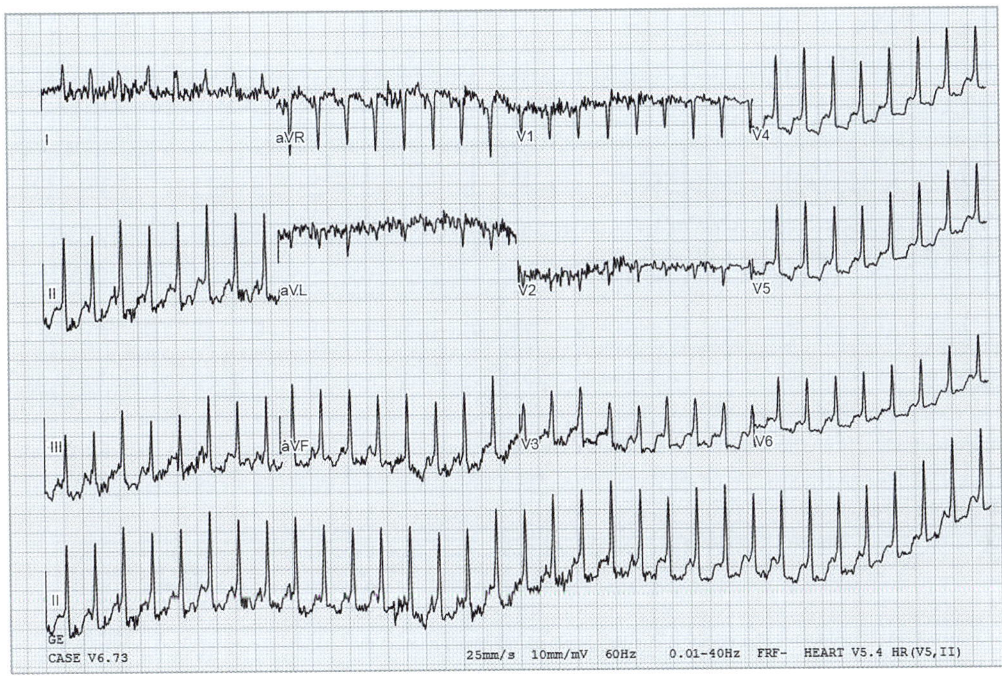

Fig. 12: Pre-excitation persists at peak exercise suggesting a possible high-risk pathway

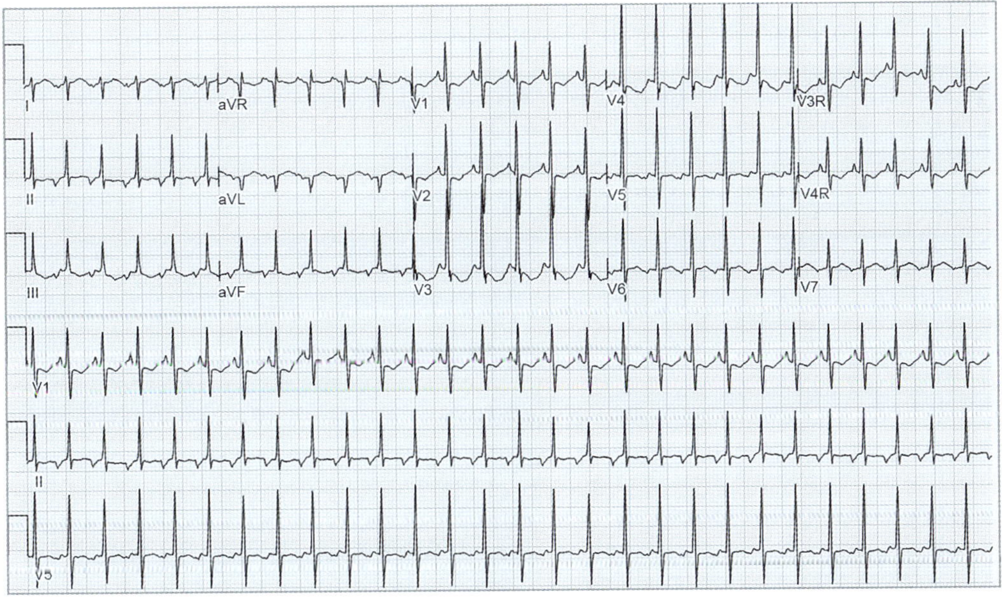

Fig. 13: Permanent junctional reciprocating tachycardia (note the negative P waves in leads II, III and aVF)

Transcatheter ablation is effective in approximately 80% of the patients with EAT and can be performed at any age but is associated with lower a risk of complications in patients who weigh more than 20 kg.[24]

About a third of patients who have EAT present with tachycardia-induced cardiomyopathy, the risk of which is the highest in children with a heart rate percentile for age >130%, PR index (PR/RR interval during tachycardia)

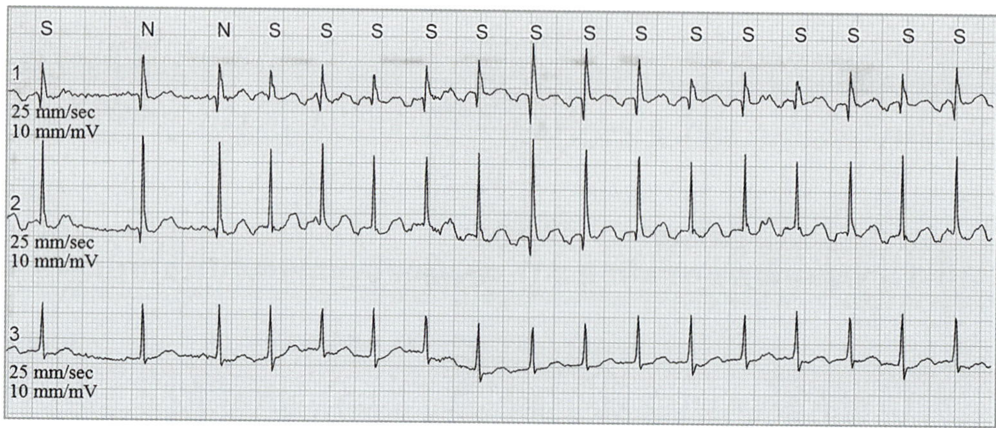

Fig. 14: Holter tracing from the patient whose ECG is shown in Figure 13. The PJRT starts with a sinus beat rather than a PAC

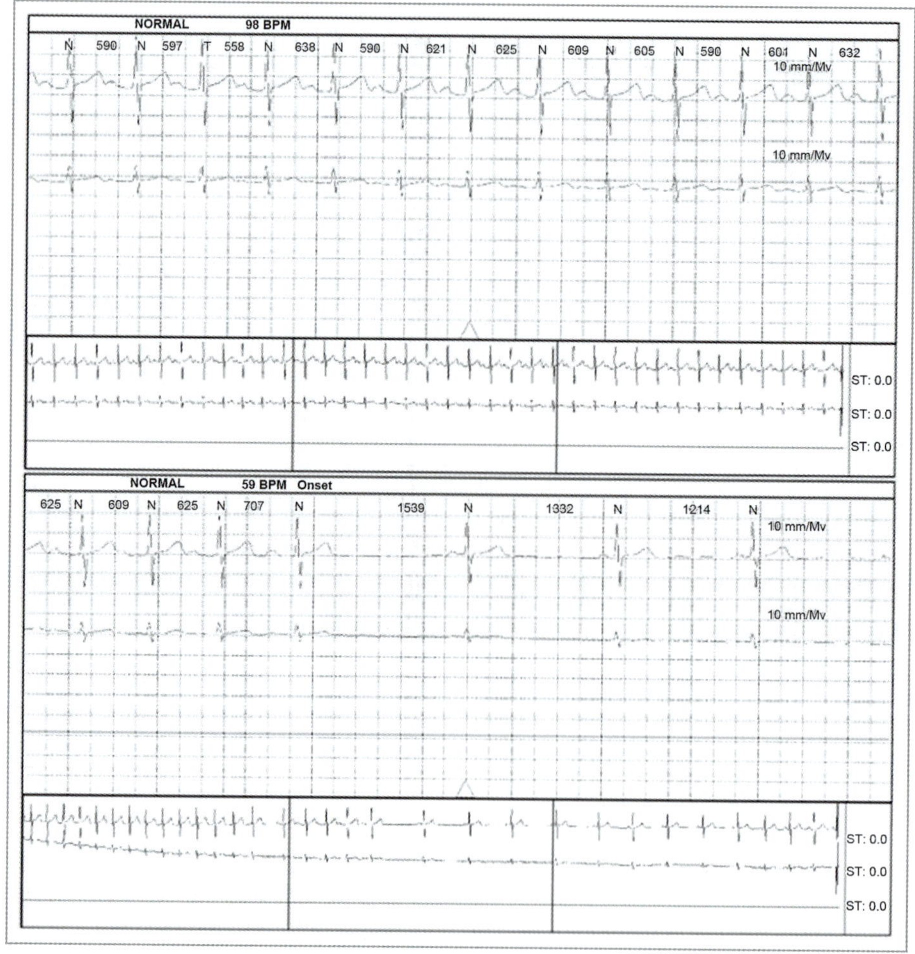

Fig. 15: A slow long RP tachycardia (ectopic atrial tachycardia) is noted on this Holter tracing during sleep. Note the long PR and RP intervals during the tachycardia. The tachycardia terminates spontaneously and the last 3 beats on this tracing are sinus beats which have a shorter PR interval

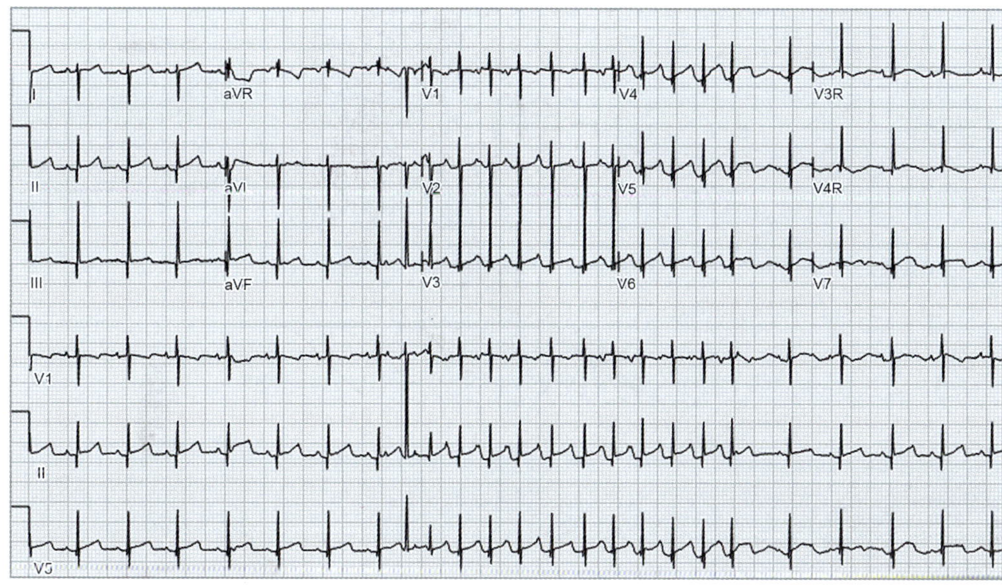

Fig. 16: A newborn with ectopic atrial tachycardia. Note the change in P wave morphology during the tachycardia (P waves are best seen in lead V1). The tachycardia terminates spontaneously and the rest of the ECG shows sinus rhythm

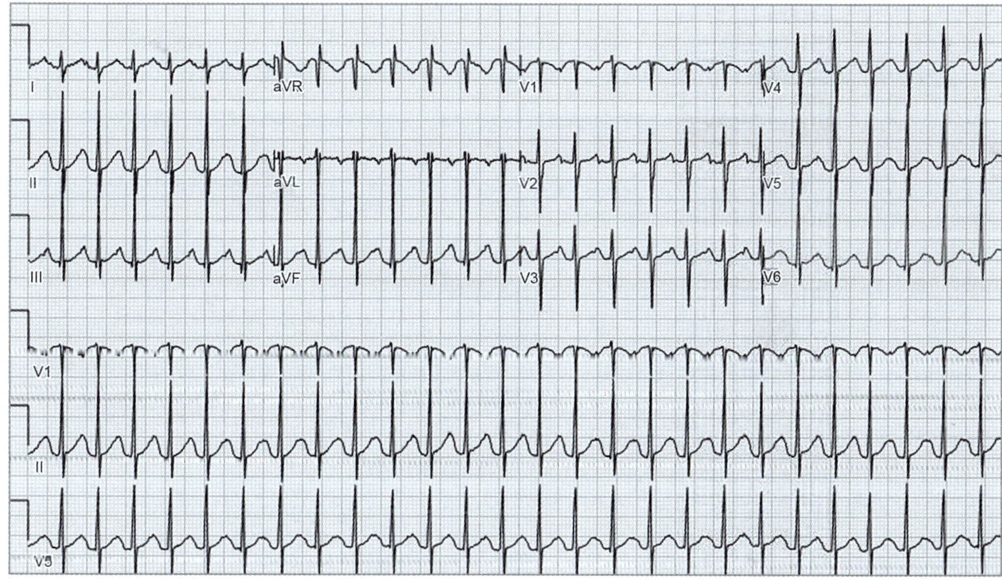

Fig. 17: This 12-lead ECG shows a long RP tachycardia (P waves are best seen in lead V1). This 14 year-old girl presented with tachycardia-induced cardiomyopathy. Note the prolonged PR interval during tachycardia. The Holter tracing in Figure 15 is from the same patient

>30%, and non-sinus P wave morphology. The prognosis in young children is good and spontaneous resolution is seen in about a third (mostly before 3–4 years of age).[24] The spontaneous resolution rates are higher in infants but, less frequent in older children.

Multifocal Chaotic Atrial Tachycardia

Multifocal chaotic atrial tachycardia (MAT) is a rare arrhythmia, which is mostly seen in newborns and infants. It is usually idiopathic, although it can be associated with respiratory syncytial virus infection and other respiratory

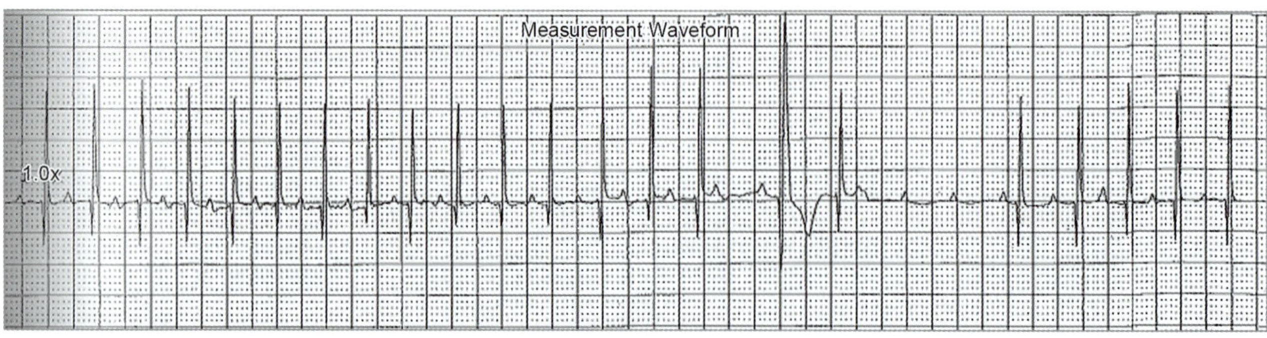

Fig. 18: Spontaneous second-degree heart block is noted in this 14 year-old girl with ectopic atrial tachycardia. The presence of heart block rules out an accessory pathway mediated reentry mechanism

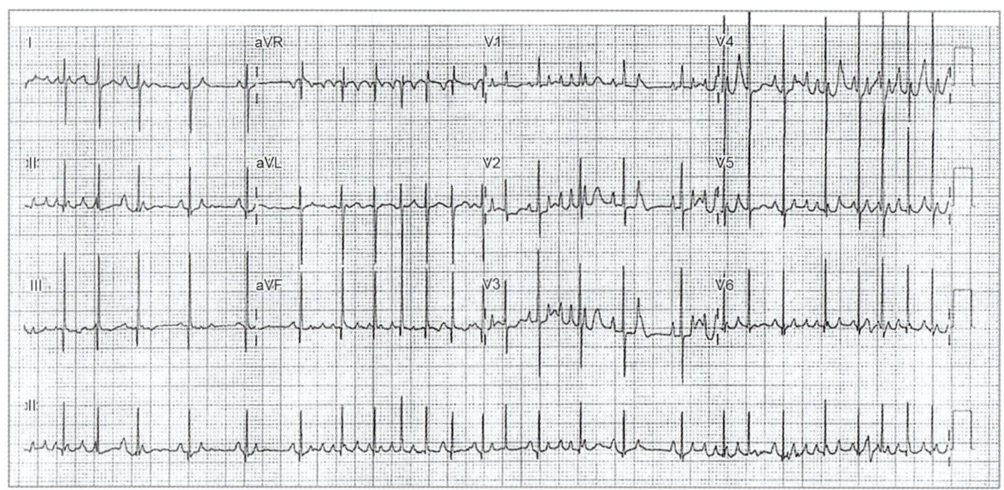

Fig. 19: Multifocal chaotic atrial tachycardia in a newborn. Note the different P wave morphologies and irregularity in both the atrial and the ventricular rate (*Courtesy*: Dr Chenni Sriram, Children's Hospital of Michigan, Wayne State University School of Medicine)

comorbidities such as bronchopulmonary dysplasia. The majority of children with MAT are healthy infants under 1 year of age. About 40% of patients with MAT have underlying structural heart diseases, another 40% or so have structurally normal hearts and no other comorbid conditions and the rest have a variety of comorbidities.[25]

Diagnosis

Clinical manifestations vary from a benign asymptomatic arrhythmia to heart failure and sudden death. Characteristic ECG findings include multiple (at least 3) distinct P-wave morphologies; irregular P–P intervals; isoelectric baseline between P-waves and occasionally a rapid ventricular rate (**Fig. 19**). First- and second-degree AV blocks cause variable PR and RR intervals, and a relatively slow heart rate has also been reported in patients with MAT. The arrhythmia is often incessant.

Treatment

Treatment is recommended for symptomatic children. Cardioversion is not effective. Digoxin, sotalol, flecainide, and propafenone have been tried with variable results. Amiodarone is the drug of choice in patients with ventricular dysfunction. Spontaneous resolution has been reported in a high proportion of patients with neonatal and infantile-onset MAT.

Atrial Flutter (AF)

Neonatal AF is rare (0.03% of neonates) and usually idiopathic (**Fig 20**). In 12% to 33% of patients, it is

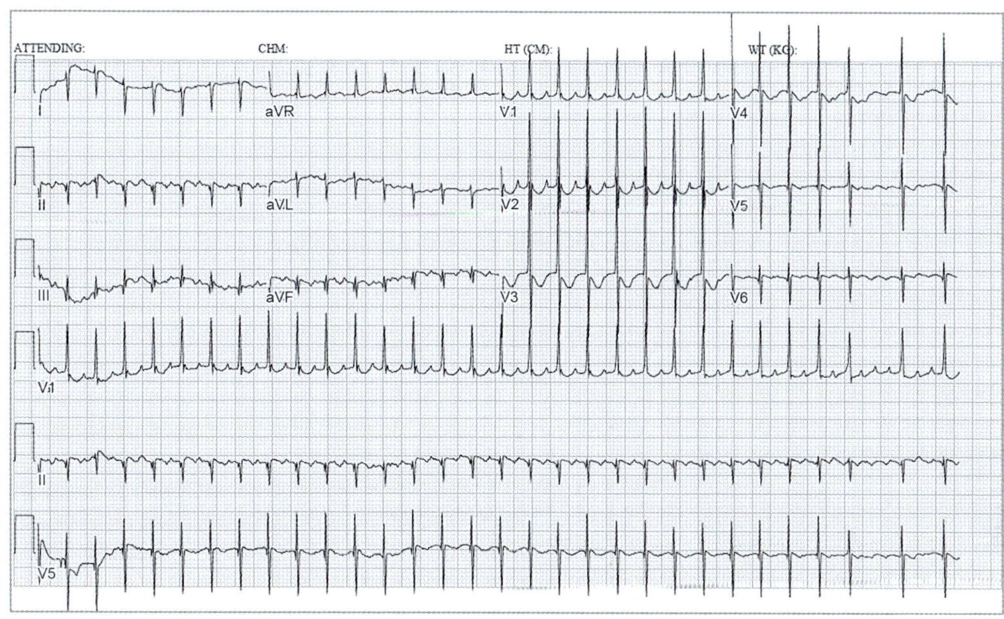

Fig. 20: Atrial flutter in a newborn with 2:1 AV conduction
(*Courtesy:* Dr Chenni Sriram, Children's Hospital of Michigan, Wayne State University School of Medicine)

associated with the presence of an accessory pathway. In contrast, AF is common in patients with congenital heart disease, particularly when right atrial hypertrophy or dilation is present.

Pathophysiology

The arrhythmia is sustained by a circular macroreentrant pathway within the atrial wall, which does not involve the AV node. Typical flutter involves counterclockwise propagation of wave front around the tricuspid annulus with a critical zone of slow conduction in the cavotricuspid isthmus (**Fig. 21**) whereas atypical flutter involves clockwise propagation of wave front around the cavotricuspid isthmus (**Fig. 22**). Atrial rates typically range between 300 and 500 bpm, 2:1 AV conduction is commonly seen leading to ventricular rates between 150 and 250 bpm. Normal or near-normal ventricular rates can be observed in AF with slower 3:1 or 4:1 AV conduction (**Figs. 21 and 22**).

Intra-atrial reentrant tachycardia (IART) is frequently seen in patients with congenital heart disease with scars from previous operations. It can be slow with 1:1 AV conduction and be barely discernible due to low amplitude P waves (**Fig. 23**). The mechanism of this arrhythmia is propagation of wave fronts around anatomic barriers and scars instead of the tricuspid annulus. Palpitations or dizziness are common symptoms at presentation. However, patients with underlying structural or hemodynamic abnormalities can present with syncope.

Diagnosis

The ECG diagnosis of AF is straightforward with saw-toothed flutter waves, which are best seen in leads II, III, and aVF. IART on the other hand, can be difficult to diagnose due to lower ventricular rates and low amplitude P waves. Fixed heart rate on telemetry or Holter monitor should always raise a concern for this arrhythmia. Vagal maneuvers or adenosine, both of which slow down AV nodal conduction and ventricular rate can help in better visualization of P waves.

Treatment

In neonates, if the AF is well-tolerated, cardioversion can be delayed as the arrhythmia can terminate spontaneously within 24 to 48 hours (26% of patients). Digoxin has been utilized during this wait period for rate control. This approach however prolongs the hospitalization and increases the cost of care.[26] For persistent AF, electrical (0.5–1.0 J/kg, synchronized) or pharmacologic cardioversion using amiodarone (5 mg/kg in 20 minutes), flecainide or propafenone can be utilized. In hemodynamically

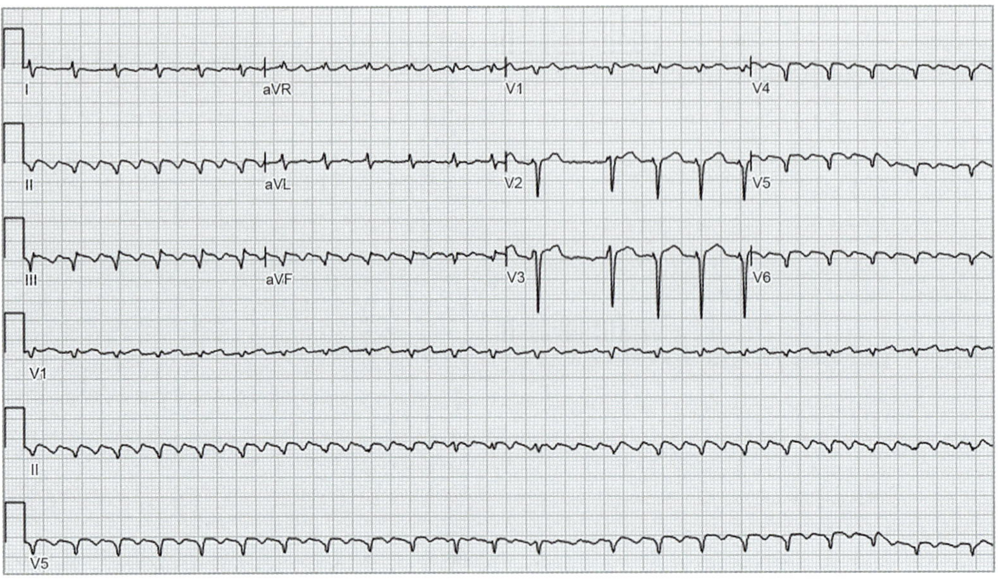

Fig. 21: Typical atrial flutter (counterclockwise loop around cavotricuspid isthmus; negative P waves in leads II, III and aVF) with variable AV conduction

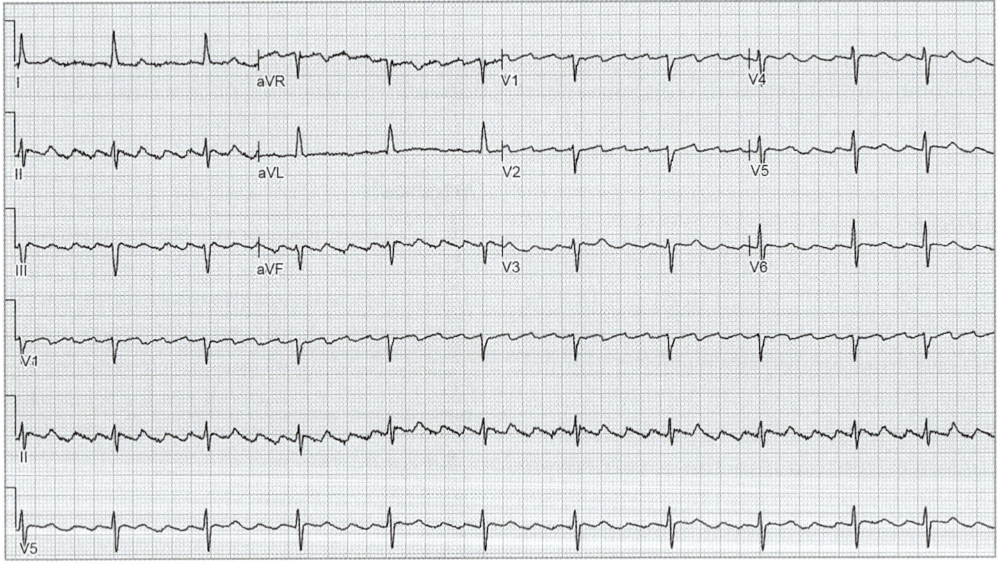

Fig. 22: Atypical atrial flutter (clockwise loop around cavotricuspid isthmus; positive P waves in leads II, III and aVF) with 3:1 atrial conduction

unstable patients, electrical cardioversion should be the first-line therapy.

For patients with AF of 48 hours' duration or longer, or when the duration of AF is unknown, anticoagulation with warfarin (INR 2.0 to 3.0), a factor Xa inhibitor, or direct thrombin inhibitor is recommended for at least 3 weeks before and at least 4 weeks after cardioversion. For patients with AF of 48 hours' duration or longer or of unknown duration who have not been anticoagulated for the preceding 3 weeks, it is reasonable to perform transesophageal echocardiography before cardioversion and proceed with cardioversion if no left atrial thrombus is identified, including in the left atrial appendage (LAA), provided that anticoagulation is achieved before transesophageal echocardiography and maintained after cardioversion for at least 4 weeks.

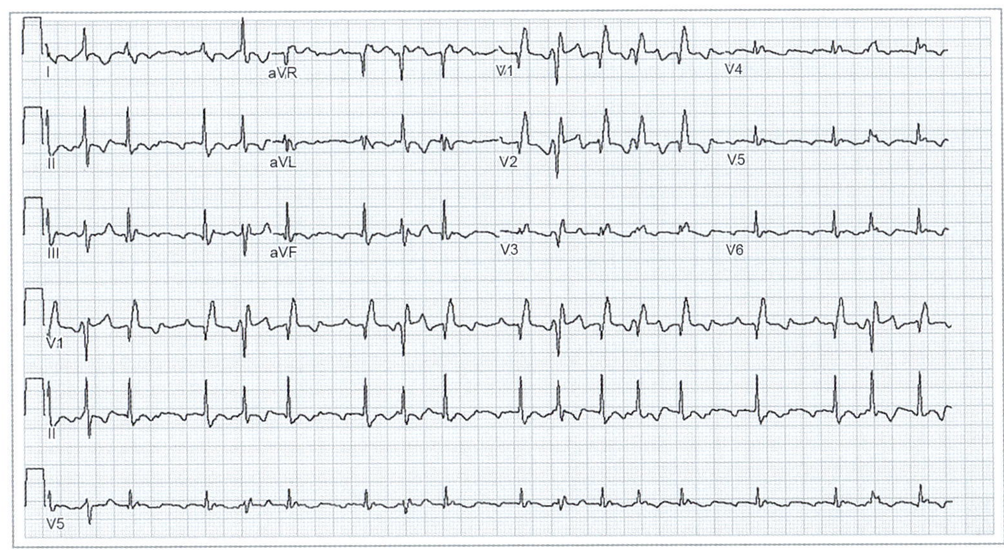

Fig. 23: Intra-atrial reentrant tachycardia in patient with Ebstein's anomaly with grouped beating/Wenckebach pattern (*Courtesy:* Dr Chenni Sriram, Children's Hospital of Michigan, Wayne State University School of Medicine)

Prognosis

In general, in neonates with no other arrhythmic substrate (e.g. accessory pathways), recurrences are unusual and long-term treatment is rarely required. AF recurrence is common in older children and prophylactic therapy is therefore needed. Class IC antiarrhythmic medications in combination with a β-blocker or class III drugs such as amiodarone or sotalol are often used in older children. The aim of the treatment is either to suppress the arrhythmia or, if that is not achieved, to slow down the ventricular rate to a more normal heart rate. In patients weighing more than 25–30 kg, transcatheter ablation is a safe and effective option.

Atrial Fibrillation

Atrial fibrillation (AFib), a common arrhythmia in adults, is extremely rare in otherwise healthy children. A significant proportion (~40%) of those with lone AF in childhood or adolescence has coexistent arrhythmias such as atrioventricular nodal reentrant tachycardia (AVNRT) or atrioventricular reentrant tachycardia (AVRT) due to an accessory pathway. Many patients have a focal trigger/triggers that lead to AFib and that ablation of such triggers may be an effective treatment for AFib.

Diagnosis

The patients typically present with abrupt onset palpitations, shortness of breath, chest discomfort or dizziness. Rapid conduction of AFib to the ventricles can present as syncope or sudden death. AFib can also be silent and only be detected on cardiac monitors. Prolonged AFib is known to predispose to thromboembolism, which can present as stroke, acute coronary syndrome, mesenteric or renal ischemia. AFib is classified as paroxysmal (episodes spontaneously terminate in 7 days), persistent (episodes last >7 days and require intervention to restore sinus rhythm), long-standing persistent (continuous atrial fibrillation lasting >12 months) and permanent (interventions to restore sinus rhythm have either failed or have not been attempted).[27]

The ECG is characterized by irregularly irregular heart rate and the absence of P waves. The QRS complex can be wide if there is rate-dependent or permanent bundle branch block. (**Figs. 24 to 26**). Other arrhythmias that can be confused with AFib include sinus rhythm with frequent PACs, AF and EAT.

Treatment

For persistent AFib, electrical (0.5–1.0 J/kg, synchronized) or pharmacologic cardioversion using amiodarone (5 mg/kg in 20 minutes), flecainide or propafenone can be utilized. In hemodynamically unstable patients, electrical cardioversion is the first-line therapy. Anticoagulation therapy and indications remain the same as described for atrial fflutter in the previous sections.

Long-term suppression of AFib can be achieved with antiarrhythmics (class IA or IC agents, class III agents)

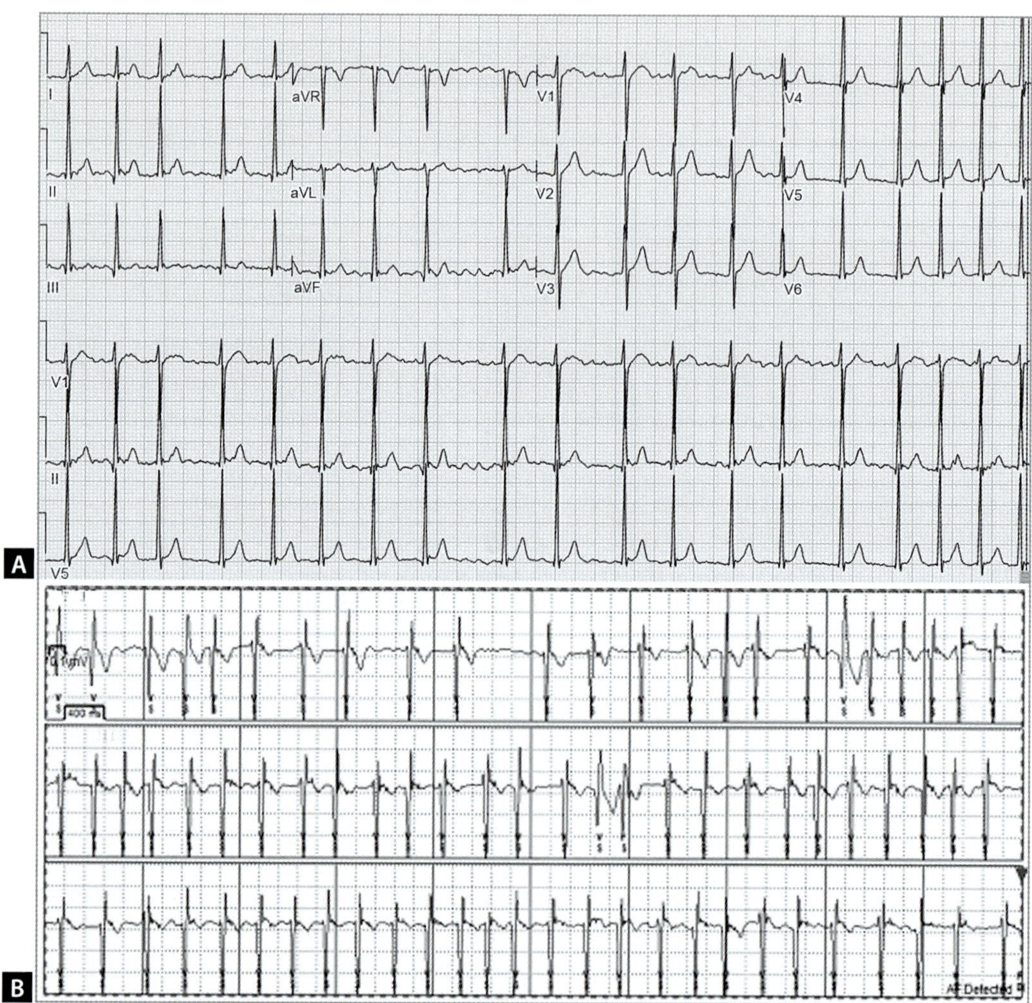

Figs. 24A and B: (A) Atrial fibrillation in a 16-year-old boy. Irregularly irregular tachycardia with no discernable P waves is noted; (B) Subcutaneous implantable loop recorder transmission from the same patient

or with catheter ablation which leads to symptomatic improvement in 70% of the patients. Bleeding and thromboembolic risk should be used to guide long-term anticoagulation in each individual patient.[27]

Junctional Ectopic Tachycardia

Junctional ectopic tachycardia (JET) is fairly common (up to 15% patients) after open heart surgical procedures, especially operations involving ventricular septal defect closure, right ventricular outflow tract muscle bundle resection or reconstruction. The mechanism of arrhythmia has been postulated to be injury and inflammation near the proximal conduction system in the postoperative period.

Diagnosis

Postoperative JET is characterized by onset of rapid heart rate, usually between 160 and 250 bpm within the first 24 to 48 hours. It may lead to marked hemodynamic instability. Congenital JET, if untreated, can lead to tachycardia-induced cardiomyopathy and can therefore present with symptoms and signs of heart failure. Sudden death due to AV block has been reported in association with congenital JET. On the 12-lead ECG, as with VT, AV dissociation is generally present but with a narrow QRS. However, in neonates and infants, a 1:1 ventriculoatrial retrograde conduction with negative P waves in inferior leads can be seen owing to a lower effective refractory

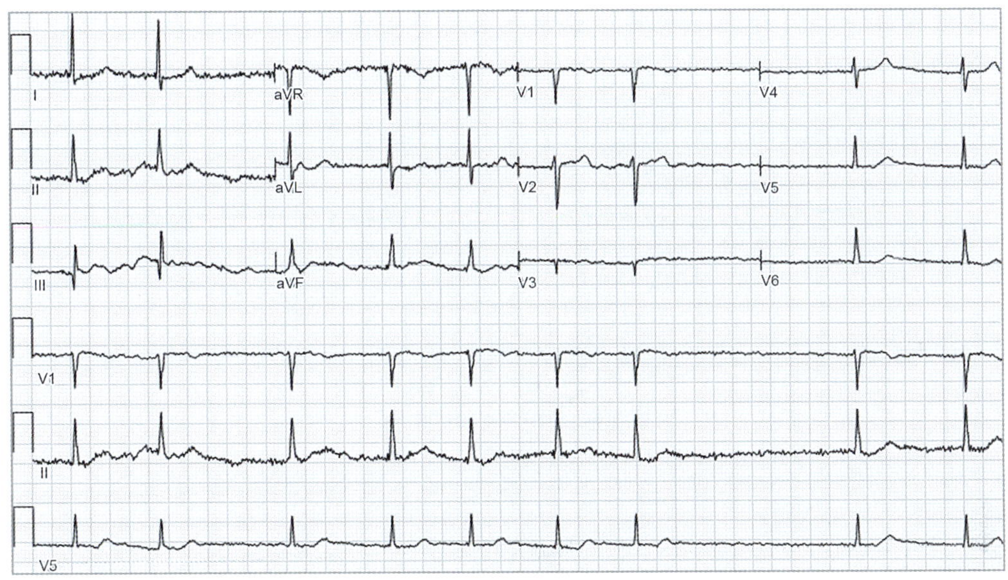

Fig. 25: Atrial fibrillation with slow ventricular response

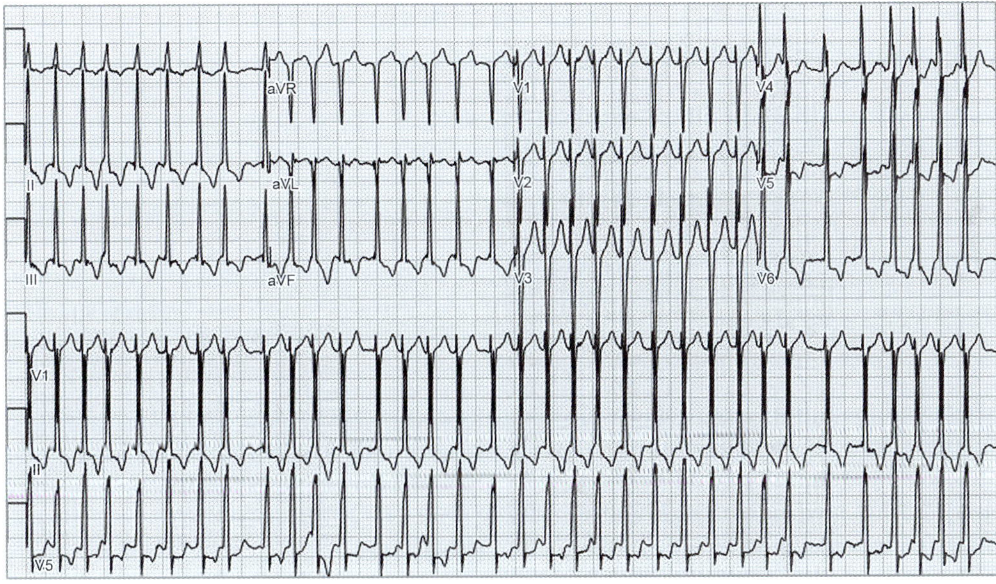

Fig. 26: Atrial fibrillation with rapid ventricular response

period of AV node this subgroup of pediatric patients. The heart rate is between 160 and 250 bpm, and often changes with variation in autonomic tone and body temperature. Another characteristic feature of JET and other automatic arrhythmias is a "warming-up" phase at its onset and a "cooling-down" phase at its termination (**Figs. 27 and 28**).[12]

The JET can be confused with SVT, particularly if the P waves are buried within the QRS and are not visualized well.

Treatment

Both congenital and postoperative JET, like other automatic arrhythmias are highly catecholamine sensitive. The goal of treatment for both postoperative and congenital JET is to decrease the arrhythmia rate to <150 bpm or to achieve sinus rhythm if possible.[8] Adequate sedation, paralysis, pain management, and therapeutic hypothermia also play an important role in the management of this arrhythmia. Amiodarone is one of the most widely used and effective

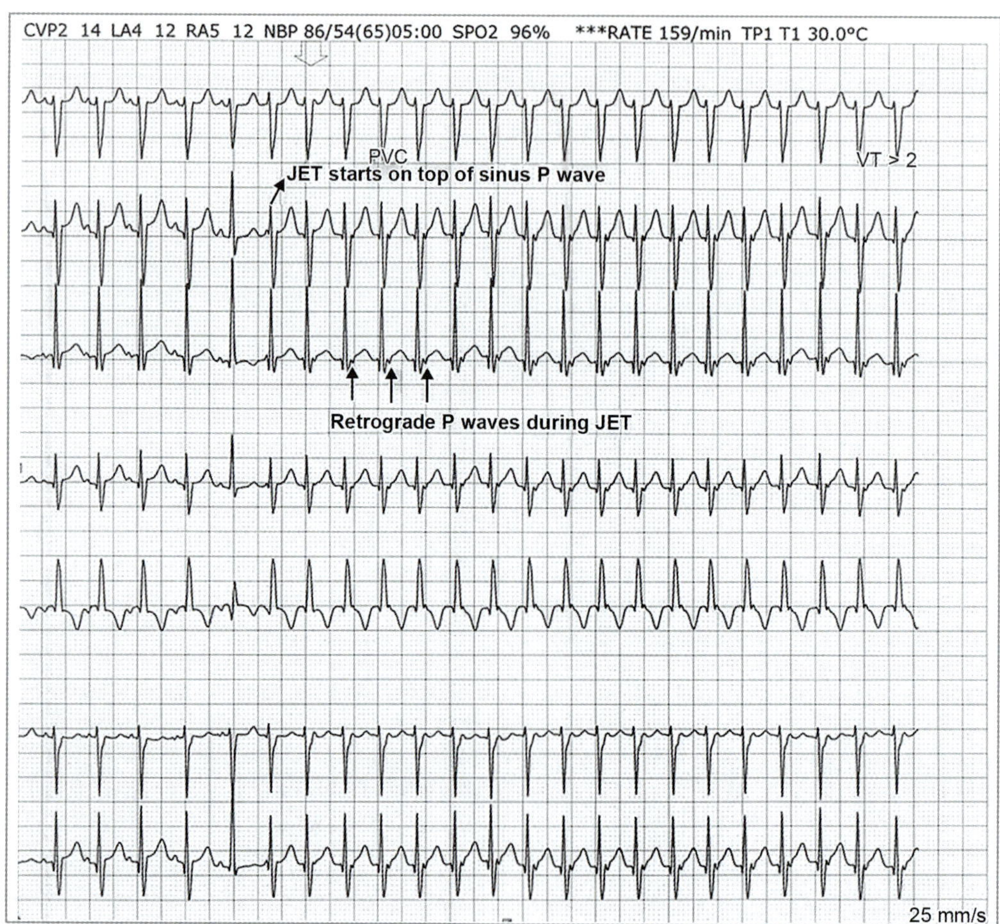

Fig. 27: Postoperative JET (*Courtesy*: Dr Chenni Sriram, Children's Hospital of Michigan, Wayne State University School of Medicine)

drugs for management of both postoperative and congenital JET (intravenous amiodarone 10 mg/kg in two 5 mg/kg increments, followed by an infusion of 10–15 mg/kg/day for 48–72 hours).[28] Other medications which have been tried with good results include intravenous flecainide (1- to 2-mg/kg bolus [mean dose 1.6 ± 0.5 mg/kg] over 10 minutes followed by a continuous infusion of 0.40 mg/kg per hour), intravenous landiolol hydrochloride (initial dose of 3–5 μg/kg/min before gradually increasing to the maintenance dose of 3–10 μg/kg/min or 40 μg/kg/min for loading and gradually decreasing to the recommended maintenance dose of 10–40 μg/kg/min), a combination of intravenous amiodarone and flecainide, intravenous sotalol (1 mg/kg IV bolus to be given over 1 hour), ivabradine (0.1 to 0.28 mg/kg per day in two divided doses) and intravenous nifekalant. Once the JET rate decreases, sequential AV pacing is often employed to generate AV synchrony. Extracorporeal membrane oxygenation support might be required if other measures fail.

Prognosis

Postoperative JET is usually a self-limited arrhythmia, which tends to resolve in a few days; therefore, the prognosis is good. Congenital JET on the other hand can be difficult to control and is associated with a mortality as high as 35% (mostly sudden death which is sometimes related to high grade or complete AV block). In addition, cardiomegaly and/or heart failure are present in approximately 60% of the patients. Adverse clinical outcomes in congenital JET are related to the ventricular rate rather than the time of onset.

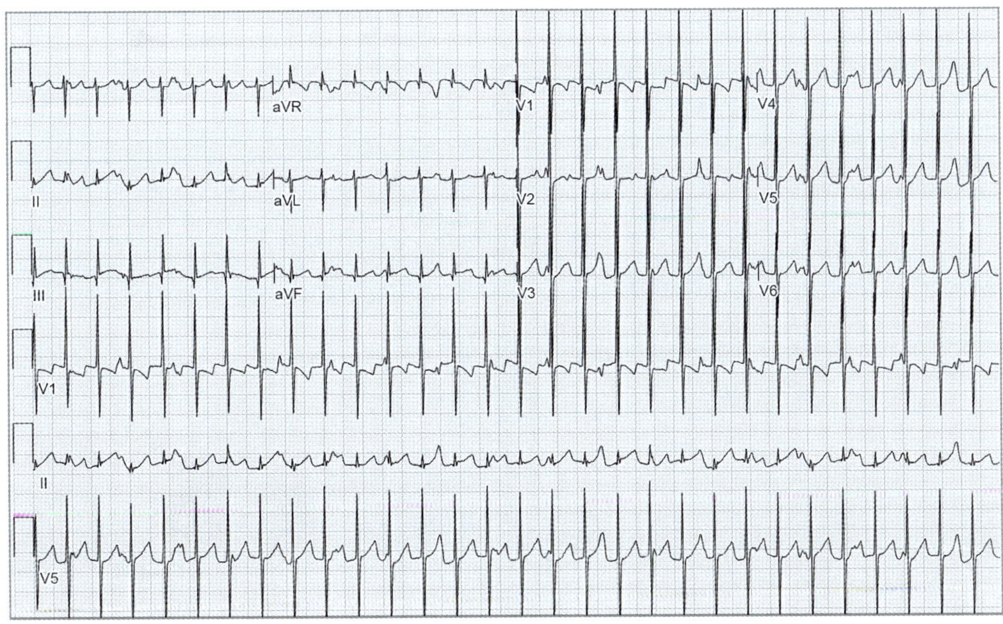

Fig. 28: Congenital JET. The ventricular rate is faster than the atrial rate and AV dissociation is noted

MONOMORPHIC VENTRICULAR TACHYCARDIA

Idiopathic VT is distinctly uncommon in children with a structurally normal heart (0.2–0.8/10,000), tends to self-resolve, and carries an overall good prognosis.

Classification

Four broad types of monomorphic VT are identified in children with structurally normal hearts. By far the commonest is the (a) *right ventricular outflow tract* VT (RVOT VT) (**Fig. 29**) which is mostly mediated by triggered activity related mechanisms but can sometimes be mediated by enhanced automaticity and reentry. RVOT VT accounts for 60–80% of all VTs seen in children with a structurally normal heart. Other VT types include (b) *incessant VT of infancy* which mostly arises from the left ventricle and is mediated by enhanced automaticity, (c) *intrafascicular verapamil sensitive* VT which is mediated by reentry and accounts for 10–15% of pediatric VTs (**Fig. 30**) and (d) *bundle branch reentrant* VT which as a rule is seen in association with left ventricular failure and dilation but has rarely been reported in patients with myotonic dystrophy with a structurally normal heart.

Sustained monomorphic VT is more common in patients with underlying structural heart disease and/or ventricular dysfunction and is often related to areas of dense fibrosis after surgical incisions, patch material, and the valve annuli, which can form regions of conduction block. These regions can define reentry circuit borders and create intervening anatomical isthmuses consisting of conducting myocardium.[29] More than 80% of all treated VTs in patients with repaired tetralogy of Fallot who received ICDs for primary and secondary prevention were fast monomorphic VTs with a median heart rate of 212 bpm.[30] These fast VTs can be fatal, even in the presence of a preserved cardiac function. Monomorphic VTs have also been described after ventricular septal defect closure and repair of d-transposition of great arteries.

Types of monomorphic VT

- **Idiopathic RVOT VT** has two distinct subtypes. The more common subtype is characterized by VT at rest or during recovery which is completely suppressed or decreases during exercise. A less common subtype presents with longer runs of monomorphic VT triggered by exercise. The RVOT VT is more common in females and the mean age of presentation is approximately 8 years. The arrhythmia is sometimes exacerbated during menstrual periods. Palpitations and near-syncope have been reported in ½ to ⅔ of patients with RVOT VT; syncope, however is unusual and should prompt careful evaluation for an underlying cardiomyopathy.

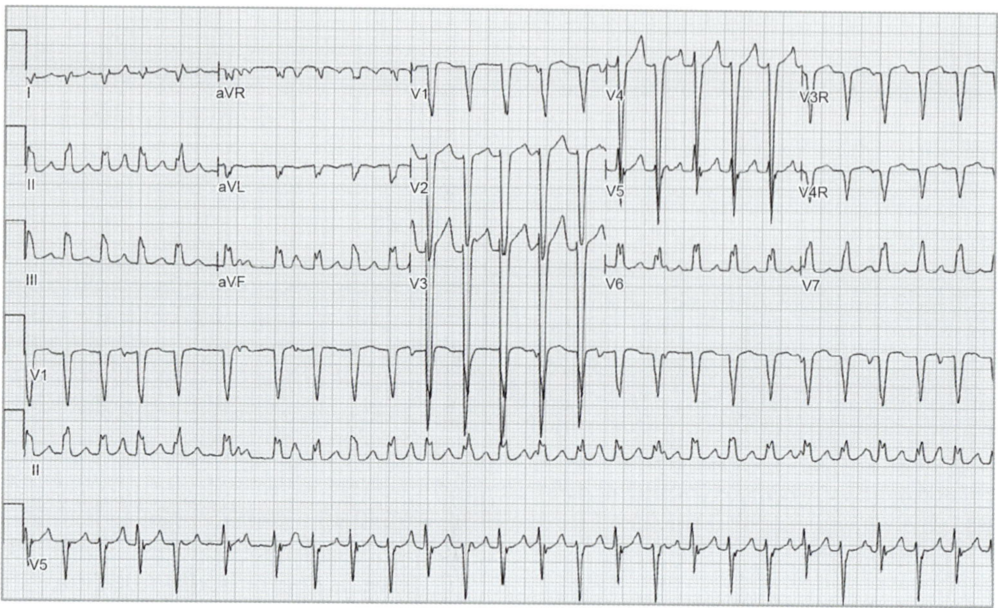

Fig. 29: Monomorphic idiopathic RVOT VT. VA dissociation can be seen in lead V1

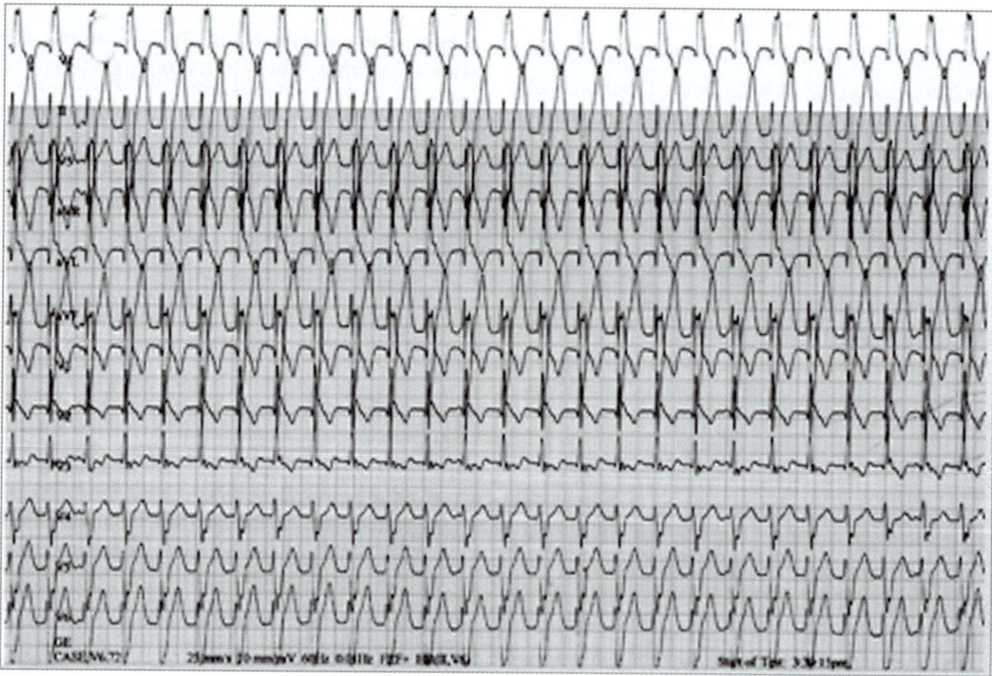

Fig. 30: This ECG is obtained from a14-year-old asymptomatic male who presented for pre-participation sports screening. The ECG shows a wide complex tachycardia with RBBB pattern and superior axis which is characteristic of verapamil sensitive intrafascicular VT (*Courtesy:* Dr Brojendra Agarwala, The University of Chicago Pritzker School of Medicine)

- **Incessant VT in infancy**, as the name suggests, presents with persistent VT with heart rates greater than 200 bpm. These patients often develop tachycardia-induced cardiomyopathy and present with symptoms of heart failure.
- **Intrafascicular verapamil sensitive VT** is more common in males and presents with runs of sustained or non-sustained VT (rate 150–250 bpm) which are triggered by stress or exercise. These episodes of are usually well tolerated with only mild symptoms (palpitations or dizziness).
- **Bundle branch reentrant VT** presents with palpitations or dizziness in children with normal left ventricular function whereas severe symptoms such as syncope or collapse have been reported in children with decreased cardiac function.

Diagnosis

The electrocardiographic hallmark of VT is a wide QRS tachycardia with ventriculoatrial (VA) dissociation. Sinoatrial capture beats or fusion beats can sometimes be seen (**Fig. 29**). Differentials of VT include other wide complex tachycardias which include SVT with bundle branch block type aberrancy and antidromic SVT. In addition to VA dissociation, sinoatrial capture beats, and fusion beats, additional ECG findings which favor a diagnosis of VT over SVT in a patient with wide complex tachycardia include absence of typical right bundle branch block or left bundle branch block type morphology, extreme axis deviation (northwest axis, QRS positive in leads aVF and aVR and negative in lead I), very wide QRS complexes (>160 msec), positive or negative concordance throughout the precordial (chest) leads (leads V1-V6 show entirely positive (R) or entirely negative (QS) complexes, with no RS complexes seen), the time from the onset of the QRS complex to the nadir of the S-wave >100 ms (*Brugada sign*), notching near the nadir of the S-wave (*Josephson sign*) and RSR′ complexes with a taller R (*Marriott sign* which is considered to be the most specific sign to differentiate wide-complex SVT from VT).[31]

Treatment

Any *hemodynamically unstable patient* with a wide complex tachycardia should be assumed to be in VT and should immediately undergo synchronized cardioversion (1st cardioversion: 0.5–1.0 J/kg, following cardioversions: 2 J/kg) as per the PALS protocol.

For hemodynamically stable patients with monomorphic VT, a dose of adenosine [0.1 mg/kg IV or IO (6 mg maximum)] should be considered as common idiopathic VTs in children sometimes respond to adenosine. Other medications that are recommended in PALS protocol include amiodarone (5 mg/kg intravenous or intraosseous over 20 to 60 minutes) or procainamide (15 mg/kg intravenous or intraosseous over 30 to 60 minutes). However, since an overwhelming majority of VTs in children is benign, an effort should be made to obtain a 12-lead ECG in stable pediatric patients with monomorphic wide-complex tachycardia to diagnose the specific type of tachycardia.

The RVOT VT carries a benign prognosis with spontaneous resolution in a vast majority of children. In fact, spontaneous resolution is the rule in infants. However, the VT might persist in some older children.[9] Treatment is only indicated in children with symptoms or decreased ventricular function due to frequent runs of tachycardia. For acutely symptomatic, hemodynamically stable children with RVOT VT, adenosine can be tried as mentioned above. Since β-blocker are quite effective and are recommended as the first line of therapy for RVOT VT, the next step should be trial of a rapid acting β-blocker such as esmolol. Those who respond to esmolol can be discharged home on an oral β-blocker. Calcium channel blockers are also effective but are contraindicated in children less than 12 months of age due to a risk of heart failure, hypotension and conduction problems.[9] A lack of response to β-blockers should prompt treatment with antiarrhythmics such as lidocaine, flecainide, amiodarone and sotalol. Catheter ablation is indicated and quite effective in those who are refractory to drug therapy.[9]

The PALS protocol should be followed for an unstable patient with incessant VT of infancy. Antiarrhythmics are often required for therapy of patients with incessant VT of infancy. These patients should be hospitalized for initiation and monitoring of antiarrhythmic therapy with medications such as β-blockers, lidocaine (can be converted to oral mexiletine if response to lidocaine is documented), flecainide, sotalol and amiodarone (**Table 1**).[9]

Intrafascicular VT of is acutely highly sensitive to intravenous verapamil[9] which should therefore be the first line therapy in these patients. However, 20% of the patients fail to respond to oral verapamil and require other medications such as β-blockers and amiodarone. Catheter ablation is an option in children with intrafascicular VT who have severe symptoms despite maximal medical therapy.[9]

It is important to emphasize that all children with a documented wide-complex tachycardia should be hospitalized after acute management in the ER as they often require further investigations and evaluation including serial electrocardiograms, telemetric monitoring, blood tests such as serum C-reactive protein, serum ESR, complete blood count, comprehensive metabolic panel, troponin, creatine phosphokinase-MB to evaluate for myocarditis, exercise stress testing (if stable), cardiac MRI or echocardiogram to evaluate for structural abnormalities, a careful family history and review of other family members' ECGs. In addition, hospitalization is recommended for initiation and monitoring of several antiarrhythmic drugs.

Acute management of monomorphic VT in patients with repaired congenital heart disease is broadly similar to patients with idiopathic monomorphic VT and a structurally normal heart. However, class IC antiarrhythmic drugs such as flecainide should be avoided in patients with structural heart disease. Children with repaired or unrepaired congenital heart disease, cardiomyopathies or significant hemodynamic abnormalities constitute a high-risk group, which is likely to require additional investigations such as an electrophysiology study and cardiac catheterization. An implantable-cardioverter defibrillator may be indicated in some of the children in this subgroup for prevention of sudden cardiac death.

POLYMORPHIC VENTRICULAR TACHYCARDIA

Pathophysiology

Polymorphic VT is rare in children but is often associated with marked hemodynamic perturbations and can quickly degenerate into ventricular fibrillation if sustained. It often indicates an underlying global myocardial electrical abnormality which can be associated with reversible conditions such as dyselectrolytemia, acidosis, hypoxia, ischemia, hypothermia or hyperthermia, or with inherited abnormalities such channelopathies (CPVT, LQTS, Brugada syndrome, SQTS) or cardiomyopathies (DCM, Restrictive CMP, HOCM).

Clinical Features

Patients with short runs of polymorphic VT may report palpitations but are often asymptomatic. Longer, more sustained runs are associated with symptoms such as dizziness, syncope, seizures or sudden death. The syncopal episodes either have a brief prodrome or are not preceded by a prodrome at all (malignant syncope).

Diagnosis

Polymorphic VT is characterized by a fast wide QRS rhythm with variation in QRS morphology (amplitude, axis and/or duration) or from beat to beat (**Figs. 31 and 32**).[32] Torsades de pointes (TdP), a type of polymorphic VT, is characterized by a gradual change in amplitude and twisting of the QRS complexes around an isoelectric line on the electrocardiogram. TdP is associated with QTc prolongation, which is the heart rate adjusted lengthening of the QT interval. A QTc is considered long when it is greater than 450 ms in males and 460 ms in females. A QTc greater than 500 ms has been associated with a two- to three-fold increase in risk for TdP. The rhythm may terminate spontaneously or may degenerate into ventricular fibrillation (**Figs. 33 and 34**).

Bidirectional VT is characterized by beat-to-beat alternation in the QRS frontal plane axis. It is associated with digitalis toxicity, Andersen-Tawil syndrome (LQTS7; periodic paralysis, electrical abnormalities and characteristic physical deformities) (**Fig. 35**) or CPVT.

Sustained polymorphic VT often degenerates into ventricular fibrillation, which is characterized by disordered electrical ventricular activation without identifiable QRS complexes (**Fig. 36**).

Non-sustained runs of polymorphic VT in asymptomatic children including TdP do not require defibrillation. Patients who are acutely symptomatic with documented polymorphic VT should be immediately defibrillated as per the PALS protocol. Every effort should be made to look for a reversible (dyselectrolytemia, acidosis, hypo or hyperthermia, ischemia, hypoxia, myocarditis) or an inherited cause (channelopathies, cardiomyopathies) as the episodes tend to be recurrent and can become more sustained and degenerate into ventricular fibrillation.

It is critical to obtain a 12-lead ECG during atrial or sinus rhythm without delay as the changes can be transient. The EKG can help identify long QT syndrome (LQTS), short QT syndrome, Brugada syndrome (Coved type ST elevation >2 mm in leads V1 and V2), and malignant early repolarization. Disorders of acid-base, temperature regulation, hypoxia, and ischemia also produce characteristic changes on 12- lead ECG such

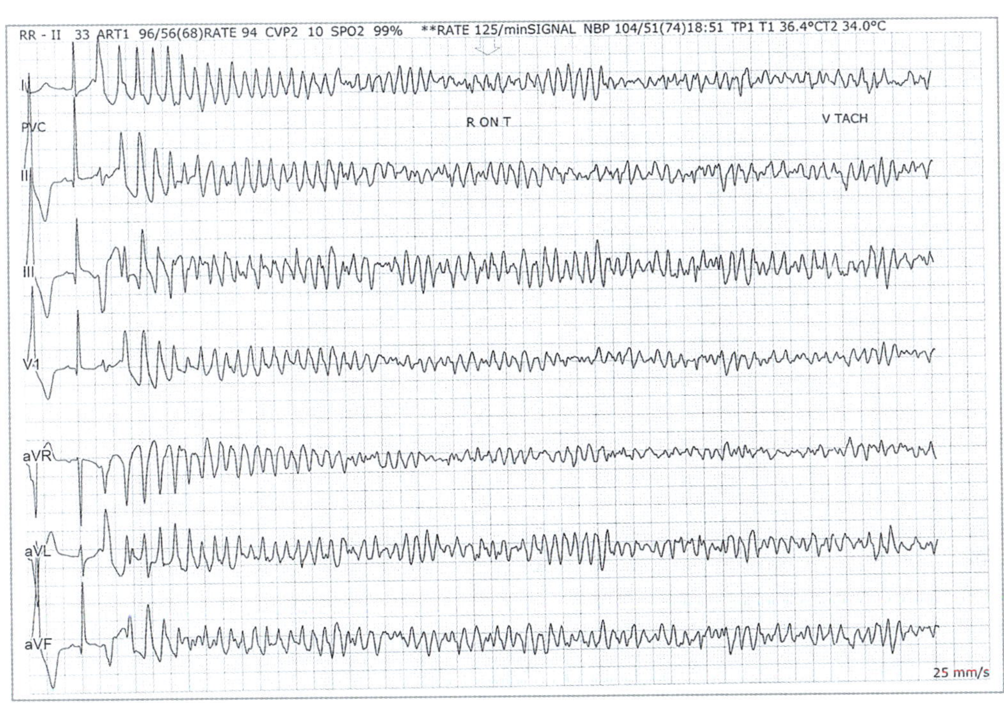

Fig. 31: Ischemic polymorphic VT which degenerates into ventricular fibrillation in a 13-year-old girl following unroofing of the anomalous right coronary artery. The VT is initiated by a short-coupled PVC (R-on-T phenomenon) (*Courtesy*: Dr Chenni Sriram, Children's Hospital of Michigan, Wayne State University School of Medicine).

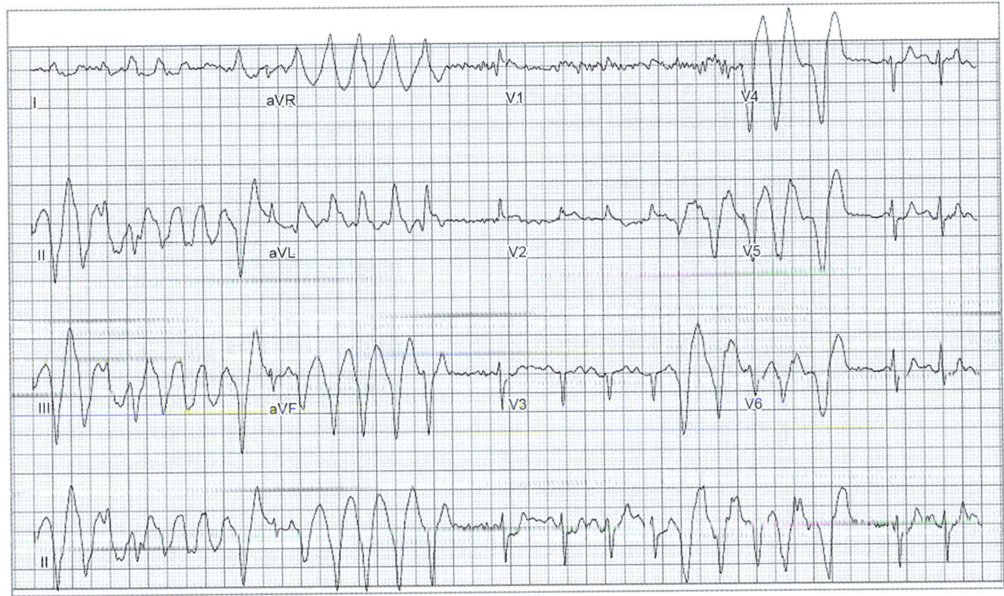

Fig. 32: Runs of non-sustained polymorphic VT are seen during exercise stress testing in a patient with dilated cardiomyopathy

as short QTc (acidosis and hypercalcemia), prolonged QTc (hypokalemia and hypocalcemia), J point elevation (hypothermia), and ST segment elevation or depression (ischemia, infarction, myopericarditis or profound hypoxia). All children with documented polymorphic VT should be hospitalized in an intensive care unit.

Fig. 33: Several runs of Torsades de pointes are seen on telemetry in a 26-year-old male with marked QT prolongation (QTc>600 msec)

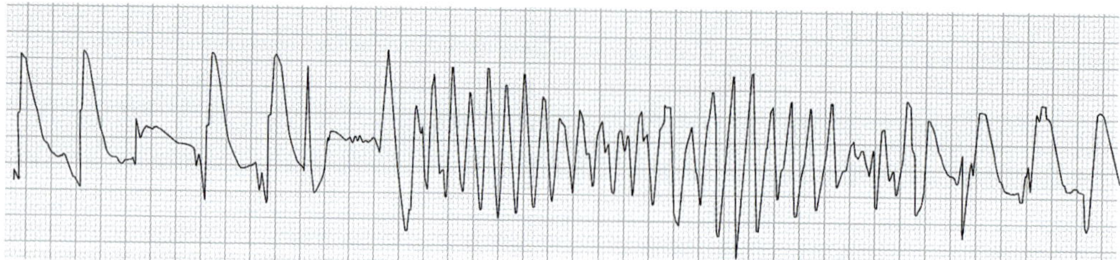

Fig. 34: A run of Torsades de pointes is noted in a 17-year-old boy with seizure disorder

Treatment

Further management of patients with polymorphic VT depends on the underlying predisposing condition and is detailed in **Table 1**. A subset of patients with inherited channelopathies or cardiomyopathies present with VT storm (>3 episodes of VT in a 24-hour period). These patients are at a very high risk of dying and should therefore be admitted to a cardiac intensive care unit or an equivalent unit where extracorporeal membrane oxygenation is available as a therapeutic option. The acute management of VT storm and long-term management of patients with inherited arrhythmia syndromes is detailed in **Table 1**. Catheter ablation is in general not effective in management of patients with polymorphic VT or ventricular fibrillation

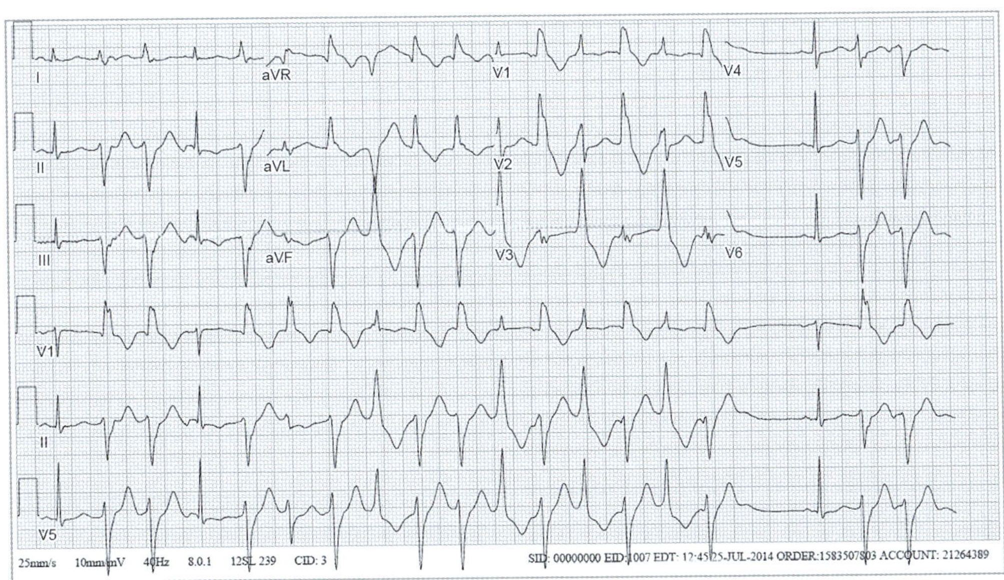

Fig. 35: A short run of bidirectional VT is noted at rest in a 25 year old woman with Andersen-Tawil syndrome (*Courtesy*: Dr Chenni Sriram, Children's Hospital of Michigan, Wayne State University School of Medicine)

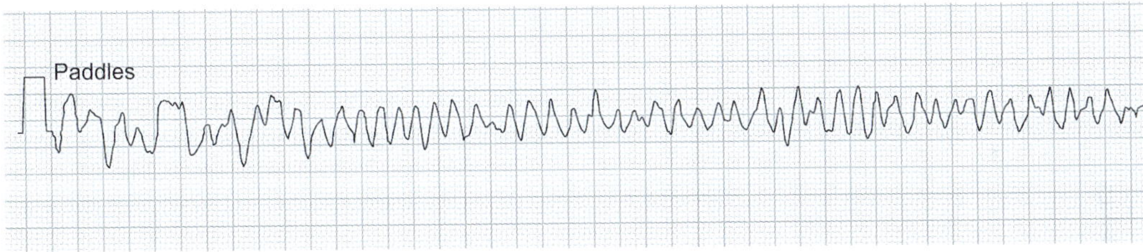

Fig. 36: Ventricular fibrillation is seen on AED tracings from a 16-year-old male who suddenly collapsed while playing with his friends

with a few exceptions such as Brugada syndrome and PVC triggered ventricular fibrillation where modification of the substrate or catheter ablation of the inciting PVC have been shown to be effective in preventing further episodes.[33]

Any patient who presents with TdP should be assumed to have a prolonged QT interval and drugs such as procainamide and amiodarone, which are recommended in the PALS protocol, should be avoided as they can further prolong the QT interval and precipitate incessant TdP and ventricular fibrillation. A comprehensive list of medications, which prolong QT interval, is available on *www.crediblemeds.org*. These medications should be avoided in all patients with prolonged QTc or documented TdP. Sodium channel blockers such as procainamide should not be administered to patients with Brugada syndrome as they can precipitate refractory ventricular fibrillation.

Polymorphic VT due to reversible causes is usually associated with a good long-term prognosis. Prognosis is more variable for polymorphic VT due inherited channelopathies and cardiomyopathies.

BRADYARRHYTHMIAS

First-Degree Heart Block and Mobitz Type 1 Second-Degree Heart Block (Wenckebach)

Both first-degree heart block and Mobitz type 1 second-degree heart block (Wenckebach) are common in otherwise healthy adolescents. They are also common during sleep when the vagal tone is high. Pathological conditions such as acute rheumatic fever, ischemia, drug effect or toxicity (calcium channel blockers, β-blockers, cardiac glycosides and cholinesterase inhibitors), dyselectrolytemia and myocarditis can also present with first-degree heart block and Mobitz type 1 second-degree heart block (Wenckebach). First-degree heart block is characterized by a PR interval, which is prolonged for age. Mobitz type 1 second-degree heart block is characterized by successive prolongation of PR interval and shortening of RR interval before a missed beat. The PR interval following the missed beat is shorter than the PR interval preceding the missed beat (**Fig. 37**). These blocks occur at the AV nodal level, are typically benign, do no progress to a higher grade block, and therefore, do not require any treatment. Ongoing monitoring is recommended in patients with a trifascicular block (first-degree heart block, right bundle branch block and left anterior fascicular block or left posterior fascicular block). In addition, medications that can slow down conduction should be avoided in these patients.

Mobitz Type 2 Second-Degree Heart Block

Mobitz type 2 second-degree heart block (**Fig. 38**) is caused by disease of distal conduction system (His-Purkinje system) and is characterized by intermittently non-conducted P waves. Unlike Mobitz type 1 second-degree heart block, the PR interval does not vary for conducted P waves. This heart block can progress to complete heart block and if there is no ventricular escape rhythm, the patient can present with malignant syncope or sudden cardiac death. In an acutely symptomatic patient, atropine or isoproterenol can be tried as temporizing measures until a temporary pacemaker is placed. Definitive treatment of Mobitz type 2 second-degree heart block is implantation of a permanent pacemaker. The indications are similar to indications for permanent pacing in a patient with complete heart block.[12,34]

2:1 Heart Block

A 2:1 heart block is characterized by 2 P waves for every QRS complex. It is difficult to differentiate between Mobitz type 1 and type 2 2:1 second-degree heart blocks. However, this distinction is important as patients with Mobitz type 2, 2:1 second-degree heart block have significant infranodal disease and require a pacemaker. The Wenckebach pattern typically improves during exercise whereas infranodal blocks (Mobitz type 2 second-degree heart block) usually worsen during exercise. In addition, Mobitz type 1 second-degree heart block is often associated with a long PR interval and a narrow QRS complex whereas Mobitz type 2 second-degree heart block is associated with a short PR interval but a wide QRS complex. Sometimes, a higher grade second-degree heart block pattern is noted upon telemetric monitoring in patients with Mobitz type 2 second-degree 2:1 heart block (**Fig. 39**). 2:1 heart block can sometimes be associated with congenital LQTS.

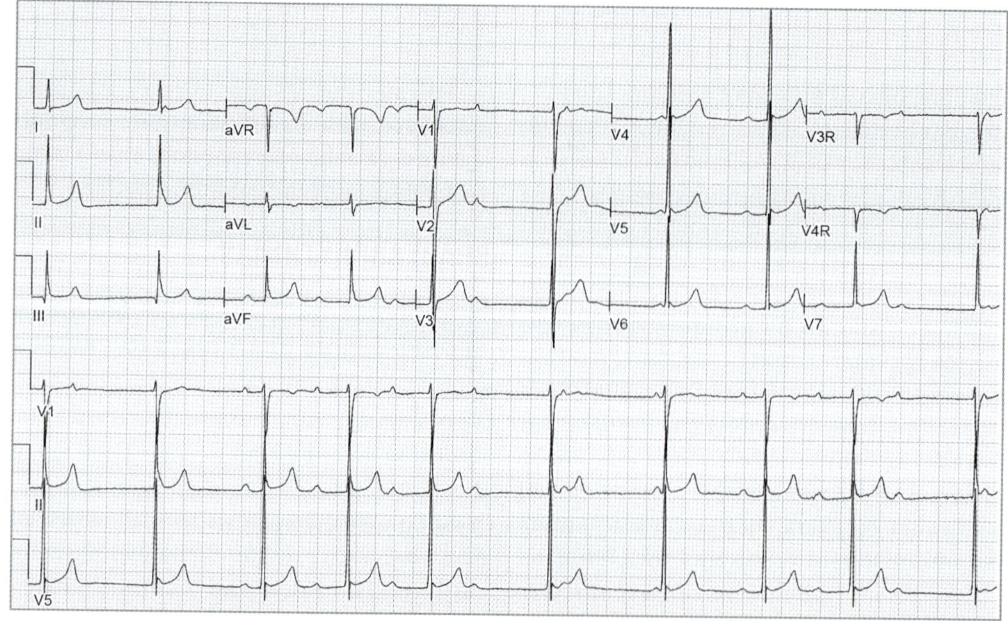

Fig. 37: Both first-degree and Mobitz type 1 second-degree heart blocks are seen on this ECG

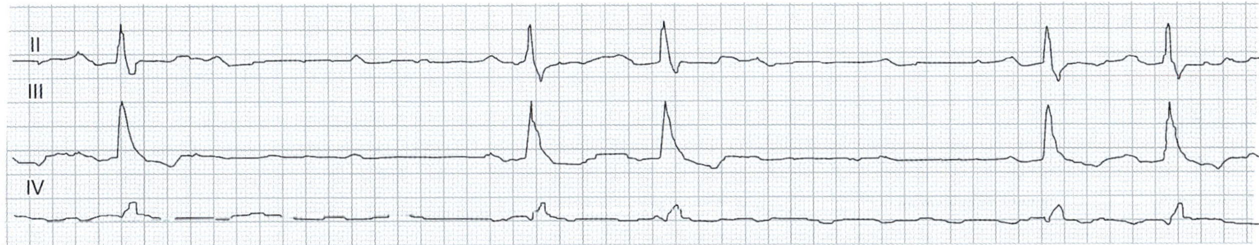

Fig. 38: Mobitz type 2 second-degree heart block

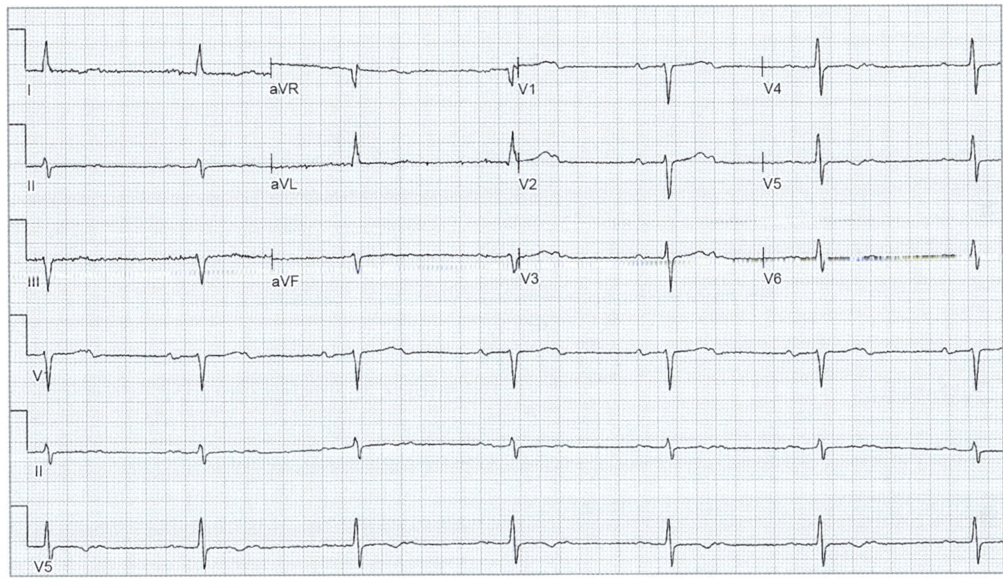

Fig. 39: 2:1 heart block

Complete Heart Block

Complete heart block is characterized by complete failure of atrioventricular conduction, which manifests as AV dissociation (**Fig. 40**). The symptoms depend upon the underlying junctional or ventricular escape rhythm-patients with an absent, slow or unreliable escape rhythm can present with syncope, cardiac arrest, or sudden death. Patients with complete heart block are also predisposed to ventricular dilation and cardiomyopathy and can present with symptoms of heart failure. Common causes in pediatric age group patients include maternal SLE and damage to cardiac conduction system after surgical repair of congenital heart disease. Rare causes include Lyme carditis and myocarditis. Patients with heterotaxy syndrome (polysplenia) and corrected transposition of great arteries (risk 1–2%/year) have abnormal conduction systems and are also predisposed to spontaneous complete heart block.[10]

For acute onset, complete heart block with an inadequate escape rhythm, atropine, isoproterenol, transcutaneous pacing and temporary transvenous pacing can be tried as temporizing measures. Unless the cause is reversible (myocarditis, Lyme carditis), permanent pacing is indicated. In asymptomatic infants with congenital complete heart block, pacing is indicated if the heart rate is less than 55 bpm with a structurally normal heart or less than 70 bpm with significant structural abnormalities. Permanent pacing is also indicated in asymptomatic infants if a wide QRS escape rhythm, complex ventricular ectopy, abrupt pauses in ventricular rate that are 2–3 times the basic cycle length or ventricular dysfunction are noted. All symptomatic infants with congenital complete heart block require a permanent pacemaker. Postoperative complete heart block that is expected to persist or that does not resolve in 7 days after cardiac surgery is also an indication for permanent pacemaker placement.[12,34]

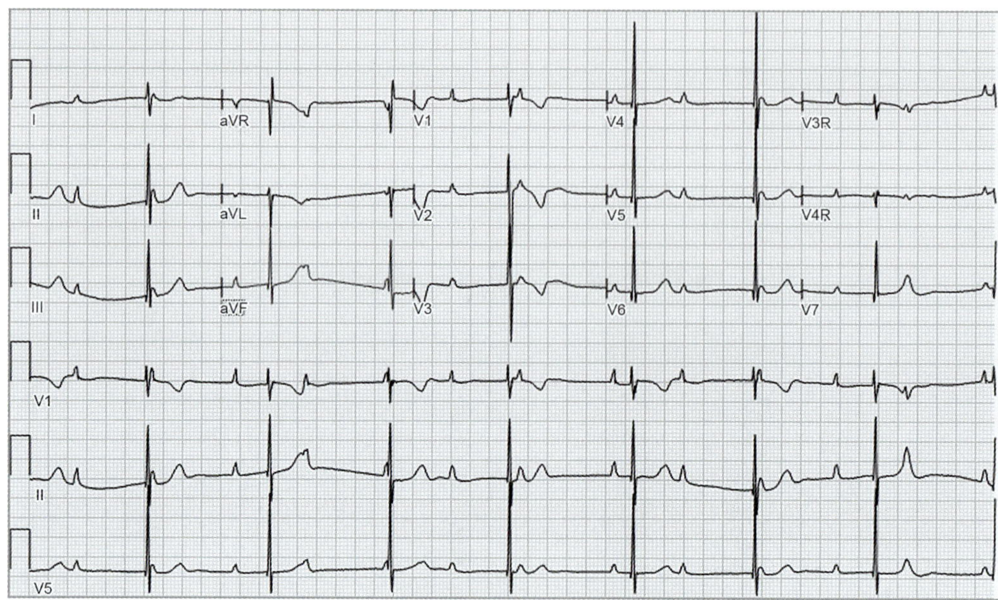

Fig. 40: Congenital complete heart block in a 4-year-old boy

Sinus Node Dysfunction

Sinus node dysfunction is a broad term, which encompasses several different bradyarrhythmias such as sinus bradycardia, sinus pauses, junctional bradycardia, tachycardia-bradycardia syndrome and chronotropic incompetence without any other identifiable cause. ECG criteria for the diagnosis of sinus node dysfunction include sinus bradycardia, sinus pauses of greater than 3 seconds, and a slow escape rhythm (**Figs. 41 and 42**).[12]

Pathophysiology

Sinus node dysfunction can be due to (1) non-cardiac causes (neurologic or metabolic disorders) or (2) intrinsic anomalies of sinus node function. Sinus bradycardia, sinus pauses, and junctional escape beats can occur in 20% to 90% of normal neonates and are more common in preterm or low weight babies. In neonates, sinus pauses of 800 to 1000 msec can be present but pauses of longer than 2000 msec are considered pathologic. A junctional rhythm can be present in healthy neonates as well. Transient bradycardia and QT interval prolongation (≤470 msec) can be the result of a stressful delivery, but usually these forms normalize in 48 to 72 hours.[12] Familial forms of primary sinus bradycardia and sinus node dysfunction have been associated with several genetic mutations, including mutation in the hyperpolarization-activated cyclic nucleotide-gated potassium channel 4 (*HCN4*) gene, the sodium channel voltage gated type V alpha subunit (*SCN5A*) gene, and the ankyrin 2, neuronal (*ANK2*) gene. In addition, sinus node dysfunction can complicate channelopathies such as Brugada syndrome and CPVT (*RYR2* mutations).

Sinus node dysfunction can also be associated with unrepaired congenital heart disease such as atrial septal defects, AV canal defects, Ebstein anomaly or a single ventricle but is more common after cardiac surgical procedures such as Fontan, Mustard, and Senning operations.[14]

Treatment

Patients with sinus atrial node dysfunction can be completely asymptomatic or may suffer from weakness, pallor, presyncope/syncope or heart failure.[12] If acute support is needed, atropine (0.02–0.04 mg/kg intravenous), isoproterenol, adrenaline (0.01 mg/kg intravenous), or, if necessary, transcutaneous or transvenous pacing are suggested. When associated with symptoms, pacemaker implantation is strongly indicated.[12]

Secondary sinus bradycardia can be a consequence of sepsis, central nervous system anomalies, hypothermia, hypopituitarism, intracranial hypertension, meningitis, maternal assumption of drugs, obstructive icterus,

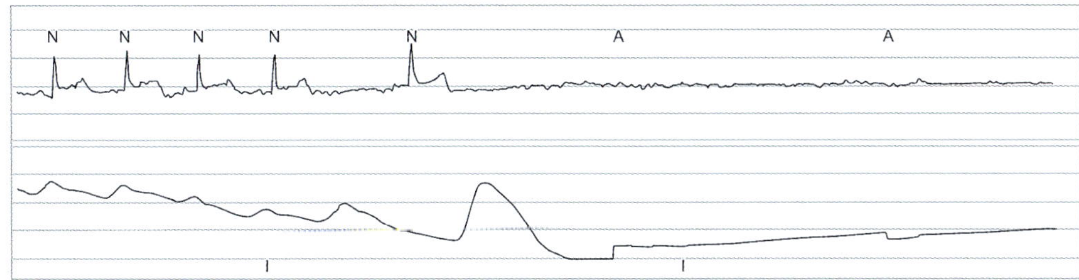

Fig. 41: Sinus arrest in a patient with sinus node dysfunction

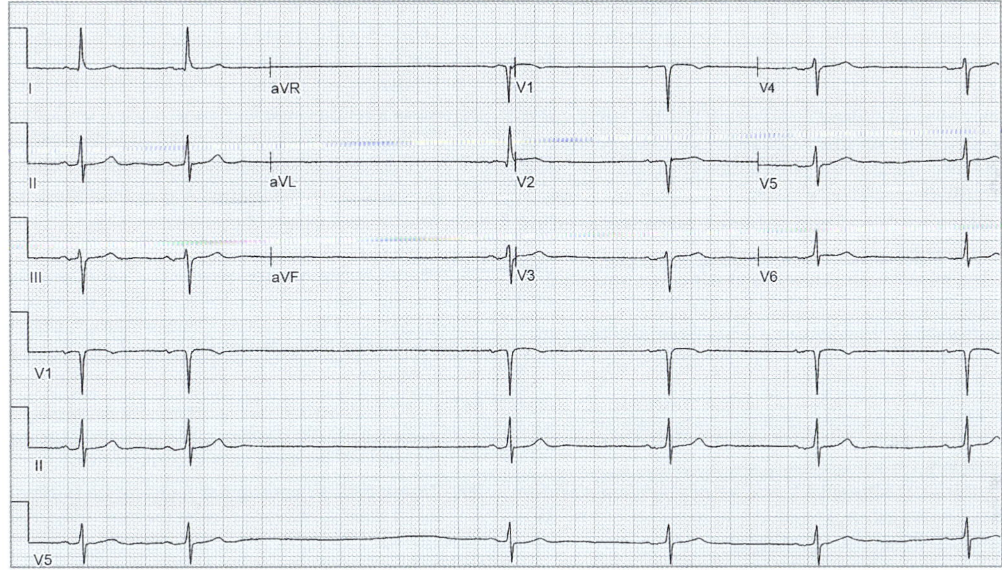

Fig. 42: Severe sinus bradycardia and an abrupt sinus pause are seen in a patient with sinus node dysfunction

hypothyroidism, electrolytes or metabolic alterations, maternal autoimmune diseases, and rarely conditions such as myocarditis and congenital long QT syndrome.

KEY MESSAGES

- Heart rhythm abnormalities are common in children. However, a vast majority of these abnormalities is benign and tend to self-resolve.
- Supraventricular arrhythmias are more common than ventricular arrhythmias which are infrequently seen in children with a structurally normal heart.
- First-degree heart block and Mobitz type 1 second-degree heart block are commonly seen in healthy children with high vagal tone and do not progresses to higher grade heart blocks.
- Pacemaker implantation is recommended for postoperative high grade or complete heart block that persists for longer than 7 days.
- Sinus node dysfunction can be seen in patients with repaired congenital heart disease but is distinctly uncommon in children with a structurally normal heart.
- A hemodynamically unstable child with a tachyarrhythmia should be cardioverted or defibrillated without delay.
- A hemodynamically unstable child with a bradyarrhythmia should be stabilized with atropine, adrenaline, isoproterenol and temporary transcutaneous or transvenous pacing if hemodynamic instability persists.

REFERENCES

1. Sacchetti A, Moyer V, Baricella R, *et al.* Primary cardiac arrhythmias in children. Pediatr Emerg Care. 1999;15:95-8.
2. Hoffman TM, Wernovsky G, Wieand TS, *et al.* The incidence of arrhythmias in a pediatric cardiac intensive care unit. Pediatr Cardiol. 2002;23:598-604.

3. Nagashima M, Matsushima M, Ogawa A, *et al.* Cardiac arrhythmias in healthy children revealed by 24-hour ambulatory ECG monitoring. Pediatr Cardiol. 1987;8:103-8.
4. Losek JD, Endom E, Dietrich A, *et al.* Adenosine and pediatric supraventricular tachycardia in the emergency department: Multicenter study and review. Ann Emerg Med. 1999;33:185-91.
5. Poutiainen AM, Koistinen MJ, Airaksinen *et al.* Prevalence and natural course of ectopic atrial tachycardia. Eur Heart J. 1999; 20:694-700.
6. Francis J. Junctional ectopic tachycardia. Indian Pacing Electrophysiol J. 2010;10:288-91.
7. Moak JP, Arias P, Kaltman JR, *et al.* Postoperative junctional ectopic tachycardia: Risk factors for occurrence in the modern surgical era. Pacing Clin Electrophysiol. 2013;36:1156-68.
8. Sarubbi B, Vergara P, D'Alto M, Calabro R. Congenital junctional ectopic tachycardia: Presentation and outcome. Indian Pacing Electrophysiol J. 2003;3:143-7.
9. Crosson JE, Callans DJ, Bradley DJ, *et al.* PACES/HRS expert consensus statement on the evaluation and management of ventricular arrhythmias in the child with a structurally normal heart. Heart Rhythm. 2014;11:e55-78.
10. Jaeggi E, Ohman A. Fetal and neonatal arrhythmias. Clin Perinatol. 2016;43:99-112.
11. Lee AKY, Deyell MW. Premature ventricular contraction-induced cardiomyopathy. Curr Opin Cardiol. 2016;31:1-10.
12. Drago F, Battipaglia I, Di Mambro C. Neonatal and pediatric arrhythmias: Clinical and electrocardiographic aspects. Card Electrophysiol Clin. 2018;10:397-412.
13. Ergul Y, Koca S, Akdeniz C, *et al.* Electroanatomic mapping-guided catheter ablation of supraventricular tachycardia in children with Ebstein's anomaly. Pediatr Cardiol. 2018;39: 1445-52.
14. Sorbo MD, Buja GF, Miorelli M, *et al.* The prevalence of the Wolff-Parkinson-White syndrome in a population of 116, 542 young males. G Ital Cardiol. 1995;25:681-7.
15. Savini E, Capone PL. Wolff-Parkinson-White, a study on the prevalence of the site of accessory pathways: Relations between stability of pre-excitation, symptoms, cardiac arrhythmias and association of mitral valve prolapse with localization of pre-excitation. Minerva Cardioangiol. 1994;42:339-43.
16. Watanabe S, Yoshida Y, Suzuki T, *et al.* Successful catheter ablation using real-time ultrasound-assisted 3-D electroanatomical mapping system for atrioventricular accessory pathway in a. Heart Rhythm Case Rep. 2016;2:351-5.
17. Hernandez-Madrid A, Sanchez I, Matia R. Multiple accessory pathways in a patient with congenitally corrected transposition of the great arteries and severe malformation of the coronary sinus. Europace. 2014;16:108.
18. Chavan C, Rao HB, Badani RS, *et al.* Ablation of incessant orthodromic reciprocating tachycardia in a child with congenitally corrected transposition of great arteries and ebsteinoid malformation of left atrioventricular valve. J Interv Card Electrophysiol. 2008;23:149-52.
19. Un H, Dogan M, Uz O, *et al.* Novel vagal maneuver technique for termination of supraventricular tachycardias. Am J Emerg Med. 2016;34:118.e5-7.
20. Deal BJ, Keane JF, Gillette PC, *et al.* Wolff-Parkinson-White syndrome and supraventricular tachycardia during infancy: Management and follow-up. J Am Coll Cardiol. 1985;5: 130-5.
21. Sanatani S, Potts JE, Reed JH, *et al.* The study of antiarrhythmic medications in infancy (SAMIS): A multicenter, randomized controlled trial comparing the efficacy and safety of digoxin versus propranolol for prophylaxis of supraventricular tachycardia in infants. Circ Arrhythm Electrophysiol. 2012;5: 984-91.
22. Kohli U, Pumphrey KL, Ahmed A, *et al.* Pre-excitation induced ventricular dysfunction and successful berlin heart explantation after accessory pathway ablation. J Electrocardiol. 2018;51:1067-70.
23. Dalili M, Vahidshahi K, Aarabi-Moghaddam MY, *et al.* Exercise testing in children with Wolff-Parkinson-White syndrome: What is its value? Pediatr Cardiol. 2014;35: 1142-6.
24. Kang KT, Etheridge SP, Kantoch MJ, *et al.* Current management of focal atrial tachycardia in children: A multicenter experience. Circ Arrhythm Electrophysiol. 2014;7:664-70.
25. Bouziri A, Khaldi A, Hamdi A, *et al.* Multifocal atrial tachycardia: An unusual cause of cardiogenic shock in a newborn. Tunis Med. 2011;89:59-61.
26. Prasad D, Steinberg J, Snyder C. Cost-effectiveness of digoxin, pacing, and direct current cardioversion for conversion of atrial flutter in neonates. Cardiol Young. 2018;28:725-9.
27. Zimetbaum P. Atrial fibrillation. Ann Intern Med. 2017;166: ITC33-48.
28. Laird WP, Snyder CS, Kertesz NJ, *et al.* Use of intravenous amiodarone for postoperative junctional ectopic tachycardia in children. Pediatr Cardiol. 2003;24:133-7.
29. Zeppenfeld K. Ventricular tachycardia in repaired congenital heart disease. Herzschrittmacherther Elektrophysiol. 2016;27: 131-6.
30. Khairy P, Harris L, Landzberg MJ, *et al.* Implantable cardioverter-defibrillators in tetralogy of Fallot. Circulation. 2008 Jan 22;117:363-70.
31. Kaiser E, Darrieux FCC, Barbosa SA, *et al.* Differential diagnosis of wide QRS tachycardias: Comparison of two electrocardiographic algorithms. Europace. 2015;17:1422-7.
32. Buxton AE, Calkins H, Callans DJ, *et al.* ACC/AHA/HRS 2006 key data elements and definitions for electrophysiological studies and procedures: A report of the American College of Cardiology/American Heart Association Task Force on Clinical Data Standards (ACC/AHA/HRS Writing Committee to Develop Data Standards on Electrophysiology). Circulation. 2006;114:2534-70.
33. Shah AJ, Hocini M, Denis A, *et al.* Polymorphic ventricular tachycardia/ventricular fibrillation and sudden cardiac death in the normal heart. Card Electrophysiol Clin. 2016;8: 581-91.
34. Epstein AE, Dimarco JP, Ellenbogen KA, *et al.* ACC/AHA/HRS 2008 guidelines for device-based therapy of cardiac rhythm abnormalities: Executive summary. Heart Rhythm. 2008; 5:934-55.

CHAPTER

23

Emergencies in Congenital Heart Disease

Amber Kumar, Mahesh Maheshwari

INTRODUCTION

Cardiac emergencies in children comprise a spectrum of conditions that includes manifestations of undiagnosed, unoperated and palliated congenital heart diseases (CHD) and wide range of arrhythmias. The incidence of CHD reported across the world as 8–10/1000 live births,[1] whereas nearly one third to half of these are critical CHD requiring intervention in the first year of life.[2] The prevalence of CHD reported in various series across India range from 2.25 to 5.2/1000 live births.[3] The pediatrician posted in the emergency services should have the essential knowledge of the wide spectrum of cardiac disease to diagnose cardiac emergencies and to provide appropriate therapy and early referral, as they are the first line of care in any emergency.

The most challenging scenarios of cardiac emergencies in children present in the following four ways:

1. Cyanosis
2. Cardiogenic shock
3. Congestive heart failure (CHF)
4. Arrhythmias.

Duct dependent congenital heart disease is the most common cause of emergency admission in neonatal age group and will appear with cyanosis and shock. In children less than 2 years of age, cyanotic spells is the presenting symptom in emergency room in cases of CHD with decreased pulmonary blood flow situations (TOF physiology). Whereas CHF either due to pump failure or volume overload and respiratory tract infections are the most common presentations of CHD with increased pulmonary blood flow situation. In a patient with cardiogenic shock, the result of outflow obstruction and/or pump failure, the infant may appear mottled and ashen, which is not the usual finding in left-to-right shunt lesions and congestive heart failure scenarios.

Structural congenital heart disease is usually divided into cyanotic and acyanotic groups. Acyanotic category is further divided into lesions with left-to-right shunt and lesions with left ventricular outflow obstruction **(Flowchart 1)**. The cyanotic heart disease can be divided into increased and decreased pulmonary blood flow situation **(Flowchart 2)**. This chapter will focus on the cardiac emergencies that usually present in the neonatal, infantile and childhood period.

EMERGENCIES IN NEONATAL PERIOD

Deoxygenated hemoglobin is blue and the presence of noticeable cyanosis means that there is 3 to 5 g/dL of deoxyhemoglobin in the blood, corresponding with the room air saturation of 70% to 85%. The presence of anemia might mask clinically apparent cyanosis, because the oxygen carrying capacity is based on the amount of hemoglobin available to carry oxygen. An infant who is polycythemic, cyanosis can be detected at around 80–85% saturation, whereas in anemic child (Hb-6 g/dL), cyanosis usually appears at a saturation of 45–50% or below.

Hyperoxia test: This is used to differentiate between cardiac and non-cardiac causes of cyanosis. Pulse oximetry and an arterial blood gas determination from right radial artery should be performed initially on room air as baseline and then on 100% oxygen. Neonates with pulmonary or

Flowchart 1: Classification of acyanotic heart disease

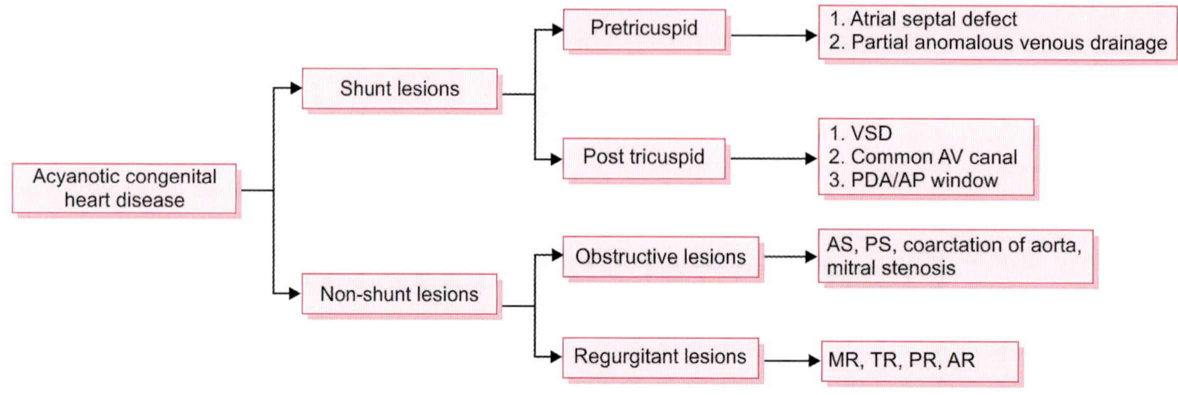

Flowchart 2: Classification of cyanotic heart disease

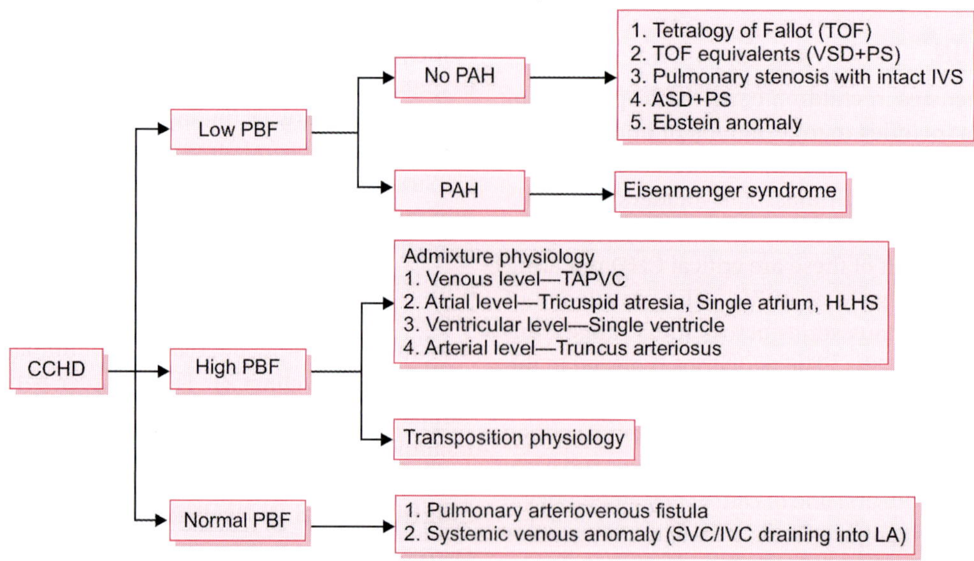

neurological causes of cyanosis reveals significant rise in partial pressure of oxygen (PO_2 > 300 mm Hg). Cyanotic heart disease can be ruled out reliably with PO_2 > 300 mm Hg. An arterial PO_2 < 100 mm Hg is indicator of intracardiac right to left shunt and especially in the absence of respiratory illness; it reliably points towards duct dependent congenital cyanotic heart disease. Prostaglandin infusion is indicated in these neonates until the confirmation of echocardiographic diagnosis.[4-5] The third group of children having an arterial PO_2 between 100 and 300 mm Hg may have congenital heart disease with increased pulmonary blood flow situations like admixture lesions[4] **(Table 1)**.

Duct dependent circulations ***(Flowchart 3)***: Infants with severe congenital heart disease can have a relatively normal physical examination prior to discharge from the newborn unit, due to patent ductus arteriosus (PDA). The PDA used to close normally in initial two weeks of life, but it may take up to 2 months. Neonates with duct dependent lesions, constriction of duct may lead to severe cyanosis and/or shock. It is imperative to realize that any infant under 2 month of age, who presents in profound circulatory compromise and/or deep cyanosis might be the result of duct constriction in a right or left sided obstructive cardiac condition.[6]

Neonate Presenting with Circulatory Collapse (Duct Dependent Systemic Circulation)

These include the congenital heart disease with left-sided obstructive lesions like critical aortic stenosis, severe coarctation of the aorta and hypoplastic left heart syndrome (HLHS), where systemic circulation is dependent on the patent ductus arteriosus for survival. PDA closure in HLHS results in systemic hypoperfusion leading to circulatory collapse and shock. Signs of critical coarctation of the aorta are weak or absent femoral pulses with upper limb hypertension, reflecting the gradient across the stenotic aortic segment. The patient will present with signs of systemic hypoperfusion/shock and/or cardiac failure. Prostaglandin infusion is indicated here to reopen and maintain the patency of PDA apart from timely initiation of basic resuscitative measures like airway, breathing and circulation.

Table 1: Hyperoxia test

Hyperoxia test (Right radial ABG in air and after 10 min of 100% O_2)	
Result	*Interpretation*
$PaO_2 > 300$ mm Hg	Excludes cyanotic CHD
$PaO_2 > 100$ <300 mm Hg	Unlikely to be cyanotic CHD (NB: False negative in TAPVC-Unobstructed)
$PaO_2 < 100$ mm Hg (usually lower)	Likely to be cyanotic CHD Differentials: Severe lung disease (high $PaCO_2$), Persistent pulmonary hypertension of newborn (PPHN)

Medical management

The management of these neonates starts with basic resuscitative measures like airway, breathing and circulation. Establishing stable vascular access followed by correction of metabolic acidosis and treatment of shock should be the top priority. Mainstay of therapy is the infusion of prostaglandin E1 (alprostadil) to reopen the PDA and maintain its patency. The starting dose of PGE1 is usually 0.05 μg/kg/minute intravenous

Flowchart 3: Classification of duct dependent lesions

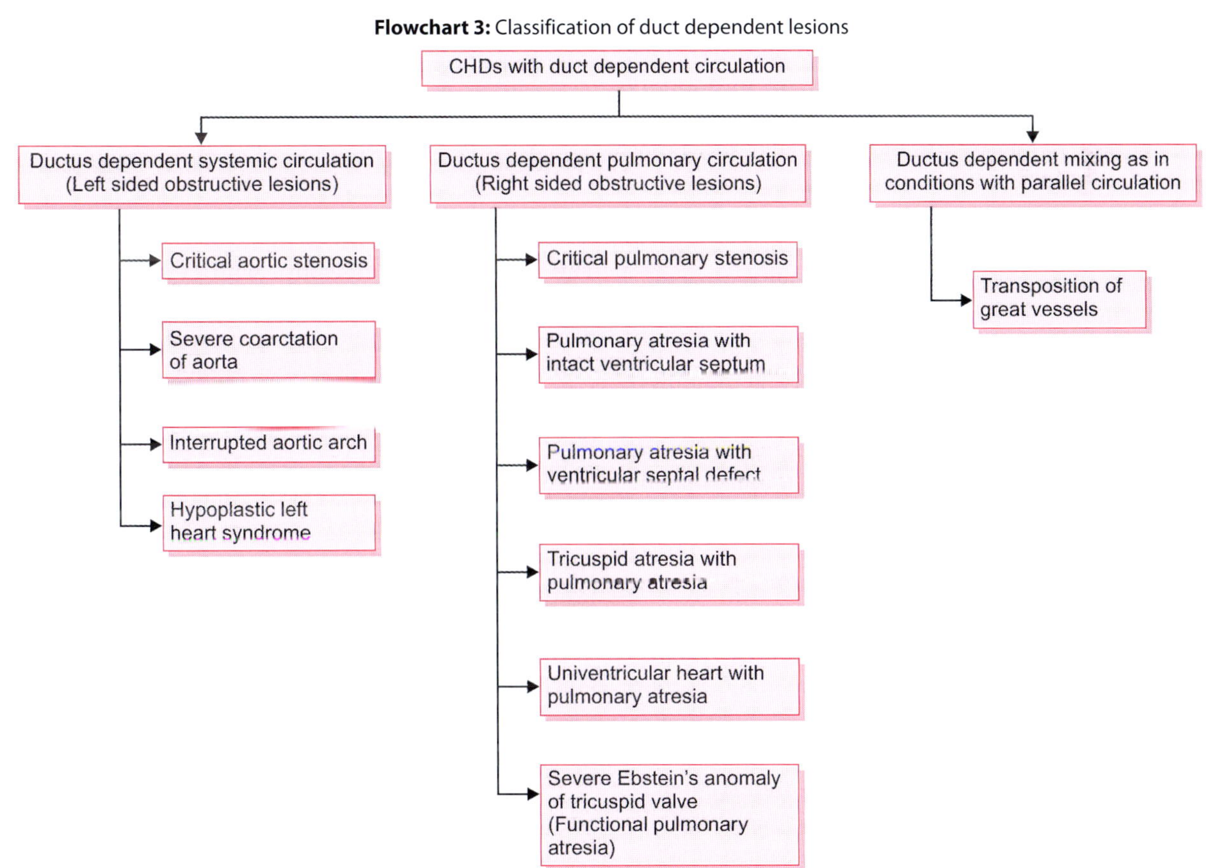

infusions and that can be increased to 0.1 µg/kg/minute to achieve the desired effect of normal perfusion. Dose should be gradually reduced to 0.01 µg/kg/minute after establishment of normal perfusion. Continuous cardiorespiratory monitoring is required during infusion, as the most common serious adverse effect of PGE1 is apnea (may occur in 10–12% of cases), usually within 6 hours of infusion. Other important side effects in decreasing order of frequency are fever (14%), flushing (10%), bradycardia (7%) and seizures (4%).[7]

It is imperative to use oxygen judiciously considering the underlying cardiac anatomy and expected oxygen saturation for the congenital heart defect, as it can even harm the patient. In hypoplastic left heart syndrome, oxygen administration to achieve 100% saturation would be detrimental for the infant as the reduction in pulmonary vascular resistance with oxygen ultimately compromises the systemic perfusion.[8] In patients with critical coarctation of aorta, the lower limbs blood supply will be extremely compromised, so venous access should be established either in right upper limb or in scalp veins for appropriate management of shock. It is crucial to maintain a balance between systemic and pulmonary blood flow and since the systemic perfusion is dependent on pulmonary vascular resistance (PVR), so any medications and/or any maneuver that reduces pulmonary vascular resistance should be avoided. Judicious use of inotropes to increase the systemic vascular resistance (SVR) and avoidance of hyperventilation to achieve PO_2 between 40 and 50 mm Hg (oxygen saturation in range of 70–80%) should be the target to manage these cases. At centers without intensive care facility, prostaglandin E2 (dinoprostone) in a dose of 25 µg/kg orally or through nasogastric tube every 30 minutes–1 hour is an alternative option. Oral prostaglandin E2 is a safe alternative and it will not harm even in cases of wrong interpretation of cyanotic CHD. Prostaglandins may be used for reopening of PDA in neonatal period (up to one month of age).

Definitive treatment

Balloon dilatation of aortic valve is preferred in neonates with critical aortic stenosis having duct dependent systemic circulation with adequate left ventricular size which can handle systemic circulation on echocardiography evaluation.[9] Surgery is preferred over balloon dilatation in neonates with coarctation of aorta, as balloon procedure has high risk of restenosis (>80%). Although balloon dilatation is an alternate option with immediate good result in sick babies having severe sepsis or organ dysfunction.[10] Surgery is the only available option in case of interrupted arch. The treatment of hypoplastic left heart syndrome is Norwood staged operation whereas cardiac transplantation is the last resort.[11]

Neonates Presenting with Cyanosis (Duct Dependent Pulmonary Circulation)

Right-sided obstructive lesions are severe tetralogy of Fallot and pulmonary atresia with intact ventricular septum, which depends on patent duct to maintain pulmonary blood flow. Infants usually develop rapid cyanosis, unresponsive to oxygen administration with progressive constriction of duct. Unrecognized cases land up in severe hypoxemia, respiratory distress, metabolic acidosis that ultimately leads to death. As evident by the physiology of duct dependent pulmonary circulation, systemic perfusion is not affected till the very end. The progression of cyanosis is dependent on rate of reduction in pulmonary blood flow with constriction of the duct.

Echocardiography helps in establishing correct anatomy of congenital heart lesion and in its absence, physiological diagnosis should be made with the help of history, clinical findings, blood gas analysis, electrocardiography, chest X-ray, and hyperoxia test.

Management

The treatment of a newborn with cyanosis starts with correction of metabolic abnormalities like acidosis, dehydration and hypoglycemia. Baby should be initiated on PGE1 infusion (as described earlier), if the saturation drops below 70%. Definitive surgery of two ventricle repair or single ventricle palliation pathway in staged repair has to be decided based on the size of right ventricle, which can be easily assessed on echocardiography.

Obstructed Total Anomalous Pulmonary Venous Connection

This is a type of surgical cardiac emergency. These cases usually presents in neonatal age group with severe cyanosis and respiratory distress.

EMERGENCIES IN INFANTS AND CHILDREN

See the chapter numbers 21 and 22 for Congestive Heart Failure and Arrhythmias.

CYANOTIC SPELL (TET SPELL; HYPERCYANOTIC SPELL)

Definition

A typical spell begins with paroxysmal hyperpnea (progressive increase in rate and depth of respiration), increasing cyanosis followed by limpness, syncope, convulsions, cerebrovascular accident and even death. The spells are usually self-limited usually within 30 minutes. During the spell, the ejection systolic murmur (ESM) of infundibular stenosis, which is heard along the left sternal border, may disappear or diminish in intensity. Classical cyanotic spells are common in; tetralogy of Fallot, transposition of great arteries with pulmonary stenosis (PS), double outlet right ventricle with VSD with PS, tricuspid atresia with VSD with PS, single ventricle with PS.

Pathophysiology

The interplay between systemic vascular resistance and the severity of pulmonary stenosis determines the degree of cyanosis and onset of cyanotic spell in a case of tetralogy of Fallot (TOF). There is equalization of pressure between left and right ventricle in a typical case of TOF, whereas in cases of mild pulmonary stenosis the shunt is usually left to right. In a case of TOF with cyanotic spells, the systemic vascular resistance is low, resulting in right to left shunt across the VSD that leads to progressive cyanosis. The vicious cycle of cyanotic spell starts with hypoxemia causing stimulation of the carotid receptors and the brainstem nuclei, which leads to hyperpnea in a child resulting in increased venous return to the right atrium and thus more right to left shunt of deoxygenated blood across the unrestrictive VSD. Timely interruption of vicious cycle of spell prevents the progressive worsening of the hemodynamic condition of the baby **(Flowchart 4)**.

Following theories as a possible explanation for the cause of cyanotic spells have been proposed by various scientists:

1. *Wood's theory*[12]: Wood's believes that the hypoxemic spells are initiated by the infundibular spasm of right ventricle, which leads to increased right to left shunt resulting in hypoxemia and metabolic acidosis.
2. *Catecholamine theory*: Any cause like irritability or crying causes rise in catecholamine levels, which leads to increased myocardial contractility and increased infundibular stenosis.

Flowchart 4: Schematic representation of vicious cycle of cyanotic spell as described by Guntheroth et al

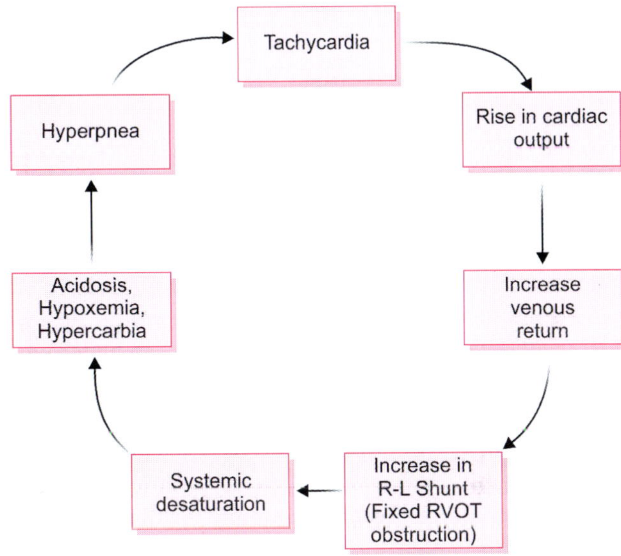

3. *Morgan theory*: Spells are common in early morning or on waking up from the sleep. Respiratory center is sensitive to prolonged sleep, which reacts to rise in cardiac output provoked by feeding, crying and straining, which initiate the vicious cycle by increasing the right sided venous return and so more right to left shunt across the VSD.
4. *Guntheroth's theory*[13]: He proposed paroxysmal hyperpnea is the underlying cause rather being the effect of cyanotic spells. Increased systemic venous return with increase in rate and depth of respiration leads to more right to left shunt of deoxygenated blood.
5. *Kothari theory*[14]: They propose the role of stimulation of mechanoreceptors present in the right ventricle to be the underlying cause of spells.

Clinical Manifestations

Typically cyanotic spells occur early in the morning when the systemic vascular resistance is lowest and similarly on waking up from the day time sleep. It commonly occurs in infants between 2 months to 1 year of age. The triggers of cyanotic spells are fever, irritability, crying, straining, anemia, sepsis or even spontaneously without any cause. The theory behind this mechanism is drop of systemic vascular resistance with increase in left to right shunt during exercise.

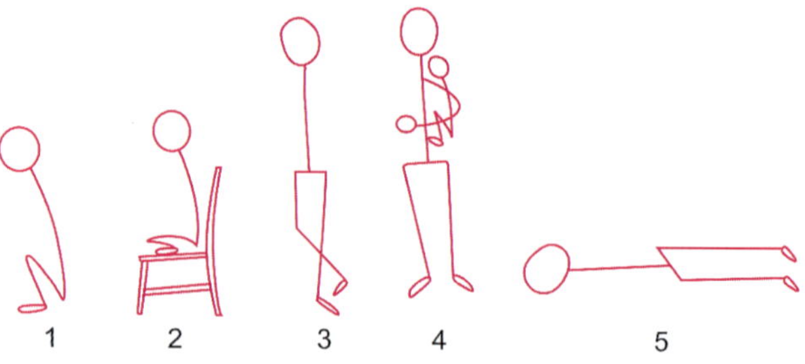

Fig. 1: Squatting equivalents

An infant with typical cyanotic spell would appear fussy with inconsolable cry, that progresses to hyperpnea and deep cyanosis, which characterizes the spell.

Mechanisms postulated for the less occurrence of the spell after the age of 2 years could be: The child learns to squat by habit, maturation of the respiratory center by this age, collaterals development and/or fibrosis of the infundibulum, which prevents it from developing a spasm.

Flowchart 5: Squatting mechanism in relieving cyanotic spell

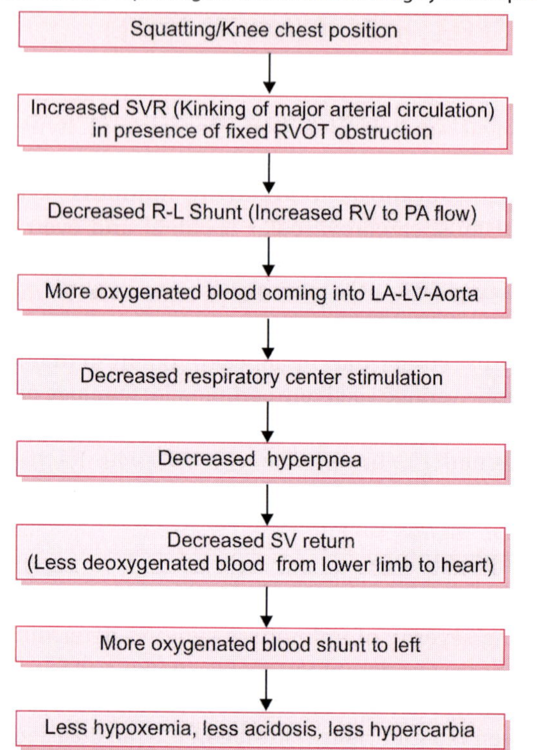

Management

1. *Knee chest position/Squatting* ***(Fig. 1)***: The initial step of management of cyanotic spell in a conscious child is to put him/her in a knee chest position against the mother's shoulder and squatting position in older children, which increases the systemic vascular resistance resulting in decrease right to left shunt across the VSD level **(Flowchart 5)**.
2. *Oxygen*: Oxygen has a little effect on arterial saturation, as the shunt is a central right to left shunt. Here the limited pulmonary blood flow is causing the hypoxemia; hence oxygen may be of little benefit. Oxygen may be administered, but it should be stopped if this agitates the child, as the agitation will worsen the spell more.
3. *Hydration*: Hydration increases the right ventricular preload and thus might increase the right ventricular output. Intravenous fluid boluses of isotonic saline 10–20 mL/kg are indicated in cyanotic spell. TOF physiology is not prone for CHF because of restrictive RV physiology.
4. *Acidosis correction*: Acidosis stimulates the respiratory center, so metabolic acidosis correction by slow intravenous infusion of sodium bicarbonate in a dose of 1–2 mEq/kg is indicated in cyanotic spell.
5. *Morphine*: Morphine in a dose of 0.1 to 0.2 mg/kg IV, SC or IM can be given with ventilation backup. The various possible mechanisms by which morphine helps in breaking the vicious cycle of spell are as follows:
   - Morphine induced respiratory center depression abolishes the hyperpnea.
   - Morphine induced relaxing effect on subpulmonary infundibulum via central or through peripheral vagotonic effect.
   - Morphine induced sedation reduces the release of norepinephrine.
   - Respiratory center depression also decreases the systemic venous return.
6. *Inj Metoprolol*: Injection metoprolol 0.1 mg/kg over 5 min under BP and ECG monitoring followed by repeat dose every 5 minutes with total of 3 doses can be given. Infusion metoprolol at the rate of 1–5 μg/kg/min can be considered afterwards. Once stable can be switched to oral propranolol. Injection esmolol is an alternative short acting beta-blocker which is recommended in a dose of 0.5 mg/kg over 1 min followed by 50 μg/kg/min over 4 min. The various possible mechanisms by which

β-blockers helps in breaking the vicious cycle of spell are as follows:

- Reduce dynamic RV outflow obstruction by reducing infundibular spasm.
- Decrease in heart rate (Less R→ L Shunt).
- Slight increase in systemic vascular resistance.
- Blunting of hyperpnea response.

Few authors recommend the cardiac pacing facility in cases of drug-induced bradycardia with beta blockers. It is rarely seen with metoprolol. Metoprolol in comparison to propranolol is short acting, so mere stopping the infusion of metoprolol in case of bradycardia, will reverse the effect within one hour. Isoproterenol is the antidote of beta-blocker overdose.

7. *Phenylephrine hydrochloride*: It increases the systemic vascular resistance (SVR), and the recommended dose is 0.01 mg/kg slow IV or 0.1 mg/kg SC/IM. The dose has to be titrated to achieve the target BP. Alternatively, methoxamine 0.1 mg/kg IV can be given over 5 minutes which leads to similar increase in SVR.
8. *Ketamine*: Ketamine 0.5–1.0 mg/kg IV or IM has dual benefit of causing sedation and increasing the SVR.
9. *Transfuse PRBC's*: 5–10 mL/kg PRBC can be transfused over 4–5 hr if hemoglobin is less than 12 g/dL.
10. *Correct tachyarrhythmia*: This will improve the diastolic filling and cardiac output.
11. *Emergency systemic-to-pulmonary artery shunt (Blalock-Taussig shunt)* is rarely required for refractory spells.

Prevention of Spell

Propranolol (1–4 mg/kg), orally in divided doses is highly effective in deferring the surgery till the time child is older (>1 year of age) and the risk of surgery is low, although current strategy is early intracardiac repair to prevent development of right ventricular dysfunction. Repeated spells also leads to brain damage and mental retardation and hamper the growth of the child. Prolonged hypoxic spells may lead to cerebral venous sinus thrombosis.

CONGESTIVE HEART FAILURE (CHF)

Duct dependent lesions usually present after duct closure within the first two weeks of life, other CHD usually present in 4 to 6 weeks after birth with the fall in pulmonary vascular resistance like ventricular septal defect or patent ductus arteriosus.[15] Large left to right shunt lesions lead to increased pulmonary blood flow, volume overload of left atrium and left ventricle and finally congestive heart failure. These infants with CHF usually manifest with poor feeding, tachypnea, and forehead sweating resulting in malnutrition/failure to thrive. Following cardiac conditions can lead to CHF in pediatric age group: large left to right shunt lesions (e.g. VSD, PDA), congenital cardiomyopathies more of dilated cardiomyopathy (both acquired and non-compacted type), ALCAPA (anomalous left coronary artery from the pulmonary artery) and/or arrhythmias.

The ALCAPA typically presents when the pulmonary artery (PA) pressure declines at around two months of age and they usually die within the first year of life, if left untreated. They typically present with episodic irritability (angina pain), sweating during the feed (increase in myocardial oxygen consumption) and signs of CHF because of myocardial ischemia (anterolateral infarct pattern).[16] Timely diagnosis of ALCAPA and early surgical correction has excellent results with gradual improvement in myocardial function with time. See chapter 21 for management of CHF.

Arrhythmias

See Chapter 22.

COMPLICATIONS OF PALLIATED CONGENITAL HEART DISEASE

Single ventricle physiology, TOF physiology or pulmonary atresia patients born with the obstruction of pulmonary blood flow receive an aortic to pulmonary artery shunt, usually a modified Blalock-Taussig shunt (BT shunt) or underwent PDA stenting. Modified BT shunt material made up of Gore-Tex graft usually connects the subclavian artery with ipsilateral pulmonary artery.[17] The most feared, and most fatal, complication in patients with palliated shunts or PDA stents is an occlusive thrombus within the Gore-Tex graft or intraluminal stent. Severe cyanosis and respiratory distress are the usual presenting features of severely obstructed PDA stent or BT shunt and rapid hemodynamic deterioration is the rule in these cases, ultimately leads to cardiac arrest in the absence of timely diagnosis in emergency situation. A continuous murmur of the BT shunt or PDA stent should normally be audible on auscultation. Absence or faintly audible murmur is a classical sign of obstructed BT shunt or PDA stent, and the management starts with care of airway, breathing, circulation as per basic life support protocol. In cases of suspected obstructed shunt or PDA stent, heparin should be initiated early to prevent the progression of the thrombus, especially in cases of acute events. Transcatheter shunt opening by interventional pediatric cardiologist or shunt revision by cardiac surgeon is the definitive treatment in emergency settings. Patients with uncorrected or palliated cyanotic congenital heart disease may present with cerebrovascular accidents (CVAs) and brain abscess, which is supposed to be caused by intracardiac right to left shunt. Prevention and timely treatment of iron deficiency anemia and dehydration may prevent CVA of infancy and early childhood. Timely palliative or complete corrective surgery is the only means to decrease the frequency of CVA by preventing severe hypoxemia and polycythemia.

KEY MESSAGES

- Neonates with critical CHD usually present with either severe cyanosis and cardiogenic shock or acute heart failure situation which can mimic neonatal sepsis or lung disease. Nearly everyone will require catheter or surgical intervention in the first month of life.
- The hyperoxia test is a basic screening tool to differentiate cardiac and non-cardiac causes of cyanosis.
- Prostaglandin, an essential life-saving drug, should be commenced as early as possible in case of suspicion of critical CHD. Prostaglandin therapy to reopen and maintain the patency of duct is indicated for both duct-dependent pulmonary blood flow situations and duct-dependent systemic blood flow situations.
- Judicious use of oxygen is recommended for congenital heart lesions having usual saturations of around 75% to 85%.
- Management of an acutely obstructed shunt involves first the basic life support and heparin infusion should be commenced early to prevent the progression of the thrombus.

REFERENCES

1. Abdulla R. What is the prevalence of congenital heart diseases? Ped Cardiol. 1997;18:268.
2. Hoffman JI, Kaplan S. The incidence of congenital heart disease. J Am Coll Cardiol. 2002;39:1890-900.
3. Saxena A. Congenital heart disease in India: A status report. Indian J Pediatr. 2005;72:595-8.
4. Gardner TH. Cardiac emergencies in the newborn period. Radio Clin North Am. 1971;9:385-97.
5. Wechsler SB, Wernovsky G. Cardiac disorders. In: John PC, Ann RS, editors. Manual of Neonatal Care—Joint Program in Neonatology. Philadelphia: Lippincott-Raven; 1998.
6. Colletti JE, Homme JL, Woodridge DP. Unsuspected neonatal killers in emergency medicine. Emerg Med Clin North Am. 2004;22:929-60.
7. Coceani F. Prostaglandins and the central nervous system. Arch Interm Med. 1974;133:119.
8. Schamberger MS. Cardiac emergencies in children. Pediatr Ann. 1996;25:339-44.
9. Lee C, Mason LJ. Pediatric cardiac emergencies. Anesthesiol Clin North Am. 2001;19:286-309.
10. Gewitz M, Vetter V. Cardiac emergencies. In: Fleisher GR, Ludwig S, editors. Text Book of Pediatric Emergency Medicine. Philadelphia: Lippincott, Williams and Wilkins; 2000.
11. Norwood WI, Kirklin JK, Sanders SP. Hypoplastic left heart syndrome: Experience with palliative surgery. Am J Cardiol. 1980;45:87-91.
12. Wood P. Attack of Deeper cyanosis and loss of consciousness (syncope) in Fallot's Tetralogy. Br Heart J. 1958;20:282-6.
13. Guntheroth WG, Morgan BC, Mullins GL. Physiologic studies of paroxysmal hyperpnea in cyanotic congenital heart disease. Circulation. 1965;31:70.
14. Kothari SS. Mechanism of cyanotic spells in tetralogy of Fallot--the missing link? Int J Cardiol. 1992;37:1-5.
15. Massin MM, Malekzadeh-Milani SG, Van Aerschot I, *et al.* Management of cardiac emergencies in children. Minerva Pediatr. 2009;61:163-73.
16. Park MK. Pediatric Cardiology for Practitioners, 5th edition. Missouri: Mosby; 2008. pp. 62-4; 314-5.
17. Blalock A, Taussig HB. Landmark article May 19, 1945: The surgical treatment of malformations of the heart in which there is pulmonary stenosis or pulmonary atresia. JAMA. 1984;251: 2123-38.

CHAPTER

24

Hypertensive Emergencies

Christy Cathreen Thomas, Aditi Sinha

Severe hypertension, also called hypertensive crisis, is uncommon in children. It is a potentially life-threatening emergency that calls for immediate medical attention to prevent or limit end-organ damage. While the level of blood pressure determines the gravity of situation, the rapidity of rise of blood pressure and end-organ damage are more important than the absolute level of blood pressure.

DEFINITION

Hypertension in children is classified based on age, gender and height percentiles and were recently revised in the guidelines provided by the American Academy of Pediatrics (**Table 1**).[1,2] **Severe hypertension** is defined as stage II hypertension that is accompanied by symptoms, with or without abnormalities on examination or biochemistry.[3] Usually, a diastolic blood pressure of more than 110 mm Hg in an adolescent is considered as severe hypertension.

Traditionally, hypertensive crises are further classified as **hypertensive emergencies** and **hypertensive urgencies.**[4] **Hypertensive emergency** is defined as severe hypertension with target organ damage and life-threatening complications. **Hypertensive urgency** is characterized by severe hypertension with no or mild symptoms and no target end organ damage. Hence, hypertensive emergencies can have encephalopathy, cardiac failure, retinal hemorrhage and renal dysfunction, while severe hypertension in the absence of clinical or laboratory evidence of end-organ damage is referred as hypertensive urgency. If left untreated, hypertensive urgency may progress to an emergency. However, the distinction is not absolute, and is based on clinical judgment.

ETIOLOGY

An increasing proportion of children with hypertension, particularly adolescents in developed countries, are diagnosed to have essential or primary hypertension.[5] However, essential hypertension rarely presents as an emergency. The majority of children with hypertensive crisis have secondary hypertension, and kidney disease is the most common etiology. Hypertensive emergencies may accompany acute kidney injury, particularly rapidly progressive glomerulonephritis or atypical hemolytic syndrome. It is not uncommon for children to present with severe hypertension and then be diagnosed with renovascular stenosis, or with advanced chronic kidney disease (CKD) with fluid overload. Hypertensive crisis also occur in context of known hypertension, due to non-compliance to antihypertensive medications (**Table 2**). Patients with CKD stage 5 on dialysis may

Table 1: Definition and staging of hypertension in children

Elevated blood pressure	SBP or DBP 90–95th percentile
Hypertension	SBP or DBP > 95th percentile
Stage I hypertension	SBP or DBP between 95th percentile and 95th percentile + 12 mm Hg
Stage II hypertension	SBP or DBP >95th percentile + 12 mm Hg

(SBP: systolic blood pressure; DBP: diastolic blood pressure)

Table 2: Important causes of severe hypertension
Renal
Parenchymal: Acute glomerulonephritis, hemolytic uremic syndrome, chronic glomerulonephritis, obstructive uropathy, reflux nephropathy, hypodysplasia
Vascular: Renal artery stenosis (Takayasu aortoarteritis, fibromuscular dysplasia), polyarteritis nodosa, other vasculitis
Cystic: Polycystic kidney disease
Neoplastic: Wilms tumor, neurofibromatosis
Monogenic causes (e.g. glucocorticoid remediable hypertension)
Cardiovascular: Coarctation of aorta, aortoarteritis
Endocrine: Pheochromocytoma, neuroblastoma, Cushing disease, Conn syndrome
Miscellaneous: Therapy with corticosteroids or calcineurin inhibitors, Guillain-Barré syndrome, medication non-compliance in known hypertensive patient, abuse of illicit substance (e.g. cocaine)
"Rebound" hypertension due to rapid withdrawal of clonidine or beta-adrenergic blockers

develop hypertensive crisis due to inadequate dialysis and/or poor compliance to salt and water restriction.

PATHOGENESIS

The rapidity of onset, degree of elevation and duration of persistence of elevated blood pressure have critical role in the pathogenesis of hypertensive emergency. Endothelial dysfunction, oxidative stress, dysregulation in renin angiotensin aldosterone system and/or sympathetic system, and fluid overload appear to mediate the effects of severe hypertension.[6] Various humoral and myogenic mechanisms mediate autoregulation of blood pressure in cerebral, renal and cardiovascular circulation (**Fig. 1**). Elevation of blood pressure beyond the threshold of autoregulatory limits causes hypertensive changes to be transmitted to the distal circulation leading to damage of vasculature.

CLINICAL FEATURES

Hypertensive emergencies are typically associated with a rapid rise in blood pressure. The presentation varies widely, from totally asymptomatic state to symptoms suggesting a primary cardiac, neurological or ocular disorder.[7] Common clinical features include nausea, headache, vomiting, blurred vision, confusion, agitation or frank encephalopathy, manifest as seizures and altered sensorium. However, elevated blood pressure may be present without such symptoms and, therefore, blood pressure should be evaluated in all unwell children. Newborns and infants may present with atypical

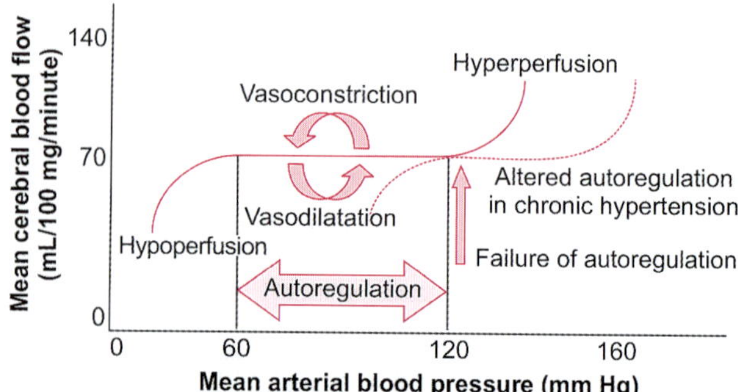

Fig. 1: Altered cerebral autoregulation in chronic severe hypertension

presentations like apnea, cyanosis, extreme irritability or hypotonia. Chronic elevation of blood pressure is surprisingly well tolerated, particularly in neonates.

The presentation may also provide leads to diagnosis. Asymmetry of pulses suggests Takayasu aortoarteritis. Cutaneous markers of neurofibromatosis may be present. Children with renovascular hypertension may sometimes present with polyuria, weight loss, hyponatremia and hypokalemic metabolic alkalosis, termed the hyponatremic hypertensive syndrome.

Evidence of end-organ damage includes left ventricular hypertrophy, congestive cardiac failure and hypertensive retinopathy. Rarely, severe hypertension may trigger thrombotic microangiopathy, characterized by features of anemia, thrombocytopenia and acute kidney injury. Other rare complications include myocardial infarction or aortic dissection.

Encephalopathy is common and represents a severe form of hypertensive emergency.[4] The condition is caused by a failure of the autoregulation of cerebral blood flow, leading to impaired cerebral perfusion. Symptoms include headache, vomiting, lethargy, confusion, altered sensorium, stupor, seizures and ataxia.[8] Focal neurological deficits such as hemiparesis, blindness and facial nerve palsy may be present.[9] Magnetic resonance imaging detects characteristic findings of leukoencephalopathy, predominantly affecting the parieto-occipital white matter. These changes are potentially reversible with correction of hypertension.[10]

Clinical presentation influences the management strategy. Children presenting with severe symptoms need more aggressive blood pressure control than those who are asymptomatic. Presence of papilledema, retinal hemorrhages, congestive heart failure and pulmonary edema indicate hypertensive crisis.

EVALUATION

It is extremely rare for primary or essential hypertension to result in hypertensive emergency in children. Hence, a thorough evaluation for the underlying cause should be carried out after initial management of blood pressure. Important investigations include renal function tests, serum electrolytes, venous blood gas, abdominal ultrasound and Doppler evaluation of renal vessels, urinalysis, electrocardiography, and often, a dimercaptosuccinic acid (DMSA) scan or digital subtraction angiography to rule out reflux nephropathy and renal artery stenosis, respectively. All patients with severe hypertension require evaluation to assess for target organ damage. Abnormal neurological examination or suggestive history is an indication for neuroimaging. Fundus and cardiac evaluation are necessary. **Flowchart 1** indicates a plan for evaluation and management.

Flowchart 1: Plan of management of hypertensive crisis

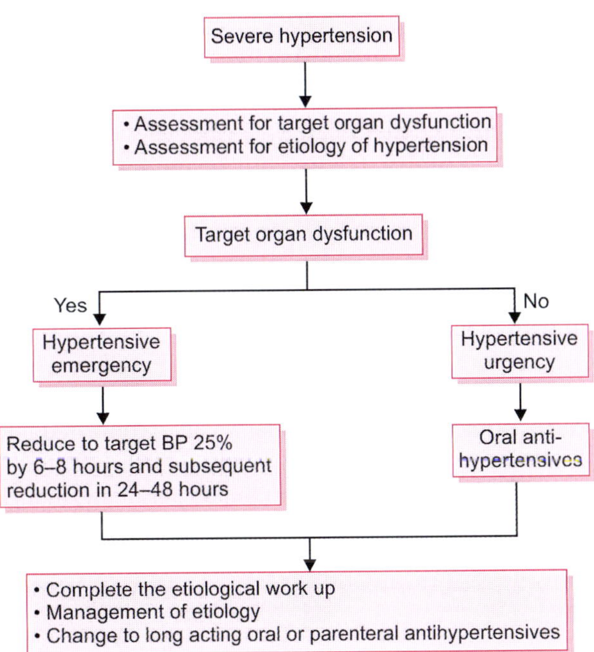

MANAGEMENT

Adequate lowering of blood pressure is essential to prevent serious sequelae. However, overzealous therapy may be hazardous in patients with long-standing severe hypertension. In chronic severe hypertension, a gradual shift in cerebral autoregulation protects the brain from excessive perfusion in the hypertensive state (**Fig. 1**).[11] Ischemic complications are likely to occur if the blood pressure is reduced abruptly, causing it to fall below the new lower threshold of autoregulation. Hence, the aim of treatment of hypertensive crises is to minimize hypertension-related adverse effects by a controlled reduction of blood pressure, allowing preservation of target organ function and minimizing complications of therapy, such as ischemic neuropathy of the optic nerve, transverse ischemic myelopathy and acute kidney injury. Therapeutic success is achieved by slow and controlled reduction of blood pressure.[12]

However, robust evidence to guide the evaluation and management of children with acute severe hypertension is lacking. The principles of managing hypertensive crises in children are adapted chiefly from studies conducted in adults, including rate of blood pressure change and medications choices. The aim is to decrease the blood pressure by no more than 25% of the planned blood pressure reduction over the first 6–8 hours, followed by gradual decline in blood pressure to the upper limit of normal (95th percentile) over the next 24–48 hours.[8,12]

Management should be done in an intensive care unit setting, or an emergency department with appropriate monitoring, nursing and physician support. Careful neurological and cardiovascular assessment should be undertaken throughout the initial treatment.

Choice of Antihypertensive

The choice of antihypertensive medication depends on the etiology of hypertension, rapidity of onset of action, the half-life, safety and efficacy of the drug, as well as the experience of the care provider. The drugs used for treating hypertensive emergency should be short-acting and administered by intravenous (IV) route, which allows easy modification of dose according to the therapeutic response. In patients with less severe symptoms, oral agents can be used.

Invasive arterial blood pressure monitoring is desirable when using IV antihypertensive agents. The agents usually chosen for IV infusion include sodium nitroprusside, nitroglycerin, hydralazine, labetalol and nicardipine (**Table 3**). Patients with severe acute kidney injury or advanced chronic kidney disease with fluid overload might benefit from initiation of dialysis to enable adequate control of hypertension.

Sodium nitroprusside

The drug of choice for hypertensive emergencies is sodium nitroprusside.[12] It is metabolized to nitric oxide, a potent venous and arteriolar vasodilator that reduces both preload and afterload. Hence, it is especially useful in case of congestive cardiac failure with severe hypertension. The hypotensive action begins within seconds after the infusion is started, and disappears rapidly when it is discontinued. Because of its potent hypotensive effect, nitroprusside should be administered in an intensive care unit with blood pressure recording done continuously or at least every 5 minutes. The drug should be shielded from light to prevent degradation. The metabolic product of sodium nitroprusside is cyanide, which is converted into thiocyanate in the liver and almost exclusively removed by the kidneys. Thiocyanate or cyanide poisoning, though rare, may occur in patients with renal or hepatic injury and in those in whom nitroprusside infusion is given for prolonged duration (>24-48 hours). Co-administration of thiosulfate or hydroxocobalamin minimizes this risk. Overt toxicity requires discontinuation of nitroprusside infusion, treatment with administration of amyl nitrate and sodium nitrate, and hemodialysis. Tachyphylaxis is another problem associated with prolonged use of nitroprusside.

Hydralazine

Hydralazine is a direct arteriolar vasodilator. It can be administered intramuscularly when IV access is not available immediately. It does not affect coronary arteries or venous smooth muscle. Its effects on arteriolar smooth muscle stimulate the sympathetic nervous system, leading to side effects like tachycardia, increased renin activity, and sodium retention. Patients treated with IV hydralazine can be easily converted to oral dosing; additionally, oral

Table 3: Drugs used in management of hypertensive emergencies

Agent	*Dose*	*Onset*	*Duration of effect*	*Adverse effects*
Intravenous route				
Sodium nitroprusside	0.5–10 µg/kg/min (in 5% dextrose)	0.5–2 minutes	3–5 minutes	Tachyphylaxis; nausea, vomiting; headache; tachycardia; cyanide toxicity (dizziness, confusion, seizures, jaw stiffness, lactic acidosis)
Hydralazine	0.1–0.4 mg/kg per dose	5–15 minutes	3–8 hours	Tachycardia
Labetalol	Bolus: 0.25–1 mg/kg q 5–15 min in increasing doses (max. total of 40 mg) Infusion: 1–3 mg/kg/hour	5–10 minutes	3–6 hours	Bradycardia; bronchospasm; heart failure; orthostatic hypotension; pallor; abdominal pain; diarrhea
Esmolol	100–500 µg/kg/min	Within seconds	10–20 minutes	Bradycardia, bronchospasm
Nicardipine	Bolus: 30 µg/kg dose (max 2 mg) Infusion: 0.5–4 µg/kg/min (max. 5 mg/hour)	1–10 minutes	2–6 hours	Tachycardia; flushing; phlebitis
Enalaprilat	0.005–0.01 µg/kg/min	15 minutes	6 hours	Renal dysfunction; hyperkalemia
Sodium nitroglycerin	0.1–3 µg/kg/min	1–2 minutes	5–10 minutes	Methemoglobinemia; headache; tachycardia
Phentolamine	0.1–0.2 mg/kg (max 5 mg) q 2–4 hours	2 minutes	5–15 minutes	Reflex tachycardia
Diazoxide	Bolus: 1–3 mg/kg q 5–15 min Infusion: 0.3–5 µg/kg/min	3–5 minutes	6–24 hours	Nausea; salt and water retention; hypotension, hyperglycemia
Oral route				
Clonidine	2–6 µg/kg	10 minutes	2–4 hours	Dry mouth, sedation
Hydralazine	0.25–0.6 µg/kg	20–30 minutes	3–7 hours	Tachycardia
Minoxidil	0.1–0.2 mg/kg	5–10 minutes	8 hours	Fluid retention
Isradipine	0.05–0.1 mg/kg	1 hour		Rapid fall in blood pressure
Nifedipine	0.1–0.2 mg/kg	20–30 minutes	4–6 hours	Rapid fall in blood pressure
Labetalol	0.2–1 mg/kg	10 minutes	2–4 hours	Rapid fall in blood pressure

hydralazine may be useful in patients with less severe hypertension who are able to tolerate oral drugs.

Labetalol

Labetalol has both alpha and beta-adrenergic blocking activity and is an effective and safe agent for use in hypertensive emergency.[12] It causes vasodilatation without significantly altering cardiac output. It is important to note that the alpha-to-beta blocking ratio of the IV preparation is 1:7, whereas it is 1:3 for the oral preparation. Hence, the infusion should be avoided in patients with asthma, acute left ventricular failure and heart block. It can be used safely in patients with renal dysfunction.

Esmolol

Esmolol is a cardioselective β-blocker. It is particularly useful after the repair of congenital heart disease and in presence of severe tachycardia. However, it can cause congestive heart failure, bradycardia, and bronchospasm. Its rapid metabolism by an intracytoplasmic red blood cell esterase is independent of both renal and hepatic metabolism, making it well-suited for critically ill patients with multiorgan failure.

Fenoldopam

Fenoldopam, administered at 0.2–0.8 µg/kg/min, is the first available peripheral dopamine receptor (DA1) agonist. It is a vasodilator with its greatest effect in the renal and splanchnic arterial beds, with less effect in the cerebral and coronary circulation. It leads to vasodilatation by increasing cAMP, which promotes smooth muscle cell relaxation. Through the inhibitory effects of cAMP on the sodium-hydrogen exchanger and the sodium/potassium-ATPase pumps in the renal tubule, the agent also maintains or increases renal perfusion and is associated with short-term increase in urine output and creatinine clearance. Its toxicities are relatively limited but include reflex tachycardia and tachyphylaxis. Surprisingly, the magnitude of blood pressure reduction with fenoldopam in children was significantly smaller than reported in adults.[13]

Nicardipine

The use of this dihydropyridine calcium channel blocker is relatively recent. It is an arteriolar vasodilator with prompt hypotensive effect that can be titrated by adjusting the infusion rate.[11] Its onset of action and efficacy is comparable to nitroprusside. Selective vasodilatation of the cerebral and coronary vasculature makes it more useful in a setting of myocardial ischemia, but should be avoided in patients with raised intracranial pressure and head trauma. The risk of thrombophlebitis is another disadvantage.

Sodium nitroglycerin

This drug has been used as an alternative to nitroprusside in children with myocardial dysfunction. Its rapid onset and short duration of action allow easy titratability of IV dose. Adverse effects include headache, tachycardia and methemoglobinemia. Tachyphylaxis is noted with prolonged use.

Diazoxide

This drug causes direct vasodilatation by increasing vascular smooth muscle cell permeability to potassium that interrupts voltage-gated calcium transport. A mini-bolus frequent dosing regimen is recommended to avoid the significant hypotension associated with administration of large doses. However, the blood pressure reduction is unpredictable and hyperglycemia is a concern.[14]

Phentolamine

This agent is used in the setting of pheochromocytoma, and is given 1–2 hours prior to surgery to control the blood pressure perioperatively. Because of its ultra-short acting, cardioselective alpha-1 adrenergic blockade, esmolol is well suited as an IV infusion, especially for management of intraoperative hypertension.[15]

IV enalaprilat

This agent is useful in patients with renin mediated hypertension. However, given the high incidence of renovascular hypertension in children, the lack of safety information in pediatric population, and the reported adverse effects like prolonged hypotension and oliguria, it is an unlikely first choice for management of hypertensive emergency in children.[16] The agent should be avoided in neonates and in presence of renal insufficiency or hyperkalemia.

Other IV Agents

Intravenous furosemide is helpful in lowering blood pressure in patients with salt and water retention (e.g. acute glomerulonephritis) and adequate renal function.

Clevidipine is an ultra-short-acting dihydropyridine calcium channel blocker with a high specificity for vascular smooth muscle. Its action is seen within 2 minutes of infusion initiation, and the effect lasts only a few minutes beyond discontinuation.[17] Tachycardia is uncommon and it can be used in renal and hepatic dysfunction without need for dose modification. Efficacy in adults is comparable to nitroprusside; studies in pediatric population are awaited.

Urapidil is a peripheral postsynaptic alpha-adrenoceptor antagonist with a central agonistic action at serotonin 5-HT receptors. Its rapid onset of action, along with strong vasodilating properties, such that it does not increase myocardial oxygen demand, heart rate and intracranial pressure, give this drug an edge over other vasodilators. Its efficacy is proven in adults with hypertensive emergencies, perioperative hypertension and eclampsia.[18] However, pediatric experience with this drug is limited.

IV Bolus Administration

If continuous infusion of an antihypertensive agent is not immediately available/feasible, IV bolus dosing of labetalol, enalaprilat and hydralazine can be used for management. However, boluses provide less minute to-minute control of blood pressure compared with continuous infusion therapies. Hydralazine, which interferes with intracellular calcium metabolism to cause arterial vasodilation by unclear mechanisms, may be administered IV or intramuscularly as a bolus. Adverse effects include reflex tachycardia, and sodium and fluid retention.

Oral Agents used in Management of Severe Hypertension

Agents with relatively rapid onset of action when administered orally may be used in management of severe hypertension, particularly in hypertensive urgencies and where IV administration is not possible. These include nifedipine, clonidine, minoxidil, labetalol, isradipine and hydralazine (**Table 3**).

Sublingual nifedipine has been widely used for treatment of hypertensive urgency and emergency. Oral administration is equally effective. Sublingual administration is by puncturing and squeezing the contents of the 5 mg capsule under the tongue. The dose may be repeated twice at 10 minute intervals. There is some concern about sublingual absorption of nifedipine, with reports suggesting that the absorption occurs predominantly after swallowing.[19] The overall response rate to the first dose of nifedipine is 70–75%. The use of immediate release of nifedipine for hypertensive emergencies has been criticized in adults for its unpredictable effect, and association with an increased risk for adverse cardiovascular outcomes, such as myocardial infarction and arrhythmia, in adults. In children, however, nifedipine seems to be effective and safe for management of hypertensive emergencies except those with hypertensive encephalopathy.[20]

Clonidine is a centrally acting $\alpha 2$ adrenergic agonist that decreases cerebral sympathetic output. It can be used in renal failure. Excessive use can cause sedation and dry mouth. Minoxidil is a direct arteriolar vasodilator that causes potassium efflux from smooth muscle cells, leading to smooth muscle relaxation. It is renally excreted and easily removed by dialysis; therefore, dose adjustment may be needed in patients with severe renal insufficiency, and should be dosed after dialysis. Minoxidil is effective in children with severe chronic hypertension refractory to other oral agents, and in children with chronic hypertension experiencing acute blood pressure elevations. Prolonged use can result in hirsutism and pericardial effusion.

Monitoring and Supportive Care

Children with hypertensive emergency should preferably be managed in an intensive care unit under continuous blood pressure monitoring. Pupillary reactions, sensorium and neurological findings should be monitored carefully. In case hypotension occurs, IV saline should be promptly infused.

At presentation, an assessment of volume status is essential. Volume status can be depleted (due to decreased oral intake and pressure natriuresis), causing stimulation of the renin-angiotensin system, worsening the hypertension. Volume repletion may lower renin levels, help restore tissue perfusion, and prevent a precipitous fall in blood pressure that may occur with antihypertensive therapy.

Therapy with oral antihypertensive agents should be commenced as soon as patient can take orally, in order to permit IV therapy to be withdrawn over the next 24 hours. Oral drugs such as sustained release of nifedipine, angiotensin converting enzyme inhibitors and beta-blockers may be used.

Therapy for Hypertensive Urgency

There is no consensus for a first agent in hypertensive urgencies. Hypertensives urgencies can be managed outside an intensive care setting with oral medication. An observation period of 24 to 48 hours is optimal. Reflux hypertensive crisis can develop when patient is non-compliant or upon stopping the agent. An initial slow reduction of blood pressure should be followed by restoration of the normal dosage.

Special Situations

The treatment of severe hypertension has to be modified in special situations. Sodium nitroprusside and labetalol are recommended and safe in patients with neurological impairment. Nicardipine should be used with caution in patients with intracranial space occupying lesions and atelectasis. The drugs of choice for hypertensive crisis due to pheochromocytoma are phentolamine, sodium nitroprusside with beta-blockers and labetalol. Patients with unilateral renovascular disease benefit from use of angiotensin converting enzyme inhibitors. In patients with mineralocorticoid excess and rare endocrine disorders including Liddle syndrome, severe hypertension may not respond adequately to any therapy other than triamterene or amiloride. Patients with end stage renal failure with volume overload show blunted response to antihypertensive agents and require repeated dialyses to remove excess fluid.

KEY MESSAGES

- Severe systemic hypertension is rare in childhood and is usually secondary to a renal or renovascular etiology.
- Presence of end organ damage is termed as hypertensive emergency and requires more aggressive management, preferably with an intravenous agent.
- Oral antihypertensive agents can be used as initial therapy for hypertensive urgencies, i.e. severe hypertension without end-organ damage.
- Both uncontrolled hypertension and overzealous correction of blood pressure are dangerous. Hence, in patients with hypertensive emergency or urgency, the blood pressure should be reduced in a controlled manner under close monitoring.
- Simultaneous evaluation to determine underlying etiology is essential to enable specific management.

REFERENCES

1. Bagga A, Jain R, Vijaykumar M, *et al.* Evaluation and management of hypertension. Indian Pediatrics. 2007;44:103-21.
2. Flynn JT, Kaelber DC, Baker-Smith CM, *et al.* Clinical Practice Guideline for screening and management of high blood pressure in children and adolescents. Pediatrics. 2018; e20171904.
3. Stein DR, Ferguson MA. Evaluation and treatment of hypertensive crises in children. Integr Blood Press Control. 2016;9: 49-58.
4. Marik PE, Varon J. Hypertensive crises: Challenges and management. Chest. 2007;131:1949-62.
5. Flynn JT. Hypertension in childhood and adolescence. In: Kaplan NM, editor. Kaplan's Clinical Hypertension, 9th edition. Philadelphia: Lippincott-Williams and Wilkins; 2005;465-88.
6. Patel HP, Mitsnefes M. Advances in the pathogenesis and management of hypertensive crisis: Curr Opin Pediatr. 2005; 17:210-4.
7. Hari P, Bagga A, Srivastava RN. Sustained hypertension in children. Indian Pediatr. 2000;37:268-74.
8. Seeman T, Hamdani G, Mitsnefes M. Hypertensive crisis in children and adolescents. Pediatr Nephrol. 2018; doi: 10.1007/s00467-018-4092-2.
9. Baracco R, Mattoo TK. Pediatric hypertensive emergencies. Curr Hypertens Rep. 2014;16:456.
10. Schwartz RB, Jones KM, Kalina P, *et al.* Hypertensive encephalopathy: Findings on CT, MR imaging, and SPECT imaging in 14 cases. AJR Am J Roentgenol. 1992;159:379-83.
11. Rose JC, Mayer SA. Optimizing blood pressure in neurological emergencies. Neurocrit Care. 2004;1:287-99.
12. Yang WC, Lin MJ, Chen CY, *et al.* Clinical overview of hypertensive crisis in children. World J Clin Cases. 2015;3:510-3.
13. Hammer GB, Verghese ST, Drover DR, *et al.* Pharmacokinetics and pharmacodynamics of fenoldopam mesylate for blood pressure control in pediatric patients. BMC Anesthesiol. 2008; 8:6.
14. Grossman E, Ironi AN, Messerli FH. Comparative tolerability profile of hypertensive crisis treatments. Drug Saf. 1998;19: 99-122.
15. Adamson PC, Rhodes LA, Saul JP, *et al.* The pharmacokinetics of esmolol in pediatric subjects with supraventricular arrhythmias. Pediatr Cardiol. 2006;27:420-7.
16. Wells TG, Bunchman TE, Kearns GL. Treatment of neonatal hypertension with enalaprilat. J Pediatr. 1990;117:664-7.
17. Nordlander M, Sjöquist PO, Ericsson H, *et al.* Pharmacodynamic, pharmacokinetic and clinical effects of clevidipine, an ultrashort-acting calcium antagonist for rapid blood pressure control. Cardiovasc Drug Rev. 2004;22:227-50.
18. Woisetschläger C, Bur A, Vlcek M, *et al.* Comparison of intravenous urapidil and oral captopril in patients with hypertensive urgencies. J Hum Hypertens. 2006;20:707-9.
19. van Harten J, Burggraaf K, Danhof M, *et al.* Negligible sublingual absorption of nifedipine. Lancet. 1987;11:1363-5.
20. Calvetta A, Martino S, von Vigier RO, *et al.* What goes up must immediately come down! Which indication for short-acting nifedipine in children with arterial hypertension? Pediatr Nephrol. 2003;18:1-2.

CHAPTER

25

Acute Kidney Injury

Jitendra Meena, Arvind Bagga

Acute kidney injury (AKI) is common in hospitalized children, occurring often in the setting of multiorgan dysfunction. AKI is a clinical syndrome characterized by rapid decline in renal function resulting in accumulation of nitrogenous waste, and disturbance in fluid and electrolyte homeostasis. The term acute renal failure was used before, with variable definitions and was therefore difficult to compare across centers. The diagnosis of AKI is based on blood level of creatinine and urine output. Its management requires knowledge of fluid-electrolyte homeostasis and an understanding regarding renal replacement therapy. AKI is associated with several short- and long-term complications, and an increased risk of mortality.[1,2]

DEFINITION AND CLASSIFICATION

A uniformly accepted definition of AKI in the last decade has helped understand the burden of illness and its impact on outcome. A definition of AKI based on blood level of creatinine and urine output, proposed by the Acute Dialysis Quality Initiative in 2004, was modified by the Acute Kidney Injury Network in 2007.[3,4] In an attempt to harmonize differences in definitions, the Kidney Disease: Improving Global Outcome (KDIGO) proposed a unified definition of AKI in 2012 **(Table 1)**, which is now widely accepted.[5] AKI is defined by increase in serum creatinine >0.3 mg/dL within 48 h or ≥1.5 fold rise in serum creatinine from baseline in 7 days, or decrease in urine output <0.5 mL/kg/h for 6–12 h. If urine output and serum creatinine do not correspond to the same stage, KDIGO recommends the use of the higher stage for classification. For neonatal AKI, the lowest available creatinine is considered as reference value; serum creatinine level of >2.5 mg/dL is considered to represent stage 3 AKI, instead of >4 mg/dL for older children.[5]

Table 1: Acute kidney injury definitions proposed by pediatric RIFLE (pRIFLE) and KDIGO

*pRIFLE**			*KDIGO*		
Class	*Estimated CrCl*	*Urine output*	*Stage*	*Serum creatinine*	*Urine output*
Risk	eCrCl decreased by ≥25%	<0.5 mL/kg/h for ≥8 h	1	Rise in blood creatinine 1.5 to <1.9 times from baseline within 7 days *or* Increase in blood creatinine >0.3 mg/dL from baseline within 48 h	<0.5 mL/kg/h for 6-12 h
Injury	eCrCl decreased by ≥50%	< 0.5 mL/kg/h for ≥16 h	2	Rise in blood creatinine 2 to 2.9 times from baseline	<0.5 mL/kg/h for ≥12 h
Failure	eCrCl decreased by ≥75% *or* eCrCl <35 mL/min/1.73 m^2	<0.3 mL/kg/h for 24 h *or* anuria for 12 h	3	Rise in blood creatinine ≥ 3 times from baseline *or* Increase in blood creatinine > 4 mg/dL from baseline *or* Initiation of renal replacement therapy *or* eGFR < 35 mL/min/1.73 m^2	<0.3 mL/kg/h for ≥24 h *or* anuria ≥12 h

*L Persistent failure (F) more than 4 weeks, E Persistent failure more than 3 months
(eCrCl: estimated creatinine clearance; KDIGO: Kidney Disease: Improving Global Outcome; eGFR: estimated glomerular filtration rate)

The KDIGO definition has few limitations. The serum creatinine level is affected by muscle mass, age, volume status and metabolic state. Urine output needs to be related to the hydration status. Secondly, the KDIGO criteria defines AKI irrespective of etiology; while in adults, the usual cause is acute tubular necrosis, this is not always true for children. Finally, the duration of injury is not included in the definition but is associated with long-term outcome. Patients in whom AKI persists beyond 7 days but less than 3-months, are classified as acute kidney disease. Patients with injury that persists beyond 3-months are defined as having chronic kidney disease.

EPIDEMIOLOGY

The incidence of AKI in children is not precisely known. A systematic review that used KDIGO-equivalent definition of AKI, showed a pooled prevalence of 33.7% in hospitalized children and AKI associated mortality of 14%.[6] Recent studies, using the KDIGO definition, suggest that AKI is common in hospitalized children and its incidence depends on the studied population. In a large multicentric epidemiological study "AWARE", 26% of critically ill children developed AKI, including 11.6% with severe AKI.[7] Patients with severe AKI show higher mortality. In another multicenter study in neonates (AWAKEN), the incidence of AKI was almost 30%.[8] Patients undergoing surgery for repair of congenital heart disease are also at high risk of AKI, with an estimated incidence of 30% to 65%.[9]

The AKI is common in non-critically ill hospitalized patients with reported incidence of 4% to 6%. Exposure to nephrotoxic drugs **(Table 2)** is another important risk factor. AKI is reported to develop in 25% patients using aminoglycosides for more than 3 days. While AKI in the developed world predominately occurs in hospital settings and is associated with multiple risk factors (e.g. sepsis, hypotension, following surgery), in developing countries AKI is chiefly community acquired and secondary to a single illness, e.g. gastroenteritis, dengue, leptospirosis and malaria. A recent global study confirmed that patients with community acquired stage III AKI had high mortality in low-income countries, compared to high-income countries.[10] Preventive measures are therefore likely to be effective in low-income countries.

ETIOLOGY

The etiology of AKI is traditionally classified as *prerenal*, *renal* (intrinsic) causes and *post-renal* **(Table 3)**. Since

Table 2: Commonly used nephrotoxic drugs in children

Antimicrobial agents	*Chemotherapeutic agents*
Acyclovir	Cisplatin
Aminoglycosides	Ifosfamide
Amphotericin B	Methotrexate
Cidofovir, tenofovir	Mitomycin-C
Indinavir	
Beta-lactams	*Calcineurin inhibitors*
Foscarnet	Tacrolimus
Ganciclovir	Cyclosporine
Quinolones	
Rifampicin	*Diuretics*
Sulfonamides	Loop diuretics
Vancomycin	Triamterene
Analgesics	*Others*
Acetaminophen, aspirin	Proton pump inhibitors
NSAIDs (naproxen, ibuprofen)	Allopurinol
	Phenytoin
Antihypertensive medications	Pamidronate
Angiotensin-converting enzyme inhibitors, angiotensin receptor blockers	Zoledronic acid
	Iodinated radiocontrast media

(NSAIDs: nonsteroidal anti-inflammatory drugs)

AKI is a heterogeneous syndrome due to multiple pathophysiological pathways, the primary mechanism resulting in renal injury is not same for all causes. Prerenal causes include dehydration, where serum creatinine rises due to functional adaptive drop in the glomerular filtration rate (GFR) and is fluid responsive. In other prerenal causes, including congestive cardiac failure or nephrotic syndrome, acute tubular necrosis may be present and administration of fluids in such setting may be detrimental to patient outcome. Differentiation between fluid responsive prerenal cause and other prerenal causes of acute tubular necrosis is important, since it helps in reducing further renal injury.

The chief causes of AKI in the developing world are diarrhea, septicemia, endemic infections such as malaria, leptospirosis, and use of nephrotoxic agents. The use of appropriate antibiotics has led to decline in post-infectious glomerulonephritis. The etiology of AKI in intensive care units is multifactorial, secondary to sepsis, hypovolemia, and use of nephrotoxic agents or radiocontrast agents.[10,11]

Neonatal AKI

Prerenal causes, including perinatal hypoxia, hypovolemia and hypotension, contribute to ~85% of neonatal AKI, while intrinsic and post-renal causes are uncommon.

More than one-half of the neonates with severe birth asphyxia may show AKI. Hypovolemia, secondary to dehydration, intraventricular hemorrhage, twin-twin transfusion syndrome, placental hemorrhage and increased insensible losses (use of radiant warmer, phototherapy), are also important causes.[12]

Congenital malformation of kidney and urinary tract can initially manifest as AKI in neonatal age. Since neonates have high levels of renin and angiotensin, they are more sensitive to therapy with angiotensin converting enzyme (ACE) inhibitors and show increased risk of developing AKI. Risk factors for renal vein thrombosis include maternal diabetes, perinatal asphyxia, polycythemia, umbilical vein catheterization, dehydration and sepsis. Patients with renal vein thrombosis should be screened for protein C and S deficiency, homocystinuria and rare hereditary prothombotic disorders.[13]

DIAGNOSTIC EVALUATION

Clinical Evaluation

A careful history provides clues to the underlying etiology. In a patient with history of oliguria, history includes questions on prerenal causes: vomiting, diarrhea, blood and volume loss, and fluid intake in the last 24-hr. Acute tubular necrosis is the chief cause of AKI in hospitalized children, and can occur in multiple settings, i.e. sepsis with capillary leak, burns, cardiac dysfunction and inadequate fluid replacement. Attention is given to fluid balance; negative balance suggests dehydration and hypovolemia contributing to AKI, while progressive increase in weight indicates fluid accumulation. History is obtained for features of the underlying cause: edema, hematuria, hypertension (glomerulonephritis); dysentery, pallor, petechiae (hemolytic uremic syndrome); sudden onset pallor, jaundice, cola-colored urine (intravascular hemolysis); rash and arthritis (SLE, vasculitis).

A history of abdominal colic with hematuria and dysuria suggest nephrolithiasis, while an interrupted urinary stream and palpable urinary bladder indicates obstruction of lower urinary tract. Urine output is preserved in patients with AKI secondary to nephrotoxic medications and radiocontrast agents **(Table 3)**. Anuria may occur in patients with urinary tract obstruction, cortical necrosis, bilateral vascular occlusion and severe glomerulonephritis. Polyuria is observed in patients with partial ureteral obstruction, AKI with pre-existing tubular disorders, and hyperglycemia induced osmotic diuresis. Patients with AKI may present with altered sensorium and seizures, secondary to severe hypertension, uremia or hyponatremia. Metabolic acidosis manifests with rapid and deep breathing. Patients may present with features of fluid overload (pulmonary edema, heart failure).

Renal Angina Index

Due to lack of curative therapy for AKI, its prompt identification helps in early institution of preventive measures that reduce further renal injury. Analogous to

Table 3: Important causes of acute kidney injury in children

Prerenal	*Hypovolemia*: Acute gastroenteritis, vomiting, hemorrhage, bleeding, nasogastric drainage and diuretic use *Third space loss*: Nephrotic syndrome, sepsis and burns *Congestive cardiac failure, hepatorenal syndrome* *Medications*: NSAIDs, ACE, ARBs, calcineurin inhibitors
Intrinsic (renal)	*Vascular*: Renal vein or artery thrombosis, renal artery stenosis, hemolytic uremic syndrome, thrombotic thrombocytopenic purpura, malignant hypertension, disseminated intravascular coagulation *Glomerular*: Rapidly progressive GN (ANCA associated vasculitides, immune mediated disease, anti-glomerular basement membrane disease) Immune mediated GN: Postinfectious, IgA nephropathy, lupus, membranoproliferative *Acute tubular necrosis*: Hypoxic/ischemic injury, drug-induced (aminoglycosides, amphotericin B, acyclovir, cisplatin, radiocontrast), exogenous toxin (ethylene glycol methanol, heavy metals), intrinsic toxins (myoglobin, hemoglobin, tumor lysis syndrome), any prolonged prerenal cause can lead to acute tubular necrosis *Interstitial nephritis*: Drug induced, idiopathic *Infections*: Pyelonephritis, malaria, leptospirosis
Post-renal	Posterior urethral valve, urethral stricture Bilateral pelviuretric junction obstruction *Ureteral obstruction:* Stenosis, stone, ureterocele

(ACEI/ARB: angiotensin converting enzyme inhibitors/angiotensin receptor blockers; ANCA: antineutrophil cytoplasmic antibodies; GN: glomerulonephritis; NSAIDs: nonsteroidal anti-inflammatory drugs)

Table 4: Renal angina index

Risk		*Injury*		
Risk factor	*Score*	*Reduced creatinine clearance*	*Fluid overload (%)*	*Score*
Sepsis or ICU admission	1	No change	≤5	1
Stem-cell or solid organ transplant	3	0–24.9%	5–9.9	2
Mechanical ventilation and inotropic support	5	25–49.9%	10 to 14.9	4
		>50%	≥15	8

$$\text{Fluid overload (\%)} = \frac{\text{(Fluid in)} - \text{(fluid out)}}{\text{Weight (kg)}} \times 100$$

concept of cardiac angina, where myocardial infarction is identified by precordial pain the concept of renal angina has been proposed for early identification of AKI. This is a collection of clinical risk factors and features of AKI that are used for stratification of patients at risk **(Table 4)**.

Renal angina index = Risk factor for AKI × Evidence of kidney injury

Renal angina index score ranges from 1 to 40; score of <8 has a negative predictive value of 92% for predicting severe AKI on day 3 of ICU admission. This prediction tool is utilized for identification of high-risk patients who would benefit from further testing with biomarkers of kidney injury. The combination of renal angina index with biomarkers enables early diagnosis of AKI.[14,15]

Biomarkers

The diagnosis of AKI depends on serial monitoring of serum creatinine. Efforts have been made to identify biomarkers that detect structural injury of renal tissue, including neutrophil gelatinase-associated lipocalin (NGAL), kidney injury molecule-1 (KIM-1), interleukin-18 (IL-18) and liver-type fatty acid-binding protein (L-FABP). Due to paucity of evidence, biomarkers have limited role in diagnosis of AKI. Further studies are required before these biomarkers are used as point of care test for making clinical decision in children.[14]

Laboratory Evaluation

Investigations are necessary to confirm the underlying etiology, assess severity of AKI and detect complications. Differentiating the prerenal cause from intrinsic causes is of utmost importance utmost importance. In established acute tubular necrosis in setting of hypoperfusion, there is diminished tubular functions resulting in high urinary sodium (>40 mEq/L) and dilute urine (urine osmolality <300 mOsm/kg). In prerenal state in the setting of hypovolemia, GFR is reduced but tubular reabsorption is normal, hence urine sodium is low (<20 mEq/L), fractional excretion of sodium is low (<1%), and there is increased ratio of blood urea to creatinine (>20). Fractional excretion of sodium is most reliable, but these indices have limited role in non-oliguric renal failure.

Table 5: Investigations in acute kidney injury

Urine	Protein, albumin Cells; red and white cells; casts
Blood	Creatinine, urea, protein, albumin Potassium, sodium, calcium, phosphate; pH, bicarbonate Complete blood count Coagulation profile* Antinuclear antibody, antineutrophil cytoplasmic antibody, C3
Imaging	Abdominal ultrasonography Chest X-ray, electrocardiogram Doppler study*
Renal biopsy*	Diagnosis of glomerulonephritis, interstitial nephritis

*Investigations required, if suggested clinically, to determine cause of acute kidney injury

Investigations in a patient with AKI are listed in **Table 5**. Peripheral smear should be examined for evidence of hemolytic anemia and thrombocytopenia (hemolytic uremic syndrome). Urinalysis helps in evaluation of acute glomerulonephritis, as indicated by presence of proteinuria, hematuria and red cell casts. Presence of renal epithelial cells and muddy brown tubular casts suggests the diagnosis of ATN. Serum C3 and ASO titer is required in patients with suspected post-infectious glomerulonephritis.

An ultrasound scan is the most important radiological investigation for evaluating etiology of AKI. Ultrasound scan allow delineation of kidney anatomy, and identification of congenital anomalies of kidney and urinary tract. Loss of corticomedullary differentiation and small kidney size are suggestive of chronic kidney disease. Doppler ultrasonography can identify reduced renal blood flow and ischemic causes of AKI.

Patients with AKI should be simultaneously screened, for associated complications, including fluid overload that is calculated as follows:

$$\text{Percent fluid overload} = \frac{\text{(Fluids in)} - \text{(Fluids out)}}{\text{Admission weight (kg)}} \times 100$$

Clinical evaluation should focus on detection of hypertension, signs of fluid overload, acidosis and anemia. Laboratory investigations include blood levels of electrolytes, urea, creatinine, bicarbonate and hemoglobin. Electrocardiogram is done to look for features of potassium excess and chest X-ray for features of fluid overload.

Most patients with AKI do not require renal biopsy. A biopsy is considered in patients where the histology is likely to modify therapy and enable recovery of renal function, as in patients with rapidly progressive glomerulonephritis, acute interstitial nephritis and vasculitis. Renal biopsy should be considered if the etiology of AKI is unclear, and with prolonged course of AKI lasting more than 3–4 weeks.

MANAGEMENT

In a patient with suspected prerenal AKI, especially oligoanuria, assessment of intravascular volume is necessary. Correction of intravascular volume with IV fluids leads to better renal perfusion and increase in urine output. Hypovolemia is initially corrected by administration of 20 mL/kg of isotonic solution over 45 to 60 minutes. During fluid administration, vital signs and central venous pressure should be monitored to determine adequacy of fluid replacement and to avoid overhydration, which may be detrimental in AKI. If hypovolemia does not improve despite two fluid boluses, therapy with vasopressors should be initiated. If urine output is less than 1 mL/kg/hr after 2 hr and there are no signs of intravascular volume deficit, furosemide is administered at a dose of 1–2 mg/kg. If therapy with furosemide fails to increase urine output an intrinsic cause for AKI is suspected.[16] All patients with AKI should undergo ultrasonography to evaluate kidney size and exclude urinary tract obstruction.

Principles of management of established AKI comprise of supportive care with attention to fluids and nutrition, treatment of complications, therapy of the underlying disorder, and renal replacement therapy if indicated. Patients with obstruction of lower urinary tract, e.g. posterior urethral valves require appropriate management.

Therapy of Complications

Patient presenting with AKI and oligoanuria should be screened for life-threatening complications including hyperkalemia, hypertension, pulmonary edema and metabolic acidosis. Hyperkalemia is an important complication and can result in arrhythmias and sudden death. Urgent treatment is instituted depending on serum potassium levels and ECG changes. Hyponatremia in AKI is chiefly related to hypotonic fluid administration and is best managed by restriction of fluid intake. Patients with sodium level >125 mEq/L are usually asymptomatic; those with symptomatic hyponatremia require therapy with 3% saline. Therapeutic measures for complications are summarized in **Table 6**. Patients showing metabolic complications should be considered for early renal replacement therapy.

Specific Therapy

Immunosuppressive therapy with intravenous methylprednisolone and cyclophosphamide is indicated in patient with crescentic glomerulonephritis and lupus nephritis. Plasmapheresis is recommended in patients with pauci-immune crescentic glomerulonephritis and atypical hemolytic uremic syndrome. Patient with interstitial nephritis show satisfactory response to oral corticosteroid therapy. Patients with urinary tract obstruction often require bladder catheterization, or urinary tract diversion through interventional radiology or surgery.

Management of Fluid and Electrolytes

Fluid overload >10–15% has been shown to be associated with an increased risk of mortality. Fluid management should therefore be meticulous in order to mitigate this complication. Daily fluid intake should be restricted to insensible losses (400 mL/m^2 body surface area) and ongoing losses. Insensible losses should be replaced with 10% dextrose while urine and extrarenal losses with 0.45% saline in 5% dextrose. Oral route is preferred, since it enables appropriate nutrition. In fluid overloaded patients, less than the total urine output should be replaced to promote negative balance. Daily fluid prescription should be guided by strict input output monitoring, daily weight, physical examination and serum sodium. Judicious fluid administration with appropriate composition should allow 0.5–1% weight loss per day in these patients. Low serum sodium, hypertension and failure to lose weight suggest excessive fluid intake, whereas excessive weight loss and increasing sodium concentration suggest inadequate free water replacement.

Patients with oligoanuria are at risk of hyperkalemia; potassium containing fluids should be avoided. Sodium intake should be restricted to 2–3 mEq/kg/day to avoid hypernatremia and fluid retention. In the setting of

Table 6: Therapies for complications of acute kidney injury

Fluid overload	Fluid restriction to 400 mL/m^2 plus urine output and losses; 5% dextrose for insensible loss and N/2 for urine output; prefer oral to intravenous fluid		
Pulmonary edema	Oxygen, IV furosemide 2–4 mg/kg, fluid restriction, dialysis		
Hypertensive emergency	Infusion of sodium nitroprusside (0.5–8 µg/kg/min) or labetalol (0.25–3 mg/kg/hr); furosemide if fluid overload; 25% of desired blood pressure reduction should be done within 8 h, with remainder reduction over 12–24 h		
Metabolic acidosis	If bicarbonate <18 mEq/L: Sodium bicarbonate oral or IV; monitor for fluid overload and hypernatremia		
Hyponatremia	Restrict fluid intake If altered sensorium or seizures: 3% saline 6–12 mL/kg over 30–90 minutes		
	Hyperkalemia		
Medication	*Dose*	*Onset*	*Remarks*
Calcium gluconate, 10%	1 mL/kg IV over 3–5 minutes; repeat after 10 minutes	5 minutes	Stabilizes cell membrane and prevents arrhythmias; give under cardiac monitoring
Salbutamol	5–10 mg through nebulization over 10 minutes	30 minutes	Shift potassium into cells
Insulin with dextrose	0.1 U/kg of insulin with 0.5 g/kg glucose IV over 30 minutes	20 minutes	Shifts potassium into cells, monitor for hypoglycemia
Sodium bicarbonate, 7.5%	1–2 mL/kg IV over 5–10 minutes	15–60 minutes	Shifts potassium into cells, do not give with calcium gluconate
Calcium or sodium resonium	1 g/kg/d orally, per rectal	2 hr	Slow action with variable efficacy

non-oliguric AKI patients may lose excessive fluid and electrolytes, and need potassium and sodium supplements. Patients with prolonged duration of AKI may develop hyperphosphatemia, which is managed with phosphate restriction and phosphate binders.

Pharmacological Therapy for AKI

There is limited data on the efficacy of pharmacological agents for therapy of AKI. While dopamine in low doses improves renal blood flow and sodium excretion, this effect is short lasting and quite variable. There is no evidence that use of low-dose dopamine or of fenoldopam prevents or improves renal recovery in AKI. Intravenous furosemide may increase urine output in some patients but there is no evidence that it improves renal recovery or long-term prognosis of patients with AKI. Single dose of theophylline (5–8 mg/kg/day) has been shown to reduce incidence of severe AKI in term neonates with severe birth asphyxia.[17]

Nutrition

Patients with AKI have increased metabolic requirements and are usually catabolic. Adequate nutritional supplementation is thus a crucial component of management. Since children with AKI are critically ill with increased protein catabolism, the initial protein intake should be 0.8–1.2 g/kg/day. The daily intake is increased to 1.0–1.5 g/kg in patients on peritoneal or hemodialysis. Patients should receive 60–70 Calorie/kg/day, which is 20–30% above the basal needs. While on dialysis, patients require supplementation of water soluble vitamins and other micronutrients. Enteral feeding should be preferred for patients with AKI.[18,19]

Renal Replacement Therapy

Acute dialysis is an effective therapy for management of AKI and can be provided safely to children of all ages. It is recommended that acute dialysis be used early to avoid complications of AKI, and facilitate renal recovery. Indications for renal replacement therapy include:[20]

- Fluid overload (>10–15%)
- Hyperkalemia (>7 mEq/L)
- Symptomatic hyponatremia and hypernatremia
- Severe metabolic acidosis (TCO_2 <10–12 mEq/L)
- Seizures or altered sensorium secondary to azotemia
- Uremic pericarditis
- Patients in whom adequate nutrition intake is not achieved due to fluid restriction.

Emphasis is given to detect fluid overload and start acute dialysis early, as prospective observational studies show that fluid overload is an independent risk factor for mortality and prolonged hospital stay. Patients with AKI and fluid overload exceeding 10–15% should be considered for initiating acute dialysis. Fluid overload is calculated as follows:

$$\text{Fluid overload} = \frac{\text{(Fluids in)} - \text{(Fluids out)}}{\text{Admission weight (kg)}} \times 100$$

Modalities for renal replacement therapy in children include peritoneal dialysis (PD), intermittent hemodialysis (IHD) and continuous renal replacement therapy (CRRT) **(Table 7)**. There are number of factors need to considered while choosing optimal modality for dialysis:

- Primary goal of dialysis: Rapid solute clearance, fluid and toxin removal
- Hemodynamic status of the child
- Expertise of medical staff and available infrastructure
- Coagulopathy and need of anticoagulation
- Feasibility of vascular access, compared to peritoneal access
- Patient size.

Peritoneal dialysis

In resource limited settings like India, PD is the chief modality in sick hemodynamically unstable children. PD requires less expertise to perform, and is cost-effective. Temporary soft peel-away catheters are preferred for obtaining peritoneal access for acute dialysis. Soft catheters are easily available and associated with fewer complications than stiff catheters. PD prescription (duration of therapy, composition of dialysate, frequency and duration of exchange) is chiefly governed by patient clinical condition. PD fluid is hyperosmotic (350–360 mOsm/kg) and designed to correct metabolic and electrolyte disturbances.[20]

Prescription for peritoneal dialysis

- *Session length*: In the setting of AKI, patients require continuous removal of fluid and solute to support ongoing nutritional and therapeutic interventions. The PD prescription is initially planned for 24 hr, since patients require frequent monitoring of the clinical state.
- *Dwell volume*: The dwell volume per cycle varies from 800 to 1100 mL/m^2, depending on the clinical condition. Patients with respiratory distress tolerate smaller dwell volumes. In order to achieve better solute clearance and ultrafiltration, the optimal tolerable dialysate volume should be prescribed.
- *Dwell time*: The dwell time is variable. Initial cycles may be short ~30 minutes, especially in patients with refractory hyperkalemia, fluid overload and metabolic acidosis; patients with azotemia require longer duration cycles (60–90 minutes).
- *Dextrose*: The dialysate dextrose concentration is chiefly responsible for generating the osmotic gradient during PD. Commercially available dialysate contains 1.7% dextrose. Its concentration may be increased by adding glucose, when required for extra fluid removal.
- *Additives*: Once serum potassium level is ~3.5 mEq/L, 1.5–2 mL of 15% potassium chloride is added to the dialysate. Heparin, 500–1000 Units/L, is added to the dialysate to prevent catheter blockade.

The dialysate effluent is examined for clarity and cell counts, to diagnose peritonitis early. With use of soft catheter and automated cycler devices, the rate of peritonitis has reduced significantly. Other complications associated chiefly with a stiff catheter include bowel and

Table 7: Modalities for renal replacement therapy in acute kidney injury

	Peritoneal dialysis (PD)	*Hemodialysis (HD)*	*Continuous renal replacement therapy (CRRT)*
Advantages	• Easy to perform • Gentle fluid removal • Less hemodynamic instability • No need for anticoagulation	• Highly efficient solute and fluid clearance • Short duration of therapy • Reliable fluid removal if hemodynamically stable	• Effective solute clearance in hemodynamicaly unstable patients • Fluid removal possible with less hemodynamic instability • Better clearance of cytokines, toxins
Disadvantages	• Less efficient in solute clearance • Variable rate of fluid removal • Can worsen respiratory distress • Risk of peritonitis, catheter related complications	• Need technical expertise • Equipment is expensive • Not suitable in patients with hemodynamic instability • Need anticoagulation	• Need for expensive equipment and technical expertise • Require team with enough experience • High risk of bleeding • Limited data on drug dosage adjustment

bladder injury, bleeding and blockage of catheter, and incomplete emptying.

Intermittent hemodialysis

Intermittent hemodialysis (IHD) is the preferred modality in older children, as it is more efficient for fluid removal and solute clearance. The modality is still not widely available for children in India as equipment for hemodialysis is expensive and requires expertise. IHD requires satisfactory vascular access to achieve optimal blood flow (5–8 mL/kg/hr). A double lumen venous catheter is inserted in one of the larger central veins (internal jugular or femoral). The catheter size is determined by bodyweight of the child: 5–7 Fr for <6 kg, 8 Fr for 6–15 kg, 9 Fr 15–30 kg and 10–11.5 Fr for >30 kg. Dialyzers are also available in variable sizes; the surface area of the dialyzer should approximate (~80%) of the body surface area of the patient. Extracorporeal blood volumes of the dialyzer and its tubings should not excess 10% of the patient's blood volume. The dialysate concentration should be similar to extracellular fluid, except low potassium and higher concentration of bicarbonate to correct hyperkalemia and metabolic acidosis, respectively. The sodium concentration of the dialysate can be adjusted as per patient requirements. The dialysate flow rate is kept at 1.5–2 times the blood flow rate to achieve optimal solute clearance.[20]

The first session of dialysis should be brief (60–90 minutes) to avoid dialysis disequilibrium. Subsequent duration of sessions is approximately 4-hr, three times a week. Metabolically active and young children may require more frequent sessions. Unfractionated heparin is used for anticoagulation of the dialysis circuit; loading dose of 30–50 units/kg is followed by 20–25 units/kg/hr, to maintain activated clotting time around 150% of baseline. In patients with coagulopathy or bleeding, IHD may be done without anticoagulation. However, these patients require frequent flushing of the dialyzer with saline to avoid clotting. Common complications observed during IHD are hypotension, chills, rigors and vomiting during the procedure, and the rare occurrence of dialysis disequilibrium syndrome.

Sustained low efficiency dialysis (SLED) is a comparatively recent form of renal replacement therapy that can be safely used in patients with hemodynamic instability. SLED is a form of prolonged intermittent renal replacement therapy that involves slow and low efficiency IHD done over a period of 6 hours or longer. SLED combines the advantage of CRRT and IHD using low blood and dialysate flow rates, with slow continuous solute and fluid clearances for 6–12 hr. During SLED, the blood flow rate is 3–5 mL/kg/hr and dialysate flow rate is ~200 mL/min or twice the blood flow rate.

Continuous renal replacement therapy

Advancements in technology have led to development of several forms of CRRT, including continuous venovenous hemodialysis (CVVHD), venovenous hemofiltration (CVVH), or venovenous hemodiafiltration (CVVHDF). While CVVH depends on convection, CVVHD relies on diffusion and CVVHDF uses combination of both techniques. These mechanisms can be manipulated to selectively influence solute clearance. CRRT require expensive equipment and expertise. It is however the preferred modality for managing AKI with heart failure, septic shock and pulmonary edema. Patients with tumor lysis syndrome, hyperammonemia and hypercatabolic state are better managed with CRRT.[20]

Use of Medications

Medications that may worsen renal injury or delay recovery, e.g. aminoglycosides, NSAIDs, ACE inhibitors, amphotericin B and radiocontrast media should be avoided. Drug dosing should be adjusted as per residual renal function to avoid their accumulation and mitigate renal injury. Drugs excreted through the kidney require dose modification once the GFR is <50% of normal. Many drugs are cleared during dialysis and CRRT; drug levels should be monitored, if available.

Outcome

Despite advancements in renal replacement therapy, the mortality related to AKI has not improved significantly. The outcome is chiefly determined by the etiology of AKI. While diarrheal dehydration, intravascular hemolysis and nephrotoxin related AKI has favorable prognosis, the course is less satisfactory in patients with crescentic GN, sepsis and multiorgan failure. Overall mortality rates of 30–80% are reported in low-middle income countries, with poor survival in critically ill children. A recent worldwide study reported 7-day mortality of ~10% in hospitalized patients with incident AKI; the mortality was almost double in resource limited settings. In another prospective study on patients admitted to the PICU, the 28-day mortality among critically sick children and young adults was 13%.[11]

Long-term Sequelae

Patients who survive an episode of AKI are at risk of CKD and ESRD.[21,22] Maladaptive repair and inflammation, reduced capillary density and increased interstitial myofibroblasts might result in progression to CKD. A recent meta-analysis on patients with AKI showed 9-fold risk of CKD and 3.3 fold risk of ESRD. A meta-analysis of pediatric studies showed increased incidence of proteinuria (13.2%), hypertension (6.6%) and CKD (28%), confirming high risk of adverse outcomes. It is recommended that patients of AKI should be carefully followed up, for proteinuria, hypertension and decline in GFR.[23] The first assessment is done at 2–3 months, and then 3–6 monthly based on risk factors and degree of recovery from AKI.

KEY MESSAGES

- Acute kidney injury (AKI) is common in critically sick children and contributes to poor outcomes.
- Utilization of standardized definition, the KDIGO criteria, allows better understanding of the epidemiology of AKI, and monitoring progress. Clinical tools, e.g. renal angina index and furosemide stress test allow early recognition of severe degree of AKI.
- AKI results in serious metabolic complications, which should be anticipated and appropriately managed.
- Fluid overload is an important cause for mortality in children with AKI. Monitoring of fluid balance is necessary; patients showing >10% fluid overload should be considered for early initiation of renal replacement therapy.
- AKI might not always be short-term self limiting process; a significant proportion is at risk of chronic kidney disease and requires long-term follow-up.

REFERENCES

1. Lameire NH, Bagga A, Cruz D, *et al.* Acute kidney injury: An increasing global concern. Lancet. 2013;382(9887):170-9.
2. Macedo E, Cerda J, Hou J, *et al.* Recognition and management of acute kidney injury in children: The ISN 0by25 Global Snapshot study. PLoS One. 2018;13(5):e0196586.
3. Bellomo R, Ronco C, Kellum JA, *et al.*; Acute Dialysis Quality Initiative workgroup. Acute renal failure - definition, outcome measures, animal models, fluid therapy and information technology needs: The Second International Consensus Conference of the Acute Dialysis Quality Initiative (ADQI) Group. Crit Care. 2004;8(4):R204-12.
4. Mehta RL, Kellum JA, Shah SV, *et al.* Acute Kidney Injury Network: Report of an initiative to improve outcomes in acute kidney injury. Crit Care. 2007;11:R31.
5. Kidney Disease: Improving Global Outcome (KDIGO) acute kidney injury work group. KDIGO clinical practice guideline for acute kidney injury. Kidney Int Suppl. 2012;2:124-38.
6. Susantitaphong P, Cruz DN, Cerda J, *et al.*; for the Acute Kidney Advisory Group of the American Society of Nephrology. World incidence of AKI: A meta-analysis. Clin J Am Soc Nephrol. 2013;8:1482-93.
7. Kaddourah A, Basu RK, Bagshaw SM, *et al.*; AWARE Investigators. Epidemiology of acute kidney injury in critically ill children and young adults. N Engl J Med. 2017;376(1):11-20.
8. Jetton JG, Boohaker LJ, Sethi SK, *et al.* Incidence and outcomes of neonatal acute kidney injury (AWAKEN): A multicentre, multinational, observational cohort study. Lancet Child Adolesc Health. 2017;1(3):184-94.
9. Lameire N, Van Biesen W, Vanholder R. Epidemiology of acute kidney injury in children worldwide, including developing countries. Pediatr Nephrol. 2017;32(8):1301-14.
10. Cerdá J, Bagga A, Kher V, *et al.* The contrasting characteristics of acute kidney injury in developed and developing countries. Nat Clin Pract Nephrol. 2008;4(3):138-53.
11. Feehally J. The ISN 0by25 global snapshot study. Ann Nutr Metab. 2016;68 Suppl 2:29-31.
12. Jetton JG, Askenazi DJ. Update on acute kidney injury in the neonate. Curr Opin Pediatr. 2012;24(2):191-6.
13. Mian AN, Askenazi DJ, Mhanna MJ. Therapeutic options for neonatal acute kidney injury (AKI). Curr Treat Options Pediatr. 2016;2(2):69-81.
14. Ciccia E, Devarajan P. Pediatric acute kidney injury: Prevalence, impact and management challenges. Int J Nephrol Renovasc Dis. 2017;10:77-84.
15. Goldstein SL, Chawla LS. Renal angina. Clin J Am Soc Nephrol. 2010;5(5):943-9.
16. Koyner JL, Davison DL, Brasha-Mitchell E, *et al.* Furosemide stress test and biomarkers for the prediction of AKI severity. J Am Soc Nephrol. 2015;26(8):2023-31.
17. Doyle JF, Forni LG. Update on sepsis-associated acute kidney injury: Emerging targeted therapies. Biologics: Targets and Therapy. 2016;10:149-56.
18. Li Y, Tang X, Zhang J, *et al.* Nutritional support for acute kidney injury. Cochrane Database of Sys Rev. 2012;8:CD005426.
19. Sethi SK, Maxvold N, Bunchman T, *et al.* Nutritional management in the critically ill child with acute kidney injury: A review. Pediatr Nephrol. 2017;32(4):589-601.
20. Blanco FC, Ortega G, Qureshi FG. Renal replacement therapy in children. Semin Pediatr Surg. 2015;24(1):25-31.
21. Mammen C, Al Abbas A, Skippen P, *et al.* Long-term risk of CKD in children surviving episodes of acute kidney injury in the intensive care unit: A prospective cohort study. Am J Kidney Dis Off J Natl Kidney Found. 2012;59(4):523-30.
22. Sigurjonsdottir VK, Chaturvedi S, Mammen C, *et al.* Pediatric acute kidney injury and the subsequent risk for chronic kidney disease: Is there cause for alarm? Pediatr Nephrol. 2018;33(11):2047-55.
23. Mehta R, Bagga A, Patibandla R, *et al.* Detection and management of AKI in the developing world: The 18th Acute Disease Quality Initiative (ADQI) International Consensus Conference. Kid Int Rep. 2017;2(4):515-8.

CHAPTER

26

Hematuria

Anil Vasudevan, Arpana Iyengar

INTRODUCTION

Hematuria is a common presenting feature of diseases or abnormalities of genitourinary system and systemic diseases like coagulation disorders. It rarely could be factitious. It is not uncommon for children to present to the emergency room with hematuria. The prevalence of gross hematuria, based on a retrospective review of children seen in an emergency clinic was 0.13%.[1]

The goals for the physician attending to a child with hematuria in the emergency are: (i) to recognize and confirm the finding of hematuria, (ii) to identify common etiologies for hematuria and differentiate between benign and serious causes (iii) to recognize children with serious causes who warrant immediate referral for further evaluation and management.

An orderly, comprehensive approach can simplify the diagnosis and ensure appropriate management. The chapter highlights the common causes of hematuria in children and suggests a systematic approach to evaluation of these children.

Hematuria is defined as more than 5 red blood cells (RBCs) per high-power field in the urinary sediment.[2] Blood in the urine that is visible without microscopy is *gross hematuria* and finding RBCs in urine on microscopy is termed *microscopic hematuria*. Hematuria can result from non-renal, and glomerular and extraglomerular abnormalities. Asymptomatic microscopic hematuria is unlikely to be encountered in emergency clinics and is not discussed further.

The list of common causes of hematuria is given in **Table 1**.

CATEGORIZING PATIENTS WITH HEMATURIA

Children with hematuria may come to the emergency room with following presentations:

Gross Hematuria

Gross hematuria is a frightening experience for the child and parents. A cause is identified in almost half the cases.[3] The common causes of gross hematuria include acute glomerulonephritis (e.g. poststreptococcal and IgA nephropathy), benign familial hematuria and bleeding disorders, which are usually painless. Urinary tract infections, idiopathic hypercalciuria, hemorrhagic cystitis, ureteropelvic junction obstruction, calculi, trauma and meatal stenosis with ulceration may present with painful gross hematuria. Hematuria associated with minor trauma may unmask an underlying congenital anomaly. Recurrent hematuria with complete clearing of hematuria or persistent microscopic hematuria between the episodes of gross hematuria is seen in IgA nephropathy, Alport syndrome and benign familial hematuria. Among hematological causes, hematuria (both microscopic and macroscopic) is the most frequent complication of sickle cell trait.

An important but underdiagnosed cause of gross hematuria is idiopathic hypercalciuria and the child may have gross or microscopic hematuria with symptoms of dysuria, frequency and urgency. Wilms tumor typically presents with a flank mass and macroscopic hematuria and is the most common urological malignancy

Table 1: Causes of hematuria

Glomerular	*Non-glomerular*
Acute postinfectious glomerulonephritis IgA nephropathy* Benign familial hematuria*† Systemic infections (malaria, leptospirosis, infective endocarditis) Membranoproliferative glomerulonephritis Focal segmental glomerulosclerosis Systemic lupus erythematosus Hemolytic uremic syndrome† Henoch-Schonlein purpura Alport syndrome*†	Nephrolithiasis*† Hypercalciuria*† Viral hemorrhagic cystitis Urinary tract infection@ Vascular abnormalities Renal vein or artery thrombosis@ A-V malformations Ureteropelvic obstruction@ Renal cystic disease†@ Bleeding, clotting disorders *Medications:* cyclophosphamide, anticoagulants, NSAIDs Idiopathic hypercalciuria, Wilm tumor

* Causes of recurrent hematuria
† Hematuria with familial association
@ Common in newborns

in children. Strenuous exercise alone can cause hematuria but is uncommon in children.

Clinical symptoms with microscopic hematuria: Many of the conditions mentioned above may also manifest with symptomatic microscopic hematuria. The clinical symptoms may be related to systemic illness or to the genitourinary tract.

Hematuria secondary to trauma: Traumatic hematuria is seen due to injury to genitourinary system following vehicle accidents, fall or sports injuries. In fact, after the brain, the kidney is the most frequently injured internal organ in children. The degree of hematuria however is not a reliable indicator of severity of injury.

Blood spotting on diaper or underwear (urethrorrhagia): Usually seen in pre-pubertal children.

EVALUATING A CHILD WITH HEMATURIA

A detailed history, comprehensive physical examination and relevant laboratory tests are indispensable to the evaluation of hematuria (**Flowchart 1**).

Presenting history: Child may present with clinical manifestation that is general (e.g. fever, upper respiratory complaints, malaise), unrelated to urinary tract (e.g. rash, arthritis, bleeding from other sites), symptoms of upper urinary tract (e.g. facial puffiness, limb edema, decreased urine output, breathlessness secondary to fluid overload, headache or altered sensorium, seizures due to severe hypertension) or lower urinary tract (dysuria, urgency, frequency and flank pain).

Drug history: Many drugs (analgesics, cyclophosphamide, anticoagulants and quinine) can cause hematuria, hence a detailed history of drugs used by the child is useful.

Family history: History of deafness, recurrent hematuria and kidney disease in family members should be enquired into.

Physical examination: Blood pressure should be measured and skin examined for rashes, bruises and palpable purpuric spots. Abdomen should be inspected for flank masses and bladder. Evaluation is not complete without examination of urethral meatus in males and vaginal introitus in females.

Clues from History and Physical Examination

- An important step in evaluation is to distinguish bright red-urine from "cola-colored" urine as it indicates the source of bleeding (glomerular vs. lower urinary tract). The characteristics that help in distinguishing the two conditions are given in **Table 2**.
- Initial gross hematuria suggests a problem in the distal urethra, while hematuria throughout urination indicates upper urinary tract or bladder disease.
- Edema, decreased urine output, hypertension and cola-colored urine with a history of pyoderma or pharyngitis few weeks prior to onset of symptoms indicate poststreptococcal glomerulonephritis.

Flowchart 1: Algorithm for evaluation of hematuria

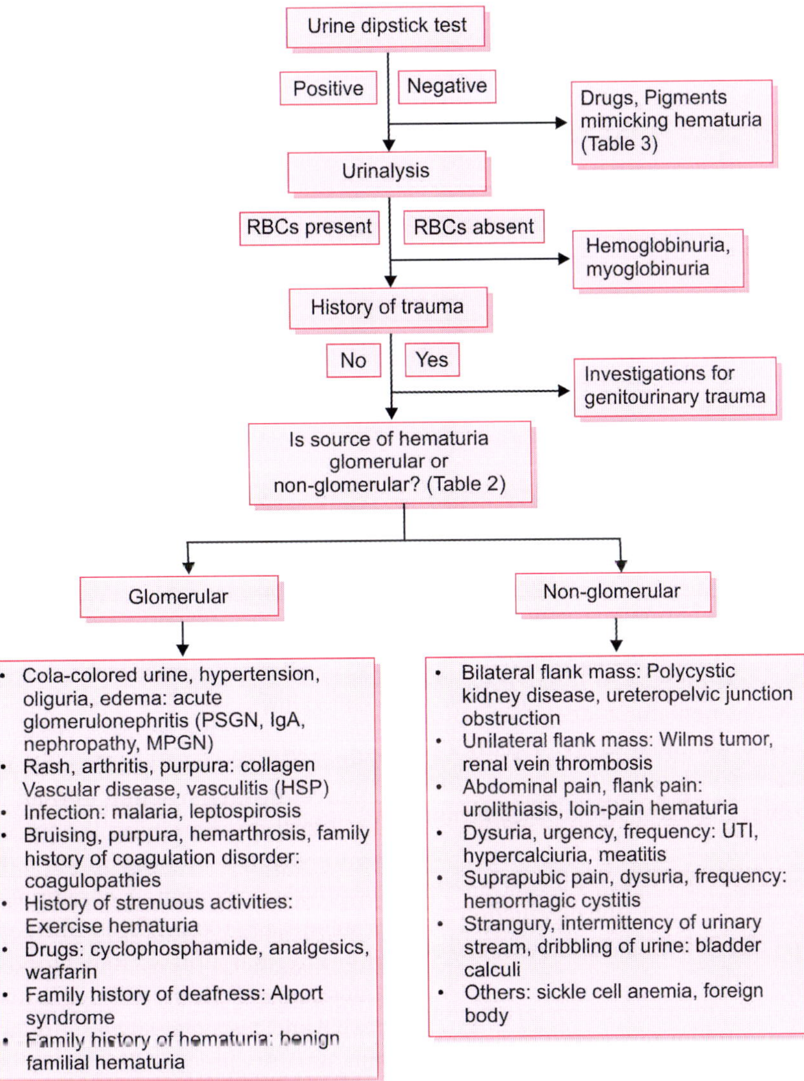

(PSGN: post-streptococcal glomerulonephritis; MPGN: membranoproliferative glomerulonephritis; HSP: Henoch Schonlein purpura).

- History of upper respiratory infection followed within a few days by hematuria also suggests renal parenchymal disease
- Bleeding or coagulation disorder should be suspected in a presence of bruising, purpura, hemarthrosis or positive family history of similar disorder.
- A history of joint pains, skin rashes and prolonged fever in adolescents is suggestive of a collagen vascular disorder.
- Dysuria, urgency and frequency in older children are often seen in urinary tract infection or hemorrhagic cystitis.
- Family history of hematuria may be present in patients with stones, polycystic kidney disease, sickle cell disease or hearing loss.
- Flank pain with hematuria may indicate calculi, pelviureteric junction obstruction, renal vein or artery thrombosis or very rarely loin-pain hematuria syndrome.

Table 2: Differentiating glomerular and non-glomerular hematuria

Features	*Glomerular diseases*	*Non-glomerular causes*
History of dysuria	Absent	Present in urethritis and cystitis
Systemic complaints	Edema, fever, pharyngitis, rash, arthralgia	Fever (urinary infection), pain (calculi)
Family history	Deafness, hematuria (Alport syndrome)	Positive with calculi and hypercalciuria
Hypertension, edema	Usually present	Less common
Abdominal mass	Absent	Present in Wilms tumor, obstructive uropathy
Rash, arthritis	Lupus erythematosus, Henoch Schonlein purpura	Absent, unless part of drug induced interstitial nephritis
Urinalysis		
Color	Brown, tea, cola	Bright red, clots may be present
Proteinuria	2+ or more	Less than 2+
Dysmorphic RBCs	More than 80%	Less than 20%
RBC casts	Common	Absent

- History of strenuous activities like participation in athletic events or exercise suggests exercise hematuria.
- Strangury, intermittency of urinary stream and dribbling of urine indicates an obstructive process.
- The diagnosis of genitourinary trauma must be considered if a child has hematuria, decreased urine output, unexplained abdominal mass or pain and tenderness, penetrating abdominal trauma, fracture pelvis, blood at urethral meatus or scrotal swelling and hematoma.
- Wilms tumor (in younger children), polycystic kidney disease and pelviureteric junction obstruction are the differential diagnosis in a child presenting with a flank mass and hematuria.
- Blood spotting the underwear of an otherwise normal prepubertal child with dysuria and microscopic hematuria suggest idiopathic urethritis.

Investigations

Urine dipstick: The first step is to inspect the urine and perform a dipstick test as many substances may discolor urine and mimic hematuria (**Table 3**). It is important to briefly dip the strip in the urine, tap off excess urine, and read the strip at the recommended time (usually one minute). Dipsticks have a sensitivity of 100% and a specificity of 99% in detecting one to five red blood cells (RBCs) per high power field.[4] The dipstick test will also be positive in hemoglobinuria and myoglobinuria. False positive test is obtained if urine is alkaline or in presence of oxidizing agents like povidone iodine.

Table 3: Substances that color urine and mimic hematuria

Red or pink urine: Hemoglobinuria, myoglobinuria, beets and red dyes in food, porphyrins, chloroquine, phenazopyridine
Dark brown or black: Methemoglobinemia, homogentisic acid, bile pigments
Dark yellow or orange: Rifampicin, concentrated urine, pyridium

Urinalysis: Hematuria is confirmed by microscopy. A positive dipstick reaction and an absence of RBCs and RBC casts on examining the urinary sediment suggest hemoglobinuria or myoglobinuria. The urine is also tested for protein excretion. A combination of hematuria and proteinuria (>100 mg/dL) indicates a significant disease of glomerular illness. Red blood cell casts is usually diagnostic of glomerulonephritis. White blood cells (WBC) and casts may suggest urinary tract infection or an inflammatory process. Examining red cell morphology by phase contrast microscopy may help to locate the site of bleeding. Presence of greater than 80% dysmorphic RBCs is suggestive of glomerular hematuria with a sensitivity of 96% and specificity of 93%.[5]

Ultrasonography: Ultrasonography should be performed in children with abdominal trauma, pelvic fracture, signs of obstruction of the urinary tract or in the presence of renal mass. Ultrasound is known to miss some small stones (<3 mm) and hence CT imaging may be indicated in children with strong suspicion of stones.

X-ray KUB: A plain X-ray of kidney and urinary bladder (KUB) region in erect posture may be advised in suspected cases of genitourinary trauma or in children with renal colic.

Other investigations: Obtaining blood for levels of urea, creatinine and electrolytes should be individualized. Hemogram, platelet count and coagulation profile are obtained in suspected cases of coagulopathies or bleeding disorders. Urine sample for culture is taken if a urinary infection is suspected and measurement of spot urine calcium-creatinine ratio is helpful in establishing hypercalciuria as a cause of hematuria. Serologic tests (C3, antinuclear antibodies) and ASLO titer may be requested in systemic lupus and poststreptococcal glomerulonephritis, respectively.

Children with history of abdominal, groin, perineal trauma and urine demonstrating >50 RBC/HPF should undergo imaging with an abdominal CT scan.

MANAGEMENT

A hemodyamically unstable or sick child with hematuria should be stabilized before specialist consultation is sought. A child with severe hematuria and passing clots should be catheterized, except in cases of urethral trauma. Children with evidence of acute nephritis, azotemia, severe acute kidney injury or complicated UTI should be admitted and managed appropriately. Treatment of hematuria in the emergency is based on the diagnosis.[6]

Children who require admission include those with acute nephritis, renal failure, trauma, severe systemic manifestations or bleeding manifestations, infections requiring intravenous antibiotics and obstructive calculi. Children with asymptomatic isolated gross hematuria and a normal physical examination can follow-up in outpatient setting for further evaluation. Children with trauma, stones, mass in abdomen and congenital anomalies require a pediatric surgery or urology consult. Patients with family history of deafness or nephritis, recurrent episodes of hematuria, systemic complaints like arthritis, rash and fever and isolated gross hematuria need to be referred for specialist opinion.

KEY MESSAGES

- The goals for the physician attending to a child with hematuria in the emergency are: (i) to recognize and confirm the finding of hematuria, (ii) to identify common etiologies for hematuria and differentiate between benign and serious causes (iii) to recognize children with serious causes who warrant immediate referral for further evaluation and management.
- Hematuria is defined as more than 5 red blood cells (RBCs) per high-power field in the urinary sediment.[2] Blood in the urine that is visible without microscopy is gross hematuria and finding RBCs in urine on microscopy is termed microscopic hematuria. Hematuria can result from non-renal, and glomerular and extra-glomerular abnormalities.
- Investigations include urine dipstick test, complete microscopic, examination of urine, urine culture, ultrasonography, renal function, coagulation profile, and serological tests for immune etiology.
- A child with severe hematuria and passing clots should be catheterized, except in cases of urethral trauma.

REFERENCES

1. Ingelfinger JR, Davis AE, Grupe WE. Frequency and etiology of gross hematuria in a general pediatrics setting. Pediatrics. 1977;59:557-61.
2. Phadke KD, Vijayakumar M, Sharma J, *et al.*; Indian Pediatric Nephrology Group, Indian Academy of Pediatrics. Consensus statement on evaluation of hematuria. Indian Pediatr. 2006; 43:965-73.
3. Greenfield SP, Williot P, Kaplan D. Gross hematuria in children: A ten-year review. Urology. 2007;69:166-9.
4. Moore GP, Robinson M. Do urine dipsticks reliably predict microhematuria? The bloody truth! Ann Emerg Med. 1988; 17:257-60.
5. Stapleton FB. Morphology of urinary red blood cells: A simple guide in localizing the site of hematuria. Pediatr Clin North Am. 1987;34:561-9.
6. Pade KH, Liu DR. An evidence-based approach to the management of hematuria in children in the emergency department. Pediatr Emerg Med Pract. 2014;11:1-13.

CHAPTER 27

Acute Seizure

Sangeetha Yoganathan, Rangan Srinivasaraghavan

INTRODUCTION

Seizures are common pediatric emergency that often results from various etiologies, thus making it a diagnostic challenge. A seizure is defined as "a transient occurrence of signs and/or symptoms due to abnormal excessive or synchronous neuronal activity in the brain".[1] A single seizure episode does not necessarily mean that a child has epilepsy. Epilepsy is considered if there are "at least two unprovoked or reflex seizures >24 h apart or one unprovoked or reflex seizure and a probability of having another seizure similar to the general recurrence risk after two unprovoked seizures (≥60%) over the next 10 years, or an epilepsy syndrome".[2] Status epilepticus (SE) is defined as condition that results "either from the failure of the mechanisms responsible for seizure termination or from the initiation of mechanisms which lead to abnormally prolonged seizures (after time point t1)".[3] Time point t2 refers to the limit beyond which patients may have long-term consequences such as neuronal network alteration and injury to neurons resulting in neuronal death.[3] The time frame (t1 and t2) for tonic-clonic SE are 5 min and 30 min. The time frame (t1 and t2) for focal SE with impaired awareness are 10 min and 60 min respectively. Febrile seizures are the most common convulsive events in children less than 5 years of age. Simple febrile seizures are "seizures accompanied by a fever without CNS infection".[4] Simple febrile seizures occur in children between 6 and 60 months of age. This chapter focuses on the practical approach to children with acute seizure in terms of detailed history taking, clinical examination, appropriate investigations and treatment. Also, this chapter discusses the management protocol for status epilepticus in children.

CLASSIFICATION OF SEIZURES

Classification of seizures is crucial for the clinicians and researchers as it not only provides an insight into the diagnosis but also improves the understanding and communication and helps in optimizing the treatment options. The classification of seizures was described by the International League Against Epilepsy (ILAE) in 1981, 1985, 1989 and 2017. The ILAE in 2017 has classified the seizures based on the onset as focal, generalized, unknown and unclassified.[5] The classification of seizures based on onset is shown in **Figure 1**. The generalized and partial seizures are reclassified in the recent ILAE classification as generalized and focal seizures.

Focal Seizures

If the abnormal electrical activity originates on one region of brain, it results in focal seizures which may or may not spread to other side.[6] Simple and complex partial seizures have been replaced by the terms focal

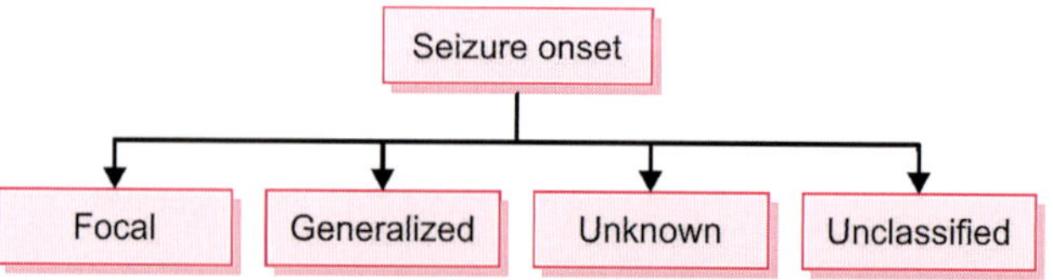

Fig. 1: Classification of seizures based on onset

seizures with awareness or impaired awareness.[5] The term impaired awareness cannot be used exchangeable with loss of consciousness. The focal-onset seizures can either be motor or non-motor. The focal motor seizures include automatisms, atonic, clonic, epileptic spasms, hyperkinetic, myoclonic and tonic while the focal non-motor seizures include autonomic symptoms, behavioral arrest, cognitive, emotional and sensory symptoms as listed in **Table 1**.[6]

Generalized Seizures

If the abnormal electrical activity originates simultaneously from bilateral cerebral hemispheres and spreads through neuronal networks, it results in generalized seizures.[6] Seizures with the focal onset and secondary generalization are now reclassified as focal to bilateral tonic-clonic seizures. The generalized motor seizures include tonic, clonic, tonic-clonic, myoclonic, atonic, epileptic spasms, myoclonic-tonic-clonic and myoclonic-atonic while the generalized non-motor seizures are typical absence, atypical absence, myoclonic absence, and eyelid myoclonia as listed in **Table 2**.[6]

Unknown or Unclassified Seizures

If the seizure event cannot be classified with confidence even after all available clinical and supporting information, it must be categorized under unknown onset, or if the available information is incomplete, it is categorized as unclassified.

Table 1: Focal onset seizure types

Motor onset	*Non-motor onset*
• Atonic • Clonic • Hyperkinetic • Myoclonic • Tonic • Epileptic spasms • Automatisms	• Sensory • Cognitive • Emotional • Autonomic • Behavioral arrest

Table 2: Generalized onset seizure types

Motor onset	*Non-motor onset*
• Tonic-clonic • Tonic • Clonic • Atonic • Myoclonic • Myoclonic-atonic • Myoclonic-tonic-clonic • Epileptic spasms	• Typical absence • Atypical absence • Myoclonic absence • Absence with eyelid myoclonia

Classification of Status Epilepticus (SE)

The four-axis used in the classification of SE are semiology, etiology, electroencephalography (EEG) correlates and age.[3] The classification of SE is depicted in **Table 3**.[3]

ETIOLOGY OF SEIZURES AND EPILEPSY

Seizures are one of the most common pediatric emergencies. The incidence of status epilepticus was determined to be 6.6% in an Indian study.[7] The etiologies for acute seizures in children are diverse, and the causes of acute seizures in children are summarized in **Table 4**.[8] In a retrospective study of 236 children with new-onset seizures presenting as status epilepticus (SE), about one-quarter were acute symptomatic seizures.[9] Based on the etiology, seizures can be classified as unprovoked and acute symptomatic seizures.[10]

- **Acute symptomatic seizures** refer to seizures that occur in "close temporal relationship with an acute CNS insult, which may be metabolic, toxic, structural, infectious, or due to inflammation."[10] The time interval between the acute CNS insult and the occurrence of clinical seizures may vary depending upon the cause.
- **Unprovoked seizures** refer to "seizures occurring in the absence of a potentially responsible clinical condition or beyond the interval estimated for the occurrence of acute symptomatic seizures."[10] Unprovoked seizures

Table 3: Classification of status epilepticus

Axis	*Description*
Axis 1	Semiology: • Convulsive or non-convulsive SE
Axis 2	Etiology: • Symptomatic: acute, remote, progressive, SE in children with epilepsy syndromes • Cryptogenic
Axis 3	EEG correlates: • Location • Morphology • Pattern of discharges • Modulation • Time-related features such as frequency, duration, and dynamics • Effect of medication on EEG
Axis 4	Age: Neonatal (<30 days) Infancy (1–24 mon) Childhood (2–12 y) Adolescence and adults (13–59 y) Elderly (>60 y)

(SE: status epilepticus; EEG: electroencephalography)

Table 4: Causes of acute seizures in children

Category	*Causes*
Infective	Meningitis, encephalitis, brain abscess, neurocysticercosis, tuberculoma
Traumatic	Intracranial bleed
Metabolic	Hypoglycemia, hypomagnesemia, hyponatremia, inborn error of metabolism
Vascular	Hemorrhagic or ischemic stroke
Structural	Cortical malformations
Drugs or toxins	Oral hypoglycemic drugs, antidepressants, isoniazid, antipsychotics, camphor ingestion
Inflammatory	Acute disseminated encephalomyelitis, autoimmune encephalitis
Others	Hypoxic ischemic encephalopathy

must be considered in children without an immediate or identified provoking cause.

The etiology of epilepsy may be placed in one of the six categories as shown in **Table 5**.[5]

Table 5: ILAE task force defined etiology categories of epilepsy

Category	*Description*
Structural	Findings on the neuroimaging implicated to cause seizures due to concordant clinical and EEG findings
Genetic	Pathogenic variants in gene or copy number variants with typical clinical and EEG findings with or without family history
Infectious	Refers to patients with epilepsy due to an underlying infective etiology such as neurocysticercosis, toxoplasmosis or post meningitic sequelae Patients with acute seizures due to infection are not placed in this category
Metabolic	Refers to patients with epilepsy due to an underlying metabolic disorder such as pyridoxine dependent epilepsy Transient metabolic disturbances are not placed in this category
Immune	Patients with epilepsy due to an underlying autoimmune encephalitis
Unknown	Patients with epilepsy of unknown etiology

(EEG: electroencephalography)

DIAGNOSTIC EVALUATION

History

The standard tools to establish the diagnosis are structured history taking and analysis of video record of paroxysmal events. The history must be obtained from the parents or caretakers who have directly witnessed the events. The important points to be ascertained while eliciting history in a child presenting with seizures are:[8]

- Age at onset of seizures
- Provoking factors (fever, sleep deprivation, prolonged fasting, toxins, trauma)
- Description of the pre-ictal period (description of aura)
- Description of ictal event
- Description of post-ictal period
- Classify the seizures as focal, generalized, unknown or unclassified onset
- Exclude seizure mimics
- Record seizure frequency
- Duration of seizures
- Exposure to drugs or toxins
- If known patient of epilepsy on treatment, check for compliance and response to treatment
- Family history of febrile seizures, epilepsy, neuro-metabolic disorders
- Antenatal or neonatal risk factors
- Developmental history
- Immunization history
- Document comorbidities such as hyperactivity, attention deficits, aggressive behavior, autistic traits, and learning disabilities.

Focused Examination

If a convulsing child is brought to the emergency room, a rapid assessment of appearance, work of breathing, and circulation must be done using the pediatric assessment triangle.[11] Clinical evaluation and treatment must go on simultaneously in the emergency room. A meticulous general examination must be carried out to look for the neurocutaneous markers such as ash-leaf macules, adenoma sebaceum, shagreen patch, café-au-lait macules, epidermal nevus, port wine stain, and pigmentary mosaicism.[8] Other specific findings that are to be checked in the general examination are facial dysmorphism, exanthems, BCG scar, anemia, petechiae or purpura, generalized lymphadenopathy, icterus and signs of avitaminosis. Anthropometric parameters must be documented to exclude microcephaly, macrocephaly, and failure to thrive.

Neurological examination in a child presenting with altered sensorium includes assessment of the level of consciousness using Glasgow coma scale, assessment of pupillary size, symmetry and reaction to light, fundus examination, elicitation of Doll's eye reflex and also to look for facial asymmetry, hemiparesis and signs of

Table 6: Salient features in general and neurological examination of a convulsing child

General examination		*Neurological examination*
Clinical findings	Etiology	GCS score Pupillary size, symmetry, reaction to light Fundus examination Doll's eye movement Facial symmetry Focal motor deficits Signs of meningeal irritation Cranium: microcephaly, macrocephaly, craniosynostosis Spine: spinal dysraphism, gibbus
Ash-leaf macules, adenoma sebaceum, shagreen patch, café-au-lait macules, epidermal nevus, port wine stain and pigmentary mosaicism	Neurocutaneous syndrome	
Facial dysmorphism Coarse facies	Chromosomal disorders Storage disorders	
Icterus	Hepatic encephalopathy	
Anemia, petechiae, purpura, generalized lymphadenopathy	Lymphoreticular malignancy Meningococcal meningitis	
Cyanosis, polycythemia	Congenital cyanotic heart disease	
Failure to thrive, generalized lymphadenopathy, candidiasis	Primary or secondary immunodeficiency	
Exanthems	Viral exanthematous illness	
Sketelal dysostosis	Storage disorders	
Glossitis, knuckles and oral pigmentation, pallor	Nutritional-vitamin B_{12} deficiency	

(GCS: Glasgow coma scale)

meningeal irritation. The salient features in the general and neurological examination are summarized in **Table 6**.

DIFFERENTIAL DIAGNOSIS

The first important step in the management of seizures is to confirm the diagnosis of seizure and differentiate the paroxysmal event from non-epileptic events. The non-epileptic events and their identification during the various stages of development are summarized in **Tables 7 and 8**.[8,12-15]

PATHOPHYSIOLOGY

The abnormal electrical discharges resulting from the excitation of the cortical neurons lead on to seizures. Under normal circumstances, only a single action potential could pass from one neuron to another neuron through a normal synapse.[16] An aberration in the ions, receptors, cells, a network of the brain and focal or diffuse structural malformations results in seizures.[16] Few examples include defect at the level of ions such as sodium or calcium channel mutations, acetylcholine receptor defects in autosomal dominant frontal lobe epilepsy and aberrant cell proliferation may result in self-excitation that might occur in temporal lobe epilepsy. The excitation of susceptible cortical neurons leads to synchronous discharges of a larger connecting group of neurons resulting in seizures. Also, an imbalance of excitatory and inhibitory neurotransmitters occurs in these patients.[16]

If the seizure does not terminate in some instances, depending on the etiology, it results in status epilepticus. Understanding the pathophysiology is crucial for the decision of drug therapy in patients with SE. The possible explanations for prolonged seizures are:[17]

- Receptors trafficking at the cellular level that results in internalization of GABA receptors
- Increase in the glutaminergic receptors at the level of cell surface
- GABA-mediated currents may turn excitatory due to changes in extracellular chloride ion concentration
- Energy failure resulting from mitochondrial dysfunction
- Increased blood brain barrier permeability that stimulates an inflammatory process.

MANAGEMENT

The diagnostic approach to a child with acute seizures may be discussed under two categories namely management at the emergency department and ongoing care at the ward or pediatric intensive care unit. The goals of management while dealing with a child with active seizures are:[11]

- Maintain airway, breathing, and circulation
- Identify and correct hypoglycemia and dyselectrolytemia
- Rapid control of clinical and electrographic seizures by an appropriate drug therapy
- Treat fever and infection with analgesics and antibiotics
- Appropriate investigations to identify the etiology
- Manage the systemic complications.

Table 7: Non-epileptic events in neonates and infancy

Paroxysmal events	*Description*
Jitteriness	Rapid oscillations of limbs, equal in amplitude and frequency which are not associated with autonomic disturbances. Jitteriness occurs in awake state and these events are decreased by restraining
Benign sleep myoclonus	Repetitive myoclonic jerks that occurs in non-rapid eye movement (NREM) sleep
Breath holding spells	Cyanotic and pallid spells are the two types of breath holding spells. Events are initiated on denial of demands, fright or pain. Events are characterized by vigorous cry, forced expiration, apnea, cyanosis and loss of consciousness with or without clonic seizures
Gratification behavior	Episodes of tonic posturing with flushing, sweating, grunting, irregular breathing and copulatory movements
Night terrors	Events are characterized by arousal in stage 3 or 4 of NREM sleep and screaming spells. Child appears fearful and inconsolable. These episodes are followed by sleep and amnesia for these events
Sandifer syndrome	Occurs in the postprandial period of children with gastroesophageal reflux disease and the events are characterized by tonic extension of neck, dystonic posturing of trunk and limbs
Hyperekplexia	Exaggerated startle with or without loss of muscle stiffness and loss of posture
Stereotypies	Involuntary, repetitive and rhythmic movements that occur in a predictable pattern and location
Drug reactions	Oculogyric crisis that occurs in children with metoclopramide overdose
Shuddering attack	Sudden flexion of head and trunk with shuddering movements

Table 8: Non-epileptic events in older children and adolescents

Paroxysmal events	*Description*
Syncope	Transient loss of consciousness that results from decreased cerebral perfusion
Psychogenic non-epileptic events	Events are typically precipitated by stressors. Events are characterized by forced eye closure, absence of tongue injury, bladder or bowel incontinence, vocalization during events and preserved consciousness. These events typically occur in awake state, in the presence of witnesses. Events are variable in semiology and duration
Tics	Brief rapid movements affecting single, localized or multiple muscle groups
Childhood periodic syndromes	Cyclical vomiting syndrome is considered if there are at least 5 attacks over any interval or at least 3 attacks in 6 months period. Intense nausea and vomiting episodes lasting from 1 h–10 d and the frequency of vomiting during attacks must be at least 4 per hour. Children return to baseline in between the events
Paroxysmal dyskinesias	Dystonia, chorea, athetosis or ballismus that are precipitated by sudden movements, exercises, caffeine, alcohol, stress and sleep
Migraine variants	

The management of convulsing child in the emergency room begins with the maintenance of airway, breathing, and circulation. Simultaneous focused history and examination must be performed to assess the cardiopulmonary status and etiology.

Maintain Airway, Breathing and Circulation

The steps to be considered in the management of airway, breathing, and circulation are:[11]

- Proper positioning to maintain the airway patency and suction the nasopharyngeal secretions
- If adequate respiratory efforts are observed, provide oxygen via a nonrebreathing mask
- If there are poor respiratory efforts, poor oxygenation, cyanosis or desaturation, initiate bag, and mask ventilation
- Endotracheal intubation must be considered in case of refractory status epilepticus, shock, raised intracranial pressure and in children with the need for a prolonged bag and mask ventilation
- Establish intravenous access and administer fluid boluses if shock is identified.

Investigations

The investigations are directed to identify the etiology and to monitor the complications of status epilepticus. The summary of investigations in children with new-onset seizures or status epilepticus is given in **Box 1**.[18] In case of breakthrough or withdrawal seizures in a patient with epilepsy while on treatment, the drug levels must be measured.

Appropriate Drug Therapy

On arrival to the emergency room, after stabilization of airway, breathing, and circulation, check for hypoglycemia and dyselctrolytemia. The steps involved in the management of status epilepticus is described in **Table 9**.[17,19-22]

Specific Treatment

In children with bacterial meningitis, IV ceftriaxone (100 mg/kg/d in 2 divided doses) is recommended for 10–14 days. Acyclovir (60 mg/kg/d in 3 divided doses) is recommended in children with viral encephalitis awaiting the CSF viral PCR reports. The duration of treatment in confirmed cases ranges from 14 to 21 days.[23]Cysticidal therapy must be considered in children with non-calcified granuloma of neurocysticercosis (NCC). Albendazole 15 mg/kg/d is given as a single dose for 7–28 days after an ophthalmological examination.[8] Cysticidal therapy must be administered from the third day of steroid such as oral prednisolone 1 mg/kg/d or dexamethasone 0.15 mg/kg/dose every 6 hourly. Cysticidal therapy is contraindicated if there are multiple granulomas, ocular cysticercosis, intraventricular or spinal granulomas.

In children with proven autoimmune encephalitis, simultaneous administration of intravenous immunoglobulin 400 mg/kg/d for 5 days and intravenous pulse dose of methyl prednisolone 30 mg/kg/d for 5 days followed by oral prednisolone are recommended.[24] If the clinical response is adequate, the tapering schedule of steroid must be planned. If there is poor clinical response, rituximab infusion 375 mg/m^2 once in a week for 4 weeks must be considered. Tumor surveillance is mandatory in all children with autoimmune encephalitis. Intravenous pulse doses of methyl prednisolone 30 mg/kg/d for 5 days followed by a tapering schedule of oral prednisolone is recommended in the management of children with ADEM.[25] Intravenous immunoglobulin or plasma exchange may be considered if there is no significant clinical response with steroid.

DOMICILIARY MANAGEMENT

The most important part of the management of children with acute seizures is counseling the parents to reduce their fear and anxiety.[8] The parents must be counseled regarding the risk of recurrence, need for long-term antiepileptic medications, adverse effects of drugs, long-term outcome and domiciliary management of seizures. The parents must adhere to the following instructions in case of breakthrough seizures:

- Place the child in the left lateral position
- Do not administer any oral medications
- Suctioning of airway if possible
- Intranasal midazolam 0.2 mg/kg/dose (max dose 10 mg) to be administered into the nostrils
- Seek medical care at the earliest.

COMPLICATIONS OF STATUS EPILEPTICUS

The SE is one of the common neurological emergencies in children with high morbidity and mortality and the reported mortality in these patients varies from 3–40%.[26] The acute systemic complications in SE result from prolonged seizures, effects of antiepileptic medications and the underlying etiology. The long-term consequences result from the neuronal injury and neuronal death. The acute systemic complications of status epilepticus are summarized in **Box 2**.

LONG-TERM OUTCOME

The predictors of morbidity in children with SE are etiology, younger age, super refractory status epilepticus, presence of specific EEG patterns such as periodic discharges, burst suppression, multifocal discharges and suppression of background activity.[27] The long-term consequences in SE are an intellectual disability, learning disabilities, memory deficits, linguistic deficits, motor deficits, behavioral problems, and epilepsy.[20] Children with developmental delay, neurocutaneous syndrome, genetic epilepsies, metabolic disorders, inflammatory granulomas, progressive myoclonic epilepsies, epilepsy syndromes, and cortical malformations are candidates for long term antiepileptic medications.

KEY MESSAGES

- Seizures result from abnormal synchronous electrical discharges due to cortical excitation.
- The etiologies for acute seizures in children are often diverse and may be classified in to acute symptomatic or unprovoked seizures.
- Based on the onset, the seizures can be classified in to focal, generalized, unknown and unclassified.

Box 1: Investigations in children with status epilepticus

- Blood glucose
- Serum electrolytes: sodium, calcium, magnesium
- Complete blood count
- C-reactive protein
- Blood culture
- Liver function test
- Renal parameters
- Toxin screening
- Screening for inborn error of metabolism: ammonia, arterial lactate, tandem mass spectrometry, urine gas chromatography mass spectrometry
- Lumbar puncture
- Routine: CSF cell count, protein, sugar
- Specific for metabolic disorders: lactate, amino acid, neurotransmitters
- Specific for infection: bacterial culture, latex agglutination, viral PCR, TB PCR and MGIT, fungal culture
- Others: Oligoclonal bands in children with suspected ADEM, autoimmune encephalitis panel
- CT brain/MRI brain with contrast
- Electroencephalography
- PET or SPECT brain in children with suspected structural malformations

(CSF: cerebrospinal fluid; PCR: polymerase chain reaction; MGIT: mycobacteria growth indicator tube; ADEM: acute disseminated encephalomyelitis; PET: positron emission tomography; SPECT: single-photon emission computed tomography)

Table 9: Drug therapy in status epilepticus

Timeline	*Drugs*
On arrival	**IV access established:** Lorazepam (0.1 mg/kg; Max 4 mg) over 1 min or midazolam (0.1 mg/kg; Max 5 mg) over 1 min or diazepam (0.2 mg/kg; Max 10 mg) **IV access not established:** Intranasal/buccal/intramuscular midazolam (0.2 mg/kg) or rectal diazepam (0.2–0.5 mg/kg)
5 min	Repeat 2nd dose of benzodiazepine
10 min	Loading dose of phenytoin 20–30 mg/kg diluted in normal saline @ 1 mg/kg/min (max rate of infusion 50 mg/min)
Shift to pediatric intensive care unit	
30 min	If seizures persists after phenytoin infusion, consider 3rd anticonvulsant: Valproate (20–40 mg/kg IV diluted in normal saline) @ 5 mg/kg/min (must be used in caution in metabolic disorders and contraindicated in severe thrombocytopenia and liver dysfunction) Levetiracetam (20–40 mg/kg IV diluted in normal saline) @ 5 mg/kg/min or Phenobarbitone (20–30 mg/kg IV diluted in normal saline) @ 2 mg/kg/min
Refractory SE	IV midazolam bolus of 0.2 mg/kg followed by infusion @ 1 μg/kg/ min and increase once in every 5–10 min till the clinical and electrographic seizures are controlled or up to a max dose of 36 μg/kg/min; monitor hemodynamic status and consider continuous EEG recording. Taper midazolam @ 1 μg/kg/min if burst-suppression is maintained for 24 hours under continuous EEG monitoring for at least 24 h after withdrawal of midazolam If midazolam is not tolerated, consider bolus of thiopentone 5 mg/kg IV followed by an infusion up to max dose of 5 mg/kg/h Other drug options are topiramate, lacosamide and propofol
Super-refractory SE	Other drugs that may be considered are: Ketamine: loading dose of 0.5–4 mg/kg IV followed by infusion up to a max dose of 5 mg/kg/h (extrapolated from data in adult studies) Pyridoxine: 100 mg IV in children less than 2 years of age; 30 mg/kg Magnesium: 50 mg/kg IV over 30 min to target serum magnesium level of 3.5 mmol/L Methylprednisolone pulse dose of 30 mg/kg/d for 3 days followed by oral prednisolone 1 mg/kg/d Intravenous immunoglobulin 0.4 g/kg/d for 5 days Ketogenic diet 1:1 to 4:1 ratio Hypothermia 30–36°C Inhalational anesthetics Vagus nerve stimulation Tailored resection in focal lesion or hemispherotomy in hemispherical lesions

Box 2: Acute systemic complications of SE.

- Respiratory failure
- Neurogenic pulmonary edema
- Hypotension
- Stress cardiomyopathy
- Hypoglycemia
- Metabolic acidosis
- Thermal dysregulation
- Infection
- Hypoxic brain injury
- Raised intracranial pressure
- Rhabdomyolysis
- Renal dysfunction
- Hepatic dysfunction
- Paralytic ileus
- Acute pancreatic damage
- Bone fractures

- The standard tools to establish the diagnosis are structured history taking and analysis of video record of paroxysmal events. Always exclude seizure mimics.
- Correct hypoglycemia and dyselectrolytemia. Administer appropriate antiepileptic drugs according to standard protocols.

REFERENCES

1. Fisher RS, van Emde Boas W, Blume W, *et al.* Epileptic seizures and epilepsy: Definitions proposed by the International League Against Epilepsy (ILAE) and the International Bureau for Epilepsy (IBE). Epilepsia. 2005;46:470-2.
2. Fisher RS, Acevedo C, Arzimanoglou A, *et al.* ILAE official report: A practical clinical definition of epilepsy. Epilepsia. 2014;55:475-82.
3. Trinka E, Cock H, Hesdorffer D, *et al.* A definition and classification of status epilepticus—Report of the ILAE Task Force on Classification of Status Epilepticus. Epilepsia. 2015; 56:1515-23.
4. Subcommittee on Febrile Seizures; American Academy of Pediatrics. Neurodiagnostic evaluation of the child with a simple febrile seizure. Pediatrics. 2011;127:389-94.
5. Falco-Walter JJ, Scheffer IE, Fisher RS. The new definition and classification of seizures and epilepsy. Epilepsy Res. 2018; 139:73-9.
6. Brodie MJ, Zuberi SM, Scheffer IE, *et al.* The 2017 ILAE classification of seizure types and the epilepsies: What do people with epilepsy and their caregivers need to know? Epileptic Disord Int Epilepsy J Videotape. 2018;20:77-87.
7. Gulati S, Kalra V, Sridhar MR. Status epilepticus in Indian children in a tertiary care center. Indian J Pediatr. 2005;72: 105-8.
8. Gulati S, Kaushik JS. How I treat a first single seizure in a child. Ann Indian Acad Neurol. 2016;19:29-36.
9. Kravljanac R, Jovic N, Tadic BV, *et al.* New-onset seizure presenting as status epilepticus: Etiology and clinical characteristics in a cohort of 236 children. Seizure. 2018;63: 79-84.
10. Beghi E, Carpio A, Forsgren L, *et al.* Recommendation for a definition of acute symptomatic seizure. Epilepsia. 2010;51: 671-5.
11. Sasidaran K, Singhi S, Singhi P. Management of acute seizure and status epilepticus in pediatric emergency. Indian J Pediatr. 2012;79:510-7.
12. Obeid M, Mikati MA. Expanding spectrum of paroxysmal events in children: potential mimickers of epilepsy. Pediatr Neurol. 2007;37:309-16.
13. Cross JH. Differential diagnosis of epileptic seizures in infancy including the neonatal period. Semin Fetal Neonatal Med. 2013;18:192-5.
14. Mikati MA, Obeid M. Conditions that mimics seizures. In: Robert Kliegman, Richard E Behrman, Bonita Stanton, Joseph W St. Geme (III), Nina Felice Schor, editors. Nelson Textbook of Pediatrics, 20th edition. Elsevier; 2016. p. 2857-63.
15. Friedman N, Ghosh D, Moodley M. Syncope and paroxysmal disorders other than epilepsy. In: Swaiman K, Ashwal S, Ferriero D, Schor N, editors. Swaiman's Pediatric Neurology Principles and Practice, 5th edition. Elsevier; 2012. p. 905-25.
16. Huff JS, Fountain NB. Pathophysiology and definitions of seizures and status epilepticus. Emerg Med Clin North Am. 2011;29:1-13.
17. Shorvon S, Ferlisi M. The treatment of super-refractory status epilepticus: a critical review of available therapies and a clinical treatment protocol. Brain. 2011;134:2802-18.
18. Riviello JJ, Ashwal S, Hirtz D, *et al.* Practice parameter: diagnostic assessment of the child with status epilepticus (an evidence-based review): Report of the Quality Standards Subcommittee of the American Academy of Neurology and the Practice Committee of the Child Neurology Society. Neurology. 2006;67:1542-50.
19. Mishra D, Sharma S, Sankhyan N, *et al.* Consensus guidelines on management of childhood convulsive status epilepticus. Indian Pediatr. 2014;51:975-90.
20. Abend NS, Gutierrez-Colina AM, Dlugos DJ. Medical treatment of pediatric status epilepticus. Semin Pediatr Neurol. 2010; 17:169-75.
21. Rossetti AO. Which anesthetic should be used in the treatment of refractory status epilepticus? Epilepsia. 2007;48 Suppl 8:52-5.
22. Arayakarnkul P, Chomtho K. Treatment options in pediatric super-refractory status epilepticus. Brain Dev. 2019;41:359-66.
23. Sharma S, Mishra D, Aneja S, *et al.* Consensus guidelines on evaluation and management of suspected acute viral encephalitis in children in India. Indian Pediatr. 2012;49: 897-910.
24. Dalmau J, Lancaster E, Martinez-Hernandez E, *et al.* Clinical experience and laboratory investigations in patients with anti-NMDAR encephalitis. Lancet Neurol. 2011;10:63-74.
25. Pohl D, Alper G, Van Haren K, *et al.* Acute disseminated encephalomyelitis: Updates on an inflammatory CNS syndrome. Neurology. 2016;87:S38-45.
26. Sutter R, Dittrich T, Semmlack S, *et al.* Acute systemic complications of convulsive status epilepticus: A systematic review. Crit Care Med. 2018;46:138-45.
27. Kravljanac R, Jovic N, Djuric M, *et al.* Outcome of status epilepticus in children treated in the intensive care unit: A study of 302 cases. Epilepsia. 2011;52:358-63.
28. Ostrowsky K, Arzimanoglou A. Outcome and prognosis of status epilepticus in children. Semin Pediatr Neurol. 2010; 17:195-200.

CHAPTER

28

Approach to a Comatose Patient

Rajeshwari Nataraj, Suchitra Ranjit

INTRODUCTION

A child presenting with coma is one of the most difficult diagnostic and management problems that may be encountered by a pediatrician in an emergency setting. We need a systematic approach to a child with coma, considering wide range of etiology and a constant fear of further neurological damage. Regardless of the etiology, initial management includes immediate attention to the ABCs in order to sustain life and prevent loss of brain function.

DEFINITIONS

Coma is a pathological state of consciousness with significant alteration in awareness and variable degree of wakefulness. Consciousness is divided into two components: wakefulness (arousal) and awareness of self and environment. Coma is characterized by complete absence of arousal and awareness with lack of sleep wake cycle. Wakefulness is a function of reticular activating system located in the brainstem; whereas, awareness is a cortical function. Various states of consciousness have been enumerated in **Table 1**.

This state of altered consciousness needs to be differentiated from an acute onset, rapidly fluctuating confusional state called delirium. It also needs to differentiate from those with injury to ventral pons, where the patient will be mute and flaccid with preserved wakefulness and awareness (Locked in syndrome).

Comatose states may be caused by supratentorial lesions affecting deep diencephalic structures, sub-tentorial lesions affecting the brainstem or metabolic lesions diffusely affecting brainstem function[1] (**Table 2**).

Sequelae of coma: Coma is a transient phase, and the consequences are recovery, death or progress to persistent vegetative state.

ETIOLOGY

Although it is common practice to divide the etiology of coma as metabolic and structural causes, strict compartmentalization is not always possible as structural causes of coma may be associated with metabolic dysfunction, e.g. the syndrome of inappropriate antidiuretic hormone secretion (SIADH) complicating head injury. **Table 3** provides a simple scheme for remembering the causes of coma in children presenting to emergency room.

EVALUATION OF A CHILD IN COMA

Immediate Considerations

1. Assess and optimize **A**irway, **B**reathing and **C**irculation in order to ensure that the brain is being adequately perfused.
2. Obtain an immediate bedside capillary blood glucose level and correct if low.

Table 1: Various states of consciousness

Arousal	*Awareness*	*Brainstem reflex*	*State of consciousness*
Absent	Absent	Absent	Brain dead
Absent	Absent or suboptimal	Preserved	Coma
Preserved	Suboptimal	Preserved	Minimally conscious state
Preserved	Absent	Preserved	Vegetative state

Table 2: Differentiating characteristics of structural and metabolic coma

Supratentorial lesions	*Infratentorial lesions*	*Toxic, metabolic or infectious processes*
Initial signs focal	Initial signs of brainstem dysfunction	Confusion/stupor often precede motor signs
Rostrocaudal progression seen	Sudden onset coma	Symmetrical neurological findings
Asymmetric neurological signs at onset	Cranial nerve abnormalities common	Pupillary reactions preserved
Seizures may be present	Respiratory patterns often altered	Respiratory rate often altered

Table 3: Etiology of coma in children

The mnemonic "TIPS from the Vowels" is a useful method to remember the most common of the wide range of possible causes.

Conditions	*Comments*	
T	Trauma, head injury	Shaken baby syndrome: May present with nonspecific history, retinal hemorrhages
I	Intussusception Insulin-hypoglycemia	Mental status changes may precede abdominal finding Hypoglycemia secondary to accidental ingestion of oral hypoglycemic agents Ketotic hypoglycemia following prolonged fasting in thin built children
	Inborn errors of metabolism	Coma may be associated with vomiting and seizures
P	Psychogenic	Common in adolescents
S	Seizures Shock, stroke Shunt Snake bite	Postictal states, non-convulsive status may masquerade as undifferentiated coma Autoimmune encephalitis ADEM, Coma secondary to poor brain perfusion, arterial and venous infarcts Blocked or infected ventriculo-peritoneal shunts Snake bite can mimic coma
A	Alcohol ingestion, Abuse (Battered baby)	
E	Electrolytes Encephalopathy	Disturbances of sodium, calcium, magnesium Hypertension, Reye syndrome, hepatic failure, urea cycle defects, lead poisoning
I	Infections	Encephalitis, meningitis, malaria
O	Overdose: opioids, barbiturates benzodiazepines, ingestion, etc. Drug abuse: Cocaine, methanol, etc.	Consider with unexplained loss of consciousness
U	Uremic encephalopathy	

3. Brief relevant history of chronic and recent illnesses, trauma, medications in the home.
4. Consider naloxone 0.1 mg/kg in suspected narcotic ingestions.

Secondary Considerations

A complete neurological examination is necessary with particular attention to five physiological variables. These may give valuable information about the level of the lesion in the brain, nature of involvement and direction of progression of the disease process.

- The level of consciousness
- Pattern of respiration
- Size and reactivity of the pupils
- Spontaneous and induced eye movements
- Motor responses.

Level of consciousness

Numerous scoring systems have been developed to assess the level of consciousness. By far the most useful is the **Glasgow Coma Score** (GCS), which was originally used to predict the outcome after head injury in adults. The **modified GCS** is applicable to younger patients and is the most frequently used general means of neurological assessment[2] (**Table 4**). GCS scoring becomes difficult among children who are intubated (verbal component) or those on neuromuscular blockade (motor component). Although GCS is commonly used, the FOUR score has been validated and it provides a more detailed neurological examination. FOUR scores are especially useful for serial monitoring and for assessment of therapeutic intervention (**Fig. 1**). An alternative simple method for assessing the level of consciousness is the **AVPU** score. This score, like the GCS, is also useful for the serial observation of the trends in the level of coma. AVPU stands for **A**: alert, **V**: responds to voice, **P**: responds to pain, **U**: unresponsive

Respiratory pattern

The control of respiration is governed by centers located in the brainstem (lower pons and medulla) and modulated by forebrain cortical centers. Respiratory pattern abnormalities signify either metabolic derangements or neurologic insult. There are several characteristic respiratory patterns that exist in comatose patients. *Cheyne Stokes respiration (CSR)* is a pattern of periodic breathing where hyperpnea alternates with apnea. The depth of breathing alters from breath to breath with a smooth rise to a peak and a smooth fall (decrescendo). CSR results from deep hemispheric or diencephalic dysfunction and may also be seen in children with metabolic abnormalities. *Central neurogenic hyperventilation* refers to sustained regular, rapid and deep respiration, which is seen in children with brainstem dysfunction. *Apneustic breathing* is a pattern of breathing that is characterized by inspiratory pauses lasting 2–3 seconds often alternating with end-expiratory pauses. Apneustic breathing is characteristic of pontine infarction and anoxic encephalopathy.

Pupillary size and reactivity

Pupillary reactions are controlled by a balance between the sympathetic and parasympathetic nervous system. As brainstem centers controlling consciousness are anatomically adjacent to those controlling pupils, pupillary changes are a valuable guide to the presence and location of brain lesions.

Additionally, metabolic disturbances affect pupillary pathways late. Consequently, the presence or absence of the papillary reaction to light is one of the single most important differentiating features to distinguish between structural and metabolic disorders (**Fig. 2**). Children with metabolic encephalopathy will have preserved reactive pupils.

Induced eye movements

Two specific eye movements are helpful in evaluating comatose children. One is the ***oculocephalic*** or ***the***

Table 4: The Glasgow coma score

(< 5 years)	*(>5 years)*	
Eye opening response		
Spontaneous	Spontaneous	4
To speech	To speech	3
To pain	To pain	2
None	None	1
Verbal response		
Alert, coos, words – normal	Oriented	4
Irritable cry	Confused	3
Cries to pain	Inappropriate words	2
Moans to pain	Incomprehensible sounds	1
No response to pain	None	
Motor response		
Normal spontaneous movements	Obeys commands	6
Localizes (>9 months)	Localizes to supraorbital stimulus	5
Withdraws	Withdraws	4
Abnormal flexion (decorticate posturing)	Abnormal flexion (decorticate posturing)	3
Abnormal extension (decerebrate response)	Abnormal extension (decerebrate response)	2
None	None	1

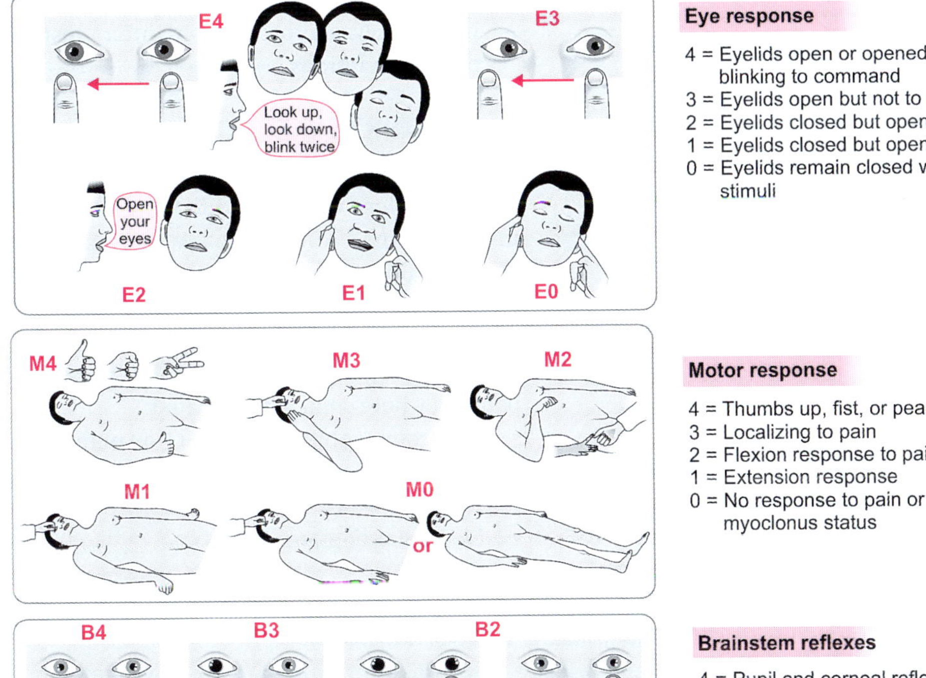

Eye response

4 = Eyelids open or opened, tracking or blinking to command
3 = Eyelids open but not to tracking
2 = Eyelids closed but opens to loud voice
1 = Eyelids closed but opens to pain
0 = Eyelids remain closed with pain stimuli

Motor response

4 = Thumbs up, fist, or peace sign
3 = Localizing to pain
2 = Flexion response to pain
1 = Extension response
0 = No response to pain or generalized myoclonus status

B4 B3 B2 or B1 B0

Brainstem reflexes

4 = Pupil and corneal reflexes present
3 = One pupil wide and fixed
2 = Pupil or corneal reflexes absent
1 = Pupil and corneal reflexes absent
0 = Absent pupil, corneal, or cough reflex

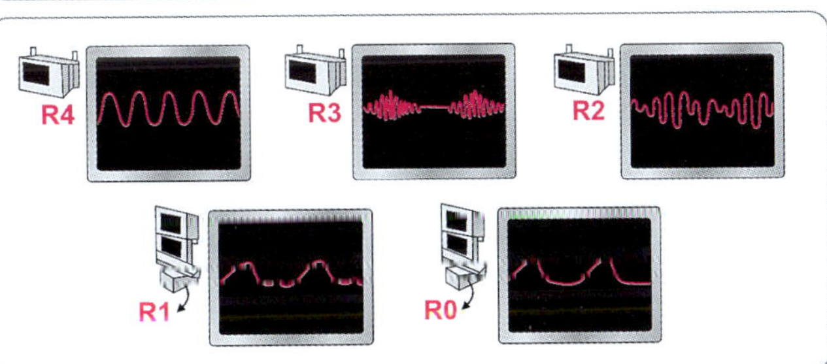

Respiration

4 = Regular breathing pattern
3 = Cheyne-Stokes breathing pattern
2 = Irregular breathing
1 = Triggers ventilator or breathes above ventilator rate
0 = Apnea or breathes at ventilator rate

Fig. 1: FOUR score Neurological scale in coma[3]
Adapted from Wijdicks FM, Annals of Neurology 2005

doll's eye response. This is performed by holding the eyelids open end rotating the head from side to side. When there is a conjugate deviation of the eyes in the opposite direction to which the head is turned, the dolls eye response is considered preserved. This indicates "integrity of brainstem". Hence, if the dolls eye response is "not preserved", it indicates compromise of brainstem functions. Other tests for brainstem integrity includes ***oculovestibular or the calorie test*** which is performed by elevating the patient's head to 30° and slowly injecting 50 mL of ice water with a syringe. A perforated eardrum, wax in canal, or fracture base of skull should be excluded before performing this test. The classical mnemonic "COWS" refers to fast component of nystagmus.

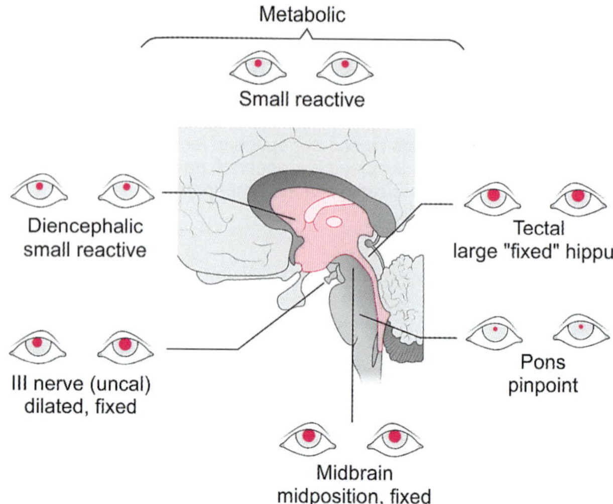

Fig. 2: Pupillary abnormalities based on site of lesion
Adapted from Plum F, Posner JB. The diagnosis of stupor and coma[4]

Hence, when right ear is irrigated with cold water, fast component will be towards left and slow nystagmus will be towards right. Clinically it is difficult to visualize the fast component; what we usually see is a slow component. Hence in a normal awake patient, nystagmus with the slow component will be towards the irrigated ear and fast component towards midline. Hence in a comatose patient, if the eyes move towards stimulus and remain tonically deviated for >1 minute, it indicates brainstem integrity. *In an unconscious patient with brainstem dysfunction/ brain dead patient, there is* no response to stimuli, i.e. eyes remain in the midline.

Motor examination

Assessment of muscle strength, tone and tendon reflexes should be assessed for normality and symmetry. The ability of the patient to localize stimuli as well as the presence or absence of abnormal posturing helps in the assessment of severity of the neurological derangement.

- **Decorticate posturing** with flexion of the upper extremities and extension of the lower extremities suggests involvement of the cerebral cortex and preservation of brainstem function.
- **Decerebrate posturing** with rigid extension of the arms and legs is indicative of cortical and brainstem damage.
- The **flaccid patient** with no response to painful stimuli has the gravest prognosis with injury sustained to deep brainstem lesions.

LABORATORY EVALUATION

Laboratory evaluation of a patient in coma of indeterminate etiology may be divided into routine and specific investigations.[5] Routine Investigations includes white blood count, coagulation screen, arterial blood gas, glucose, electrolytes, calcium, magnesium; serum and urine osmolality; urine for sugar, ketones, pH; infection screen, virology; chest X-ray. Specific investigations can be planned where clinically indicated:

- Electroencephalogram (EEG) is paramount in coma of unknown etiology, as some comatose children may have non-convulsive seizures
- Electrocardiogram (ECG)
- CT scan
- CSF analysis if features of raised intracranial tension (ICT) not present
- Serum ammonia, lactate, pyruvate in suspected metabolic disorders
- Liver, renal function tests
- Drug levels in suspected drug abuse and intoxication.

Additional tests, where appropriate includes thyroid function tests, lead level, skeletal survey, and contrast studies of gastrointestinal tract.

MANAGEMENT OF A COMATOSE PATIENT

The main goals of care include optimizing cerebral blood flow (CBF)/cerebral perfusion pressure (CPP) and minimizing factors that can aggravate neuronal injury or trigger intracranial pressure (ICP) elevation.

Assessment

Assess the airway, breathing and circulation (ABCs)

The airway should be stabilized and an assessment made for the need for intubation. Even if spontaneously breathing with normal gas exchange, many comatose children will benefit from intubation, especially if they have intracranial hypertension. Early intubation, ventilation and deep sedation are often overlooked as key interventions for ICP control.

A GCS below 8 has been the standard indication for intubation. Recent literature however states that intubation should be considered in patients with a GCS below 12. Other indications for intubation include deterioration in the level of consciousness, evidence of herniation and irregularities in respiration[6] (**Table 5**).

The blood pressure should be kept at the higher range of normal (for age). This requires ensuring appropriate fluid and inotrope management.

Assess and treat for immediately correctable cause of coma

Perform bedside capillary glucose test and correct if low, send samples to lab for routine hematological and biochemical testing.

Assessment of the depth of coma

The standard assessment tool is the GCS in older children and modified GCS in children <5 years old or the AVPU.

Treatment of Raised ICP

The focus of contemporary ICP management has changed in recent years in two important aspects.

Firstly, increasing emphasis on CPP (cerebral perfusion pressure) management in addition to ICP control.

Secondly, the increasing recognition of the potential for overzealous hyperventilation to aggravate cerebral ischemia by reducing cerebral blood flow (CBF).[6,7]

CPP = Mean arterial pressure (MAP) – Intracranial pressure (ICP)

Cerebral ischemia may result when CPP is lowered, either from raised ICP or lowered MAP (hypotension) When the ICP is critically raised, herniation syndromes (uncal, central or medullary herniation) can occur, which, along with hypoxic-ischemic damage from reduced CPP, are the most important causes of death. **Table 5** describes the signs of herniation.

If raised ICP is clinically suspected, therapeutic measures should be immediately instituted as papilledema may not be seen in acutely elevated ICP and fatal herniation can occur even after a "normal" CT scan.

- *Role of hyper-osmotherapy*: Osmotherapy requires an intact blood-brain barrier. In areas of disrupted barrier, equilibration occurs and these agents work by removing water from normal brain tissues.

Table 5: Signs of cerebral herniation

Types of herniation	*Key feature*
Central or transtentorial	Glasgow coma scale <8, abnormal pupil (from reactive pupil to fixed dilated pupil), absent doll's eye movement (loss of brainstem integrity), decorticate progressing to decerebrate posturing, respiratory abnormality from neurogenic hyperventilation to Cheyne stokes respiration to ataxic breathing, Cushing triad (hypertension, bradycardia, irregular respiration)
Uncal herniation	Altered consciousness with unilateral dilated pupil (third nerve palsy) with or without hemiparesis
Subfalcine herniation	Altered consciousness with monoparesis of contralateral lower limb extremity

- *Mannitol*: Mannitol is indicated acutely for patients in whom there is a strong clinical suspicion of raised ICP or imminent herniation (**Table 6**). Mannitol has two distinct effects.
  - The immediate effect is related to its rheologic properties (first-pass effect in brain resulting in decreased blood viscosity) resulting in a transient increased CBF followed by a more sustained fall in CBF.
  - The delayed osmotic effects occur after 15–30 minutes and last for 4–6 hours. Urinary fluid losses should be replaced with isotonic crystalloids to avoid volume depletion.
  - Mannitol can be used in focal pathological conditions associated with mass effects such as contusion, intracranial bleed, tumor and infarcts.

Hypertonic saline (HTS). HTS acts like mannitol by establishing a constant osmolar gradient in order to draw fluid from the brain parenchyma but without the risks of dehydration and tubular damage as in the case of mannitol. Maintain serum sodium of 145–150 mEq/L. In the hypotensive/hypoperfused patient, HTS may be the osmotherapy of choice for reducing ICP while maintaining MAP/CPP. The beneficial effects of HTS with a low frequency of side effects have been described in the setting of pediatric traumatic brain injury and cerebral edema occurring during diabetic ketoacidosis treatment in children.

Anti-seizure medications: Convulsions can cause massive increases in CBF, consequent increase in ICP, can lead to secondary brain damage and may precipitate or be precipitated by cerebral herniation. Apart from generalized tonic-clonic seizures (GTCS), some comatose children may have non-convulsive seizures (NCS) manifesting with subtle signs such as eyelid twitching, eye deviation or nystagmus. A bedside EEG may be informative. If in doubt, empiric treatment of seizures may be justified and can result in improvement of consciousness.

Temperature control: Hyperthermia worsens ICP and brain damage in ischemia. Hence, hyperthermia should be strictly avoided. There is no potential benefit of hypothermia in pediatric studies. However, like in adult population, mild hypothermia is found to be beneficial in out of hospital arrest and in ventricular arrhythmia associated cardiac arrest.[8]

Consider an antidote

Flumazenil and naloxone can be used in benzodiazepine and opioid toxicity respectively. Specific antidotes should be considered in drug intoxication.

Neuroimaging

Urgent imaging is indicated in afebrile coma and the presence of focal signs or papilledema, as the diagnosis includes stroke, intracranial bleed, tumor or hydrocephalus. However, any child who does not have a very obvious metabolic/toxic cause for the coma generally requires to be imaged.

A CT scan may provide information about the cause of altered mental status and the presence of intracranial hypertension, however a normal CT scan does not rule out raised ICP (**Table 7**).

An MRI may be more specific for early changes of herpes simplex encephalitis (where CT may be normal), posterior fossa and white matter pathology (**Table 8**). A cranial ultrasound may miss subdural collections or even extensive infarcts and a CT or MRI is an essential investigation in a deeply comatose infant even when the anterior fontanelle is open.

Lumbar puncture (LP) in a comatose child

The potential benefits of early LP include making an early diagnosis of CNS infection and identification of the pathogen and drug sensitivities. Contraindications to LP include signs of cerebral herniation, low GCS, focal neurological signs, or cardiorespiratory compromise. In an unconscious child with potential raised ICP, the decision is controversial with some authors stating that the risk of herniation far outweighs the benefit of knowing the pathogen from an early LP.

Choice of empiric antimicrobials

If a CNS infection is suspected in a febrile child presenting in acute coma and seizures, empiric antimicrobial

Table 6: Mannitol: Concerns and contraindications

Concerns	*Effects*	*How/when to avoid*
Excess diuresis	Osmotic diuresis /hypovolemia Fall in CPP	Lower doses 0.25–0.5 g/kg (1.2–2.5 mL/kg of a 20% solution) repeated 4–6 hourly* Mannitol should be reserved for features of severely increased ICP or impending herniation Use on an as-needed basis (Avoid scheduled dosages). Limit use to less than 48–72 hours Use smaller doses. Avoid concurrent hypotonic IV fluid or dilute enteral feeds or during hypotension
Rebound effect: challenging to prove if osmolarity is maintained	Mannitol may cause "selective debulking" of normal brain parenchyma with increase in midline shift and theoretic risk of worsening edema after discontinuation (although not clinically significant)	
Contraindications Risk of renal failure		Renal failure Hypotension Serum osmolality > 320 mOsm/kg

*Emergency therapy for herniation syndromes: 1.0–1.5 g/kg of 20% mannitol, Subsequent doses: 0.2.5–0.5 g/kg Q4–6H, measure serum osmolality.
(ICP: intracranial pressure; CPP: cerebral perfusion pressure).

should include acyclovir in addition to a third generation cephalosporin and vancomycin until further confirmatory tests are available. The need for empiric antimalarials, as well as antimicrobials to cover scrub typhus and mycoplasma infections should be carefully assessed based on the prevalence of these infections in the community.

Fluid therapy

There is accumulating data that hypovolemia worsens outcome in children with meningitis, malaria and severe head injury. Hypovolemia (fluid restriction, diuretics) can lower the CPP and lead to worse ICP due to autoregulatory vasodilation. What must be restricted are hypotonic fluids such as N/5 saline in 5% dextrose (Isolyte P). The dextrose will be metabolized with a resultant hypotonic fluid that can exacerbate cerebral edema and ICP. Adult and pediatric literature stress the importance of avoiding both hyperglycemia as well as hypoglycemia since the former can also worsen neurological outcome. Enteral feeds should be started at the earliest.

Management of Persistent Coma and Raised ICP in the ICU

If despite the above treatment, the patient continues to show evidence of raised ICP, further measures to tackle refractory raised ICP must be instituted. Specific surgically correctible lesions should be attended to.

While steroids should not be used for ICP related to infarcts, hemorrhage or trauma, the use of dexamethasone for vasogenic edema related to tumors, granulomas and abscesses can lead to dramatic reduction in lesion volume.

Table 7: CT findings in comatose patients

Computed tomography (CT) findings	*Radiological differentials*
Diffuse cerebral edema	Traumatic brain injury with diffuse axonal injury, menigoencephalitis, post-cardiac arrest, acute liver failure
Dilated ventricles with presence of periventricular hypodensity (obstructive hydrocephalus)	Obstructed CSF pathways – Pineal tumors, bleed, etc.
Intraventricular hemorrhage	Arteriovenous malformation (AVM)
Cerebral infarcts	Vasculitis, coagulopathy, thrombotic thrombocytopenic purpura
Hemorrhagic infarcts	Cerebral venous thrombosis
Cerebellar, pontine or occipital hemorrhage	Hypertension, AVM and cavernous malformation
Basal cistern hemorrhage	Aneurysmal sub-arachnoid hemorrhage, cocaine abuse

Table 8: MRI findings in a child with coma

MRI findings	*Radiological differentials*
Lesions in white matter, corpus callosum	TBI, viral encephalitis
T2 hyperintensities in temporal/frontal lobe with hemorrhage	Herpes encephalitis
T2 hyperintensity in thalamus, substantia nigra and basal ganglia	Japanese encephalitis
Hyperintensities – White matter, and/or basal ganglion	Acute demyelinating encephalomyelitis (ADEM) Metabolic leukodystrophy Posterior reversible encephalopathy syndrome (PRES)
Caudate and putamen lesions	Carbon monoxide and methanol toxicity
Pontine lesions	Pontine myelinosis
Midbrain, pons, medulla lesion with dentate nucleus of cerebellum	Enterovirus (EV 71 virus)
Occiput, thalamus, brainstem lesions	Basilar artery narrowing

Head end elevation by 30° (provided patient not hypotensive) and avoidance of neck kinking are important. Fever, agitation and seizures must be assiduously controlled as they can cause massive increases in CBF and CPP. If ventilated, the $PaCO_2$ should be maintained between 30 and 35 mm Hg in order to prevent cerebral ischemia. More extreme hypocapnia can be employed as a short-term temporizing measure for acute deterioration.

Barbiturate coma and/or mild hypothermia are used in order to reduce the cerebral metabolic rate for oxygen ($CMRO_2$) and thus the cerebral blood flow, although most references pertain to adults. Hypotension during barbiturate use may require vasopressors to optimize the MAP/CPP.

In ICP refractory to medical measures, surgical decompression has been shown to improve survival and functional outcome.

PROGNOSIS

The prognosis of a child in coma depends on the cause of altered mental status. In general, children have a better prognosis than adults. Prolonged coma after hypoxic-ischemic insult carries a poor prognosis, but children sustaining intoxication have good prognosis. Infectious encephalopathies also have a reasonably good outcome. Cortical blindness often recovers.

Prognosis for coma recovery in children has been most studied for hypoxic-ischemic encephalopathy (HIE) and traumatic brain injury.[9] For HIE: GCS <5 and absent spontaneous breathing at 24 hours have a very high predictability of severe disability or death, however, drowning is an exception.

Neuro-prognostication should be done at the end of 72 hours after return of circulation in post-arrest situations after excluding confounders such as sedation, electrolyte imbalance, etc. A careful clinical exam is key in prognostication however, multimodal monitoring is appropriate to avoid false poor prognosis.

Indicators of good prognosis after in a comatose patient following cardiac arrest:

- Presence of a continuous or nearly continuous EEG within 12 hours from ROSC;
- Presence of EEG reactivity to auditory stimuli; and
- Absence of diffusion weighted imaging (DWI) abnormalities on MRI within 1 week of ROSC.

KEY MESSAGES

- The main goals of care include optimizing cerebral blood flow (CBF)/ cerebral perfusion pressure (CPP) and minimizing factors that can aggravate neuronal injury or trigger intracranial pressure (ICP) elevation.
- The blood pressure should be kept at the higher range of normal (for age). This requires ensuring appropriate fluid and inotrope management.
- The focus of contemporary ICP management has changed in recent years in two important aspects. Firstly, increasing emphasis on CPP (cerebral perfusion pressure) management in addition to ICP control and Secondly, the increasing recognition of the potential for overzealous hyperventilation to aggravate cerebral ischemia by reducing cerebral blood flow (CBF).
- Hypertonic saline acts like mannitol by establishing a constant osmolar gradient in order to draw fluid from the brain parenchyma but without the risks of dehydration and tubular damage as in the case of mannitol.
- There is accumulating data that hypovolemia worsens outcome in children with meningitis, malaria and severe head injury. Hypovolemia (fluid restriction, diuretics) can lower the CPP and lead to worse ICP due to autoregulatory vasodilation.
- What must be restricted are hypotonic fluids such as N/5 saline in 5% dextrose (Isolyte P) rub to be avoided.

REFERENCES

1. Strange GR, Cooper A, editors. Altered Level of Consciousness. APLS: The Pediatric Emergency Medicine Course. American Academy of Pediatrics; 1998. p. 159-66.
2. Tatman A, Warren A. Development of a modified paediatric coma scale in intensive care practice. Arch Dis Child. 1997;77: 519-21.
3. Wijdicks EF. The bare essentials: Coma. Pract Neurol. 2010; 10:51-60.
4. Plum F, Posner JB, editors. The Diagnosis of Stupor and Coma, 4th edition. New York: Oxford University Press; 2007.
5. Larsen GY, Vernon DD, Dean JM. Evaluation of the comatose child. In: Rogers MC, editor. Textbook of Pediatric Intensive Care, 3rd edition. Baltimore: Williams and Wilkins; 1996. p. 735-45.
6. Kirkham FJ. Non-traumatic coma in children. Arch Dis Child. 2001;85:303-12.
7. Ranjit S. Emergency and intensive care management of a comatose patient with intracranial hypertension: Current concepts. Indian Pediatr. 2006;43:409-15.
8. Hutchison JS, Ward RE, Lacroix J, *et al.* Hypothermia therapy after traumatic brain injury in children. N Engl J Med. 2008;358: 2447-56.
9. Sandroni C, D'Arrigo S, Nolan JP. Prognostication after cardiac arrest. Critical Care. 2018;22:150.

CHAPTER

29

Febrile Encephalopathy

Priyanka Madaan, Naveen Sankhyan

INTRODUCTION

Acute febrile encephalopathy (AFE) is a common medical emergency in children. It is a syndromic diagnosis, commonly used for a clinical presentation of fever, with altered cognition or personality, and altered consciousness and/or seizures. Acute febrile encephalopathy may occur as a result of gamut of causes. These include—direct infections of the intracranial structures (such as encephalitis, complicated meningitis, focal infections like abscess, empyema), systemic infections with secondary central nervous system involvement (such as typhoid, malaria, sepsis associated encephalopathy), infections/unknown agent triggering possible immune mediated/inflammation mediated encephalopathy (such as demyelination, autoimmune encephalitis, etc.), toxic-metabolic (such as metabolic and electrolyte disturbance, intoxication), and heat stroke (**Table 1**). Besides these, infection may also trigger organ failure or metabolic crisis (such as Reye syndrome, inborn error of metabolism, hemolytic uremic syndrome—thrombotic thrombocytopenic purpura, etc.) which may present as acute febrile encephalopathy. The varied etiology makes the diagnosis and management of this entity very challenging.[1]

Acute encephalitis syndrome (AES) is a related terminology used by the World Health Organization (WHO) for syndromic surveillance, especially for Japanese B encephalitis. WHO defines a case of AES as a person of any age, at any time of year with acute onset fever and altered mentation (including symptoms such as confusion, disorientation, come, or inability to talk) and/or new onset seizures (excluding simple febrile seizures).[2] Hence, AES is similar to AFE in terms of case definition. Also, the duration of illness that should be classified as acute is not clear. It was proposed to be less than 14 days by an expert consensus group.[3] However, encephalitis classically refers to inflammation of brain parenchyma. Many non-encephalitic causes such as infection associated encephalopathies are classified as AES despite having a different underlying pathophysiology and requiring different management strategies. Therefore, non-encephalitic causes need to be aptly distinguished.

EPIDEMIOLOGY AND ETIOLOGY

The exact incidence of AES is not known in Indian children. Besides, epidemiology of the specific encephalitic syndromes is also not well defined due to lack of a robust surveillance system. The etiological profile of AES available is based on either outbreak investigations studies or few studies from tertiary care hospitals. In the year 2017, 13,672 cases and 1097 deaths were reported due to AES to the National Vector Borne Diseases Control Programme (NVBDCP) and JE contributed to around one-fifth of the cases and deaths.[4]

Infections contribute to almost half of the cases of AES in children while the etiology remains unknown in 40–50% cases with viral infections being the most common cause (**Table 2**).[5] In immunocompromised hosts, other

Table1: Etiology of acute febrile encephalopathy in children

1. Direct infection of the intracranial structures
   - Meningitis: Bacterial, viral, tubercular, parasitic, fungal, etc.
   - Encephalitis: viral, parasitic (cysticercal)
   - Focal infection (brain abscess, subdural empyema)
2. Systemic infections with secondary CNS involvement
   - Enteric fever
   - Malaria
   - Dengue
   - Scrub typhus
   - Septic encephalopathy
3. Infection/unknown trigger to possible immune mediated/inflammation mediated encephalopathy
   - Demyelinating: Acute disseminated encephalomyelitis (ADEM)
   - Autoimmune encephalitis
   - Infection associated encephalopathies which include
     - Acute leukoencephalopathy with restricted diffusion (ALERD)
     - Acute necrotizing encephalopathy (ANEC)
     - Mild encephalopathy with reversible splenial lesion
     - Febrile infection related epilepsy syndrome
     - Infantile hemiconvulsion hemiplegia epilepsy syndrome
4. Infection triggering organ failure or metabolic crisis
   - Reye syndrome
   - Inborn error of metabolism: organic acidemia, urea cycle defect
   - Hemolytic uremic syndrome, thrombotic thrombocytopenic purpura
5. Toxic-metabolic
   - Metabolic disturbance: Litchi associated encephalopathy
   - Intoxication: drugs, toxins
   - Heat stroke
6. Any cause of encephalopathy with secondary infection (e.g. aspiration pneumonia after status epilepticus)

Table 2: Selected infectious agents causing acute febrile encephalopathy

1. Viruses
   Japanese B encephalitis, enteroviruses
   Dengue, Chikungunya, Chandipura, Nipah and West Nile encephalitis
   Herpes simplex virus, Ebstein Barr virus, varicella zoster virus, Rabies virus, HIV, HHV-6
   Emerging viruses: Henipaviruses (Hendra and Nipah viruses)
2. Parasitic
   Malaria
   Protozoal : Amebic
3. Bacterial
   Pneumococcal, *Haemophilus influenzae* B, *Meningococcus*, *Staphylococcus aureus*
   Tubercular meningitis
   Spirochetal : Syphilis
   Orientia tsutsugamushi (Scrub Typhus)
4. Fungal: Cryptococcal, Aspergillus

(HIV: human immunodeficiency virus; HHV: human herpes virus)

agents like *Aspergillus, Acanthamoeba* spp., *Balamuthia, Cryptococcus* and other atypical organisms may be responsible for AES (**Figs. 1 and 2**).

Eastern Uttar Pradesh (Gorakhpur district) and Bihar (Muzaffarpur district) are endemic for acute encephalitis in children in India. In 2014, Jain P et al.[6] reported that JEV was the most commonly detected in patients with AES (16.2%) followed by Dengue virus (10%). However, there has been a recent epidemiological shift. Kumar R et al.[7] reported HSV1 (31.50%) as the commonest cause followed by adenovirus (10.95%), parvovirus (2.73%), JE virus (1.36%), enterovirus (1.36%), and EBV (1.36%) in children

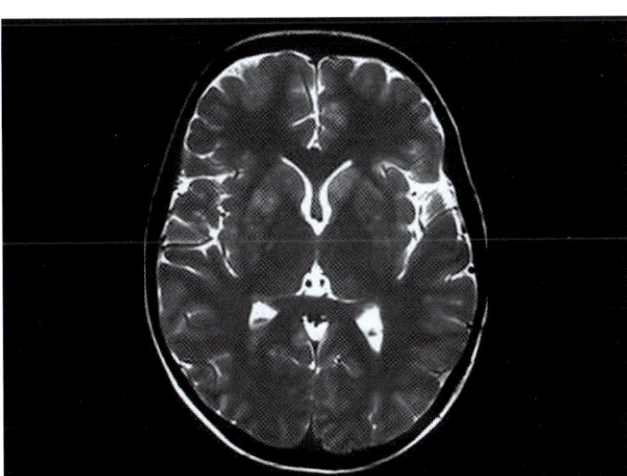

Fig. 1: MRI brain T2 weighted axial sequence showing hyperintense cysts (pseudocysts) in bilateral basal ganglia in an immunosuppressed child with cryptococcal meningitis

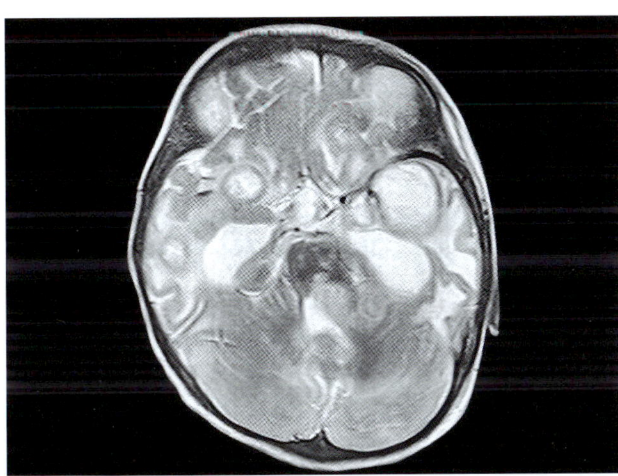

Fig. 2: MRI brain T2 weighted axial sequence showing multiple brain abscesses due to *Aspergillus* in a child with primary immune deficiency

admitted with AES at Agra. Besides these, epidemics of Chandipura virus encephalitis have been reported from Andhra Pradesh,[8] Nipah virus from Siliguri,[9] enterovirus from Karnataka and Andhra Pradesh[10] and West Nile Virus from Kerala (**Fig. 3**).[11]

Among the tropical fevers in intensive care units all over India, dengue was the most common cause (23%) followed by scrub typhus (18%), meningoencephalitis (9%) and malaria.[12] Encephalopathy was seen in 25% of the patients with scrub typhus. Scrub Typhus has been reported from all over India.[13-17] A substantial number of cases have been reported from Uttarakhand, Tamil Nadu, Puducherry,

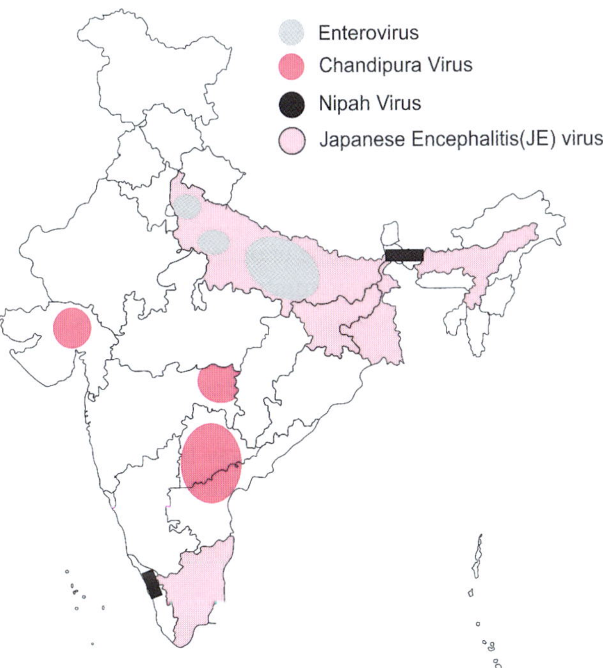

Fig. 3: Reported areas of various viral encephalitis in India. Enteroviruses have been reported from Delhi, Aligarh and Eastern UP; Chandipura Virus from Gujrat, Nagpur and Andhra Pradesh; Nipah virus from Siliguri(WB) and Kozhikode, Kerala; JE virus is endemic in Tamil Nadu, Assam, Bihar and UP. **Scrub Typhus is endemic is nearly all of India*

Assam, and Uttar Pradesh. In immunocompromised hosts, other agents like *Acanthamoeba* spp., *Balamuthia* and *Cryptococcus* may be responsible for AES.

Litchi associated encephalopathy has been reported from Muzaffarpur district of Bihar.[18,19] This encephalopathy is believed to occur as a result of a toxin "hypoglycin-A" in litchi. There have been no epidemiological studies from India for infection associated encephalopathies, and autoimmune encephalitis. These encephalopathies probably occur all over this country.

Emerging infections: Several emerging viruses (West Nile fever, influenza A, enterovirus 71, ebola virus, influenza virus, Hendra and nipah viruses, etc.) have been recognized which may pose a threat in the future.[20-24]

PATHOGENESIS/PATHOPHYSIOLOGY

The pathophysiology of acute febrile encephalopathy depends on the underlying etiology. Encephalopathy usually occurs as a result of alteration in any of the neural networks responsible for arousal and awareness.

These include the ascending reticular activating system and its thalamocortical connections (for arousal), and the cerebral cortex and its connections (for awareness).[25]

Direct neuronal damage, electrolyte abnormalities or alteration of neuronal milieu, inflammation, autoantibodies, demyelination, etc. are central to the pathogenesis of encephalopathy. Selectivity of brain dysfunction depends on the etiology for example: some viruses may have preferential involvement of certain structures like herpes virus preferentially involves medial temporal lobe, cingulate gyrus and inferior frontal lobe. Similarly, autoantibody mediated damage might depend on the antigen location in the brain. Neurons, which are more metabolically active, may be more involved during metabolic decompensation. The outcome of virus infections depends on a critical balance between disadvantages of excess inflammation and the benefits of appropriate inflammation.

DIAGNOSIS AND MANAGEMENT

Acute febrile encephalopathy is a medical emergency. Hence, initial stabilization, diagnosis and treatment should proceed simultaneously. The management begins with immediate emergency room (ER) assessment followed by a detailed assessment, investigations and treatment.

Immediate ER Assessment

A rapid, focused history and examination helps in identifying, treating and preventing catastrophic complications like herniation. Airway, breathing and circulation should be stabilized. Children with GCS less than 8 should be intubated and mechanically ventilated. Vascular access should be established and blood samples for sugar, electrolytes, hemogram, rapid diagnostic tests (malaria, dengue, etc.) and culture should be obtained, and appropriate measures should be instituted for any abnormality detected. Measures for raised intracranial pressure should be instituted in case of suspicion based on history and examination. An emergent computed tomography (CT) may be considered in children with suspicion of intracranial hemorrhage with signs of raised intracranial pressure. CT scan, although suboptimal, has the advantages over MRI. Its availability in emergent setting, ease and shorter acquisition time especially for critically ill patients are helpful. Risk of radiation exposure should always be kept in mind before ordering CT head.

CT scan should be looked for any intracranial hemorrhage, infective collections (brain abscess, subdural empyema), hydrocephalus, cerebral edema, effacement of cisterns, localized hypodensities (frontotemporal hypodensities in herpes simplex encephalitis, thalamic abnormalities in Japanese Encephalitis), ring enhancing lesions and basal exudates (CNS tuberculosis).

Empirical treatment should be initiated for treatable causes of encephalitis awaiting etiological diagnosis. A broad-spectrum antibiotic such as ceftriaxone (± vancomycin) along with intravenous acyclovir must be started. Empirical antimalarial (artesunate combined chemotherapy) should be started in endemic area and stopped if the peripheral smear and rapid diagnostic tests are negative. Similarly if there is suspicion of scrub typhus, anti-rickettsial treatment (doxycycline/azithromycin) should be started.

Detailed Assessment

After initial stabilization, a detailed history and clinical examination should be done. History should focus on the onset (acute vs. subacute), progression, duration of the illness and presence of associated symptoms such as headache, vomiting, seizures, etc. **Table 3** illustrates the key points in history and examination, which may provide clues to the underlying infectious etiology.

A detailed neurological examination should be performed to localize the neurological deficits and to look for features of raised intracranial pressure and impending herniation. Subtle ongoing seizures may indicate the need for an EEG. Presence of behavioral abnormalities, bradykinesia, movement disorder and sleep problems should prompt an evaluation for autoimmune encephalitis. Movement disorder such as dystonia (in JE), hemiballismus (CNS tuberculosis), may be seen in many infectious and noninfectious etiologies. Limb weakness, in encephalitis, may occur with enterovirus infections, poliomyelitis and JE. **Table 4** illustrates the etiological clues based on neuroimaging findings. Systemic involvement such as myocarditis (EV71 encephalitis), vomiting with transaminitis (influenza, Reye's syndrome) may also be seen. Besides infectious encephalitis, there is an entity termed as viral infection associated encephalopathies.[26] These are disorders where there is an encephalopathy associated with a viral infection (e.g. influenza) however there is no CSF pleocytosis or other evidence of encephalitis (**Figs. 4 and 5**).

Table 3: Clinical evaluation of a child with acute febrile encephalopathy

Key points in history and examination

1. *Residence:* especially for endemic areas such as Gangetic planes (JE), Muzaffarpur (litchi encephalopathy), endemic for cerebral malaria and scrub typhus
2. *Onset:* acute (for most encephalitis), subacute (such as HSV encephalitis, malaria)
3. *Progression:* monophasic, biphasic (such as dengue virus, ADEM, ALERD)
4. *Prodromal illness*: flu-like illness (Influenza), diarrhea (enterovirus, shigella encephalopathy), measles (for tubercular meningitis)
5. *Associated symptoms:*
   Rash: maculopapular (measles encephalitis), vesicular (varicella encephalitis), petechial (dengue, chikungunia), purpura (meningococcemia), eschar (scrub typhus)
   Jaundice: Leptospirosis, hepatic failure
   Severe anemia: prior blood loss/hemorrhage (dengue, cerebral malaria)
   Diarrhea, dysentery: enterovirus, JE virus, shigella encephalopathy
   Significant lymphadenopathy: Tubercular, HIV
   Parotid swelling: mumps
6. History related to intoxication: litchi intake in endemic location
7. History of animal contact or bite, drug or toxin exposure, trauma
8. Recent history of travel
9. Recent immunizations: for demyelination
10. History of recurrent episodes of encephalopathy: underlying metabolic causes such as Fatty acid oxidation defect (Reye syndrome), other inborn errors of metabolism
11. Past medical history
12. Family history
13. Risk factors for immunodeficiency – HIV risk factors, cancer treatment, steroid/immunosuppressant treatment

(HSV: herpes simplex virus; ADEM: acute disseminated encephalomyelitis; ALERD: acute leukoencephalopathy with restricted diffusion; JE: Japanese encephalitis virus)

Table 4: Clues to etiology based on neuroimaging in child with acute febrile encephalopathy

Neuroimaging findings	*Etiology*
Limbic involvement (medial temporal lobe, cingulate gyrus, orbital surface of frontal lobes)	Herpes simplex encephalitis (necrotic lesions), autoimmune encephalitis (NMDAR, VGKC)
Basal ganglia, thalamus and substantia nigra	Japanese B encephalitis, Basal ganglia encephalitis (encephalitis lethargica), Metabolic causes (leigh syndrome, Biotin thiamine responsive basal ganglia disease)
Basal ganglia microcystic lesions	Cryptococcal meningitis
Brainstem	Enterovirus 71, Rabies, West Nile virus, Listeria encephalitis, HSV (occasionally), Bickerstaff encephalitis, Demyelination (esp. Neuromyelitis optica spectrum disorder)
Hemorrhagic thalamic lesions	Dengue, Influenza, HSV, Arboviruses, ANEC
Multifocal involvement • Ring enhancing lesions with basal exudates • Ill-defined subcortical white matter, thalami, basal ganglia and brainstem • Focal subcortical, white matter, gray matter and brainstem lesions with diffusion restriction suggesting micro-infarcts from vasculitis-induced thrombosis	 Tubercular meningitis ADEM Nipah virus, tubercular meningitis (if localized to basal ganglia)
Acute hydrocephalus	Mumps encephalitis (if associated hypoglycorrhachia), tubercular meningitis

(NMDAR: NMDA receptor encephalitis; VGKC: voltage gated potassium channels; HSV: herpes simplex virus; ADEM: acute disseminated encephalomyelitis; ANEC: acute necrotizing encephalopathy)

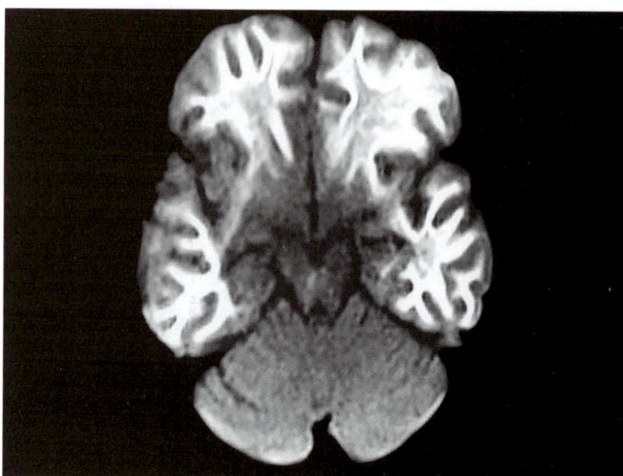

Fig. 4: MRI of the brain (diffusion weighted imaging) in a 4-year-old boy with encephalopathy and fever showing intense diffusion restriction in all of temporal and frontal white matter. He was diagnosed with acute leukoencephalopathy with restricted diffusion (ALERD) triggered by a viral infection

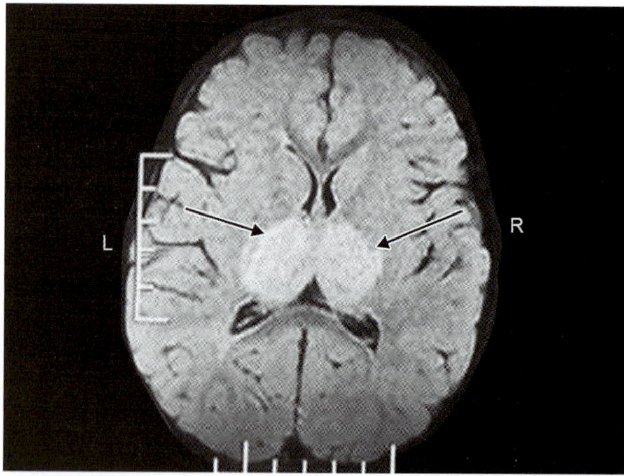

Fig. 5: MRI brain (Axial section) FLAIR sequence showing bilateral thalamic swelling with hyperintensity (arrows) in a patient with acute necrotizing encephalopathy (ANEC) of childhood, the child had fever, deep encephalopathy, transaminitis, acute kidney injury

Autoimmune encephalitis may occur in association with a systemic autoimmune disorder such as systemic lupus erythematosus, Hashimoto thyroiditis (steroid responsive encephalopathy with autoimmune thyroiditis; SREAT) or with a malignancy (onconeural antibodies in paraneoplastic syndromes). But more commonly autoimmune encephalitis occurs in association with viral encephalitis. For example, NMDAR encephalitis is reported following herpes encephalitis. Few cases of autoimmune encephalitis may occur without any clear trigger.

INVESTIGATIONS

Basic Investigations

Blood investigations including a complete blood count, electrolytes, liver and renal function tests, blood culture and arterial blood should be done to look for any abnormality. A peripheral smear for malarial parasite and rapid diagnostic test for malaria should be done in malaria endemic areas. Other rapid diagnostic test such as NS1 antigen may be done based on the season, endemicity and symptoms. Besides these, serology for scrub typhus and leptospira should also be done when they are suspected.

Lumbar Puncture (LP)

A lumbar puncture should be performed after ruling out any contraindications. The absolute contraindications for a lumbar puncture include any signs of raised intracranial pressure (decerebrate posturing, papilledema), local skin infection, obstructive hydrocephalus, cerebral edema or mass effect. Relative contraindications include hemodynamic instability, coagulation abnormality (disseminated intravascular coagulation, platelet count <50 000/mm^3, therapeutic use of warfarin), presence of focal neurological deficit, especially when posterior fossa lesion is suspected, etc. Neuroimaging should be considered before LP when the patient is unstable, or has features of raised intracranial pressure.

Cerebrospinal fluid (CSF) should be subjected to cytology and biochemistry (sugar, protein). CSF should be sent for gram stain, Ziehl-Nielsen stain for acid fast bacilli, bacterial culture, latex agglutination (for *Pneumococcus, Haemophilus influenzae*), polymerase chain reaction (PCR) for Herpes simplex virus (HSV) 1 and 2, and IgM antibodies for Japanese B encephalitis, and for Dengue virus (if suspected). CSF findings in viral encephalitis include lymphocytic cellular response, elevated protein, and usually no CSF hypoglycorrhachia. In immunocompromised cases, CSF should also be sent for India ink preparation, cryptococcal antigen and other tests to detect atypical organisms such as enterovirus in agammaglobulinemia (**Table 5**).

Table 5: Typical cerebrospinal fluid (CSF) findings and diagnostic tests in CSF in acute febrile encephalopathy

Organism/ condition	*Appearance*	*Cytology (per cumm)*	*Glucose (mg/dL; %)*	*Protein (mg/dL)*	*CSF diagnostic testing/other tests*
Bacterial meningitis	Cloudy, turbid	100–2000 polymorphs	<40; < 50%	100–500	Gram staining Culture Antigen detection (latex agglutination for *Meningococcus*, *Haemophilus* and *Pneumococcus*) Automated PCR based Panel
Tubercular meningitis	Straw colored	10–500 lymphocytes	<50	100–3000	TB PCR, GeneXpert, MGIT culture
Viral encephalitis	Clear, slightly cloudy	10–500 lymphocytes	Normal except in Mumps	50–200	CSF PCR for specific viruses: HSV, VZV, EBV, CMV, HHV Urine PCR: CMV Stool culture: enterovirus Swabs (nasopharyngeal, vesicle, throat): H1N1, enterovirus, Automated PCR based Panel
Cryptococcal meningitis	Clear	10–200 lymphocytes	Normal, slightly reduced	25–500	India Ink preparation Cryptococcal antigen in CSF

(HSV: herpes simplex virus; TB: tunberculosis; VZV: varicella zoster virus; EBV: Ebstein Barr virus; CMV: cytomegalovirus; HHV: human herpes virus)

Magnetic Resonance Imaging (MRI) Brain

MRI brain is a useful investigation, which provides clue to the underlying etiology and may help in establishing diagnosis such as in cases with acute necrotizing encephalitis (ANEC) (**Fig. 5**), acute disseminated encephalomyelitis (ADEM) (**Fig. 6**). However, its use is limited by prolonged acquisition time, difficulties in transporting critically ill children and higher cost. A contrast enhanced MRI (including T1, T2 weighted, T2 FLAIR and diffusion weighted imaging) is recommended in children with AES. **Table 4** illustrates the etiological clues based on MRI findings (**Figs. 7 to 12**). The diagnostic yield of MRI brain is around 75% in children with non-traumatic coma while a similar proportion of children have additional findings detected on MRI in comparison to CT brain.[27]

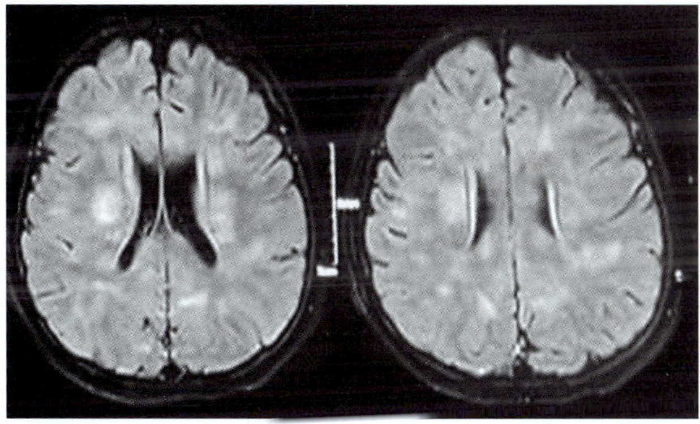

Fig. 6: MRI brain (axial section) T2 weighted sequence showing multiple patchy large ill-defined T2 hyperintensities in cerebral white matter suggestive of demyelination in a child with fever and encephalopathy. The child recovered after a course of intravenous steroids

Other Microbiological Investigations

In cases with unestablished etiology, special microbiological tests may be done. Some commercial labs offer DNA hybridization based tests for a panel of viruses [Chandipura, chikungunya, dengue, enteroviruses, HSV1, 2, human herpes virus (HHV)-6, Jap B, measles, mumps, varicella zoster virus (VZV), rubella, nipah, Rabies, West Nile virus] and bacteria using 1–2 mL CSF sample. High cost is a major limitation for these commercially available panel testing. Human immunodefeciency virus (HIV) testing should also be considered in children with encephalitis as HIV-positive children may have rare opportunistic infections such as cytomegalovirus.

Other Tests

Other supportive investigations may be useful. The electroencephalography (EEG) helps to rule out ongoing non-convulsive status epilepticus in an unconscious child.

Figs. 7A to C: MRI brain in viral encephalitis. (A) Bilateral temporal lobe (right> left) and right orbitofrontal cortex T2 hyperintensity with heterogeneous hypointensities (white arrow) in right temporal lobe (suggestive of necrosis) in patient with HSV encephalitis. The child developed anti-NMDAR encephalitis 2 weeks after this episode; (B) Bilateral thalamic hyperintensities (black arrow) in a child with Japanese B encephalitis; (C) MRI (SWI sequence) showing multiple small heterogeneous lesions (black) suggestive of extensive hemorrhages in a patient with dengue hemorrhagic fever and encephalopathy

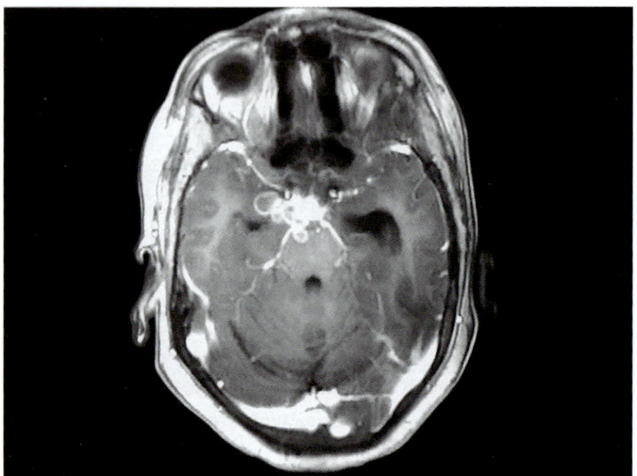

Fig. 8: A contrast enhanced MRI brain (T1 sequence) showing basal exudates and tuberculomas in a patient with tuberculous meningitis

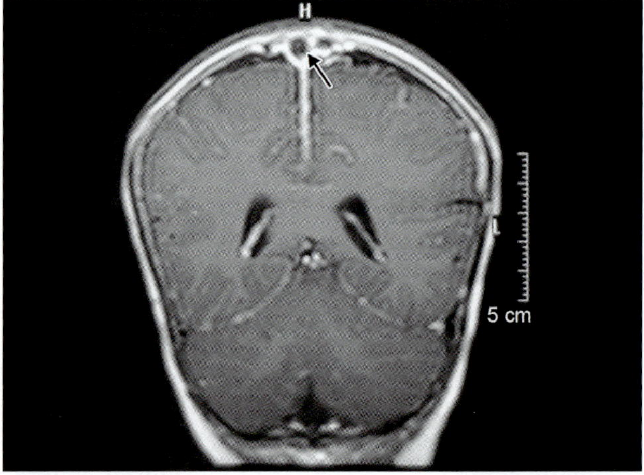

Fig. 9: MRI brain, post contrast coronal image showing sagittal sinus thrombosis evident as a filling defect (black arrow). The baby had loose stools, fever followed by encephalopathy

The presence of lateralized periodic discharges (LPDs) may be suggestive of focal encephalitis such as herpes simplex encephalitis (**Fig. 13**). The EEG may show extreme delta brushes in patients with anti-NMDA receptor encephalitis.[28]

Serological testing for autoimmune encephalitis must be considered in suspected cases. Autoantibody testing is usually done in CSF except for serum anti-glutamic acid decarboxylase (GAD). Besides these, testing for systemic autoimmune disorders (SLE, Hashimoto's thyroiditis) should be done. When suspected in young children with unexplained encephalopathy, metabolic testing including ammonia, lactate, Tandem mass spectrometry (TMS) and urine gas chromatography mass spectrometry (GCMS) should be done. A toxicology screen should be performed in cases with suspected poisoning or in the presence of a specific toxidrome. Finally, if no diagnosis has been established, a brain biopsy may be considered.

TREATMENT (TABLE 6)

Empirical treatment should be continued till the results of investigations are available to direct therapy. Supportive care is the mainstay in management of viral encephalitis. Raised intracranial pressure needs to be managed with appropriate measures. Sedation, conservative measures (minimal stimulation, head in midline and head end elevation) and osmotherapy (with hypertonic saline, mannitol) should be instituted in patients with raised intracranial pressure.

Anticonvulsants

Anticonvulsants should be promptly given in patients with ongoing seizures or history of seizures. These should also be considered in children without seizures among comatose children (GCS < 8) with features of raised intracranial pressure.[24] The clinical and neurological monitoring should be done closely to identify raised intracranial pressure, impending herniation or hemodynamic instability.

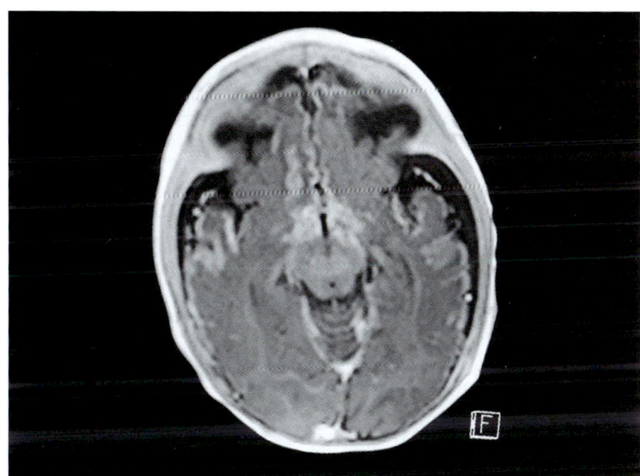

Fig. 10: MRI brain, post contrast image showing extensive meningeal enhancement and areas of cerebritis in an infant with pyogenic meningitis

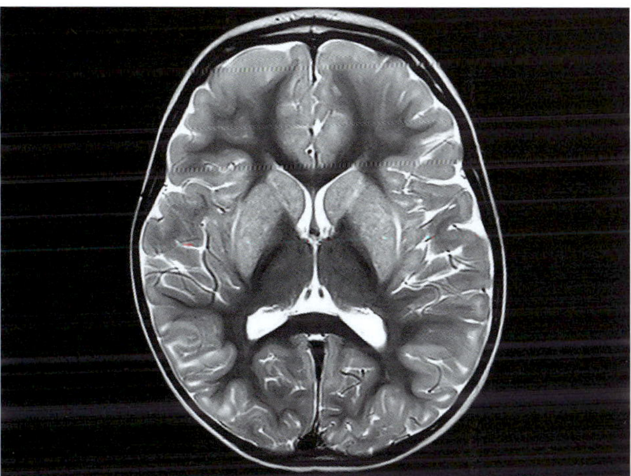

Fig. 12: T2W MRI in a child with organic acidemia showing basal ganglia and white matter hyperintensities. The child had presented with encephalopathy and fever. (*Courtesy*: Dr Gurpreet Singh Kochar)

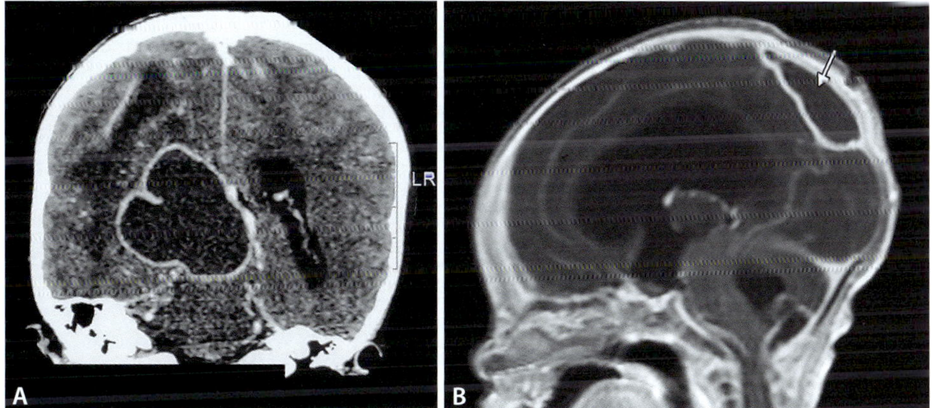

Figs. 11A and B: (A) CECT brain (coronal section) with a large brain abscess crossing the midline. The lesion is showing perilesional edema. The child had hemiparesis, altered consciousness and seizures; (B) CEMRI brain (sagittal section) showing midline subdural empyema (white arrow) in a child with bacterial meningitis

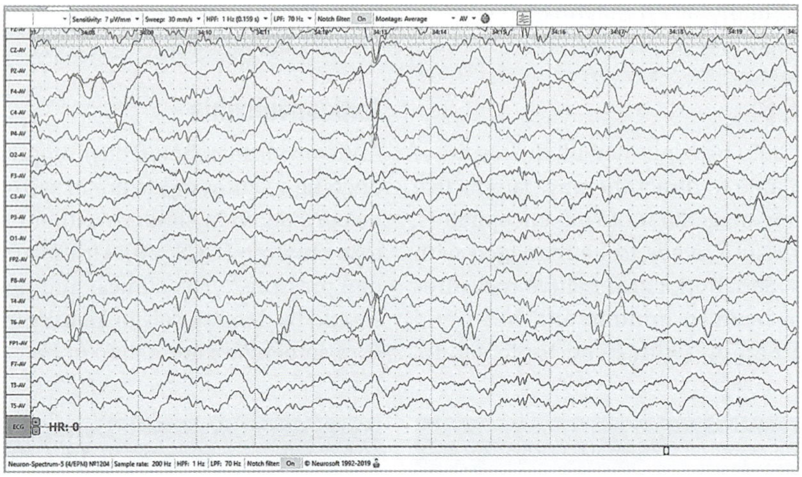

Fig. 13: EEG showing periodic discharges lateralized to right temporal electrodes (T4 and T6) occurring at an interval of 1.5–2 seconds suggestive of periodic lateralized discharges (PLDs) in a child with encephalitis. (Referential montage; sensitivity: 7 uV/mm; sweep speed: 30 mm/s)

Table 6: Selected drugs used in empirical management of acute febrile encephalopathy in children

Drugs	*Dose and duration*
Acyclovir (empirically in AFE and specifically for HSV encephalitis)	Dose: Neonates -3 months: 20 mg/kg/dose, 8 hourly 3 months to 12 years:10–15 mg/kg/dose, 8 hourly >12 years: 10 mg/kg/dose, 8 hourly Duration: 21 days
Antibiotics (empirically for bacterial meningitis) Ceftriaxone	100 mg/kg/day in two divided doses intravenously
Vancomycin	60 mg/kg/day in 4 divided doses intravenously (to be initiated if associated shock requiring ionotropes, suspicion of staphylococcal infection) Duration: 7 days (meningococcal meningitis), 10 days (*Haemophilus influenza* B meningitis), 14 days (pneumococcal meningitis), longer duration (21–28 days for staphylococcal and enterococcal meningitis)
Artesunate (for suspected cerebral malaria)	2.4 mg/kg body weight given intravenously or intramuscularly at admission then at 12h, 24h and then once a day till the child accepts orally. Following this, full course of oral artemisinin combination therapy should be given.
Azithromycin (in cases with suspected scrub typhus)	10 mg/kg/day for 3–5 days
Methylprednisolone pulse (in cases with ADEM, autoimmune encephalitis, etc.)	10–30 mg/kg/day as an infusion over 3 hours for 3–5 days
Intravenous Immunoglobulin (in cases with autoimmune encephalitis)	2 g/kg divided over 3–5 days

(ADEM: acute disseminated encephalomyelitis)

Acyclovir can be stopped after documenting a negative HSV PCR in the CSF (sensitivity of 95%), or normal MRI brain.[29,30] But these investigations may be false negative when performed very early in the disease course. Hence, these may be repeated in cases with high suspicion.

Steroids and IVIG

Corticosteroids have a controversial role in the management of viral encephalitis. They may be considered in patients with marked cerebral edema, or raised intracranial pressure.[31] However, there in a risk of active viral replication and ensuing damage. Steroid have been tried in HSV encephalitis and Japanese B encephalitis.[32,33] Steroids are the treatment of choice in immune mediated disorders like, ADEM, Hashimoto encephalopathy, and autoimmune encephalitis.

Intravenous immunoglobulin (IVIG) may be beneficial in viral encephalitis especially in immunocompromised patients. A multi-centric randomized controlled trial -"IGNITE trial" of early IVIG is in progress in children with encephalitis due to any cause[34] and will clarify their role in encephalitis.

Others

Several drugs are under trial for treating viral infections such as: Pleconaril in enterovirus encephalitis and aseptic meningitis (except EV 71), oral ribavirin and minocycline have been tried in Japanese B encephalitis but none of the drug is recommended as the standard of care in these infections.

After the acute phase, transitional care with proper care of nutrition and neurological rehabilitation is important to optimize outcomes.

KEY MESSAGES

- Acute encephalitis syndrome is a potential life-threatening emergency with significant morbidity and mortality.
- There are a gamut of causes responsible which includes: infections (viruses being most predominant), post-infectious such as acute disseminated encephalomyelitis and autoimmune encephalitis.
- Prompt recognition and appropriate treatment is essential.
- Empirical treatment for treatable causes should be initiated awaiting diagnostic workup.
- Ongoing physiotherapy and austere rehabilitative measures are important in reducing morbidity.

REFERENCES

1. Yeolekar M, Trivedi T. Febrile encephalopathy: Challenges in management. J Assoc Physicians India. 2006;54:845-7.
2. World Health Organisation. Acute Encephalitis Syndrome. Japanese encephalitis surveillance standards. From WHO-recommended standards for surveillance of selected vaccine-preventable diseases. WHO/V&B/03.01. Available from: *http://www.who. int/vaccines-documents/DocsPDF06/843.pdf.*; 2006.
3. Sharma S, Mishra D, Aneja S, *et al.* Consensus guidelines on evaluation and management of suspected acute viral encephalitis in children in India. Indian Pediatr. 2012;49: 897-910.
4. National Vector Borne Disease Control Programme, New Delhi. Acute Encephalitis/Japanese Encephalitis cases and deaths in the country since 2013. Available from: *http://www.nvbdcp.gov.in/WriteReadData/l892s/25510462041546326501.pdf.* Accessed January 10, 2019.
5. Gupta K, Purani CS, Mandal A, *et al.* Acute febrile encephalopathy in children: A prospective study of clinical features, etiology, mortality, and risk factors from western India. J Neurosci Rural Pract. 2018;9:19-25.
6. Jain P, Jain A, Kumar A, *et al.* Epidemiology and etiology of acute encephalitis syndrome in North India. Jpn J Infect Dis. 2014;67:197-203.
7. Kumar R, Kumar P, Singh MK, *et al.* Epidemiological profile of acute viral encephalitis. Indian J Pediatr. 2018;85:358-63.
8. Rao BL, Basu A, Wairagkar NS, *et al.* A large outbreak of acute encephalitis with high fatality rate in children in Andhra Pradesh, India, in 2003, associated with Chandipura virus. Lancet Lond Engl. 2004;364 :869-74.
9. Chadha MS, Comer JA, Lowe L, *et al.* Nipah virus-associated encephalitis outbreak, Siliguri, India. Emerg Infect Dis. 2006; 12:235-40.
10. George S, Yergolkar PN, Kamala H, *et al.* Outbreak of encephalitis in Bellary district of Karnataka & adjoining areas of Andhra Pradesh. Indian J Med Res. 1990;91:328-30.
11. Anukumar B, Sapkal GN, Tandale BV, *et al.* West Nile encephalitis outbreak in Kerala, India, 2011. J Clin Virol. 2014; 61:152-5.
12. Singhi S, Rungta N, Nallasamy K, *et al.* Tropical Fevers in Indian Intensive Care Units: A Prospective Multicenter Study. Indian J Crit Care Med. 2017;21:811-8.
13. Khan SA, Dutta P, Khan AM, *et al.* Re-emergence of scrub typhus in northeast India. Int J Infect Dis. 2012;16:e889-90.
14. Mittal M, Thangaraj JWV, Rose W, *et al.* Scrub typhus as a cause of acute encephalitis syndrome, Gorakhpur, Uttar Pradesh, India. Emerg Infect Dis. 2017;23:1414-6.
15. Kumar Bhat N, Dhar M, Mittal G, *et al.* Scrub typhus in children at a tertiary hospital in north India: clinical profile and complications. Iran J Pediatr. 2014;24:387-92.
16. Viswanathan S, Muthu V, Iqbal N, *et al.* Scrub typhus meningitis in South India—a retrospective study. PloS One. 2013;8:e66595.
17. Murhekar MV, Mittal M, Prakash JAJ, *et al.* Acute encephalitis syndrome in Gorakhpur, Uttar Pradesh, India - Role of scrub typhus. J Infect. 2016;73:623-6.
18. Spencer PS, Palmer VS. The enigma of litchi toxicity: an emerging health concern in southern Asia. Lancet Glob Health. 2017;5:e383-4.
19. Shrivastava A, Kumar A, Thomas JD, *et al.* Association of acute toxic encephalopathy with litchi consumption in an outbreak in Muzaffarpur, India, 2014: A case-control study. Lancet Glob Health. 2017;5:e458-66.
20. Denizot M, Neal JW, Gasque P. Encephalitis due to emerging viruses: CNS innate immunity and potential therapeutic targets. J Infect. 2012;65:1-16.
21. Britton PN, Blyth CC, Macartney K, *et al.*; Australian Childhood Encephalitis (ACE) Study Investigators, Influenza Complications Alert Network (FluCAN) Investigators, and Paediatric Active Enhanced Disease Surveillance (PAEDS) Network. The Spectrum and Burden of Influenza-Associated

Neurological Disease in Children: Combined Encephalitis and Influenza Sentinel Site Surveillance From Australia, 2013-2015. Clin Infect Dis. 2017;65:653-60.

22. Mahalingam S, Herrero LJ, Playford EG, *et al.* Hendra virus: an emerging paramyxovirus in Australia. Lancet Infect Dis. 2012;12:799-807.
23. Ong KC, Wong KT. Henipavirus encephalitis: Recent developments and advances. Brain Pathol Zurich Switz. 2015;25: 605-13.
24. Aneja S, Sharma S. Diagnosis and management of acute encephalitis in children. Indian J Pediatr. 2019;86:70-5.
25. Ashwal S. Disorders of consciousness in children. In: Swaiman KF, Ashwal S, Ferriero DM, Schor NF, Finkel RS, Gropman RL, Shevell M, Pearl PL, editors. Swaiman's Pediatric Neurology: Principles and Practice, 6th edition. Philadelphia: Elsevier Publications; 2017. p. e1741-73.
26. Mizuguchi M, Yamanouchi H, Ichiyama T, *et al.* Acute encephalopathy associated with influenza and other viral infections. Acta Neurol Scand. 2007;115:45-56.
27. Khipal J, Sankhyan N, Singhi SC, *et al.* Clinical utility of MRI brain in children with non-traumatic coma. Indian J Pediatr. 2017;84:838-42.
28. Graus F, Titulaer MJ, Balu R, *et al.* A clinical approach to diagnosis of autoimmune encephalitis. Lancet Neurol. 2016; 15:391-404.
29. Kirkham FJ. Guidelines for the management of encephalitis in children. Dev Med Child Neurol. 2013;55:107-10.
30. Kneen R, Michael BD, Menson E, *et al.* Management of suspected viral encephalitis in children - Association of British Neurologists and British Paediatric Allergy, Immunology and Infection Group national guidelines. J Infect. 2012;64:449-77.
31. Kamei S, Sekizawa T, Shiota H, *et al.* Evaluation of combination therapy using aciclovir and corticosteroid in adult patients with herpes simplex virus encephalitis. J Neurol Neurosurg Psychiatry. 2005;76:1544-9.
32. Martinez-Torres F, Menon S, Pritsch M, *et al.* Protocol for German trial of acyclovir and corticosteroids in herpes-simplex-virus-encephalitis (GACHE): A multicenter, multinational, randomized, double-blind, placebo-controlled German, Austrian and Dutch trial [ISRCTN45122933]. BMC Neurol. 2008;8:40.
33. Hoke CH, Vaughn DW, Nisalak A, *et al.* Effect of high-dose dexamethasone on the outcome of acute encephalitis due to Japanese encephalitis virus. J Infect Dis. 1992;165: 631-7.
34. Wang SM, Lei HY, Huang MC, *et al.* Modulation of cytokine production by intravenous immunoglobulin in patients with enterovirus 71-associated brainstem encephalitis. J Clin Virol. 2006;37:47-52.

CHAPTER

30

Intracranial Hypertension

Arushi Gahlot Saini

INTRODUCTION

Raised intracranial pressure (ICP) and compromised cerebral perfusion are one of the most commonly encountered neurocritical care emergencies in children. Significant elevations in the ICP are not only acutely deleterious by causing cerebral herniation, but also portend poor neurological outcomes. Raised ICP contributes to morbidity and mortality in a broad spectrum of pathological illnesses affecting the brain such as traumatic brain injury, central nervous system (CNS) infections, intracranial hemorrhages, tumors, hydrocephalous, stroke and acute liver failure.[1] Physiological principles guiding the ICP, followed by monitoring and management of raised ICP in children are briefly discussed in this chapter. Historical perspective of intracranial pressure is summarized in **Table 1**.

PHYSIOLOGICAL BASIS OF ICP

Based on the principles of Monro-Kellie doctrine, ICP is derived from the volumes of three compartments inside the fixed cranial vault: brain, blood and cerebrospinal fluid (CSF), assuming that the CSF flow is unobstructed and that the pressures are equally distributed across the compartments.[2] Brain tissue occupies nearly 80% of the intracranial volume; the remaining 20% is nearly equally shared by the blood and CSF.[3] Any increase in the volume of one compartment is compensated by a corresponding decrease in the volume of other two compartments.[2] The reduced buffering capacity in children is related to the smaller spinal CSF volume.[4]

Cerebral blood flow (CBF) depends on both the cerebral perfusion pressure (CPP) and the vascular resistance. It is calculated as the difference between mean arterial pressure (sum of diastolic blood pressure and 1/3rd of the difference of systolic and diastolic pressures) and ICP. Normal CPP in children is not exactly known, but following values have been proposed to prevent ischemia: adults >70 mm Hg, children >50–60 mm Hg and infants/toddlers >40–50 mm Hg.[5] Cerebral autoregulation is the ability of the blood vessels to change the diameter to keep constant blood flow regardless of the mean arterial pressure and it depends on metabolic, myogenic and neuronal mechanisms.[6,7] Once this compensation fails, cerebral swelling occurs secondary to oligemia or hyperemia.

The relationship between ICP and intracranial volume (pressure-volume curve) is dynamic, non-linear and follows a sigmoid curve.[8] The first part of the curve depicts a compensatory reserve due to which an extra volume in any of the compartments will be adequately accommodated by a mild increase in intracranial pressure.[9] However, with increasing volume, the compensation is lost and small further increases in volume leads to marked and rapid rise in ICP. This is depicted by the second half of the pressure-volume curve. Any further significant and/or persistent increase in the ICP will compromise the CBF

Table 1: Historical perspectives on intracranial pressure

- Alexander Monroe, a Scottish anatomist and his student George Kellie gave the concept of ICP as being a relation of the volume and compliance of each intracranial compartment
- Heinrich Quinke, a German surgeon, proposed the earliest method of measuring ICP via lumbar punctures
- Harvey Cushing, an American neurosurgeon, first described the 'Cushing triad' in relation to ICP

and cause brain ischemia and infarction.[10] A recent meta-analysis of studies that analyzed CBF autoregulation in patients undergoing ICP monitoring showed that patients with ICP ≥20 had an elevated risk of impaired cerebral autoregulation (OR 2.27, 95% CI 1.20-4.31, $p = 0.01$).[11]

The normal ICP depends on the age of the patient. In term infants, it ranges from 1.5 to 6 mm Hg, in children 3–7 mm Hg, and in older children and adults, it is <10–15 mm Hg.[12] CSF pressures between 15–20 mm Hg are considered borderline and treatment may depend on clinical presentation of raised pressure. Pressures >20 mm Hg are considered pathological and warrant urgent treatment. Severe, uncontrolled raised ICP >40 mm Hg, if persists, leads to brain herniation and irreversible loss of brain functions.[10]

CAUSES OF RAISED ICP

Based on the compartmentation of intracranial volumes, increased blood volume is primarily responsible for raised ICP in conditions such as vascular malformations, venous thrombosis, and CNS infections. Similarly, increased CSF volume accounts for raised ICP in causes such as hydrocephalus, choroid plexus papillomas producing excessive CSF and shunt dysfunctions, and altered CSF dynamics in idiopathic intracranial hypertension. Increased brain volume accounts for raised ICP in conditions such as intracranial space occupying parenchymal lesions, and, diffuse or focal cerebral edema secondary to trauma, bleed, infections, strokes and metabolic disturbances.[13] The common causes of raised ICP in children are listed in **Table 2** and these often act in combination.[14]

MONITORING OF RAISED ICP

Clinical features: Symptoms of raised ICP can be nonspecific and depend on the age of the patient, underlying etiology and the rapidity of rise of ICP. Some of the clinical signs and symptoms indicative of raised ICP in children, especially if they are accompanied by a low GCS score are tabulated in **Table 3**. A child may have one or more of these symptoms. Headache, vomiting and altered consciousness are nonspecific symptoms and are unreliable predictors of raised ICP as well as have limited value in serial monitoring. Knowledge about these clinical features helps in early recognition of raised ICP in the emergency department.[15]

ICP Monitoring Methods

Monitoring of ICP is important to recognize raised pressures in sedated or obtunded patients, for early detection of changing cerebral function and assessment of response to treatment. A single measurement of ICP is often done in routine clinical practice by attaching a manometer to the lumbar puncture needle and recorded as the "opening pressure" of CSF. As the clinical signs of raised ICP in children are nonspecific, continuous monitoring of ICP is an essential method in neurocritical patients. ICP can be measured by directly or invasive methods, which provide direct signals from a CSF space in the cranium, or by indirect or noninvasive methods where ICP is derived from related parameters.

Table 2: Causes of raised intracranial pressure in children
With mass effect compressing the normal brain:
Hydrocephalus, shunt dysfunction/block/breakage/infection, choroid plexus papilloma
Intracranial space occupying lesions: tumors, metastasis, abscesses, cysts, vascular malformation
Cerebrovascular lesions (bleed, hematoma, thrombosis, infarction)
Focal cerebral edema associated with trauma, infarction, tumor, abscess, prolonged seizure
Without mass effect:
Central nervous system infections (meningitis, encephalitis)
Status epilepticus
Traumatic brain injury
Hypoxic-ischemic catastrophe: cardiac arrest, near drowning
Metabolic encephalopathy: inborn errors of metabolism leading to intoxication, acute liver failure, uremia, Reye syndrome, diabetic ketoacidosis
Hypertensive encephalopathy, PRES*
Burns
Toxic substances (e.g., lead, heavy metals)
Craniosynostosis syndromes
Benign intracranial hypertension (disordered CSF dynamics)

*(PRES: posterior reversible encephalopathy syndrome)

Table 3: Common signs and symptoms of raised ICP in children

Common symptoms of intracranial hypertension

1. *Infants and small children:* Tense, bulging fontanel, increased sutural separation in the skull bones, prominent scalp veins, silent tachypnea, sun-setting phenomenon in the eyes, failure to thrive, persistent vomiting, irritability, progressive head growth changing the percentiles, delayed motor milestones, poor head control or pseudo-regression of milestones
2. *Older children:*
   a. Irritability, behavior or personality changes or progressive encephalopathy
   b. Recurrent vomiting, typically in the morning, associated with slight relief in pressure symptoms, cascade-like and often associated with headache and nausea
   c. Blurring of vision, double vision, recent-onset unilateral squint, restriction of eye movements in lateral gaze (sixth nerve palsy), papilledema
   d. Neck stiffness, torticollis (tilted head and possible decreased motion)
   e. Focal neurological deficit
   f. Seizures
   g. Ataxia

Impending signs of brain herniation:

1. Deterioration of consciousness
2. Sluggishly reactive pupils, asymmetrical pupils, fixed dilated pupil with light reaction
3. Restriction of eye movements
4. Focal neurological deficits
5. Hyperventilation, Cheyne-Stokes respiration
6. Decerebrate rigidity/opisthotonos
7. Babinski's sign (extensor plantar response)
8. Cushing's triad: hypertension, bradycardia and irregular or superficial respiration

Indirect methods

Computed tomography (CT): CT scan is probably the most feasible and widely available investigations in all trauma and emergency care set-ups to assess neurological and neurosurgical patients. The use of skull radiographs to demonstrate raised ICP is nearly obsolete although it may show erosion of clinoid process and separation of sutures. Several CT findings indicate raised ICP such as midline shift, ventricular dilation, sulcal effacement, loss of differentiation of gray-white matter, cistern effacement especially compressed or obliterated basal cistern and herniation.[16] It has been estimated that nearly 75% of children who has obliterated cisterns demonstrated at least one episode of raised ICP on invasive monitoring.[17] Presence of open cisterns alone does not predict normal ICP, rather it indicates a window of opportunity to initiate urgent therapeutic measures among those with raised ICP.

Optic nerve sheath diameter (ONSD) by ultrasonography: The optic nerve sheath is an extension of the cerebral dura mater and communicates with the subarachnoid space of the meninges. Hence, ICP changes are reflected in the CSF inside the optic nerve sheath and result in widening of its diameter within minutes of acute changes in ICP making optic nerve sheath diameter an important modality of non-invasive measurement/monitoring of ICP.[18] In these cases, the blood flow through the central retinal vein that passes through the sheath is impeded, resulting in papilledema.[19] An ONSD of >5 mm corresponds to an ICP of 20 mm Hg or higher.[20] Transocular ultrasonographic measurement of widened ONSD has shown a sensitivity of 80% in detecting ICP ≥ 20 mm Hg in children.[21] The technique has the advantage of feasibility, easy reproducibility, taking repeated measurements, bedside testing, economic and less requirement of expertise as compared to CT or MRI based measurements.[22-24]

Intracranial elastance: Elastance is defined as the ratio of change in pressure to change in volume ($\Delta P/\Delta V$), and an elasticity index has been determined for the brain over a range of ICPs. MRI-based analysis of CSF and blood (arterial and venous) flow dynamics are used in this technique to calculate fluctuations in intracranial volume and pressure, and elastance during a cardiac cycle and then ICP is derived from these measurements. Although useful in pediatric TBI patients, the technique is not suited for rapid diagnosis and decision-making.[25]

Transcranial Doppler (TCD): CBF can be studied by TCD as well as magnetic resonance angiography. As raised ICP leads to a greater reduction in diastolic blood flow velocity than systolic flow velocity, the Gosling pulsatility index (difference between systolic and diastolic flow velocities divided by mean flow velocity) is calculated and correlated with ICP.[26] Resistive index (difference between systolic and diastolic flow velocities, divided by systolic flow velocity) is another TCD variable which defines the correlation between ICP and CBF.[27] Blood flow velocities are commonly measured in middle cerebral artery, anterior cerebral artery, and ophthalmic artery over the acoustic window regions such as temporal region, back of the head or through the eye. An extremely good correlation has been shown between the two in early stages post injury in children, with 100% sensitivity and 82% specificity in predicting raised ICP (≥ 20 mm Hg).[28] Given the complexity of analysis and duration of assessment in neurocritical patients, MRA seems less clinically useful in pediatric TBI.

Tympanic membrane displacement (TMD): Similar to the optic nerve sheath, CSF and perilymph in the inner ear communicate with each other via the perilymphatic duct. CSF pressure is transmitted to the perilymph of the cochlea and any increase in ICP is directly transmitted to the footplate of the stapes. Stimulation of stapedial reflex causes undulation of tympanic membrane, which correlates with ICP.[29] An inward displacement suggests raised ICP whereas an outward displacement suggests normal or low ICP.[30]

Direct methods

Direct measurements of ICP require placement of a transducer within the cranial cavity such as intraventricular, intraparenchymal, epidural, subdural, or subarachnoid space. The goal of all modalities of continuous ICP monitoring is maintenance of optimal CPP.[31]

Intraventricular catheter placement was the original method used and remains the gold standard for accurate measurement of ICP and ICP-directed therapy.[32] A burr hole is created in the skull and a ventricular catheter is inserted into one of the lateral ventricles at the bedside. ICP is measured via the transducer, which remains in direct contact with the CSF and displays the fluctuations in a bedside monitor by a continuous waveform. Knowledge of normal waveforms and its variations is important for the neuro-intensivist for proper interpretation of ICP reflections. Additionally, the catheter can be used for therapeutic CSF drainage and intraventricular administration of drugs. Disadvantages include a falsely low ICP reading due to CSF leakage, risk of infection, inability to insert the catheter in a compressed or displaced ventricles and possible local trauma to the brain.[33] Subdural pressure transducers are least invasive, technically less demanding and more feasible. However, the ICP readings are less accurate and may be erroneous due to CSF block as the device transmits the readings from the CSF that fills the device after insertion.[34] Intra-parenchymal monitors are almost as accurate as the intraventricular devices but run the disadvantages of inability to drain CSF (as the tip is located in the brain parenchyma) and reflection of localized pressure more than the global ICP.[12]

MANAGEMENT OF RAISED ICP

Evidence for the most effective modes of treatment in children with raised ICP is insufficient and majority of the guidelines are based on studies in adults and consequently in children with traumatic brain injury. Majority of protocols are hospital policy-based and may vary depending on the feasibility and availability of resources.[35] Nevertheless, the main aim of the treatment of raised ICP in children is to treat the primary/underlying cause and to prevent/minimize secondary injury.[36] Secondary brain injury refers to the processes that occur after the primary injury, even up to several days, and it adds to the neurological insult. These include factors such as cerebral ischemia, cerebral edema, hypoxia, hypotension, hypertension, hypoglycemia, seizures and biochemical changes in the brain milieu including neurochemical alterations, free radical generation, and alterations in the levels of intracellular potassium and calcium.[37]

Goals of therapy are: (i) to maintain ICP <20–25 mm Hg, (ii) to maintain CPP >60 mm Hg by maintaining adequate MAP, (iii) to prevent/avoid factors that cause secondary injury and/or aggravate raised ICP.[9,38]

A broad approach to the management of raised ICP in children is presented in **Flowchart 1**.

First Line Therapy

ABCDs

Raised ICP is an important neurocritical care emergency where several interventions may have to be begun immediately. In any patient, the initial management requires maintenance of airway, breathing and circulation. A focused history and examination and a quick disability assessment needs to be done simultaneously to assess the etiology and extent of neurological deterioration and severity of raised ICP. Early intubation should be considered under rapid sequence intubation if: the patient is unarousable, has GCS ≤ 8 or has a difficulty in

Flowchart 1: Tiered approach to intracranial hypertension in children

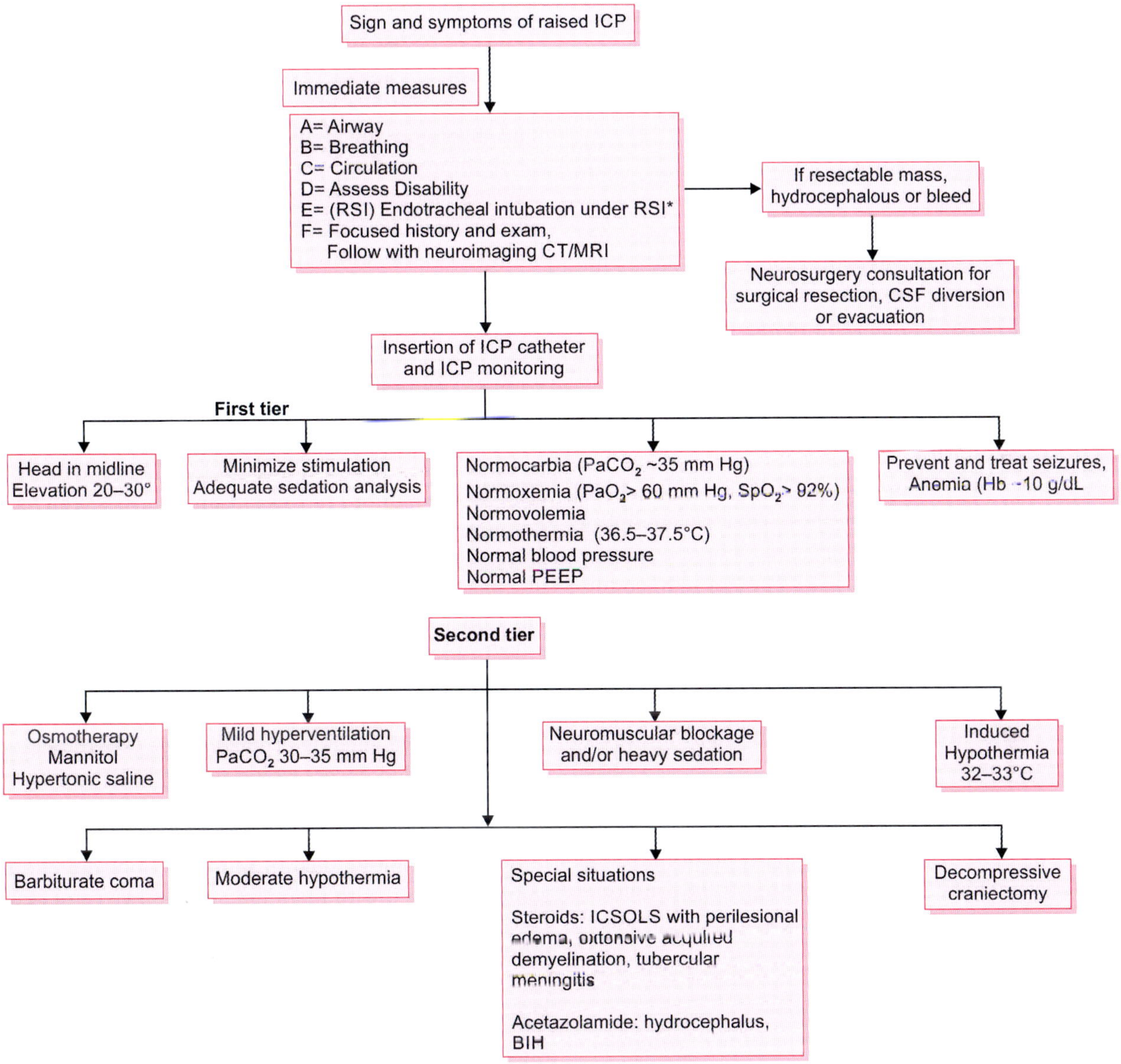

Sign and symptoms of raised ICP

Immediate measures

A= Airway
B= Breathing
C= Circulation
D= Assess Disability
E= (RSI) Endotracheal intubation under RSI*
F= Focused history and exam, Follow with neuroimaging CT/MRI

If resectable mass, hydrocephalous or bleed

Neurosurgery consultation for surgical resection, CSF diversion or evacuation

Insertion of ICP catheter and ICP monitoring

First tier

- Head in midline Elevation 20–30°
- Minimize stimulation Adequate sedation analysis
- Normocarbia ($PaCO_2$ ~35 mm Hg)
  Normoxemia (PaO_2> 60 mm Hg, SpO_2> 92%)
  Normovolemia
  Normothermia (36.5–37.5°C)
  Normal blood pressure
  Normal PEEP
- Prevent and treat seizures, Anemia (Hb ~10 g/dL

Second tier

- Osmotherapy Mannitol Hypertonic saline
- Mild hyperventilation $PaCO_2$ 30–35 mm Hg
- Neuromuscular blockage and/or heavy sedation
- Induced Hypothermia 32–33°C

- Barbiturate coma
- Moderate hypothermia
- Special situations
  Steroids: ICSOLS with perilesional edema, extensive acquired demyelination, tubercular meningitis
  Acetazolamide: hydrocephalus, BIH
- Decompressive craniectomy

maintaining a patent airway, has neurological injury at risk for decompensation, chest wall instability, abnormal respiratory pattern, loss of protections airway reflexes or upper airway obstruction.[39] Ventilations not only optimizes oxygenation but also helps manipulate carbon dioxide levels to reduce CBF. Increasing the PEEP may increase thoracic pressure and reduce venous return from the brain. Fluid resuscitation with normal saline boluses (20 mL/kg) and vasoactive drugs (increase the mean arterial pressure and try to maintain adequate CPP in the face of rising ICP) should be started based on signs of hemodynamic compromise (poor perfusion, tachycardia, prolonged capillary refill time and/or hypotension).[9]

Positioning, head in midline, minimal stimulation, sedation and analgesia

Placing the head in midline position and 20–30° elevation facilitates venous drainage.[40] After securing airway, adequate analgesia and sedation should be administered to avoid pain and frequent movements in the patient which result in surges in ICP and decrease the CPP. Benzodiazepine such as continuous midazolam infusion, propofol, and narcotics like fentanyl and morphine are the preferred medications.[9,38]

Hyperventilation

Hyperventilation, instituted by reducing the $PaCO_2$ to the range of 30–35 mm Hg, lowers the CBF by constricting cerebral blood vessels.[41,42] This is an effective and rapid method to reduce acute, sharp increase in ICP or reverse signs of impending herniation, but its effect lasts only 11–20 hours because the pH of the CSF rapidly equilibrates to the new $PaCO_2$ level. Aggressive hyperventilation can be detrimental as it can dramatically reduce CBF and induce ischemia.[41]

Normothermia, normocarbia, normo-oxia and normovolemia

Elevation in body temperature increases the metabolic demands as well as blood-brain barrier permeability, glutamate release, and free radical production, leading to worsening cerebral edema and ICP.[43] The core temperature should be maintained between 36.5° and 37.5°. Carbon dioxide has a vasodilatory effect on intracranial vessels and increases ICP. Hyperventilation aids in reducing ICP by decreasing CO_2 levels and inducing vasoconstriction. $PaCO_2$ levels should be targeted between 25 and 35 mm Hg. The oxygen saturation should be above 95%. A strict blood pressure monitoring is essential as hypotension is detrimental to the brain.

Electrolyte imbalances, especially hyponatremia secondary to either cerebral salt wasting or the syndrome of inappropriate antidiuretic hormone needs attention. These may lower the seizure threshold in the setting of CNS disease.[9]

Control of seizures, anemia and blood glucose

Blood glucose is targeted between 80 and 120 mg/dL among children with raised ICP. Both hyperglycemia and hypoglycemia are detrimental to brain. Similarly, hemoglobin levels are targeted above 10 g/dL considering the risk of increase cerebral blood flow and subsequent increase in ICP in anemic children. Seizures need to be controlled with antiepileptic drugs. Seizures are known to increase CBF and ICP leading to further neuronal injury. Among children with raised ICP and children with traumatic brain injury might benefit from short-term use of prophylactic antiepileptic drugs.[10]

Second Line Therapy

Hyperosmolar therapy

Hyperosmolar agents reduce ICP by creating an osmotic gradient across the blood brain barrier and promoting fluid shifts from the interstitial and intracellular spaces of the brain to the intravascular spaces. Mannitol has been conventionally used as an osmotic diuretic; it reduces blood viscosity, improves cerebral blood flow and oxygenation.[44] Mannitol (20% solution) is given as an initial bolus (0.25–1 g/kg over 20 minutes) followed by repeated boluses of 0.25–0.5 g/kg every 4–6 hours. The effect starts within 1–5 minutes, peaks at 20–60 minutes and may last for up to 6 hours. Mannitol therapy needs caution in children with hypotension, hypovolemia, intracranial bleed, renal failure and serum osmolality above 320 mOsmol/kg. In such cases, hypertonic saline (1.5–23.5%; commonly used as 3% solution) proves advantageous as it increases the intravascular volume by fluid shift from interstitial and intracellular spaces and causes minimal diuresis.[45] It is generally begun as 0.2 to 1.0 mL/kg/hr continuous infusion to target a serum sodium levels of 145–155 mEq/L. Gradual tapering is advised for weaning off both the therapies to prevent rebound rise in ICP or rapid fluid shifts.[46]

Other agents include acetazolamide (20–100 mg/kg/day, in 3 divided doses) which reduced CSF production and is particularly helpful in hydrocephalus, benign intracranial hypertension and high altitude illness; furosemide (1 mg/kg/day, q8 hourly) is a loop diuretic and sometimes used with mannitol; and oral glycerol (1.5 g/kg/day, q4–6 hourly) which readily crosses blood brain barrier and helps in reduction of ICP.[47,48]

Hypothermia

Elevated body temperature raised the metabolic demands, increase the blood flow to the brain in the face of impaired autoregulation as well as releases cytokines, which worsen the cerebral edema. Every 1°C reduction in core body temperature reduces brain metabolism by 5–7%. On the other hand, medically-induced hypothermia (target temperature 32–34°C) causes cerebral vasoconstriction, reduces metabolic and glucose demand and intracranial blood volume and has a neuroprotective role.[49] Complications of therapeutic hypothermia include neutropenia, infections, arrhythmias, clotting abnormalities and renal dysfunction.[50]

Neuromuscular blocking agents

Neuromuscular blocking agents reduce the overall metabolic demands of the body as well as prevent intermittent surges in ICP associated with stimulation, movements, suctioning, coughing, and sampling. Commonly used intravenous agents include pancuronium, vecuronium and atracurium.[9]

Third Line Therapy

Pentobarbital coma

Barbiturate-induced coma is generally used as a third-tier therapy for reducing the cerebral blood flow, and metabolic needs, thereby reducing the ICP.[51] The adequacy of coma is generally adjudged by attainment of a 90% burst suppression pattern (2–6 bursts per minute) on continuous EEG monitoring. A loading dose of 10 mg/kg over 20 to 30 minutes is followed by an infusion of 1 mg/kg/hr. Commonly associated adverse effects include respiratory depression, hypokalemia, hypovolemia, infections and renal and hepatic dysfunction.[52]

Decompressive craniectomy

Medically refractory raised ICP can be a nightmare for the neurocritical care team and decompressive craniectomy is now being increasing used in these cases, irrespective of the etiology. The long-term cognitive and neuromotor effects of this form of treatment in children need to be seen but it remains an effective life-saving measure in refractory or malignant cases of raised ICP, especially if there is evidence of cerebral herniation.[53,54]

KEY MESSAGES

- The prime focus of management of raised ICP in children is to treat the primary (underlying) cause.
- Second most important focus is to prevent or minimize secondary injury due to cerebral ischemia, cerebral edema, hypoxia, hypotension, hypertension, hypoglycemia, seizures and electrolyte imbalances.
- Goals of therapy are: (i) to maintain ICP <20–25 mm Hg, (ii) to maintain CPP >60 mm Hg by maintaining adequate MAP, (iii) to prevent/avoid factors that cause secondary injury and/or aggravate raised ICP.
- Decompressive craniotomy is an effective life-saving measure in refractory or malignant cases of raised ICP, especially if there is evidence of cerebral herniation.

REFERENCES

1. de Lima Oliveira M, Kairalla AC, Fonoff ET, *et al.* Cerebral microdialysis in traumatic brain injury and subarachnoid hemorrhage: state of the art. Neurocrit Care. 2014;21:152-62.
2. Mokri B. The Monro-Kellie hypothesis: Applications in CSF volume depletion. Neurology. 2001;56:1746-8.
3. Allen CH, Ward JD. An evidence-based approach to management of increased intracranial pressure. Crit Care Clin. 1998; 14:485-95.
4. Kaufman BA, Dacey RG, Jr. Acute care management of closed head injury in childhood. Pediatr Ann. 1994;23:18-20, 5-8.
5. Mazzola CA, Adelson PD. Critical care management of head trauma in children. Crit Care Med. 2002;30:S393-401.
6. Salinet AS, Panerai RB, Robinson TG. The longitudinal evolution of cerebral blood flow regulation after acute ischaemic stroke. Cerebrovasc Dis Extra. 2014;4:186-97.
7. Czosnyka M, Smielewski P, Piechnik S, *et al.* Cerebral autoregulation following head injury. J Neurosurg. 2001;95: 756-63.
8. Smith M. Monitoring intracranial pressure in traumatic brain injury. Anesth Analg. 2008;106:240-8.
9. Singhi SC, Tiwari L. Management of intracranial hypertension. Indian J Pediatr. 2009;76:519-29.
10. Sankhyan N, Vykunta Raju KN, Sharma S, *et al.* Management of raised intracranial pressure. Indian J Pediatr. 2010;77:1409-16.
11. de-Lima-Oliveira M, Salinet ASM, Nogueira RC, *et al.* Intracranial hypertension and cerebral autoregulation: A systematic review and meta-analysis. World Neurosurg. 2018; 113:110-24.
12. Raboel PH, Bartek J, Jr., Andresen M, *et al.* Intracranial pressure monitoring: Invasive versus non-invasive methods-A review. Crit Care Res Pract. 2012;2012:950393.
13. Rajesh A, Hepner MK, Krishnakumar D. Raised intracranial pressure. Paediatrics and Child Health. 2017;27:260-67.
14. Dunn LT. Raised intracranial pressure. J Neurol Neurosurg Psychiatry. 2002;73 Suppl 1:i23-7.
15. Stevens RD, Shoykhet M, Cadena R. Emergency neurological life support: Intracranial hypertension and herniation. Neurocrit Care. 2015;23 Suppl 2:S76-82.
16. Kayhanian S, Young AMH, Piper RJ, *et al.* Radiological correlates of raised intracranial pressure in children: A review. Front Pediatr. 2018;6:32.
17. Kouvarellis AJ, Rohlwink UK, Sood V, *et al.* The relationship between basal cisterns on CT and time-linked intracranial pressure in paediatric head injury. Childs Nerv Syst. 2011;27: 1139-44.
18. Gilger-Tobler C, Elsenack J, Holzmann D, *et al.* Measurement of optic nerve sheath diameter: Differences between methods? A Pilot Study. Klin Monbl Augenheilkd. 2015;232:467-70.
19. Weinmann AV, Beaucreux C, Kearns K, *et al.* Keep an eye on the intracranial pressure, thanks to the optic nerve sheath diameter. Indian J Crit Care Med. 2018;22:460-2.
20. Jeon JP, Lee SU, Kim SE, *et al.* Correlation of optic nerve sheath diameter with directly measured intracranial pressure

in Korean adults using bedside ultrasonography. PLoS One. 2017;12:e0183170.

21. Padayachy LC, Padayachy V, Galal U, *et al.* The relationship between transorbital ultrasound measurement of the optic nerve sheath diameter (ONSD) and invasively measured ICP in children. Part II: age-related ONSD cut-off values and patency of the anterior fontanelle. Childs Nerv Syst. 2016;32:1779-85.
22. Kim SE, Hong EP, Kim HC, *et al.* Ultrasonographic optic nerve sheath diameter to detect increased intracranial pressure in adults: A meta-analysis. Acta Radiol. 2019;60:221-9.
23. Wang LJ, Chen LM, Chen Y, *et al.* Ultrasonography assessments of optic nerve sheath diameter as a noninvasive and dynamic method of detecting changes in intracranial pressure. JAMA Ophthalmol. 2018;136:250-6.
24. Singh SK, Bhatia K. Ultrasonographic optic nerve sheath diameter as a surrogate measure of raised intracranial pressure in severe pregnancy-induced hypertension patients. Anesth Essays Res. 2018;12:42-6.
25. Raksin PB, Alperin N, Sivaramakrishnan A, *et al.* Noninvasive intracranial compliance and pressure based on dynamic magnetic resonance imaging of blood flow and cerebrospinal fluid flow: review of principles, implementation, and other noninvasive approaches. Neurosurg Focus. 2003;14:e4.
26. Gosling RG, King DH. Arterial assessment by Doppler-shift ultrasound. Proc R Soc Med. 1974;67:447-9.
27. Zweifel C, Czosnyka M, Carrera E, *et al.* Reliability of the blood flow velocity pulsatility index for assessment of intracranial and cerebral perfusion pressures in head-injured patients. Neurosurgery. 2012;71:853-61.
28. O'Brien NF, Maa T, Reuter-Rice K. Noninvasive screening for intracranial hypertension in children with acute, severe traumatic brain injury. J Neurosurg Pediatr. 2015;16:420-5.
29. Shimbles S, Dodd C, Banister K, *et al.* Clinical comparison of tympanic membrane displacement with invasive intracranial pressure measurements. Physiol Meas. 2005;26:1085-92.
30. Campbell-Bell CM, Birch AA, Vignali D, *et al.* Reference intervals for the evoked tympanic membrane displacement measurement: A non-invasive measure of intracranial pressure. Physiol Meas. 2018;39:015008.
31. Nwachuku EL, Puccio AM, Fetzick A, *et al.* Intermittent versus continuous cerebrospinal fluid drainage management in adult severe traumatic brain injury: Assessment of intracranial pressure burden. Neurocrit Care. 2014;20:49-53.
32. Ghajar J, Hariri RJ. Management of pediatric head injury. Pediatr Clin North Am. 1992;39:1093-125.
33. Bhatia A, Gupta AK. Neuromonitoring in the intensive care unit. I. Intracranial pressure and cerebral blood flow monitoring. Intensive Care Med. 2007;33:1263-71.
34. Poca MA, Sahuquillo J, Topczewski T, *et al.* Is intracranial pressure monitoring in the epidural space reliable? Fact and fiction. J Neurosurg. 2007;106:548-56.
35. Palmer J. Management of raised intracranial pressure in children. Intensive Crit Care Nurs. 2000;16:319-27.
36. Jha RM, Kochanek PM. A precision medicine approach to cerebral edema and intracranial hypertension after severe traumatic brain injury: Quo Vadis? Curr Neurol Neurosci Rep. 2018;18:105.
37. Roth P, Farls K. Pathophysiology of traumatic brain injury. Crit Care Nurs Q. 2000;23:14-25.
38. Kumar R, Singhi SC, Singhi P. Raised intracranial pressure (ICP): Management in emergency department. Indian J Pediatr. 2012;79:518-24.
39. Marcoux KK. Management of increased intracranial pressure in the critically ill child with an acute neurological injury. AACN Clin Issues. 2005;16:212-31.
40. Kenning JA, Toutant SM, Saunders RL. Upright patient positioning in the management of intracranial hypertension. Surg Neurol. 1981;15:148-52.
41. Godoy DA, Seifi A, Garza D, *et al.* Hyperventilation therapy for control of posttraumatic intracranial hypertension. Front Neurol. 2017;8:250.
42. Schneider GH, Sarrafzadeh AS, Kiening KL, *et al.* Influence of hyperventilation on brain tissue-PO_2, PCO_2, and pH in patients with intracranial hypertension. Acta Neurochir Suppl. 1998;71:62-5.
43. Badjatia N. Hyperthermia and fever control in brain injury. Crit Care Med. 2009;37:S250-7.
44. Freeman WD. Management of intracranial pressure. Continuum (Minneap Minn). 2015;21:1299-323.
45. Upadhyay P, Tripathi VN, Singh RP, *et al.* Role of hypertonic saline and mannitol in the management of raised intracranial pressure in children: A randomized comparative study. J Pediatr Neurosci. 2010;5:18-21.
46. Mortazavi MM, Romeo AK, Deep A, *et al.* Hypertonic saline for treating raised intracranial pressure: literature review with meta-analysis. J Neurosurg. 2012;116:210-21.
47. Thenuwara K, Todd MM, Brian JE, Jr. Effect of mannitol and furosemide on plasma osmolality and brain water. Anesthesiology. 2002;96:416-21.
48. Berger C, Sakowitz OW, Kiening KL, *et al.* Neurochemical monitoring of glycerol therapy in patients with ischemic brain edema. Stroke. 2005;36:e4-6.
49. Rosario BL, Horvat CM, Wisniewski SR, *et al.* Presenting characteristics associated with outcome in children with severe traumatic brain injury: A secondary analysis from a randomized, controlled trial of therapeutic hypothermia. Pediatr Crit Care Med. 2018;19:957-64.
50. Sandestig A, Romner B, Grande PO. Therapeutic hypothermia in children and adults with severe traumatic brain injury. Ther Hypothermia Temp Manag. 2014;4:10-20.
51. Majdan M, Mauritz W, Wilbacher I, *et al.* Barbiturates use and its effects in patients with severe traumatic brain injury in five European countries. J Neurotrauma. 2013;30:23-9.
52. Mellion SA, Bennett KS, Ellsworth GL, *et al.* High-dose barbiturates for refractory intracranial hypertension in children with severe traumatic brain injury. Pediatr Crit Care Med. 2013;14:239-47.
53. Robinson JD. Management of refractory intracranial pressure. Crit Care Nurs Clin North Am. 2016;28:67-75.
54. Berger S, Schwarz M, Huth R. Hypertonic saline solution and decompressive craniectomy for treatment of intracranial hypertension in pediatric severe traumatic brain injury. J Trauma. 2002;53:558-63.

CHAPTER

31

Acute Flaccid Paralysis

Ranjith Kumar Manokaran, Jaya Shankar Kaushik

INTRODUCTION

The term "Acute flaccid paralysis (AFP)" is defined as a clinical syndrome characterized by rapid onset (usually hours to days), progressive weakness of at least one, usually two or more limbs.[1] In addition, there may be bulbar and respiratory involvement. The term "flaccid" indicates the absence of spasticity or other signs of disordered central nervous system motor tracts such as hyperreflexia, clonus, or extensor plantar responses.

A lot of clinical entities which affect upper motor neuron (Spinal cord) and lower motor neuron (Anterior horn cell to muscle) may present as acute flaccid paralysis with diverse clinical manifestations. A systematic clinical approach followed by appropriate investigations is required to arrive at an accurate diagnosis. Accurate diagnosis of the cause of AFP is important for therapy and prognosis. If untreated, AFP may not only persist but also lead to death due to respiratory failure due to weakness of respiratory muscles. It can also cause complications like aspiration pneumonia, deep venous thrombosis, bed sores and contractures. AFP is of great public health importance because of its use in surveillance for poliomyelitis in the context of the global polio eradication initiative. In this chapter, we will elucidate the clinical approach and also discuss the latest management guidelines for various disorders presenting as acute flaccid paralysis.

EPIDEMIOLOGY

Although poliovirus no longer poses the worldwide public health threat that it once did, areas of endemic wild-type poliovirus still exist in Asia and Africa. The last case of polio from India was reported in 2011. That year, the non-polio acute flaccid paralysis (NPAFP) rate in India was 13.35/100,000, whereas the expected rate is 1–2/100,000. India completed full 5 years as a "polio-free nation" on January 13, 2016.[2]

Since the eradication of poliomyelitis, the two most common causes of acute flaccid paralysis are Guillain-Barré syndrome (GBS) and acute transverse myelitis. Enteroviruses other than wild-type polio must be considered, particularly in the current era in which polio has been eradicated in most countries. West Nile virus, a mosquito-borne flavivirus, can produce acute flaccid paralysis. Accidental reactivation of virus strains in OPV can cause paralysis in vaccinated children.[3] The Inactivated polio vaccine is known to be safer. At least in India, OPV has been blamed for causing more paralysis than the actual virus does (1% case prevalence rate). The causes of acute flaccid paralysis in children are varied. The common causes based on the neuroanatomical classification are listed in **Table 1**.

PATHOGENESIS

The pathophysiology varies according to the spectrum of causes behind acute flaccid weakness. In Guillain-Barré syndrome, there is a cell mediated immune attack on the myelin proteins. Literature indicates that it is an autoimmune disease, often triggered by a preceding viral or bacterial infection with organisms such as *Campylobacter jejuni*, cytomegalovirus, Epstein-Barr virus, or *Mycoplasma pneumoniae*. In the acute motor axonal neuropathy (AMAN) form of GBS, the infecting organisms probably share homologous epitopes to a component of the peripheral nerves (molecular mimicry)

Table 1: Causes of acute flaccid paralysis

Neuroanatomical site	*Common causes*
Muscle	Inflammatory myopathy (polymyositis, dermatomyositis) Viral myositis Periodic paralyses (hypokalemic, hyperkalemic) Metabolic derangements (hypophosphatemia, hypokalemia, hypermagnesemia)
Neuromuscular junction	Myasthenia gravis Animal toxins (snakebite especially cobra, krait; shellfish, crab, etc.) Botulism Tick paralysis Organophosphate toxicity (can also cause neuropathy) Lambert-Eaton myasthenic syndrome (LEMS)
Nerve (acute neuropathies)	Diphtheria "Dumb" rabies Porphyria Drugs and toxins (arsenic, thallium, lead, gold, chemotherapy—cisplatin/vincristine) Vasculitis (incl. lupus, polyarteritis)
Nerve roots (acute polyradiculopathies) and plexus lesions	Guillain-Barré syndrome HIV Other viruses like CMV Cauda equina syndrome (lumbar disc, tumor, etc.) Sarcoidosis Lyme disease Plexus lesions (brachial plexitis, lumbosacral plexopathy)
Anterior horn cell	Poliomyelitis Other viruses like HIV Paraneoplastic
Spinal cord	Inflammatory (Transverse myelitis) • Other myelopathies (epidural abscess or hematoma) • Anterior spinal artery syndrome

and, therefore, the immune responses cross-react with the nerves causing axonal degeneration; the target molecule in AMAN is most likely to be ganglioside GM1. In the acute inflammatory demyelinating polyneuropathy (AIDP) form, immune system reactions against target epitopes in Schwann cells or myelin result in demyelination; however, the exact target molecules in the case of AIDP have not yet been identified.[4]

Transverse myelitis (TM) is a clinical syndrome in which an immune-mediated process causes neural injury to the spinal cord, resulting in varying degrees of weakness, sensory alterations and autonomic dysfunction.[5] TM may exist as part of a multi-focal CNS disease (e.g. MS), multi-systemic disease (e.g. systemic lupus erythematosus), or as an isolated, idiopathic entity.

Viral infections can directly affecting the neuronal structures. Poliovirus and West Nile virus affect the anterior horn cells.[6] Enterovirus and other viruses like CMV can cause radiculomyelitis mimicking polio like paralytic illness or GBS like illness.

CLINICAL FEATURES

Majority of children present with one or more of the following clinical features: flaccid weakness of limbs resulting in inability to stand/lift the arm above the shoulder, get up from lying down position (truncal weakness), inability to lift the neck off the couch while lying (neck flexor), inability to swallow or alteration of voice (bulbar weakness), difficulty in breathing (respiratory involvement), drooping of eyelids (ptosis), diplopia (possible 3/4/6 CN involvement), and facial weakness.

Few clinical pearls in evaluating children with acute flaccid paralysis include: presence of asymmetry often points to acute poliomyelitis; children with GBS will have severe radicular pain; presence of ptosis/extraocular muscle involvement or presence of diurnal variation must point towards underlying myasthenia; autonomic instability often point to GBS, pupillary abnormality point towards tick paralysis; bladder involvement often points to acute cord pathology. The clinical features of disorders causing acute flaccid paralysis are summarized in **Table 2**.

APPROACH TO DIAGNOSIS

History

Following points in the history must be enquired into so as to classify the presenting pattern of weakness. This helps not only finding the underlying etiology, but also the prognosis and deciding the therapy.

- Onset and progression of weakness: sudden, acute (over hours), subacute (days to weeks)
- Duration of weakness (hours to days to weeks)
- Pattern of weakness (e.g. proximal, distal)
- Pattern of progression (e.g. onset in arms, "ascending paralysis")
- Sensory involvement (numbness, tingling, loss of balance especially in dark, pain/burning). bulbar involvement (change in voice or swallowing)
- Facial weakness (trouble chewing, sucking with straw, blowing)
- Extraocular muscle weakness (diplopia) or ptosis
- Respiratory involvement (inability to complete sentences, dyspnea, orthopnea)
- Bladder or bowel involvement
- Autonomic involvement (diarrhea, orthostatic dizziness, urinary retention, palpitations)
- Systemic symptoms (fever, weight loss, rash, joint pain)
- Recent illness or immunization (diarrheal or respiratory tract infection, anti-rabies vaccine, oral polio vaccine)
- Recent travel (endemic areas, to forest areas [tick bites])
- Recent history of dog bite/snake bites
- Precipitating factors (exertion, carbohydrate meal - with periodic paralyses)

Table 2: Clinical features of conditions causing acute flaccid paralysis

Condition	*Classical features*
Guillain-Barré syndrome	Symmetrical flaccid weakness, areflexia, cranial nerve involvement (facial) uncommon, ascending paralysis, bladder involvement uncommon; prior infection/immunization; presence of radicular pain and distal paresthesiae
Acute myelopathy (e.g. transverse myelitis, cord compression, infarct)	Hyperreflexia, extensor plantar responses (although corticospinal tract findings may be absent early); bladder retention in acute stage; history of trauma; absence of antecedent illness
Vasculitic neuropathy	Asymmetric polyneuropathy or multifocal mononeuropathies; painful, systemic symptoms (e.g. unexplained weight loss, fever rash); multiorgan involvement (e.g. joints, skin, kidney, respiratory tract)
Myasthenia gravis	Ocular (e.g. diplopia), bulbar (e.g. dysarthria), and limb weakness without sensory symptoms; fatigable, fluctuating symptoms; absence of an antecedent illness. Pattern of descending weakness
Botulism	Infants (most frequent) (e.g. foodborne, such as exposure to honey). Nausea, vomiting, constipation, diplopia, ophthalmoplegia, ptosis, blurring of vision, dysphagia, dysarthria, urinary retention. Pattern of descending weakness
West Nile encephalomyelitis	Fever, meningoencephalitis (may be mild), rash, abdominal pain, back pain; acute-onset lower motor neuronopathy. No sensory disturbance
Lyme neuroborreliosis	Endemic area during tick season; meningitis, fever, myalgias, arthralgias, facial weakness; tick bite and rash
Heavy metals (e.g. arsenic) and other toxins	Known exposure; neuropathy is accompanied by systemic symptoms (e.g. abdominal pain, diarrhea, constipation, rash, alopecia, central nervous system involvement); absence of an antecedent illness; prominent small-fiber nerve component (e.g. "burning" neuropathic pain)
Tick paralysis	Children during tick season. Ataxic gait, diplopia, dysarthria, pupillary abnormalities (dilated pupils). No sensory complaints. Tick on scalp (e.g. behind the ear) or skin (e.g. nape of the neck)
Acute intermittent porphyria	Accompanying autonomic symptoms (tachycardia, hypertension, constipation, urinary retention), abdominal pain (usually severe), psychiatric and other CNS manifestations; patient with a history of prior suggestive attacks
Diphtheria	Patient (e.g. from a developing country) with recent sore throat, fever, and multiple cranial neuropathies (e.g. diplopia, ptosis, dysarthria, dysphagia, numb tongue, gingivae and face)
HIV	GBS more common in HIV patients; occurs at seroconversion
CMV polyradiculopathy	AIDS patient, late stages. Rapidly progressive lower extremity weakness and pain (sparing upper extremities)
Poliomyelitis	Endemic area; sore throat, fever, nausea, vomiting, headache, acute-onset lower motor neuronopathy with myalgias and fasciculations
Critical illness myopathy and polyneuropathy	Quadriparesis in pediatric critical care (PICU) patients

- Fluctuation in weakness (e.g. diurnal variation, fatigability in myasthenia)
- Drug or toxin exposure (honey, pesticides, lead exposure)
- Change of urine color/Family history (porphyria).

Physical Examination

Distribution and degree of weakness looking specially for extraocular muscles, facial muscles and bulbar involvement must be determined. We need to rule out causes of pseudoparalysis like joint involvement. One must assess for fatigability (myasthenia). Sensory impairment: particular modality (vibration/proprioception vs. pain/temperature) must be determined. Presence of sensory level often points to cord pathology. Deep tendon reflexes give lot of clue. For example, reflexes can be absent in spinal shock stage, can be brisk with transverse myelitis and can be normal or diminished in muscle pathology. Few of the specific points include: autonomic features (postural fall, abnormal sweating, pupillary response, ileus) in GBS; examination of skin to look for lines on nails with arsenic poisoning (Mee's lines), ticks, photosensitivity, Gottron's papules on extensor surfaces and heliotrope discoloration over eyelids (dermatomyositis), fang marks (snake bite). Look for spinal tenderness (with epidural abscess or hematoma, spinal tumor). Also look for straight leg raise test (to look for radiculopathy), which can be present in children with GBS. Algorithmic approach to diagnosis has been depicted in **Flowchart 1**.

Investigations

It is essential to have a clinical approach as expounded above rather than relying solely on electrophysiology, lab parameters or neuroimaging to aid in the diagnosis. After the differential diagnosis is narrowed down, then the nece-ssary tests can be done to confirm diagnosis based on the clinical localization and etiological possibilities (**Table 3**).

Acute flaccid myelitis (AFM): Acute flaccid myelitis has been defined as acute onset focal weakness with MRI spine showing predominantly gray matter lesions in the spinal cord. Recently outbreaks of enterovirus D68 associated AFM have been reported from United States.[7] Children following an enterovirus related URTI developed acute flaccid weakness and MRI showed central gray matter involvement. Neurological involvement in these children was flaccid asymmetric limb weakness, bulbar weakness and cranial nerve dysfunction. Majority of proportion of children with AFM had residual motor deficits.

MANAGEMENT

General Measures

Any child presenting with acute flaccid paralysis should be reported according to the AFP surveillance protocol. Emergency management includes

- *Respiratory weakness*: Careful monitoring for respiratory rate, oxygen saturation, single breath count (SBC) and chest expansion should be done. Because of profound respiratory muscle or diaphragmatic weakness, these children may have significant respiratory acidosis without tachypnea or respiratory distress. Blood gas measurement may be required for monitoring. Early elective intubation and respiratory support (both invasive and noninvasive depending on the clinical situation) are critical.
- *Bulbar weakness*: Recent onset hypophonia, weak cry, pooling of secretions, swallowing difficulty and nasal regurgitation may suggest bulbar dysfunction. Protection of airway and prevention of aspiration are important. Elective and planned airway protection is must for those children who have bulbar weakness.
- *Toxins and snakebites*: Snake envenomation and organophosphorus poisoning are important causes of AFP in children. Every child should be evaluated for a possible toxin exposure. Flaccid paralysis, respiratory weakness, miotic pupils and fasciculation suggest an organophosphorus exposure. Sudden onset flaccid paralysis, respiratory weakness, ptosis and external ophthalmoplegia suggest possibility of snake envenomation. Empirical management including anti-snake venom should be considered if there is a high index of suspicion.
- *Electrolyte abnormalities*: Periodic paralysis and hypokalemia are important causes of flaccid paralysis in children. Assessment of electrolytes should be done in all patients with AFP.
- *Compressive myelopathy*: If there is a history of trauma or symptoms and signs suggestive of spinal cord compression (asymmetric weakness, spinal deformity, sensory and bladder dysfunction, fever), an urgent MRI spine and neurosurgical opinion are required in these children. Immediate spinal stabilization and intravenous steroid administration is necessary to prevent long-term morbidity.

Flowchart 1: Algorithmic approach to a child with acute flaccid paralysis

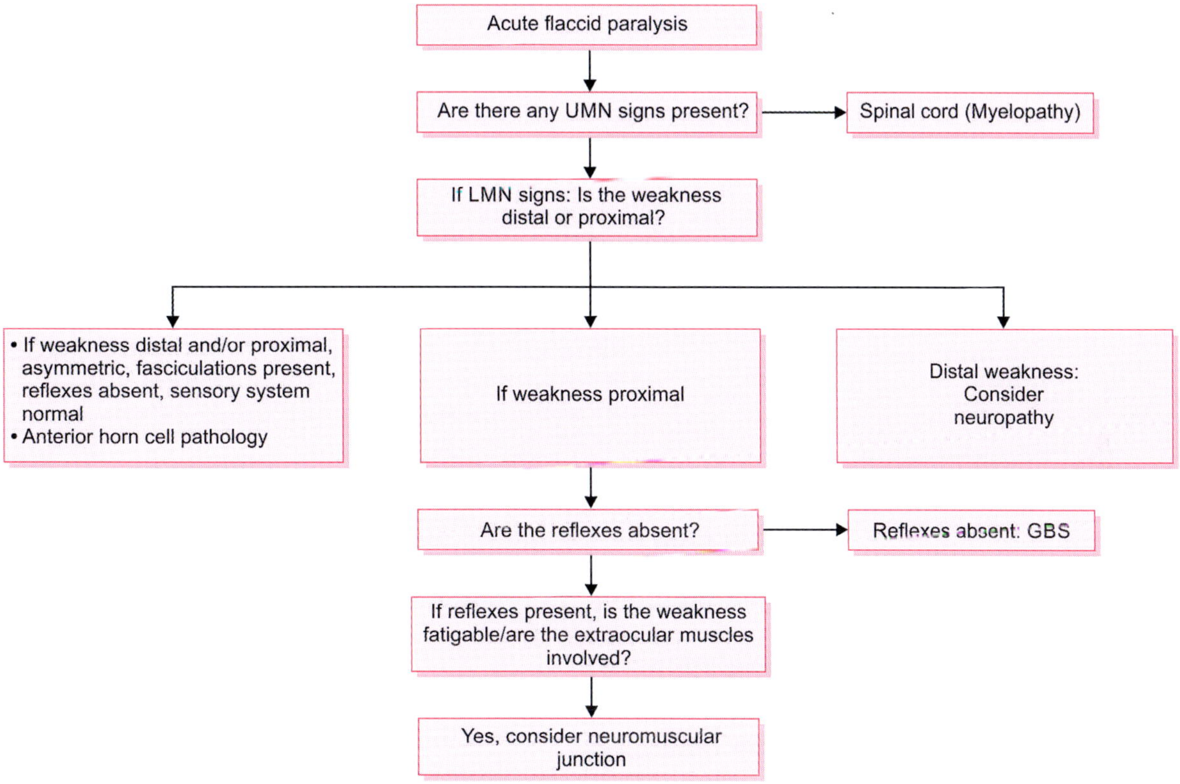

(UMN: upper motor neuron; LMN: lower motor neuron)

Treatment in Specific Causes

Guillain-Barré syndrome

IVIg or plasmapheresis are equally effective in reversing the condition.[8] However, considering the side effect profile, IVIg is better. IVIg is given in dose of 400 mg/kg/day for 5 days while plasmapheresis can be done on alternate day for 5–6 sessions depending on the response. Indications for IVIg include rapidly progressive weakness and presence of respiratory or bulbar involvement. Air way protection, cardiovascular monitoring for autonomic dysfunction, enteral feeding if oropharyngeal dysfunction present, nutrition and daily fluid balance in PICU patients, correction of electrolyte imbalance and conditions like SIADH, prevention of bed sores and early rehabilitation are key additional measures which are mandatory to prevent complications.

Transverse myelitis

The management consists of immunosuppression and supportive care. Methylprednisolone is given in a dose of 10–30 mg/kg/d (max: 1 g/d) for 5 days followed by oral prednisolone 1–2 mg/kg/day for 2 weeks and then tapered over subsequent 2–4 weeks. Outcome is guarded as about 40–50% children tend to have persistent motor and bladder dysfunction.[9]

Myasthenia gravis crisis

IVIg (400 mg/kg/day × 5 days) or plasmapheresis is indicated if patient presents in crisis or impending crisis. Presence of respiratory distress defines the presence of crisis.

Hypokalemic periodic paralysis

Correction should start with oral therapy of 15 mL solution of KCl (diluted) and can be given as frequent as 30 minutes till improvement starts. IV replacement is usually not necessary and indicated if there is swallowing difficulty or vomiting. Long-term therapy consists of acetazolamide in doses from 250–1000 mg/day.

Supportive measures for other conditions like poliomyelitis, West Nile virus myelitis, post-diphtheritic

Table 3: Investigations and their findings in conditions causing acute flaccid paralysis

Disease	*Investigation*
Guillain-Barré syndrome	Nerve conduction study will show either acute demyelinating polyradiculoneuropathy or acute motox axonal polyneuropathy according to the subtypes. CSF analysis will show albumino-cytological dissociation
Acute myelopathy (e.g. transverse myelitis, cord compression, infarct)	MR imaging of spine or cauda equina is indicated to exclude spinal cord or cauda equina structural lesion
Vasculitic neuropathy	Serologic markers (e.g. elevated sedimentation rate, rheumatoid factor); absence of an antecedent illness. Normal CSF. Axonal polyneuropathy on electrodiagnostic testing
Myasthenia gravis	Serological testing (Anti-acetylcholine receptor antibody) Abnormal CMAP decrement on slow RNS studies
Botulism	Abnormal CMAP decrement on slow RNS studies. Abnormal CMAP facilitation on fast RNS
West Nile encephalomyelitis	CSF pleocytosis and viral PCR. Lower motor neuronopathy on electrodiagnostic testing
Lyme neuroborreliosis	CSF pleocytosis and Lyme serology. Axonal polyradiculoneuropathy on electrodiagnostic testing
Heavy metals (e.g. arsenic) and other toxins	Blood levels of toxic metals. Axonal polyneuropathy on electrodiagnostic testing
Tick paralysis	Low CMAPs and normal SNAPs on electrodiagnostic testing
Acute intermittent porphyria	Urinary porphobilinogen levels. Axonal polyradiculoneuropathy or neuronopathy, often asymmetric. CSF resembles GBS with cytoalbuminological dissociation
Diphtheria	CSF resembles GBS with cytoalbuminological dissociation. Axonal polyradiculoneuropathy on electrodiagnostic testing
HIV	Demyelinating polyradiculoneuropathy on electrodiagnostic testing. CSF pleocytosis
CMV polyradiculopathy	CSF pleocytosis. Axonal polyradiculopathy on electrodiagnostic testing
Poliomyelitis	CSF pleocytosis. Lower motor neuronopathy on electrodiagnostic testing
Critical illness myopathy and polyneuropathy	Elevated CPK levels. Myopathic and/or axonal neuropathic features on electrodiagnostic testing

paralysis and traumatic neuritis, the treatment is essentially supportive.

KEY MESSAGES

- Acute flaccid paralysis in children is a medical emergency.
- Acute flaccid paralysis is a clinical condition with diverse etiologies.
- The common causes of AFP are Guillain-Barré syndrome, viral myelitis and acute transverse myelitis.
- AFP can lead to respiratory failure.
- Emergency management including airway protection measures and respiratory support are crucial to prevent mortality.
- Every case of AFP should be reported for surveillance.

REFERENCES

1. Singhi SC, Sankhyan N, Shah R, *et al.* Approach to a child with acute flaccid paralysis. Indian J Pediatr. 2012;79:1351-7.
2. Thacker N, Vashishtha VM, Thacker D. Polio eradication in India: The lessons learned. Pediatrics. 2016;138:e20160461.
3. Polio is not yet gone: It prevails in India. BMJ. 2018;361:2077.
4. Van den Berg B, Walgaard C, Drenthen J, *et al.* Guillain-Barre syndrome: Pathogenesis, diagnosis, treatment and prognosis. Nat Rev Neurol. 2014;10:469-82.
5. Krishnan C, Kaplin AI, Deshpande DM, *et al.* Transverse myelitis: Pathogenesis, diagnosis and treatment. Front Biosci. 2004;9:1483-99.
6. A Arturo Leis, Dobrivoie S stokic. Neuromuscular manifestations of West Nile virus infection. Front Neurol. 2011;3:37.
7. Holm-Hansen CC, Midgley SE, Fischer TK, *et al.* Global emergence of enterovirus D68: A systematic review. Lancet Infect Dis. 2016;16:e64-75.
8. Raphaël JC, Chevret S, Hughes RA. Plasma exchange for Guillain-Barré syndrome. Cochrane Database Syst Rev. 2012;7:CD001798.
9. Scott TF, Frohman E, De Seze J. Evidence-based guideline: Clinical evaluation and treatment of transverse myelitis. Neurology. 2011;77:2128-34.

CHAPTER

32

Acute Bacterial Meningitis

Satinder Aneja, Kausalya Raghuraman

Acute bacterial meningitis (ABM) remains a common life-threatening condition in children. In a multicentric survey in India, ABM constituted 1.5% of admissions in pediatric wards, and the mean case fatality was 16%.[1]

EPIDEMIOLOGY

Acute bacterial meningitis is primarily a disease of young children. The annual incidence of bacterial meningitis was estimated at 105 (53–173) cases per 1,00,000 children in South Asia.[2] Even though the mortality on account of this formidable disease has decreased over the years with the availability of potent antibiotics, a significant number of patients are left with neurological sequelae.[3] Poor socioeconomic condition, overcrowding recent colonization with pathogenic bacteria, cerebrospinal fluid (CSF) communications (congenital or acquired) across the mucocutaneous barrier are some of the host factors which increase the risk of meningitis.[4] Exposure to cigarette smoke has been demonstrated to increase the risk of ABM.[5] The widespread use of conjugate vaccine against *Haemophilus influenzae* type b (Hib) in many countries has led to marked decline in number of cases of meningitis. In countries with routine Hib vaccination, the median age of ABM has shown an increase, with proportionately more cases occurring in adults.[6] Before the introduction of pentavalent vaccine, Hib was found to be the predominant cause of bacterial meningitis in young children aged less than 2 years in India.[7] Hib conjugate vaccine reduced the number of cases of Hib meningitis and probable meningitis within the first 2 years of its introduction.[8]

The preliminary data from hospital-based surveillance network shows *S. pneumoniae* as the most common cause of meningitis following the universal Hib vaccination.[9] India has introduced Pneumococcal vaccination in national immunization schedule since May 2017 and is currently being given in six states. With universal immunization with PCV, the epidemiology of meningitis may show increase in the median age of bacterial meningitis.

Most cases of ABM are sporadic except meningococcal meningitis, which often occurs in an epidemic form especially in sub-Saharan Africa and Indian subcontinent. Meningococcal meningitis occurs most frequently in young children with peak attack rates in 6–12 months infants. A second peak occurs in adolescence. Clusters of meningococcal disease among adolescents and young adults have been reported with increasing frequency in the last decade. Disease rates in adolescents are high because this group has the highest percentage of carriage of *Meningococcus*.

In acute meningitis and encephalitis syndrome surveillance from four provinces in China, a total of 19,423 cases were reported from 2006–2013. The study revealed an estimated incidence of *Neisseria meningitidis, Streptococcus pneumoniae, Haemophilus influenzae b* meningitis in children <5 years old was 0.46/100,000–0.71/100,000, 0.34/100,000–0.83/100,000 and 0.32/100,000–0.57/100,000 respectively; the estimated incidence of *Neisseria meningitidis* and *Streptococcus pneumoniae* meningitis in children aged 5–9 years was 0.59/100,000–1.14/100,000 and 0.50/100,000–1.66/100,000 respectively.[10]

ETIOLOGY

Any organism can potentially cause meningitis but the usual causative agents of ABM vary with age, immune system and immunization status of the patient. Lack of bactericidal or opsonic antibody is one of the significant risk factors for meningitis resulting from *Pneumococcus*, group B *Streptococcus*, and *Escherichia coli*. During the first 2 months of life, *Escherichia coli* K1, gram-negative enteric bacilli, *Streptococcus agalactiae*, and *Listeria monocytogenes* are the usual offending organisms. In unimmunized children between 2 months to 12 years, bacterial meningitis is primarily due to *H. influenzae* type b, *Streptococcus pneumoniae*, and *Neisseria meningitidis*. Meningitis in infants between the ages of 1–3 months may be due to pathogens found in both neonates and older children.

In a meta-analysis conducted to determine the frequency of organism known to cause ABM, it was observed that *Streptococcus pneumoniae* (25.1–45.2%) and *Neisseria meningitidis* (9.1–36.2%) were the most common etiology in all age groups.[11] There is a marked reduction in the incidence of ABM following the introduction of vaccination against Hib and pneumococcal in both vaccinated, and unvaccinated children. Hence, there is a predicted trend of changing epidemiology with the introduction of pentavalent and conjugate pneumococcal vaccine in the universal immunization program of Government of India. Launch of Mission Indradhanush (2014) and the introduction of pneumococcal vaccine (2017) in the Universal Immunization program is likely to reduce the incidence of invasive diseases like meningitis.

There is a concern that nonvaccine serotypes, which currently cause invasive pneumococcal disease may become a predominant causative organism. Non-PCV-13 serotypes could probably trend in the causation of ABM. A retrospective study from Vellore has shown that nonvaccine serotypes are causative agents in nearly one-third of invasive pneumococcal disease. [12] In children with severe malnutrition, compromised immunity or anatomical defects, the infection can occur with other microbes like *Staphylococcus, Salmonella,* and *Pseudomonas* species. The risk factors for acute bacterial meningitis include poverty, malnutrition, daycare attendance, recent travel/ exposure, unimmunized or partly immunized child, primary immunodeficiency, HIV infection, asplenia, sickle cell anemia, and cochlear implant. Nosocomial meningitis has been reported among those with skull base fracture, neurosurgical procedure, CSF leak, penetrating head trauma, and open meningomyelocele.

PATHOGENESIS

The mucosal surfaces in the nasopharynx are the initial site of colonization for the common meningeal pathogens. The exact mechanism by which bacteria invade CNS is not clear. For some organisms, specific surface components as K1 polysaccharide antigen of *E. coli* are essential for attachment to the mucosal surface and specific virulence. Bacteria penetrate through or between mucosal epithelial cells and enter subepithelial blood vessels to enter the bloodstream. The bacteria survive in the bloodstream if it is able to counter the host defense mechanism. From the bloodstream, the pathogen may cross the blood-brain barrier to induce ABM. To get across the blood-brain barrier, pathogens attach to brain microvascular endothelial cells [human brain microvascular endothelial cells (HBMEE)] which are facilitated by receptors for meningeal pathogens found on endothelium in choroid plexus. Blood-brain barrier receptors used by organisms include OmpA (*E. coli*), Vip (*Listeria*), and PilQ/PorA (*Meningococcus*). After attaching itself to HBMEE, the pathogen gains entry to CSF space either by transcellular or paracellular route.[13]

Toll-like receptors (TLR) signals are responsible for immune recognition in meningitides. The effect of the immune response and the bacterial invasion responsible for pyogenic meningitis. TLR2, TLR4 and TLR9 are responsible for immune recognition in *Streptococcus pneumoniae* and *N. meningitidis*. TLR2, TLR7, TLR 8 are for *S. agalactiae* and TLR 2 and 5 recognize the LTA and flagellin in *Listeria monocytogenes.*[14]

Once inside the CSF space, the bacteria multiply freely because of the relative lack of host defense mechanism in this space. The release of bacterial components during this process of replication stimulates the release of pro-inflammatory cytokines. With the induction of inflammation, neutrophils migrate into CSF, there is the release of reactive oxygen species and nitric oxide, and all this adds to the deleterious effect of inflammation on the brain.

The fundamental pathological change in ABM is inflammation of leptomeninges with meningeal exudates of varying thickness encasing the brain. These exudates can compress the cranial nerves. The exudates extend into Virchow-Robin spaces along with penetrating vessels. Inflammation of meninges can lead to vasospasm, thrombosis of cerebral arteries or cerebral vein. Involvement of vessels leads to phlebitis or arteritis and softening or necrosis of corresponding vascular territory. Cerebral edema develops early in the course of ABM and together with acute hydrocephalus may be responsible for intracranial hypertension. Intracranial pressure (ICP) is maximally increased within the first 48 hours. This, in turn, impedes cerebral perfusion resulting in neuronal injury. Nearly 30% of infants and children with ABM have decreased cerebral blood flow ranging from 30–70%. Transcranial Doppler studies on patients with meningitis show disease related arterial narrowing in approx 50% of cases and this correlates with neurologic impairment.[15]

CLINICAL FEATURES

Early symptoms of meningitis in young children are often vague and ill-defined. In general, younger the infant the more nonspecific are the symptoms. History suggestive of upper respiratory infection may be noted in nearly 75% of patients. Intercurrent viral infection plays a key role in invasive pneumococcal infections by generating local inflammatory factors that upregulate platelet-activating factor receptor. The main symptoms which are highly suggestive of a diagnosis of ABM in infants are fever or hypothermia (with or without vomiting), alteration of behavior (infant becomes lethargic or drowsy, irritable, feeds poorly), a high pitched cry, seizures (15–35%) and a full or tense anterior fontanelle. Specific signs of meningeal irritation are hardly ever present in infants below the age of one year. In older children, classical signs and symptoms of meningitis like fever, headache, vomiting, photophobia, neck stiffness, and the meningeal signs are likely to be present. Neck stiffness is the most important of all meningeal signs, present in nearly 75% of children with meningitis and earliest to appear. It becomes more marked if tested while the patient sits up with knees extended. Kernig's sign and Brudzinski's sign are other meningeal signs. The meningeal signs are due to reflex muscle spasm in reaction to pain on stretching of contents of the spinal cord. These signs may be absent in comatose patients or infants younger than one year.

The second mode of presentation is acute and fulminant in which manifestations of sepsis and meningitis develop rapidly associated with severe brain edema and raised ICP. This type of presentation is seen most often with *N. meningitidis.* Petechial hemorrhages appearing on the skin, which rapidly coalesce producing areas of purpura are considered the hallmark of this disease, although they may be seen in meningitis due to other organisms also. Profound hypotension and fatal shock has been reported.[16]

Seizures occur in about 30–40% of cases of ABM. A high concentration of tumor necrosis factor (TNF) has been associated with the occurrence of seizures.[17] Alterations of mental status and reduced level of consciousness are common and may be due to increased ICP, cerebritis or hypotension. Papilledema is uncommon in uncomplicated acute meningitis and when present suggests a more chronic process such as the presence of an intracranial abscess, or subdural empyema. Focal neurologic signs may be due to vascular occlusion, subdural collection or cortical infarction. Overall 14% of children of bacterial meningitis have focal neurological signs.[3] Reactive thrombocytosis is common during recovery from meningitis and implies favorable prognosis for survival.[18]

COMPLICATIONS

Complications of ABM can develop early in the course of illness or later after several days of therapy or may be noticed on follow-up (**Table 1**).

Table 1: Complications and sequelae of acute bacterial meningitis

Complication

Neurological
- Increased intracranial pressure
- Seizures
- Subdural effusion/empyema
- Ventriculitis
- Cranial nerve palsies
- Hemi/quadriparesis
- Hearing loss
- Hydrocephalus

Systemic
- Peripheral circulatory failure
- Disseminated intravascular coagulation
- Syndrome of inappropriate antidiuretic hormone secretion
- Arthritis

Sequelae
- Epilepsy
- Sensorineural hearing loss
- Visual impairment
- Behavioral problems
- Motor deficits
- Hydrocephalus
- Learning disabilities

Systemic Complications

Complications of ABM are enumerated in **Table 1**. Peripheral circulatory failure is a life-threatening complication of meningitis. It occurs most commonly with meningococcal infection but can accompany other types of infection. About 15% of children with pneumococcal meningitis have been reported to present with shock.[19]Antibiotic therapy may initially aggravate hypotension. Hence, intensive monitoring is required in the initial period.[20] Other manifestations of acute bacterial sepsis may be seen as coagulopathy, acidosis, and hypoglycemia. Pneumonia, pericarditis, and arthritis occur occasionally. Prolonged fever (>10 days) is seen in some cases due to intercurrent viral infection, secondary bacterial infection, thrombophlebitis or a drug reaction. Secondary fever that is seen after an initial afebrile period is usually due to nosocomial infection.

Neurological Complications

Increased intracranial pressure (ICP) is present in almost all cases of ABM initially though only 1–3% of cases have persistent hydrocephalus. Raised ICP is a complication of ABM that should be anticipated and treated promptly. When ICP is very high, herniation of brain tissue may occur at the incisura or at the foramen magnum and may lead to sudden respiratory arrest, sudden death or persistent vegetative state. Cerebral herniation following lumbar puncture (LP) is an important contributor to overall mortality.[21] Lumbar puncture should therefore not be done in children with clinical evidence of raised ICP.

Seizures occur in about 30–40% of children with meningitis. Generalized seizures occurring within the first 4 days are of no prognostic significance. Seizures that present after the 4th day and those that are difficult to treat and those that appear late in the course of meningitis are associated with poor prognosis. Children with focal convulsions are more likely to have neurologic sequelae of meningitis. Causes of late-onset seizures include cerebritis, subdural effusion, vascular thrombosis, and abscess formation.

Subdural effusions develop in 10–30% of patients with meningitis and are more common in *H. influenzae* meningitis. These effusions are mostly asymptomatic. Effusions usually resolve spontaneously, and aspiration is required only in case of increased ICP or a depressed consciousness. Subdural empyema requires more aggressive treatment in the form of aspiration.

Transient cranial nerve dysfunction and motor deficits may be seen during the acute phase of the illness. Hearing loss is the most common sequel of ABM. Nearly 10–25 % of survivors are left with a permanent sensorineural loss.[3,22] All patients of ABM should have audiologic evaluation after recovery. Cochlear enhancement on GdMRI is associated with the occurrence of labyrinthitis and sensorineural hearing loss (SNHL).[23]

DIAGNOSIS

The diagnosis of ABM is based on documenting the inflammatory response of meninges (e.g. CSF cell count, protein, sugar) and on tests that demonstrate the specific causative bacterial agent in CSF (Gram stain, culture, tests for bacterial antigen/DNA). Since the clinical features of ABM are nonspecific especially in infants, LP should be performed whenever there is suspicion of meningitis. Lumbar puncture must be postponed in cardiorespiratory compromise, signs of increased ICP and infection at the LP site. Clinical sign of raised ICP is a more reliable indicator to withhold a lumbar puncture since even a normal CT scan does not exclude the imminent risk of coning. In case LP is deferred, empirical treatment should be started after taking blood culture.

LP in Children with Febrile Seizures

A seizure associated at the onset of meningitis may not be distinguishable from simple febrile convulsion. It is therefore advocated that LP be routinely done in all infants/young children after an initial febrile seizure to exclude cases of occult meningitis. Lethargy, irritability, vomiting, and presence of complex febrile seizures are strong indicators of meningitis in febrile infants with seizures. LP in infants with seizure and fever should only be withheld if the patient is well and alert on examination and can be observed for the next few hours. In patients who have been pretreated with antibiotics or anticonvulsants, the signs are masked, and hence they must be subjected to LP.

CSF Examination

The CSF opening pressure above 200 mm is common among children with ABM. However, pressures above 300 mm could increase the risk of central herniation. CSF examination includes a naked eye examination, pressure, microscopy—total and differential leukocyte count, Gram-stain, estimation of proteins and glucose and CSF culture. The CSF should be examined immediately after doing the LP since the cell count tends to fall over some time and may be falsely low after 30–60 min. The normal CSF of children contains less than 6 WBCs/mm,[3] and in 95% of cases, there are no polymorphonuclear (PMN) leukocytes.[24] Hence, the presence of even a single polymorphonuclear leukocyte in a child 6 weeks of age is suggestive of ABM. However, CSF lymphocytosis may be a predominant feature in 10–13% of cases.[25] CSF lymphocytosis is believed to represent an early phase of infection and repeat CSF examination in these cases will show a PMN predominance. Prior antibiotic therapy also results in lymphocytosis. Patients on steroids might have normal cellularity. Majority of children with ABM will have TLC more than 1000 cells/cumm with neutrophilic predominance.

Proteins in CSF are elevated, usually more than 100 mg/dL (normal 20–40 mg/dL); CSF sugar is decreased to <40 mg/dL (>40 mg/dL); and ratio of CSF blood sugar is decreased (<60%) in acute bacterial meningitis. **Table 2** differentiates the CSF findings of bacterial, viral and tubercular meningitis.

Gram-stain of the smear is one of the most simple, cheap and rapid diagnostic bedside tool useful for detection of etiological organism. In a series of patients with pneumococcal meningitis, Gram stains of CSF were positive in 90% cases.[18] Its yield in *Meningococcus* is 80%, gram-negative organism is 50% and 33% of those with *Listeria*. Centrifugation of CSF increases the positivity. Fluorescent staining of bacterial DNA with acridine orange may show the bacterial morphology in cases where Gram stain is negative.

Acridine orange staining is superior to Gram stain in pretreated patients.[26] CSF culture provides confirmatory evidence of ABM and is essential for selecting appropriate antibiotic for the etiological organisms. The rate of bacterial isolation is affected by antibiotic use before lumbar puncture; further rate of isolation is increased if direct plating of CSF is done at the bedside. CSF cultures are considered to become sterile within 2–4 hours of intravenous antibiotics.

In case LP is traumatic, it is recommended to do the cell count and then lyse RBCs with acetic acid and repeat cell count. The ratio of WBCs to RBCs (normal 1:500 to 1:750) can give some indication of the total cell count though it is rather cumbersome. Besides, the biochemical parameters and the Gram stain culture are not affected by blood in CSF. CSF from a traumatic LP should therefore be interpreted on a combination of factors.

Rapid Diagnostic Tests

Various rapid diagnostic tests including counter-immuno-electrophoresis (CIE), latex particle agglutination (LPA), and enzyme-linked immunosorbent assay (ELISA) are used to detect bacterial antigen. These tests are especially useful among those pretreated with antibiotics, where Gram stain and cultures were negative despite the biochemical findings consistent with bacterial meningitis. Of these, the results of CIE and LPA can be available within 1–2 hours but ELISA takes a longer time. LPA is more sensitive than CIE. The sensitivity of CIE can be improved by screening multiple body fluids. LPA kits are commercially available for detecting antigen of *Haemophilus* spp, pneumococci and meningococci. LPA is more sensitive for detection of Hib than *Pneumococcus* and *Meningococcus*. Ultrasound enhanced LPA has been developed which is more sensitive than conventional LPA.[27] A negative test for bacterial antigen cannot exclude bacterial meningitis, since these tests are limited to a few specific pathogens. Due to high cost, these tests should be reserved for patients who have received antibiotics if Gram stain is negative.[28]

The PCR of CSF has been employed to detect microbial DNA in patients with ABM. Primers are available for simultaneous detection of the common organisms. There is a trend towards molecular PCR-based assays and DNA sequencing which allows accurate detection of organisms. PCR-based technology can almost detect all aerobic, anaerobic bacteria, viruses and fungi despite

Table 2: CSF findings in common causes of meningitis

CSF	*Bacterial meningitis*	*Viral meningitis*	*Tubercular meningitis*
Cells	>1000 cells/cumm	10–500 cells/cumm	100–500 cells/cumm
Protein	>100 mg/dL	50–100 mg/dL	>100–200 mg/dL
Glucose	<10 mg/dL	>40 mg/dL	10–40 mg/dL

prior antibiotic administration. There are PCR-based panels in CSF covering main bacteria, viruses, and fungus like *Cryptococcus*. PCR-based techniques can detect the organism with only a few DNA copies. It can deliver the results within a few hours of testing. The main disadvantage of only PCR-based diagnosis is the lack of antibiotic sensitivity patterns that are useful. Hence, these advances can be an adjunct to conventional CSF Gram stain and cultures and cannot replace them.

The PCR-based detection of meningococcal antigen in CSF is useful in patients who have been pretreated with antibiotics as bacterial DNA remains in CSF 2–3 days after treatment.[29] Panbacterial nested PCR targeting 16S ribosomal RNA gene sequencing has demonstrated the high sensitivity of 97.2% for the diagnosis of acute bacterial meningitis.[30] Other newer experimental techniques for identification of pathogen include loop-mediated isothermal amplification (nucleic acid amplification technique that can be read with the naked eye), extraction of DNA by microarray or biochip and immunochromatographic test.

Various nonspecific markers of inflammation such as C-reactive proteins, CSF lactate, CSF CPK, heparin binding protein, TNFα, and interleukins have been investigated to differentiate bacterial meningitis from aseptic meningitis and as a marker of severity of ABM with relation to outcome.[31] CSF lactate is a sensitive marker to differentiate bacterial from aseptic meningitis provided other neurological disorders where raised CSF lactate are not considered, and the patient has not been pretreated with an antibiotic. However, these tests do not help in confirming the diagnosis and are of no value in the choice of therapy.

Despite advancements in laboratory techniques, the routine culture of CSF, blood, and Gram stain of CSF remain the standard methods of establishing the etiological agent of ABM. LPA and PCR-based tests are useful in patients pretreated with antibiotics. These tests can also help identify the serotype of meningococci in an outbreak situation.

Blood culture: Blood culture is positive in two-third cases of ABM and should be done in all cases. It is especially useful in cases in which LP cannot be done or is traumatic.

Smear of petechiae: Smear of the petechial lesion (if present) after puncture with a lancet should be made and subjected to Gram stain for meningococci.

Indications for Repeat Lumbar Puncture

If lumbar puncture is deferred on admission, it should be performed after the patient is stable and an attempt made to demonstrate the organism on Gram stain or by LPA. A repeat spinal tap is not indicated in most of the cases of ABM. It should be done in case of poor clinical response to therapy of 48–72 hours, persistent fever, unusual etiological organism or suspicion of bacterial resistance. Similarly, end of therapy LP is not routinely required if the patient is well and afebrile for the preceding 5 days.

Radiological Evaluation

Cranial sonography is the investigation of choice in infants and neonates and can detect early structural changes. Sonography should be done in all neonates and infants less than 2 months since the risk of complications is higher. Contrast-enhanced MRI brain is the preferred modality if subdural empyema or parenchymal damage is suspected. CT brain is preferred in emergent situations with features of raised intracranial pressure. In nonemergent condition, MRI is preferred over CECT brain considering the risk of radiation exposure in the latter. Neuroimaging is preferred before lumbar puncture when the child has a focal neurological deficit, new onset seizures, altered sensorium, or a severely immunocompromised state. Antibiotics must be commenced empirically irrespective of delay in getting the neuroimaging. However, in uncomplicated meningitis radiological evaluation by CT is not necessary.[32] These investigations should be considered in patients with (i) signs of raised ICP, (ii) focal neurologic deficits, (iii) persistent fever, (iv) recurrent/focal seizures, (v) prolonged coma and (vi) increasing head circumference.

DIFFERENTIAL DIAGNOSIS

Several diseases, particularly aseptic meningitis, tuberculous meningitis, cerebral malaria, brain abscess and lead encephalopathy present with signs and symptoms similar to ABM. A careful examination of CSF, which shows pleocytosis with polymorphonuclear predominance with reduced CSF sugar is highly suggestive of ABM. Gram stain and culture confirm the diagnosis. Pre-treatment of meningitis with oral or systemic antibiotics often poses a diagnostic problem since CSF is rapidly sterilized though cell count, and CSF biochemical abnormalities persist. In any case of clinically suspected ABM, empiric therapy for ABM should be immediately started.

TREATMENT

Treatment can be broadly categorized into (1) antibiotic therapy; (2) supportive care and (3) adjuvant therapy.

Antibiotic Therapy

Selection of initial antibiotic therapy

The antibiotic regimen should be such that it covers all the likely pathogens according to the age of the child, the combination should not be antagonistic, and it should achieve bactericidal concentration in the CSF. Later the treatment can be modified depending upon the result of Gram stain and CSF culture. Various antibiotics used in initial therapy and subsequent treatment are shown in **Tables 3 and 4**. In a study from Vellore, it was reported that penicillin resistance amongst pneumococcal meningeal isolates increased from 9.5% in 2008 to 42.8% in 2016, whereas cefotaxime non-susceptibility increased from 4.7% in 2008 to 28.5% in 2016. Serotypes 14, 19F, 6B, 6A, 23F, 9V and 5 were the most common serotypes causing meningitis, with the first five accounting for over 75% of resistant isolates.[33] Penicillin can no longer be recommended as empiric therapy when pneumococci is a likely pathogen since this therapy may not be effective for meningitis caused by penicillin-resistant strains. Considering the emergence of resistance of *Pneumococcus* to ceftriaxone and other third-generation cephalosporins, it is strongly recommended to add vancomycin to ceftriaxone in the empirical treatment of ABM. Meropenem has been reported to be as efficacious and safe as cefotaxime as initial therapy for meningitis in a prospective study and can be considered as an alternative treatment.[34] Addition of rifampicin should be considered in highly resistant strains. There are anecdotal reports of cefotaxime or ceftriaxone failure in the management of pneumococcal meningitis.[35] Meropenem has been used for the treatment of penicillin-resistant pneumococci and multi-drug resistant *Pseudomonas meningitis*.[36] Newer fluoroquinolones—levofloxacin and sparfloxacin are effective against invasive *S. pneumoniae* isolates, though their routine use in ABM has not been studied well.[37]

Drug of choice for bacterial meningitis as based on culture sensitivity is depicted in **Table 3**. Alternative drugs for resistant organisms include meropenem, cefepime, linezolid, and moxifloxacin. European Society of Clinical Microbiology and Infectious Diseases guidelines recommend antibiotics to be administered within one hour of hospital admission (door to antibiotic time).[38] The odds of unfavorable outcome may increase up to 30% per hour of treatment delay.[39]

Fortunately, resistance to 3rd generation cephalosporins among *Haemophilus* spp. has not emerged. There are reports of meningococcal resistance to penicillin. Chloramphenicol resistance in meningococci has been reported from Vietnam and France.[40] Chloramphenicol is often not used in the present era.

Duration of therapy

The duration of antimicrobial therapy is based on the causative agent, and clinical response (**Table 3**). In children with rapid initial recovery, 4 days of ceftriaxone was found to be adequate.[41] However, this cannot be recommended as a standard duration of therapy. Longer duration of treatment is required in cases of complications such as subdural empyema, prolonged fever, the persistence of meningeal signs or development of nosocomial infections. In such cases, discontinuation of antimicrobial therapy is individualized. In principle, we plan for 14 days if the organism is not identified, 10 days for Hib, 14 days for *Streptococcus pneumoniae*, 7 days for *N. meningitidis*, 3 weeks for *Staphylococcus* and *Pseudomonas*.

Supportive Therapy

The first 3–4 days of treatment are critical because life-threatening complications of meningitis occur most frequently during this period. It is advisable to manage infants and children with meningitis in hospitals that have staff with expertise in caring for infants and children who are critically ill. Vital signs of patients should be monitored regularly during the first 24–28 hours of treatment. The patient should be kept nil orally to prevent aspiration. Neurological examination should be performed initially and daily throughout hospitalization. Blood urea, sugar, gases, serum electrolytes, urine osmolality, and urine output, and body weight should be monitored closely.

Hypovolemia and hypotension should be aggressively treated with normal saline and inotropic support. Maintenance of systemic blood pressure is critical to maintaining cerebral blood flow. The concurrence of shock and cerebral edema is a therapeutic challenge. The treatment of shock with fluids and inotropes takes priority in such cases. Hyponatremia is a frequent finding in patients with meningitis most often due to SIADH.[42] However, it may be due to volume contraction rather

Table 3: Choice and duration of antibiotic therapy for acute bacterial meningitis

Organism	*Antibiotic*	*Duration*
Streptococcus pneumonia Penicillin sensitive Penicillin resistant Cephalosporin susceptible (MIC<0.2 μg/mL) Cephalosporin resistant (MIC>0.2 μg/mL)	 Penicillin Ceftriaxone or cefotaxime Ceftriaxone or cefotaxime Ceftriaxone/cefotaxime with vancomycin or rifampicin	 10–14 days
Neisseria meningitidis Penicillin sensitive Penicillin resistant	 Penicillin Ceftriaxone or cefotaxime	 7 days
Listeria monocytogenes	Ampicillin or penicillin	21 days
Haemophilus influenzae Beta lactamase negative Beta lactamase positive	 Ampicillin Ceftriaxone or cefotaxime	 7–10 days
Staphylococcus aureus Methicillin sensitive Methicillin resistant Vancomycin resistant	 Cloxacillin Vancomycin Linezolid	 14 days
Pseudomonas	Ceftazidime	21 days
Acinetobacter	Meropenem	21 days

Ampicillin: 300 mg/kg/24 hours, in 4 divided doses
Ceftriaxone: 100 mg/kg/24 hours, in 2 divided doses
Cefotaxime: 200 mg/kg/24 hours, in 4 divided doses
Cefepime: 150 mg/kg/24 hrs in 3 divided doses
Ceftazidime: 150 mg/kg/24 hrs in 3 divided doses
C. Penicillin: 300,000 units/kg/24 hours, in 4–6 divided doses
Vancomycin: 60 mg/kg/24 hours, in 3–4 divided doses
Meropenem: 120 mg/kg/24 hours, in 3 divided doses
Amikacin: 15 mg/kg/24 hours, in 2 divided doses
Linezolid 10–15 mg/kg/dose 8–12 hrourly

Table 4: Initial or empirical antibiotic therapy in bacterial meningitis

Age	*Initial antibiotic*	*Alternative*
0–2 months	Cefotaxime plus amikacin	Ampicillin plus cefotaxime
2 months—5 years	Ceftriaxone or cefotaxime plus vancomycin	Meropenem plus vancomycin

than water retention.[43] While optimizing the fluid therapy, it is important to recognize that hyponatremia may be due to dehydration or water retention as in SIADH. The circulatory compromise caused by hypovolemia is as dangerous as cerebral edema caused by water retention. Therefore, the cause of hyponatremia should be assessed along with clinical signs of volume depletion and biochemical parameters, i.e. serum and urine osmolality.

In normovolemic patients, fluids are conventionally restricted to two-third of maintenance initially until raised ICP and SIADH are excluded. Fluid administration may be returned to normal when serum sodium level has normalized. There is insufficient evidence to guide practice as to whether maintenance fluids should be chosen over restricted fluids in the treatment of acute bacterial meningitis.[44] Fluid therapy should be guided based on the clinical condition of the patient.

Intracranial pressure can be reduced by elevating the head end of the bed by 30° to maximize venous drainage. Osmotic diuretics such as mannitol (0.5-1 g/kg) and oral glycerol can be used to reduce ICP. Hyperventilation to maintain the arterial pCO_2 between 27 and 30 mm of Hg may also be used to reduce ICP. Aggressive hyperventilation may be counterproductive as it causes reduction of already compromised CBF with resultant ischemic damage.

Seizures are common during the course of bacterial meningitis. Metabolic complications like hyponatremia, hypocalcemia, and hypoglycemia must be excluded and specific therapy instituted, if present. Immediate management of seizures include intravenous diazepam (0.1–0.2 mg/kg/dose) or lorazepam (0.05 mg/kg/dose). This is followed by a loading dose of phenytoin (15 mg/kg) and the maintenance dose of 5 mg/kg/24h for further control of seizures. Phenytoin is preferred over phenobarbitone because it causes less CNS depression and allows assessment of sensorium. Anticonvulsants can be discontinued after a few days unless there is evidence of persistent seizure activity.

Adjunct Therapy

Improvement in our understanding of the pathophysiology of ABM has led to the development of therapeutic approaches to modulate the inflammatory cascade to reduce the incidence of sequelae and death. Adjunctive anti-inflammatory agents, which may be of benefit in the treatment of bacterial meningitis, include corticosteroids and newer anti-inflammatory drugs.

Steroids

Corticosteroids have been used with the objective of blocking the secondary release of cytokines and toxic intermediaries from the brain cells and are also presumed to stabilize altered vascular permeability. Several trials were conducted in the last two decades to evaluate the role of dexamethasone (0.15 mg/kg every 6 hours for 2–4 days). The benefit of dexamethasone use in these studies was only moderate and limited to a decrease in the frequency of audiologic sequelae in *Haemophilus* meningitis.[45-46] Concerns with use of dexamethasone in ABM include reduced CSF penetration of vancomycin, increased risk of flare-up of bacterial infection, and possible fear of neuronal injury. According to a recent Cochrane review in all-cause meningitis, use of corticosteroids decreases the incidence of severe hearing loss and reduces short-term neurological sequelae in high-income countries.[47] However in low-income countries, no beneficial effect of adjunctive dexamethasone treatment in ABM was observed. Data from two randomized controlled trials suggest that some reduction in death and hearing loss may result from the use of adjunctive steroids alongside standard antibiotic therapy for the treatment of patients with neonatal meningitis. [48]

In a prospective, randomized, double-blind trial comparing adjuvant dexamethasone or oral glycerol or both with placebo in children aged from 2 months through 16 years in Latin America, glycerol and dexamethasone plus glycerol reduced severe neurological sequelae, compared with placebo. Dexamethasone plus glycerol was not more effective than glycerol alone.[48] Glycerol is a hyperosmolar agent that is cheap, easily available, safe and can be used as adjunctive therapy for children with ABM.

Anti-endotoxin antibodies have been produced by monoclonal antibody technology and appear to have a beneficial role in ABM caused by gram-negative organisms. Monoclonal antibodies against TNF, IL-IB and against CD 18 cells may help in reducing inflammation as shown in experimental studies. Role of indomethacin (nonsteroidal inflammatory agent), pentoxyphylline (phosphodiesterase inhibitor) is still at experimental stage, and further trials are required to define their use in meningitis in humans.[49] There is no proven role of acetaminophen infusion, hypothermia, intravenous immunoglobulin in the treatment of children with ABM.

Since the bacterial cell wall products are potent inducers of inflammation, initiation of therapy with non-bacteriolytic antimicrobial agents such as rifampicin has been suggested. In a pilot study, a single dose of rifampicin given 30 mins before ceftriaxone in children with bacterial meningitis was reported to reduce the CSF levels of TNF alpha.[50] Initiation of therapy with a protein synthesis-inhibiting antibacterial and continuation of therapy with a combination that includes a β-lactam has been suggested as a strategy to decrease inflammation and subsequent neuronal injury in bacterial meningitis.

PROGNOSIS

The prognosis of a patient with pyogenic meningitis depends on many factors including age, causative microorganism, bacterial density, the intensity of the host's inflammatory response and time taken to sterilize the CSF. Case fatality is reported to be 3–6% in developed countries, but higher mortality (16%) is reported from developing countries.[1] Most deaths occur within the first 48–72 hours. Early fatality is most often due to septic shock. Close monitoring for signs of septic shock and brain herniation should be done in first 2–3 days of hospitalization. Neurodevelopment sequelae are seen in 10–20% of patients.[4] Baraff *et al.*[3] in a meta-analysis of 19 reports estimated that 83.6% of patients had no sequelae. A recent systematic review reported that risk of at least one major sequela (cognitive deficit, bilateral hearing loss, motor deficit, seizures, visual impairment, hydrocephalus) was 12.8% (7.2–21.1%) and of at least one minor sequela (behavioral problems, learning difficulties, unilateral hearing loss, hypotonia, diplopia) was 8.6% .[51]

The sequelae of bacterial meningitis may improve with time and even resolve completely. The potential for recovery is attributed to the plasticity of the brain. Focal neurological signs at admission are reliable predictors of permanent sequelae especially later epilepsy.[52] Persistence of fever, neck rigidity and reluctance to leave the supine position beyond the first week was associated with risk of neurologic complication or sequelae.[53] Prognosis is poorest among infants less than 6 months, in those with delayed sterilization of the CSF, seizures beyond 4th day of hospital stay, coma, (Glasgow Coma Scale <8), focal neurological signs on presentation and infection with pneumococci, and other organisms like *Salmonella* or *Pseudomonas*.

PREVENTION

Prevention of ABM is possible with (i) Prevention of secondary cases with antibiotic chemoprophylaxis of index case and close contacts, and (ii) Vaccination of susceptible population with specific vaccines. Vaccination is not a substitute for chemoprophylaxis because secondary cases develop within 2–7 days of presentation of index case and vaccination is not effective in that stage.

Chemoprophylaxis

Rifampicin prophylaxis for *H. influenzae* is recommended (20 mg/kg daily for 4 days) for all household contacts, if there is an infant (<12 months) in the household or when a child 1–3 years who is inadequately immunized resides in the household.[54] Prophylaxis for index case is not required for those treated with cefotaxime or ceftriaxone.

For *N. meningitidis,* chemoprophylaxis is recommended for all close contacts (household contacts, day care contacts and any one exposed to oral secretions) regardless of age and immunization status. Chemoprophylaxis should be provided even if the close contact has received meningococcal vaccine because currently licensed vaccines are not 100% effective.

Routine prophylaxis is not recommended for health-care personnel unless they have had intimate exposure to respiratory tract secretions, such as occurs with unprotected mouth-to-mouth resuscitation, intubation, or suctioning before or less than 24 hours after antimicrobial therapy was initiated. Rifampicin (10 mg/kg every 12 hours for 2 days) can be given. There is concern about the emergence of resistance to rifampicin among strains of meningococci.[55] This has to be monitored closely with obvious implication for prophylaxis. Ceftriaxone (250 mg intramuscularly as a single dose) and ciprofloxacin (single dose 500 mg) are other effective chemoprophylactic agents. No prophylaxis for *S. pneumoniae* is required for normal hosts.

Vaccination

Immunization with *H. influenzae* type b vaccine as a part of pentavalent is now a part of routine vaccination in India. The universal access to the pentavalent vaccine has resulted in a decline of meningitis due to Hib. In a study from Chennai, Hib vaccination has reduced the number of cases of meningitis by nearly 79% and cases of probable meningitis by 44%.[8] Mass immunizations with a quadrivalent meningococcal vaccine against serogroup A, C, Y and W135 have been used to control epidemics. The current epidemiology and burden of meningococcal diseases in India do not justify routine use of meningococcal vaccines. Meningococcal vaccines are recommended only for certain high-risk conditions and areas. A quadrivalent (A, C, W135, Y) meningococcal conjugate vaccine using diphtheria toxin as carrier protein (A, C, W135, Y-D), is licensed in India and has been recommended for use in high-risk children and high-risk areas.[56] Interference with PCV13 immune responses was noted when MenACWY-D and PCV13 were administered simultaneously in patients with asplenia. It is recommended that at least one-month interval should be kept between PCV13 and MenACWY-D, and PCV13 should be administered first. Early recognition and treatment of meningococcal infection is another way to reduce morbidity and deaths due to this disease.

Pneumococcal vaccine (PCV7) was introduced in the year 2000 in around 142 countries that resulted in the reduction of incidence of invasive pneumococcal disease. In the year 2017, India introduced the pneumococcal vaccine (PCV 13) in the universal immunization program in selected districts. Three doses of PCV13 are recommended to be given in UIP. In Unites States, the impact of PCV-13 vaccine had revealed around 48,000 hospitalizations in the age group of 0–1 year and 17,000 in the age of 2–4 years were averted since PCV-13 was introduced from the year 2010–2014.[57]

Besides giving immunity to the individual patient, vaccination can interrupt the transmission of antibiotic-resistant organisms belonging to the serotypes included in the vaccine and thus hold the promise of reducing the frequency of ABM caused by antibiotic-resistant strains.[58]

Future Indian studies on the impact of universal immunization with PCV13 is likely to depict the burden of invasive pneumococcal disease particularly meningitis. In the meantime, development of new and effective antimicrobial drugs against the ever-increasing resistant pathogens is urgently needed.[59]

KEY MESSAGES

- The clinical features of ABM are often nonspecific in infants, LP should be performed whenever there is suspicion of meningitis.
- Routine culture of CSF, blood, and Gram stain of CSF remain the standard methods of establishing the etiological agent of ABM. Polymerase chain reaction (PCR) based detection of microbial DNA in cerebrospinal fluid (CSF) are useful for diagnosis of acute bacterial meningitis in patients pretreated with antibiotic.
- A combination of third-generation cephalosporin and vancomycin is recommended for empirical treatment of acute bacterial meningitis pending the culture sensitivity pattern of the isolate in CSF.
- As per current evidence there is no benefit of adjunctive corticosteroids in the management of acute bacterial meningitis in low middle income countries.
- Neurodevelopment sequel may be seen in 10–20% of patients. Patients should be evaluated for neuropsychological deficits, and SNHL.

REFERENCES

1. Kabra SK, Kumar P, Verma IC, *et al.* Bacterial meningitis in India—an IJP survey. Indian J Pediatr. 1991;58:505-11.
2. Ali M, Chang BA, Johnson KW, *et al.* Incidence and etiology of bacterial meningitis among children aged 1-59 months in South Asia: Systematic review and meta-analysis. Vaccine. 2018;36:5846-57.
3. Baraff LJ, Lee SI, Schriger DL. Outcomes of bacterial meningitis in children: A meta-analysis. Pediatr Infect Dis J. 1993;12: 389-94.
4. Prober CG. Central nervous system infections. In: Kleigman RH, Jenson HB, Behrman RE, Stanton BF, Nelson WE, Vaughan VC, editors. Nelson Textbook of Pediatrics, 18th edition. India: Elsevier; 2008. p. 2513-24.
5. Stanwell-Smith RE, Stuart J, Hughes AO, *et al.* Smoking, the environment and meningococcal disease: A case control study. Epidemiol infect. 1994;112:315-28.
6. Schuchat A, Robinson K, Wenger JD, *et al.* Bacterial meningitis in United States in 1995; Active surveillance team. New Eng J Med. 1997;337:970-6.
7. Ramachandran P, Fitzwater SP, Aneja S, *et al.* Prospective multi-centre sentinel surveillance for *Haemophilus influenza* type b and other bacterial meningitis in Indian children. Indian J Med Res. 2013;137:712-20.
8. Fitzwater SP, Ramachandran P, Kahn GD, *et al.* Impact of the introduction of the *Haemophilus influenza* type b conjugate vaccine in an urban setting in Southern India. Vaccine. 2019;37:1608-13.
9. Jayaraman Y, Veeraraghavan B, Purushothaman GKC, *et al.* Burden of bacterial meningitis in India: Preliminary data from a hospital based sentinel surveillance network. PLoS One. 2018;13:e0197198.
10. Wu D, Li YX, Shao ZJ, *et al.* Acute meningitis and encephalitis syndrome surveillance disease burden in four China prefectures. Zhonghua Yu Fang Yi Xue Za Zhi. 2019;53:164-8.
11. Oordt-Speets AM, Bolijn R, van Hoorn RC, *et al.* Global etiology of bacterial meningitis: A systematic review and meta-analysis. PLoS One. 2018;13:e0198772.
12. John J, Varghese R, Lionell J, *et al.* Non-vaccine pneumococcal serotypes among children with invasive pneumococcal disease. Indian Pediatr. 2018;55:874-6.
13. Leib SI, Tauber MG. Pathogenesis of bacterial meningitis. Infect Dis Clin North Am. 1999;13:527-48.
14. Hanke ML, Kielian T. Toll- like receptors in health and disease in the brain: Mechanisms and therapeutic potential. Clin Sci (Lond). 2011;121:367-87.
15. Tuomanen EL. The biology of pneumococcal infection. Pediatr Res. 1997;42:253-8.
16. Talukdar B, Khalil A, Sarkar R, *et al.* Meningococcal meningitis: Clinical observations during an epidemic. Indian Pediatr. 1988;125:329-34.
17. Arditi M, Manogue KR, Caplan M, *et al.* Cerebrospinal fluid cachectin /tumor necrosis factor and platelet activating factor concentration and severity of bacterial meningitis in children. J Infect Dis. 1990;162:139-47.
18. Kilpi T, Anttila M, Markker JT, *et al.* Thrombocytosis and thrombocytopenia in childhood bacterial meningitis. Pediatr Infect Dis J. 1992;11:456-60.
19. Arditi M, Mason EO, Bradley JS, *et al.* Three year multicenter surveillance of pneumococcal meningitis in children: Clinical characteristics and outcome related to penicillin susceptibility and dexamethasone use. Pediatrics. 1998;102:1087-97.
20. Klein JO, Feigin RD, McCracken GH Jr. Report of the task force on diagnosis and management of meningitis. Pediatrics. 1986; 78(Suppl):959-82.
21. Horwitz SJ, Boxer Baum B, O'bell J. Cerebral herniation in bacterial meningitis in childhood. Ann Neurol. 1980;7:524-8.
22. Damodaran A, Aneja S, Malhotra VL, *et al.* Sensorineural hearing loss following acute bacterial meningitis. A prospective evaluation. Indian Pediatr. 1996;33:763-6.
23. van Loon MC, Hensen EF, de Foer B, *et al.* Magnetic resonance imaging in the evaluation of patients with sensorineural hearing loss caused by meningitis: Implications for cochlear implantation. Otol Neurotol. 2013;34:845-54.
24. Portnoy JM, Olson LC. Normal cerebrospinal fluids values in children: Another look. Pediatrics. 1985;75:484-7.
25. Powers WJ. Cerebrospinal fluid lymphocytosis in acute bacterial meningitis. Am J Med. 1985;79:216-20.
26. Kleiman M, Reynolds J, Watt N. Superiority of acridine orange stain versus gram stain in partially treated bacterial meningitides. J Pediatr. 1984;104:401-4.

27. Gray SJ, Sobanski MA, Kachmarski EB, *et al.* Ultrasound-enhanced latex immunoagglutination and PCR as complementary method of non-culture based confirmation of meningococcal disease. J Clin Microbiol. 1999;37:1797-801.
28. Finlay FO, Witherow H, Rudd PT. Latex agglutination testing in bacterial meningitis. Arch Dis Child. 1995;73:160-9.
29. Borrow R, Clause H, Guiver M, *et al.* Non-culture diagnosis and serogroup determination of meningococcal B and C infection by a sialytransferase (siaD) PCR ELISA. Epidemiol Infect. 1997; 118:111-7.
30. Lal H, Agarwal A, Singh AK, *et al.* Nested polymerase chain reaction targeting 16S r RNA gene in diagnosis of acute bacterial meningitis. J Acad Clin Microbiol. 2018;20:77-83.
31. Jain M, Aneja S, Mehta G, *et al.* CSF interleukins, tumor necrosis factor and free radicals production in relation to clinical outcome in acute bacterial meningitis. Indian Pediatr. 2000;37:608-14.
32. Archer BD. Computed tomography before lumbar puncture in acute meningitis. A review of the risk and benefits. Can Med Assoc J. 1993;148:961-5.
33. Verghese VP, Veeraraghavan B, Jayaraman R, *et al.* Increasing incidence of penicillin and cefotaxime resistant *Streptococcus pneumoniae* causing meningitis in India: Time for revision of treatment guidelines? Indian J Med Microbiol. 2017;35: 228-36.
34. Odio CM, Puig JR, Ferris JM, *et al.* Prospective, randomized investigator-blinded study of the efficacy and safety of meropenem vs cefotaxime therapy in bacterial meningitis in children. Meropenem Meningitis Study Group. Pediatr Infect Dis J. 1999;18:581-90.
35. Bradley JS, Connor JD. Ceftriaxone failure in meningitis caused by *Streptococcus pneumoniae* with reduced susceptibility to beta lactamase antibiotics. Pediatr Infect Dis J. 1991;10:871-7.
36. Rhomberg PR, Jones RN. Summary trends of meropenem yearly test information collection program: A 10-year experience in United States (1999-2008). Diagn Microbiol Infect Dis. 2009;65: 414-26.
37. Oncu S, Punar M, Eraksoy H. Comparative activities of beta-lactam antibiotics and quinolones for various *S. pneumoniae* isolates. Chemotherapy. 2009;50:98-100.
38. van de Beek D, Cabellos C, Dzupova O, *et al.* ESCMID guideline: Diagnosis and treatment of acute bacterial meningitis. Clin Microbiol Infect. 2016;22 Suppl 3:S37-S62.
39. Køster-Rasmussen R, Korshin A, Meyer CN. Antibiotic treatment delay and outcome in acute bacterial meningitis. J Infect. 2008;57:449-54.
40. Galimand M, Gerbaud G, Guibourdenche M, *et al.* High-level chloramphenicol resistance in Neisseria meningitis. N Engl J Med. 1988;339:868-74.
41. Roine I, Ledermann W, Foncea LM, *et al.* Randomized trial of four vs. seven days of ceftriaxone treatment for bacterial meningitis in children with rapid initial recovery. Pediatr Infect Dis J. 2000;19:219-22.
42. Patwari AK, Singh BS, Deb M. Inappropriate secretion of antibiotic hormone in acute bacterial meningitis. Ann Trop Pediatr. 1995;15:179-83.
43. von Vigier RO, Colombo SM, Stoffel PB, *et al.* Circulating sodium in acute meningitis Am J Nephrol. 2001;21:87-90.
44. Maconochie IK, Bhaumik S. Fluid therapy for acute bacterial meningitis. Cochrane Database Syst Rev. 2016;11:CD004786.
45. Lebel MH, Freij BJ, Syrogiannopoulos GA, *et al.* Dexamethasone therapy for bacterial meningitis. Results of 2 double blind, placebo controlled trials. N Eng J Med. 1988;319:964-71.
46. Schaad VB, Lips U, Gneham HE, *et al.* Dexamethasone therapy for bacterial meningitis in children. Lancet. 1993;342: 457-61.
47. Brouwer MC, McIntyre P, Prasad K, *et al.* Corticosteroids for acute bacterial meningitis. Cochrane Database Syst Rev. 2015; 9:CD004405.
48. Ogunlesi TA, Odigwe CC, Oladapo OT. Adjuvant corticosteroids for reducing death in neonatal bacterial meningitis. Cochrane Database Syst Rev. 2015;11:CD010435.
49. Saez-Llorens X, McCraken GH Jr. Antimicrobial and anti-inflammatory treatment of bacterial meningitis. Infect Dis Clin North Amer. 1999;13:619-36.
50. Uppal L, Singhi S, Singhi P, *et al.* Role of rifampin in reducing inflammation and neuronal damage in childhood bacterial meningitis: A pilot randomized controlled trial. Pediatr Infect Dis J. 2017;36:556-9.
51. Edmond K, Clark A, Korczak VS, *et al.* Global and regional risk of disabling sequelae from bacterial meningitis: A systematic review and meta-analysis. Lancet Infect Dis. 2010;10:317-28.
52. Pomeroy SL, Holmes SJ, Dodge PR, *et al.* A prospective evaluation of the neurologic sequelae of bacterial meningitis in children with special emphasis on late seizures. N Eng J Med. 1990;323:1651-7.
53. Antilla M. Clinical criteria for estimating recovery from childhood bacterial meningitis. Acta Paediatr. 1994;83:63-7.
54. American Academy of Pediatrics. *Haemophilus influenzae* infections. In: Kimberlin D, Brady MT, Jackson MA, editors. Red book: 2018 report of the Committee on Infectious Diseases, 31st edition. Elk Grove Village, IL: American Academy of Pediatrics; 2018. p. 367-74.
55. Almog R, Block C, Gdalevich M, *et al.* First recorded outbreaks of Meningococcal disease in the Israeli defence Force Three cluster due to serogroup C and the emergence of resistance to rifampicin. Infection. 1994;22:69-71.
56. Balasubramaniam S, Shah A, Pemde H, *et al.* Indian Academy of Pediatrics (IAP) Advisory Committee on Vaccines and Immunization Practices (ACVIP) Recommended Immunization Schedule (2018-19) and Update on Immunization for Children aged 0 through 18 Years. Indian Pediatr. 2018;55: 1066-74.
57. Lessa FC, Michael (Trey) Spiller, Elizabeth Soda, *et al.* Impact of introduction of infant vaccination with 13-valent pneumococcal conjugate vaccine (PCV13) on pneumonia and invasive pneumococcal disease (IPD) in the United States, 2005–2014. Available from: *https://www.cdc.gov/vaccines/acip/meetings/downloads/slides-2018-10/Pneumococcal-04-Lessa-508.pdf.* Accessed August 17, 2019.
58. Dagan R, Givon-Lavi N, Zamir O, *et al.* Reduction of nasopharyngeal carriage of *Streptococcus pneumoniae* after administration of a 9-valent pneumococcal conjugate vaccine to toddlers attending day care centres. J Infect Dis. 2002;185: 927-36.
59. Saez-Llorens, McKracken Jr GH. Bacterial meningitis in children. Lancet. 2003;361:2139-48.

CHAPTER

33

Acute Encephalitis

Sheffali Gulati

INTRODUCTION

Encephalitis is an inflammatory process that affects brain tissue. Encephalopathy implies cerebral dysfunction due to circulating toxins, poisons, abnormal metabolites or intrinsic biochemical disorders affecting neurons but without inflammatory response. Encephalitis is almost always accompanied by inflammation of the adjacent meninges, thus the term meningoencephalitis. Both entities may be caused by a wide variety of agents.[1] Some of the causes are self-limiting, while others may rapidly lead to death or severe neurological damage.

Diagnosis of encephalitis with absolute certainty is only possible by microscopic examination of brain tissue. Practically, the diagnosis is made based on neurological manifestations, recovery of infectious agent, serologic evidence of infection and relevant epidemiological findings.

Acute encephalitis is more common in children (more than 16 cases per 100,000 patient years) than in adults (between 3.5 and 7.4 cases per 100,000 patient years). In the United States, about 1000–2000 cases of viral encephalitis are reported to the Centers, for Disease Control, Atlanta annually.[2] Its incidence in India is not known.

ETIOLOGY

Common etiologic agents of acute encephalitis and acute meningoencephalitis are detailed in **Table 1**. Infectious causes of encephalitis in immunocompromised patients are also mentioned in **Table 1**. Although evidence of an infectious etiology is presumed in most cases, often no causative agent can be identified. Of 412 patients with encephalitis under 16 years of age (1968–1987), the chief causes included measles, mumps and rubella in 30.4%, herpes group in 24.1%, respiratory viruses (adenovirus, parainfluenza virus, respiratory syncytical virus and influenza A and B viruses) in 18.3%, enteroviruses in 9.7%, *Mycoplasma pneumoniae* in 13.1%, more than one virus in 2.9%, post-vaccination encephalitis (measles-mumps-rubella, polio) in 1.0%.[3] No agents were identified in 32%. In India, Japanese B encephalitis (JE) is probably the commonest form of viral encephalitis and occurs in epidemics over large parts of the country. Non-JE viral encephalitis is emerging as an important cause of acute viral encephalitis since widespread use of JE vaccine in endemic area. There have been reports of Nipah virus encephalitis from Siliguri, West Bengal, West Nile virus encephalitis in Kerala, and outbreaks of Chandipura virus encephalitis in Gujarat. Rabies also poses a public health problem in this country. There is paucity of data from our country on the etiologic importance of other agents.

EPIDEMIOLOGY

Several factors such as age, geographical location, season, climate and host immunocompetence effect the epidemiology of viral encephalitis. The incidence of encephalitis differs greatly in different countries and in different seasons of the year. This is due to the seasonal variation in the incidence of common viral infections such as enteroviruses and mumps, as well as the geographical restriction of arboviral infections influenced by the

Table 1: Common etiologic agents in acute encephalitis and acute meningoencephalitis

Viruses	*Bacteria**
Spread person to person only	*H. influenzae, N. meningitidis, S. pneumoniae, M. tuberculosis*
Herpes simplex 1 and 2+	***Spirochetes.*** *Borrelia, Leptospira, Treponema pallidum*
Varicella zoster virus+	
Mumps virus	
Measles virus+	***Others***
Variola	*Chlamydia*
Epstein-Barr virus	*Rickettsia*
Cytomegalovirus	*Mycoplasma*
Influenza virus	
Enteroviruses+	
Rubella virus+	
Rotavirus	***Fungi***
Adenovirus	*Cryptococcus neoformans*+, Coccidioidomycosis+, Blastomycosis+,
Human herpesvirus 6+	Histoplasmosis+, *Aspergillus*+, *Candida*+
Spread to people by mosquitoes or ticks	
Japanese B encephalitis virus	
Kyasanur forest disease	***Protozoal***
Dengue virus	*Plasmodium falciparum,* Trypanosomes,
West Nile virus	*Naegleria*+, *Acanthamoeba*+,
Equine encephalitis viruses	Toxoplasma+
St Louis encephalitis virus	
Chandipura virus	
Spread by warm blooded mammals	***Helminths***
Rabies	*Schistosoma*
Lymphocytic choriomeningitis virus Others	
Human immunodeficiency virus	
Slow virus infections, prion diseases	

*Often have an encephalitic component
+Infectious causes of encephalitis in immunocompromised patients; JC (polyoma) virus produces progressive multifocal leukoencephalopathy in patients with HIV infection.

activity of their insect vectors. JE is transmitted in our country by female mosquitoes *Culex tritaeniorhynchus* and *Culex vishnui.* Herpes tends to occur worldwide with little seasonal variation.[4] Mumps, measles and rabies encephalitides have been eradicated from many developed countries.[2] Scrub typhus has been reported in up to 20% of all acute encephalitis syndrome (AES) cases presenting in Gorakhpur region of Uttar Pradesh in India, with range from 14% to 60% in other areas. This an arthropod vector borne infection caused by mosquito bite and is becoming increasingly common following rapid urbanization of rural areas. It has also now been isolated at cities in Tamil Nadu, Uttrakhand and Lucknow city of Uttar Pradesh. The recently discovered Zika virus, transmitted by *culex* mosquitoes, is now WHO category 2 for India after confirmed cases have been reported from Gujarat and Chennai. However, AES is not a presenting feature for the same. Neurological complications associated with Zika virus include Guillain-Barré syndrome and myelitis. Recently, litchi encephalitis has been reported in epidemic forms in regions of Bihar, Uttar Pradesh and West Bengal. The incriminating toxins, hypoglycin A and methylenecyclopropylglycine (MCPG), result in severe fatty acid oxidation inhibition and hypoglycemia.

PATHOGENESIS

Acute encephalitis may; be (i) primary—direct invasion and replication of the virus leading to tissue necrosis, encephalitis due to herpes simplex, arboviruses and rabies; (ii) para infectious—a postinfectious inflammatory response characterized by immune mediated central nervous system (CNS) damage, demyelination with preservation of neurons and their axons. Clinical manifestations in such a type of injury are variable and recovery is likely. Distinction between primary infection and parainfectious is however, difficult.[5] The reactions of brain tissue to viral invasion are similar in all forms of encephalitis. Many viruses cause widespread inflammation, cerebral edema and necrosis. Some such as herpes and rabies have a predisposition to involve specific areas of the brain namely temporal lobes and basal structures, respectively.[2,4] Most neuronal destruction is probably due to direct viral invasion, whereas the hosts tissue response induces demyelination and vascular and perivascular destruction.

CLINICAL FEATURES

The clinical findings in encephalitis are determined by:

- The severity of involvement and anatomic localization of the affected portions of the nervous system
- The inherent pathogenicity of the offending agent
- The immune and other reactive mechanisms of the patient.

A wide variety of clinical manifestations may occur ranging from inapparent, mild abortive type of illness, or aseptic meningitis syndrome to severe encephalomyelitis with or without radiculitis.

The onset of encephalitis usually is acute, but signs and symptoms of CNS involvement often are preceded by a nonspecific, acute febrile illness. Presenting symptoms in older children are headache and malaise; infants typically are irritable and lethargic. Fever, nausea, vomiting, neck pain, and photophobia are common. Alteration of level of consciousness ranges from mild lethargy and confusion to coma. Evidence of brain parenchymal involvement is the hallmark of encephalitis.[1] Children with encephalitis may demonstrate evidence of diffuse disease such as behavioral or personality changes; decreased consiousness; and generalized seizures or localized changes, such as focal seizures, hemiparesis, movement disorders, cranial nerve deficits and ataxia.[6] The most common cause of focal encephalopathic findings is *Herpes simplex* virus. Nuchal rigidity is often not as pronounced as in purely meningitic illness. Neurological abnormalities may be stationary, progressive or fluctuating. Unprovoked emotional bursts and loss of bowel and bladder control may occur.

Sudden severe rise of intracranial pressure may result in decerebration, cardiorespiratory insufficiency, hyperventilation and autonomic dysfunction. Uncontrolled cerebral edema may lead to herniation at tentorial hiatus, compression of the midbrain causing deterioration in consciousness, pupillary abnormalities, ptosis, sixth nerve palsy, ophthalmoplegia, paralysis of upward gaze, Cheyne-Stoke breathing, hyperventilation and bradycardia. Herniation of cerebellum through the foramen magnum causes distortion and compression of the medulla oblongata with severe disturbances of vital centers leading to respiratory or cardiac arrest. The course of encephalitis varies from that of the fulminating type, ending in death in 2 to 4 days, to that of a mild form in which the illness subsides in 1 or 2 weeks with complete recovery. Typically this stage lasts for 7–10 days after which there is gradual recovery with or without sequelae.

There is tropism of a variety of viruses for different CNS cell types (e.g. polioviruses for motor neurons; rabies virus for neurons of the limbic system; mumps virus for ependymal cells of newborn). Demyelination follows the destruction of oligodendroglias, whereas the involvement of ependymal cells can result in hydranencephaly. Certain specific clinical features of viral encephalitides are shown in **Table 2**.

DIAGNOSIS

The diagnosis of viral encephalitis is usually made on the clinical presentation of a nonspecific prodrome followed by progressive CNS symptoms. The immediate goals are to identify focal features that may imply herpes simplex encephalitis (HSE) and to detect other disorders that may mimic encephalitis.[2] History is taken for prior viral infections, exanthem (e.g. echovirus, coxsackievirus, *Varicella zoster* virus, measles, rubella) or recent vaccination. History of a bite from a potentially rabid animal, travel history, exposure to mosquitoes, rodents and ticks, the season in which illness occurs, and the diseases prevalent in the community may provide clues to the diagnosis.

Patients with fever and altered neurological function require a prompt neurodiagnostic evaluation that typically includes an electroencephalogram (EEG), a neuroimaging study computed tomography (CT) or magnetic resonance imaging (MRI)], and a lumbar puncture. Patients with suspected viral encephalitis require a detailed microbiological evaluation. In the acute stage, blood counts usually show a polymorphonuclear leukocytosis.

Positive identification of viral infection in the CNS helps to curtail investigations, rationalize treatment, and improve the reliability of prognosis. Though the identification of etiology is difficult, a rational use of various diagnostic studies may result in etiological diagnosis in approximately 60% patients.[6]

Table 2: Clinical features of viral encephalitides

Agent	*Typical findings/history*
Enterovirus	Herpangina, myocarditis, pleurodynia, rhombencephalitis*
Herpes simplex type I	Symptoms due to focal necrosis of orbital or temporal regions#, focal neurological symptoms
Japanese B encephalitis	Extrapyramidal signs, respiratory difficulties, vasomotor instability
Varicella zoster	Characteristic rash, cerebellar ataxia, hemiparesis
Rabies	History of animal bite, autonomic dysfunction, hydrophobia
Mumps	Parotitis
Lymphocytic	History of exposure to rodents choriomeningitis virus
Adenovirus	Acute respiratory disease, conjunctivitis, keratoconjunctivitis
Influenza	Acute respiratory disease, opisthotonous, ataxia, transverse myelopathy
Epstein-Barr virus	Encephalomyelitis, meningoencephalitis

*Myoclonic jerks, ataxia, brainstem signs
#Anosmia, aphasia temporal lobe seizures, memory loss, disordered behavior, olfactory or gustatory hallucinations

Cerebrospinal Fluid

The cerebrospinal fluid (CSF) pressure is normal or slightly elevated. There is usually lymphocytic pleocytosis (5–500 cells/mm^3); rarely more than 1,000 cells/mm^3 may be seen in conditions like eastern equine encephalitis and lymphocytic choriomeningitis. Early in the disease, the cells might be polymorphonuclear; later mononuclear cells predominate. This change in cellular type is often demonstrated in CSF samples obtained as little as 8–12 hours apart. However, CSF pleocytosis is found in only half of patients with clinically suspected encephalitis.[7] Some patients with HSE may show a xanthochromic or bloody CSF, usually with less than 500 red blood cells/mm^3. CSF pleocytosis can be absent in conditions like Chandipura and measles viral encephalitis

The protein content is mildly elevated (50–200 mg/dL). The concentration of proteins may be high in some patients with HSE and extensive brain destruction. The CSF glucose content is normal or slightly decreased. Neonates with HSE tend to have mild hypoglycorrhachia (Low CSF glucose). A small proportion of patients with mumps encephalitis may have CSF sugar lower than 40 mg/dL.

Microbiological Evaluation

The CSF should be cultured for viruses, bacteria, fungi and mycobacteria; in some instances when suspected, special examinations are indicated for protozoa, mycoplasma and other pathogens.

Various laboratory methods involved in diagnosing viral infections of the CNS include isolation of virus, detection of viral antigen or its nucleic acids and serology. Workup includes viral culture of respiratory secretions, throat swab, CSF, blood, urine, stool, swab from skin rash and brain tissue taken as early as possible in the illness.[7] Appropriate transport media should be used. These specimens should, if possible, be taken within four days of the onset of the illness and sent quickly to the laboratory on ice, but should not be frozen. Detection of viral antigen can be done in brain tissue or CSF (leukocytes or soluble antigen). Detection of antibodies in CSF and the CSF to blood ratio of specific IgG can be helpful in diagnosing HSV infection. Single serum IgM value or paired sera (acute and convalescent phase) to show rising titers of IgG are also useful. Polymerase chain reaction to detect viral nucleic acids in CSF is promising and is likely to provide a rapid, accurate diagnosis in future.

Measurement of interferon α in CSF provides evidence of active viral infection in the CNS but this test is not widely available. IgG index, which is derived by calculating the ratios of IgG and albumin in CSF and serum is another indicator of intrathecal synthesis of antibodies. A raised IgG index and the presence of oligoclonal bands in CSF suggest intrathecal synthesis of IgG.[7] Various virologic and serologic tests are detailed in **Table 3**.

Table 3: Virologic and serologic studies in viral encephalitis

Agent	*Virologic studies*	*Serologic studies*
HSV	Culture—CSF, brain biopsy; Antigen detection-brain biopsy (IFA)*; PCR-CSF (method of choice)	Acute, convalescent sera; CSF antibody detection (less useful); CSF: serum antibody ratio
Arboviruses	Culture—CSF, brain; Antigen detection—brain, CSF (IFA)	IgM (isotype antibody capture immunoassay)# CSF, serum (very useful); Acute, convalescent sera-IgG
Cytomegalovirus	Culture—CSF, brain; PCR-CSF	Acute, convalescent sera (little diagnostic value)
Epstein-Barr virus	Rarely cultured; PCR-CSF	Acute sera for antibody profile (serology most useful)
Varicella zoster virus	Culture—skin vesicles, CFS; DFA**—skin, brain; PCR-CSF	Acute, convalescent sera; Antibody in CSF (IgA, IgG)
Rabies	Fluorescence microscopy or culture-corneal smear, skin biopsy, muscle biopsy (nape of neck), saliva, CSF; Antigen detection/culture-brain	Serology (possible); CSF antibody detection
Adenovirus	Culture—CSF, brain, urine, nasal or conjunctival swab	Acute, convalescent sera-IgG
Enteroviruses	Culture—stool, CSF, urine, blood, brain biopsy; PCR-CSF	Acute, convalescent sera (not useful)
Influenza	Culture—respiratory secretions	Acute, convalescent sera-HAI• antibody
Paramyxoviruses	Culture—CSF; PCR-CSF	Acute, convalescent sera; elevated CSF globulin
Rubella		Serology—IgM
Human immunodeficiency virus	Culture/PCR-CSF, brainbiopsy; p24 antigen-blood	Serology—ELISA, western blot (>18 months age)
Lymphocytic choriomeningitis virus	Culture—CSF, blood, urine, pharyngeal secretions; RT-PCR°-CSF	Serology—IgM CSF

*IFA indirect immunofluorescent antibody; #Also known as MAC-ELISA (enzyme linked immunosorbent assay) or IgM capture test; **DFA: Direct fluorescent antibody; •HAI: Hemagglutination inhibition; °RT-PCR: reverse transcriptase PCR)

Electroencephalogram

Electroencephalogram (EEG) may be useful in patients with (i) Markedly altered neurological function, where EEG helps in detecting seizures and monitoring the efficacy of anticonvulsant therapy; (ii) Suspected HSV infection where characteristic periodic sharp waves repeating every 0.5 to 4 seconds are found (**Fig. 1**). Such EEG abnormalities may be diffuse or temporofrontal, unilateral or bilateral, and are always accompanied by diffuse or temporally accentuated excess delta activity.[8]

Neuroimaging

It can help to separate viral encephalitis from metabolic or toxic disorders and acute disseminated encephalomyelitis (ADEM). Early viral encephalitis is characterized by low density lesions on CT, and prolonged T1 and T2 relaxation times on MRI. MRI appears to be significantly more sensitive.[9]

Japanese B encephalitis

In JE, CT shows non-enhancing low-density areas in the thalamus, basal ganglia, midbrain, pons and medulla.

Fig. 1: EEG showing bilateral independent lateralized discharges recurring at regular intervals of 1 second, moreover the left hemispheric EEG leads

MRI show extensive involvement of the thalamus, midbrain, cerebrum and cerebellum (**Fig. 2**). Classically, the lesions are hyperintense on T2-weighted images and hypointense on T1-weighted images. In 70% patients, they are hemorrhagic. Bilateral hemorrhagic thalamic involvement is characteristic of JE in endemic areas.[10]

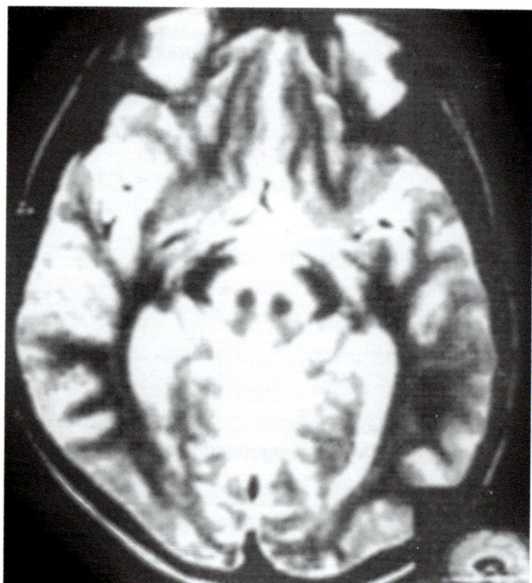

Fig. 2: Axial MRI on T2-weighted sequence through midbrain showing bilaterally symmetrical hyperintensity signals in midbrain typically sparing substantia nigra and red nucleus (Panda's eye sign) in a child with Japanese B encephalitis

Herpes simplex encephalitis

CT abnormalities are usually not found before the fifth day of illness. MRI and single photon emission CT (SPECT) studies are more sensitive early in the course of the disease. MRI with greater spatial resolution than SPECT is the modality of choice. The characteristic CT findings in HSE are poorly defined areas of low density in the anteromedial portion of the temporal lobe with extension to the insular cortex but sparing of the lentiform nucleus. A gyral pattern of contrast enhancement is frequently seen. MRI shows prolonged T1 and T2 relaxation times in the medial temporal lobe, the insular cortex, and the orbital surface of the frontal lobe, particularly the cingulate gyrus (**Figs. 3 and 4**).[11]

Acute disseminated encephalomyelitis (ADEM)

CT and MRI show moderate to large areas of demyelination, characterized by low density lesions on CT and prolonged T1 and T2 relaxation times on MRI. The MRI findings in this condition are more extensive, appear to be of the same age, are frequently bilateral and reveal abnormalities of the deep cerebral nuclei in 50% children.[12] The white matter lesions are asymmetrical and predominantly involve subcortical areas (**Fig. 5**).

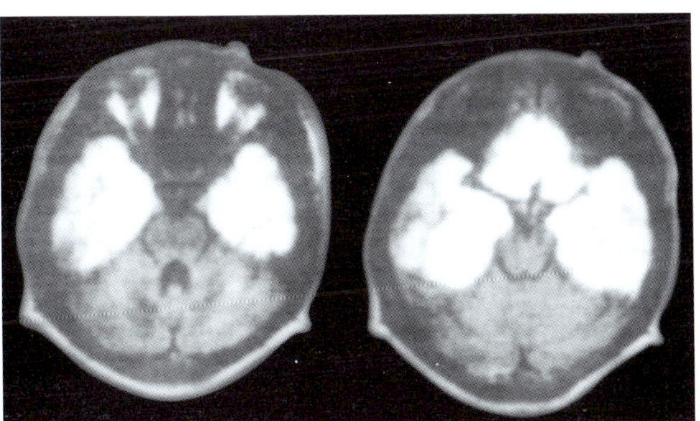

Fig. 3: Axial FLAIR MRI sequence showing bilaterally symmetrical hyperintensity signals in basifrontal and temporal lobes characteristic of herpes simplex encephalitis. (FLAIR: fluid-attenuated inversion recovery; MRI: magnetic resonance imaging)

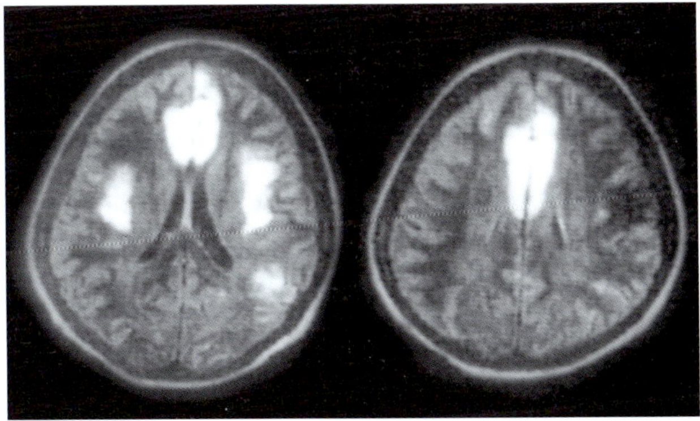

Fig. 4: Axial FLAIR MRI sequence (at a level higher than Fig. 3) showing extension of signal abnormalities in bilateral medial frontal lobes and insular cortex, which are pathognomonic of herpes simplex encephalitis. (FLAIR: fluid-attenuated inversion recovery; MRI: magnetic resonance imaging)

DIFFERENTIAL DIAGNOSIS

Viral encephalitis should be considered in a patient with acute onset of fever and altered consciousness. A wide range of CNS disorders would need careful exclusion. The sequence of tests are dictated by the clinical features. A wide differential diagnosis is illustrated in a case series, in which 50% patients with presumed viral encephalitis were found to have other disorders.

In India, viral encephalitis should be distinguished from other CNS infections such as bacterial or tuberculous meningitis, cerebral malaria, encephalitis or meningoencephalitis due to *Leptospira* spp., *Mycoplasma pneumoniae* or *Acanthamoeba* and brain abscess. Patients with bacterial infection of the CNS usually appear more acutely ill than those with viral infection. However, meningitis caused by *Streptococcus pneumoniae*, *Neisseria meningitidis* and *Haemophilus influenzae* type b may be insidious in onset. CNS infection caused by less virulent bacteria, such as *Mycobacterium tuberculosis*, *Treponema pallidum* may also be clinically indolent. If CSF shows pleocytosis, acute bacterial meningitis should be carefully excluded. If CSF is normal, then disorders like cerebral malaria, Reye syndrome and enteric encephalopathy need to be differentiated. Clinical findings distinguish patients with encephalitis from viral meningitis; the latter usually have nuchal rigidity, headache, photophobia, irritability, fever and the sensorial loss is usually not severe.[4] Cerebral venous thrombosis, electrolyte and metabolic encephalopathies, drug ingestion, postinfectious disease including Guillain-Barré syndrome and acute cerebellar ataxia, brain tumors, and cerebral vascular disorders should be excluded. Autoimmune encephalitis including NMDA receptor and VGKC receptor encephalitis must be considered with predominant neuropsychiatric manifestations, autonomic instability and normal findings on neuroimaging.

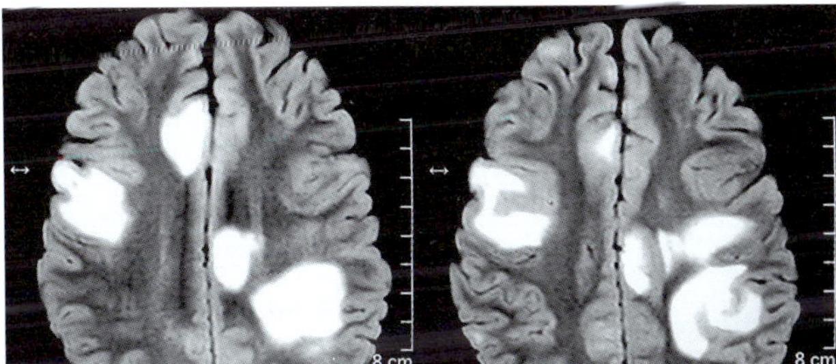

Fig. 5: Axial FLAIR MRI sequence showing multiple large asymmetrical foci of T2/FLAIR hyperintensity which are seen in ADEM. (FLAIR: fluid-attenuated inversion recovery; MRI: magnetic resonance imaging)

Acute Disseminated Encephalomyelitis

A distinction should be made between acute viral encephalitis and acute disseminated encephalomyelitis (ADEM) or postinfectious encephalomyelitis, since the outcomes are quite different.[12] ADEM involves autoimmune responses that are directed, at least in part, against myelin antigens. Before wide- spread vaccination, postinfectious encephalomyelitis most commonly occurred after smallpox and measles infections. In recent years, the disease has been associated with various viral and bacterial infections. Patients may have a history of an exanthem or a nonspecific respiratory or gastrointestinal illness 1 to 3 weeks before onset of neurological symptoms. Neurologic findings vary and reflect the areas of the brain involved. The clinical features include multifocal neurological signs, lethargy, coma and seizures, which often implicate widespread areas of the brain, spinal cord, and optic nerves.[12] Acute cerebellar ataxia is a form of acute postinfectious encephalomyelitis following varicella infection.

CSF pressure may be slightly elevated and white cells are mild to moderately increased to 15 to 250 cells/mm^3 with lymphocytes predominating. CSF protein is normal or slightly elevated (35–150 mg/dL) and glucose levels are normal. Oligoclonal bands are usually negative and Myelin basic protein level is usually increased in the CSF. EEG is abnormal in most cases, with high voltage slow frequency waves. The EEG abnormalities may persist for several weeks after apparent clinical recovery. Neuroimaging findings have been described above.

TREATMENT

Until a bacterial cause is excluded by culture of blood and CSF, parenteral antibiotic therapy should be given. Patients with presumed virus encephalitis require treatment strategies that are tailored to the severity of the illness and the availability of specific antiviral therapy. Such patients require frequent assessment of their level of consciousness and anticipatory care for the potential complications of encephalitis like seizures, increased intracranial pressure, hyperpyrexia, adequate respiratory exchange, disturbed fluid and electrolyte balance, aspiration and asphyxia, and cardiac or respiratory arrest of central origin.

The three immediate steps are to give intravenous acyclovir promptly if focal features suggest HSE, to search for other treatable causes of an acute encephalopathy and to protect the child's brain against further insult.

Principles of Treatment

The main objectives of treatment of a child with viral encephalitis are to reduce intracranial pressure (ICP), to optimize systemic arterial pressure to maintain adequate cerebral perfusion pressure and prevention of secondary complications. Increased ICP contributes greatly to the morbidity and mortality. Dangerous elevations in ICP are manifested by rapid deterioration in clinical status as detailed earlier and by radiographic changes such as obliteration of the lateral ventricles or basal cisterns on CT. The most important step is early identification. Most therapeutic measures fail if they are instituted late, as irreversible cerebral damage has already occurred. The control of raised ICP involves:

- Avoiding situations that increase the ICP
- Therapeutic measures to decrease ICP.

In patients with evidence of increased ICP, placement of a pressure transducer in the epidural space may be indicated for monitoring of ICP. Although the ICP can be monitored from the ventricle, brain parenchyma, subarachnoid space, subdural space and epidural space, it is important to realize that the pressure is not equal throughout the intracranial space. Although role of invasive ICP monitoring has been seen in cases with traumatic brain injury, no evidence for the same is as yet available for acute encephalitis (non-traumatic).

Control of Factors Aggravating Intracranial Pressure

Positioning and general care of patient: A 15°–30° head up tilt with head kept in the midline position facilitates venous return from the head, decreases ICP and improves cerebral perfusion pressure.[13,14] Hyperflexion, hyperextension or turning the neck which can elevate ICP, as can inordinately tight tracheostomy ties, should be avoided. Increase in ICP with suctioning can be minimized with gentle suctioning and intravenous lidocaine. Elevations in ICP from indirect transmission of elevated intrathoracic pressure to the intracranial vessels can be avoided by sedation and decreasing the inspiratory phase of the respirator.

Temperature control: Aggressive treatment of fever is essential as increased temperature increases ICP by increasing cerebral metabolism, cerebral blood flow and cerebral edema. Temperature control may be accomplished with cooling mattresses and the administration of paracetamol.

Role of sedation: Pain and arousal cause elevated ICP by increasing cerebral blood flow. Sedatives play an important role in the prevention of worsening of ICP by this mechanism. Conventionally, sedatives were avoided (except for seizure control), due to the fear of clouding the neurological examination. Midazolam may be tried initially as a first step. Inadequate sedation in the ventilated patient is clearly detrimental. The ideal sedative should have a rapid and smooth onset, decrease ICP, preserve autoregulation and vasoreactivity to carbon dioxide and allow easy titration of effect during neurological assessment. Propofol causes a decrease in cerebral blood flow and ICP, and maintains a degree of autoregulation. Barbiturates are no longer used as long-term sedatives because of their prolonged effects.

Seizures control: Normal blood levels of glucose, magnesium and calcium should be maintained to minimize the threat of seizures. Seizures increase ICP by increasing cerebral metabolism and cerebral blood flow. Midazolam or diazepam is effective for emergency use. Phenytoin, which does not have the depressant effects of barbiturates, should be considered for acute treatment. Management of seizures is discussed elsewhere.

Fluid and Electrolyte Management

The patient should be kept nil orally for first 24 hours. Thereafter the decision to start oral feeds depends upon the sensorium. The patient should receive intravenous fluids as N/2 in 5% dextrose in normal maintenance requirements, except in shock when a fluid bolus with normal saline or Ringer's lactate is required. The syndrome of inappropriate antidiuretic hormone secretion (SIADH) is quite common in acute CNS disorders. If there is clinical or laboratory evidence that the patient is suffering from SIADH, two-thirds of maintenance fluids are started and symptomatic management for hyponatremia instituted. Full maintenance requirements of sodium should be given as hyponatremia impairs cerebrovascular reactivity. There may be cerebral salt wasting with a combination of hypovolemia, hyponatremia, excessive renal sodium losses and marked elevation of plasma atrial natriuretic hormone. Treatment includes volume-for-volume replacement of urinary sodium losses and oral sodium supplementation after discharge from the hospital to correct and maintain normal fluid balance.

Measures to Decrease Intracranial Pressure

Hyperventilation: Hyperventilation after endotracheal intubation with maintenance of $PaCO_2$ between 25 and 30 mm Hg effectively reduces ICP by causing cerebral vasoconstriction. The drop in ICP occurs within 1 to 5 minutes of initiation of hyperventilation. ICP can be satisfactorily controlled in two-thirds of patients using a combination of a hyperosmolar agent and hyperventilation. Hyperventilation should not be prolonged beyond 1–2 days, following which it is gradually discontinued. Failure to reduce ICP with hyperventilation is a grave prognostic sign.

The potential deleterious effects of hyperventilation include an elevation of mean airway pressure and diminished cardiac filling pressures, resulting in barotrauma and hypotension. Although hyperventilation is useful in acutely decreasing ICP, prolonged hyperventilation, in fact, worsens the outcome. Chronic aggressive hyperventilation might result in areas of oligemia in marginally perfused brain tissue.

Mannitol

Mannitol is the most commonly used agent for control of raised ICP. Mannitol acts by two different mechanisms. While vascular mechanism is the explanation for the rapid (acute) effect of mannitol, diuresis explains the more prolonged effect of mannitol. On intravenous administration, it leads to an abrupt increase in intravascular osmolality relative to the brain compartment. This osmotic gradient facilitates a fluid shift from the brain into the vascular space. The dose is 0.25 to 1.0 g/kg body weight every 4 to 6 hours, or 20% mannitol 5 mL/kg over 5–10 minutes followed by 3 mL/ kg 6 hourly till 48 hours, beyond which mannitol loses its efficacy. The onset of action is within 1–5 minutes and duration 2–3 hours. Complications include dehydration and electrolyte imbalance especially hypernatremia.

Other Medications

Acetazolamide in dose of 20–50 mg/kg/day in 3 to 4 doses, oral glycerol 1 mL/kg/dose 8 hourly may be used if ICP is elevated beyond 48 hours. Furosemide can be given in a dose of 1 mg/kg intravenously every 12 hours. It may be added if response to mannitol is poor. Furosemide has a synergistic effect with mannitol in terms of reducing the ICP by virtue of decreasing free water. Barbiturates, e.g. pentobarbital and thiopentone reduce cerebral metabolism which leads to reduction in cerebral blood flow and intracranial volume and the ICP. Barbiturates are generally used only when standard therapy consisting of osmotic agents, hyperventilation and head position has failed to control the ICP. They should be used only in intensive care setting. Complications include hypotension in 50%, pneumonia and hyponatremia. The use of corticosteroids to reduce ICP or decrease toxic effects of inflammatory cytokines is controversial. They probably should not be used in acute viral diseases because of risk of potentiation of the viral infection.

CSF removal by an external ventricular drain: It has a therapeutic potential by allowing CSF removal once the ICP has reached dangerous levels.[14] After all medical measures for ICP control have been exhausted and barbiturate coma therapy is being considered, CSF removal may produce dramatic reduction in ICP. It may also provide temporary relief for elevated ICP in patients with acute hydrocephalus.

Supportive Management

Maintenance of cerebral perfusion: It is essential to prevent secondary cerebral ischemia. In conditions where cerebral autoregulation is impaired, cerebral perfusion depends exclusively on the cerebral perfusion pressure. The normal cerebral perfusion pressure in infants is in the range of 30 mm Hg. Hence, it is important that the cerebral perfusion pressure should be maintained above 30 mm Hg in infants less than 6 months age, above 40 mm Hg in older children and above 60 mm Hg in adolescents. Considering the fact that the clinical signs appear when ICP is usually above 15–20 mm Hg, it is imperative to maintain a mean arterial pressure above 75 mm Hg in mild and moderate grade coma and more than 85 mm Hg in severe grade coma.

Feeding: Feeding should be started once the sensorium improves.

Monitoring: The patient should be managed in an intensive care unit. The aim is to evaluate cardiorespiratory stability and detect acute life-threatening neurological complications at the earliest. Vitals including temperature, pulse, respiratory rate, blood pressure, neurological status, head size, body weight and urine output are recorded carefully.

Antiviral Therapy

Despite intensive clinical and laboratory investigations, relatively few viruses can be treated with specific antiviral chemotherapy (**Table 4**). Specific therapy is recommended in encephalitis due to herpes group of viruses.

Herpes simplex encephalitis

In some centers in the west, acyclovir treatment is started as soon as viral encephalitis in suspected even without evidence of localization. We recommend that specific therapy for HSE should be given early, if the diagnosis is suspected, e.g. in patients with localizing clinical signs, focal EEG changes, neuroimaging showing focal involvement of temporal lobes, or CSF examination showing red cells. Early therapy is mandatory, even before virological confirmation is obtained. Patients with suspected or confirmed HSE should receive acyclovir as detailed in **Table 4**. Because HSV-induced thymidine kinases effectively phosphorylate the drug to its more active form, acyclovir which has a relatively specific action on virus-infected cells and few side effects. Relapse after acyclovir therapy has been described in a small proportion of cases. Strains of HSV resistant to acyclovir have been isolated from immunocompromised patients who have received several courses of the drug. Should acyclovir therapy fail to arrest the disease, a trial of intravenous foscarnet is recommended at a dosage of 60 mg/kg every 8 hours intravenously for 14 days.[15]

Varicella zoster encephalitis

Although controlled studies have not been conducted, current data indicates that acyclovir can be used in dose regimens similar to those for HSE.

Japanese B encephalitis

No effective treatment exists for JE. Treatment with oral or parenteral corticosteroids is not indicated. Interferon α has been used in a small number of patients and larger trials are awaited.

Therapy for acute disseminated encephalomyelitis

Many agents have been used, including corticosteroids, adrenocorticotropic hormone, intravenous immunoglobulin (IVIG) and cyclosporine. Most patients respond to corticosteroid treatment. The clinical response is observed within hours of initiation of treatment with intravenous corticosteroids (15–20 mg/kg methyl-prednisolone or 5 mg/kg dexamethasone for 7 days). There are however, no clear guidelines regarding the appropriate steroid dosage and length of therapy. Corticosteroid dependency may occur during tapering necessitating a slower taper.

Table 4: Antiviral chemotherapy for viral encephalitis

Virus	*Drug*	*Dose*	*Toxicity*
HSV	Acyclovir	10 mg/kg (500 mg/m^2 of body surface area for children < 12 years) every 8 hours intravenously for 14 to 21 days⁺	Local-bullous inflammatory reaction, nephrotoxicity (renal tubular crystalluria with elevation of serum creatine), leukopenia, tremor, confusion, rarely, seizures, encephalopathy
Varicella zoster virus	Acyclovir	10 to 15 mg/kg (500 mg/m^2) every 8 hours intravenously for 7–10 days	As above
Cytomegalovirus	Ganciclovir	7.5 mg/kg/day in 3 divided doses* for 14 to 20 days	Myelosuppression, nausea, vomiting, CNS irritability, liver dysfunction
Influenza[18]	Amantadine	100 mg twice daily orally (<40 kg, 1–10 years: 5 mg/kg/d orally in 2 divided doses; maximum 150 mg/d) for 5 to 7 days	Depression, congestive heart failure, vomiting, CNS irritability, confusion
	Rimantadine	<14 years not recommended, ≥14 years 100 mg orally twice daily	

⁺ In the form of a 20 mg/mL solution, administered over an hour. A higher dose, such as 15 mg/kg every 8 hours, or a longer duration of therapy may occasionally be required.[4]

*Alternative regimens using ganciclovir and CMV immune globulin have been proposed : Ganciclovir (7.5 mg/kg/24 hr I/V in three divided doses for 14 days) and CMV immune globulin 400 mg/kg on days 1,2,7 and 200 mg/kg on day 14 or Ganciclovir (7.5 mg/kg/24 hr I/V in three divided doses for 20 days) and CMV immune globulin 500 mg/kg every other day for 10 doses.[17]

In cases resistant to high doses of corticosteroids, IVIg or cyclosporine may be used. Patients in coma from ADEM have been successfully treated with plasma exchange or plasmapheresis.

OUTCOME AND PROGNOSIS

The prognosis in all encephalitides is guarded with respect to immediate outcome and sequelae. Sequelae involving the CNS include intellectual, motor, psychiatric, epileptic, visual or auditory manifestations.

Clinical features are helpful in predicting the outcome. Young age, lower Glasgow coma score, abnormal oculocephalic responses, focal neurological signs, reduction in cerebral perfusion pressure (difference between systolic blood pressure and ICP), abnormal neuroimaging study and unilateral hyperperfusion on SPECT suggest a poor prognosis.[6,7,16]

Case fatality rate of 34% was reported among 338 children under 3 years of age with acute encephalopathies in a study by Madge *et al.,* which was similar whether or not encephalitis was diagnosed.[17] At 10 years follow-up, almost half the survivors had motor dysfunction and educational problems, one-third had neurological dysfunction and one-fifth had behaviour problems. High mortality has been reported in some recent outbreaks of encephalitis. In a study of 462 children under 17 years of age the mortality and serious morbidity of encephalitis were 2.8% and 6.7%, respectively. An increased risk of adverse outcomes was observed after *Mycoplasma pneumoniae* encephalitis and HSE.[6]

Mortality rate has been reported between 10 and 50 including mental retardation, neurological deficits and/ or epilepsy have been reported in 45% and minor motor deficits, behavioral problems and/or scholastic backwardness in 25%. Diagnosis and appropriate treatment. In 90% of survivors there is complete recovery. The exception is measles, in which sequelae may occur in 20% to 50% of patients.

Supportive and rehabilitative efforts are important after patients recover. Motor incoordination, seizure disorders, deafness, visual and behavioral disturbances may appear only after an interval of time. Neurodevelopmental and audiologic evaluation should be a part of routine follow-up of such children. Overall, the prognosis is good in ADEM.

KEY MESSAGES

- Acute encephalitis is an emergency – timely and effective management can change the course of illness and long-term outcome of the patient.
- Always look for infectious causes and treat appropriately, early CSF studies prior to antibiotic initiation are most informative for the same.
- Even if CSF does not give a diagnosis, neuroimaging and EEG are good ancillary investigations which may provide clues for certain etiologies like HSV encephalitis.
- Prevention is better than cure, more so for neurological infections, which can have lifelong morbidity. Ensuring vaccination, especially in endemic areas can go a long way in achieving disease control.
- In context of no infectious agent, poor response to antibiotics and persisting encephalopathy, keep autoimmune encephalitis as a possibility and investigate appropriately.

Case Definitions

Acute Encephalitis Syndrome

Case of any age, at any time of the year presenting with acute onset fever and change in mental status (such as confusion, irritability, disorientation, coma or inability to talk) AND/OR new onset seizure (excluding simple febrile seizures).

Japanese B Encephalitis

Laboratory confirmed JE: Case of suspected AES laboratory confirmed to be JE by any one of the following:

- Presence of JE IgM positivity in serum and/or CSF
- Four-fold change in paired antibody sera for IgG
- Virus isolation from brain tissue
- Antigen detection by immunofluorescence
- Nucleic acid detection by PCR

Probable JE: A suspected case of JE that occurs in close geographical or temporal relationship to lab confirmed case of JE or in an epidemic.

World Health Organization. Acute Encephalitis Syndrome. Japanese encephalitis surveillance standards. January 2006. From WHO-recommended standards for surveillance of selected vaccine-preventable diseases. WHO/V&B/03.01. Available from: http://www. who. int/vaccines-documents/DocsPDF06/843.pdf. Accessed on 8 August, 2012

REFERENCES

1. Cherry JD, Shields WD. Encephalitis and meningoencephalitis. In: Feign RD, Cherry JD, editors. Textbook of Pediatric Infectious Diseases, 4th edition. Philadelphia: Saunders; 1998. p. 457-68.
2. Bale JF. Viral encephalitis. Med Clin N Am. 1993;77:25-41.
3. Koskiniemi M, Vaheri A. Effect of measles, mumps, rubella vaccination on pattern of encephalitis in children. Lancet. 1989;1:31-4.
4. Whitley RJ. Viral encephalitis. N Engl J Med. 1990;323:242-9.
5. Johnson RT. The pathogenesis of acute viral encephalitis and postinfectious encephalomyelitis. J Infect Dis. 1987;155: 359-61.
6. Rautonen J, Koskiniemi M, Vaheri A. Prognostic factors in childhood acute encephalitis. Pediatr Infect Dis J. 1991;10: 441-6.
7. Kennedy C. Acute viral encephalitis in childhood. Br Med J. 1995;310:139-40.
8. Chien LT, Boehm RM, Robinson H, *et al.* Characteristic early electroencephalographic changes in herpes simplex encephalitis. Arch Neurol. 1977;34:361-4.
9. Koelfen W, Freund M. Guckel F, *et al.* MRI of encephalitis in children: Comparison of CT and MRI in the acute stage with long-term follow-up. Neuroradiology. 1996;38:73-9.10
10. Kalita J, Misra UK. Comparison of CT scan and MRI findings in the diagnosis of Japanese encephalitis. J Neurol Sci. 2000; 174:3-8.
11. Misra UK, Kalita J. A comparative study of Japanese and herpes simplex encephalitides. Electromyogr Clin Neurophysiol. 1998;38:41-6.
12. Kesselring J, Miller DH, Robb SA, *et al.* Acute disseminated encephalomyelitis: MRI findings and the distinction from multiple sclerosis. Brain. 1990;113:291-302.
13. Grant IS, Andrews PJD. Neurologic support. Br Med J. 1999;319: 110-3.
14. Kapoor R. Raised intracranial pressure. Pediatr Today. 2000; 3:361.
15. Wutzler P. Antiviral therapy of herpes simplex and varicella zoster virus infections. Intervirology. 1997;40:343-56.
16. Klein SK, Hom DL, Anderson MR, *et al.* Predictive factors of short-term neurologic outcome in children with encephalitis. Pediatr Neurol. 1994;11:308-12.
17. Madge N, Diamond J, Miller D, *et al.* The National Childhood Encephalopathy Study: A 10-year follow-up. A report on the medical, social, behavioural and educational outcomes after serious acute neurologic illness in early childhood. Dev Med Child Neurol. 1993;68:1-118.
18. American Academy of Pediatrics: Arboviruses. In Peter G, Elk Grove Village IL editors: 1997 Red Book : Report of the Committee on Infectious Diseases, 24th edition, American Academy of Pediatrics, 1997;11:308-12.

CHAPTER

34

Metabolic Encephalopathies

Mahesh Kamate

INTRODUCTION

Inborn errors of metabolism (IEM) refer to a group of disorders resulting from the deficiency of activity of one or more specific enzymes or defects in the transportation of proteins. As of now, more than 500 disorders are known, and their estimated prevalence is 2–3/1000. Though rare, early recognition of IEM is of immense importance for prompt treatment and a better outcome. Many of the IEMs present to the intensive care in crisis precipitated by infections, stress and other factors. Irrespective of the cause, delay in initiation of appropriate treatment leads to death or irreversible brain damage. IEMs can present with nonspecific symptoms and resembles other common acquired conditions like sepsis, hypoxic-ischemic encephalopathy (HIE). Hence, it is important to consider IEM as an important clinical differential to these common conditions. As is the dictum in medicine, it is very important not to miss a treatable disorder, though rare.

When to Suspect IEM

The recognition of IEM in clinical practice is based on the following simple principles:[1]

- Think of IEM in the pediatric intensive care unit, when we have a child with altered sensorium where differentials of sepsis, hypoxic-ischemic encephalopathy, intoxication, encephalitis and brain tumors are considered and investigate accordingly.
- When common conditions causing encephalopathy are being treated, if few of the symptoms persist and remain unexplained after the initial treatment and the usual investigations have been performed, consider IEMs.
- All neonatal/infant deaths presumed to be due to sepsis, should be thought of as due to an underlying IEM. Do a biochemical autopsy and send necessary investigations.
- Not to confuse a symptom (such as peripheral neuropathy, retinitis pigmentosa, cardiomyopathy, etc.) or a syndrome (such as Reye syndrome, Leigh syndrome, sudden infant death, etc.) with etiology.
- There is no age bar to consider IEM; IEMs can affect individuals of all ages from fetal life to old age.
- Absence of family history should not rule out the possibility of IEM in a given scenario. Though IEMs are hereditary and transmitted as recessive disorders, in many cases there is no significant family history.
- Always think of IEMs, which are amenable to treatment (mainly those that cause intoxication). Presume IEMs and treat accordingly awaiting the final reports.
- Screen all sick children with few simple biochemical investigations (lactate, ammonia, blood gases, electrolytes, blood sugar, ketone bodies and liver/renal function tests) that can diagnose treatable IEMs.
- Do not hesitate to collaborate with specialized centers working on IEMs for investigations, guidance and treatment advice.
- Go through in detail, all the available reports (biochemical, histopathological, clinical autopsy) of the siblings who have died in the family and see if it can suggest an IEM.

DIAGNOSIS

Initial Investigations

Appropriate screening biochemical investigations like random blood sugar, arterial lactate, ammonia, liver function tests, renal function tests, serum electrolytes, ketones and reducing sugar in the urine, should be sent at presentation and not after the routine investigations are inconclusive. If IEM is a strong suspect or if we get positive clues on screening biochemical tests, then further confirmatory tests like tandem mass spectrometry (TMS), plasma and urine amino-acidogram, organic acids by urine gas chromatography/mass spectrometry (U-GCMS) should be considered.[2-4] **Flowchart 1** gives a simple

Flowchart 1: Approach to infant/young child with suspected metabolic disorder[2-4]

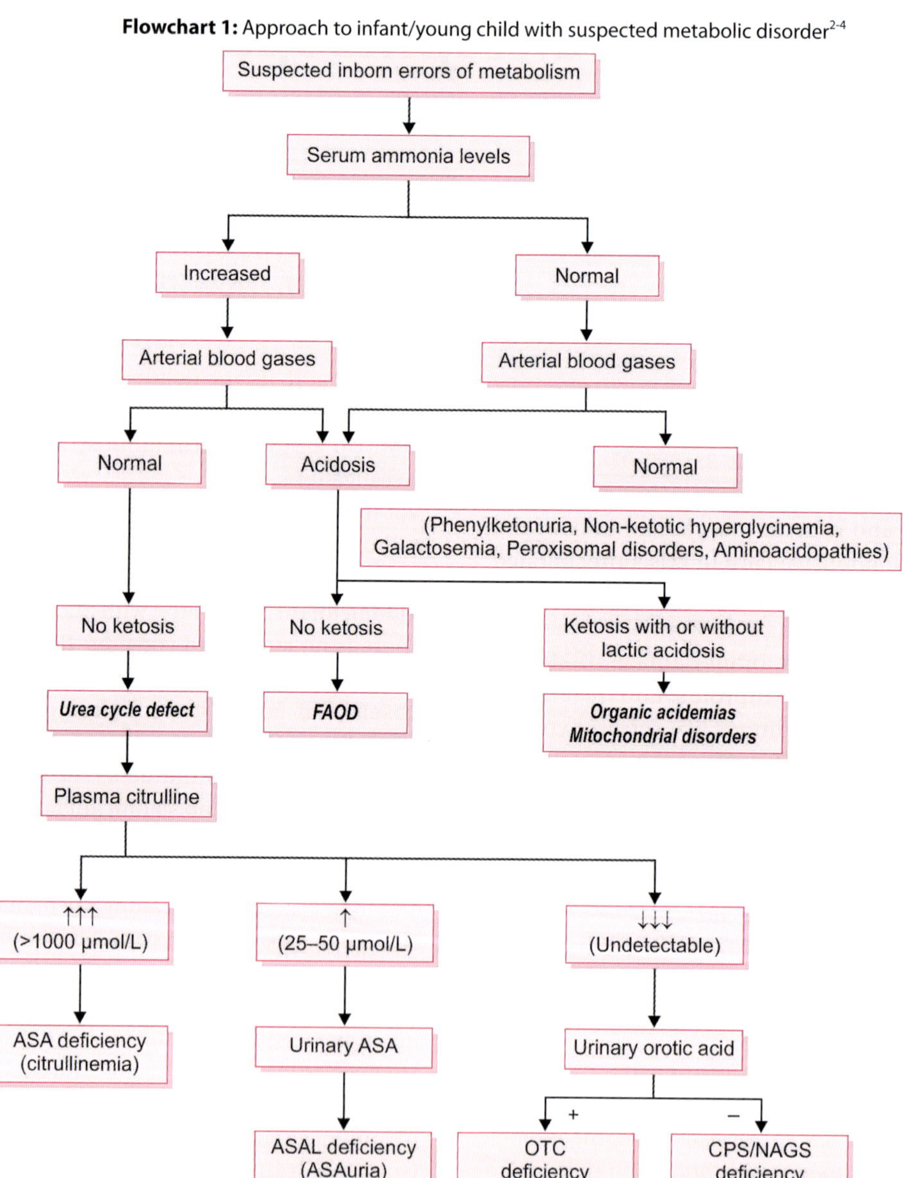

(FAOD: fatty acid oxidation defects, PKU: phenylketonuria, NKH: nonketotic hyperglycinemia, ASA: argininosuccinic acid, OTC: ornithine transcarbamoylase, CPS: carbamoylphosphate synthetase I; NAGS: N-acetylglutamate synthetase, THAN: transient hyperammonemia of newborn, ASAL: argininosuccinic acid lyase)

algorithm which helps in most neurometabolic disorders. Neuroimaging in the form of magnetic resonance imaging (MRI) of the brain with spectroscopy (MRS) also gives important clues for IEM and should be considered in every child with suspected IEM.[5] As we order for different tests, concurrently emergency treatment should be started. Based on the availability of reports the treatment can be subsequently modified later. There should not be any delay in treatment as delay leads to worse outcomes. Genetic tests based on next-generation sequencing (NGS) can also be used for confirmation and counseling for future pregnancies.

Clinical Scenarios Where IEMs are Very Likely

At all ages, consider IEM in children with neurological deterioration, liver failure, hypoglycemia, cardiac failure, hyperlactatemia in the absence of shock, sepsis, and intractable seizures. In older children, IEM should be considered in any type of coma, acute onset of psychiatric symptoms; gastrointestinal complaints like repeated admissions for unexplained dehydration, abdominal pain; muscle pain with or without myolysis and peripheral neuropathy. Unexplained deterioration after a period of apparent normalcy, parental consanguinity, family history of death in early childhood and rapidly progressive encephalopathy of obscure etiology, peculiar odor to body/urine are other strong pointers to IEM in a given scenario.

Among the various IEMs, disorders resulting from intoxication and energy metabolism disorders can present in intensive care units while most disorders involving complex molecules do not present acutely.

EMERGENCIES IN IEM

Encephalopathy with Biochemical Abnormalities

1. *Hyperammonemia*: Urea cycle defects, organic acidemia and rarely fatty acid oxidation defects.[6]
2. *Metabolic acidosis*: Acidosis secondary to lactic acid accumulation can be seen in mitochondrial and pyruvate metabolic defects and in organic acidemias like methylmalonic acidemia, proprionic acidemia, isovaleric acidemia and multiple carboxylase defects.[7]
   - *Metabolic acidosis with ketosis*: Glycogen storage disorders, fructose 1,6 diphosphatase deficiency, beta-ketothiolase deficiency, maple syrup urine disease (MSUD), organic acidemia and sometimes medium chain acyl CoA dehydrogenase deficiency.
   - *Metabolic acidosis without ketoacidosis*: When there is metabolic acidosis with moderate to severe lactic acidosis but without ketosis, then conditions like pyruvate dehydrogenase (PDH) deficiency, fatty acid oxidation disorders (FAOD), and few disorders of gluconeogenesis can be considered. Other than PDH deficiency, FAODs and gluconeogenesis disorders will have concomitant fasting hypoglycemia. Fructose-1,6-diphosphatase (F-1,6DP) deficiency usually presents with ketoacidosis, but during hypoglycemia, some of them can have low concentrations of ketone bodies. Patients who have normal anion gap metabolic acidosis without hyperlactatemia or hypoglycemia, the most frequent cause is renal tubular acidosis (RTA) type I or II.
3. *Hypoglycemia*: If hypoglycemia occurs shortly after feeds then it suggests hyperinsulinism; if after few hours of feed then glycogen storage disorders and if after prolonged fasting >8 hrs then it could be due to fatty acid oxidation defects. Hypoglycemia is prominently seen children in hereditary fructose intolerance, F-1,6DP deficiency, and galactosemia. **Flowchart 2** gives an approach to a child with severe or recurrent hypoglycemia.

Encephalopathy without Biochemical Abnormality

Some IEMs do not have positive results on initial screening. Examples include nonketotic hyperglycinemia, maple syrup urine disease (rarely ketosis and hypoglycemia), molybdenum cofactor deficiency/isolated sulfite oxidase deficiency, peroxisomal disorders and refractory seizures secondary to glucose transporter-1 deficiency syndrome (GLUT 1 DS), pyridoxine dependency, pyridoxal phosphate deficiency, folinic acid responsive seizures.

Presentation as Refractory Seizures

Biotinidase deficiency, methylmalonic acidemia, hyperhomocysteinemia, pyridoxine dependency and pyridoxal phosphate deficiency (in children <3 years), GLUT-1 deficiency syndrome, serine synthesis disorders, creatine synthesis disorders, purine metabolic defects, GABA transaminase deficiency, carbohydrate deficiency glycoprotein disorders, and few of the progressive myoclonic epilepsies [(myoclonic epilepsy with ragged red fibers (MERRF)] can present as difficult to control seizures.

Flowchart 2: Approach to child with persistent/recurrent hypoglycemia and suspected IEM[1-3]

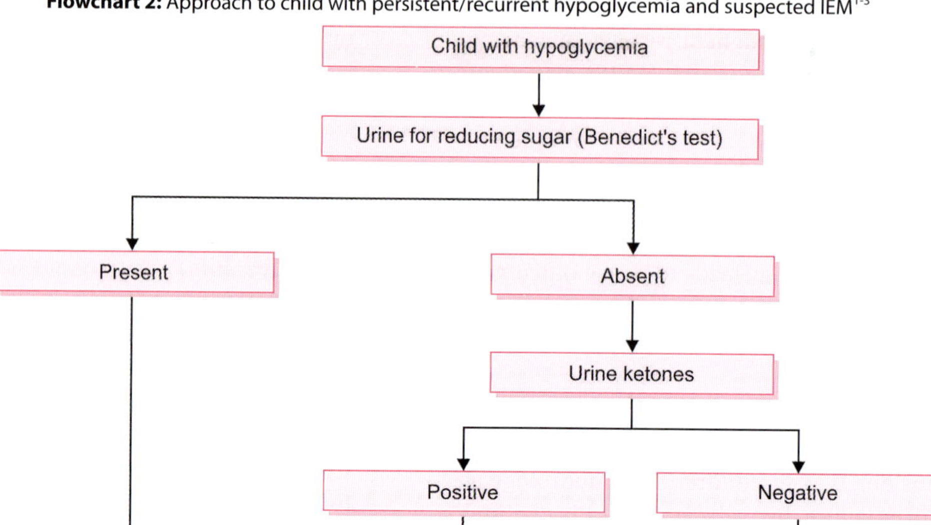

APPROACH TO DIAGNOSIS

Presenting Features

The IEMs presenting with acute encephalopathy (metabolic encephalopathy) is a common problem in intensive care units. IEM is a possibility in children with coma, including those who have focal neurological signs. Children with IEMs can present to the intensive care unit following an intercurrent event (infection, stress) or may present without an overt cause. All conditions that enhance protein catabolism in the body like increased protein intake, prolonged fasting, prolonged exercise may exacerbate such decompensations. It is important to elicit this history in all children with IEMs and educate the parents to avoid future recurrences. IEMs can have involvement like hepatic, gastrointestinal, neurological, and psychiatric system. Presence of specific organ involvement should not deter us from considering IEM. Few IEMs can improve spontaneously or with just supportive care while others progressively worsen resulting in death. The encephalopathy in some IEMs may be accompanied by focal neurological deficits like dystonia in organic acidemia, stroke-like presentation in mitochondrial encephalopathies, homocystinuria and urea cycle disorders.[1]

The IEMs can sometimes mimic presentations of encephalitis, basilar migraine, intoxication, poisoning, or cerebral thrombophlebitis. The presence of associated moderate ketoacidosis, hyperlactatemia, or hyperammonemia should make IEMs a strong possibility. Children with IEM can have premonitory symptoms like acute ataxia, persistent anorexia, chronic vomiting, failure to thrive, hypotonia, and progressive developmental delay. These premonitory symptoms can be seen in urea cycle disorders, respiratory chain defects, and organic acidurias. Repeated episodes consisting of acute onset ataxia, abnormal posturing of limbs with pain due to dystonia and weakness in limbs due to peripheral neuropathy can be seen in some late-onset forms of pyruvate dehydrogenase (PDH) deficiency.

Clinical Pointers

Though many IEMs do not have characteristic features some of them have clinical findings which could suggest a particular IEM. Abnormal twisting posturing of the limbs suggesting dystonia with a large head in an otherwise normal infant could suggest glutaric aciduria type I; organic acidemias present with repeated episodes of unexplained dehydration precipitated by infections; and hepatomegaly in a child with altered sensorium is important although inconsistent finding in F-1,6DP deficiency. During the acute phase, many of the organic acidemia like propionic acidemia, methylmalonic acidemia, and isovaleric acidemia can have severe hematologic manifestations and recurrent infections due to associated leukopenia. Disorders of cobalamin or folate metabolism can show macrocytic anemia on peripheral smear examination. When encephalopathy is associated with hepatic dysfunction, Reye syndrome secondary to urea cycle defects and FAODs should be considered. Similarly, hepatic coma with liver failure and hyperlactatemia can suggest the possibility of respiratory chain disorders. Wilson disease can present in a varied manner as hepatic coma with cirrhosis, chronic hepatic dysfunction, hemolytic jaundice, and various neurological signs (psychiatric, extrapyramidal). Acute psychiatric symptoms may be the predominant presentation of late-onset forms of urea cycle defects like ornithine transcarbamylase deficiency, maple syrup urine disease, acute intermittent porphyria, and homocysteine remethylation defects.

Recurrent episodes of dehydration secondary to polyuria, hyperventilation or excessive sweating can be a presentation of few IEMs like organic acidemia, cystinosis, and Fanconi-Bickel syndrome. In such clinical scenarios, accompanying findings like severe diarrhea, salt wasting, ketoacidosis, failure to thrive, Fanconi syndrome can be pointers to IEMs as a cause of dehydration.

Investigations

As mentioned earlier, whenever there is clinical suspicion of an IEM, general supportive measures and laboratory investigations should be undertaken simultaneously.

Biochemistry

Simple screening biochemical tests (arterial blood gases, serum ammonia, glucose, arterial lactate, urine ketone bodies with reducing sugars, electrolytes, liver and renal functional tests) should be considered in all cases of suspected IEM. Abnormal urine odors can be a useful clue for IEM. It may not be appreciated on a freshly voided urine sample. Abnormal odor can be detected by opening a container of urine, which has been closed at room temperature for a few minutes or on a drying filter paper. Normally, young infants do not excrete ketone bodies in urine and if there is Ketonuria in a neonate or a young infant, it is always abnormal and suggests IEM.[4] The simple bedside urine test, dinitrophenylhydrazine (DNPH) test screens for the presence of alpha-keto acids in urine and if positive could suggest a possibility of MSUD.

Unlike renal tubular acidosis, the metabolic acidosis of organic acidurias is usually associated with an increased anion gap. Urine pH should be below 5 in organic acidemia in contrast to renal tubular acidosis where it is generally above 5. It is important to appreciate that lactic acidosis up to 5 mmol/L can be seen with a normal blood pH value; only beyond 5 mmol/L, the pH will decrease. In the absence of infection, shock and tissue hypoxia, lactic acidosis suggests IEMs. Moderate elevations (3–6 mmol/L) are often observed in organic acidemias and hyperammonemias; levels greater than 10 mmol/L are frequent in hypoxia. In most anoxic lactic acidoses, ketosis is absent. Hyperammonemia seen in urea cycle defects induces respiratory alkalosis; hyperammonemia with ketoacidosis can be seen in organic acidemia (OA). At times isolated hyperammonemia can occur.

Hematology

Hematologic abnormalities can be seen in IEMs. Severe organic acidemia like propionic acidemia, methylmalonic acidemia, and isovaleric acidemia can induce granulocytopenia and thrombocytopenia. This is one of the reasons why many of these conditions might be mistaken for sepsis at presentation. Similarly, transaldolase deficiency and some forms of mevalonate kinase deficiency (early onset) can present with severe recurrent hemolytic anemia.

Caution in interpretation

The results of the various metabolic tests in IEMs need careful interpretation. They change with the condition of the patient (fasting or fed), the severity of the disease and with treatment. Many of the symptoms like acidosis and ketosis can be transient and can disappear with appropriate treatment. In untreated patients who are decompensated, many nonspecific abnormalities (respiratory acidosis due to the altered sensorium, severe lactic acidosis, secondary hyperammonemia) can complicate the original metabolic profile. This typically happens in fatal IEMs like urea cycle disorders, in which the initial finding of hyperammonemia with respiratory alkalosis shifts turns into a rather non-specific picture of acidosis and hyperlactatemia.[6] Hence, it is important to look at the initial biochemical blood reports and observe the trends rather than absolute values.

Ketosis can be physiological when it occurs during fasting, catabolism, repeated vomiting, following the use of medium-chain triglyceride enriched or other ketogenic diets. This usually does not produce metabolic acidosis and is not associated with lactic acidosis or hypoglycemia. Disorders of Ketolysis like succinyl-CoA transferase and 3-ketothiolase deficiencies usually have persistent moderate ketonuria occurring mainly in the fed state at the end of the day. When there is moderate to severe fasting ketonuria without acidosis with marked hepatomegaly, it could suggest glycogen storage disorder III.

Increased lactate does not always suggest an underlying IEM and is frequently seen in intensive care units in children with shock, hypoxia, and in other conditions involving failure of cellular respiration. It is prudent that these acquired conditions must be excluded before an inborn error of lactate-pyruvate oxidation is considered. Similarly, persistently increased lactate levels can also result from many acquired conditions, like diarrhea, persistent infections (mainly urinary tract infections), hyperventilation, and liver cell failure. It is important to note that when tissue hypoxia causes lactic acidosis, ketosis is absent, while it is a nearly constant finding in most IEM (except in PDH deficiency, glycogen storage disorder type-I and FAODs). The serum levels of lactate do not suggest acquired cause or IEMs. Some acquired disorders like shock can be associated with very high levels, whereas in IEMs of lactate-pyruvate metabolism there could be just moderate lactic acidosis.

MANAGEMENT

The treatment in IEMs should not wait for the confirmation of diagnosis. As soon as the diagnosis of IEM is considered, an emergency management plan should be in place. Emergency treatment for IEM should be started concurrently along with the workup and as and when the results of biochemical tests arrive, the treatment can be subsequently modified accordingly.[8]

Stabilization and Initial Treatment

Many times, treatment may have to be instituted empirically without a specific diagnosis. Treatment mainly consists of supportive care in the form of ventilation and circulatory support, careful rehydration, correction of electrolyte, calcium and phosphate imbalance, prevention, early recognition and if present treatment of infection/ septicemia with antibiotics.

Patients with a metabolic encephalopathy frequently suffer from septicemia, that results in persistent catabolism and lead to therapeutic failure. Hence, it is prudent that while managing IEMs, infections must be prevented, thoroughly investigated for and, if present, treated appropriately. Acidosis correction is important and bicarbonate can be used if pH is less than 7.1. When pH is more than 7.1, correction of dehydration, hypoglycemia and providing adequate calories/proteins will suffice. Excessive bicarbonate when given intravenously can cause paradoxical CNS acidosis and cerebral edema; hence, bicarbonate should be used with caution. When possible, oral supplementation of sodium bicarbonate is encouraged as it is safe and does not cause sudden changes in pH. When required, IV sodium bicarbonate can be given at 0.35–0.5 mEq/kg/hr (max: 1–2 mEq/kg/hr). Sodium bicarbonate alkalizes the urine and increases the excretion of organic acids. Diuretics can be used if urine output is less than 3–4 mL/kg/day. Metronidazole is used in children with propionic acidemia and methylmalonic acidemia (MMA) as 20% propionic acid comes from gut bacteria. In some cases of MMA, forced alkaline diuresis can be used.

Nutrition in IEM

Nutritional management needs priority irrespective of the underlying disease. Nutritional supplements and dietary modifications are two important steps in the nutritional management of IEM. It is important to provide adequate calories (At least the age-related recommended daily energy: 100–120 kcal/kg/day). Otherwise, there would be catabolism and worsening of the metabolic crisis. We need to correct the metabolic imbalance and that can be done by restricting (or supplementing) one or more nutrients or dietary components depending on the type of IEM. Treatment should be started as early as possible and should preferably be oral if the condition and clinical status allow. Start IV 10% dextrose at glucose infusion rate of 8–10 mg/kg/ min. Calorie requirement can be met by giving oral (NGT) or parenteral administration of glucose 15–30 g/kg/day and lipids 2–4 g/kg/day (once fatty acid oxidation disorders are ruled out). Feeding should be either by continuous enteral feeding or total parenteral nutrition (TPN). TPN is used if there is intestinal intolerance and there is a need for high-energy or high-glucose requirements or invasive techniques required.[1]

Insulin

To counter hyperglycemia secondary to high glucose infusions and due to its anabolic effect insulin is used to suppress severe catabolism. Prerequisite for its use is dehydration and acidosis should be corrected. Can be started as infusion of 0.05–0.3 IU/kg/h if RBS >150 mg/dL. The dose is adjusted frequently to control glycemia. Once there is sustained normalization of glucose then slowly withdraw insulin.

Proteins

For maintenance of anabolism, not only energy, even all the essential amino acids should be provided. For patients who have a restriction of specific amino acids, such as in propionic acidemia, early introduction of a metabolic formula with gastric drip-feeding can be used. For disorders with limitation of overall protein intakes, such as urea cycle defects or organic acidemias, protein should be restricted up to 24–48 hours. The requirement for essential amino acids should still be fulfilled. Otherwise, this will induce catabolism with more severe protein catabolism. A first practical approach can be to provide a medical food containing essential amino acids via gastric feeding or drip-feeding. If all enteral feedings are not possible, then intravenous protein should be given without delay to provide the essential amino acids.

Mode of nutrition

Total parenteral nutrition: This is the method of choice in the acute state as usually there is higher risk of gastric intolerance in the initial stages. To avoid exacerbation of existing hyperammonemia, usually the amino acid free TPN solution is suitable for the first 2 days. Later on, protein must then be added using a commercially available amino acid-solution as early as possible. The recommended daily requirement of the amino acids should be met with TPN.

Enteral feeding: As the condition of the baby stabilizes, an attempt to switch from parenteral to enteral nutrition should be made. This shift has to be gradual and done over a 4-day to 5-day period, using continuous nasogastric tube feeding. Because of the risk of gastric intolerance, initially, small volumes are given and then increased every 24 h until the full fluid requirement is met. As the amount of enteral feeds is gradually increased, the parenteral infusion rate is decreased reciprocally. To prevent vomiting which is commonly seen, antiemetic drugs like ondansetron can be given. The general principles of enteral nutrition include progressively increasing the protein intake to reach the recommended daily requirements using human milk or infant formula; slow addition of calories using either carbohydrates (glucose polymer) and lipids, and supplementation of micronutrients (minerals and vitamins). It is important to ensure that the prescribed diet provides 130–150 kcal/kg/day. If a high osmolar diet is given, it can result in diarrhea and dehydration. If the underlying IEM is known then, the appropriate amino acid mixture can be added to cover the protein requirement. After the serum ammonia (NH_3 < 100 micromols/L) and acidosis are corrected, natural proteins are introduced using measured amounts of infant formula (0.5 g/kg/day).

Specific Therapy

It can be used for certain disorders. To enhance the excretion of toxic metabolites, substrates that enable the excretion of ammonia by alternate pathways like sodium benzoates and acceleration of removal of the substrate can be used. Cofactor replacement is an important step in many IEMs (**Table 1**).[3] Carnitine is supplemented to compensate for secondary carnitine deficiency caused by urinary excretion of carnitine bound organic acids. Replacement of product that is not produced is also important in some IEMs like creatine monohydrate in guanidinoacetate methyltransferase deficiency, arginine in arginino-succinicaciduria, and L-Serine in 3-phosphoglycerate dehydrogenase deficiency.

Children with mild hyperammonemia/acidosis

Most of these children have signs of dehydration and rehydration should be done over 24 hours. Meanwhile, a procedure for toxin removal has to be arranged. Rehydration can be done using a standard 5–10% glucose solution containing 34 mmol/L of Na^+, and 20 mmol/L of K^+. Simultaneously to avoid ongoing catabolism, high-calorie, protein-free nutrition should be started using carbohydrates and lipids to provide 100 kcal/kg/day. For the first 24–36 hours, because of gastric intolerance, parenteral and enteral nutrition can be used together. However, to avoid acute protein malnutrition, the

Table 1: Cofactors in inborn errors of metabolism

Cofactor	*Disorders*
Thiamine	MSUD, PDH deficiency and complex I deficiency
Riboflavin	Glutaric aciduria Type I and II, complex I deficiency
Pyridoxine	Homocystinuria, pyridoxine dependency, xanthurenic aciduria, primary hyperoxaluria type I
Pyridoxal PO_4	Pyridoxamine 5-phosphate oxidase deficiency
Cobalamin	Methylmalonic acidemia
Folic acid	Some cases of homocystinuria
Folinic acid	Hereditary orotic aciduria, methionine synthase deficiency, cerebral folate transporter deficiency, Kearns-Sayre syndrome
Biotin	Biotinidase deficiency, holocarboxylase synthetase deficiency
Pantothenic acid	3-methylglutaconic aciduria Type III
Nicotinamide	Hartnup disease
Coenzyme Q10	CoQ10 deficiency, mitochondrial cytopathies
Ascorbic acid	Hawkinsuria, tyrosinemia type III
Vitamin E	Abetalipoproteinemia, glutathione synthetase deficiency
Tetrahydrobiopterin	Disorders of BH4 synthesis, BH4 responsive forms of PKU

protein-free diet should not be used for more than 2 days. As the levels of toxic metabolites like ammonia, lactate has decreased, natural proteins are introduced using calculated amounts of infant formula.[6,7]

Children with severe hyperammonemia/acidosis

It is important to note that children with severe keto-acidosis have intracellular dehydration that is often underestimated. Over-zealous rehydration with hypotonic fluids and alkalization can cause or exacerbate pre-existing cerebral edema in such situations. Hence, intravenous fluids should be given slowly over a 48-h period, with an infusion of less than 150 mL/kg/24 h, that contains an average concentration of 70–85 mmol/L of sodium, 30–40 mmol/L of potassium and 5% dextrose. The associated acidosis usually improves with the first measures of toxin removal. However, if does not improve or it is severe (pH<7.10) then it can be partially corrected with IV bicarbonate or oral bicarbonate supplementation. Aggressive therapy with repeated boluses of IV bicarbonate can be harmful as it causes hypernatremia, cerebral edema, and rarely, even cerebral hemorrhage. As a general rule, to compensate for bicarbonate consumption, 25–50% of the calculated sodium requirements can be given as sodium bicarbonate during the first 6–12 h of fluid therapy.[6,7]

Removal of Toxin(s)

To facilitate the elimination of accumulated ammonia, sodium benzoate and/or sodium phenylacetate is given at 250–500 mg/kg/day in 4 divided doses. Sodium benzoate and sodium phenylacetate provide alternative pathways for nitrogen elimination by conjugation with glycine and glutamine, respectively. In all urea cycle disorders (except arginase deficiency), because of the block in the enzymatic pathway, L-arginine is not produced, and it becomes an essential amino acid. Hence, in these conditions, it is important to supplement L-arginine at a dose of 250–500 mg/kg/day. As intravenous preparation is not available in India, sodium benzoate can be given orally through a nasogastric tube.

In cases of hyperammonemia due to N-acetylglutamate synthetase deficiency, N-carbamyl glutamate has to be given. N-carbamyl glutamate is also helpful in hyper-ammonemia seen in severe organic acidemia where the accumulating acyl-coenzyme A inhibits N-acetylglutamate synthetase enzyme.

Extracorporeal procedures

When the above measures fail or if the serum ammonia levels are very high then dialysis (hemofiltration, hemo-dialysis) and peritoneal dialysis can be considered. However, peritoneal dialysis is not very effective.

Role of L-carnitine in Neurometabolic Disorders

L-carnitine supplementation at doses of 100–150 mg/kg/day in 3–4 divided doses helps to compensate losses of carnitine that occurs due to urinary excretion of carnitine bound organic acids. L-carnitine supplementation never worsens these disorders and as a rule in the acute stage, there is no harm is giving carnitine. L-carnitine supplementation should be avoided in children with suspected long chain fatty acid oxidation defect. In this condition, carnitine supplementation leads to acute accumulation of toxic long-chain acyl carnitines and increases the risk of a fatal cardiac arrhythmia.

Specific Conditions: Organic Acidemias

These disorders are also treated on the same lines as hyperammonemia. Along with supportive care, dietary measures and carnitine (100–200 mg/kg/day in 3–4 divided doses), biotin (10–40 mg per day) and in isovaleric acidemia and methylcrotonyl CoA carboxylase deficiency, glycine 250 mg/kg/day oral or intravenous can be given.

Primary Lactic Acidosis (Mitochondriopathies)

Treatment includes supportive care with hydration, sepsis treatment, ventilation; avoiding sodium valproate; treatment of acidosis if pH <7.1 with sodium bicarbonate (0.35–0.5 mEq/kg/hr, maximum:1–2 mEq/kg/hr); supplementing thiamine up to 300 mg/day in 4 divided doses, riboflavin 100 mg/day in 4 divided doses, coenzyme Q10 at 5–15 mg/kg/day, biotin 10–20 mg twice a day, and L-carnitine at 100–150 mg/kg/day.

Refractory Seizures

Treatment includes trial of pyridoxine 100 mg IV or oral 20–50 mg/kg/day, pyridoxal phosphate 10 mg/kg 6th hourly and if seizures persist, then biotin 10–40 mg/day and folinic acid 15 mg/day (0.5–1 mg/kg). Glucose transporter-1 defect (where CSF sugar ≤1/3rd blood sugar) is usually treated with ketogenic diet.

KEY MESSAGES

- Inborn errors of metabolism can present like meningoencephalitis, toxic encephalopathy, status epilepticus, or hepatic/renal encephalopathy.
- Initial investigations should include blood sugar, serum electrolytes, lactate, ammonia, arterial blood gases, ketone bodies and liver/renal function tests for all children.
- Treatment should be started immediately presuming IEMs pending the metabolic investigations and modified as and when the reports are available. If treatment is instituted early, better outcomes can be expected.
- Main principles of treatment include stabilization including supportive measures, dietary interventions, specific treatment with cofactors and use of extracorporeal measures to remove accumulating toxins.
- Always attempt to confirm the correct diagnosis in a case and genetic confirmation, so that parents can be offered prenatal diagnosis.

REFERENCES

1. Fernandes J, Saudubray JM, van den Berghe G, Walter JH, editors. Inherited Metabolic Diseases-Diagnosis and Treatment, 4th edition Heidelberg: Springer Medizin Verlag; 2006.
2. Childs B, Valle D, Jimenez-Sanchez. The Inborn error and biochemical variability. In: Scriver CR, Beaudet AL, Sly WS, Valle D, editors. The Metabolic and Molecular Basis of Inherited Disease, 8th edition, New York: McGraw-Hill, 2001. p.155-66.
3. Clarke JTR. A Clinical Guide to Inherited Metabolic Diseases, 3rd, edition. Cambridge: Cambridge University Press; 2006.
4. Cataltepe SU, Levy HL. Inborn errors of metabolism. In: Cloherty JP, Eichenwald EC, Stark AR, editors. Manual of Neonatal Care, 6th edition. Philadelphia: Lippincott Williams & Wilkins; 2008. p. 558-73.
5. Blaser S, Feigenbaum A. A neuroimaging approach to inborn errors of metabolism. Neuroimag Clin N Am. 2004;14:307-29.
6. Leonard JV, Morris AAM. Urea cycle disorders. Semin Neonatol. 2002;7:27-35.
7. de Baulny HO, Saudubray JM. Branched-chain organic acidurias. Semin Neonatol. 2002;7:65-74.
8. Saudubray JM, Sedel F, Walter JH. Clinical approach to treatable inborn metabolic diseases: An introduction. J Inherit Metab Dis. 2006;29:261-74.

CHAPTER 35

Acute Diarrhea and Dehydration

Ashok K Patwari

INTRODUCTION

Diarrhea is one of the leading causes of childhood mortality, accounting for approximately 8% of all deaths among children under the age of 5 years, worldwide in 2016.[1] Oral rehydration therapy (ORT), one of the greatest scientific achievements in the last century, has revolutionized management of diarrheal dehydration and led to a significant reduction of diarrhea-related deaths. For children aged 1–15 months, the mortality rate from diarrhea reduced from 9·4 per 1000 livebirths in 2000 to 3·2 per 1000 livebirths in 2015,[2] even though the prevalence of diarrhea has not significantly reduced.[3] Eighty percent of these deaths occur in the first 2 years of life; main causes being dehydration, complications associated with dysentery, malnutrition, and serious co-infections such as pneumonia. Most of the diarrheal episodes occur during the first 2 years of life (highest incidence 6–11 months), in low socioeconomic status, in non-breastfed infants, and in association with measles, severe malnutrition and immunodeficiency.

Dehydration, the immediate consequence of diarrheal diseases, remains the primary focus in case management. Dehydration is a frequent and a serious consequence of acute watery diarrhea (acute episode of diarrhea lasting <2 weeks) including cholera, but some cases of dysentery (clinical syndrome characterized by the presence of visible blood and mucus in the stools, abdominal cramps and fever) and persistent diarrhea (an episode that lasts for ≥14 days, often associated with growth failure) may also present with variable degree of dehydration. Prolonged and recurrent episodes of diarrhea adversely affect the nutritional status of a child and thereby significantly contribute to vicious cycle of malnutrition and infection.[4]

DIARRHEAL DEHYDRATION

Young children are more susceptible to develop dehydration due to limited urinary concentration capacity of the kidneys, more insensible losses of water through skin and lungs owing to large surface area and rapid breathing, and their dependence on adults to replace their fluid losses. Loss of water and electrolytes in the diarrheal stool results in depletion of the extracellular fluid volume (ECFV), electrolyte imbalance and clinical manifestations of dehydration. Even though both intracellular and extracellular fluid compartments are depleted in diarrhea, the measurement of ECFV show mostly a depletion of this compartment. The reason is that ECFV contracts in "two directions" – out in the stools and into the cell – so that the net measured loss of volume appears to come chiefly from the ECFV. Continued ECFV contraction is at the root of all the physiological changes taking place in dehydration and reversion to normal is more readily accomplished by solutions more nearly approximating that of the extracellular fluid.

The first symptom of dehydration appears after fluid loss of about 5% of body weight. When fluid loss reaches 10%, shock often sets in and the cascade of events that follows can culminate in death unless there is immediate intervention. Without treatment, severe episodes literally wring out body fluids from the patient faster than they can be replaced. Rehydration, whether given orally or intravenously, is the only effective therapy.

COMPENSATORY MECHANISMS IN ACUTE DIARRHEA

Contraction of the ECFV, consequent upon loss of water and electrolytes in diarrheal stools, leads to increase in renin, angiotensin, aldosterone and antidiuretic hormone (ADH), and fall of glomerular filtration rate (GFR). All these changes lead to compensatory retention of salt and water but proportionately more of the latter. The first response to ECFV contraction is thirst, and if water is administered, it will be mostly retained due to the effect of ADH. In addition, water may also be generated internally by steroids and catecholamines. Therefore, retention of water by these mechanisms results in isotonic or hypotonic dehydration. Pre-existing or uncorrected potassium deficiency can also perpetuate hypotonicity.

Comparison of various intravenous regimens containing high or low sodium have shown that rational treatment should reverse all the compensatory events by restoring volume quickly, correcting acidosis and reducing potassium deficit with solutions approximating the composition of the extracellular fluid. The more hypotonic the fluid is with respect to sodium, the less well it can quickly correct the ECFV contraction.

CLINICAL FEATURES

Most enteropathogens can cause diarrhea by more than one mechanism. Hence, the clinical presentation depends upon the underlying pathophysiological changes taking place in the gastrointestinal tract. Three clinical types of diarrhea have been defined, each reflecting a different mechanism.

1. *Secretory diarrhea*: It is characterized by acute watery diarrhea with profound losses of water and electrolytes due to sodium pump failure as a result of the action of identified toxins [e.g. cholera, enterotoxigenic *Escherichia coli* (*ETEC*)]. This group is at risk of rapid development of dehydration and electrolyte imbalance.
2. *Invasive diarrhea (Dysentery)*: Intestinal mucosal cells are invaded by the microorganisms, which set up an inflammatory reaction clinically presenting with blood and mucus in the stools [*Shigella, Salmonella,* enteroinvasive *Escherichia coli* (EIEC), *Campylobacter jejuni,* rotavirus, *Entamoeba histolytica*]. This group is also prone to develop other complications like intestinal perforation, toxic megacolon, rectal prolapse, convulsions, septicemia and hemolytic uremic syndrome.
3. *Osmotic diarrhea*: Injury to enterocytes may result in brush border damage [*Giardia lamblia,* Rotavirus, Enteropathogenic *E. coli* (EPEC), *Y. enterocolitica*] and destruction leading to decreased mucosal disaccharidase activity (*Y. enterocolitica*). Clinical presentation in these cases is characterized by passing of large, frothy, explosive and acidic stools. High osmolar solutions given orally (e.g. fruit juices, carbonated soft drinks and ORS with high sugar content) can also result in osmotic diarrhea. Besides worsening of the hydration status of the child, there is also a serious danger of developing hypernatremia in these cases.

APPROACH TO CASE MANAGEMENT

In order to institute an appropriate treatment plan, a patient with acute diarrhea should be assessed and managed as per following approach:

- Determine nature and pattern of diarrhea
- General assessment of the child
- Assessment of hydration status and administration of appropriate fluids for prevention and treatment of dehydration
- Correction of electrolyte and acid-base imbalance
- Proper feeding to provide normal nutritional requirements
- Zinc supplementation
- Treatment of associated infection
- Nutritional rehabilitation
- Prevention of diarrhea.

ASSESSMENT OF DEHYDRATION

Loss of water and electrolytes in the stools can produce varying degree of dehydration. Thirst and irritability are the earliest symptoms, which appear by the time an infant has already lost about 5% of body weight. Extreme degree of dehydration presents with alteration in consciousness, shock, acidosis and renal failure. Several clinical signs and symptoms can help in detecting dehydration. However, a simple assessment chart suggested by Integrated Management of Neonatal and Childhood Illness (IMNCI)[5]

Table 1: Assessment of dehydration in a patient with diarrhea[5]

Clinical signs			
General condition	Well, alert	Restless, irritable	Lethargic or unconscious
Eyes	Normal	Sunken	Sunken
Thirst	Drinks normally, not thirsty	Drinks eagerly, thirsty	Drinks poorly, not able to drink
Skin pinch	Goes back quickly	Goes back slowly	Goes back very slowly
Decide hydration status	The patient has *No Dehydration*	If the patient has two or more above signs, there is *Some Dehydration*	If the patient has two or more Above signs, there is *Severe Dehydration*
Treatment plan	Plan A	Plan B	Plan C

can be referred for quick assessment of dehydration (**Table 1**). According to the assessment chart, a patient may be grouped as "no dehydration" (when there are less than two signs of dehydration), "some dehydration" (presence of at least two of the signs) and "severe dehydration" (presence of two or more signs of dehydration in this category). Depending upon the state of hydration, patients with "no dehydration" (Plan A) or "some" dehydration (Plan B) can be successfully treated with ORT, and the ones with "severe dehydration" should be initially rehydrated by intravenous therapy (Plan C) and supplemented by/changed over to ORT as soon as the child is able to take orally (**Table 2**). ORT alone may not successfully rehydrate a child with "some dehydration" in certain situations such as high purge rate (watery stools >15 mL/kg/hour), persistent vomiting (≥4 episodes/hour), inability to drink (due to severe stomatitis, fatigue, central nervous system depression induced by antiemetics or antimotility drugs), and glucose malabsorption. Such cases need to be rehydrated with intravenous therapy as per Plan C if they fail to rehydrate after a trial of Plan B.

ORAL REHYDRATION THERAPY

The ORT is the main mode of treatment of diarrheal diseases. The term ORT includes (i) Oral rehydration salt (ORS) solution of WHO-recommended composition, (ii) Food-based solutions (with appropriate concentration of salt), and (iii) Plenty of water along with continued feeding.

The use of ORS to treat diarrhea stems from the discovery during 1960s of coupled active transport of glucose and sodium in the small bowel resulting in the passive absorption of water and other electrolytes even during copious diarrhea. The standard WHO/UNICEF formulation saved millions of lives in late 20th century, but did not decrease diarrheal duration or stool output. Additionally, there was a concern among pediatricians that there was a risk of hypernatremia with standard WHO-ORS when given to children with non-cholera diarrhea. Reduced osmolarity of ORS achieved by reducing the glucose and salt concentrations of the solution, to avoid possible adverse effects of hypertonicity on net fluid absorption, has been found to be safe and efficacious in treating children with diarrhea. Because of the improved effectiveness of reduced osmolarity ORS solution, WHO and Indian Academy of Pediatrics recommend use of reduced osmolarity ORS (**Table 3**) as the universal solution for treatment and prevention of dehydration for all causes of diarrhea, and at all ages.[6-8]

INTRAVENOUS FLUID THERAPY

Ringer's lactate given rapidly as 30 mL/kg followed by 70 mL/kg for deficit therapy is considered the treatment of choice for severe dehydration (**Table 2**). However, in order to encourage oral feeding, the child should be offered ORS (5 mL/kg/h) along with intravenous infusion as soon as he is able to drink orally. It is imperative to closely watch the child for passage of urine after plasma expansion has been achieved by rapid intravenous therapy. If the child fails to pass urine even after 2 hours of administering Ringer's lactate, acute renal failure should be suspected and managed accordingly.

Rehydration of Children Having Severe Malnutrition

Rehydration of children having severe malnutrition deserves special attention owing to certain pathophysiological changes in water and electrolyte balance peculiar to protein energy malnutrition (PEM). Children with severe PEM have an increase in total body water and

Table 2: Rehydration therapy in acute diarrhea

Treatment plan	*Plan A*	*Plan B*	*Plan C*
State of hydration	No dehydration	Some dehydration	Severe dehydration
Percentage of body weight loss	<5	5–10	>10
Estimated fluid deficit (mL/kg)	<50	50–100	>100
Goals of management	Replacement of ongoing losses of fluid and electrolytes	Correction of existing deficits of fluid and electrolytes	Urgent replacement of existing deficits of fluid and electrolytes
Fluid therapy	Oral rehydration therapy	Oral rehydration therapy	Intravenous fluid therapy
Treatment facility	Home	Health facility	Health facility
Rehydration fluid	Homemade solutions/ORS	ORS	Ringer's lactate*
Amount of rehydrating fluid	For every loose stool: 10 mL/kg body wt or *Children < 2 years:* (50–100 mL) *Children 2–10 years:* (100–200 mL) *Older children and adults*: as much as desired **plus** Free access to drinking water	50–100 mL/kg body wt (average 75 mL/kg) over 4 hours** **plus** *Non-breastfeed infants less than 6 months:* 100–200 mL of clean drinking water *Older children and adults:* Free access to plain water in addition to ORS	*Infants:* 30 mL/kg over 1 hour followed by 70 mL/kg over 5 hours *Older children and adults:* 30 mL/kg over ½ hour followed by 70 mL/kg over 2 ½ hours **plus** ORS (5 mL/kg/hour) to be started orally as soon as the child is able to drink
Monitoring	Watch for vomiting, early signs of dehydration, blood in the stools, etc. **Reassess** after 2 days or earlier	Monitor every hour and reassess after 4 hours: - If still in Plan B, repeat as above - If rehydrated shift to *Plan A* on ORS	Monitor ½ hourly and reassess after 6 hour (infants), or 3 hour (older children): - If still in Plan C, repeat as above - If rehydrated shift to Plan B or A as per hydration status

* Normal saline (0.9% NaCl) or half strength Darrow's solution may be used if Ringer's lactate is not available.
** Severely malnourished children should be rehydrated slowly over 6–12 hours.
(ORS: oral rehydration salt solution)

sodium while potassium stores in the body are depleted. The renal concentration capacity is poor, and thus they cannot conserve water efficiently. Moreover, they cannot handle excessive fluid and salt load, and can develop fluid retention. On the one hand, malnourished children are more prone to diarrheal dehydration, but if given excessive fluids, they run a risk of developing cardiac failure. This risk is further increased by the fact that it is often difficult to judge the extent of dehydration in these children owing to absence of subcutaneous fat. Assessment of hydration status is also difficult because a few signs that are normally used are unreliable in the presence of malnutrition. Marasmic children normally have sunken eyes, and the diminished skin turgor may be masked by edema in children with kwashiorkor. In both types of patients, irritability or apathy makes assessment of mental state difficult. Signs that remain useful for assessing hydration status in severe PEM include: eagerness to drink (sign of some dehydration); very dry mouth and tongue, cool and moist extremities, and weak or absent radial pulse (signs of severe dehydration). It is often difficult to distinguish between some and severe dehydration in severely malnourished children, and it is best to assume at least some dehydration if they have acute watery diarrhea.

Table 3: Reduced osmolarity ORS formulation recommended by WHO/UNICEF

Reduced osmolarity ORS	*g*	*mOsm*	*L*
Sodium chloride	2.6	Sodium	75
Glucose, anhydrous	13.5	Chloride	65
Potassium chloride	1.5	Glucose, anhydrous	75
Trisodium citrate	2.9	Potassium	20
		Citrate	10
Total osmolarity 245 mOsm/L			

The WHO recommends special ORS [Rehydration Solution for Malnutrition (ReSoMal)] for children with severe malnutrition. Several workers have reported a high incidence of hyponatremic dehydration in malnourished children and found low osmolarity ORS to be safe in these children. However, it is recommended that rehydration of severely malnourished children should be carefully monitored and preferably take place in a hospital. Rehydration with ORS solution should be preferred because IV fluids can easily cause overhydration and heart failure. Rehydration should take place slowly in children with severe malnutrition giving 70–100 mL of ORS solution per kg body weight over 6–12 hours (5 mL/kg every 30 minutes for first 2 hours, then 5–10 mL/kg/hour for the next 4–10 hours).[9] The exact amount depends on how much the child wants, volume of stool loss, and whether the child is vomiting. Feeding should begin as soon as possible, preferably along with dehydration correction, and supplemental potassium should be provided for 2 weeks.

ELECTROLYTE DISTURBANCES

Hypernatremia

Some children with diarrhea, especially young infants, develop hypernatremic dehydration, which usually follows use of hypertonic drinks (canned fruit juices, carbonated cold drink, incorrectly prepared ORS or salt and sugar solutions). Children with hypernatremic dehydration (serum sodium >150 mEq/L, osmolality >295 mOsm/kg) are extremely thirsty, out of proportion to the other signs of dehydration, and sometimes have convulsions. Patients with hypernatremic dehydration have a total body deficit of sodium, even though the concentration of this cation in serum and extracellular fluid is abnormally high. Therefore, infants with overt diarrheal dehydration of the hypernatremic variety can be successfully treated with reduced osmolarity ORS solution. Rapid absorption of this solution during the rehydration phase leads to expansion of intravascular compartment and increases renal perfusion. Administration of plain water provides free water for the infant's renal physiologic mechanism with which to carry out further homeostasis. However, if the child is unable to drink orally, Ringer's lactate can be initially given to treat shock and later switch over to ORT with ORS alternating with plain water.

Hyponatremia

Patients who ingest only large amount of water or watery drinks that contain very little salt, may present with hyponatremia (serum sodium <130 mmol/L, osmolality < 275 mOsm/kg water), which may be clinically associated with lethargy and seizures. ORS solution is safe and effective therapy for hyponatremia also. However, in the treatment of hyponatremia, administration of ORS alone without extra water has been observed to be superior because of higher sodium intake. For children who are unable to drink orally, IV infusion of Ringer lactate can effectively treat hyponatremia.

Hypokalemia

Inadequate replacement of potassium losses during diarrhea can lead to potassium depletion and hypokalemia (serum potassium <3 mEq/L), which may result in muscle weakness,[10] paralytic ileus, renal impairment and cardiac arrhythmias. Severe potassium depletion, particularly in malnourished children, may lead to acute onset flaccid paralysis ranging from neck flop to quadriparesis and even respiratory paralysis.[11] The potassium deficit can be corrected by using ORS solution for rehydration therapy and by feeding potassium rich foods (e.g. banana) during and after diarrhea. Oral potassium supplementation (2 mEq/kg/ day) is indicated in malnourished children. In transient flaccid paralysis due to hypokalemia, potassium can be administered parenterally by using 15% solution of potassium chloride (1 mL = 2 mEq of potassium) but not exceeding 40 mEq/L of IV fluids after ensuring adequate renal function.

Metabolic Acidosis

During acute diarrhea, large amounts of bicarbonate may be lost in the stools. If the kidneys continue to function normally, most of the lost bicarbonate is replenished, and a serious base deficit does not develop. Metabolic acidosis tends to correct spontaneously in most of the cases as the child is properly rehydrated. WHO/UNICEF ORS solution contains adequate bicarbonate/citrate to counter acidosis in less severe cases. However, in severe dehydration, compromised renal function leads to rapid development of base deficit and metabolic acidosis. Hypovolemic shock, as a consequence of rapid loss of water and electrolytes in severe diarrhea, results in excessive production of lactic acid, which may further contribute to metabolic acidosis. Rapid intravenous infusion of Ringer's lactate, which contains 28 mEq/L of lactate (metabolized to bicarbonate), is recommended in severe dehydration. However, in the presence of circulatory failure, bicarbonate precursors (e.g. citrate, lactate) may not be readily metabolized in the body.

If the patient presents with severe metabolic acidosis (pH <7.20, serum HCO_3^- <8 mEq/L), sodium bicarbonate in a bolus dose of 2–3 mEq/kg may be administered to correct acidosis. If facilities for blood gas estimation are available, accurate dose of bicarbonate can be calculated by the formula: bicarbonate dose (mEq) = (desired HCO_3^- – observed HCO_3^-) × 0.6 × body weight in kg. It is preferable to increase the bicarbonate level only up to 12 mEq/L to prevent overshoot metabolic alkalosis. Attention should be paid to serum potassium concentration as correction of acidosis in a patient with low potassium can lead to life-threatening severe hypokalemia.

ZINC SUPPLEMENTATION

Zinc deficiency is common in children from developing countries because of intake of predominant vegetarian diets and the high content of dietary phytates. Increased fecal losses during episodes of diarrhea aggravate pre-existing zinc deficiency. WHO and Indian Academy of Pediatrics recommend zinc supplementation as an adjunct to ORS in the treatment of diarrhea. All children aged between 6 months and 5 years and suffering from diarrhea should receive a uniform dose of 20 mg of elemental zinc as soon as diarrhea starts and continued for a total of 14 days. Children aged 2 to 6 months should be advised 10 mg per day of elemental zinc for a total period of 14 days. Zinc not only decreases the stool frequency and duration of the acute episode; it also prevents episodes of diarrhea in next 6 months.[12,13]

INDICATIONS FOR ANTIBIOTICS

Diarrhea in young children is often infective in origin. The organisms most frequently associated with acute diarrhea in young children in developing countries include rotavirus, ETEC, *Shigella, Campylobacter jejuni, Cryptosporidium, Vibrio cholerae,* non-typhoidal *Salmonella* and EPEC. However, it is important to remember that most of these infections are self-limiting, and antibiotic therapy does not significantly alter the clinical course. Antibiotic therapy in most of these cases, therefore, is not only unnecessary but may lead to undesirable side effects and consequences. Antibiotic therapy should be reserved for cases of dysentery and suspected cholera only. Therefore, every case of diarrhea needs to be carefully evaluated for presence of visible blood in the stools, which indicates dysentery; and to identify cases of suspected cholera (high purge rate with severe dehydration in a child above 2 years in an area where cholera is known to be present).

For the management of dysentery, it is assumed that the cause is shigellosis and therefore an oral antibiotic to which *Shigella* are sensitive should be prescribed. Indian Academy of Pediatrics Task Force recommends ciprofloxacin (15 mg/kg per dose twice a day for 3 days) as first line drug for treatment of uncomplicated dysentery. Switch to oral cefixime, if there is no response in 48 hours. This may be continued for 5 days. The stool microscopy for trophozoites of *E. histolytica* needs to be performed, if the child does not respond after 48 hours of cefixime. For proven as well as suspected cases of cholera, single dose doxycycline (5 mg/kg) is recommended in children aged more than 2 years.[14] Other alternatives include single dose administration of ciprofloxacin or azithromycin.

Antibiotics in Severely Malnourished Children

In severe malnutrition, systemic infections are common in children presenting with diarrhea, and the usual signs of infection such as fever may be absent. Hypoglycemia and hypothermia are often signs of severe infection. Therefore, it is assumed that all malnourished children presenting with diarrhea have an underlying infection, and should be treated with broad-spectrum parenteral antibiotics like ampicillin with gentamicin.[9]

RISK FACTORS FOR DIARRHEAL MORBIDITY AND MORTALITY

Early home therapy with ORT at the onset of a diarrheal episode remains the treatment of choice in almost all cases of diarrhea. However, it may be necessary to identify on the first day of an episode of diarrhea, signs and symptoms, which indicate an increased likelihood of developing dehydration. Alteration in thirst (increased in a normal child and decreased in a dehydrated child as his hydration worsens), 6 or more loose stools, presence of fever, vomiting and a reduction in appetite[15] are some of the clinical features, which help to recognize potentially severe cases who should be kept under close surveillance. Associated major infections (pneumonia, septicemia or meningitis), severe wasting and severe stunting have been reported as risk factors for fatal diarrhea[16] and hence such children need to be identified and targeted for intensive intervention.

NUTRITIONAL MANAGEMENT

Diarrhea is a major cause of malnutrition owing to low food intake during the illness, reduced nutrient absorption in the intestine, and increased nutrient requirements as a result of the infection. Poor appetite, vomiting and the common practice of withholding or diluting food are some of the reasons for poor intake during an episode of diarrhea. Therefore, food intake should never be restricted during or following diarrhea. Rather, the goal should be to maintain the intake of energy and other nutrients at as high a level as possible. When this is done, even with only 80–95% carbohydrates, 70% fat and 75% nitrogen being actually absorbed during acute diarrhea, sufficient nutrients can be absorbed to support continued growth and weight gain. Continued feeding also speeds the recovery of normal intestinal function, including the ability to digest and absorb various nutrients. In contrast, children whose food is restricted or diluted usually lose weight, have diarrhea of longer duration, and recover intestinal function more slowly.[17]

During an episode of diarrhea, specific recommendations for feeding are determined by the child's age and feeding pattern before the illness and the state of hydration. If the child is dehydrated, *during the rehydration phase,* breastfeeding should be continued and normal feeding resumed after rehydration is completed. However, in severely malnourished children, some food should also be offered as soon as possible during the rehydration period.[18] *After the rehydration phase*, the recommendations for dietary management are: (i) For breastfed infants and children, continue breastfeeding as often as the child wishes; (ii) Young infants who take animal milk should continue to take undiluted milk as before; (iii) Children 6 months of age and older should receive energy-rich mixture of soft complementary foods in addition to breast milk or animal milk; (iv) Energy-rich food (thick preparations of staple food with extra vegetable oil or animal fats), potassium rich foods (legumes, banana) and carotene containing foods (dark green leafy vegetables, red palm oil, carrots, pumpkins) should be given to the child in sufficient quantity. In young children, these foods should be particularly well-cooked and soft or mashed to aid digestion. Owing to loss of appetite or vomiting, children may need considerable encouragement to eat. It is helpful to give food frequently in small amounts, i.e. 6 times per day or more.

After an episode of diarrhea, a child should receive more food than usual for at least two weeks after diarrhea stops. During this period, the child may consume up to 150 kcal/kg of body weight per day. A practical approach is to give the child at least one extra meal each day with energy rich foods.[18]

PREVENTION

Comprehensive diarrhea prevention package includes vaccines, nutritional interventions and improving hygiene and sanitation. Rotavirus accounts for 30–50% of all hospitalizations for acute diarrhea. Natural protection against a subsequent infection with rotavirus has been reported only in 40% children after a single natural infection. Therefore, immunization of young children with a rotavirus vaccine is an effective way of preventing at least episodes of severe watery diarrhea in young children. Effective vaccines against rotavirus are commercially available. Improving measles vaccine coverage also results in reduction in the prevalence of postmeasles diarrhea.

Promotion of exclusive breastfeeding, zinc and vitamin A supplementation and management of undernutrition are key nutritional interventions for preventing diarrhea in children. Handwashing, safe disposal of stools, preventing water contamination and food-borne transmission, discouraging bottle feeding and fly control are some of the effective measures for improving hygiene and sanitation.

KEY MESSAGES

- Acute watery diarrhea is a self-limiting disorder and is successfully managed with ORT, zinc supplementation and continued feeding.
- Acute watery diarrhea is frequently caused by rotavirus, ETEC, EPEC and *Cryptosporidium*.
- Dehydration in severely malnourished children needs to be carefully assessed and managed.
- Oral rehydration therapy is the cornerstone of management of acute watery diarrhea.
- Intravenous fluid therapy is indicated only in severe dehydration and in the presence of high purge rate, persistent vomiting, inability to drink and glucose malabsorption.
- Antibiotics do not have any beneficial role in majority of children with diarrhea, and are recommended only in cases of dysentery (visible blood in stools), cholera and severe malnutrition.
- Feeding should be started as soon as the child is rehydrated. Feeding should be started during rehydration phase in children with severe malnutrition.

REFERENCES

1. UNICEF. Diarrheal Disease. June 2018. *https://data.unicef.org/topic/child-health/diarrhoeal-disease.* Accessed on January 27, 2019.
2. Million Death Study Collaborators. Changes in cause-specific neonatal and 1-59-month child mortality in India from 2000 to 2015: A nationally representative survey. Lancet. 2017; 390(10106):1972-80.
3. National Family Health Survey (NFHS-4, 2015-2016) India Fact Sheet. India-Key Indicators: Treatment of Childhood Diseases (children under age 5 years). International Institute for Population Science, Mumbai, December 2017.
4. Patwari AK. Diarrhoea and malnutrition interaction. Indian J Pediatr 1999;66:S124-34.
5. Government of India. Integrated Management of Neonatal and Childhood Illness. Chart Booklet for Physicians. Ministry of Health and Family Welfare, 2009.
6. WHO/UNICEF Statement. Oral Rehydration Salts (ORS): A New Reduced Osmolarity Formulation. World Health Assembly, New York. 2002
7. Bhan MK. Current concepts in management of acute diarrhea. Indian Pediatr 2003;40:463-76.
8. Bhatnagar S, Bhandari N, Mouli UC, Bhan MK. Consensus statement of IAP National Task Force: Status Report on Management of Acute Diarrhea. Indian Pediatr 2004;41:335-48.
9. World Health Organization. Management of the Child with a Serious Infection or Severe Malnutrition. WHO/ FCH/ CAH/00.1, WHO, Geneva, 2000;1-146.
10. Shah SH, Thakur DM, Damle AS, Mehta NC. Hypokalemic myopathy complicating acute gastroenteritis. J Assoc Physician India 1990;38:677.
11. Chhabra A, Patwari AK, Aneja S. Neuromuscular manifestations of diarrhea related hypokalemia. Indian Pediatr 1995;32:409-15.
12. Lazzerini M, Ronfani L. Oral zinc for treating diarrhea in children. Cochrane Database of Systematic Reviews 2008;3: CD005436,DOI:10.1002/14651858
13. Mazumdar S, Taneja S, Bhandari N, *et al.* Effectiveness of zinc supplementation plus oral rehydration salts for diarrhea in infants aged less than 6 months in Haryana state, India. Bull World Health Organ 2010; 88:754-60.
14. Government of India. Integrated Management of Neonatal and Childhood Illness. Training Modules for Physicians. Ministry of Health and Family Welfare, 2003.
15. Victora CG, Kirkwood BR, Fuchs SC, *et al.* Is it possible to predict which diarrhea episodes will lead to life-threatening dehydration. Int J Epidemiol 1990;19:736-41.
16. Sachdev HPS, Kumar S, Singh KK, *et al.* Risk factors for fatal diarrhea in hospitalized children in India. J Pediatr Gastroenterol Nutr 1991;12:76-81.
17. Brown KH, Gastanaduy AS, Saavedra JM. Effect of continued oral feeding on clinical and nutritional outcome of acute diarrhea in children. J Pediatr 1988; 112:191-200.
18. Jelliffe DB, Jelliffe EFP. Dietary management of Young Children with Acute Diarrhea, 2nd edition. Geneva, WHO/ UNICEF, 1991.

CHAPTER

36

Acute Liver Failure

Neelam Mohan, Maninder Dhaliwal

INTRODUCTION

Acute liver failure (ALF) in children is characterized by acute deterioration of liver function, leading to a complex clinical syndrome with deranged liver function and coagulopathy. The varying etiologies among different age groups, diverse clinical manifestations and unclear pathophysiology make ALF a constant challenge to a clinician. Over the last few decades, ALF has retransformed from a condition with a near fatal outcome, to one where advanced intensive care protocols are now applied, and also urgent liver transplantation is an established available treatment option, leading to overall improved outcomes. Mortality in ALF is usually related to coexistent sepsis, coagulopathy, cerebral edema and multiorgan dysfunction. Neonatal liver failure is reported rarely; the identification requires high index of suspicion and carries high mortality if not treated promptly. Newer liver support devices like molecular adsorbent recirculating system (MARS) and extracorporeal liver assist device (ELAD) also help buy time for transplantation or as a bridge to recovery.

DEFINITION

There are several proposed definitions for ALF. Trey and Davidson in 1970 defined fulminant hepatic failure (FHF) as a potentially reversible condition as a consequence of severe liver injury in which encephalopathy develops within 8 weeks of the onset of first symptoms in the absence of pre-existing liver disease.[1] O'Grady, *et al.*[2] used the terms hyper-acute liver failure, acute liver failure and subacute liver failure for patients presenting with encephalopathy within 7 days, 8–28 days and 5–12 weeks of onset of jaundice, respectively. The International Association of Study of Liver Disease (IASL 1999) accepts the definition of acute liver failure as onset of encephalopathy within 4 weeks of jaundice and sub-acute hepatic failure from 4 weeks to 6 months.[3]

The above-mentioned definitions are more apt for adults and have various shortcomings for applicability in children. Early stages of encephalopathy are difficult to assess in infants, and encephalopathy may not be apparent until terminal stages of ALF. Also, duration of illness can be difficult to assess, particularly in infants, who present with ALF in the first few weeks of life. ALF also may be the first manifestation of an underlying unrecognized metabolic problem, which is usually associated with variable degree of chronic liver injury, such as Wilson's disease and inborn errors of metabolism. The Pediatric Acute Liver Failure (PALF) study group, after analyzing data from 24 pediatric liver centers, has defined ALF in children as biochemical evidence of liver injury in a child with no known history of chronic liver disease, and coagulopathy uncorrected by vitamin K administration in form of prothrombin time, international normalized ratio (INR) greater than 1.5 if the patient has encephalopathy, or greater than 2 if the patient does not have encephalopathy.[4]

But above-mentioned definition of PALF is also controversial to apply for neonatal liver failure as INR of normal newborn extends up to 2 and normal preterm newborn may have INR ≥2. So some authors suggest that NLF should be defined as abnormal coagulation with INR of ≥3 in an infant 60 days old or younger.[5]

The term *"acute on chronic liver failure"* (ACLF) is used widely in adults; however, there is no clear consensus on its definition.[6] It is generally used to indicate rapid deterioration of a pre-existent chronic liver disease (CLD) and has high mortality in short-term.[7]

ETIOLOGY

Acute liver failure affects children worldwide and the etiology remains age- and region-dependent, with viral hepatitis probably the most common identifiable cause in all age groups overall. ALF is a clinical syndrome, and can have several etiologies: infective, metabolic, toxic, autoimmune, hematological malignancy, vascular and indeterminant. GALD-NH (Gestational alloimmune liver disease - Neonatal hemochromatosis) is the most common cause of liver failure in neonatal period followed by infective and metabolic liver disease. In infants, metabolic disease is the most frequent cause of ALF, whereas beyond infancy, viral hepatitis (in low- and middle-income countries of Asia and Africa) and drug-induced ALF (in North America and United Kingdom) are most frequently seen.[8-10] ALF of indeterminate cause is also frequently observed; 40% of ALF among patients younger than 3 years and 60% in those age 3 years and older (**Table 1**). With extensive latest investigations, the rate of undetermined causes of ALF has decreased, but still remain a challenge in resource-limited settings.

PATHOGENESIS (FIG. 1)

The specific pathogenesis of the liver injury is dependent mostly on the etiology. But irrespective of etiology, it is now clear that ALF is not one disease of the liver but rather one consequence of multiple organ dysfunctions at various levels. Characteristically, hepatocellular injury is central to pathogenesis of ALF. The initial direct insult and subsequent interplay of cytokines released both locally in liver or spillage in systemic circulation, lead to hepatocyte necrosis or apoptosis.[11,12] And results in compromised glucose hemostasis, increased lactate production with reduced clearance of endotoxin and other substrates, leading to an intense systemic inflammatory response syndrome (SIRS)[13] with distant organ damage. The existence of compensatory anti-inflammatory response syndrome (CARS)—mediated by anti-inflammatory cytokines—is not only insufficient to counter the response, but it acts to predispose bacterial and fungal sepsis during evolution of ALF.[14]

Hepatic encephalopathy that occurs in ALF is complex and multifactorial. Exact pathogenesis is still

Table 1: Etiology of acute liver failure in children

Age	*Infectious disease*	*Cardiovascular*	*Drugs/Toxins*	*Metabolic*	*Vascular*	*Malignancy*	*Immune*
Neonates and infants	Herpes simplex, Parvovirus B19, Adenovirus, Echovirus, Hepatitis B, Measles, HHV6, Varicella, Septicemia	Birth asphyxia, Myocarditis, Congenital heart disease, Hypoplastic left heart, Coarctation of aorta, Congestive heart failure Cardiac surgery	Valproate, TMP/SMX, Paracetamol overdose, Isoniazid Nitrofurantoin	Galactosemia Tyrosinemia Fatty acid defects Mitochondrial defects Hereditary fructose intolerance Niemann-Pick disease type -C	Hepatic venous outflow tract obstruction, Hemangioma	Congenital leukemia Hemophago-cytic histiocytosis	Gestational Alloimmune liver disease/ Neonatal hemochro-matosis
Children/ Adolescents	Hepatitis A, B, C, D, E Leptospirosis, Epstein-Barr virus, Cytomegalovirus, Dengue fever, Sepsis	Cardiomyopathy Budd-Chiari syndrome Myocarditis Congestive heart failure Heat stroke Shock	Rifampicin, TMP/SMX, Valproate, INH Halothane, Paracetamol, Phenytoin Methotrexate, Minocycline, Creon, Pravastatin Poisonous mushrooms	Wilson's disease Leukemia Hereditary fructose intolerance Hemophagocytic syndrome Mitochondrial defects	Hepatic venous outflow tract obstruction	Lymphoma Leukemia Hemophago-cytic histiocytosis	Autoimmune liver disease

(HHV: human herpes virus; TMP/SMX: trimethoprim/sulfamethoxazole; INH: isoniazid)

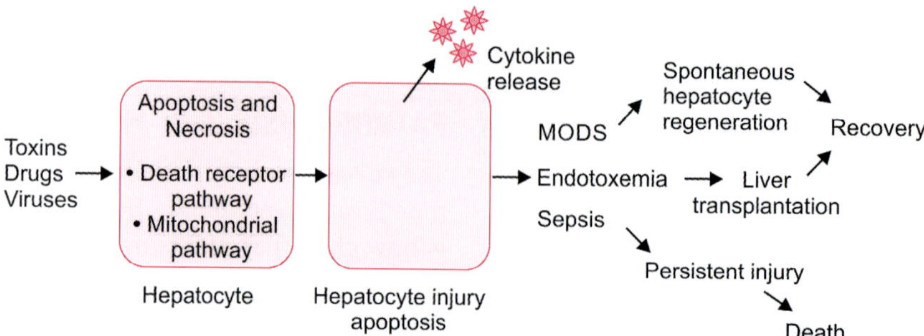

Fig. 1: Pathogenesis of acute liver failure

not completely known and various hypotheses have been suggested.[15,16] Hyperammonemia, increased levels of false neurotransmitters and neuroinhibitory GABA along with various other cytokines and chemicals, infections, and hyponatremia are believed to contribute to cerebral edema and dysregulation of metabolism in the brain leading to hepatic encephalopathy.

Ammonia that reaches the brain is converted to glutamine by astrocytes, which then accumulates, and in high concentrations exert an osmotic effect leading to cerebral edema. SIRS and sepsis further cause oxidative injury and endothelial damage leading to increased permeability of cerebral circulation, adding further to brain swelling and raised intracranial pressure (ICP).

CLINICAL FEATURES

The clinical presentation varies with etiology but essentially there is hepatic dysfunction with hypoglycemia, coagulopathy and encephalopathy. A detailed history with physical examination is must for assessment of a child with ALF. In viral etiology, jaundice is preceded by symptoms such as fever, myalgia, arthralgia and nausea. Jaundice may be a late feature, particularly in metabolic disease and the infant may present with nonspecific symptoms such as vomiting and altered general condition. The clinical onset may be within hours or weeks. ALF eventually represents a multiple organ dysfunction syndrome (MODS) involving the kidneys, lungs, bone marrow, circulatory system and brain. Therefore, the initial examination and biochemical investigations must evaluate hepatic, cerebral, cardiovascular, respiratory, renal and acid base status. On examination, a rapidly shrinking liver with falling liver enzymes and rising bilirubin suggest massive hepatocellular necrosis and are indicators of poor prognosis. Ascites is mostly seen in ACLF, except for Budd-Chiari syndrome. Hepatic encephalopathy may be absent in spite of severe liver dysfunction or may develop after few days to weeks from onset of liver failure in children. Hepatic encephalopathy is classified into four grades of increasing severity (**Table 2**).

Table 2: Grades of hepatic encephalopathy

Grade	Features
I	Reversal of sleep rhythm, personality and intellectual changes, euphoria, lack of concentration
II	Confusion, drowsiness, inappropriate behavior, asterixis (flapping tremors)
III	Stupor, incoherence, unresponsive to verbal commands, hyperreflexia, positive Babinski sign (extensor plantar)
IV	Comatose, gradually more unresponsive, decerebrate posturing, seizures

DIAGNOSIS

Diagnosis of ALF and its cause is established by a combination of clinical and biochemical features and specific diagnostic tests. Biochemical features demonstrate marked conjugated hyperbilirubinemia, elevated aminotransferases, raised plasma ammonia and coagulopathy. Initially laboratory tests should be focused in two areas:

1. *General laboratory investigations* to assess liver dysfunction, sepsis, hematological, renal status, etc. (**Table 3**).
2. *Etiological tests* – prioritize for age and history (**Table 4**).

Wilson's disease in ALF needs special consideration, as it may be difficult to diagnose because low ceruloplasmin level can be present in most patients with ALF, regardless of etiology. Kayser-Fleischer (KF) ring is not uniformly present and result of serum copper levels may take several

Table 3: General laboratory investigations in acute liver failure

Category	*Laboratory investigations*
Hematological	Complete blood cell count with platelet count PT – International normalized ratio, aPTT fibrinogen, D – dimer, blood group, cross match
Electrolytes	Blood glucose, lactate, arterial ammonia, serum osmolarity Blood gas with pH, sodium, potassium, calcium, magnesium, bicarbonate, creatinine
Sepsis	Procalcitonin, urinalysis, blood culture, urine culture, tracheal culture (if intubated)
Imaging and other testing	Chest radiograph, electrocardiogram, abdominal ultrasound with Doppler study of the liver, hepatic and portal venous systems
CNS	Electroencephalography, bispectral index, intracranial pressure monitoring

Table 4: Specific diagnostic tests to evaluate etiology of acute liver failure

Cause	*Test*
Hepatitis A infection	Anti-HAV antibody (IgM)
Hepatitis B infection	HbsAg, Anti-core antibody (HbcAb IgM)
Hepatitis D infection	Anti-hepatitis D virus antibody (IgM)
Hepatitis C infection	Anti-hepatitis C virus antibody (IgM)
Other infections	HHV-1, 2; CMV; EBV; VZV; echovirus; parvovirus B19; malaria; dengue; leptospirosis
Autoimmune hepatitis	Autoantibodies ANA, ASMA, anti-LKM1, immunoglobulins IgG
Hemophagocytic lymphohistiocytosis	Bone marrow aspiration (typical cells), raised ferritin, raised TGs, low/absent NK cell activity
Neonatal hemochromatosis/ Congenital alloimmune hepatitis	Buccal mucosal biopsy, raised ferritin, high transferrin saturation
Veno-occlusive disease/ Malignancies	Doppler ultrasonography/ venography imaging (computed tomography/ magnetic resonance imaging) and histology
Toxicology screen and drug panel	Acetaminophen, opiates, barbiturates, cocaine, alcohol
Metabolic Liver Disease	
Galactosemia	Galactose-1-phosphate uridyl transferase assay (provided child not received blood transfusion in last 3 months)
Tyrosinemia	Urinary succinylacetone
Wilson's disease	Urinary copper (>100 µg/day), Kayser–Fleischer ring, Coombs negative hemolytic anemia, low serum ceruloplasmin (<10 mg/dl)
Urea cycle defect	Plasma aminoacidogram, Orotic acid estimation in urine to diagnose supplementation OTC deficiency
Fatty acid oxidation defect	Carnitine - acyl carnitine profile
Mitochondrial hepatopathies	Muscle and liver biopsies for quantitative assay of respiratory chain enzymes, tandem mass spectroscopy

(HHV: human herpesvirus; EBV: Epstein-Barr virus; CMV: cytomegalovirus; VZV: varicella zoster virus; ANA: antinuclear antibody; ASMA: anti-smooth muscle antibody; LKM: liver kidney microsomal antigen; NK: natural killer; OTC: ornithine transcarbamylase)

days to obtain. In these cases, the following tests can aid in making a diagnosis of Wilson's disease in ALF:

1. Coombs-negative hemolytic anemia
2. Very low serum alkaline phosphatase or uric acid levels
3. Ratio of serum alkaline phosphatase to total bilirubin below 4 and Serum AST to ALT above 2.2.[17]

Hepatic Doppler ultrasound is essential to assess liver parenchyma (nodularity, texture, etc.), varices, splenomegaly, features of portal hypertension, and patency of hepatic veins, portal veins and hepatic artery.

MANAGEMENT

There is no specific therapy for ALF, except hepatic replacement. Management therefore is directed towards organ supportive care, prevention and treatment of complications, and early consideration for liver transplantation. With advances in critical care medicine and liver transplantation, mortality has considerably reduced.

Principles of Management

1. Monitor and support the patient and organ systems.
2. Identify and treat complications.
3. Treat the patient to maximize chances of spontaneous recovery and maintain optimal clinical condition for best post-transplant survival.

Although these principles appear straightforward, their practical applications are more complex. Due to the rapidity of the illness and potentially devastating course, the patient requires close observation in a suitable facility where mechanical ventilation, rapid availability of blood products, ICP monitoring (if deemed beneficial), and renal replacement therapy are available. Typically, this level of support warrants referral to transplant center where emergency liver transplantation, if needed, is available. Early transfer to a pediatric liver transplant center before development of clinical encephalopathy is associated with improved outcomes; few criteria for referral have been listed in **Table 5**.[18,19]

General Measures (Table 6)

The nursing of the patient should be in a quiet environment, and one must avoid excessive stimulation and pain. Sedation should ideally be avoided. A central venous catheter will enable simultaneous administration of blood products, intravenous fluids, high concentration infusions (e.g. 25% Dextrose or 3% NaCl) and drugs with added advantage of facilitating repeated blood sampling. An open nasogastric tube is put in with regular gentle saline lavage to detect upper gastrointestinal bleeding, and to prevent aspiration. The urinary bladder should be catheterized, and strict output record is to be maintained. Care should be taken for prevention of bed sores. Baseline biochemical and other investigations are performed. Frequency of monitoring will depend on the severity of illness ranging from daily in mild cases to 4–6 hourly in patients with stage III and IV coma. Vitamin K should be administered to all patients but may be avoided in G6PD deficient cases due to risk of hemolysis. Fluid therapy is a dynamic clinical decision, with aim to maintain hydration and renal function, while not causing cerebral edema and fluid overload. Restrict fluids to 2/3rd maintenance, provided child is hemodynamically stable. Children are frequently hypovolemic due to inadequate fluid intake and due to associated vomiting and diarrhea. The hemodynamic profile of ALF patient is hyperdynamic circulation with low systemic vascular resistance, usually necessitating fluids followed by inotropic agent (norepinephrine is preferred).[20] Bedside echocardiography can guide fluid therapy, by assessing pre-load, contractility and ejection fraction. Insert arterial line in patients with cardiopulmonary instability or in whom ICP monitoring is planned. In refractory hypotension, hydrocortisone may be beneficial as adrenal insufficiency can occur in ALF.

Hypoglycemia

It is present in most of patients with ALF, which can worsen hepatic encephalopathy; and thus intravenous glucose

Table 5: Criteria for referral of cases of ALF to specialist ICU and liver units[19]

Paracetamol and hyperacute etiology	*Non-paracetamol*
Arterial pH <7.30 or HCO_3 <18	pH <7.30 or HCO_3 <18
INR >3.0 day 2 or >4.0 thereafter	INR >1.8
Oliguria and/or elevated creatinine	Oliguria/renal failure or Na <130 mmol/L
Altered level of consciousness	Encephalopathy, hypoglycemia or metabolic acidosis
Hypoglycemia	Bilirubin >300 µmol/L (17.6 mg/dL)
Elevated lactate unresponsive to fluid resuscitation	Shrinking liver size

(ALF: acute liver failure; ICU: intensive care unit; INR: international normalized ratio)

Table 6: Target specific therapy of underlying ALF

Cause	*Treatment*
Acetaminophen poisoning	Activated charcoal 1 g/kg orally
	N-acetylcysteine 150 mg/kg IV in 15 min, then maintenance dose 50 mg/kg over 4 h, followed by 100 mg/kg administered over 16 hours
Herpes simplex virus	Acyclovir 10 mg/kg 8 hourly or 150 mg/m²/day IV
Neonatal hemochromatosis	Deferoxamine 30 mg/kg/day IV in 3 doses Selenium 2–3 μg/kg/day IV N-acetyl-cysteine 140 mg/kg, then 70 mg/kg orally or IV tocopherol polyethylene glycol succinate 20 U/kg/day orally
Mushroom poisoning	Penicillin G 300,000–1 million units/kg/day IV Silymarin 30–40 mg/kg/day IV or orally
Hepatitis B	Interferon – α - 2b for children > 1 years of age Lamivudine or entecavir for children >2 years of age
Autoimmune hepatitis	Methylprednisolone 1–2 mg/kg IV (max 60 mg) Azathioprine may be added to steroids

infusion (6–8 mg/kg/min) is recommended in patients who develop hypoglycemia. One single bolus of 2 mL/kg of 25% dextrose can be administered through peripheral line, if hypoglycemia is present. However, for continuous infusion of dextrose infusion concentration greater than 12.5%, central venous catheters are preferred.

Fluid and electrolytes

Usually, the sodium should be maintained between 145 and 155 mEq/L, especially in patients with hepatic encephalopathy. Potassium should be maintained between 3.5 and 5 mEq/L as hypokalemia may worsen encephalopathy.

Hepatic Encephalopathy and Cerebral Edema

Hepatic encephalopathy and cerebral edema represent two different neurological complications of ALF. Careful observation is necessary to detect their onset and progression.

The first line of treatment is to minimize aggravating conditions that can increase ICP. Therefore, any precipitating events that can result in hyperammonemia or raised ICP should be avoided. The usual standard line of treatment of encephalopathy in ALF is the following:

- Lower endogenous nitrogen intake (by limiting bleeding and controlling infection) or exogenous nitrogen intake (avoiding unjustified fresh frozen plasma administration).
- Maintain electrolytes, sugar and oxygenation.
- Raise the head end of bed to 20–30°, provided there is no shock. Avoidance of neck rotation additionally helps to reduce cerebral edema.
- There is insufficient evidence for use of lactulose, lactitol, ornithine aspartate, rifaximin or sodium benzoate in ALF.[21] Role of N-acetyl-cysteine in non-paracetamol induced ALF is also controversial.[22,23]
- *Hyperosmolar therapy* acts by raising blood osmolarity, thereby reducing astrocyte swelling in brain. Mannitol is often the first-line therapy (2 mL/kg/dose of 20% mannitol), and can be repeated as boluses. It is effective if serial serum osmolality is below 320 mOsm/L. In patients with significant kidney injury or shock, its use is limited. Hypertonic saline can be used with a goal of achieving sodium of 145 to 155 mEq/L, provided serum osmolality remains below 360 mOsm/L.[24,25]
- Spontaneous hyperventilation, which is usual in patients with ALF, should not be treated. However, prophylactic hyperventilation is not recommended in patients with ALF because vasoconstriction can reduce cerebral oxygen utilization. Acute transient hyperventilation (reduce PCO_2 to 30–34 mm Hg for <20 min) is however recommended as an emergency rescue therapy of patients with evidence of diencephalic herniation.[26]
- Hypothermia (core body temperature 32–33°C) was reported to improve outcome in small case series but was not found to confer benefit in two randomized trials.[27,28]

- Barbiturate coma is used to reduce brain metabolism; although, incremental benefit is unclear if the patient is already in stage 4 encephalopathy with coma. Continuous EEG is recommended till burst-suppression is achieved. Thiopental levels should be done frequently.
- *Seizures*: Seizures in ALF are treated with phenytoin or levetiracetam as seizures cause spikes in ICP. Prophylactic anti-epileptics in ALF are not recommended.[29]
- Elective intubation and ventilation are undertaken when patients progress to grades II – III and become unmanageable. Profofol and fentanyl are suggested for analgesia and sedation. Positive end-expiratory pressure (PEEP) may increase ICP and should be used carefully.

More than 75–80% of patients, especially in stage IV encephalopathy, develop cerebral edema and raised ICP – the primary cause of death. Clinical signs of raised ICP include systemic hypertension, bradycardia, pupillary abnormalities, decerebrate posturing, epileptiform activity and brainstem respiratory patterns. However, most of these clinical signs are nonspecific and may develop in patients in hepatic grade IV encephalopathy without intracranial hypertension. Computed tomography/Magnetic resonance imaging/Positron emission tomography are unreliable in diagnosis of intracranial hypertension in ALF patients. The most accurate method of diagnosis of intracranial hypertension is ICP monitoring.

ICP monitoring and significance: Direct monitoring of ICP helps to diagnose and manage cerebral edema in ALF.[30] Epidural devices have a lower complication rate than subdural or parenchymal monitoring. The goal in the medical management of ALF patients with intracranial hypertension is to maintain ICP below 20 mm Hg and cerebral perfusion pressure (CPP) above 70 mm Hg (Maintain CPP >50 mm Hg for children <4 years, > 55 mm Hg for children 4–10 years, and >60 mm Hg for children >10 years). Cerebral ischemia occurs if CPP is less than 40–50 mm Hg and liver transplantation should be contra-indicated if CPP remains below 40 mm Hg for two hours.

No consensus exists on the use of invasive ICP monitoring.[19] The risk of intracranial hemorrhage and absence of evidence of improved survival are the major reasons against its routine use. But some centers do practice insertion of ICP monitors, indications being hyperacute liver failure with grade 4 encephalopathy, patient listed for liver transplantation, and patient on vasopressors.[31]

Coagulopathy

Overt bleeding is not very common in patients with ALF, and this reflects a rebalanced hemostasis; therefore, prophylactic correction of coagulopathy in ALF patients should not be done without overt bleeding.[32] Also, unnecessary FFP will interfere with the evaluation of liver function as prothrombin time is essential for monitoring disease progression and for assessment of prognosis in ALF. Other disadvantages associated with unnecessary FFP include fluid and protein overload and hyperviscosity syndrome. An exception to this would be if an invasive procedure is planned or there is marked coagulopathy with INR >7. Cryoprecipitate is recommended in a bleeding patient who has significant hypofibrinogenemia (less than 100 mg/dL).[33] In presence of gastrointestinal bleeding, which is mostly due to stress-induced gastric ulcer, coagulopathy and thrombocytopenia should be corrected. Use of H_2 antagonists or proton pump inhibitors may reduce this complication.

Respiratory System and Ventilation

Many respiratory problems can complicate ALF. These include respiratory depression, hypoventilation, aspiration, pneumonia, ARDS, intrapulmonary hemorrhage, and intrapulmonary shunt.

Oral intubation is preferred by modified RSI (rapid sequence intubation), with a cuffed ETT (endotracheal tube), due to risk of bleeding and aspiration. Indications of intubation are: >grade 2 encephalopathy, raised intracranial pressure, rapidly deteriorating course, respiratory failure, and cardiovascular collapse. Aim is to oxygenate (SpO_2 >90%) and maintain normocarbia ($PaCO_2$ 35–45 mm Hg).

Infections

Patient with ALF are prone to infections. Empirical administration of broad-spectrum antibiotics is recommended, especially in advanced state (III/IV) hepatic encephalopathy, persistent hypotension, presence of systemic inflammatory response syndrome (SIRS), and patients listed for liver transplant.[34] Prophylactic systemic antifungal therapy may be particularly warranted in patients who are listed for liver transplant, those with renal failure, and in those who show poor response to antibacterial therapy.

Acute Kidney Injury

The incidence of acute kidney injury (AKI) in acute liver failure varies from 30–85% depending on the etiology. The aim is to maintain optimal circulating blood volume and ensure good urine output (>1 mL/kg/h). An early fluid challenge followed by a trial of diuretic is indicated in patients who develop oliguria. Where available and when needed, early continuous renal replacement therapy (CRRT), pre-empting standard indication is worth considering. Starting RRT in ALF serves dual purpose: for the AKI which sets in ALF plus a detoxification mechanism for the high ammonia, lactate and other metabolic disturbances of ALF. Experts recommend CRRT for hyperammonemia >200 μmol/L, grade 3 or 4 encephalopathy with high ammonia, metabolic disarray, and fluid overload. Continuous RRT rather than intermittent dialysis is advisable in ALF.[35]

Nutrition

There is a need for nutritional supplementation in ALF because these patients are catabolic and enteral nutrition should be administered whenever possible, with higher caloric density feeds preferred. Normal protein intake is recommended till stage I and II encephalopathy and thereafter restriction (0.5–1 g/kg/day) is recommended.[36,37] Metabolic liver disease presenting as ALF needs special nutrition plan, as diet modification in early stages can be life saving.

Liver Support Systems

An extracorporeal support for short period to replace the acutely failing liver seems a reasonable approach, while the native liver recovers or a liver transplant becomes available. The ideal replacement for the failing liver would detoxify, metabolize and synthesize; in short, perform all the liver's many functions. A variety of systems has been tested to date, with no certain evidence of efficacy. Currently available liver support systems are not recommended outside of research trials.[38]

Plasmapheresis or Plasma Exchange

Adults case reports and case series have suggested that plasma exchange can serve as a bridge to recovery for liver transplantation if applied on the first 3 days of admission to intensive care. It acts by clearance of mediators, replacement of plasma derived factors, and improving coagulation and other biochemical parameters.[39] In patients with Wilson's disease presenting with ALF and hemolytic anemia, plasma exchange may serve to remove toxic levels of copper and stabilize the hemolytic process before liver transplant.[40] Studies and data in children are currently under evaluation with promising results.

Emergency Liver Transplantation

Emergency liver transplantation remains the only treatment for poor prognosis group in ALF. This decision to transplant or to wait remains fraught with uncertainty; although, a number of prognostic scores have been described. The most commonly used transplantation criteria are King's College[41,42] and Clinchy Criteria[43] (**Table 7**). A recent study in non-acetaminophen-induced ALF in children documented that INR >4, bilirubin >13.74 mg/dL, age <2 years and WBC > 9 × 10^9/L are associated with poor outcome without liver transplantation and the group so recommends using an INR >4 or factor V concentration of <25% as the best available criteria for listing for liver transplantation in the present era.[19,44,45] There always remains a need for clinical judgment in any decision to proceed with liver transplantation, keeping in mind the dynamicity of disease progression.

In children, etiology is also a critical determinant of outcome. Fulminant Wilson's disease with encephalopathy, Wilson's disease index IQ is the worst prognosis and require emergency liver transplantation.[46,47] In Wilson's disease without encephalopathy (**Table 8**), a score is used and a score of ≥11 indicates need for liver transplantation. Liver transplantation may be contraindicated in congenital lymphohistiocytosis. Other contraindications are uncontrolled sepsis, fixed dilated pupils and severe respiratory failure.

Family support

Liver transplantation in west is usually cadaveric. However, in India and other LMICs, mostly living related liver transplant (LRLT) are performed. The outcome in LRLT setting is superior to cadaveric transplant, probably due to decrease in waiting time for recipient, and better quality of graft in an LRLT setting. Liver transplantation is now available in India, and excellent outcomes have been reported.[48]

Table 7: King's college hospital and Clichy liver transplantation criteria for fulminant hepatic failure

King's college criteria[41,42]	
ALF secondary to acetaminophen overdose	pH less than 7.30 (irrespective of encephalopathy grade), following volume resuscitation >24 hours post overdose Or Hepatic encephalopathy III–IV, PT over 100 seconds (INR > 6.5), and Serum creatinine over 300 μmol/L (3.4 mg/dL) Or The extended KCH criteria Serum lactate > 3.5 mmol/L after early resuscitation Serum lactate > 3.0 mmol/L 24 hours post overdose and adequate volume resuscitation
ALF with other causes	Prothrombin time over 100 seconds (INR > 6.5) (irrespective of encephalopathy grade), Or Any three of the following (irrespective of encephalopathy grade) Age under 10 or over 40 years Non-A, non-B hepatitis or drug-induced origin Duration of jaundice before encephalopathy over 7 days Serum bilirubin greater than 300 μmol/L (17.6 mg/dL) Prothrombin time over 50 seconds (INR > 3.5)
Clichy criteria[43]	
Presence of confusion or coma (stage III–IV Hepatic encephalopathy) associated with Factor V level lower than 20% of normal in patients aged less than 30 years Factor V level lower than 30% of normal in patients aged over 30 years	
EASL and IAP *(accepted, not validated)*[19,44]	
INR >4 and total bilirubin >300 μmol/L (17.6 mg/dL) irrespective of HE	

Table 8: Wilson disease index

Score	*Bilirubin (mg/dL)*	*Aspartate transaminase (UI/L)*	*INR*	*White cell count (10^9/L)*	*Albumin (g/ L)*
0	< 5.8	<100	<1.29	0–6.7	>45
1	5.9–8.8	100–150	1.3–1.6	6.8–8.3	34–44
2	8.9–11.7	151–300	1.7–1.9	8.4–10.3	25–33
3	11.8–17.5	301–400	2.0–2.4	10.4–15.3	21–24
4	>17.5	>401	>2.5	>15.4	<20

Families need good amount of psychological support and counseling to assimilate the seriousness of their child's condition. They are naturally devastated by the rapid development of potentially fatal, acute organ failure in their child. The possibility and the urgency of emergency liver transplantation adds further stress to the family in terms of donor availability, finances and need for long-term immunosuppression.

KEY MESSAGES

- Acute liver failure (ALF) in children is defined when liver dysfunction along with coagulopathy (INR >2.0 without encephalopathy and INR>1.5 in presence of encephalopathy) occurs in a child with no evidence of pre-existing liver disease.
- The most common causes of ALF in neonates are neonatal hemochromatosis and sepsis/hypoxia, whereas in older children and adolescents, the most common causes are hepatitis viruses, hepatotoxic drugs and toxins.

- Children with ALF should be managed in intensive care unit with facilities for ventilation, dialysis and prompt referral to a liver transplant unit.
- Management of ALF is directed towards organ supportive care (respiratory, renal, central nervous system), and prevention and treatment of complications such as hypoglycemia, hyponatremia and cerebral edema.
- Emergency liver transplantation may be required in patients with severe coagulopathy (INR >4.0) or fulminant hepatic failure due to Wilson disease.

REFERENCES

1. Trey C, Davidson C. The management of fulminant hepatic failure. In: Popper H, Schaffner F, editors. Progress in Liver Disease. New York: Grune and stratton; 1970. p. 282–98.
2. O'Grady JG, Schalm SW, Williams R. Acute liver failure: Redefining the syndromes. Lancet Lond Engl. 1993;342 (8866):273-5.
3. Tandon BN, Bernauau J, O'Grady J, *et al.* Recommendations of the International Association for the Study of the Liver Subcommittee on nomenclature of acute and subacute liver failure. J Gastroenterol Hepatol. 1999;14:403-4.
4. Squires Jr RH, Shneider BL, Bucuvalas J, *et al.* Acute liver failure in children: The first 348 patients in the pediatric acute liver failure study group. J Pediatr. 2006;148:652-8.
5. Ciocca M, Álvarez F. Neonatal acute liver failure: A diagnosis challenge. Archivos Argentinos de Pediatria. 2017;115:175-80.
6. Sarin SK, Kedarisetty CK, Abbas Z, *et al.* Acute-on-chronic liver failure: Consensus recommendations of the Asian Pacific Association for the study of the liver (APASL). Hepatol Int. 2009;3:269-82.
7. Jalan R, Yurdaydin C, Bajaj JS, *et al.* World Gastroenterology Organization Working Party. Toward an improved definition of acute-on-chronic liver failure. Gastroenterology. 2014;147: 4-10.
8. Durand P, Debray D, Mandel R, *et al.* Acute liver failure in infancy: A 14-year experience of a pediatric liver transplantation center. J Pediatr. 2001;139:871-6.
9. Black DD. The continuing challenge of "indeterminate" acute liver failure in children. J Pediatr. 2009;155:769-70.
10. Sartorelli MR, Comparcola D, Nobili V. Acute liver failure and pediatric ALF: Strategic help for the pediatric hepatologist. J Pediatr. 2010;156:342.
11. Lee WM, Squires Jr RH, Nyberg SL, *et al.* Acute liver failure: summary of a workshop. Hepatology. 2008;47:1401-15.
12. Hawker F. Liver dysfunction in critical illness. Anaesth Intensive Care. 1991;19:165-81.
13. Antoine DJ, Jenkins RE, Dear JW, *et al.* Molecular forms of HMGB1 and keratin-18 as mechanistic biomarkers for mode of cell death and prognosis during clinical acetaminophen hepatotoxicity. J Hepatol. 2012;56:1070-9.
14. Shubin NJ, Monaghan SF, Ayala A, *et al.* Anti-inflammatory mechanisms of sepsis. Contrib Microbiol. 2011;17:108-24.
15. Wright G, Jalan R. Management of hepatic encephalopathy in patients with cirrhosis. Best Pract Res Clin Gastroenterol. 2007;21:95-110.
16. Bhatia V, Singh R, Acharya SK. Predictive value of arterial ammonia for complications and outcome in acute liver failure. Gut. 2006;55:98-104.
17. Korman JD, Volenberg I, Balko J, *et al.* Screening for Wilson disease in acute liver failure by serum testing:a comparison of currently used tests. Hepatology. 2008;48:1030-2.
18. Devictor D, Desplanques L, Debray D, *et al.* Early transfer to a pediatric liver transplant center before development of clinical encephalopathy is associated with improved outcomes. Hepatology. 1992;16:1156-62.
19. Wendon J, Cordoba J, Dhawan A, *et al.* EASL Clinical Practical Guidelines on the management of acute (fulminant) liver failure. J Hepatology. 2017;66:1047-81.
20. Eefsen M, Dethloff T, Frederiksen HJ, *et al.* Comparison of terlipressin and noradrenaline on cerebral perfusion, intracranial pressure and cerebral extracellular concentrations of lactate and pyruvate in patients with acute liver failure in need of inotropic support. J Hepatol. 2007; 47:381-6.
21. Alba L, Hay JE, Angulo P, *et al.* Lactulose therapy in acute liver failures. J Hepatol. 2002;36:33.
22. Lee WM, Hynan LS, Rossaro L, *et al.* Intravenous N-acetylcysteine improves transplant-free survival in early stage non-acetaminophen acute liver failure. Gastroenterology. 2009;137:856-64.
23. Squires RH, Dhawan A, Alonso E, *et al.* Intravenous N-acetylcysteine in pediatric patients with non-acetaminophen acute liver failure: A placebo-controlled clinical trial. Hepatology. 2013;57:1542-9.
24. Francony G, Fauvage B, Falcon D, *et al.* Equimolar doses of mannitol and hypertonic saline in the treatment of increased intracranial pressure. Crit Care Med 2008;36:795-800.
25. Koenig MA, Bryan M, Lewin JL 3rd, *et al.* Reversal of transtentorial herniation with hypertonic saline. Neurology 2008;70:1023-9.
26. Coles JP, Minhas PS, Fryer TD, *et al.* Effect of hyperventilation on cerebral blood flow in traumatic head injury: Clinical relevance and monitoring correlates. Crit Care Med. 2002;30:1950-9.
27. Bernal W, Murphy N, Brown S, *et al.* A multicentre randomized controlled trial of moderate hypothermia to prevent intracranial hypertension in acute liver failure. J Hepatol. 2016;65:273-9.
28. Karvellas CJ, Todd Stravitz R, Battenhouse H, *et al.* Therapeutic hypothermia in acute liver failure: A multicenter retrospective cohort analysis. Liver Transpl. 2015;21:4-12.
29. Bhatia V, Batra Y, Acharya SK. Prophylactic phenytoin does not improve cerebral edema or survival in acute liver failure—a controlled clinical trial. J Hepatol. 2004;41:89-96.
30. Vaquero J, Fontana RJ, Larson AM, *et al.* Complications and use of intracranial pressure monitoring in patients with acute liver failure and severe encephalopathy. Liver Transpl. 2005; 11:1581-9.
31. Bernal W, Hall C, Karvellas CJ, *et al.* Arterial ammonia and clinical risk factors for encephalopathy and intracranial hypertension in acute liver failure. Hepatology. 2007;46:1844-52.
32. Agarwal B, Wright G, Gatt A, *et al.* Evaluation of coagulation abnormalities in acute liver failure. J Hepatol. 2012;57:780-6.
33. Stravitz RT, Lisman T, Luketic VA, *et al.* Minimal effects of acute liver injury/acute liver failure on hemostasis as assessed by thromboelastography. J Hepatol. 2012;56:129-36.

34. Vaquero J, Polson J, Chung C, *et al.* Infection and the progression of hepatic encephalopathy in acute liver failure. Gastroenterology. 2003;125:755-64.
35. Deep A, Stewart CE, Dhawan A, Douiri A. Effect of continuous renal replacement therapy on outcome in pediatric acute liver failure. Crit Care Med. 2016;44:1910-9.
36. Walsh TS, Wigmore SJ, Hopton P, *et al.* Energy expenditure in acetaminophen-induced fulminant hepatic failure. Crit Care Med. 2000;28:649-54.
37. Plauth M, Cabré E, Riggio O, *et al.* ESPEN guidelines on enteral nutrition: liver disease. Clin Nutr. 2006;25:285-94.
38. Liu J, Gluud L, Als-Nielsen B, *et al.* Artificial and bioartificial support systems for liver failure. Cochrane Database Syst Rev 2004; 1:CD003628.
39. Larsen FS, Schmidt LE, Bernsmeier C, *et al.* High-volume plasma exchange in patients with acute liver failure: An open randomised controlled trial. J Hepatol. 2016;64: 69-78.
40. Kiss JE, Berman D, Van Thiel D. Effective removal of copper by plasma exchange in fulminant Wilson's disease. Transfusion. 1998;38:327-31.
41. McPhail MJ, Wendon JA, Bernal W. Meta-analysis of performance of King's College Hospital Criteria in prediction of outcome in non-paracetamol-induced acute liver failure. J Hepatol. 2010;53:492-9.
42. Craig DG, Ford AC, Hayes PC, *et al.* Systematic review: Prognostic tests of paracetamol-induced acute liver failure. Aliment Pharmacol Ther. 2010;31:1064-76.
43. Bernuau J, Rueff B, Benhamou JP. Fulminant and subfulminant liver failure: Definitions and causes. Semin Liver Dis. 1986; 6:97-106.
44. Bhatia V, Yachha SK, Bavdekar A. Management of Acute Liver Failure in Infants and Children: Consensus Statement of the Pediatric Gastroenterology Chapter, Indian Academy of Pediatrics. Indian Pediatr. 2013;50:477-82.
45. Shanmugam NP, Dhawan A. Selection criteria for liver transplantation in paediatric acute liver failure: The saga continues. Pediatr Transplant. 2011;15:5-6.
46. Nazer H, Ede RJ, Mowat AP, *et al.* Wilson's disease: Clinical presentation and use of prognostic index. Gut. 1986;27:1377-81.
47. Dhawan A, Taylor RM, Cheeseman P, *et al.* 37-year experience and revised King's score for liver transplantation. Liver Transpl. 2005;11:441-8.
48. Mohan N, Karkra S, Rastogi A, *et al.* Outcome of 200 pediatric living donor liver transplantations in India. Indian Pediatr. 2017;54:913-8.

CHAPTER

37

Gastrointestinal Bleeding

Rishi Bolia, Anshu Srivastava, Surender K Yachha

INTRODUCTION

Gastrointestinal (GI) bleeding is one of the most alarming emergencies in childhood. It is potentially life-threatening and due to its frightening nature, medical attention is sought early, which is helpful in its prompt management. Diagnosis and treatment of GI bleeding requires a multidisciplinary approach involving various pediatric specialties (gastroenterology, emergency medicine, intensive care), radiology (diagnostic and interventional) and surgery. The bleeding can occur from anywhere in the gastrointestinal tract (GIT) and is broadly divided into upper gastrointestinal bleeding (UGIB) and lower gastrointestinal bleeding (LGIB). UGIB is more common than LGIB in children, and often massive.[1]

UPPER GI BLEEDING

Upper GI Bleeding is defined as bleeding from a site proximal to the ligament of Treitz (at the level of duodenojejunal flexure).

Epidemiology and Etiology

The incidence of UGI bleeding is not well-established in children and there is scarcity of data from India. A population-based French study estimated that UGIB occurred in 1–2 per 10,000 children per year (77% required hospitalization), and that exposure to nonsteroidal anti-inflammatory drugs (NSAIDs) played a role in one-third of these cases.[2] Ibuprofen and aspirin were the most common incriminated drugs. UGIB is common in children in intensive care unit (ICU) as a result of stress-related mucosal erosions/ulcerations. Children requiring mechanical ventilation have a higher incidence of UGIB, especially if they need high pressure ventilatory setting or have organ failure.[3]

The etiology of UGIB varies in different parts of the world, reflecting geographical differences in disease prevalence. Extrahepatic portal venous obstruction (EHPVO) being most common in India and ulcer disease in the West. **Table 1** illustrates the data from across the world in comparison to that from India.[4-17] The etiology of UGIB can be categorized by age groups **(Table 2)** and as more/less common causes.

Clinical Features

Depending on severity, UGIB can be classified as *major* and *minor*. When an episode of UGI bleeding is associated with hemodynamic instability, significant drop in hemoglobin (<8 g/dL/or drop of >2 g/dL) or hematochezia, it is called *major* UGIB. Depending on the site, rate and etiology of hemorrhage, the following terms are used to describe manifestations of UGIB:

- *Hematemesis* refers to passage of bright red or altered coffee ground blood in vomiting and suggests an UGI site of bleeding.
- *Melena* refers to passage of black tarry stools and suggests an UGI or small bowel site of bleeding. At least 60 mL blood is required to produce melena and blood should stay in the intestine for ≥6 h.
- *Hemobilia* refers to bleeding from biliary tree.
- *Hemosuccus pancreaticus* is a bleeding from the pancreas.

Table 1: Etiology of upper gastrointestinal bleeding in children

	North and South America	*Europe*	*Middle- East and Asia*	*India*
Varices	10.6%	15.6%	23.4%	52.7%
Erosive esophagitis	0.6%	–	0.2%	0.3%
Peptic-ulcer disease	43.5%	12.5%	23.6%	1.2%
Vomiting-induced#	1.2%	12.5%	0.2%	–
Esophagitis, gastritis or duodenitis	27.3%	34.3%	34.3%	23.8%
No etiology found	12.4%	9.3%	18.4%	21%

Source: References 4–17
includes prolapse gastropathy (submucosal hemorrhage caused by retching) and Mallory-Weiss tear

Table 2: Etiology of upper gastrointestinal bleeding categorized by age groups

Neonates/Infants	*Children > 2 years*
Esophagitis *Gastritis* Gastric ulcer ** Duodenal ulcer** *Vitamin K deficiency* *Sepsis* Vascular malformation Trauma (NG tube) CMPA Gastrointestinal duplication Coagulation disorders	*Esophagitis* *Esophageal varices*** Mallory-Weiss syndrome *Gastritis* Gastric ulcer ** Gastric antral vascular ectasia Portal hypertensive gastropathy Gastric varices** Dieulafoy lesion** *Duodenitis* *Duodenal ulcer*** Hemobilia** Hemosuccus pancreaticus** Aortoenteric fistula ** Coagulation disorders Caustic ingestions Foreign bodies *NSAIDs use* Polyps Crohn's disease Gastrointestinal duplication Henoch-Schonlein purpura Tumor – Leiomyoma, lymphoma

CMPA: cow-milk protein allergy; NSAIDs: nonsteroidal anti-inflammatory drugs.
** Often large volume bleeding
Common causes are highlighted in Italics

Hematemesis is the most common mode of clinical presentation seen in ~ 80–96%; some children may present with only melena or hematochezia.

Differential Diagnosis

It is important to differentiate GI bleed from epistaxis, hemoptysis or oromucosal bleeding by history and examination. Certain foods may mimic the appearance of blood in vomitus (e.g. beetroot, tomato skin, drugs like rifampicin), while substances like iron, spinach and charcoal may be mistaken for melena. Testing the vomitus or stool for occult blood will solve this dilemma. In newborns, swallowed maternal blood during delivery or from cracked nipples may be confused with UGIB. An alkali denaturation test (i.e. the Apt-Downey test) can differentiate neonatal from maternal blood.

Approach to Diagnosis

A detailed history and examination help to confirm the site of bleed (UGI *vs.* LGI), and list the likely differential etiology in any given case. Thereafter, investigations help to establish the site, severity and cause of bleeding.

Identify the site of bleeding, i.e. UGIB versus LGIB

Presence of hematemesis and melena suggests an UGI source while passage of bright red blood in stools points to LGIB. But sometimes brisk or massive bleed from an UGI source may also manifest as hematochezia. Nasogastric (NG) aspiration helps to confirm the presence of intragastric blood, determine the rate of gross bleeding, check for ongoing or recurrent bleeding, clear the gastric field for subsequent endoscopic visualization, and prevent aspiration of gastric contents. However, absence of blood in the NG aspirate does not rule out a UGI source of bleed.

Determine the severity of bleeding

Presence of features of major bleed as detailed above suggests significant bleed. Hemoglobin and hematocrit measured immediately after a bleed may be falsely high due to hemoconcentration and should be rechecked after fluid resuscitation.

Table 3: Findings on history and examination that help in identifying the cause of UGIB

Diagnosis	*Findings on history and examination*
Chronic liver disease with varices	Splenomegaly# with jaundice, ascites or other stigmata of liver disease
Extra hepatic portal vein obstruction	Splenomegaly# without other signs of liver disease
Medication-induced ulceration	Ingestion of drugs (aspirin, NSAID, steroids or anticoagulants)
Esophagitis or peptic ulcer disease	Presence of heart burn, regurgitation, epigastric pain or family history of peptic ulcer
Mucosal erosions and ulcerations or fistulization into vessels in retained foreign body	Foreign body ingestion or corrosive intake
Stress ulcers	Concurrent major illness (sepsis, etc.)
Hemobilia	Recent liver biopsy, endoscopic retrograde cholangiopancreatography, or percutaneous cholangiogram
Hemosuccus pancreaticus	History of acute or chronic pancreatitis
Coagulopathy*, thrombocytopenia@	Easy bruising, bleeding from multiple sites, petechiae, ecchymosis.
Vascular malformation	Vascular malformations (hemangioma, telangiectasia) on skin
Henoch-Schonlein purpura Other vasculitis	Abdominal pain, purpuric rash, arthritis, hematuria

In portal hypertension with variceal bleed the spleen may reduce in size, just after a bout of massive hematemesis and thus missed on examination
@Thrombocytopenia may occur in hyper-splenism, disseminated intravascular coagulation (DIC), drug related thrombocytopenia
* May be deranged in DIC/liver disease

Determine the cause of bleeding

A detailed history and examination help in pointing towards the cause of the bleeding **(Table 3)**. The following investigations help in confirming the cause of UGIB:

- Platelet count, coagulation profile, liver function tests, urea, creatinine, and electrolytes should be checked simultaneously. Additional evaluation then depends on clinical suspicion of a particular diagnosis.
- *Endoscopy:* UGI endoscopy is extremely useful for finding the cause and site of bleeding and offering therapy. A complete examination of esophagus, stomach and duodenum with retroflexion to inspect the fundus and gastroesophageal junction detects the etiology in 85–90% cases. The endoscopic appearance of some of the common causes of UGIB is shown in **Figures 1A to D**.

  Single dose of prokinetic (erythromycin or metoclopramide) before endoscopy helps to clear the stomach.[18] Emergency endoscopy (<12 hours) is indicated for patients who require ongoing circulatory support, have large volume hematemesis or melena, or are known to have esophageal varices.
- *Ultrasound abdomen* helps in confirming presence of portal hypertension (PHT) and its likely etiology such as chronic liver disease or EHPVO. It is also helpful in children with hematemesis and associated mass lesions. It confirms biliary or pancreatic disease in patients with suspected hemobilia or hemosuccus pancreaticus.
- *CT angiography:* When endoscopy does not identify a bleeding site and the patient is hemodynamically stable with evidence of active bleeding, multiphasic CT angiography (CTA) is performed. It is playing a growing role in the management of acute GI bleeding by localizing the source of bleeding, differentiating the underlying disease processes and aiding decisions to proceed to endovascular therapy for many causes of GI bleeding. CTA detects bleeding rates as slow as 0.3 mL/min compared with 0.5–1.0 mL/min for conventional angiography.

Hemosuccus pancreaticus and hemobilia can be identified by CTA. *Hemosuccus pancreaticus* occurs as a complication of chronic or acute pancreatitis. Splenic (60–65%) and gastroduodenal (20–25%) arteries are commonly involved. *Hemobilia* occurs when there is a fistula between the splanchnic circulation and the biliary tree. It usually follows liver trauma (direct or after procedures) but may occur as a result of infections (hydatid disease, liver abscess, ascariasis) or bleeding disorders.

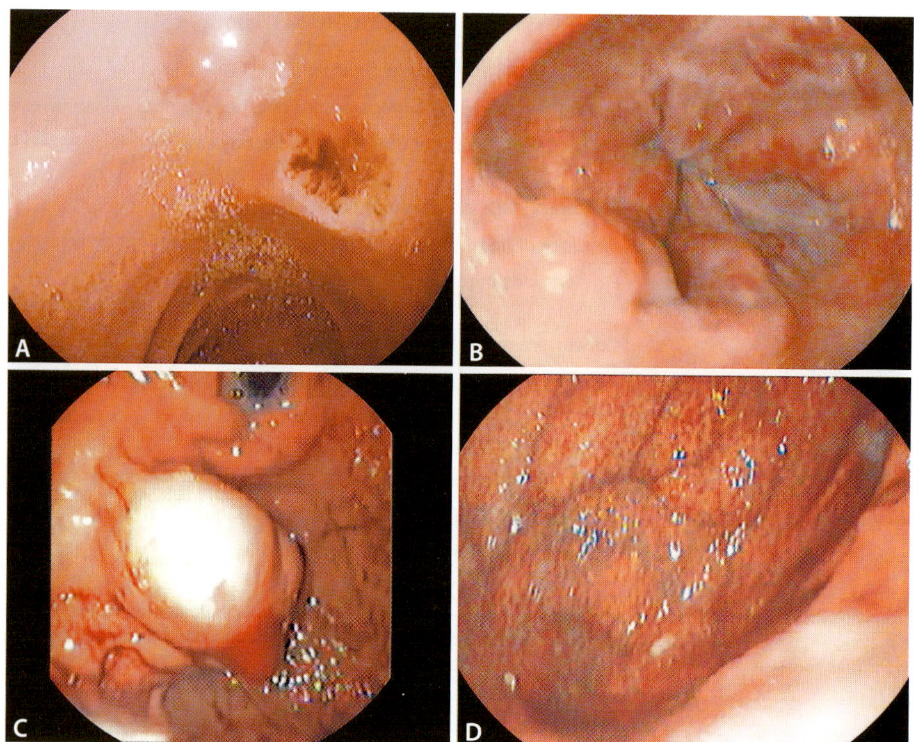

Figs. 1A to D: Endoscopic appearance of common causes of upper gastrointestinal bleeding. (A) Duodenal ulcer with bleed; (B) Esophageal varices with red color signs; (C) Gastric varices with ongoing ooze; (D) Diffuse gastritis

Once the site of bleeding is identified on CTA, conventional angiography and embolization (coil/fibrin/glue) of the arterial branches supplying the lesion is done. If a patient has massive GI bleeding with hemodynamic instability, direct conventional angiography is done.

LOWER GI BLEEDING

It is defined as bleeding from a site distal to ligament of Treitz. Patients are classified as having *small bowel bleeding* if the source of bleeding is distal to the ampulla of Vater and proximal to the ileocecal valve.

Epidemiology and Etiology

The epidemiology of LGIB has not been well-studied in children. In a series of more than 40,000 patients presenting to pediatric emergency, bleeding per rectum was the chief complaint in 0.3% cases, which seems to have further increased in recent years.[19]

Age is an important factor in differentiating the etiology of LGIB and the causes are divided into two groups: neonatal–infants and older children as shown in **Table 4**.[20-23] In the west, allergic colitis is most common in infancy, while enteric infections and anorectal fissures constitute the most common causes in older children.[20] Among low- and middle-income countries (LMIC), infectious colitis (13–24%) and polyps (49–64%) are the most common causes.[21]

- *Small bowel bleeding* (SBB) is uncommon and accounts for ~ 5–10% of all patients with GIB. The common causes of SBB are Meckel's diverticulum, vascular malformation, Crohn's disease, tuberculosis, polyps, small bowel varices, duplication cyst and anastomotic ulcers.
- *Obscure GI bleed* (OGIB) is defined as patients not found to have a source of bleeding after performance of standard upper and lower endoscopy, small bowel evaluation with video capsule endoscopy and/or enteroscopy, and radiographic testing.

Clinical Features

The clinical presentation of LGIB varies with the anatomic source of the bleeding. *Hematochezia* is passage of bright

Table 4: Causes of lower gastrointestinal bleeding in children[21-23]

Neonates/Infants	*Children > 2years*
Anorectal fissure *Infectious colitis* *Allergic colitis* Necrotizing enterocolitis Hirschsprung's enterocolitis *Intussusception* Duplication cyst** Arteriovenous malformation** Rectal prolapse *Meckel's diverticulum*** Coagulopathy, disseminated intravascular coagulopathy, Hemorrhagic disease of the newborn	*Polyps* *Anal fissure* *Infectious colitis* Solitary rectal ulcer syndrome (SRUS) Rectal varices/colopathy Inflammatory bowel disease (ulcerative colitis, Crohn's disease) ** *Meckel's diverticulum*** Pseudomembranous colitis Hemorrhoids Henoch Schonlein purpura Hemolytic uremic syndrome Arteriovenous malformation** Duplication cysts** Coagulopathy, disseminated intravascular coagulopathy

** Often large volume bleeding. Common causes in India in Italics

red blood in stools and usually originates from left colon. The site of bleeding may also be from small bowel if the bleeding is brisk. *Maroon stools* are generally seen in bleed from the distal small bowel or right side of the colon. The presentation of LGIB varies depending on the etiology. It can be mild and intermittent, as with polyp or anal fissure, or moderate to severe, as in Meckel's diverticulum. Associated symptoms depend on the etiology and include abdominal or anorectal pain, colitis, constipation and digital evacuation as shown in **Table 5**.

Differential Diagnosis

It is important to ensure that menstrual bleeding and hematuria is not confused with LGIB. Because many substances can mimic blood in stools, it is useful to test stools for presence of blood in doubtful cases.

Approach to Diagnosis

The approach to investigate the causes of LGIB, is to take a focused history and have a differential diagnosis based on

Table 5: Clinical pointers in identifying the common causes of lower gastrointestinal bleeding

Amount of blood	*Appearance of blood*	*Characteristic of stool*	*Pain*	*History*	*Underlying condition*
Small	Red	Hard	Yes (anorectal)	Constipation	Anal fissure
Small	Red	Hard	Variable	Straining at stools and digital evacuation	Solitary rectal ulcer syndrome
Small to moderate	Red	Loose	Variable	• Infant on cow's milk, eczema • Acute onset in a previously well child • Recurrent abdominal pain, diarrhea, weight loss, aphthous ulcers, joint pain, anal tag • Recent antibiotic exposure	Allergic colitis Infectious colitis IBD Pseudomembranous colitis
Small to moderate	Red	Normal, coated with blood	No	±Mass felt on P/R examination	Polyp
Moderate	Red to tarry	Normal	Yes (abdominal)	Skin lesions (palpable purpura)	Henoch Schonlein purpura
Moderate	Red to tarry, currant jelly	Normal	Yes (abdominal)	Visible or palpable abdominal mass	Intussusception
Moderate	Red	Normal	No	• Typical cutaneous lesions • Skin hemangiomas	Blue rubber bleb nevus syndrome Vascular malformations
Moderate	Red to tarry	Loose	Yes (abdominal)	Delayed passage of meconium followed by constipation	Hirschsprung's disease enterocolitis
Large	Red to tarry	Normal	No		Meckel's diverticulum

the child's age, presence or absence of colitis, associated complaints, and amount of blood in stool. The points that help in identifying the common causes of LGIB are summarized in **Table 5**.

Laboratory Investigations

These aim to localize the site of bleeding, i.e. small bowel or colon, and to determine the etiology.

- *Hemogram* may show anemia, raised ESR with thrombocytosis in inflammatory bowel disease (IBD) and neutrophilic leukocytosis in infectious colitis.
- *Complete stool examination* for trophozoites, stool culture and sensitivity and *Clostridium difficile* toxin.
- *Ultrasound* abdomen confirms the diagnosis of intussusception. It can show features suggestive of abdominal TB (necrotic lymph nodes, loculated ascites) and GI lymphoma (mass, lymph nodes).
- *Endoscopy*: Hematochezia associated with hemodynamic instability may be indicative of an UGIB source, and an upper endoscopy should be performed. Colonoscopy is the investigation of choice for nearly all patients presenting with acute LGIB.[24] It has a diagnostic yield of ~ 80%.[25] Unprepared colonoscopy is not recommended as it is often difficult to get a proper view in subjects with active bleeding. In patients with high-risk clinical features and ongoing bleeding, a rapid bowel purge should be initiated following hemodynamic resuscitation and a colonoscopy should be done within 24 hours of presentation. Examination of the terminal ileum should be attempted to detect active bleeding from the small bowel. Proctosigmoidoscopy is useful for detecting presence of colitis, polyps, solitary rectal ulcer syndrome (SRUS), hemorrhoids and rectal varices. An enema is administered 20–30 minutes before the procedure. Many of the lesions can be treated in the same session. The endoscopic appearance of some of the common causes of LGIB is shown in **Figures 2A to D**.

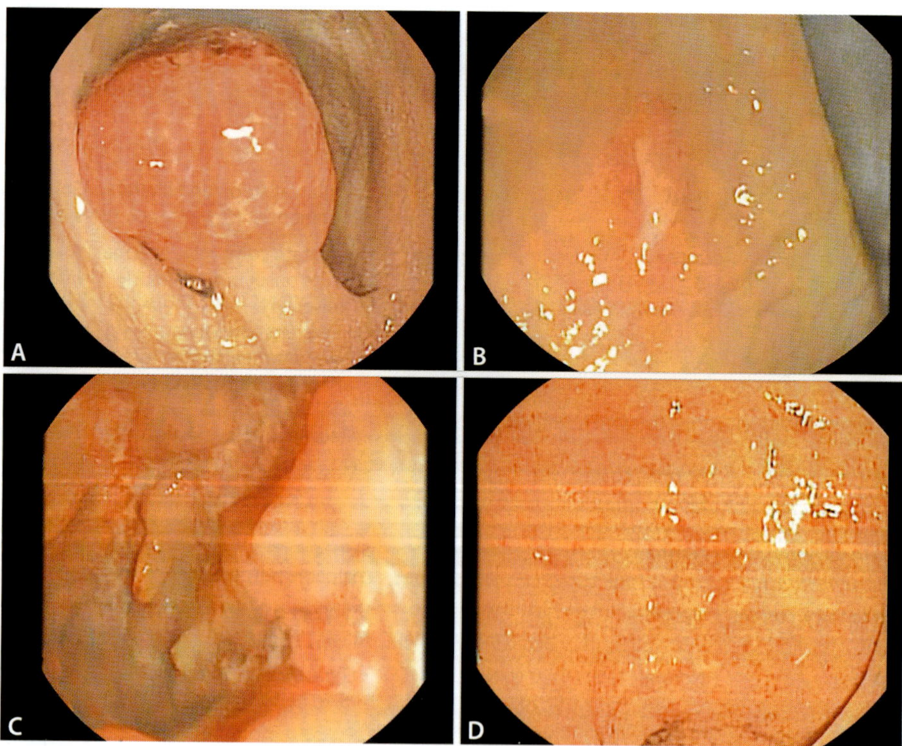

Figs. 2A to D: Endoscopic appearance of common causes of lower gastrointestinal bleeding. (A) Large pedunculated polyp; (B) Solitary rectal ulcer syndrome; (C) Deep longitudinal ulcers in Crohn's disease; (D) Erythema, lack of vascular pattern, erosions in ulcerative colitis

- *Nuclear scans*: Two types of scans are available for evaluation of LGIB:
  Technetium 99m (Tc^{99m}) pertechnetate scan is done to detect ectopic gastric mucosa in Meckel's diverticulum or enteric duplication cyst. As 90% of the bleeding Meckel's has gastric mucosa, it is very useful. Ranitidine (oral or IV), given for 24 h prior to the scan, enhances the sensitivity of this test.[26]
  Tc^{99m} tagged red blood cell scan (Tc RBC scan) detects ongoing bleed if the rate of bleed is ≥0.1 mL/min. Presence of Tc activity in the gut suggests the site of bleeding and can guide selective angiography, i.e. superior mesenteric or inferior mesenteric territory.
- *CT angiography (CTA)*: In patients who continue to have active bleeding *CTA* is performed. The sensitivity of CT in localizing the LGIB is more in patients with active bleed (70–90%) than in patients with occult hemorrhage (55%).[27] Once we have a positive CTA or Tc RBC scan, *conventional angiography* (CA) is performed.[28] However, in patients who are hemodynamically unstable and acutely bleeding, CA should be performed directly. Transcatheter embolization is done after location of the bleeding site.

Small bowel endoscopy

- *Wireless capsule endoscopy* (WCE) should be considered as a first-line investigation for SB evaluation after upper and lower GI sources have been excluded in patients who have a sub-acute ongoing bleed. However, it does not have much role in acute management of LGIB. WCE can be done safely even in children 2–3 years of age. WCE is contraindicated in subjects with suspected intestinal obstruction as the capsule can get impacted. The disadvantage of WCE is the inability to perform therapeutic interventions.
- *Double balloon enteroscopy (DBE) or single balloon enteroscopy* is a useful diagnostic and therapeutic tool for SB bleeding in children. The DBE has two balloons that are used to grip the intestinal wall, and this helps in pleating of bowel over the scope and visualization of the entire SB. DBE allows for tissue sampling and endoscopic therapy. The diagnostic yield can be increased if WCE is done before enteroscopy.
- *Exploratory laparotomy and peroperative enteroscopy* is the last resort and it is done at the time of surgery in patients who continue to bleed significantly and investigations have not revealed the cause.

MANAGEMENT OF GASTROINTESTINAL BLEEDING

General Management

Once the cause of bleeding is identified, the management is done accordingly. The condition of the child dictates the rapidity and approach to diagnosis. In a child with minor bleed, the priority is towards determining the cause of bleed electively whereas in a child with massive bleed, hemodynamic stabilization is the priority, followed by diagnostic and therapeutic procedures.

The steps in the management of an acute GI bleed are as follows:

Hemodynamic assessment

The priority is to assess the airway, breathing and circulation. Heart rate, blood pressure, pulse volume, peripheral perfusion, peripheral cyanosis and urine output should be monitored. The best clinical indicator of blood loss is orthostatic changes in heart rate (increase in pulse rate by ≥20 beats/min) and blood pressure (decrease in systolic blood pressure of ≥10 mm Hg) upon changing the position from supine to sitting. It suggests a blood loss of ~15–20%.[29] If the child has features of shock, i.e. tachycardia, supine hypotension or poor capillary refilling, it indicates a blood loss of 25–30%.

General supportive measures

- Good venous access (2 intravenous lines in subjects with massive bleed), intake output monitoring, oxygen inhalation and charting of vitals.
- Hemodynamic resuscitation with blood transfusion and crystalloid/colloid infusion for maintenance and to replace the ongoing losses. Over-transfusion should be avoided. Hemoglobin should not exceed 7–9 g/dL. This can increase the portal venous pressure and impair clot formation.
- Correction of coagulopathy and thrombocytopenia by fresh frozen plasma (international normalized ratio >1.5 or abnormal partial thromboplastin time) and/or platelet transfusion (platelet< 50×10^9/L).[30] Parenteral vitamin K should be administered empirically while awaiting results of coagulation profile.
- Correction of electrolytes and acid base abnormalities.
- In UGIB, nasogastric tube insertion with gastric lavage and free drainage should be done.

- Short-term (7 days) intravenous antibiotic prophylaxis is required in patients with cirrhosis and GI hemorrhage.

SPECIFIC MANAGEMENT OF UPPER GASTROINTESTINAL BLEEDING

It can be broadly subdivided into two groups: variceal and non-variceal.

Variceal Bleeding

Apart from esophageal varices (EV), the other causes of UGIB in a child with PHT include gastric varices, congestive gastropathy and gastric antral vascular ectasia.

Pharmacological therapy

Pharmacological therapy should be started at the earliest in all cases. Octreotide is the drug of choice for VB and acts by decreasing splanchnic blood flow. Pediatric studies have shown that it controls VB in up to 70% cases.[31] Dose is shown in **Table 6** and main adverse effect is hyperglycemia. Somatostatin is also used for control of active bleed. Side effects include abdominal discomfort, flushing, nausea, bradycardia and steatorrhea. Terlipressin is a synthetic analogue of vasopressin and acts by reducing portal pressure and blood flow through collaterals. Pediatric data on its use are scarce. Studies have not shown any difference between the efficacy of these drugs and either of these can be used depending on the unit's preference.[32] The medication should be continued for 2–5 days.

Endoscopic therapy

Esophageal varices: The diagnosis of a VB is definite when active bleeding from a varix is observed or there are sign of recent bleeding (white nipple) or if no other source is identified in a child with varices and UGIB. Endoscopic variceal ligation (EVL) is preferred in esophageal VB. The procedure is well-tolerated;10–15% children complain of transient retrosternal pain. If EVL is not feasible (children <2 years), endoscopic sclerotherapy (EST) is an alternative. In EST, a flexible needle is inserted through the endoscope to inject a sclerosant (1% polidocanol, 0.5–1% sodium tetradecyl sulfate) into the varix. EST is effective in controlling acute bleeding in ~90% of cases. However, complications are more likely following EST and include ulceration, mediastinitis, esophageal perforation, and pneumothorax. Overall EVL is better than EST as it requires lesser number of sessions, has lower re-bleeding and complication rate.

Table 6: Drugs and their dosages for gastrointestinal bleeding

Drug	*Dosage*
Proton pump inhibitors (PPI)	Omeprazole 0.7–3.3 mg/kg/day single or 2 divided doses PPI infusion for ulcer bleed: intravenous pantoprazole 2 mg/kg (max 80 mg) loading followed by 0.2 mg/kg/h infusion (max 8 mg/h)
Ranitidine	2–4 mg/kg/day PO q 8–12 h, max 10 mg/kg/d (300 mg per day) 2–4 mg/kg/day IV q 8–12 h
Octreotide	1 μg/kg bolus and then 1 μg/kg/h infusion, max 5 μg /kg/h
Somatostatin	250 μg bolus and then 250 μg/h infusion.
Terlipressin	20 μg/kg (max 2 mg) intravenous injection every 4 hours till a bleed free period of 24–48 hours
Anti *H. pylori* therapy [Triple therapy (PPI, AMO, CLA) for 14 days]*	PPI (esomeprazole or omeprazole) Esomeprazole 15–24 kg: 20 mg BD, 25–34 kg: 30 mg BD, >35 kg: 40 mg BD Omeprazole 0.7–3.3 mg/kg/day 2 divided doses Amoxicillin (AMO) 15–24 kg: 500 mg BD, 25–34 kg:750 mg BD, >35 kg: 1000 mg BD Clarithromycin (CLA) 15–24 kg: 250 mg BD, 25–34 kg: 250–500 mg BD, >35 kg: 500 mg BD Metronidazole (MET) 15–24 kg; 250 mg BD, 25–34 kg: 250–500 mg BD, >35 kg: 500 mg BD

*Outcome of anti–*H. pylori* therapy should be assessed at least 4 weeks after completion of therapy using noninvasive methods (13C-urea breath or stool antigen test). If not available a repeat UGIE should be performed to document ulcer healing and eradication.
In case of treatment failure with PPI, AMO, and CLA switch to PPI, AMO, and MET

Gastric varices (GV): These bleed less often but more severely than EV. Endoscopic injection of tissue adhesive (glue, N-butyl 2 cyanoacrylate) that hardens within 20 seconds of contact with blood is used for GV. Nearly 14% patients may develop re-bleeding due to ulceration after glue injection.[33]

Balloon tamponade

In a child who continues to have VB despite pharmacologic and endotherapy, balloon tamponade may be used to stabilize the patient. An appropriate-sized, pediatric Sangstaken-Blakemore tube is passed through the nose and allowed to reach the stomach, gastric balloon is then inflated with 75–150 mL of air depending on the size of the patient, and tube is gently pulled outwards till it sits snugly against the upper dome of stomach and diaphragm. If the bleeding persists, the esophageal balloon is inflated with an air pressure of 20 mm Hg (monitored with the help of a sphygmomanometer). It has one perforated distal end, which helps in aspiration of the stomach contents. Plain X-ray should be taken after placement to check the position of gastric balloon in the stomach. Risks associated with balloon tamponade include aspiration, esophageal rupture and ulcers, and airway obstruction. The tube should never be kept inflated for a duration of >12 h in children. Linton tube has a larger gastric balloon and is used for tamponade of GV.

Self-expandable, covered esophageal metal stent may be an effective and safer alternative to balloon tamponade. It has only been used in adults till date but may be potentially useful in adolescents.

Interventional radiology

Transjugular intrahepatic portosystemic shunt (TIPS): This is an interventional radiology technique that establishes a communication between the portal vein and the hepatic vein and decompresses the portal system. In the adult population, TIPS is indicated in acute variceal hemorrhage refractory to standard therapy or bleeding from ectopic varices. Development of encephalopathy and stent dysfunction are major drawbacks of TIPS. In children, this procedure is technically difficult but has good success rates when done by experts. With the use of covered expanded polytetra-fluoroethylene (ePTFE) endografts, stent block rates have reduced.[34]

Balloon occluded retrograde trans-venous obliteration (BRTO): This can be used for treatment of acutely bleeding fundal GV. The technique involves retrograde cannulation of the left renal vein by the jugular or femoral vein, followed by balloon occlusion and slow infusion of sclerosant to obliterate the gastro-/splenorenal collateral and fundal varices. There is limited pediatric experience with BRTO.

Surgical management

Emergency surgery is required in patients who fail all the above measures. Decompressive surgical shunt should be considered in patients with variceal bleed and cirrhosis with Child's A status or noncirrhotic portal hypertension. In cirrhotics who are likely to be a future transplant candidate, peripheral shunt (proximal/distal splenorenal shunt) is preferable to portocaval shunt. If suitable shuntable veins are not available or in advanced cirrhotics to obviate the high incidence of encephalopathy following shunts, devascularization may be the only option.

Non-variceal Bleeding (NVB)

Intravenous proton pump inhibitors (PPI) should be initiated in any patient suspected to have NVB from the upper GI tract as it promotes clot stability and facilitates hemostasis by raising the intragastric pH **(Flowchart 1)**. Various preparations (e.g. omeprazole, pantoprazole, esomeprazole) are available with no current consensus about the drug of choice **(Table 6)**.

Endoscopic therapy

An early and meticulous UGI endoscopy done after resuscitation is essential for finding the cause of NVB and offering therapy. Depending on the findings, various therapeutic modalities can be used to achieve hemostasis. These include injection (diluted epinephrine), thermal (heater probes, argon plasma coagulation), and mechanical therapy (clips including over the scope clips or band ligation).

If bleeding continues even after standard endoscopic therapy, topical hemostatic spray (an inert nanopowder [Hemospray] that causes immediate hemostasis when sprayed onto active bleeding) can be used as salvage endoscopic therapy. In a pediatric study, the hemostatic spray achieved 100% initial hemostasis with 18% rebleeding rate.[35] If bleeding occurs even after a second

Flowchart 1: Approach to a child with upper gastrointestinal bleeding

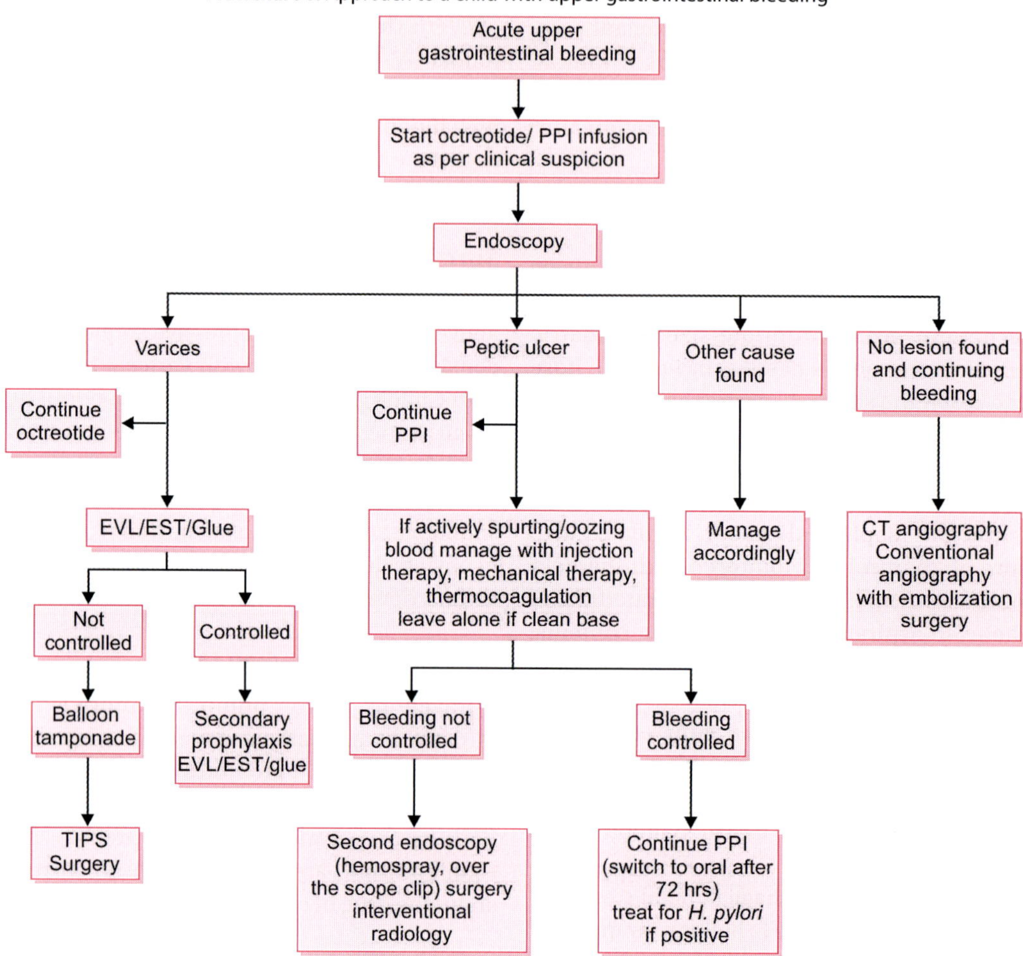

endoscopic therapeutic session, surgery or transcathether arterial embolization is recommended.

Peptic ulcer disease

Peptic ulcer disease (PUD) is the commonest cause for NVB in children, seen mainly in the second decade of life. Most common causes in children are *H. pylori* infection and NSAIDs. About 20% patients have a family history of duodenal ulcers. Ulcers with active spurt/ooze, visible vessel or clot adherent to ulcer base need endotherapy. Endoscopic treatment of peptic ulcer should not be carried out with epinephrine injection alone but in combination with thermal or mechanical techniques. Antral and corpus biopsies are taken for diagnosis of *H. pylori* that includes tissue diagnosis using combination of rapid urease test, culture, gram staining and histology. In patients who are started on a PPI infusion, treatment is changed to oral PPI after 72 hours provided there is no re-bleeding. Anti- *H. pylori* medications **(Table 6)** are prescribed for eradication of infection to prevent ulcer recurrence in subjects with *H. pylori* related ulcer.[36] PPI therapy can be stopped after the demonstration of *H. pylori* eradication. However, in patients with idiopathic (non- *H. pylori*, non-NSAID) ulcers, long-term PPI therapy is recommended.

Other causes of NVB

Other causes of NVB, and their management is summarized in **Table 7**.

Table 7: Etiology-based management of non-variceal and non-ulcer upper gastrointestinal bleeding

Cause	*Management*
Mallory–Weiss lesion	If actively bleeding: endoscopic hemostasis (clip, injection) If not actively bleeding: PPI
Dieulafoy lesion	Mechanical (hemoclip or band ligation), or combination therapy (dilute epinephrine injection combined with contact thermal or mechanical therapy)
Upper GI angioectasias	Contact thermal therapy (Argon plasma coagulation)
CMPA	Milk and milk product free diet
Polyp	Endoscopic polypectomy
Hemobilia Hemosuccus pancreaticus	Interventional radiology with transcathether arterial embolization

(CMPA: cow's milk protein allergy; PPI: proton pump inhibitors)

Table 8: Management strategies for lower gastrointestinal bleeding in children as per etiology

Management strategy	*Diagnosis*
Withdrawal of milk/milk products	Allergic colitis
Antibiotics, supportive therapy	Necrotizing enterocolitis (and surgery if needed), Hirschprung's disease with enterocolitis (followed by definitive surgical treatment), amebic dysentery (Metronidazole), bacillary dysentery (Cefixime/ Ceftriaxone)
Stop offending antibiotic, vancomycin or metronidazole	Pseudomembranous colitis
Immunosuppression	Inflammatory bowel disease, Henoch-Schönlein purpura
Beta blockers (Propranolol)	Arteriovenous malformation, portal colopathy/rectal varices
Vitamin K	Hemorrhagic disease of the newborn
Treatment of constipation	Anal fissure (and/or local nitroglycerin ointment application, sitz bath), Solitary rectal ulcer syndrome (and/or 5 ASA, sucralfate enema, argon plasma coagulation)
Banding, injection	Portal colopathy/rectal varices (and shunt surgery), hemorrhoids
Polypectomy	Polyps
Surgical excision	Duplication/Meckel's diverticulum, rectal prolapse (if persists after treating precipitating cause), intussusception (if radiological intervention fails)

SPECIFIC MANAGEMENT OF LOWER GASTROINTESTINAL BLEEDING

For LGIB, the supportive treatment is similar to that of UGIB. Specific treatment is dependent upon the cause as shown in **Table 8**. A stepwise approach for the management of LGIB is summarized in **Flowchart 2**.

OUTCOME

In a large multicenter study from USA of 19,528 children with GIB, the overall mortality was 0.37%. In children with UGIB, presence of multiple complex chronic conditions, no endoscopy during the admission and no PPI therapy during the first 2 days of admission were associated with poor outcome.[37]

In most cases of LGIB, the bleeding is self-limiting, with majority (80%) cases in the emergency department undergoing routine discharge.

PREVENTION

Endoscopic surveillance for varices in children with chronic liver disease should be performed at diagnosis. Various scores based on spleen size, platelet count, AST, etc. are available to identify the high-risk group.[38]

Secondary prophylaxis with EVL/EST reduces the risk of re-bleeding from EV. As there is a risk of esophageal variceal recurrence (~10%), appearance of new GV and/ or portal hypertensive gastropathy, these patients should be under regular follow-up even after variceal eradication.

Flowchart 2: Approach to a child with lower gastrointestinal bleeding

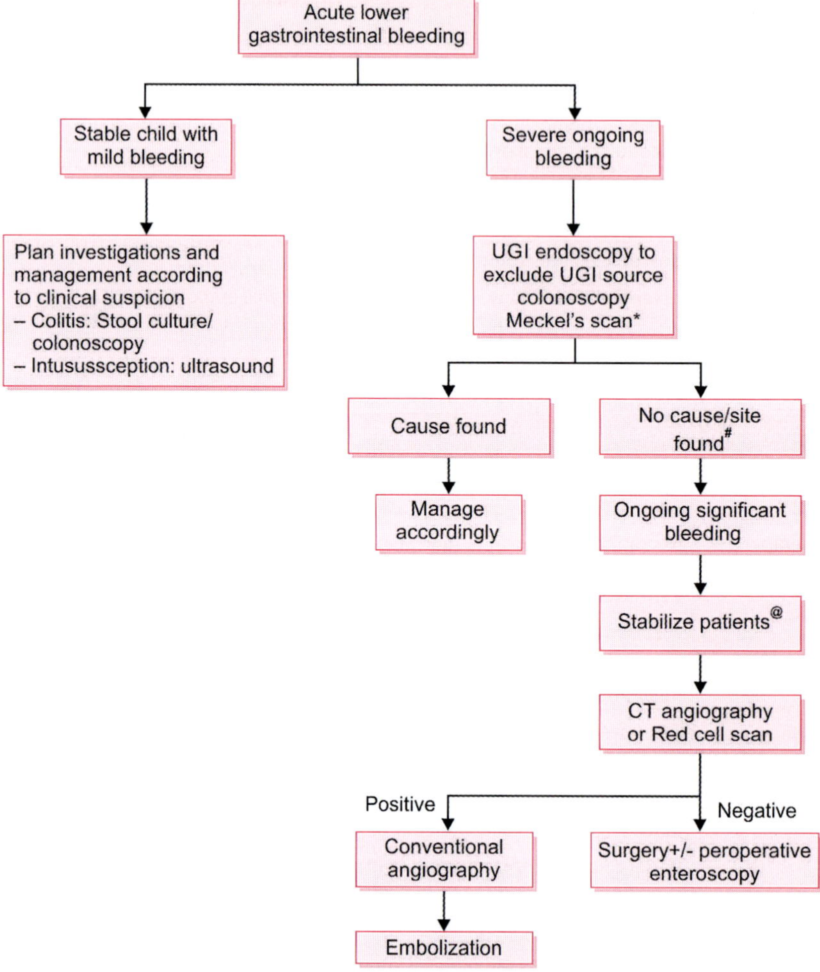

*Meckel's scan is done before colonoscopy if high suspicion of bleeding from Meckel's diverticulum [Painless, maroon colored in a young (usually <5 years) child]
If high suspicion of Meckel's diverticulum, child should be taken directly for a laparotomy as the scan may be false negative
@ Conventional angiography should be performed emergently for hemodynamically unstable patients

Pediatric data on efficacy of propranolol for secondary prophylaxis is limited. Until more evidence is available, a cautious use of beta blockers in select situations may be offered.

Meso Rex bypass (MRB) is done by placement of a jugular auto graft between the left branch of portal vein and superior mesenteric vein in children with EHPVO. It has the advantage of maintaining the hepatopetal blood flow. Children with EHPVO should be offered MRB for secondary prophylaxis of VB if appropriate expertise and favorable anatomy is present.

NSAIDs should be used cautiously, i.e. correct dose for the minimum duration and avoided in patients with known varices or ulcer disease. Prophylactic PPI/H2RA in critically ill children with risk factors (coagulopathy, mechanical ventilation, major comorbidities) in the PICU will reduce the risk of bleeding.

- *H. pylori* eradication therapy to prevent recurrence of peptic ulcer.
- Proper hygiene, sanitation and hand washing can reduce the incidence and prevent transmission of amoebic and bacillary dysentery.

- Identification and early use of laxatives in children with constipation can prevent the formation of anal fissures.

KEY MESSAGES

- Gastrointestinal (GI) bleeding can occur from anywhere in the gastrointestinal tract and is broadly divided into upper GI bleeding and lower GI bleeding. Most children have a good outcome if managed appropriately.
- The most common cause of clinically significant UGIB is esophageal varices.
- Polyps and infectious colitis are the commonest causes of LGIB in Indian children.
- Treatment aims at maintaining hemodynamic stability, identifying the cause of bleed, and providing specific treatment.
- Over transfusion should be avoided with target Hb of 7–9 g/dL.
- In cases of significant UGIB, either octreotide or proton pump inhibitor infusion should be initiated immediately based on clinical suspicion of variceal or non-variceal bleed.
- Upper GI endoscopy and colonoscopy are the preferred diagnostic modalities for the UGI and LGI tract with a yield of 85–90% and ~ 80% respectively.
- Commonly employed therapeutic endoscopic modalities include EVL/EST for varices, adrenaline injection/clips and thermocoagulation therapies for ulcers and polypectomy for polyps.
- If a bleeding source is not identified on UGI/LGI endoscopy and active bleeding continues, a CTA is performed. Meckel's scan should be done before CTA in a young child with maroon color stools.
- Explorative laparotomy with or without peroperative enteroscopy is the last resort and is done if the patient continues to bleed despite all interventions.

REFERENCES

1. Gultekingil A, Teksam O, Gulsen HH, *et al.* Risk factors associated with clinically significant gastrointestinal bleeding in pediatric ED. Am J Emerg Med. 2018;36(4):665-8.
2. Grimaldi-Bensouda L, Abenhaim L, Michaud L, *et al.* Clinical features and risk factors for upper gastrointestinal bleeding in children: A case-crossover study. Eur J Clin Pharmacol. 2010; 66(8):831-7.
3. Deerojanawong J, Peongsujarit D, Vivatvakin B, *et al.* Incidence and risk factors of upper gastrointestinal bleeding in mechanically ventilated children. Pediatr Crit Care Med. 2009; 10:91-5.
4. Yachha SK, Khanduri A, Sharma BC, *et al.* Gastrointestinal bleeding in children. J Gastroenterol Hepatol. 1996;11(10): 903-7.
5. Mittal SK, Kalra KK, Aggarwal V. Diagnostic upper GI endoscopy for hematemesis in children: Experience from a pediatric gastroenterology centre in north India. Indian J Pediatr. 1994;61(6):651-4.
6. El Mouzan MI, Abdullah AM, Al-Mofleh IA. Yield of endoscopy in children with hematemesis. Trop Gastroenterol. 2004;25(1): 44-6.
7. Dehghani SM, Haghighat M, Imanieh MH, *et al.* Upper gastrointestinal bleeding in children in Southern Iran. Indian J Pediatr. 2009;76(6):635-8.
8. Akasaka Y, Misaki F, Miyaoka T, *et al.* Endoscopy in pediatric patients with upper gastrointestinal bleeding. Gastrointest Endosc. 1977;23(4):199-200.
9. Houben CH, Chiu PWY, Lau JYW, *et al.* Duodenal ulcers dominate acute upper gastrointestinal tract bleeding in childhood: A 10-year experience from Hong Kong. J Dig Dis. 2008;9(4):199-203.
10. Huang IF, Wu TC, Wang KS, *et al.* Upper gastrointestinal endoscopy in children with upper gastrointestinal bleeding. J Chin Med Assoc. 2003;66(5):271-5.
11. Quak SH, Lam SK, Low PS. Upper gastrointestinal endoscopy in children. Singapore Med J. 1990;31(2):123-6.
12. Prolla JC, Diehl AS, Bemvenuti GA, *et al.* Upper gastrointestinal fiberoptic endoscopy in pediatric patients. Gastrointest Endosc. 1983;29(4):279-81.
13. Tedesco FJ, Goldstein PD, Gleason WA, *et al.* Upper gastro-intestinal endoscopy in the pediatric patient. Gastroenterology. 1976;70(4):492-4.
14. Ament ME, Christie DL. Upper gastrointestinal fiberoptic endoscopy in pediatric patients. Gastroenterology. 1977;72(6): 1244-8.
15. Cox K, Ament ME. Upper gastrointestinal bleeding in children and adolescents. Pediatrics. 1979;63(3):408-13.
16. Liebman WM. Fiberoptic endoscopy of the gastrointestinal tract in infants and children. I. Upper endoscopy in 53 children. Am J Gastroenterol. 1977;68(4):362-6.
17. Nasher O, Devadason D, Stewart RJ. Upper gastrointestinal bleeding in children: A tertiary United Kingdom children's hospital eperience. Children (Basel). 2017;4(11):95.
18. Barkun AN, Bardou M, Martel M, *et al.* Prokinetics in acute upper GI bleeding: A meta-analysis. Gastrointest Endosc. 2010;72(6):1138-45.
19. Pant C, Olyaee M, Sferra TJ, *et al.* Emergency department visits for gastrointestinal bleeding in children: Results from the Nationwide Emergency Department Sample 2006-2011. Curr Med Res Opin. 2015;31(2):347-51.
20. Sahn B, Bitton S. Lower gastrointestinal bleeding in children. Gastrointest Endosc Clin N Am. 2016;26(1):75-98.
21. Khurana AK, Saraya A, Jain N, *et al.* Profile of lower gastro-intestinal bleeding in children from a tropical country. Trop Gastroenterol. 1998;19(2):70-1.
22. Bai Y, Peng J, Gao J, *et al.* Epidemiology of lower gastrointestinal bleeding in China: Single-center series and systematic analysis of Chinese literature with 53,951 patients. J Gastroenterol Hepatol. 2011;26(4):678-82.
23. Mandhan P. Sigmoidoscopy in children with chronic lower gastrointestinal bleeding. J Paediatr Child Health. 2004; 40(7):365-8.
24. Strate LL, Gralnek IM. ACG Clinical guideline: Management of patients with acute lower gastrointestinal bleeding. Am J Gastroenterol. 2016;111(5):755.

25. Wu CT, Chen CA, Yang YJ. Characteristics and diagnostic yield of pediatric colonoscopy in Taiwan. Pediatr Neonatol. 2015; 56(5):334-8.
26. Rerksuppaphol S, Hutson JM, Oliver MR. Ranitidine-enhanced 99m technetium pertechnetate imaging in children improves the sensitivity of identifying heterotopic gastric mucosa in Meckel's diverticulum. Pediatr Surg Int. 2004;20(5):323-5.
27. Chan V, Tse D, Dixon S, *et al.* Outcome following a negative CT angiogram for gastrointestinal hemorrhage. Cardiovasc Intervent Radiol. 2015;38:329-35.
28. Kennedy DW, Laing CJ, Tseng LH, *et al.* Detection of active gastrointestinal hemorrhage with CT angiography: A 4(1/2)-year retrospective review. J Vasc Interv Radiol. 2010;21(6): 848-55.
29. Singhi S, Jain P, Jayashree M, *et al.* Approach to a child with upper gastrointestinal bleeding. Indian J Pediatr. 2013;80(4):326-33.
30. Romano C, Oliva S, Martellossi S, *et al.* Pediatric gastrointestinal bleeding: Perspectives from the Italian Society of Pediatric Gastroenterology. World J Gastroenterol. 2017;23(8): 1328-37.
31. Eroglu Y, Emerick KM, Whitingon PF, *et al.* Octreotide therapy for control of acute gastrointestinal bleeding in children. J Pediatr Gastroenterol Nutr. 2004;38(1):41-7.
32. Seo YS, Park SY, Kim MY, *et al.* Lack of difference among terlipressin, somatostatin, and octreotide in the control of acute gastroesophageal variceal hemorrhage. Hepatology. 2014;60(3):95-63.
33. Poddar U, Borkar V, Yachha S, *et al.* Endoscopic management of bleeding gastric varices with N-butyl, 2-cyanoacrylate glue injection in children with non-cirrhotic portal hypertension. Endosc Int Open. 2016;4(10):E1063-7.
34. Vo NJ, Shivaram G, Shivariam G, *et al.* Midterm follow-up of transjugular intrahepatic portosystemic shunts using polytetra-fluoroethylene endografts in children. J Vasc Interv Radiol. 2012;23(7):919-24.
35. Thomson M, Urs A, Narula P, *et al.* The use and safety of a novel haemostatic spray in the endoscopic management of acute nonvariceal upper gastrointestinal bleeding in children. J Pediatr Gastroenterol Nutr. 2018;67(3):e47-e5.
36. Jones NL, Koletzko S, Goodman K, *et al.* Joint ESPGHAN/ NASPGHAN Guidelines for the Management of Helicobacter pylori in Children and Adolescents (Update 2016). J Pediatr Gastroenterol Nutr. 2017;64(6):991-1003.
37. Attard TM, Miller M, Pant C, *et al.* Mortality associated with gastrointestinal bleeding in children: A retrospective cohort study. World J Gastroenterol. 2017;23(9):1608-17.
38. Adami MR, Kieling CO, Schwengber FP, *et al.* Noninvasive methods of predicting large esophageal varices in children with intrahepatic portal hypertension. J Pediatr Gastroenterol Nutr. 2018;66(3):442-6.

CHAPTER 38

Hematological Emergencies

Vineeta Gupta, Priyanka Aggarwal

INTRODUCTION

Hematological emergencies are defined as acute life-threatening conditions seen in benign hematological disorders due to the disease per se or as a result of their treatment. These emergencies can occur as initial presentation or can arise in a patient with an established diagnosis. Early diagnosis and proper management of acute complications is the key to successful outcome. They can be encountered in all medical settings ranging from primary healthcare facility to the emergency department of various sub-specialties. Therefore, it is of paramount importance that all pediatricians have a working knowledge of potential hematological emergencies that may be encountered in their practice and they are equipped with the expertise to deal with them effectively. This chapter deals with the most common hematological emergencies and provides practical guidance for the initial management of these patients.

SICKLE CELL CRISIS

Sickle cell anemia (SCA) is an autosomal recessive hemoglobinopathy where valine substitutes glutamic acid at position 6 of beta globin chain in the hemoglobin resulting in production of defective hemoglobin S. Patients with homozygous HbS gene have sickle cell anemia (HbSS) and those with heterozygous HbS gene have sickle cell trait (HbAS). In India, sickle cell disease (SCD) is common in Odisha, Maharashtra, Madhya Pradesh and Jharkhand. However, it is encountered in other states also, although not very commonly.

Presence of HbS results in conformational change in the hemoglobin tetramer. During deoxygenated state, HbS molecules form rigid polymers which give rise to the characteristic "sickled shape" of the RBCs. These sickled RBCs are less deformable and obstruct the post-capillary venules causing mechanical obstruction leading to tissue hypoxia and further aggravation of sickling.[1] Patients with sickle cell anemia can present with serious complications of the disease. It is prudent to be aware of the several crises associated with sickle cell anemia, which can present as hematologic emergencies.

Fever with Sickle Cell Anemia

Fever in a child with sickle cell disease requires prompt evaluation and management. The risk of bacteremia is high in this situation and a delay in administration of antibiotics can lead to adverse outcome. Young infants with sickle cell anemia have an abnormal immune function even in early infancy due to splenic infarcts. Complete functional asplenia can develop by 5 years of age due to repeated splenic infarcts. These patients are at increased risk of developing infections due to encapsulated organisms such as *Streptococcus pneumoniae*, *Haemophilus influenzae* type B and *Neisseria meningitidis*.[2] Infections cause more morbidity, disseminate more rapidly and are more difficult to eradicate because of impaired clearance of bacteria from the circulation and opsonization of bacteria.

Table 1: Indications for admission in sickle cell disease with fever

1.	Sick looking child
2.	Severe pain
3.	High grade fever (>40°C)
4.	High white cell count (>30,000/mm^3)
5.	Low platelet count (<1,00,000/ mm^3)
6.	Low hemoglobin (<5.0 g/dL)
7.	Poor perfusion
8.	Hypotension: systolic blood pressure <70 mm Hg at one year of age, or <70 mm Hg + 2 x age in years in children >1 year of age
8.	Features of dehydration
9.	Features of pneumonia
10.	History of previous admission for sepsis

Management

Although treatment strategies may vary in different hospital settings, outpatient management can be considered in a febrile child with sickle cell disease who has low risk of bacteremia. However, any child who has received intravenous ceftriaxone or other cephalosporins must be observed for 24 hours as they can develop severe, life-threatening immune hemolysis. Children with high risk of bacteremia must be admitted to the hospital. They should receive intravenous fluids if there is history of poor oral intake, oxygen inhalation if hypoxic and broad-spectrum antibiotics such as third generation cephalosporins. Patient should undergo a complete blood count, radiographic imaging of the chest, and blood culture as initial work up. High-risk features include sick appearance, temperature more than 40°C (>104°F), white cell count >30,000/mm^3 or <5,000/mm^3, low hemoglobin (<5.0 g/dL), previous history of sepsis, severe pain, features of dehydration and abnormal radiograph of chest **(Table 1)**. Other indications for admission may be a child from far off area where a poor follow-up is expected. It is prudent to admit such a child for 24 hours in the hospital.

Vaso-occlusive Crisis

A vaso-occlusive crisis occurs due to obstruction of microcirculation by sickled cells resulting in tissue hypoxia.[3] It can be precipitated by physical stress, dehydration, hypoxia, systemic acidosis or exposure to cold. Pain is the major presenting feature. Although pain can occur in any part of the body, it most often occurs in the chest (acute chest syndrome), abdomen (acute abdomen) and extremities (dactylitis and hand foot syndrome). There is painful swelling of fingertips, hands and feet. Painful episodes are abrupt causing severe discomfort to the child and prompting a visit to the emergency department. Patients have approximately one painful episode per year.

Management

Treatment of pain is the most important aspect of management. Specific therapy for pain may vary but generally includes use of paracetamol, or a non-steroidal anti-inflammatory agent. They should be used early in the course of the disease to relieve symptoms. Therapy can be escalated to analgesics such as hydrocodone or other short or long acting opioids. Availability of opioids may be a constraint in Indian scenario but if available should not be withheld for fear of opioid dependency.

Acute Chest Syndrome

There are episodes of acute lung injury, which manifest with fever, cough, chest pain, tachypnea and hypoxia. Acute chest syndrome may occur due to sickling of red blood cells in the microvasculature which may cause pulmonary infarction or emboli.[2] This is more common in children less than 2 years of age. Incidence is more in patients with history of asthma or previous episode of acute chest syndrome. There may be radiographic evidence of infiltrates in lung fields. Infection may precipitate acute episodes.

Management

Child should be managed with oxygen inhalation especially if hypoxic. Bronchodilators are used in patients with history of asthma. Broad-spectrum antibiotic coverage should be provided as it is very difficult to differentiate between acute chest syndrome caused by infection or infarction. Macrolide antibiotics are also given to cover atypical organisms. Transfusion may be required if patient has low hemoglobin and persistent hypoxia. However, it should be given with caution if hematocrit is high. An exchange transfusion may be indicated in such situation. Positive pressure ventilation may be needed in intensive care setting for severe hypoxia. Some studies have suggested beneficial role of inhaled nitric oxide in severe hypoxia.

Acute Splenic Sequestration

This is a life-threatening complication, which is often seen in infants and young children with sickle cell anemia. Sickled red cells block the splenic outflow resulting in pooling of blood in engorged spleen. There is rapid enlargement of spleen resulting in left-sided abdominal pain, fall in hemoglobin and profound anemia. It can also lead to hypovolemia. Reticulocytosis and a decrease in platelet count may also be associated. Sequestration may be precipitated by fever, bacteremia, or viral infections. Repeated episodes of sequestration are common and can occur in two-thirds of the patients. They have a tendency to recur within 6 months of the previous episode.

Management

Early intervention and maintenance of hemodynamic stability with isotonic fluids and blood transfusion is recommended. Blood transfusion is given carefully to treat both sequestration and anemia. Blood transfusion stops the sickling of red cells in the spleen and also releases the blood trapped in the spleen into the circulation often raising the hemoglobin to values above baseline. Therefore, only small amount of transfusion of 5 mL/kg of red cells is recommended. If the hemoglobin rises above 10 g/dL with blood transfusion, it may put the patient at the risk of hyperviscosity syndrome as the blood may be released within the spleen. Splenectomy is an option for preventing recurrent episodes of splenic sequestration. Although blood transfusion therapy has been used in an effort to reduce recurrent episodes, it has not been very successful when compared to no transfusion strategy. Moreover, prophylactic blood transfusions may put the patient at risk of hyperviscosity syndrome. As mentioned earlier, blood transfusion is given cautiously during an acute episode of splenic sequestration.

Aplastic Crisis

Patients with sickle cell anemia can have infection with human parvovirus B19 resulting in temporary red cell aplasia. This results in reticulocytopenia and severe anemia. Any child of sickle cell anemia with fever, severe anemia and reticulocytopenia should be considered to have parvovirus B19 infection.

Management

Child should be managed conservatively with red blood cell transfusion. Such patients are also contagious and appropriate infection control measures should be taken to prevent the nosocomial spread of infection.

BLOOD TRANSFUSION RELATED ADVERSE EVENTS

Acute blood transfusion reactions can cause most severe adverse reactions. An adverse reaction or event is defined as an undesirable response or effect in a patient, which is temporally associated with the administration of blood or blood components.[4] With better management of chronic hematological disorders, increasing number of thalassemia and hemophilia units are coming up transfusing several units of blood components to pediatric patients. Awareness about the various acute and delayed blood transfusion reactions is the key to proper management. It is not possible to elaborate on all the transfusion reactions in this chapter. We have discussed some of the important transfusion reactions here.

Acute Hemolytic Transfusion Reactions

A hemolytic transfusion reaction occurs due to the increased red cell destruction caused by transfusion. They can be either immune mediated or non-immune mediated. In the immune-mediated hemolytic reactions, there is interaction of recipient's preformed antibodies with the donor's red cell antigens resulting in immediate destruction of the transfused red cells in the circulation. This can happen in a situation of mismatched transfusion. Symptoms start within minutes of starting the transfusion. Investigations reveal hemoglobinemia, hemoglobinuria, decreased serum haptoglobin, unconjugated hyperbilirubinemia and increased lactic dehydrogenase levels. Non-antibody mediated acute hemolytic reactions are benign and include mechanical hemolysis of serologically compatible red blood cells due to freezing, pressure infusion pumps and osmotic hemolysis.

Management

- Transfusion should be stopped immediately. Patient's name tag and the bag number must be rechecked. Blood bank should be informed about the severe reaction and the component unit sent back to blood bank for rechecking

- Vital signs to be monitored with establishment of intravenous access
- Intravenous crystalloids: normal saline 10–20 mL/kg
- Intravenous furosemide
- Low-dose dopamine 2–5 μg/kg/min
- Maintain urine output >1 mL/kg/hour
- Severe reactions may cause acute kidney injury requiring hemodialysis
- Supportive treatment of DIC with hemostatic components: platelets, plasma, cryoprecipitate.

Febrile Non-hemolytic Transfusion Reactions

Unexplained rise in temperature of at least 1°C during or shortly after transfusion characterizes febrile non-hemolytic transfusion reactions (FNHTR). These are more common in multi-transfused patients such as thalassemia patients. Also they are more often seen after transfusion of platelets (up to 30% of platelet transfusion) than red blood cells as the platelets are stored at room temperature which promotes leukocyte activation. Patient presents with fever, chills and rigors. Other causes of fever should be excluded before making a diagnosis of FNHTR. Antipyretics may mask fever but not chills and rigor as they are usually due to cytokine mediated systemic mediated inflammatory response.

Management

- Treatment is symptomatic.
- *Antipyretics*: Paracetamol 10–15 mg/kg/dose PO (30–60 min before starting transfusion)
- *Antihistamine*: Diphenhydramine 1–1.5 mg/kg/dose PO or IV (1 hour before starting transfusion)
- Patients should receive leukoreduced blood products. Bedside filters can be used. However, pre-storage laboratory leukoreduction is more effective than bedside leukoreduction.

Transfusion Related Acute Lung Injury

Transfusion related acute lung injury (TRALI) is defined as acute respiratory distress developing during or within 6 hours of transfusion of blood product in a patient without pre-existing pulmonary disease. Other features are: hypoxia with $PaO_2/FiO_2 \leq 300$ or $SpO_2 < 90\%$ on room air, bilateral pulmonary edema on chest radiograph, no evidence of left atrial hypertrophy and no alternative risk factor for acute lung injury.[5] It is a clinical diagnosis and laboratory investigations only help in making a diagnosis. All plasma-containing components including whole blood, platelets, red blood cells, fresh frozen plasma and cryoprecipitate have been implicated in TRALI. It is an antibody mediated event involving transfusion of donor leukocyte antibody through plasma-containing components into the patient causing microvascular injury to the lung. Another proposed mechanism is neutrophil activation leading to pulmonary endothelial damage, capillary leakage and pulmonary edema.

Patients may develop fever, dyspnea, hypoxia which may be severe, hypotension and pulmonary edema. Acute hemolytic transfusion reaction should be ruled out by clinical and hematological investigations. A chest X-ray is obtained to rule out transfusion associated circulatory overload (TACO).

Management

Management is supportive in form of oxygen inhalation, intubation/mechanical ventilation depending on degree of hypoxia, and vasopressors to support blood pressure.

HYPERLEUKOCYTOSIS

A high initial WBC count, i.e >100 × 10^6/L is defined as hyperleukocytosis. It is more often observed with acute myeloid leukemia (AML) (25%) compared to acute lymphoblastic leukemia (ALL) (10%). The early morbidity (20–40%) and mortality risk with hyperleukocytosis is higher with AML as the blasts are bigger and stickier to each other as well as endothelium.[6]

Clinical Presentation

- *Pulmonary symptoms*: Dyspnea, cough, tachypnea.
- *CNS symptoms*: Headache, confusion, behavioral and mental status changes, altered sensorium, speech problem, ataxia and blurred vision, and risk of intracranial hemorrhage.
- *Genitourinary symptoms*: Oliguria, anuria, renal failure, priapism in boys.
- *Gastrointestinal symptoms*: Severe abdominal pain, melena.

Complications

- *Disseminated intravascular coagulation (DIC)*: Due to high turnover and associated high levels of released tissue factors which triggers extrinsic pathway via Factor VII.

- *Tumor lysis syndrome*: Metabolic emergency as a result of spontaneous or treatment induced cell death.

Management

- *Adequate hydration*: 1.2 to 1.5 times the maintenance intravenous fluids, preferably 5% dextrose normal saline without potassium
- Avoid packed cell transfusion (If necessary, use a dose of 5 mL/kg)
- Correct coagulopathy
- Maintain hemoglobin between 8 and 10 g/dL
- Regular monitoring for respiratory distress, sensorium and urine output.

FEBRILE NEUTROPENIA

Febrile neutropenia (FN) is defined as a single oral temperature of 38.3°C (101°F) or 38.0°C (100.4°F) over 1 hour with neutrophil count less than 500 neutrophils/mm^3, or less than 1,000/mm^3 with a predicted decline to 500/mm^3 over the next 48 hours.

Diagnosis

A detailed history and examination should be undertaken. The physician should search for focal areas of pain or disruption of mucosal barriers like gums, pharynx, perineum and anus. Also attention should be given to fundus, palpation of maxillary and frontal sinus as well as inspection of vascular access.[7] Avoid per rectal examination. At least 2 sets of blood cultures should be withdrawn. If an intravascular device is present, one sample should be obtained from that route, and ideally through each lumen of a multiple port catheter. Urine analysis and cultures should also be sent. Chest X-ray can be done to evaluate respiratory symptoms.

Management

Empirical broad spectrum antibiotics may be started based on individual patient risk assessment. **Table 2** gives causative organisms in febrile neutropenia.

Risk stratification: According to Infectious Disease Society of America (IDSA), febrile neutropenia can be stratified as follows **(Flowchart 1)**:

High risk

If any of the following are present:

- Hemodynamic instability or comorbidity.

Table 2: Causative organisms in febrile neutropenia

Gram positive	*Staphylococcus aureus, Staphylococcus epidermidis* (indwelling catheter), *Streptococcus pneumoniae, Streptococcus pyogenes, Streptococcus viridans, Enterococcus faecalis*
Gram negative	*Escherischia coli, Klebsiella* species, *Pseudomonas aeruginosa*
Fungal	Although candida is the most common fungal infection, *Aspergillus* and *Zygomycetes* are more feared because of their angioinvasive predilection
Anaerobes	*Bacteroides fragilis*
Virus	Herpes, Cytomegalovirus

- Prolonged severe neutropenia (ANC<100/mm^3) or duration >7 days.
- Pneumonia or other focus of infection at time of presentation.
- Severe mucositis (grade 3 or 4).
- Hepatic or renal insufficiency.
- Altered sensorium.

Low risk

- No comorbidities or focus of infection.
- ANC >100/mm^3 and short duration (<7 days) of severe neutropenia.
- For high-risk patients, monotherapy with a fourth generation cephalosporin like cefepime, or carbapenem or piperacillin tazobactam can be considered. Vancomycin may be added if there is soft tissue infection, pneumonia, or suspicion of infected device, but never as monotherapy. Antifungal agents can be considered if they remain febrile after 4–7 days of broad-spectrum antibiotics.

For a low-risk patient, appropriate strategy would be, if the child has not received any quinolone prophylaxis, an oral empiric therapy with ciprofloxacin and amoxicillin clavulanate. If patient has fever even after 48 hours, child must be hospitalized and given IV antibiotics. Antibiotics should be continued until ANC > 500/mm^3.

BLEEDING CHILD

Easy bruising and epistaxis are commonly encountered clinical problems in children. Only cases with excessive bleeding following a commonly encountered challenge need to be further investigated. Normal hemostasis requires interaction of normal endothelium, platelets and the

Flowchart 1: Management of febrile neutropenia

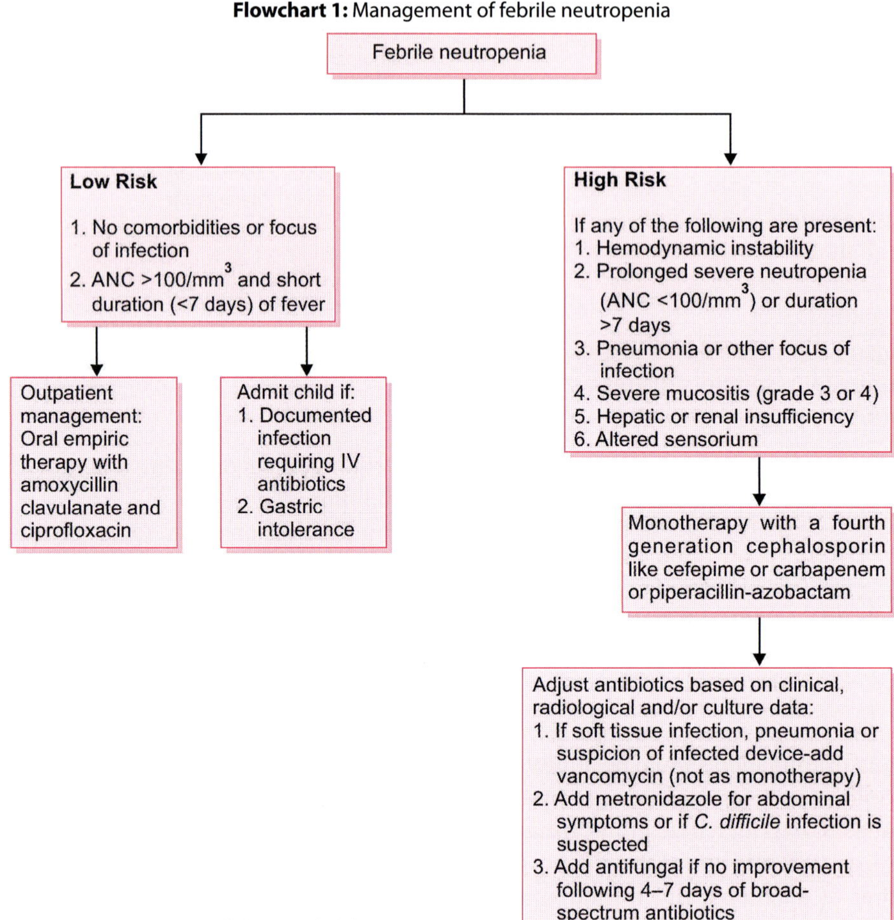

clotting cascade. Thus, assessment of these children is a diagnostic challenge because of wide range of possible causes.

Etiology

Bleeding disorders can be inherited or acquired. These include coagulation factor deficiencies, platelet deficiency and/or dysfunction as well as abnormalities of the fibrinolytic system. A detailed clinical history, physical examination and family history of bleeding disorder is required for evaluation and investigation for a possible bleeding disorder.

History should include the (i) age of onset, (ii) site, duration and severity of bleed, (iii) whether the bleed is spontaneous or induced, (iv) does bleed occurred following major surgical procedure, (v) any history of drug intake (aspirin, warfarin, NSAIDs, etc.), (vi) history of menorrhagia in an adolescent female and (vii) family history of bleeding disorder.

A careful physical examination is essential in the diagnosis of hemostatic disorders. Disorders of primary hemostasis present with mucocutaneous bleeding, i.e. epistaxis, gum bleeding, petechiae, etc. Deep hematomas, hemarthrosis, intramuscular bleed in males suggests Hemophilia. Acquired bleeding defect usually occurs in context of a coexisting illness. Presence of lymphadenopathy and/or hepatosplenomegaly may point towards malignancy or a storage disorder.

Laboratory Evaluation

Laboratory screening for a suspected bleeding disorder includes complete blood count (CBC), general blood picture (GBP) and PT/aPTT. These tests provide additional diagnostic indicators that direct more specific investigations. A simple algorithm may aid in evaluation of a bleeding disorder as depicted in **Flowchart 2**.

Flowchart 2: Algorithm for approach to bleeding child

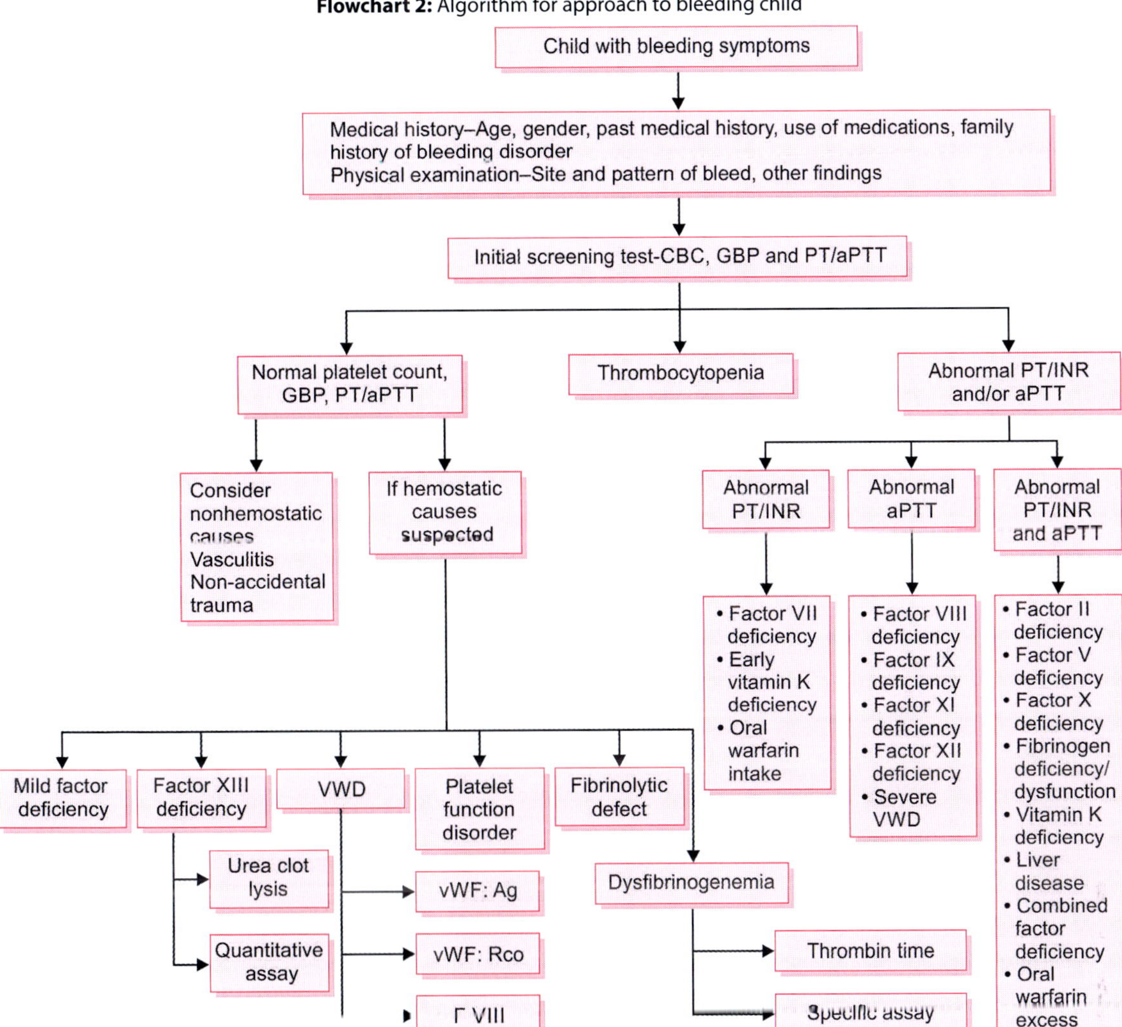

Platelet Disorders

Various defects in platelet function as well as number can result in profuse bleeding in a child. Differential diagnosis of thrombocytopenia have been presented in **Flowchart 3**. The defects of platelet function have been shown in **Flowchart 4**. Platelet aggregation test as well as platelet function assay using platelet function analyzer (PFA-100) helps in detecting qualitative defects in platelet function.

Thrombocytopenia

The normal platelet count is 1.5–4.5 × 10^6/mm^3. Thrombocytopenia refers to reduction in platelet count to less than 1.5 × 10^6/mm^3. It may occur due to decreased production either congenital or acquired, increased destruction of normally synthesized platelets via immune or nonimmune mechanism, or sequestration into enlarged spleen or another organ.

Idiopathic (Immune) thrombocytopenic purpura: The most common cause of thrombocytopenia in otherwise healthy child is ITP. It usually occurs 1–4 weeks after exposure to common viral infection with the peak age of onset being 1–4 years. Only 70–80% children experience spontaneous resolution within 6 months. <1% children with ITP may develop intracranial hemorrhage. Only 20% children presenting as acute ITP go on to have chronic ITP.

Flowchart 3: Differential diagnosis of childhood thrombocytopenia

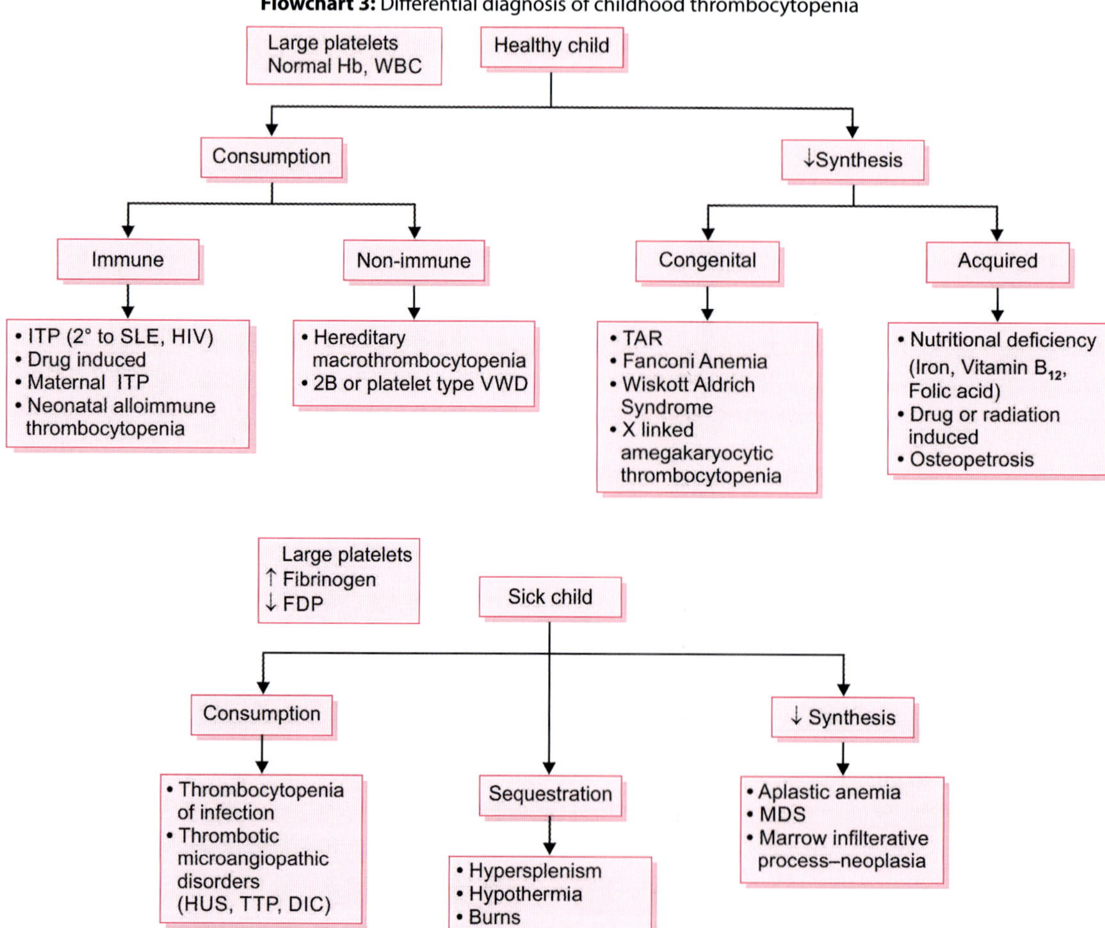

(ITP: immune thrombocytopenic purpura; TAR: thrombocytopenia with absent radii; HUS: hemolytic uremic syndrome; TTP: thrombotic thrombocytopenic purpura; MDS: myelodysplastic syndrome; VWD: von Willibrand disease)

Flowchart 4: Defects of platelet function

Congenital	Acquired
• **Bernard-Soulier disease** (Decreased platelet adhesion involving GpIb receptor for VWF) • **Glanzmann's thrombasthenia** (Decreased platelet aggregation involving glycoprotein IIb/IIIa for fibrinogen) • **Gray platelet syndrome** (Defective platelet release)	• Drugs (NSAIDs, lipid lowering agents, volume expanders, valproic acid) • Liver disease • Uremia • Disorder that trigger increased fibrinogen degradation products

Management

Platelet transfusion is contraindicated unless there is life-threatening bleed. In minimal, mild, moderate symptoms only family counseling is needed. As per the American Society of Hematology (ASH) Guidelines: "A single dose of IVIg [intravenous immunoglobulin] (0.8–1.0 g/kg) or a short course of corticosteroids should be used as first-line treatment." Short course of corticosteroids, i.e prednisolone ranging from 2 to 4 mg/kg/day have being used. Usually prednisolone at 2 mg/kg/day for 2 weeks followed by tapering over 1 week is used. IVIg at a dose of 0.8–1.0 g/kg/day for 1–2 days induces a rapid rise in platelet count (usually >20 × 10^9/L) in 95% of patients within 48 hr. IVIg appears to induce a response by down regulating the Fc-mediated phagocytosis of antibody-coated platelets. IV anti-D at a dose of 50–75 µg/kg in Rh-positive patients, causes a rise in platelet count to >20 × 10^9/L in 80–90% of patients within 48–72 hr. RBC-antibody complexes bind to macrophage Fc receptors thereby interfering with platelet destruction and causing a rise in platelet count. IV anti-D is ineffective in Rh-negative patients. It induces a mild hemolytic anemia when given to Rh-positive individuals.

Coagulation Defects: Hemophilia

Hemophilia occurs in 1:5000 with 85% having factor VIII deficiency. Clinically it presents in the form of hemarthrosis (most common), intramuscular hematomas, easy bruising. Only 2% of the neonates with hemophilia manifest with intracranial hemorrhage and 30% of male infants bleed with circumcision. The hemostatic level for factor VIII is >30–40% while for factor IX is >25–30%. According to International Society of Thrombosis and Hemophilia (ISTH), hemophilia A is classified as:

- Severe hemophilia—less than 1% activity.
- Moderate hemophilia—factor levels of 1–5%.
- Mild hemophilia—factor levels >5%.

Management

Factor replacement is the mainstay of treatment in hemophilia A and hemophilia B. In case of mild or moderate bleeds, level should be raised to 30–35%, whereas in case of life-threatening bleeds level should be raised to 100%.

Dose of rVIII (IU) = % desired (rise in rVIII) × body weight × 0.5

In case of mild factor VIII deficiency, Desmopressin may be used which helps in the release of factor VIII.

Dose of rIX (IU) = % desired (rise in plasma F IX) × body weight × 1.4

Von Willebrand Disease

Von Willebrand disease (VWD) is the most common bleeding disorder. It occurs due to quantitative or qualitative defect in the von Willebrand factor (vWF). vWF tethers collagen as well as platelets to the injured subendothelium and acts as a carrier for FVIII, protecting factor VIII from degradation in the plasma.

The VWD typically presents with mucosal bleeding. Epistaxis, petechiae, menorrhagia in females are common complaints. Surgical bleeding during dental extraction and adenotonsillectomy is another common presentation. Type 3 VWD may present with hemarthrosis. Family history of bleeding is present in most of the patients.

Treatment

The treatment depends on the type of VWD and the reason for treatment. Type I VWD may be treated with desmopressin 0.3 µg/kg IV (max 20–30 µg/day), or 150 µg intranasal in <50 kg and 300 µg intranasal in >50kg, except in cases who lack response to desmopressin and type IC. For type 2 and 3, replacement with vWF concentrates remain the treatment of choice. Apart from these, antifibrinolytics like tranexamic acid may be used for all types of VWD.[8-10]

BLEEDING NEONATE

Bleeding in neonates admitted to NICU is a common finding. It is more commonly seen in LBW babies and is due to decreased activity of several clotting factors, diminished platelet function and suboptimal defense against clot formation. Physiologic levels of many coagulation proteins are decreased in neonates. Also, the hemostatic system is dynamic and age dependent.

A detailed history including (i) family history of bleeding disorder (bleeding in previous siblings, history of menorrhagia in mother), (ii) maternal medications, i.e. anticonvulsants like phenytoin, phenobarbitone, valproic acid, antitubercular drugs, aspirin, heparin, etc, (iii) antenatal history suggestive of SLE, ITP, TORCH infection, (iv) vitamin K prophylaxis and use of antibiotics. A big cephalhematoma following normal delivery is suspicious of inherited bleeding disorder. **Table 3** illustrates the laboratory evaluation of a bleeding neonate. Algorithm suggesting approach to a bleeding neonate has been depicted in **Flowchart 5**.

ACUTE HEMOLYSIS

Acute hemolysis presents with sudden onset of anemia, jaundice, dark urine or hemoglobinuria, back and/or abdominal pain along with splenomegaly. A recent history of infections, vaccination or exposure to drugs, or signs of immune disease suggest secondary autoimmune hemolytic anemia (AIHA). Peripheral blood picture (**Flowchart 6**) remains an important tool to confirm and diagnose the cause of hemolysis. Intravascular and extravascular hemolysis can be differentiated as shown in **Table 4**. Treatment is supportive with removal of all precipitating factors. A trial of steroids may improve hemolysis in few cases of autoimmune hemolytic anemia.

DISSEMINATED INTRAVASCULAR COAGULATION

It is an acquired and systemic disorder of hemostasis that causes both thrombosis and hemorrhage. It is always associated with an underlying illness, which leads to widespread endothelial damage and release of inflammatory cytokines thereby causing systemic activation of the coagulation cascade. The resultant widespread thrombosis causes organ failure and

Table 3: Laboratory evaluation of a bleeding neonate

Clinical evaluation	*Platelets*	*Pt*	*Ptt*	*Likely diagnosis*
"SICK"	Decreased	Increased	Increased	Disseminated intravascular coagulation
	Decreased	N	N	Platelet consumption
	N	Increased	Increased	Liver disease
	N	N	N	Vascular anomaly
"HEALTHY"	Decreased	N	N	Neonatal alloimmune thrombocytopenia, autoimmune thrombocytopenia
	N	Increased	Increased	Hemorrhagic disease of newborn
	N	N	Increased	Hereditary clotting factor deficiencies
	N	N	N	Trauma, von Willebrand disease, factor XIII deficiency

Flowchart 5: Approach to bleeding neonate

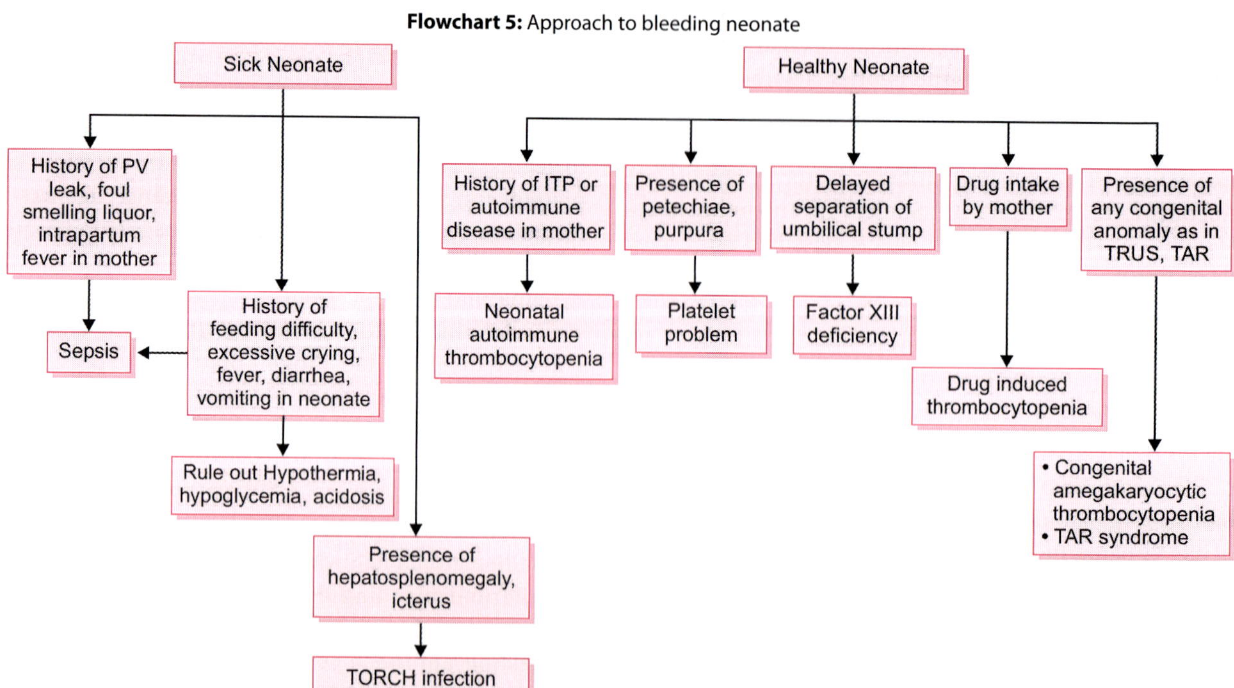

Flowchart 6: Role of peripheral blood picture in diagnosis of acute hemolysis

Peripheral blood picture

- Spherocytes → • Hereditery spherocytosis • Autoimmune hemolytic anemia • Clostridial sepsis • Severe hypophosphatemia • Severe burn, thermal injury
- Schistocytes → Microangiopathic hemolytic anemia
- • Sickle cells • Howell Jolly bodies → Sickle cell anemia
- Heinz bodies → G6PD deficiency
- Spur cells → Liver disease
- Agglutination → Cold agglutinin disease

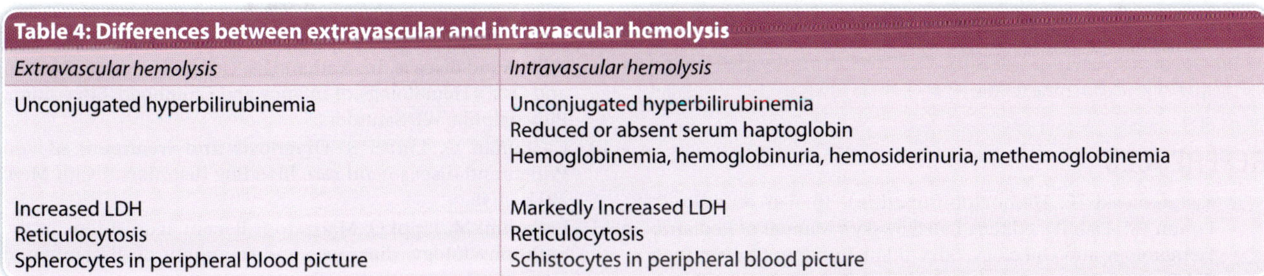

Table 4: Differences between extravascular and intravascular hemolysis

Extravascular hemolysis	*Intravascular hemolysis*
Unconjugated hyperbilirubinemia	Unconjugated hyperbilirubinemia Reduced or absent serum haptoglobin Hemoglobinemia, hemoglobinuria, hemosiderinuria, methemoglobinemia
Increased LDH Reticulocytosis Spherocytes in peripheral blood picture	Markedly Increased LDH Reticulocytosis Schistocytes in peripheral blood picture

Table 5: Differential diagnosis of DIC

PT / aPTT	*Platelet count*	*Fibrinogen level*	*Diagnosis*
Increased	Low	Low	DIC
Increased	Low	Normal	Liver disease
Increased	Normal	Normal	Vitamin K deficiency
Normal	Low (with MAHA)	Normal	TTP

(aPTT: activated partial thromboplastin time; DIC: disseminated intravascular coagulation; MAHA: microangiopathic hemolytic anemia; PT: prothrombin time; TTP: thrombotic thrombocytopenic purpura)

microangiopathic hemolytic anemia. It also depletes platelets, clotting factors and anticoagulant proteins leading to bleeding.

Diagnosis

A complete blood count may reveal anemia and thrombocytopenia related to thrombotic microangiopathy. PT/aPTT are raised due to consumption of coagulation proteins. "DIC panel" that includes fibrinogen level, fibrin degradation product (FDP) and D-dimer test also aid in diagnosis of DIC. In DIC, fibrinogen levels are low due to consumption whereas FDP and D-dimer are raised (**Table 5**).

Treatment

Treatment of the underlying cause is the mainstay. Symptomatic management of bleeding or thrombosis is dictated by clinical scenario. Fresh frozen plasma or cryoprecipitate and platelet transfusion are warranted in case of active bleeding or high risk of bleeding.

Low molecular weight heparin is suggested in the thrombotic phase of DIC but its use is controversial. Some may consider anti-thrombin III (ATIII) replacement in those with low ATIII levels and severe DIC.[11] The prognosis of patients with DIC is primarily dependent on the outcome of treatment of the primary disease and prevention of end-organ damage.

KEY MESSAGES

- The risk of bacteremia is high in a child having fever with sickle cell disease and thus requires prompt administration of antibiotics.
- Any child of sickle cell anemia with fever, severe anemia and reticulocytopenia should be considered to have parvovirus B19 infection.
- Febrile non-hemolytic transfusion reaction are more often seen after transfusion of platelets than red blood cells as the platelets are stored at room temperature which promotes leukocyte activation.
- Platelet transfusion is contraindicated for immune thrombocytopenic purpura unless there is life-threatening bleed.
- In case of mild Factor VIII deficiency, desmopressin may be used which helps in the release of factor VIII.

REFERENCES

1. Kwiatkowski JL. Hemoglobinopathies. In: Lanzkowsky P, Lipton JM, Fish JD, editors. Lanzkowsky's Manual of Pediatric Hematology and Oncology, 6th edition. London: Elsevier Inc.; 2016. p. 166-80.
2. DeBaun MR, Frei-Jones MJ, Vichinsky EP. Hemoglobinopathies. In: Kliegman RM, Stanton BF, St Geme JW, Schor NF. Nelson Textbook of Pediatrics, 1st South Asian edition. New Delhi: Reed Elsevier India Pvt Ltd.; 2016. p. 336-45.
3. Meier ER, Rampersad A. Pediatric sickle cell disease: Past successes and future challenges. Pediatr Research. 2017;81: 249-54.
4. Wong ECC, Luban NLC. Blood banking principles and practices. In: Lanzkowsky P, Lipton JM, Fish JD. Lanzkowsky's Manual of Pediatric Hematology and Oncology, 6th edition. London: Elsevier Inc.; 2016. p. 700-3.
5. Halfdanarson TR, Hogan WJ, Madsen BE. Emergencies in hematology and oncology. Mayo Clin Proc. 2017;92:609-41.
6. Lewis MA, Hendrickson AW, Moynihan TJ. Oncologic emergencies: Pathophysiology, presentation, diagnosis, and treatment. Cancer J Clin. 2011;61:287-314.
7. Freifeld AG, Bow EJ, Sepkowitz KA, *et al.* Clinical practice guideline for the use of antimicrobial agents in neutropenic patients with cancer: 2010 Update by the Infectious Diseases Society of America. Clin Infect Dis. 2011;52:427-31.
8. Blanchette VS, Breakey VR, Revel-Vilk S, editors. Sick Kids Handbook of Pediatric Thrombosis and Hemostasis. Basel, Karger, 2013, p. 14–22.
9. Montgomery RR, Gill JC, Scott JP. Hemophilia and von Willebrand disease. In: Nathan DG, Orkin SH, editors. Nathan and Oski's Hematology of Infancy and Childhood, 5th edition. Philadelphia: WB Saunders.
10. Castaman G, Linari S. Diagnosis and treatment of von Willebrand disease and rare bleeding disorders. J Clin Med. 2017;6:E45.
11. Franchini M, Lippi G, Manzato F. Recent acquisitions in the pathophysiology, diagnosis and treatment of disseminated intravascular coagulation. Thromb J. 2006;4:4.

CHAPTER

39

Oncological Emergencies

Sunil Bhat, Pooja P Mallya

INTRODUCTION

In the last few years, there has been a dramatic increase in the survival rate of pediatric cancer patients. This has been accomplished with increased awareness in the population, early detection, newer treatment modalities and most importantly improved supportive care, which importantly includes managing oncological emergencies. A child with cancer can present with emergencies, which requires early recognition, and timely treatment as these can be life-threatening. These emergencies can be because of the disease itself, or as a consequence of treatment. They can affect multiple organ systems and may be rapidly progressive. Most of the times, these patients present initially to the pediatrician, or to the emergency department. Hence, awareness of these complications and urgent referral to the oncologist is the need of the hour. Management of these emergencies requires a multidisciplinary approach with involvement of the pediatricians, pathologists, hematologists, pediatric surgeons, radiation oncologists, radiologists and other clinical specialties.

Oncological emergency is defined as an acute condition that is caused by cancer or its treatment, requiring rapid intervention to avoid death or severe permanent damage.[1] The common oncological emergencies are enlisted in **Table 1**. Few of these shall be discussed in this chapter.

Table 1: Common pediatric oncological emergencies

- *Structural compromise secondary to tumor*
  Superior mediastinal/vena cava syndrome
  Spinal compression syndrome
  Raised intracranial pressure
  Pericardial effusion and cardiac tamponade
  Massive hepatomegaly
- *Hematological emergencies*
  Hyperleukocytosis and leukostasis
  Thrombotic events
  Anemia
  Thrombocytopenia
  Veno-occlusive disease
- *Treatment related complications*
  Febrile neutropenia
  Typhilitis
  Pancreatitis
  Vesicant infiltration
  All trans retinoic acid syndrome
  Allergic reaction to chemotherapeutic drugs or blood products
- *Metabolic complications*
  Tumor lysis syndrome (electrolyte disturbances included)
  SIADH
  Hypercalcemia of malignancy

STRUCTURAL EMERGENCIES

SUPERIOR MEDIASTINAL SYNDROME OR SUPERIOR VENA CAVA SYNDROME

The presence of a mass in the anterior mediastinum can cause compression of the superior vena cava, tracheobronchial tree, or the heart and pulmonary vessels. Superior vena cava syndrome (SVCS) denotes the compression, obstruction and thrombosis of the superior vena cava. Superior mediastinal syndrome (SMS) has been used to denote the combination of great vessel and tracheobronchial tree compression. Because these two phenomena are mostly overlapping, the terms SMS and SVCS have been used interchangeably.

Etiology

Neoplasms that present as anterior mediastinal masses commonly present with SMS or SVCS include non-Hodgkin's lymphoma (NHL), acute lymphoblastic leukemia (ALL), Hodgkin's lymphoma, neuroblastoma, germ cell tumors, sarcoma, thyroid cancer and many others.

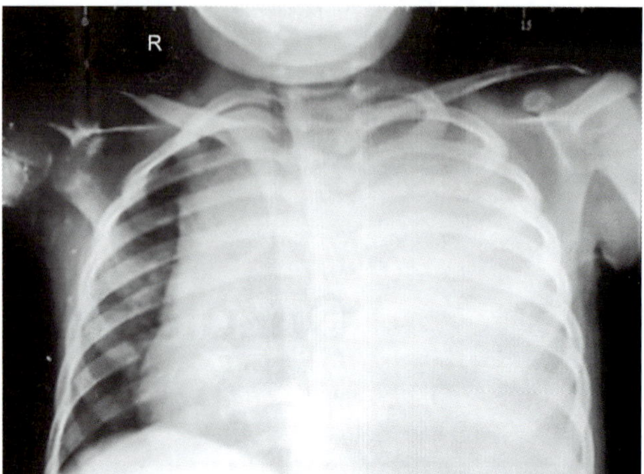

Fig. 1: Chest radiograph showing an anterior mediastinal mass

Pathophysiology

Enlargement of structures in the thorax can easily compress the SVC as the vessel is thin walled with blood flowing at low pressures. Hence, the compression or obstruction of SVC will restrict the blood return to the right atrium and impair the venous drainage from the head, neck and upper extremities. Compression of the trachea and bronchi will cause respiratory compromise especially in children where the intraluminal diameter is small and these structures are relatively easily compressible. Symptoms are more in the supine position because of the decreased thoracic volume, diaphragm position and increased blood flow to the mass.

Clinical Presentation

The presenting features are secondary to compression of the SVC and airway obstruction. These are swelling, plethora and cyanosis of the head, neck and upper extremities, hoarseness of voice, cough, wheezing, stridor, orthopnea, syncope, altered mental status, chest pain and dysphagia. The symptoms are exaggerated in the supine position.

Complications: Cardiac compromise with shock and respiratory failure can occur in malignancies with higher growth fraction such as B-lymphoblastic, or T-lymphoblastic, or mature B-cell lymphomas.

Diagnosis

The investigations comprise of:

1. Chest radiograph (include lateral view also) to identify the anterior mediastinal mass and pleural and pericardial effusion (**Fig. 1**).
2. Computed tomography of the thorax enables detailed anatomical information and opportunity for biopsy of the mass. Patients with less than 50% of the expected tracheal cross sectional area are found to be a high risk group.
3. Definitive diagnosis of the cause:
   - Complete blood count, peripheral smear and if abnormal bone marrow examination.
   - Serum α-fetoprotein or β-human chorionic gonadotropin for germ cell tumors.
   - If pleural effusion: Pleural fluid aspiration and fluid for evaluation.
   - Biopsy of the mediastinal mass (CT guided).
   - Echocardiogram for cardiac function, anesthesia risk and possible intravascular thrombus.

The diagnostic evaluation depends on the patient's condition. Pediatric population may require sedation and are at greatest risk for anesthetic complications including cardiopulmonary compromise and death.

Management

Most of the times because of the anticipated risk of the diagnostic procedures, empirical therapy to reduce the mass may have to be initiated. The following steps are to be followed in the management of such a child:

1. Supportive care which included oxygenation, semi-recumbent position and venous access (avoid upper limb veins).
2. The main treatment modalities are radiation, steroids and combination chemotherapy.

Radiation therapy: This is used as an emergency modality because lymphomas are radiosensitive. In view of post-radiation respiratory distress secondary to tracheal swelling, concurrent steroids are used. Intravenous dexamethasone at a dose of 0.5–2 mg/kg in divided doses every 6 hours needs to be initiated.

Chemotherapy: Intravenous steroids or combination chemotherapy is used. Steroid therapy should be used to manage proven or presumed acute lymphoblastic leukemia (ALL) or lymphoblastic lymphoma. Based on the chemotherapy protocols for ALL, intravenous methylprednisolone at a dose of 60 mg/m^2 divided in two divided doses needs to be started. Steroids also have a potent anti-inflammatory effect. Cyclophosphamide, vincristine and anthracyclines are the other agents used in the management.

Both radiation and steroids may obscure the diagnosis, hence, every attempt should be made to obtain a histological diagnosis prior to treatment when possible.

SPINAL COMPRESSION SYNDROME

The incidence of this complication is 5% in pediatric cancer and usually presents at diagnosis. It is the second most common neurological emergency after brain metastasis and requires urgent intervention to prevent neurological sequelae.

Etiology

Seventy one percent of the tumors causing spinal compression are extradural.[2] The most common tumors being neuroblastoma, rhabdomyosarcoma, soft tissue sarcomas and Ewing's sarcoma. Other tumors are osteosarcoma, Wilm's tumor, metastasis from brain tumors and acute myelogenous leukemia.

Pathophysiology

Damage to the spinal cord occurs by direct compression causing demyelination, axonal damage and secondary vascular complications.

Clinical Presentation

Back pain is the most common presentation and was present in 94% of pediatric patients.[2] Recurrent back pain without any history of trauma or neurological findings requires evaluation. Local pain may gain a radicular pattern and referred pain can also be seen. Pain may aggravate with movement, coughing and straining. Neurological findings will depend on the level of the spinal lesion and the degree of compression. Localized spine tenderness is the most reliable clinical finding. Muscle weakness is the most common motor deficit followed by sensory deficit. Bowel and bladder disturbance can also occur based on the site and severity of compression.

Differential Diagnosis

Benign musculoskeletal diseases (muscle spasm, intervertebral disc diseases), infectious diseases like epidural abscess, radiation myelopathy and metastatic disease with spinal metastasis should be considered in the differential diagnosis of spinal compression syndrome (SCC).

Investigations

1. *Spinal radiography*: Paraspinal soft tissue mass (dumb-bell appearance, with calcification in neuroblastoma), lytic bone lesions, enlargement of neural foramina.
2. *Magnetic resonance imaging (MRI) with contrast enhancement*: This gives a detailed delineation of the lesion. The whole spine needs to be imaged.

Treatment

The best choice of initial therapy depends on the clinical scenario of the patient. The main goal of treatment is to prevent further loss of neurological function and treat the underlying condition. Treatment options are:

1. *Surgery*: Laminectomy helps to stabilize or improve lost neurologic function. This procedure will also allow procurement of tumor tissue for diagnosis. However, this may not provide an advantage over chemotherapy and poses risk of surgical procedure and long-term orthopedic sequelae.[3]
2. *Chemotherapy*: It has been used successfully in neuroblastoma, germ cell tumors, Ewing's sarcoma, leukemia and lymphomas which are causing SCC. It is important to establish a pathological diagnosis before initiating chemotherapy. It is noninvasive and is a tumor-specific treatment modality. In the setting of a relapsed disease, the decision of chemotherapy rather than surgery or radiation for palliation can be used. The choice of chemotherapy regimen must be based on the underlying malignant process.
3. *Steroids*: Dexamethasone is recommended throughout literature for the treatment of pediatric SCC.

This reduces the swelling of the cord and minimizes the damage to the spinal cord. Detrimental effects with the routine use of Dexamethasone in acute SCC have been observed.[3] Increased rates of infection and delayed wound healing are often seen. SCC caused by tumor and any neurological compromise, rapid administration of intravenous dexamethasone at 1–2 mg/kg over 30 minutes is recommended. In the absence of neurological symptoms, a lower oral dose of 0.25–0.5 mg/kg every 6 hours needs to be initiated. Gastric protectants like proton pump inhibitors/H2 blockers are to be given along with dexamethasone.

4. *Radiation therapy*: This is very effective treatment modality as there is a rapid response and is non-invasive method. Post-radiation therapy may also warrant administration of steroids. Radiation therapy, however, has long-term effects especially in the pediatric population like stunted growth, scoliosis, cord damage and risk of secondary malignancies.

PERICARDIAL EFFUSION AND CARDIAC TAMPONADE

Malignant pericardial effusion restricts the diastolic filling of the heart and hence reduces the cardiac output and this result in cardiac tamponade.

Etiology

Common pediatric cancers causing pericardial effusion and tamponade are leukemia and non-Hodgkin's lymphoma. Rarely, primary tumors of the pericardium can also cause this complication.

Clinical Presentation

Most of the patients are asymptomatic. Symptoms of pericarditis may precede tamponade. Chest discomfort, dyspnea, orthopnea and cough are the common symptoms. Classical presentation of cardiac tamponade includes tachycardia, pulsus paradoxus, Beck's triad of hypotension, elevated jugular venous pressure and muffled heart sounds.

Investigations

1. *Chest radiograph*: Cardiomegaly and classical water bottle cardiac silhouette are seen.
2. *Electrocardiography*: Low voltage and electrical alternans is seen.
3. Echocardiography is the definitive test, which reveals the presence and quantity of pericardial effusion and demonstrates the right ventricular collapse during diastole.
4. Diagnostic and therapeutic pericardiocentesis can be done.
5. CT and MRI can provide detailed information of the effusion and the tumor.

Treatment

Pericardiocentesis helps to relieve the pressure by removal of the fluid. For prolonged drainage, a continuous draining catheter or creating a pericardial window are other methods of treatment. Radiation can also be considered with a caution regarding post-radiation pericarditis. Chemotherapy will be required to treat the underlying malignancies. Supportive care in the form of oxygenation and fluids need to managed simultaneously.

HEMATOLOGICAL EMERGENCIES

HYPERLEUKOCYTOSIS AND LEUKOSTASIS

Hyperleukocytosis is defined as a total white cell count (WBC) higher than 100×10^9/L. It is estimated to occur in 5–20% of childhood leukemias. Stasis of leukemic cells in the blood vessels and migration of blasts into tissues leads to leukostasis.

Etiology

It is most commonly seen in infant acute lymphoblastic leukemia (ALL), T-cell ALL, acute myelogenous leukemia (AML) and chronic myelogenous leukemia (CML). Hyperleukocytosis is more in ALL and leukostasis in AML (especially M4 and M5).

Pathophysiology

Hyperleukocytosis causes leukemic aggregates, increases the packed leukocyte volume, thrombus which leads to increase in blood viscosity. Myeloblasts are larger, have increased viscosity and form more aggregates.[4]

Clinical Presentation

This can affect any system in the body. Most commonly involves the lung and brain. Symptoms are based on the system involved.

Pulmonary: Dyspnea, tachypnea, hypoxia, respiratory failure.

Central nervous system: Headache, blurred vision, tinnitus, seizures, stroke, stupor, delirium and coma.

Renal: Oliguria, anuria, priapism.

Vascular: Disseminated intravascular coagulation, retinal hemorrhage, myocardial infarction.

There is always a risk of associated tumor lysis syndrome.

Investigations

A complete blood count, peripheral smear and bone marrow examination are needed for the definitive diagnosis of etiology. Investigations are based on the organ system involved. Chest radiograph may show diffuse interstitial or alveolar infiltrates. Neuroimaging is needed if neurological complications are present.

Treatment

The definitive treatment is early initiation of induction chemotherapy after obtaining the diagnosis. Measures to deal with tumor lysis syndrome, which include adequate hydration, medications to deal with hyperuricemia and other dyselectrolytemia (refer the section on tumor lysis syndrome), need to be initiated. Red blood cell transfusion should be avoided as this will increase the blood viscosity. Cytoreduction with hydroxyurea, leukapheresis and exchange transfusion can be done. Patients weighing less than 12 kg may safely undergo exchange transfusion. There has been a mean reduction of 50–60% in the WBC after exchange transfusion and leukapheresis as observed in many pediatric studies.[5] Leukapheresis is avoided in acute promyelocytic leukemia because of the risk of hemorrhage. Based on the patient's condition, more than one modality of treatment may be used.

VENOUS THROMBOEMBOLISM

Etiopathogenesis

The incidence of venous thromboembolism (VTE) depends on the cancer type and is highest among patients diagnosed with metastatic disease. The risk factors of VTE can be both disease related and treatment related. Disease related factors being the hypercoagulable state secondary to malignancy. Treatment related factors being chemotherapeutic drugs, post-surgery, prolonged immobilization and importantly central venous access devices.

Clinical Presentation

A child with VTE may present with swelling and pain of the affected limb. Patient can present with dry cough, hemoptysis, chest pain and dyspnea if pulmonary embolism is present. Signs include tachycardia, tachypnea, hypotension and pleural effusion.

Investigations

1. *Chest radiograph*: Oligemia of the affected segment, pleural effusion, atelectasis
2. *Arterial blood gas*: Hypoxemia, hypocarbia
3. Ultrasound Doppler of the affected limb
4. CT thorax and CT pulmonary angiogram
5. Ventilation-perfusion scan
6. *CT/MRI venography*: Cortical venous thrombus may be secondary to L-asparaginase therapy.

Treatment

Low molecular or unfractionated heparin are the treatment options. Enoxaparin 1 mg/kg/dose twice a day subcutaneously to be given for a duration of 3 to 6 months. Use of inferior vena cava filter and thrombectomy may be used in patients with recurrent thromboembolism.

TREATMENT-RELATED EMERGENCIES

FEBRILE NEUTROPENIA

Introduction and Classification

Fever is defined as a single oral temperature measurement of >38.3°C (101°F) or a temperature of >38°C (100.4°F) sustained over a one hour period. Neutropenia is the absolute neutrophil count (ANC) of 500 cells/mm^3 or an ANC that is expected to decrease to 500 cells/mm^3 during the next 48 hours.[6] Profound neutropenia is ANC less than 100 cells/mm^3. Febrile neutropenia (FN) is a complication of patients with cancer treated with chemotherapy and post-hematopoietic stem cell transplantation. These patients can be classified as high risk and low risk (**Table 2**) to determine inpatient or outpatient treatment, oral or intravenous antibiotic and the duration of treatment to given.

Table 2: Classification of febrile neutropenia patients

High-risk patients	*Low-risk patients*
Anticipated prolonged (>7 days) duration Profound neutropenia Comorbid conditions—hemodynamic instability, oral or gastrointestinal mucositis that interferes with swallowing or causes severe diarrhea, intravascular catheter infection, pneumonia or neurologic changes	Anticipated brief (<7 days) duration neutropenic periods No or few comorbidities

Approach to Febrile Neutropenia

1. *Detailed history*: Symptoms, antimicrobial prophylaxis, infection exposures, prior cultures, other non-infectious causes of fever, e.g. blood transfusion and any underlying comorbid conditions.
2. *Physical examination*: Detailed head to toe examination is required to detect subtle signs and symptoms of infection. Special attention must be given to the skin at the catheter site, surgical or procedure site. Also need to specifically examine the oropharynx and perineum.
3. *Investigations*
   - Blood cultures at the onset of FN. Obtain peripheral blood cultures concurrent with central venous catheter (from all lumens). Blood culture volumes should be limited to <1% of the total blood volume.[7]
   - Culture from sites of suspected infection as clinically indicated (e.g. stool, urine, CSF, skin, respiratory secretions).
   - Chest radiograph in patients with respiratory symptoms.
   - Other tests based on the patient, e.g. Serum galactomannan, imaging studies.

Treatment

These patients with febrile neutropenia need to be started on empirical antibiotics. There are special situations where antifungal and antiviral drugs also need to be administered. The epidemiology of neutropenic infection varies among different treatment centers. Only in 10–30% of the patients a culture may be found to be positive. The most important is supportive care with intravenous fluids, oxygenation, etc.

- High-risk patients require in-patient admission for intravenous antibiotics for a longer duration
- Low-risk patients can be managed on an outpatient basis with oral antibiotics for a shorter duration.

The first line of antibiotics should be based on the organisms encountered and the sensitivity pattern at a particular center. Institution based guidelines then need to be framed. The most common infections in most of centers in India are gram negative organisms, e.g. *Pseudomonas aeruginosa*, *E. coli*, *Klebsiella pneumonia* and *Acinetobacter* spp.

According to Infectious Diseases Society of America (IDSA 2018) Guidelines monotherapy with antipseudomonal β-lactam, a fourth generation cephalosporin, or a carbapenem is used as an empirical therapy in high-risk FN. A second gram negative agent is added to unstable patients, resistant infections, or at centers with a high rate of resistant organisms. However, no significant differences in treatment failure, infection-related death, or adverse events were observed while comparing anti-pseudomonas penicillin ± aminoglycoside regimen, with carbapenem monotherapy in a meta-analysis.[8] Piperacillin-Tazobactam with amikacin is being used as the first line therapy our unit at Bengaluru. Gram positive cover needs to be added if there is hemodynamic instability, pneumonia, suspected catheter related infection, skin or soft tissue infection or a positive culture. In patients who are stable and responding to the initial therapy, double coverage for gram negative infection can be discontinued. Those patients who are unstable will require escalation of antibiotics and may require addition of antifungal agents. Antibiotics can be modified based on the sensitivity pattern on culture (**Flowchart 1**). Empirical antifungals are given to patients at high risk for invasive fungal disease, these are acute myeloid leukemia, relapsed acute leukemia, high risk leukemia and children undergoing allogeneic transplant.[9] Antiviral acyclovir treatment (20 mg/kg/dose, three times a day) for herpes simplex virus or varicella zoster virus infection is only indicated if there is any clinical or laboratory evidence of active viral disease.

NEUTROPENIC ENTEROCOLITIS

It is also called as typhlitis, is a life-threatening complication associated with chemotherapy-associated neutropenia. This occurs secondary to the bowel wall

Table 3: Cairo Bishop classification

Variable	*Value*	*Change from baseline value*
Uric acid	≥8 mg/dL (476 mmol/L)	25% increase
Potassium	≥6.0 mEq/L (or 6 mmol/L)	25% increase
Phosphorus	≥4.5 mg/dL (1.45 mmol/L) for adults and ≥ 6.5 mg/dL (2.1 mmol/L) for children	25% increase
Calcium	≤7 mg/dL (1.75 mmol/L)	25% decrease

damage caused by the chemotherapy together with drug-induced neutropenia. This causes mucosal damage, ulceration and at times perforation. The most common symptoms are abdominal pain, fever, diarrhea, abdominal distension, nausea and vomiting. Radiograph and CT of the abdomen will reveal dilated cecum and ascending colon filled with liquid, gas, small bowel dilation and at times a pneumoperitoneum. Conservative management consists of fluid resuscitation, bowel rest, abdominal decompression, blood component support and broad-spectrum antibiotics. Surgery is indicated for intestinal perforation.

DIFFERENTIATION SYNDROME

This is a life-threatening complication of therapy with differentiating agents [all-*trans* retinoic acid (ATRA) or arsenic trioxide (ATO)] in patients with acute promyelocytic leukemia (APML). This is attributed to a hyperinflammatory response with vasoactive cytokines. It is characterized by unexplained fever, acute respiratory distress with interstitial pulmonary infiltrates, capillary leak syndrome leading to acute renal failure. At the earliest suspicion of differentiation syndrome (DS), ATRA or ATO should be stopped and intravenous dexamethasone should be administered until symptoms and signs resolve (minimum, 3 days). The recommended adult dose of dexamethasone is 0.25 mg/kg/dose intravenous or oral twice a day (maximum single dose of 10 mg).

METABOLIC COMPLICATIONS

TUMOR LYSIS SYNDROME

Tumor lysis syndrome (TLS) describes the metabolic derangement that occurs as a result of spontaneous or treatment/therapy related breakdown of cells.[3] The classical manifestations include hyperkalemia, hyperuricemia, hypocalcemia and hyperphosphatemia.

The Cairo Bishop Grading Classification can be used for defining TLS (**Table 3**).

Etiology

The TLS is commonly associated with initiation of treatment for cancers with high tumor burden and high proliferative index like ALL and non-Hodgkin's lymphoma (especially Burkitt's lymphoma). The risk of TLS is highest within 12 to 72 hours after initiating therapy, however, TLS can occur prior to initiation of therapy, or even 7 days later. Pathophysiology is depicted in **Flowchart 2**.

Flowchart 1: Management of high-risk febrile neutropenia

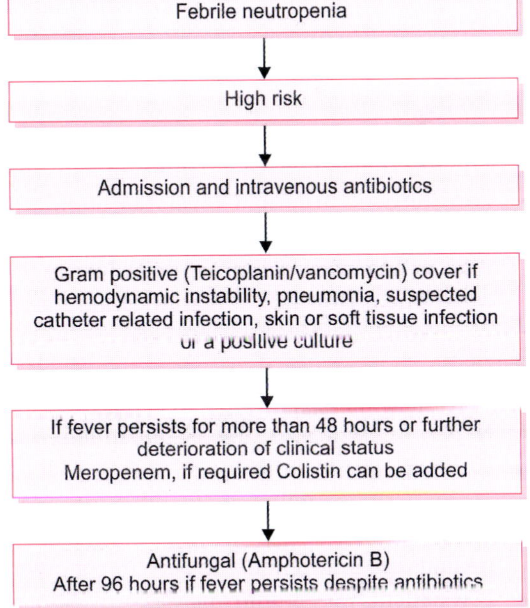

Antibiotics to be modified based on culture sensitivity reports
Piperacillin-Tazobactam (100 mg/kg/dose, three times a day)
Amikacin (15 mg/kg/day, once a day)
Vancomycin (10 mg/kg/dose, four times a day)
Teicoplanin (10 mg/kd/dose BD for three doses then once a day)
Meropenem (80–120 mg/kg/day, in three divided doses)
Colistin (60,000 IU/kg stat followed by 30,000 IU/kg, three times a day)
Amphotericin B (1 mg/kg/day)

Clinical Presentation

Nausea, cardiac arrhythmias, seizures, altered consciousness, muscle cramps, tetany, oliguria or anuria.

Management

The main principles of treatment are hydration and diuresis, careful monitoring and management of electrolyte abnormalities.

1. *Hydration*: Potassium free intravenous fluid needs to be started at 125 mL/m^2/hour.
2. *Diuresis*: It is important to maintain urine output at 100 mL/m^2/hour. Furosemide, 0.5–1 mg/kg or mannitol (0.5 g/kg) for low urine output in the absence of hypovolemia.
3. *Alkalinization of urine*: Not recommended as this may increase the precipitation of calcium phosphate in the renal tubules.
4. *Uric acid reduction*
   - *Allopurinol (xanthine oxidase inhibitor):* 100 mg/m^2/dose thrice a day or 10 mg/kg/day in three divided doses by mouth.
   - *Rasburicase (recombinant urate oxidase):* 0.2 mg/kg intravenously dissolved in 50 mL normal saline infused over 30 minutes given once daily for up to 5 days.
   - Febuxostat is a selective xanthine oxidase inhibitor and has shown to have a significant and superior control over uric acid levels as compared to allopurinol. There are only few studies in children and hence the recommended dosage is not mentioned. However, few studies have given 40 mg to children above 6 years of age.
5. *Metabolic abnormalities*
   - *Hyperkaemia*: Correction of hyperkalemia.
   - *Hyperphosphatemia*: Use of phosphate binders like Sevelamer hydrochloride (400 mg twice a day).
   - *Hypocalcemia*: Asymptomatic hypocalcemia does not need correction. Symptomatic hypocalcemia is treated with intravenous/oral calcium gluconate.
   - Few patients may require dialysis.

SYNDROME OF INAPPROPRIATE ANTIDIURETIC HORMONE SECRETION (SIADH)

Syndrome of inappropriate antidiuretic hormone secretion (SIADH) is a paraneoplastic condition due to excessive secretion of vasopressin by the tumor cells. This leads to hyponatremia. Patients can present with lethargy, confusion, seizures, muscle cramps and weakness. Management includes treating the underlying malignancy, fluid restriction, diuretics and use of vaptans.[10]

Flowchart 2: Pathophysiology of tumor lysis syndrome

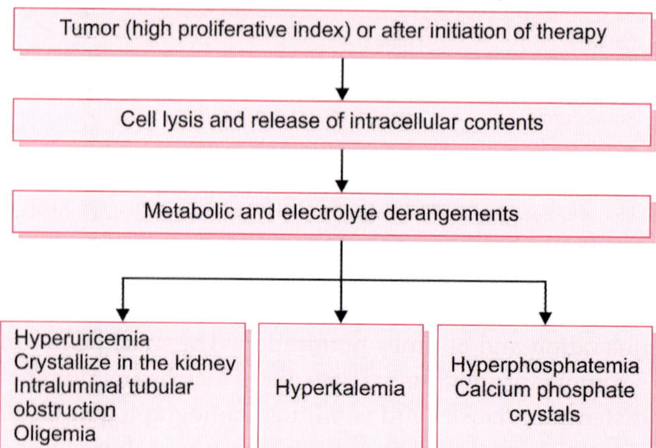

THROMBOCYTOPENIA

This is one of the most common complications of chemotherapy and can at times cause severe bleeding. Patients can present with petechiae, purpura, mucosal bleeds, gastrointestinal bleeds and very rarely intracranial bleeds. Severe thrombocytopenia (platelet count <10,000 cells/mm^3) or any bleeding needs treatment with platelet transfusion. Platelet transfusion at a dose of 6 units/m^2 or 0.1 U/kg needs to be given. Irradiated single donor platelets are preferable.

KEY MESSAGES

- Pediatric oncology patients may present with life-threatening complications, which require recognition and treatment.
- These emergencies can be classified as structural, hematological, treatment related, and metabolic.
- The main treatment options are chemotherapy, surgery, steroids and radiation. However, the management depends on the clinical condition of the patient and the probable diagnosis considered.
- Initiation of broad-spectrum antibiotics within an hour of fever in patients with febrile neutropenia is essential to cut down the mortality and morbidity due to febrile neutropenia.
- Administration of sedation/anesthesia in patients with mediastinal syndrome can be life-threatening.

REFERENCES

1. Cervantes A, Chirivella I. Oncological emergencies. Ann Oncol. 2004;4:299-306.
2. Pollono D, Tomarchia S, Drut R, *et al.* Spinal cord compression: A review of 70 pediatric patients. Ped Hematol Oncol. 2003;20: 457-66.
3. Elizabeth A, Mullen, Gratias E. Oncologic emergencies. In: Orkin SH, Fisher DE. Ginsburg D, Look AT, Lux SE, Nathan DG, editors. Nathan and Oski's Hematology and Oncology of Infancy and Childhood, 8th edition. Philadelphia: Elsevier Inc; 2015. p. 2281-91.
4. Seth R, Bhat AS. Management of common oncologic emergencies. Indian J Pediatr. 2011;78:709-17.
5. Eguiguren JM, Schell MJ, Crist WM, *et al.* Complications and outcome in childhood acute lymphoblastic leukemia with hyperleukocytosis. Blood. 1992;79:871-5.
6. Freifeld AG, Bow EJ, Sepkowitz KA, *et al.* Infectious Diseases Society of America. Clinical practice guideline for the use of antimicrobial agents in neutropenic patients with cancer: 2010 update by the Infectious Diseases Society of America. Clin Infect Dis. 2011;52:e56-93.
7. Wilson ML, Clinical and Laboratory Standards Institute. Principles and procedures for blood cultures: Approved guideline. Wayne, PA: Clinical and Laboratory Standards Institute; 2007.
8. Manji A. Lehrnbecher T, Bevene J, *et al.* A systematic review and meta-analysis of anti-pseudomonal penicillins and carbopenams in pediatric febrile neutropenia. Support Care Cancer. 2012;20:2295-304.
9. Lehrnbecher T, Robinson P, Fisher B, *et al.* Guideline for the management of fever and neutropenia in children with cancer and hematopoietic stem-cell transplantation recipients: 2017 Update. J Clin Oncol. 2017;35:2082-94.
10. Aditya S, Rattan A. Vaptans: A new option in the management of hyponatremia. Int J Appl Basic Med Res. 2012;2:77-83.

CHAPTER

40

Diabetic Ketoacidosis

Anju Virmani, Preeti Anand

INTRODUCTION

Type 1 diabetes (T1D), earlier called insulin-dependent diabetes mellitus (IDDM), juvenile diabetes or childhood onset diabetes, poses an extremely high burden on the patient, family and healthcare professionals. Diabetic ketoacidosis (DKA) unfortunately continues to be the initial presentation of T1D,[1-3] even though it was shown in the 1990s that increased awareness in the general public could prevent this, an effect which persisted years later.[4,5] It continues to occur in established T1D, usually either due to omission of insulin, or inadequate insulin during an illness. It continues to be a major cause of hospital admission, morbidity[6] and mortality, with region, young age, delayed diagnosis, and low socioeconomic status being significant predictors of mortality.[7,8] However, outcomes have improved dramatically, especially if managed in specialized centers, with one death and no residual neurologic deficits in 1389 episodes of DKA in 1255 children in the PECARN DKA FLUID study.[9]

Less often, DKA can occur in type 2 diabetes (T2D), at diagnosis or later. This is becoming important with increasing rates of obesity and T2D in adolescents.[10] These patients would be obese, have evidence of insulin excess in the form of acanthosis, skin tags, etc., and family history of T2D and obesity. The initial management of DKA remains the same.

DEFINITIONS

Diabetic ketoacidosis occurs when insulin deficiency co-exists with excess of glucagon and/or other counter-regulatory hormones, resulting in the triad of:

- Hyperglycemia (Blood Glucose: BG > 200 mg/dL),
- Ketosis (ketonemia, i.e. plasma ketones > 3 mmol/L; ketonuria, i.e. urine ketones "moderate" or "large"), and
- Acidosis (pH < 7.3, plasma bicarbonate <15 mmol/L).[7]

DKA is characterized by high anion gap (AG) metabolic acidosis[11]: the levels are usually 20–30 mmol/L. AG is calculated as follows: Na – (Cl + HCO_3). The normal AG is 10–14 mmol/L. If it is >35 mmol/L, coexistent lactic acidosis should be thought of.

DKA is graded as:

- Severe if pH < 7.1, plasma bicarbonate < 5 mmol/L;
- Moderate if pH < 7.2, plasma bicarbonate < 10 mmol/L;
- Mild if pH < 7.3, plasma bicarbonate < 15 mmol/L.

All patients with severe hyperglycemia and altered sensorium or seizures may not have DKA – rarely they develop hyperglycemic hyperosmolar state (HHS, earlier called hyperosmolar nonketotic coma). The criteria for HHS are:

- Very marked hyperglycemia (BG > 600 mg/dL),
- Lesser ketosis (ketonuria small, ketonemia absent to mild),
- Lesser acidosis (venous pH >7.25; arterial pH >7.30, bicarbonate >15 mEq/L); with
- Serum osmolality >320 mOsm/kg.

ETIOLOGY

Type 1 diabetes may present initially as DKA, especially if a history of osmotic symptoms and/or weight loss in spite of normal or increased appetite is ignored. This is more likely to happen in regions where T1D is less common, so it is not thought of; in children under age 5 years; in poor families; and in remote areas.[7] Our early experience showed that DKA accounted for 91% deaths in childhood onset diabetes, within hours, weeks or months of diagnosis, and a suspicion of death before diagnosis.[8] As awareness has increased, the situation is improving, with earlier diagnosis, i.e. before DKA occurs,[12] and better outcomes, underlining the importance of prevention and high index of suspicion. Thus, every child presenting with polyuria, recent onset of bed wetting, polydipsia; unexplained weight loss; acute episode of nausea, vomiting, pain abdomen; dehydration, especially with high urine output; blurred vision; tachypnea, especially deep sighing (Kussmaul) respiration; fruity odor of breath; tachycardia; lethargy, drowsiness or unconsciousness, should have urine and/or blood tested for diabetes. Today, every emergency room and every healthcare personnel's bag should have a glucometer, given the low cost and widespread availability. In fact, low cost point-of-care (POC) devices are becoming available in India for blood ketones and HbA1c also. As their use and the quality of communication improves, it is simply a matter of time before diagnosis and monitoring of T1D and DKA become possible even in the *smallest and most remote* set-up.

DKA can also occur in a known case of diabetes, sometimes quite rapidly, usually either due to inadvertent or deliberate omission of insulin, or inadequate insulin during an illness, or use of denatured insulin (failure of the cold chain at any point in transport or usage). Any physical stress (illness, infection, trauma or surgery) can precipitate DKA. This is especially likely with poverty and illiteracy; and inadequate medical care, diabetes education, or home BG monitoring. Children who often omit insulin, are on twice daily regimens, have poor glycemic control, or have had DKA earlier, and adolescents in general, are at high risk. In India, financial issues can contribute to inadequate home and laboratory monitoring, inadequate insulin dosing, and delayed seeking of medical attention. This can be compounded by wanting to conceal diabetes from peers and relatives, and other psychological or psychiatric problems or superstitions in the patient or key family caregivers, regardless of socioeconomic or educational status. In the early days of insulin pumps, users were more prone to DKA, as any discontinuation of insulin supply (e.g. kinked or disconnected catheter) led to a rapid fall in insulin levels. However, with improved technology, the situation has reversed.[13] Therefore, meticulous diabetes education and constant reinforcement are needed to ensure patients buy insulin from reliable sources, store it properly, are aware of sick day guidelines, have access to ketone testing, and know when to reach medical care.

All patients of DKA may not be comatose at presentation. Conversely, in a child with diabetes presenting with drowsiness/unconsciousness, other causes of coma should be thought of, whether related to diabetes, such as hypoglycemia or HHS; or not, such as head injury, hepatic coma, neurological infections, and salicylate poisoning (**Table 1**).

PATHOPHYSIOLOGY

An absolute or relative deficiency of insulin, with increase in the level of counter-regulatory hormones, leads to hyperglycemia and ketosis (**Flowchart 1**).

Insulin is an anabolic hormone, which stimulates glucose utilization in the muscle and adipose tissue, and storage of food-derived glucose in the liver. Insulin deficiency leads to build up of glucose, with lipolysis, ketogenesis, glycogenolysis and gluconeogenesis to supply energy needs. The resultant increase in free fatty acids leads to the increased formation of ketone bodies.

The *counter-regulatory hormones* (glucagon, epinephrine, cortisol and growth hormone) affect catabolic

Table 1: Differential diagnosis of diabetic ketoacidosis

Parameter	*DKA*	*HHS*	*Meningoencephalitis*	*Salicylate poisoning*	*GE with acidosis*
Drowsiness	+	+	++	±	±
Respiration	Acidotic	Shallow	Central deep	Acidotic	Acidotic
Urine output	High	High	Normal	Normal	Low
Dehydration	++	+++	–	++	+++
Blood glucose	High	Very high	Normal	Normal	Normal
Ketones	+++	±	–	–	–
Bicarbonate	Low	Normal/low	Normal	Low	Low

(DKA: diabetic ketoacidosis; HHS: hyperglycemic hyperosmolar state; GE: gastroenteritis)

Flowchart 1: Pathophysiology of diabetic ketoacidosis

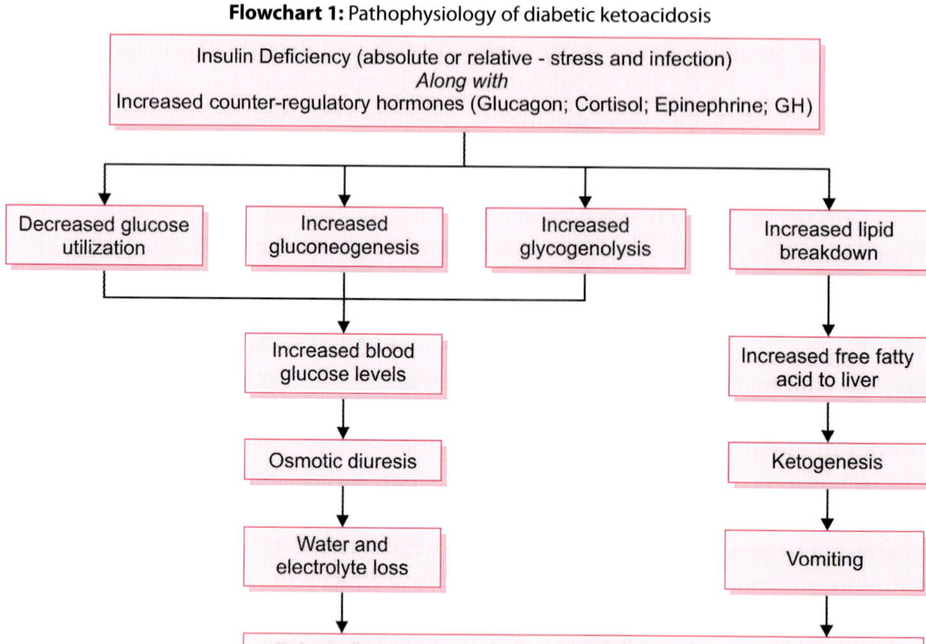

(GH: growth hormone; GFR: glomerular filtration rate)

processes directly, and indirectly by inhibiting the action of insulin. The essential paradox in DKA is that despite high BG levels there is a glucose deficit at the cellular level.

Hyperglycemia leads to osmotic diuresis, and loss of water and electrolytes, which in turn lead to dehydration, volume contraction, hyperosmolality, electrolyte imbalance and reduction in glomerular filtration rate (GFR). Vomiting caused by ketosis worsens this situation.

Sodium levels and *blood pressure* tend to be normal despite the free water loss, because the hyperosmolar state leads to a shift of intracellular water to the extracellular fluid. Factitious hyponatremia may be caused by the high triglyceride levels seen in severe DKA.

Potassium is the most severely affected electrolyte. Intracellular potassium is depleted because of transcellular shifts caused by increased osmolality (this hypertonicity causes solvent drag in which water and potassium are drawn out of the cells); acidosis; glycogenolysis and proteolysis secondary to insulin loss causing potassium to move out of the cells (**Flowchart 2**). Vomiting and osmotic diuresis cause net potassium losses, further worsened by the secondary hyperaldosteronism caused by volume depletion and dehydration. Rehydration leads to further hypokalemia due to the dilution of serum potassium, improved GFR accelerating renal losses, correction of acidosis, and therapy with insulin leading to the return of potassium into the cells.

Phosphate concentrations are also similarly affected.

Renal dysfunction and increased catabolism of protein lead to elevation of blood urea nitrogen and creatinine.

The ketoacids, beta hydroxy-butyric acid (BOHB) and acetoacetic acid (AA) are strong acids resulting in severe *metabolic acidosis*, which adversely affects the functioning of several organs. In the urine, the main component is acetoacetate; BOHB is converted to AA for excretion. Therefore, urinary levels of ketones, high during DKA, rise further initially during treatment as BOHB is cleared, and then fall. For this reason, blood ketones are more reliable than urine ketones.[14]

Serum *bicarbonate* is usually low but the deficit is decreased by peripheral metabolism of lactic acid and ketoacids into bicarbonate. Supplementation of bicarbonate is hardly ever required; it may possibly be considered in severe life-threatening hyperkalemia or severe acidosis (pH < 6.9) with cardiac dysfunction.

Hypocapnia (caused by hyperventilation) leads to cerebral vasoconstriction and reduced cerebral blood flow. Depression of the vasomotor center leads to decreased arterial smooth muscle tone and depression of myocardial contractility.

Flowchart 2: Pathophysiology of hypokalemia in DKA

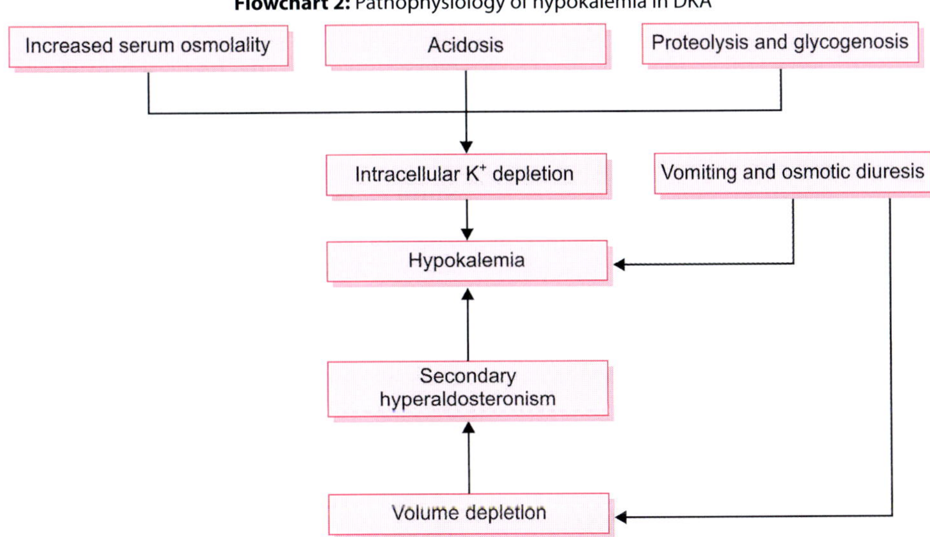

CLINICAL FEATURES

The child with DKA usually presents with a history of osmotic symptoms and weight loss, as mentioned above, Kussmaul respiration, drowsiness, and finally coma. The severity of dehydration may be difficult to assess, especially in young children, since urine output is maintained, and clinical signs may lead to overestimation.

A precipitating cause like an infection or trauma, and in a known diabetic, missed/inadequate insulin doses, must be looked for. An infection may range from the obvious, e.g. very rare rhinocerebral mucormycosis, an often-fatal opportunistic infection, to easily missed balanitis or urinary tract infection. In an infection, fever may not be present as peripheral vasodilatation causes cooling. Conversely, leukocytosis may not be due to infection, but to the DKA itself. Nausea and vomiting may suggest acute gastroenteritis, but the severity of dehydration in DKA is out of proportion to the severity of vomiting because of the continued fluid losses due to osmotic diuresis. Vomiting and abdominal pain may suggest a diagnosis of "acute abdomen", but the presence of marked hyperglycemia and ketosis should arouse suspicion; the pain improves with metabolic correction, unless a surgical condition is the precipitating cause. Ketosis and hypokalemia may cause paralytic ileus, needing the patient to be kept nil orally initially.

DIAGNOSIS

The most important step is a high index of suspicion. If looked for, the diagnosis is usually straightforward, because significant glucosuria/hyperglycemia and ketonuria/ketonemia can be estimated quickly at the bedside. Capillary glucose may be inaccurate in the presence of poor peripheral circulation and severe acidosis, and should be confirmed in the lab in a venous sample. Urine ketone strips degrade within a month of opening the bottle, and can give unreliable results unless the bottle is freshly opened. This confusion in diagnosis and monitoring may be avoided by using blood ketone strips, which are now available in India. Monitoring blood ketones has been shown to improve outcomes.[14]

Having diagnosed DKA, one must always look for a precipitating cause, e.g. infection. When sending samples urgently to the laboratory for estimation of BG, ketones, hemogram, urea, creatinine, sodium, potassium, venous blood gases, HbA1c, osmolality, calcium, phosphorus, and magnesium, and urine ketones and routine exam, it is prudent to send blood and urine cultures, and tests for any suspected precipitant. Plasma osmolality is the main determinant of severity and outcome, it can be calculated by the following formula: 2 × (plasma Na) + plasma glucose in mmol/L. To get a quick idea about potassium levels, an ECG may be useful. Residents tempted to requisition lipid profile and thyroid function tests at or soon after diagnosis should wait, as severe hypertriglyceridemia and thyroid abnormalities improve within a few weeks of recovery,[15] conversely any abnormalities which persist after metabolic control improves would need therapy. Urea and creatinine levels may be high initially because of hemoconcentration; acetoacetate also interferes with the alkaline picrate

(Jaffe) assay for creatinine, but not with enzyme-based assays.

MANAGEMENT

Where feasible, the child with severe DKA should be admitted in an intensive care unit experienced in diabetes care. However, children with mild to moderate DKA, i.e. venous pH of 7 or more, HCO_3 of 5 mmol/L or more, and potassium >2.5 mEq/L, can be effectively, safely, conveniently and very cost effectively treated, with good outcomes, in the general pediatric ward, with subcutaneous (SC) regular (soluble) insulin, and monitored less intensively.[16]

The main steps of therapy, in order of importance, are:

1. The ABC of resuscitation.
2. Correction of fluid and electrolyte abnormalities.
3. Correction of metabolic acidosis.
4. Provision of adequate insulin to prevent ketosis and reduce hyperglycemia.
5. Prevention and monitoring of complications.
6. Identification of precipitating factors and an attempt to avoid them in future.
7. Stabilization on a suitable insulin regime to achieve adequate control of hyperglycemia.
8. Reinforcement and teaching of sick day guidelines.

The ABCs

In the first few minutes, rapid physical examination should be done, including assessment of airway, breathing and circulation, of sensorium and degree of dehydration, while a brief history is taken. In the comatose child, the airway should be secured. Oxygen should be started for the child in shock. The stomach should be emptied with nasogastric suction to prevent aspiration, and also if the child has recently had sugary drinks. If possible, intubation should be avoided as it might increase the risk of cerebral edema (CE). Venous access (preferably two) should be urgently established, the blood sample sent and fluids started. Central venous lines should be avoided because these children are at risk for thrombosis. ECG monitoring for T-wave changes (reflecting potassium status) should be started. The urinary bladder should be catheterized only in the comatose or the very young child.

Capillary blood should be tested for glucose and ketones, and a sample taken for lab tests (see 'Diagnosis' above). Antibiotics should be started in the child with fever or focus of infection.

Strict monitoring and charting are key to successful management (**Table 2**). Signs of danger are onset or worsening of headache or sensorial alterations, drop in heart rate, rise in BP, drop in oxygen saturation, or rise in urea or creatinine.

Fluid Resuscitation

The degree of dehydration may be difficult to assess. Increased capillary refill time and doughy skin feel suggest at least 5% dehydration. Weak pulses, cool limbs, absent tears, oliguria and hypotension suggest severe dehydration (10% loss). The child must be weighed and current weight used for calculations of fluid (and later, insulin) needs. In an obese child, ideal body weight for height may be a better parameter than actual weight.

The aim of therapy is to replace the calculated fluid deficit over 36–48 h, and to normalize BG and serum osmolality (normal 275–295 mOsm/kg) as smoothly as possible. In almost all children, this happens within 10–15 h; potassium levels and ketonemia may take longer to normalize. The average losses of water and electrolytes during DKA are given in **Table 3**. NICE Guidelines[17] recommend maintenance fluid requirements as follows:

- Weight < 10 kg: 2 mL/kg/h
- Weight 10–40 kg: 1 mL/kg/h
- Weight > 40 kg: fixed volume of 40 mL/h.

Fluid management strategies have been changing, from the initial rapid correction of deficit in 12–24 h, to advocating slow correction over 36–48 h for fear of causing CE, to a moderate view now. The recent PECARN study concluded that whether fluid administration was slow or rapid, whether using N/2 or normal saline, there was no difference in rate of CE or neurological outcomes.[9] This reassures that where needed, somewhat rapid correction can be given.

At presentation, one bolus of 10 mL/kg of normal saline (NS) or Ringer lactate (RL) with potassium should be given over 60 minutes. If the child is anuric, potassium should be withheld till urine is passed. **Insulin should not be given initially**: fluids are enough to decrease the BG levels by 15–20%. If the child is in shock, which is unusual, 20 mL/kg of NS or RL should be given rapidly over 10–20 minutes, and repeated if peripheral pulses remain poor. Advantages of RL are the low level of chloride and the presence of lactate, which is slowly metabolized to bicarbonate; the small amount of potassium present is contraindicated only if the patient is anuric. The volume deficit, assumed to be 5–7% for moderate DKA, and 7–10%

Table 2: Diabetic ketoacidosis monitoring sheet

Hours after admission	*0*	*0.5*	*1*	*2*	*3*	*4*	*5*	*6*	*7*	*8–9*	*10–12*
Heart rate	+	+	+	+	+	+	+	+	+	+	+
Respiratory rate	+	+	+	+	+	+	+	+	+	+	+
Blood pressure	+	+	+	+	+	+	+	+	+	+	+
Neurologic status (Glasgow coma scale)	+	+	+	+				+		+	
Blood glucose using strips	+	+	+	+	+	+	+	+	+	+	+
Ketones (blood/urine)	+			+				+			+
Sodium/potassium	+							+			+
Calcium/phosphate	+							+			
Blood gases	+			+				+			+
Urea	+										
Creatinine	+							+			
Urine glucose	+										
Insulin U/kg		+		+	+		+	+			+
Fluid in		+									
Fluid out	+	+	+					+		+	+
ECG	+		+								+

Table 3: Average losses of fluids and electrolytes

Components	*Losses (mean)*	*Losses (range)*	*Maintenance needs per day*
Water	100 mL/kg	60–100	1500 mL/m^2
Sodium	6 mEq/kg	5–13	45 mEq/m^2 (3 mEq/kg)
Potassium	5 mEq/kg	4–16	35 mEq/m^2 (2 mEq/kg)
Chloride	4 mEq/kg	3–9	40 mEq/m^2 (2 mEq/kg)
Phosphate	3 mEq/kg	2–5	10 mEq/m^2 (0.7 mEq/kg)

for severe DKA, is replaced over 36–48 h, given along with maintenance fluids and replacement of ongoing losses (urinary losses are not included). Recalculation of fluids every 2–4 h, based on the child's condition, is mandatory, to safeguard against the development of fluid overload and CE. Insulin should be started only after the initial bolus is given, and shock, if present, has been corrected.

As hydration improves, any raised urea and hemoglobin begin dropping, and serum sodium rises. Initial "hyponatremia" is dilutional. The corrected sodium can be calculated as follows: (measured Na) + 2([plasma glucose in mg/dL –100]/100) mEq/L. Failure of sodium to rise or an actual fall suggests high risk for CE.

Insulin

Insulin should be started only after the first hour's bolus fluids have been given (and shock, if present, reversed), and an NS + potassium rehydration solution begun. Low dose continuous administration of soluble (regular) insulin or rapid-acting analog at the rate of 0.05–0.1 unit/kg/h is the most popular and physiological method, with close monitoring of BG and other parameters. This results in BG falling slowly, steadily and predictably by about 10% every hour, after the initial fluid bolus causes a drop of 15–20%. Initially advocated only for very young children, and in HHS, the 0.05 unit/kg/h rate is likely preferable to 0.1 unit/kg/h.[18] Ideally a solution containing 0.5–1 unit insulin/ mL of saline should be given using an infusion pump; if infusion pump is not available, a solution containing 1 unit in 10 mL can be used with a burette set. Insulin may be given through a separate line or piggybacked onto the running line using a Y-connection. The relative disadvantages of low dose IV insulin infusion are the need for micro-infusion devices, and for constant surveillance, as inadvertent discontinuation of insulin results in rapid rise in BG. **Bolus intravenous dose of insulin should not be administered**.

Therefore, as mentioned above, SC regular insulin administered intermittently has been advocated as an alternative, especially in resource limited settings, and found to be effective, safe and convenient. This needs less intensive monitoring without ICU care, as the risk of hypoglycemia is reduced. Insulin has been given 1–2 hourly, and recently 4 hourly—by dividing the total daily insulin dose (1 unit/kg) into 6 parts, testing BG and other parameters 2–4 hourly, and adjusting the insulin dose by 0.5–1 unit accordingly.[16]

The advantages of using low doses of insulin are:

- BG is reduced slowly and predictably, so there is less hypoglycemia. Rapid changes in BG may increase the risk of CE.
- Efficacy in inhibiting glycogenolysis, lipolysis and secretion of counter-regulatory hormones is the same as with higher dose infusions.
- Acidosis is corrected more slowly.
- There is less hypokalemia.
- Rates can be adjusted faster, as and when needed.

Once BG level falls < 300 mg/dL, 5% dextrose is added to the fluids. This may be increased to 10% if needed, while continuing IV or SC insulin to correct metabolic acidosis. A common mistake is to stop insulin infusion abruptly when BG drops, or when the decision to stop IV insulin is taken, resulting in a rapid rise in BG. SC insulin must be given 20–30 minutes before stopping the IV infusion. Administration of a basal insulin analog concomitant with IV insulin reduces this rebound hyperglycemia and speeds up resolution of ketoacidosis, but with an increased risk of hypokalemia.[19]

Electrolytes

Potassium

Total body potassium is always significantly depleted, though at admission serum levels may be low, normal, or high. Fluid replenishment corrects hemoconcentration; insulin drives potassium into the cells and also increases urinary losses; this can result in severe and prolonged hypokalemia.[20] Serum potassium should therefore be urgently obtained initially, and ECG monitoring reviewed periodically for evidence of hypo- or hyperkalemia. Unless the child is hyperkalemic and/or anuric, potassium chloride should be added to the initial fluid resuscitation, at a rate of 20–40 mEq/L, *before* insulin is started. It should be given throughout the period of IV therapy. Salts other than chloride (phosphate, acetate) may be used, but have not been proven to be preferable, unless there is risk of hyperchloremic metabolic acidosis. If hypokalemia is severe or persistent, the dose of insulin can be reduced. The recent trend of preferring low dose insulin (0.05 unit/kg/h), reducing the duration of IV insulin, with early refeeding, would help reduce the duration and severity of hypokalemia.

Sodium

Serum levels at diagnosis may be unreliable because of dilutional hyponatremia, with possible factitious hyponatremia due to dyslipidemia, therefore only "corrected" values should be used. With fluid and insulin administration, measured sodium rises slowly; failure to rise or too rapid a rise may warn of possible developing CE, though the relationship of sodium and CE remains controversial (see further).

Phosphate

Phosphate depletion due to osmotic diuresis is worsened by therapy with fluids and insulin. It is usually asymptomatic and not clinically important, unless the child remains "nil orally" for more than 24 hours.

Bicarbonate

Bicarbonate should not be used, as there is no evidence either for its necessity or safety, and bolus doses have been shown to be associated with CE. Its use may be considered only if there is impaired cardiac contractility in the presence of persistent shock. If used, it should be infused slowly (1–2 mmol/kg over 1h) and cautiously.

Supportive Therapy

Urine output must be carefully recorded throughout, but catheterization avoided except in the comatose patient.

Table 4: Summary of management

Time		*Aim*	*Method*
1.	Hour 0	ABC of resuscitation	Airway (intubate if comatose) Breathing Circulation
2.	First 2–5 minutes	Establish the diagnosis	Brief history Assess sensorium, pupils, vitals Establish venous access Take blood and urine samples
3.	Next 20 minutes	Volume repletion	20 mL/kg RL or NS if in shock, otherwise 10 mL/kg IV fluid infusion
4.	Next 20–30 minutes	Lowering of blood glucose Correction of ketosis	Change to NS or N/2 IV insulin infusion at 0.1 U/kg/h Add potassium: adjust according to biochemistry reports
5.	Hour 1	Fine tuning of biochemistry	Add 5% dextrose when blood glucose < 300 mg/dL Careful monitoring
6.	Hours 2–6	When blood glucose < 300 mg/dL	Careful maintenance of records

In the initial 6-8 hours, nothing should be given orally; gastric lavage may be necessary in the drowsy child who is vomiting. However, once acidosis has resolved, the child is conscious and can sit up and eat, he/she should be encouraged to do so. A long period of "nil orally" may result in hypoglycemia and hypophosphatemia, particularly in the presence of fever and hepatic or renal disease. Routine use of prophylactic antibiotics should be discouraged. If bacterial infection is suspected, every attempt should be made to identify the precipitating infection, which should then be aggressively treated using appropriate antibiotics.

The suggested protocol for management is outlined in **Table 4**.

Treatment of Complications

Severe shock

This is a very rare but important complication, as it may result in death. If BP does not improve after 1-2 h of hydration, or if acidosis is refractory, consider gram-negative sepsis.

Cerebral edema

It is a rare but dreaded complication of DKA,[21] associated with high morbidity and a mortality of 25% even in the best centers.[22] It is seen more often in severe DKA, longer duration of DKA, younger children, and those with renal compromise. Thus, there may be lower pH, lower bicarb, greater hypercapnia, higher urea and higher BG at presentation, rather than increased osmolality.

Its causes and hence, prevention remain poorly understood. Earlier CE was thought to be caused by treatment factors - large bolus doses of bicarbonate, rapid infusion of fluid, early administration of insulin, rapid fall in BG levels, or rapid fall in serum osmolality. Now it is thought that DKA causes direct brain injury, which may worsen during treatment.[23] The finding that rate of administration (rapid vs. slow) and composition (0.9% or 0.45% saline) of fluids did not alter neurologic outcomes is changing recommendations regarding fluid management in DKA; it also suggests that mechanisms apart from fluid therapy need to be explored.[9] Careful monitoring was emphasized "in patients who had more severe acidosis and a lower pCO_2" in the accompanying editorial.[24]

CE is most likely to occur in the first 24 hours of therapy or even before start of therapy, often presenting with worsening of the sensorium in spite of biochemical improvement. Warning signs and symptoms include headache, lethargy or irritability/restlessness, falling heart rate, rising BP, decreased oxygen saturation, increased intraocular pressure, unequal or dilated pupils, and eventually convulsions, papilledema and respiratory arrest. An early and sharp drop in serum osmolality or hyponatremia during treatment is ominous. Treatment should be early and aggressive:

- Reduction in rate of IV fluids, but making sure hypotension does not occur, as that would worsen brain injury;
- Elevation of the head end of the bed;

- Administration of IV mannitol (0.5–1 g/kg over 15 min) and/or 3% hypertonic saline (2.5–10 mL/kg over 20 min); and
- Intubation, if necessary.

After treatment for CE is initiated, imaging of the head should be done to look for intracranial pathology, e.g. hemorrhage, thrombosis, or any other cause of coma, which would require specific treatment.

Hyperglycemic hyperosmolar state

HHS is rare in children and adolescents, though T2D may present this way. It is more difficult to detect and treat, as symptoms are usually less dramatic; hyperglycemia, dehydration, and hyperosmolality are much more profound; and ketosis is minimal.[7] These adolescents may go into shock quickly, even with ongoing polyuria, and dehydration less apparent clinically, so IV fluids need to be given faster and in higher quantity, including replacing urinary losses (which is not needed in DKA). Potassium needs are also much higher. Insulin can be started later, as the glucose levels decrease with perfusion alone initially; and in lower doses—0.25–0.05 U/kg/h. If renal perfusion is not restored quickly, hemodialysis may be required. Central venous catheters should be avoided as these patients are prone to venous thrombosis. Rhabdomyolysis and hyperthermia can rarely occur.

Hypo/hyperkalemia

Hypokalemia at presentation and hyperkalemia later in the course of the management due to overzealous therapy, may cause arrhythmias and even cardiac arrest. Hence, therapy must be cautious and guided by frequent monitoring of serum potassium and ECG.

Severe metabolic acidosis

Prognosis worsens if pH is 6.9 or less, but bicarbonate therapy has its own problems, as discussed earlier, and should be avoided for correcting metabolic acidosis.

Acute renal tubular necrosis

This may occur due to prolonged hypotension, due to delay in reporting to hospital or inadequate fluid therapy. Urgent hemodialysis may be needed.

Stabilization to Daily Insulin Requirements

Vomiting may persist during the first 12–24 h of treatment, but most patients are well controlled within the first 6–8 h, after which they should be encouraged to take orally if they are able to, initially sips of water, and later semi-solid and then solid food. Insulin should be changed to the SC route once BG levels are stabilized below 300 mg/dL. Early co-administration of basal insulin helps achieve smoother control.[25] Pre-meal insulin, whether regular or analog, should be given at least 30 minutes before stopping IV insulin. The reason for DKA should be tackled at this time. If it was at onset of diabetes, education should begin now, with parents initially learning BG testing and insulin administration. If DKA occurred with known diabetes, prevention strategies should be discussed, including home testing of blood ketones, which has been shown to reduce hospital visits.[26]

SICK DAY GUIDELINES

Clear guidelines for sick days should be reinforced repeatedly. The main points are:

1. Never miss insulin completely, even if no food has been eaten or vomiting is present.
2. Test BG frequently, and if using continuous glucose monitoring system (CGMS), track BG on it several times a day—correct hyperglycemia with supplemental doses.
3. *Check blood ketones if hyperglycemia persists*: Urine ketones may be done in a freshly opened bottle if blood ketones are not available. Presence of ketones indicates need for extra insulin.
4. If food is not tolerated, give whatever can be tolerated, including soups, lemonade, fruit juices, etc. Plenty of oral fluids are a must.
5. Rest, avoid exertion. If hyperglycemia or ketosis persists, consult the doctor immediately.

PROGNOSIS

In developed countries, the overall mortality in uncomplicated DKA in children has been reduced but in developing countries, especially in remote areas, the situation is likely to be dismal. Hence, prevention of DKA by early diagnosis of diabetes, and effective diabetes education, assumes great importance.

KEY MESSAGES

- Even though it is theoretically totally preventable, DKA continues to be a major reason for hospital admissions, morbidity, and mortality in T1D, especially in the very young, in areas of low incidence, and with low socioeconomic status.
- Outcomes have improved dramatically in recent years, with greater awareness, earlier diagnosis, wider availability of low cost POC tests, more children on physiological insulin regimens, and more effective diabetes education.
- Those with mild to moderate DKA can be effectively managed in general pediatric wards, with 2–4 hourly SC regular insulin, and less intensive monitoring.
- Children with severe DKA continue to need intensive care. Initial adequate hydration, with lower doses of insulin started only 1–2 h later, careful correction of hypokalemia, concomitant basal analog insulin, and early oral feeding result in almost all children recovering within 12–15 h.
- Cerebral edema is rare but continues to have significant mortality.
- Prevention of DKA, especially in those with known T1D, remains crucial.

REFERENCES

1. Ganesh R, Arvindkumar R, Vasanthi T. Clinical profile and outcome of diabetic ketoacidosis in children. National Med J India. 2009;22:18-9.
2. Kanwal SK, Bando A, Kumar V. Clinical profile of diabetic ketoacidosis in Indian children. Indian J Pediatr. 2012;79:901-4.
3. Maahs DM, Hermann JM, Holman N, *et al.* Rates of diabetic ketoacidosis: International comparison with 49,859 pediatric patients with type 1 diabetes from England, Wales, the US, Austria, and Germany. Diabetes Care. 2015;38:1876-82.
4. Vanelli M, Chiari G, Ghizzoni L, *et al.* Effectiveness of a prevention program for diabetic ketoacidosis in children. Diabetes Care. 1999;22:7-9.
5. Vanelli M, Chiari G, Lacava S, *et al.* Campaign for diabetic ketoacidosis prevention still effective 8 years later. Diabetes Care. 2007;30:e12-e12.
6. Varadarajan P. Risk factors for mortality in children with diabetic ketoacidosis from developing countries. World J Diabetes. 2014;5:932-8.
7. Wolfsdorf JI, Gllaser N, Agus M, *et al.* Diabetic ketoacidosis and the hyperglycemic hyperosmolar state. ISPAD Clinical Practice Consensus Guidelines 2018. Pediatr Diabetes. 2018;19 (Suppl. 27):155-77.
8. Virmani A, Ushabala P, Rao PV. Mortality in IDDM observed in a tertiary referral hospital in India. Lancet. 1990;335:1341.
9. Kuppermann N, Ghetti S, Schunk JE, *et al.*; for the PECARN DKA FLUID Study Group. Clinical trial of fluid infusion rates for pediatric diabetic ketoacidosis. N Engl J Med. 2018;378:2275-87.
10. Klingensmith GJ, Connor CG, Ruedy KJ, *et al.* Pediatric Diabetes Consortium. Presentation of youth with type 2 diabetes in the Pediatric Diabetes Consortium. Pediatr Diabetes. 2016;17:266-73.
11. Faustino EFS, Weinzimer SA, Canarie MF, *et al.* Disorders of glucose homeostasis. In: Nichols DG, Shaffner DH, editors. Roger's Textbook of Pediatric Intensive Care, 5th edition. Baltimore: Williams & Wilkins; 2015. p. 3222-51.
12. The Indian Council of Medical Research (ICMR), India. Executive Summary: The Indian Council of Medical Research Registry of People with Diabetes with Young Age at Onset (ICMR-YDR), Phase 1 (2006-2011) report. Available from: *http://www.icmr.nic.in/sites/default/files/reports/Executive%20summary*. Accessed February 21, 2019.
13. Karges B, Schwandt A, Heidtmann B, *et al.* Association of insulin pump therapy vs insulin injection therapy with severe hypoglycemia, ketoacidosis, and glycemic control among children, adolescents, and young adults with type 1 diabetes. JAMA. 2017;318:1358-66.
14. Klocker AA, Phelan H, Twigg SM, *et al.* Blood β-hydroxybutyrate vs. urine acetoacetate testing for the prevention and management of ketoacidosis in Type 1 diabetes: A systematic review. 2013;30:818-24.
15. Rashidi H, Ghaderian SB, Latifi SM, *et al.* Impact of diabetic ketoacidosis on thyroid function tests in type 1 diabetes mellitus patients. Diabetes Metab Syndrome. 2017;11(suppl 1):557-9.
16. Cohen M, Leibovitz N, Shilo S, *et al.* Subcutaneous regular insulin for the treatment of diabetic ketoacidosis in children. Pediatr Diabetes. 2017;18:290-6.
17. NICE. NICE Guidelines [NG18]. Diabetes (type 1 and type 2) in children and young people: diagnosis and management. Available from: *https://www.nice.org.uk/guidance/ng18/chapter/1-Recommendations#diabetic-ketoacidosis-2*. Accessed July 25, 2019.
18. Nallasamy K, Jayashree M, Singhi S, *et al.* Low-dose vs standard-dose insulin in pediatric diabetic ketoacidosis: A randomized clinical trial. JAMA Pediatr. 2014;168:999-1005.
19. Barski L, Brandstaetter E, Sagy I, *et al.* Basal insulin for the management of diabetic ketoacidosis. Eur J Intern Med. 2018;47:14-6.
20. Carlotti AP, St George-Hyslop C, Bohn D, *et al.* Hypokalemia during treatment of diabetic ketoacidosis: Clinical evidence for an aldosterone-like action of insulin. J Pediatr. 2013;163:207-212.e1.
21. Shastry RM, Bhatia V. Cerebral edema in diabetic ketoacidosis. Indian Pediatr. 2006;43:701-8.
22. Lawrence SE, Cummings EA, Gaboury I, *et al.* Population-based study of incidence and risk factors for cerebral edema in pediatric diabetic ketoacidosis. J Pediatr. 2005;146:688-92.
23. Glaser N. Cerebral injury and cerebral edema in children with diabetic ketoacidosis: Could cerebral ischemia and reperfusion injury be involved? Pediatr Diabetes. 2009;10:534-41.
24. Sperling MA. Fluid composition, infusion rate, and brain injury in diabetic ketoacidosis. NEJM. 2018;378:2336-8.
25. Harrison VS, Rustico S, Palladino AA, *et al.* Glargine co-administration with intravenous insulin in pediatric diabetic ketoacidosis is safe and facilitates transition to a subcutaneous regimen. Pediatr Diabetes. 2017;18:742-8.
26. Laffel LM, Wentzell K, Loughlin C, *et al.* Sick day management using blood 3-hydroxybutyrate (3-OHB) compared with urine ketone monitoring reduces hospital visits in young people with T1DM: A randomized clinical trial. Diabet Med. 2006;23:278-84.

CHAPTER

41

Adrenal and Thyroid Emergencies

Anju Seth, Preeti Singh

ADRENAL EMERGENCIES

Adrenal Anatomy and Physiology

The adrenal is a retroperitoneal gland that has two distinct parts viz. outer cortex and inner medulla. The cells of the adrenal cortex are differentiated into three functional zones; zona glomerulosa, zona fasciculata and zona reticularis which secrete mineralocorticoids, glucocorticoids and androgens respectively. The functioning of adrenal cortex is regulated by the hypothalamo-pituitary-adrenal axis. The hypothalamus secretes the corticotropin releasing hormone (CRH) following a circadian rhythm and also under the influence of stimuli including stress, pain, hypoglycemia and hypotension. The CRH stimulates the release of adrenocorticotropic hormone (ACTH) from the corticotroph cells of the anterior pituitary. The ACTH in turn binds to its receptor in the adrenals (MC2R) to stimulate the release of cortisol, which is under the constant feedback loop via the hypothalamic-pituitary-adrenal axis.

Adrenal steroidogenesis begins with the transport of intracellular cholesterol into the mitochondria via steroidogenic acute regulatory protein (StAR) that in turn activates the cascade of steroidogenic enzymes (P450 side chain cleavage enzyme, 3β-hydroxysteroid dehydrogenase type 2, 17α-hydroxylase/17,20 lyase, 21α-hydroxylase, 11β-hydroxylase) and their co-factors to produce glucocorticoids. ACTH also triggers the zona reticularis to produce androgens. However, the mineralocorticoid (aldosterone) synthesis is regulated by the renin angiotensin system and potassium feedback loop. The inner medullary zone of the adrenal gland produces catecholamines, a process regulated by sympathetic preganglionic neurons.

ADRENAL INSUFFICIENCY

Introduction

Acute adrenal insufficiency (AI) is a life-threatening condition that warrants urgent recognition and management. It occurs due to the inability of adrenals to secrete adequate cortisol with or without deficiency of aldosterone and adrenal androgens. Both congenital and acquired disorders of adrenal, pituitary and hypothalamus can give rise to adrenal insufficiency. Dysfunction or disorders of the adrenal cortex result in primary adrenal insufficiency while the defect in the pituitary (ACTH deficiency) or hypothalamus (CRH deficiency) leads to secondary and tertiary adrenal insufficiency, respectively. Acute adrenal crisis has gained clinical importance due to widespread therapeutic use of corticosteroids in management of diverse chronic pediatric disorders including nephrotic syndrome, asthma, juvenile idiopathic arthritis and leukemia, which leads to adrenal gland suppression. Acute crisis gets precipitated in susceptible individuals by infection, trauma and surgery. The prompt identification and management of acute adrenal crisis is critical to prevent morbidity and mortality.

Primary Adrenal Insufficiency

Primary adrenal insufficiency (PAI) includes a heterogeneous group of disorders characterized by deficient production of glucocorticoids. These may be associated

Table 1: Etiology of primary adrenal insufficiency
Congenital
Defects of steroid biosynthesis • Congenital adrenal hyperplasia, aldosterone synthase deficiency, cortisone reductase deficiency
Adrenal dysgenesis • X-linked adrenal hypoplasia congenital IMAGe syndrome, Pallister–Hall syndrome
ACTH resistance • Familial glucocorticoid deficiency, Triple A syndrome
Cholesterol synthesis disorders • Wolman disease, Smith–Lemli–Opitz disease, abetalipoproteinemia
Metabolic disorders: peroxisomal defects • X-linked adrenoleukodystrophy, neonatal adrenoleukodystrophy, infantile Refsum disease and Zellweger syndrome
Acquired
Autoimmune • Isolated autoimmune adrenalitis, autoimmune polyglandular syndromes
Miscellaneous • Hemorrhage, infection, surgery/trauma, infiltration and drugs (ketoconazole, rifampicin, phenytoin, phenobarbitone)

with mineralocorticoid and adrenal androgen deficiency or androgen excess depending on the etiology. Cortisol deficiency leads to absence of negative feedback regulation to the hypothalamus pituitary axis resulting in increased ACTH release. The disruption of adrenal mineralocorticoid synthesis stimulates increased renin release by the juxtaglomerular cells of the kidneys. The diagnosis is primarily based on strong index of suspicion as the clinical features are nonspecific and confirmation requires hormonal evaluation that may not be available routinely. The presence of mineralocorticoid deficiency in PAI differentiates it from secondary adrenal insufficiency; this has clinical, diagnostic, and therapeutic implications. The causes of PAI are summarized in **Table 1**.

Congenital adrenal hyperplasia (CAH)

It is the most common cause of PAI in childhood with a worldwide incidence of 1:14,000 to 1:18,000 live births.[1] It encompasses a group of autosomal recessive disorders that develop secondary to genetic deficiencies in the enzymes and cofactor proteins required for cortisol biosynthesis. This results in accumulation of the steroid precursors proximal to the block and deficient steroids distal to the block. Based upon the defect in enzyme within the steroidogenic pathway, various combinations of adrenal steroid deficiency and excess may be observed. Nearly 90% of patients with CAH have *21-Hydroxylase deficiency*, caused by mutation in the *CYP21A2* gene encoding adrenal P450c21. The enzyme 21-hydroxylase facilitates the conversion of 17-hydroxyprogesterone to 11-deoxycortisol, and progesterone to deoxycorticosterone, respective precursors for cortisol and aldosterone. Impaired cortisol biosynthesis leads to reduced negative feedback to the hypothalamus and pituitary resulting in increased CRH and ACTH secretion. Elevated CRH and ACTH concentrations stimulate adrenal hyperplasia and redirect the steroid precursors towards sex hormone synthesis and thereby resulting in hyperandrogenism. The clinical consequences of 21-Hydroxylase deficiency, therefore, result from cortisol and aldosterone insufficiency and sex steroid excess. Three-fourths of patients with CAH due to 21-Hydroxylase deficiency have the salt wasting (SW) form (accompanying aldosterone deficiency) and are at risk of adrenal crisis from the end of the first week of life. They are associated with large gene deletions or intron mutations with no enzyme activity.[1] The other 25% cases have the simple virilizing (SV, or non-salt-wasting) form. They have point mutation with detectable enzyme activity (1–2%), are able to retain mineralocorticoid function with normal electrolyte homeostasis and have a lower risk of adrenal crisis.

Most infants with *3 βhydroxysteroid dehydrogenase deficiency* also present with salt wasting crisis in the newborn period due to the aldosterone deficiency. *Lipoid adrenal hyperplasia* (deficiency of cholesterol desmolase) is one of the rare and most severe forms of CAH, which results in deficiency of all adrenal hormones, i.e. glucocorticoids, mineralocorticoids and sex steroids.

Non-CAH inherited defects

- *Adrenal hypoplasia congenita (AHC)* is an X-linked recessive condition due to defect in adrenal development [deletion or mutation of AHC (or DAX 1/SF 1)], which is associated with deficiency of all adrenocortical hormones (aldosterone, cortisol, androgens).
- *Familial glucocorticoid deficiency* is an autosomal recessive disorder with ACTH receptor (MC2R mutation) or post receptor defect (melanocortin 2 receptor accessory protein *MRAP* mutation) characterized by isolated cortisol deficiency with a normal mineralocorticoid synthesis.

- Children who have achalasia and alacrima are classified as having *Allgrove's/Triple-A syndrome* (with classical clinical triad *Alacrima, Achalasia, and Adrenal Insufficiency)* caused due to mutations in the *AAAS* gene which encodes a nucleoporin-ALADIN.
- In *Smith-Lemli-Opitz syndrome*, adrenal insufficiency arises as a result of cholesterol biosynthesis defect (deficiency of the enzyme 7 dehydro-cholesterol reductase) accompanied with XY gonadal dysgenesis.
- *Wolman disease* is a rare autosomal dominant disorder wherein the mutation of the gene for cholesterol esterase limits cholesterol entry into the steroidogenic pathways that results in adrenal insufficiency and intestinal malabsorption.
- *X-linked adrenoleukodystrophy (ALD)* is a neurodegenerative peroxisomal disorder caused by defect in a peroxisomal membrane protein, the adrenoleukodystrophy protein (ALDP) due to mutations in the ATP binding cassette, subfamily D, member 1 gene (*ABCD1*) that leads to accumulation of very-long chain fatty acid (VLCFA). This results in demyelination of cerebral white matter and destruction of the adrenal cortex.

Acquired adrenal insufficiency

- *Autoimmune adrenalitis*: Acquired PAI is seen most often secondary to autoimmune adrenalitis, which may occur in isolation, or in association with other endocrinopathies. The antibodies to adrenal cortex and 21 hydroxylase enzyme are responsible for autoimmune destruction of adrenals and PAI. Autoimmune polyglandular syndrome (APS) type I, also called autoimmune polyendocrinopathy - candidiasis - ectodermal dystrophy (APECED), presents in early childhood and is diagnosed when 2 of the following 3 conditions are present for at least 3 months: hypoparathyroidism, chronic mucocutaneous candidiasis, and Addison's disease. Mutations in the *AIRE* gene are responsible for APS type I. Polyglandular syndrome type II is diagnosed when adrenal failure and autoimmune thyroid disease or type I diabetes mellitus are present without hypoparathyroidism or candidiasis. It is relatively more common and usually presents in adulthood or late childhood.
- *Adrenal hemorrhage*: Adrenal hemorrhage can present with signs and symptoms of acute adrenal insufficiency. It can occur at the time of birth in a newborn, in association with fulminant sepsis by *Neisseria meningitidis* (Waterhouse-Friderichsen syndrome) or as a result of trauma or bleeding diathesis.
- *Infections*: Acute adrenal insufficiency has been also associated with systemic bacterial infections by *Pseudomonas* species, streptococci, and *Staphylococcus aureus*. Among other infections TB, HIV and disseminated fungal infections including histoplasmosis, blastomycosis or *Cryptococcus* can cause PAI.
- *Drugs*: Drugs known to inhibit the cortisol synthesis like amino-glutethimide, etomidate, ketoconazole, metyrapone and suramin and some enzyme inducers that accelerate cortisol metabolism like phenytoin, barbiturates and rifampicin may precipitate adrenal insufficiency in patients with limited adrenal reserve.

Secondary Adrenal Insufficiency

Secondary adrenal insufficiency (SAI) is caused by low circulating ACTH that prevents the optimal physiological release of cortisol from adrenal gland. The most common cause is the suppression of the hypothalamic pituitary adrenal axis (HPA) by prolonged use of exogenous steroids (more than 7–10 days of supra-physiologic doses of corticosteroids). The negative feedback inhibition of hypothalamus and pituitary by administered corticosteroids results in adreno-cortical atrophy and reduced cortisol synthesis. However, the aldosterone synthesis, which is regulated by the renin angiotensin system, remains unaffected. The sex hormone and catecholamine synthesis also remain normal. Apart from systemic corticosteroids, long-term topical use of highly potent corticosteroids over large skin areas or on severely damaged skin and even long-term use of inhaled corticosteroids can precipitate adrenal crisis during stress.[2] Among the inhaled corticosteroids, fluticasone propionate (≥500 µg/d), has the highest suppressive effect on the HPA axis owing to its large volume of distribution, prolonged half-life (>10 hours) and strong affinity for glucocorticoid receptor (>18 times of dexamethasone).[3] SAI is also observed in treated cases of Cushing's syndrome where endogenous hypercortisolemia suppresses the HPA axis.

The SAI can be seen in idiopathic or acquired disorders of hypothalamus and pituitary. Isolated ACTH deficiency is uncommon. It is usually encountered as a part of multiple pituitary hormone deficiencies; either idiopathic hypopituitarism, specific gene defects, congenital malformation like septo-optic dysplasia, holoprosencephaly or in acquired causes like tumors (craniopharyngioma, germinoma, and astrocytoma), infections like TB, autoimmune hypophysitis and damage due to surgery, trauma or cranial irradiation.

Acute Adrenal Crisis

Acute adrenal crisis may be the first indication of underlying chronic adrenal insufficiency (AI) and can be life threatening if not recognized and managed promptly. The severity of the clinical presentation depends upon the underlying etiology, extent of hormone deficiency and rate at which the deficiency develops. Stress, surgery, infection or trauma may precipitate development of adrenal crisis in patients with underlying chronic insufficiency. In patients on long-term steroids, sudden omission of therapy can precipitate crisis. Adrenal crisis may be the initial presentation of infants with classical salt wasting CAH, congenital adrenal hypoplasia and adrenal hemorrhage. Fulminant infections due to meningococcemia or other bacteremia leading to endotoxic shock can also be accompanied with acute adrenal crisis. Clinical features of these and other underlying disorders should be carefully evaluated for to ascertain the etiology of AI.

Clinical features

The clinical features of adrenal crisis include hypotension and shock (disproportionate to the underlying illness), metabolic acidosis, hypoglycemia, vomiting, diarrhea and sometimes severe abdominal pain. CAH due to 21 hydroxylase defects is suspected in newborns with atypical genitals (virilization in genetically female infants) while the males have normal looking genitals and present with salt wasting crisis around 2 weeks of age.

Children with chronic AI may have a history of preceding nonspecific symptoms like fatigue, anorexia, weight loss, musculoskeletal pain, abdominal discomfort, postural hypotension, depression, and anxiety. Salt craving may be a striking clue towards diagnosis. The suspicion of PAI is also supported by the presence of progressive skin and mucosal hyperpigmentation (gums, lips, buccal mucosa, skin creases, scars, areola, and genitalia) typically seen in >90% of patients due to increased melanocyte stimulating hormone production along with increased ACTH. In children with APS type I, mucocutaneous candidiasis and hypoparathyroidism usually precede the appearance of adrenal insufficiency. In X-ALD, neurological manifestations may either precede or follow the evolution of AI.

The clinical presentation in SAI is usually milder and similar to PAI except for absence of hyperpigmentation (low ACTH), and salt wasting since the aldosterone production is unaffected. Individuals at risk for iatrogenic adrenal insufficiency often appear Cushingoid on examination, due to prior glucocorticoid therapy. Signs and symptoms of a central nervous system tumor, such as headaches, vomiting, or visual disturbances and evidence of other pituitary hormone deficiency like hypoglycemia, short stature and polyuria should be looked for, in SAI.

Diagnosis of Adrenal Insufficiency

The diagnosis of AI is based on a meticulous history and examination coupled with an accurate analysis of biochemical laboratory profile. Any child who presents with fluid unresponsive shock, and/or an abnormal electrolyte profile (low sodium, high potassium level, low glucose level, metabolic acidosis) should be suspected to have AI. Mild hyperchloremic acidosis, and increased blood urea nitrogen and creatinine levels reflect presence of dehydration. Anemia, lymphocytosis and eosinophilia are other associated laboratory findings.

Serum cortisol

Early morning cortisol (before 8 AM) is used as a screening tool in individuals suspected to have AI since it strongly correlates with peak cortisol concentrations in children beyond 6 months of age in whom the circadian rhythm is established. An 8 AM serum cortisol <5 μg/dL is strongly suggestive of AI while levels >18 μg/dL rules it out.[4] Conditions that decrease (inflammation, rare genetic disorders) or increase (estrogen, pregnancy, mitotane) cortisol binding globulin (CBG) levels need to be considered in interpretation of plasma cortisol levels because the plasma cortisol is 80% bound to CBG.[5] In cases where the serum cortisol values are equivocal (due to considerable degree of overlap between the normal cases and those with AI), a corticotropin stimulation test should be performed. This test is considered as the "**gold standard**" for the diagnosis of primary adrenal insufficiency.[4,6]

Corticotropin stimulation test

The standard short corticotropin test is performed by administration of 250 μg corticotropin (*Synacthen*, 15 μg/kg in neonates and 125 μg up to 2 years) as bolus injection IV (or intramuscular) and serum cortisol is measured at baseline and 60 minutes after the injection. A normal physiologic response is an increase in the serum cortisol levels to a peak of at least 18 μg/dL (500 nmol/L) or higher after 60 minutes. AI is confirmed if the cortisol response is subnormal, especially in the setting of stress.[6] Another variant of this test uses low dose ACTH (1 μg) which is more sensitive than the standard test in evaluation of SAI.[7]

Plasma ACTH levels

They differentiate PAI from SAI since it is elevated in PAI and normal/low in SAI. The strongest clue towards the diagnosis of PAI is plasma ACTH level more than 2-fold above the upper limit of the reference interval for the specific assay (usually >200 pg/mL) along with low cortisol <5 μg/dL (140 nmol/L).[8]

Others

Raised plasma renin activity is a sensitive test for aldosterone insufficiency, though hyponatremia and hyperkalemia are present in severe cases. The DHEAS levels are below the lower limit of normal for age and sex in PAI (except in CAH due to 21 hydroxylase and 11 beta hydroxylase deficiency).

In acutely sick patients with clinical signs and symptoms of acute adrenal crisis, treatment is not delayed awaiting test results. A blood sample for random plasma ACTH and cortisol (and 17 OH progesterone in cases with suspected CAH) levels should be drawn before starting hydrocortisone therapy (**Flowchart 1**). If required, confirmatory corticotropin testing is performed once the patient's condition is stable after initiating treatment of adrenal crisis (needs temporary cessation of glucocorticoids).

Specific tests for underlying etiology

- *Congenital adrenal hyperplasia*: 17-OH progesterone (basal/cosyntropin stimulated sometimes).
- *Autoimmune polyglandular syndrome*: 21-hydroxylase antibodies, thyroid function test, blood glucose, calcium profile.
- *Adrenoleukodystrophy*: Very long chain fatty acids.
- *Adrenal tuberculosis, Wolman disease*: CT abdomen (adrenal calcification).
- *Smith-Lemli-Opitz syndrome*: Serum cholesterol.

Management of Acute Adrenal Crisis

All patients with adrenal crisis should preferably, be managed in an intensive care unit (**Table 2**). First priority is achieving hemodynamic stability by rapid volume expansion using normal saline bolus @ 20-mL/kg and repeating if required (guided by the volume status). Thereafter, the maintenance fluids are initiated (isotonic crystalloids containing dextrose, usually 5% dextrose with normal saline) at a rate of 1.5 to 2 times the maintenance requirement. This is accompanied by hydrocortisone (HC), IV bolus @ 50–100 mg/m^2 followed by 50–100 mg/m^2/day IV divided in 6 hourly doses. The replacement dose is typically based on the severity and duration of the stressor. In infants with salt wasting crisis due to CAH are given a higher dose of hydrocortisone (HC), IV bolus @ 100 mg/m^2 followed by successive HC as one-quarter of the initial parenteral HC dose IV every 6 hourly. The parenteral HC is tapered and switched to oral regimen depending on clinical state.

Hyperkalemia must be addressed but it is usually well tolerated and corrects by sodium chloride infusions. Mineralocorticoids are not needed because HC can activate MC receptors at a dose of >50 mg/m^2. Infants with CAH need salt supplementation @1–2 g/day (divided in multiple feeds) in addition.[9] In all cases, a thorough search for a precipitating cause should be undertaken. Empiric antibiotics may be given based on the patient's clinical presentation. Reversal of coagulopathy, if present, should be attempted with fresh frozen plasma.

Long-Term Maintenance Treatment

The corticosteroid treatment in children with chronic AI is aimed at controlling the symptoms of AI, while optimizing growth and preventing side effects from steroid overdose.

- Oral HC is the drug of choice as its short half-life makes it easier to titrate and minimizes the growth suppressive adverse effects associated with long-acting potent GC.[4] Its daily replacement dose is 8 mg/m^2 usually divided into two or preferably three doses. Patients with AI due to salt wasting CAH (21OHD) have the additional burden of hyperandrogenism (not present in PAI due to other causes). To counteract this a higher dose of HC @10–15 mg/m^2/day in 3 divided doses is recommended.[1]
- Children with PAI require mineralocorticoid (MC) replacement with fludrocortisone @ typical daily dose

Flowchart 1: Diagnostic approach to a child with adrenal insufficiency

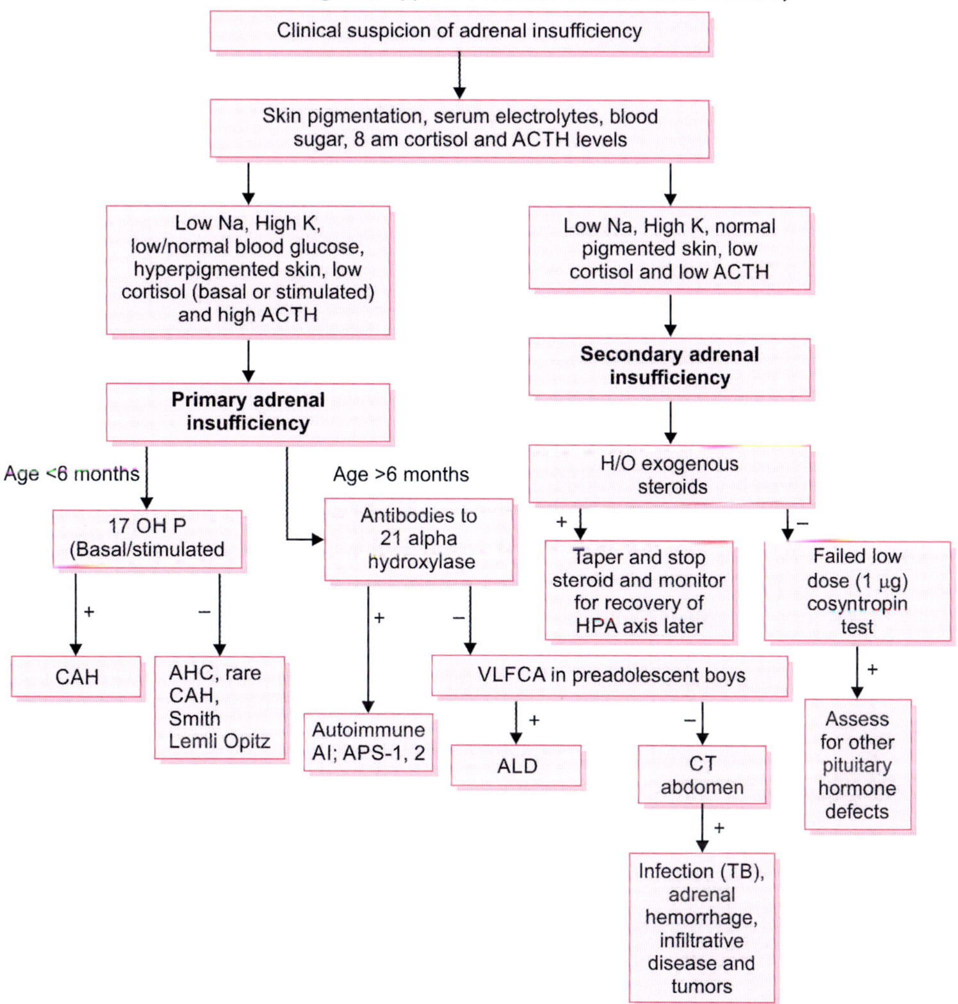

(CAH: congenital adrenal hyperplasia; AHC: adrenal hypoplasia congenita; VLCFA: very long chain fatty acids; ALD: adrenoleukodystrophy; APS: autoimmune polyglandular syndromes; CRH: corticotropin releasing hormone)

Table 2: Management of adrenal crisis

- High index of suspicion and prompt recognition based on clinical signs and symptoms
- Admission in HDU/ICU with continuous hemodynamic monitoring
- Obtain blood sample for electrolytes, glucose, cortisol, ACTH
- Rapid volume expansion using normal saline bolus @ 20-mL/kg and repeating if required (guided by the volume status) to restore cardiovascular stability. Thereafter, maintenance fluids (5% dextrose with normal saline) @1.5 to 2 times the maintenance requirement
- Management of hyponatremia at a maximal rate of 0.5 mEq/L/hour to prevent central pontine myelinosis; hyperkalemia addressed (usually corrected by saline infusions)
- For hypoglycemia—2–4 mL/kg of D25W (or 0.5–1 g/kg of dextrose or maximum single dose 25 g) is infused slowly at rate of 2 to 3 mL/min
- Stress dose steroid - Intravenous 50–100 mg/m^2 hydrocortisone bolus followed by 50–100 mg/m^2/day divided q 6 h until stable for 24 h
- Frequent monitoring of electrolytes, blood glucose, and vital signs
- A thorough search for a precipitating cause
- Empiric antibiotics may be given based on the patient's clinical presentation

Table 3: Prevention of adrenal crisis during intercurrent illness/stress in patients with adrenal insufficiency

Condition	*Intervention*
Minimal (mild upper respiratory tract infection, nonfebrile infections)	No intervention
Minor febrile illness	Home management; HC replacement doses doubled (>38°C) or tripled (>39°C) until recovery (usually 2 to 3 days); avoid fasting, increased intake of electrolyte rich fluids as tolerated
Major febrile illness (clinical condition does not permit oral intake)	HC 50 mg/m^2 IM followed by 50–100 mg/m^2/day; Infants -25 mg; school-age children -50 mg; adolescents -100 mg
Minor to moderate surgical stress	HC 50 mg/m^2 IM or oral HC replacement doses doubled or tripled
Major surgery with general anesthesia, trauma, or severe illness	HC 50 mg/m^2 IV followed by 50–100 mg/m^2/d in 6 divided doses Continuous IV fluids 0.45% NaCl with 5% dextrose (weight appropriate) HC tapered (rapid) and switched to oral regimen depending on clinical state

(HC: hydrocortisone; IM: intramuscular; IV: intravenous)

of 100 µg. The MC dose does not require adjustment by body surface area and often remains the same throughout life. Neonates and infants with CAH require higher fludrocortisone dose because of relative mineralocorticoid resistance and relatively low sodium intake. They also need sodium chloride supplementation of 1 to 2 g/d divided in several feedings.

Patients with SAI may have concurrent clinical hypothyroidism. AI must be treated before initiating thyroid hormone replacement therapy to prevent the development of an adrenal crisis. Parent education is extremely essential in children receiving chronic steroid replacement therapy to prevent adrenal crisis during inter-current illness (**Table 3**).[10] Once the acute crisis has been managed, patients with AI require follow-up with a pediatric endocrine service for monitoring, treatment compliance and dose titration.

ADRENAL RESPONSE TO CRITICAL ILLNESS

The adrenocortical response is the most critical hormonal response needed to prevent mortality in serious illness. This comprises of several fold rise in cortisol secondary to an increased production as well as decreased metabolism.[11-13] During critical illness, the elevated cortisol improves vascular tone [inhibits inducible nitric oxide synthetase (iNOS)] and enhances the inotropic and vasopressor response to catecholamines and angiotensin II, to maintain blood pressure. Hypercortisolemia is a state of insulin resistance; it accelerates glycogenolysis and gluconeogenesis in order to maintain the blood sugar. The free water clearance is increased. Finally, cortisol suppresses elements of the immune system, which may be important in preventing an over-exuberant, and potentially destructive, immune response.

Degree of cortisol response in relation to the severity of illness is an important determinant of outcome in a critical illness. Various studies have demonstrated evidence of "relative" adrenal insufficiency or "critical illness-related corticosteroid insufficiency" (CIRCI) as a risk factor for poor outcomes, primarily in the setting of septic shock.[14-16] The relative AI can possibly be explained by defect at any level of the HPA axis as well as peripheral tissue resistance to cortisol. Operational definitions and treatment guidelines for critical illness-related corticosteroid insufficiency (or "relative" AI) in children are lacking. There is conflicting evidence regarding utility of empiric therapy with corticosteroids in improving clinical outcome in critical illness.[17-18]

HYPERTENSION SECONDARY TO ADRENAL CAUSES

Endocrine hypertension in children is a medical emergency that requires prompt attention and management. Causes of hypertension attributable to adrenal glands include:

- Tumors originating from chromaffin cells (pheochromocytoma) that secrete excess catecholamines
- Disorders of adrenal cortex that result in high levels of mineralocorticoids and glucocorticoids (congenital or acquired etiology)
  - Cushing syndrome
  - Hypertensive forms of CAH
  - Primary hyperaldosteronism.

These disorders should be considered in the workup of secondary causes of hypertension in children. Work up and management of endocrine hypertension is included in the chapter on "hypertensive emergencies".

THYROID EMERGENCIES

Thyrotoxic Crisis (Thyroid Storm)

Introduction

Thyroid storm or thyrotoxic crisis is a life-threatening medical emergency that results from severe degree of thyrotoxicosis. The term "thyrotoxicosis" indicates a state of high circulating thyroid hormones, which is usually due to hyper-functioning of the thyroid gland. Thyroid storm represents an extreme form of thyrotoxicosis that results in life-threatening organ dysfunction.

Etiopathogenesis

Thyroid storm results from long standing, often untreated hyperthyroidism. Most common cause of hyperthyroidism in children is Grave's disease (GD), an autoimmune disorder, most commonly seen during adolescence in females. Other infrequent causes of thyrotoxicosis include solitary toxic adenoma and toxic multinodular goiter. Subacute thyroiditis usually causes a transient hyperthyroid state that rarely leads to thyroid storm. Thyroid storm is usually precipitated by a secondary acute insult such as infection, surgery, trauma, or discontinuation of antithyroid drugs in a patient with hyperthyroidism. The factors that lead to development of thyroid storm and their precise mechanism is not clear. The various proposed hypotheses include accelerated rate of development of thyrotoxic state, heightened responsiveness to catecholamines, and enhanced cellular responses to thyroid hormone.[19] The extent of elevation in thyroxine [T4] and triiodothyronine [T3] and suppression of thyroid-stimulating hormone [TSH]) in thyroid storm is not more severe than that seen in patients with uncomplicated thyrotoxicosis.

Clinical features

Hyperpyrexia (>39°C or 102°F) and tachycardia are seen in nearly all patients with thyroid storm. Other systemic features of decompensation pertain to neurological (agitation, lethargy, delirium, psychosis, seizure and coma), gastrointestinal (abdominal pain, vomiting, diarrhea and unexplained jaundice) and cardiac (tachyarrhythmia, usually atrial and high-output cardiac failure) systems. Dehydration and electrolyte disturbances may be observed due to fever and diaphoresis. The system-based thyroid storm score developed by Burch and Wartofsky is validated for the adult population but may be used for older pediatric patients.[20] The cumulative score achieved informs the probability of thyroid storm (unlikely, possible, or probable diagnosis).

A thorough history and meticulous clinical examination can provide critical clues to etiology of thyroid storm. Presence of heat intolerance, diaphoresis, weight loss despite good appetite, palpitations, tremors, behavioral problems (hyperactivity, emotional lability, poor school performance due to poor attention span) and sleep disturbances are some of the common symptoms observed in children with hyperthyroid state. Adolescents often complain of delayed puberty and menstrual irregularities. Other clues towards diagnosis of hyperthyroidism include a family history of thyroid or other autoimmune diseases (Type 1 diabetes mellitus or Addison disease). Physical signs are consistent with symptoms described above. The growth curve may show accelerated linear growth with concomitant weight loss. Vitals assessment reveal tachycardia, widened pulse pressure, and sometimes high blood pressure. Skin is warm and flushed with moist palms. Fine tremors and brisk DTR are usually present. Ophthalmological signs (proptosis, lid lag) are characteristic of GD but may not be always seen in children. Children with GD usually have goiter (thyroid enlargement) which is diffuse, soft, smooth and non-tender with a bruit. A solitary nodule or a multinodular goiter may be the cause of thyrotoxicosis in other patients.

Neonatal thyrotoxicosis: Neonatal thyrotoxicosis (Neonatal grave's disease) is seen in 2-3% of infants born to women with Graves' disease. The cause is trans-placental passage of thyroid-stimulating immunoglobulin (TSI) to the fetus. It may occur even when maternal hyperthyroidism is adequately treated with drugs or radioactive iodine since these women continue to have high TSI titres in their blood. The probability of neonatal/fetal toxicosis depends upon extent of elevated titres. Fetal tachycardia in the 3rd trimester is an important pointer towards presence of fetal hyperthyroidism. The affected neonates are often born premature and may have IUGR. They are restless with an anxious and alert look, poor weight gain (despite increased appetite), fever, diaphoresis, erythema and diarrhea. Thyromegaly is present in most newborns and some may have jaundice with hepatosplenomegaly. The signs and symptoms of thyrotoxicosis in the newborn may be delayed until several days if the mother received antithyroid medication.

The natural course of illness is transient, and the disease gradually dies out in 1–4 months as the maternal antibodies disappear from infant's serum. Untreated fetal and neonatal hyperthyroidism is associated with late sequelae like craniosynostosis, microcephaly, learning disorders and intellectual disability.

Diagnosis

The diagnosis of thyroid storm is based on presence of typical clinical features in a patient with evidence of thyrotoxicosis on thyroid function tests. These include elevated total and free thyroxine (T4) and triiodothyronine (T3) levels (several fold), along with a suppressed thyroid stimulating hormone (TSH). A small subset of patients might show predominant elevation of T3 with T4 in upper range of normal or minimally elevated (**T3 toxicosis**). If the etiology of thyrotoxicosis is uncertain on clinical evaluation, a thyroid scan (Radioactive iodine or the pertechnetate uptake/scan) may be done that typically shows a diffuse and high uptake of contrast in GD, while a toxic adenoma is characterized by focal uptake of contrast by the adenoma with diminished uptake in the rest of the gland. Antithyrotropin receptor antibodies or Thyroid-stimulating immunoglobulin (TSI) are elevated in most patients with GD. Other anti-thyroid autoantibodies including antithyroid peroxidase and antithyroglobulin may be detected in GD as well as autoimmune thyroiditis, which therefore cannot be used to differentiate GD from transient thyrotoxic phase of thyroiditis. An ultrasound of thyroid reveals variable findings depending upon the etiology (single or multiple nodules, diffuse large gland and high vascularity in GD and patchy appearance in thyroiditis). Neonatal Graves disease is confirmed by the presence of TSI in the mother infant pair.

The other ancillary investigations necessary in thyroid storm are serum electrolytes (including calcium), glucose, BUN, creatinine, and liver function tests to assess the end-organ dysfunction. In case of cardiac dysrhythmias and dyselectrolytemia, ECG recording is necessary for monitoring and appropriate intervention. A thorough search for any underlying infection should be undertaken that might have precipitated the thyroid crisis. Sepsis screen with complete blood count along with blood and other appropriate cultures should be obtained.

Management

Thyroid storm is an acute life-threatening condition and should be managed in an intensive care unit. Medical treatment is based on three principles: (i) counteracting the peripheral effects of thyroid hormones; (ii) inhibition of thyroid hormone synthesis and release; and (iii) treatment of systemic complications (**Table 4**).

Initial management: Initial management is aimed at patient's stabilization, i.e. maintenance of circulation, airway, breathing and temperature. Fluids administration is titrated with particular caution based upon input-output balance and serum electrolytes as patients are in a state of positive fluid balance. Tachycardia is controlled using beta-blockers (propranolol @ 0.5–2 mg/kg/day), titrated to normalize the heart rate. Propranolol has an added advantage of decreasing peripheral conversion of tetraiodothyronine (T4) to triiodothyronine (T3). Effective and prompt control of the thyrotoxic state is achieved by potassium iodide (supersaturated KI, "SSKI") or Lugol's solution.[21,22] Large doses of iodine cause an abrupt interruption of release of preformed hormone (Wolf Chaik off effect) but its effect is short lasting (up-to 2 weeks). It is typically given after at least an hour of starting an antithyroid medication so as to prevent undesired tyrosine residue iodination and building up of the thyroid hormone stores. Antithyroid drugs, which mainly comprise of methimazole (first line drug) and carbimazole are of little help during acute thyrotoxicosis. These drugs inhibit the organification of iodine by thyroid peroxidase enzyme to interfere with the hormone synthesis but do not influence the release of preformed hormone. They take at least 2 weeks for the clinical response to appear and as much as 6 weeks for the T4 and T3 levels to normalize. Corticosteroids (prednisolone @2 mg/kg/day) inhibit peripheral conversion of T4 into T3 and have been shown to improve outcomes in severe refractory cases of thyroid storm. Nutritional support is important (including vitamin replacement) and glucose levels should be closely monitored (liver glycogen stores are depleted) during thyroid storm.

Maintenance therapy: Antithyroid drugs are the mainstay of medical management in Grave's disease. The objective is to keep the thyroid hormone levels within normal range till natural remission occurs. The dose is titrated and reduced to minimum required dose to maintain euthyroid state. These patients are best followed up by a pediatric endocrinologist to monitor for remission and drug withdrawal over time or need for alternative management including radioactive iodine ablation (Iodine-131) and surgery.

Table 4: Medical management of thyroid storm

Medication	*Dose*
Antithyroid drugs (Inhibition of hormone synthesis)	
Methimazole	Neonatal: 0.2–0.5 mg/kg/day orally in 2–3 divided doses Children: 0.5-1 mg/kg/day orally in 2–3 divided doses (Max. dose: 30 mg/24 h) Daily oral dose range: Infant: 1.25 mg orally daily 1–5 years: 2.5–5 mg 5–10 years: 5–10 mg 10–18 years: 10–20 mg
Inhibition of hormone release	
Potassium iodide (supersaturated KI "SSKI") (1–2 hr. after antithyroid therapy)	Infants: 50–100 mg (one to two drops) orally every 6–8 hr Children/adolescents: 250 mg (five drops or 0.25 mL) orally every 6 hr
Lugol's solution (5% iodine and 10% potassium iodide, 126 mg of iodine per mL) (1–2 h after antithyroid therapy)	Neonates: one drop (about 8 mg)/dose orally every 8 hr Children/adolescents: Four to eight drops/dose orally every 8 hr
Inhibition of peripheral effects of excess thyroid hormone	
Propranolol	Neonates: 0.5–2 mg/kg/day oral divided every 6 to 8 hr Children: Start at 0.5–1 mg/kg/day oral divided into q6 to 8 h; increase dosage q3 to 5 days prn (dose range: 2–4 mg/kg/24 h divided q6 to 8 h) Maximum dose: 10–40 mg/24 h
Atenolol	1–2 mg/kg per day as a single daily dose or given every 12 hours

Myxedema Coma/Crisis

Introduction

Myxedema is a severe and life-threatening form of decompensated hypothyroidism triggered by an underlying precipitating factor. Despite lack of universal newborn screening in India, and often a delay in recognition and management of hypothyroidism, this clinical entity is fortunately only occasionally encountered in pediatric practice. Myxedema is more common in women and elderly and has a high mortality rate (25–60%) even with the best possible treatment.

Clinical features

Hypothermia, often profound, and unconsciousness are the hallmark features of myxedema coma. Although latter is the cardinal feature, patients may be in any stage of altered sensorium from lethargy, drowsiness progressing to stupor and comatose. In a subset of patients, hypothermia may be masked because of co-existing infection. Nevertheless, the possibility of myxedema coma should be considered in an unconscious patient who has severe hypothermia despite fulminant sepsis. Some patients may have classical stigmata of hypothyroidism such as dry, coarse, and scaly skin; sparse or coarse hair; non-pitting edema (myxedema) of the periorbital regions, hands, and feet; macroglossia; voice hoarseness; and delayed deep-tendon reflexes giving a clue towards diagnosis. In children, a useful pointer would be associated growth failure and a history of delayed development if the underlying cause is congenital hypothyroidism. A brief overview of the systemic disturbances observed in patients with myxedema is as follows:

Respiratory system: Hypoventilation is common in myxedema coma and is due to an impaired ventilatory drive of the central nervous system in response to hypoxia and hypercapnia.[23,24] In addition, enlargement and edema of the tongue or vocal cords can cause partial upper airway obstruction. The tidal volume is compromised because of the accompanying pleural effusion, ascites and obesity. These patients are susceptible to aspiration pneumonia due to hypoventilation and somnolence.

Cardiovascular system: The patients with myxedema coma are vulnerable to develop shock and fatal arrhythmias. There is cardiac enlargement either due to pericardial effusion or ventricular dilatation with decreased inotropism and chronotropism. Typical ECG findings include bradycardia; varying degrees of heart block, low-voltage, flattened or inverted T waves; and prolonged Q–T interval, which can result in *torsades de pointes* ventricular tachycardia. The cardiovascular collapse typically responds only when both a vasopressor drug such as dopamine and thyroid hormone are given.

Gastrointestinal manifestations: Oropharyngeal dysphagia and gastric atony secondary to neuropathic changes may be seen in these patients, which increases their predisposition to aspiration pneumonia. Associated coagulopathy may lead to acute GI bleed.

Renal and electrolyte disturbances: Hyponatremia is a characteristic metabolic disturbance seen in these patients. The cause is poor free water excretion due to low renal plasma flow, low glomerular filtration rate and an altered ADH secretion. Hyponatremia contributes to development of lethargy, confusion, alteration of sensorium and finally coma. Hypoglycemia can develop due to impaired gluconeogenesis, poor adrenal reserve and associated sepsis.

Hematological system: Severe hypothyroidism is associated with a high risk of bleeding due to coagulopathy related to an acquired von Willebrand syndrome and decrease in factors V, VII, VIII, IX, and X. Granulocytopenia and a decreased cell-mediated immune response can predispose these patients to severe sepsis. Anemia may develop due to hemorrhage (microcytic hypochromic) or accompanying Vitamin B_{12} deficiency (macrocytic) that also compounds the neurological deterioration.

Neuropsychiatric features: Myxedema patients have subtle features of cognitive decline, poor memory, and depressed mental state for some time before presenting in full blown psychosis and hallucinations ("myxedema madness"). Seizures may occur in 25% of patients which may be attributed to CNS dysfunction, hyponatremia, or hypoxemia due to reduced cerebral blood flow. Cerebellar signs like ataxia may be present.

Infection: Infection may be overlooked in patients with myxedema as the classical signs of sepsis like fever and tachycardia may be absent. Hence, a high index of suspicion is needed and use of broad-spectrum antibiotics justified till the culture results are negative. The host immune response is often blunted and impaired in myxedema, accounting for a high risk of mortality due to fulminant sepsis.

Diagnosis

On account of its rarity in children, diagnosis of a child with myxedema coma needs a high index of suspicion based on clinical features. It is confirmed by thyroid profile that reveals an elevated serum TSH along with very low serum total and free T4 and T3 concentrations in case of primary hypothyroid state. However, the rise in TSH may be blunted in cases of secondary hypothyroidism. Lumbar puncture done for evaluation of coma reveals high protein content in the cerebrospinal fluid. Other ancillary investigations like blood glucose, serum electrolytes, kidney function test, complete blood count with peripheral smear, ECG, arterial blood gases, coagulation profile, urinalysis and blood culture to evaluate for source of infection should be carried out in these patients.

Management

Myxedema coma is a medical emergency that warrants prompt identification and management in an ICU with continuous monitoring of vitals, cardiac and pulmonary functions (**Table 5**). Adequate airway and breathing are achieved and maintained by mechanical ventilation especially in comatose patients. This improves oxygenation and prevents hypercapnia, factors which perpetuate hypoventilation and coma. The duration of ventilation can range from 48 to 72 hours to 2–3 weeks and extubation is not attempted until full consciousness is achieved. Early thyroid hormone replacement is paramount in restoring the euthermic state. Till the effect of thyroid hormone comes into action, rewarming is achieved by elevating the room temperature and use of blankets. Overwarming should be avoided as it causes vasodilatation leading to hypotension and shock.

Fluid management: Fluid management is extremely challenging in patients with myxedema and a central venous line is essential to titrate the fluid balance. They are fraught with risk of both hypotension (requiring fluid repletion) and hyponatremia (that needs fluid restriction). The risk of mortality in cases with symptomatic hyponatremia is 60-fold higher than in those without it.[25] The fluid administration should be guided by the volume status and cardiac and renal functions. Fluid restriction may be the only desired intervention in case of asymptomatic

Table 5: Management of myxedema coma

- Prompt identification
- Admission in intensive care unit for continuous vital and temperature monitoring
- Mechanical ventilation to secure the airway and breathing especially in comatose patients
- Strict blood pressure monitoring; careful use of fluids, inotropes and corticosteroids
- Attain euthermic state, slow rewarming
- Central venous line to titrate fluids, strict input output charting
- Monitor serum electrolytes and blood glucose
- Thyroid hormone replacement- T4 @ 4 µg/kg lean body weight IV, followed by 100 µg 24 h later and then 50 µg daily, either orally or IV (if available). T3 may be initiated IV at the outset or added later @10 µg, every 8–12 hour until patient can take maintenance T4 orally.
- Dose adjustment done based on clinical and biochemical parameters

mild to moderate hyponatremia. In severe hyponatremia (serum sodium < 120 mEq/L), rate of sodium correction should not be more than 10–12 mEq/L in 24 hours. Management of hypotension is accomplished by careful volume repletion, replacement thyroid hormone therapy, vasopressor support and corticosteroids in refractory cases. Adrenal insufficiency may coexist in some patients (either in hypopituitarism or Schmidt syndrome) with severe hypothyroidism and thyroxine administration can further precipitate adrenal crisis by accelerating cortisol metabolism and clearance. In such cases, it is advocated to initiate short-term glucocorticoid therapy, which can then be tapered and discontinued when the patient is alert and stable.

Thyroid hormone replacement therapy: This is the mainstay of management of patients with myxedema coma. The goal is to attain the physiological state of thyroid hormone homeostasis without the risk of circulatory compromise and fatal dysrhythmias. There are no pediatric guidelines to recommend the preferred mode, dose and route of replacement, i.e. T4 alone (patient's endogenous deiodinase activity is utilized for conversion of T4 to T3) or to administer both T4 and T3. On account of poor peripheral conversion of T4 to T3 in myxedema patients, a few experts suggest giving both T3 and T4 for the initial few days.[26] Oral administration of T4 or T3 through nasogastric tube in the unconscious child carries the potential risk of aspiration and uncertain absorption, in the presence of gastric atony or ileus. However, parenteral preparations of T4 and T3 are not easily available, and no significant difference in outcome/survival has been observed in adult patients on oral vs IV T4 replacement.[27] One approach is to start therapy by giving T4 (loading dose 400–500 µg followed by 100–200 µg daily). Supplementation with T3 for 1–2 days may be considered if there is a suboptimal response to T4.[26] The patients need close continuous monitoring for adverse events and to titrate the dose based on clinical response (**Table 5**).

Prognosis

The outcome of patients with myxedema coma remains poor as it has a high risk of mortality (60–70%).[26] Most common causes of death are respiratory failure, sepsis, and gastrointestinal bleeding. The factors associated with poor outcome are persistent hypothermia or bradycardia, hypotension, hyponatremia, deep coma and multiorgan dysfunction (APACHE II score > 20, or SOFA score > 6).

KEY MESSAGES

- Primary adrenal insufficiency should be considered in patients presenting with shock out of proportion to underlying illness, hyponatremia, hyperkalemia or unexplained fasting hypoglycemia.
- Most common cause of secondary adrenal insufficiency is suppression of the hypothalamic pituitary adrenal axis (HPA) by prolonged use of exogenous steroids.
- Estimation of morning plasma cortisol followed by a short ACTH stimulation test helps to confirm the diagnosis of adrenal insufficiency.
- For management of acute adrenal insufficiency, replacement therapy with hydrocortisone must be started as soon as the diagnosis is suspected and continued until the diagnosis is confirmed or excluded.
- Thyroid storm is a rare state of clinical decompensation from thyrotoxicosis. The treatment includes stabilization of the airway and circulation, control of hyperthermia, judicious use of resuscitation fluids, beta-blockers and rapid control of the hyperthyroid state by potassium iodide or Lugol's solution.
- Neonatal Grave's disease occurs due to trans-placental transfer of thyroid stimulating antibodies to the newborn. Most cases spontaneously remit after 3–12 weeks. Therapy consists of anti-thyroid drug, beta-blockade and inorganic iodine.
- Myxedema is a severe form of decompensated hypothyroidism with a high risk of mortality. Diagnosis requires a high index of suspicion based on clinical features and a compatible thyroid profile.

REFERENCES

1. Speiser PW, Arlt W, Auchus RJ, *et al.* Congenital adrenal hyperplasia due to steroid 21-hydroxylase deficiency: An Endocrine Society Clinical Practice Guideline. J Clin Endocrinol Metab. 2018;103:4043-88.
2. Choi IS, Sim DW, Kim SH, et al. Adrenal insufficiency associated with long-term use of inhaled steroid in asthma. Ann Allergy Asthma Immunol. 2017;118:66-72.e1.
3. Patel L, Clayton PE. Adrenal insufficiency after treatment with fluticasone. Lowest possible dose of inhaled glucocorticoids should be given. BMJ. 2002;325:836.
4. Bornstein SR, Allolio B, Arlt W, *et al.* Diagnosis and treatment of primary adrenal insufficiency: An Endocrine Society Clinical Practice Guideline. J Clin Endocrinol Metab. 2016;101:364-89.
5. Gagliardi L, Ho JT, Torpy DJ. Corticosteroid-binding globulin: The clinical significance of altered levels and heritable mutations. Mol Cell Endocrinol. 2010;316:24-34.
6. Cho HY, Kim JH, Kim SW, *et al.* Different cut-off values of the insulin tolerance test, the high-dose short Synacthen test (250 μg) and the low-dose short Synacthen test (1 μg) in assessing central adrenal insufficiency. Clin Endocrinol (Oxf). 2014;81:77-84.
7. Dorin RI, Qualls CR, Crapo LM. Diagnosis of adrenal insufficiency. Ann Intern Med. 2003;139:194-204.
8. Kazlauskaite R, Evans AT, Villabona CV, *et al.* Corticotropin tests for hypothalamic-pituitary-adrenal insufficiency: A meta-analysis. J Clin Endocrinol Metab. 2008;93:4245-53.
9. Speiser PW, Azziz R, Baskin LS, *et al.* Congenital adrenal hyperplasia due to steroid 21-hydroxylase deficiency: An Endocrine Society clinical practice guideline. J Clin Endocrinol Metab. 2010;95:4133-60.
10. Allolio B. Extensive expertise in endocrinology: Adrenal crisis. Eur J Endocrinol.2015; 172: R115-R124.
11. Boonen E, Van den Berghe G. Endocrine responses to critical illness: Novel insights and therapeutic implications. J Clin Endocrinol Metab. 2014;99:1569-82.
12. Boonen E, Van den Berghe G. New concepts to further unravel adrenal insufficiency during critical illness. Eur J Endocrinol. 2016;175:R1-9.
13. Annane D, Sébille V, Troché G, *et al.* A 3-level prognostic classification in septic shock based on cortisol levels and cortisol response to corticotropin. JAMA. 2000;283:1038-45.
14. Marik PE. Critical illness-related corticosteroid insufficiency Chest. 2009;135:181-93.
15. Annane D, Maxime V, Ibrahim F, *et al.* Diagnosis of adrenal insufficiency in severe sepsis and septic shock. Am J Respir Crit Car Med. 2006;174:1319-26.
16. Levy-Shraga Y, Pinhas-Hamiel O. Critical illness-related corticosteroid insufficiency in children. Horm Res Paediatr. 2013;80:309-17.
17. Keh D, Trips E, Marx G, *et al.* Effect of hydrocortisone on development of shock among patients with severe sepsis: The HYPRESS randomized clinical trial. JAMA. 2016;316:1775-85.
18. Roquilly A, Mahe PJ, Seguin P, *et al.* Hydrocortisone therapy for patients with multiple trauma: The randomized controlled HYPOLYTE study. JAMA. 2011;305:1201-9.
19. Huang SA. Thyroid. In: Treves ST, editor. Pediatric Nuclear Medicine. New York, NY: Springer; 2007. p. 57-73.
20. Burch HB, Wartofsky L. Life-threatening thyrotoxicosis. Thyroid storm. Endocrinol Metab Clin N Am. 1993;22: 263-77.
21. Srinivasan S, Misra M. Hyperthyroidism in children. Pediatr Rev. 2015;36:239-48.
22. Bahn RS, Burch HB, Cooper DS, *et al.* Hyperthyroidism and other causes of thyrotoxicosis: Management guidelines of the American Thyroid Association and American Association of Clinical Endocrinologists. Endocr Pract: Official Journal of the American College of Endocrinology and the American Association of Clinical Endocrinologists. 2011;17:456-520.
23. Ladenson PW, Goldenheim PD, Ridgway EC. Prediction of reversal of blunted respiratory responsiveness in patients with hypothyroidism. Am J Med. 1988;84:877-83.
24. Birring SS, Patel RB, Parker D, *et al.* Airway function and markers of airway inflammation in patients with treated hypothyroidism. Thorax. 2005;60:249-53.
25. Pereira VG, Haron ES, Lima-Neto N, *et al.* Management of myxedema coma: Report on three successfully treated cases with nasogastric or intravenous administration of triiodothyronine. J Endocrinol Investig. 1982;5:331-4.
26. McCulloch W, Price P, Hinds CJ, *et al.* Effects of low dose oral triiodothyronine in myxedema coma. Intensive Care Med. 1985;11:259-62.
27. Dutta P, Bhansali A, Masoodi SR, *et al.* Predictors of outcome in myxoedema coma: A study from a tertiary care centre. Crit Care. 2008;12:R1.

CHAPTER 42

Management of Severely Malnourished Children

Praveen Kumar, Aman Elwadhi

INTRODUCTION

Severe acute malnutrition (SAM) or severe wasting is a serious medical condition characterized by very low weight for height [less than three standard deviation (-3SD) or more below the median according to WHO growth curves] and/or the presence of bilateral pitting edema of nutritional origin. Mid-upper-arm circumference of less than 115 mm is an additional criteria used for children aged 6 months to 5 years.[1] As per an estimate, acute malnutrition affects 8% of children i.e. 52 million across the world (1 in 12 children in this age group).[2] India is one of the countries with highest prevalence of SAM accounting for 7.5% of under-five children as per National Family Health Survey 4 (NFHS 4).[3]

Children with severe acute malnutrition have significantly higher risk of death due to common illnesses as compared to normal children. Undernutrition accounts for 45% of deaths of children younger than 5 years, and contributes to more than three million deaths every year.[4]

Why Severely Malnourished Children Need to be Treated Differently?

As malnutrition sets in, normal physiological mechanisms that adapt the organism to low food intake become pronounced called **reductive adaptation**. These affect every physiological function in the body, mobilizing nutrient reserves and decreasing energy demands. Initially beneficial as they allow the child to maintain homoeostasis but these adaptations progressively limit the body's ability to respond to stresses such as infection. More so, most cases of children with SAM are complicated by infective illnesses, like acute respiratory infection, diarrhea, urinary tract infection and gram-negative septicemia, accounting for their high case fatality rate.

Children with severe acute malnutrition need different treatment right from admission in emergency department. Some of the management practices, which are appropriate for normal children, may cause deaths in children with severe acute malnutrition like aggressive fluid therapy in dehydration or shock, use of diuretics in edema, use of albumin, etc.[1]

PROTOCOL BASED MANAGEMENT OF SAM

All sick children should be examined for presence of emergency signs and emergency treatment like administration of oxygen for children with airway and breathing problems should be started before detailed history and examination. Management of two of the emergency signs (shock and severe dehydration) is different as compared to normal children which is described here.[2]

Severe acute malnutrition may occur due to food scarcity or malabsorption or increased demand due to infections or secondary diseases. Once emergency care is provided, history and examination should be completed to detect medical complications and find out possibility of secondary causes of severe acute malnutrition like tuberculosis, HIV, liver diseases, chronic diarrhea, etc.

The World Health Organization has recommended 10 essential steps (**Fig. 1**) for management of SAM to take care of their physiological and metabolic demands, which have been adapted by the Indian Academy of Pediatrics and Ministry of Health and Family Welfare, Government of India.[5,6] Severely malnourished children also need appropriate treatment for secondary causes if any, e.g. ATT for tuberculosis, ART for HIV, and gluten free diet for celiac disease.

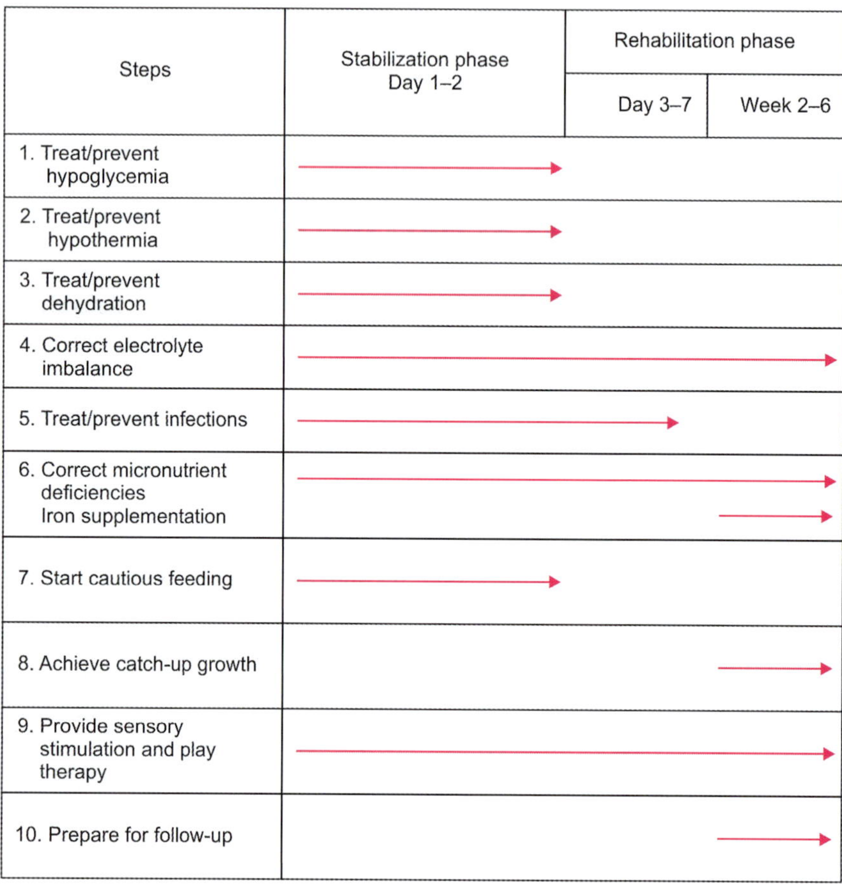

Fig. 1: WHO ten steps and two phases of management of sever acute malnutrition[5]

Step 1: Treat/Prevent Hypoglycemia

The SAM children are prone for hypoglycemia because of poor reserve hence it is important to check blood sugar of all admitted children. If blood glucose is less than 54 mg/dL, child has hypoglycemia. One should assume hypoglycemia and treat if facility for measuring blood glucose is not immediately available. If child is asymptomatic, starter feed (F-75) or 50 mL of 10% sugar solution (10% dextrose or 4 rounded teaspoons in 200 mL water) should be given followed with 2 hourly feeds. If child is unconscious, lethargic or is having seizures, 5 mL/kg of 10% dextrose intravenously should be given or 50 mL of 10% sugar solution by nasogastric tube. Blood sugar should be rechecked after 30 minutes.

Step 2: Treat/Prevent Hypothermia

Hypothermia in an SAM child is defined as axillary temperature of less than 35°C or a rectal temperature of less than 35.5°. Presence of hypothermia puts metabolic stress to these children. It is important to prevent hypothermia, the child should be covered with clothes including cap, socks and mittens in even normal environmental temperature. If child has hypothermia, then she/he should be kept near a heater but not pointing directly at the child. Child can also be put to skin to skin contact with the mother's or caregiver's chest and abdomen covered with a blanket or warm clothes (kangaroo mother care). Temperature should be monitored every 2 hours till it reaches 36.5°C. If the child has severe hypothermia (axillary temperature is less than 32°C) then he will require more intensive treatment with warm humidified oxygen, warmth by a radiant warmer till temperature rises to 35°C. Temperature should be monitored every 30 minutes in these cases till it reaches 36.5°C.

Step 3: Management of Dehydration and Shock

Diarrhea is one of the most common morbidity in children with SAM which has greater severity and increased risk of mortality as compared to children with normal nutrition.[1,5] Dehydration is often difficult to diagnose in malnourished children because the clinical signs usually used to diagnose dehydration are less reliable.[6] Skin turgor appears poor in children with SAM owing to the absence of subcutaneous fat due to which their eyes may also appear sunken. Diminished skin turgor may be masked by edema in children with edematous SAM. The child's irritability or apathy make assessment of the mental state also difficult to assess. In children with severe malnutrition, it is also often impossible to distinguish reliably between *Some* and *Severe* dehydration.

Misdiagnosis and inappropriate treatment for dehydration is the commonest cause of death in malnourished children. Malnourished children are in a state of reductive adaptation, the sodium-potassium ATPase pump that controls the balance of potassium and sodium runs slower. As a result, the level of sodium in the cells rises and potassium leaks out of the cells and is lost. Thus, there is a concern that overzealous correction of dehydration specially using intravenous fluids or oral rehydration solution (ORS) containing higher quantities of sodium may result in increased risk of fluid overload and heart failure.[5,6]

The main diagnosis can be assumed from the history rather than from the examination.

- A definite history of significant recent fluid loss—usually diarrhea in which consistency is clearly like water (not just soft or mucus) and frequent with a sudden onset within the past few hours or days.
- History of a recent change in the child's appearance.
- If the eyes are sunken then the mother confirms that these changes have occurred after onset of diarrhea.

Plan of rehydration

The SAM children with dehydration should be rehydrated slowly over 10–12 hours with close monitoring for signs of fluid overload by monitoring of their vital parameters (pulse rate and respiratory rate), liver size and auscultation for crepitations.

- It is recommended to rehydrate the child orally or by nasogastric tube even in presence of severe dehydration *unless the child is in shock* or has any other contraindication like intestinal obstruction or paralytic ileus (**Flowchart 1**).
- The amount of ORS to be given is based on the child's weight that is 5 mL/kg every 30 minutes for the first 2 hours followed by 5–10 mL/kg ORS alternating with starter diet for up to 10 hours.
- WHO recommended rehydration solution for malnourished children (ReSoMal) is not available

Flowchart 1: Fluid management in a child of SAM with diarrhea

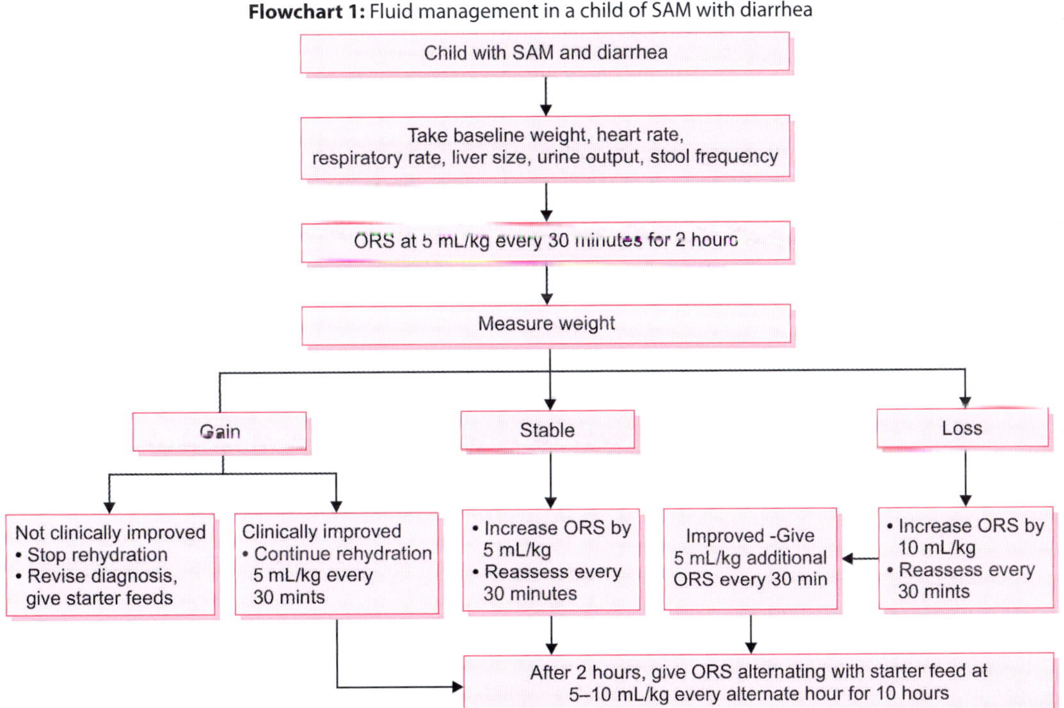

in India. WHO and IAP has recommended to use modified ORS in place of low osmolality ORS (**Table 1**). However, in case of profuse diarrhea and cholera low osmolality ORS without any modification should be used for rehydration.[1]

- Respiratory rate, pulse rate, liver size should be recorded at start and then every 30 minutes so that over hydration is prevented. Rise of respiratory rate by 5/minute along with rise of pulse rate by 15/minute indicates over hydration.

Management of shock

Shock in children with SAM is defined as cold peripheries with slow capillary refill time (>3 seconds) and weak fast pulse. Intravenous therapy is only recommended for children of SAM in shock and who are unconscious or lethargic. When resuscitating children with shock who are not malnourished, isotonic fluids bolus (R/L or NS 20 mL/kg) are given intravenously to expand the circulating volume. However, these rapid fluid boluses may cause congestive heart failure and death. High sodium and glucose free fluids are also not suitable for children with severe acute malnutrition. Guidelines recommend half-strength Darrow's solution with 5% dextrose, or Ringer's lactate solution with 5% dextrose or 0.45% saline with 5% dextrose for these children. However, half strength Darrow's solution is not commonly available in many countries, so practically Ringer lactate with 5% dextrose or the easily available 0.45% saline with 5% dextrose should be used to resuscitate these children (**Flowchart 2**).

- It is important that the child is carefully monitored every 5–10 min for signs of overhydration and signs of congestive heart failure. If signs of overhydration and congestive heart failure develop (increased respiratory rate by 5/minute or pulse rate by 15/minute) intravenous therapy should be changed to maintenance fluid and vasopressors.
- If following the bolus, the shock improves, oral rehydration with ORS alternating with starter diet should be started as described in **Flowchart 1**. Repeat IV fluid bolus, which was recommended earlier, has been removed in the updated WHO ETAT guidelines

Table 1: Preparation of modified ORS

Ingredient	*Amount*
Water	2 Liters
WHO low osmolality ORS	One packet
Sugar	50 g
Electrolyte/mineral solution*	40 mL

*in case electrolyte mineral solution is not available 45 mL of potassium chloride syrup should be added

Flowchart 2: Management in a child of SAM with shock

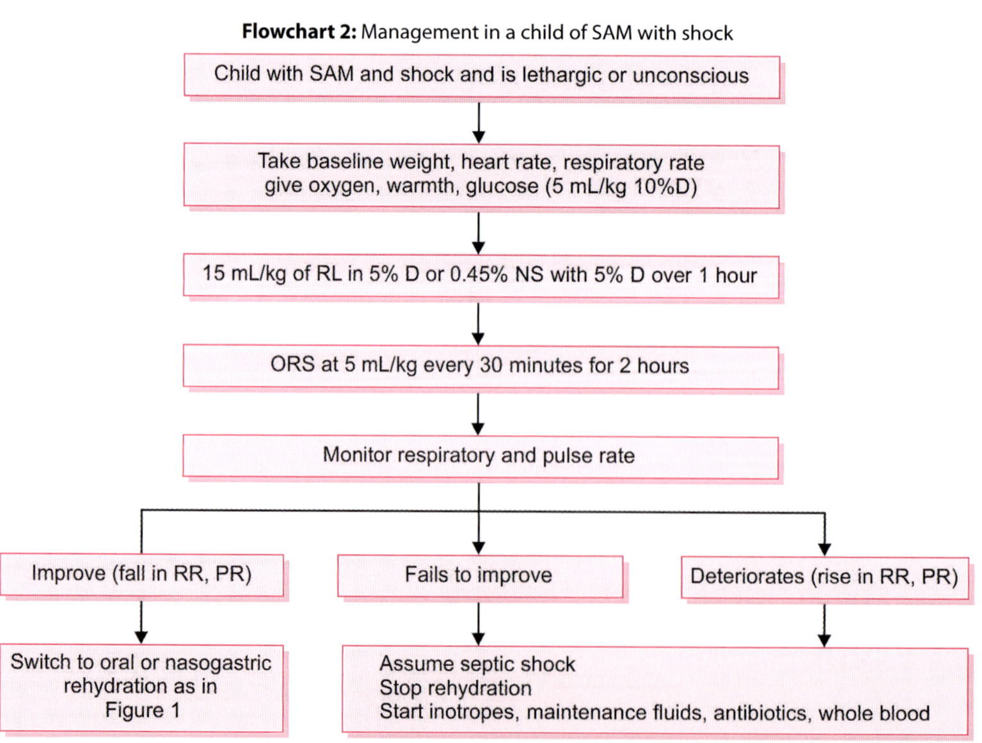

2016.[7] Repeat bolus may be given only when child has history of profuse diarrhea.

- If following the bolus, the shock does not improve, septic shock should be considered and child started on inotropes with maintenance fluids and appropriate antibiotics as described in **Table 2**.

However, few studies have raised concern regarding conservative fluid therapy. To date, the evidence supporting either benefit or harm of fluid resuscitation or rehydration is weak. This issue, however, is not unique to children with severe malnutrition; pediatric guidelines worldwide have a weak level of evidence and remain unsupported by appropriate clinical studies. The only controlled trial ever undertaken is FEAST trial (Fluid Expansion As Supportive Therapy) which was conducted in resource-poor hospitals involving 3,141 African children with severe febrile illnesses and shock, including large subgroups with sepsis and malaria but excluding children with severe malnutrition.[8] This high-quality trial provided robust evidence that fluid resuscitation increases the risk of death, leading to an excess mortality of 3 in every 100 children receiving fluid boluses, compared with controls receiving no boluses. These findings may have particular relevance to management of septic shock in children with severe malnutrition.

On other side, a recent review on use of intravenous fluid in malnourished child included four studies (two randomized controlled trials and two observational cohort studies) analyzing 883 children could not find evidence of fluid overload or other fluid-related adverse events, in children managed on more liberal rehydration protocols and concluded that children with SAM with severe dehydration, managed on WHO protocol continued to be under hydrated.[9-12] However, the review also included a large percentage (33%) of the patients who had cholera. The higher need of fluid cannot be extrapolated to non-cholera patients. At present, there are no clinical trials providing a direct assessment of the current WHO guidelines vs. IVF fluid therapy in children with SAM with diarrhea and shock. More scientific evidences are needed before any change in current conservative approach.

Table 2: Antibiotic dose and choice for various situations in children with SAM[6]

Situation	*Antibiotic*
All cases without complication and good appetite	Oral amoxicillin 15 mg/kg/dose three times a day for 5 days
Any case with complications other than shock, meningitis or dysentery	Injection ampicillin 50 mg/kg/dose 6 hourly with injection gentamicin 7.5 mg/kg once daily for 7 days
Suspected septic shock	3rd generation cephalosporins (ceftriaxone 100 mg/kg/day in 2 divided doses or cefotaxime 150 mg/kg/day in 3 divided doses) with gentamicin
Meningitis	3rd generation cephalosporins (ceftriaxone 100 mg/kg/day in 2 divided doses or cefotaxime 200 mg/kg/day in 4 divided doses) with amikacin 15 mg/kg
Dysentery	Oral cefixime 8–10 mg/kg/day for 5 days or injection ceftriaxone
On discharge	Albendazole 1–2 years – 200 mg > 2 years – 400 mg

Step 4: Management of Electrolyte Imbalance

Children with SAM usually have deficiency of potassium and magnesium and excess of sodium. Potassium is supplemented orally at 3–4 mmol/kg/day and magnesium is given at 0.3 mL/kg (maximum 2 mL) intramuscular 50% magnesium sulfate on day one followed by the same amount and preparation orally for at least 2 weeks.

Step 5: Management of Infections

- Pneumonia, bacteremia and urinary tract infection have a higher prevalence in children with SAM and are often asymptomatic.
- In children with SAM with medical complication or apparent infection, parenteral (intravenous or intramuscular) antibiotics should be given for 7 days when there is suspected sepsis, 10–14 days for culture proven sepsis, 14–21 days for meningitis and 4 weeks for deep seated infection (**Table 2**).

Step 6: Management of Micronutrient Deficiencies

All children with SAM have micronutrient deficiencies hampering their recovery and optimal weight gain, hence these need to be addressed. The micronutrients requiring supplementation are as follows:

- Vitamin A – 50,000 IU for < 6 months, 100,000 IU for 6 months 1 year or weight < 8 kg, 200,000 IU for > 1 year and > 8 kg on days 1, 2 and 15
- Folic acid – 5 mg on day 1 followed by 1 mg/day
- Elemental zinc – 2 mg/kg/day
- Copper – 0.3 mg/kg/day
- B-complex, vitamin C, vitamin D, vitamin E, vitamin K – twice the recommended dietary allowance
- Packed red cell transfusion should be given if the child is severely anemic (hemoglobin < 4 g/dL) or has

hemoglobin of 4–6 g/dL with respiratory distress. Iron therapy should be started during rehabilitation phase.

Step 7–8: Management of Feeding

Feeding in children with SAM is of paramount importance. It should be started at the earliest with low osmolality, low lactose and low protein feeds. Breastfeeding should be encouraged and night-time feeds need to be ensured. If oral acceptance is poor, nasogastric feeding should be tried. It is started with a starter diet (F-75) containing 75 calories and 0.9 g protein per 100 mL at 130 mL of feed/kg/day from the admission weight. For edematous SAM, the feed volume is reduced to 100 mL/kg/day. Initially the feed is started at 2 hourly intervals and gradually the frequency is decreased to 3 and then 4 hourly in a stepwise manner if the child accepts feed well, has no vomiting and has modest diarrhea (<5 watery stools/day). Child is then transitioned to catch-up diet (F-100) containing 100 calories and 2.9 g protein per 100 mL, which is gradually increased, starting from the same frequency and volume of the starter diet to up to 220 mL/kg of the daily weight.

For infants less than 6 months, attempt should be made to correct feeding practices including feeding by supplementary suckling technique for re-establishing lactations wherever mothers are available. In situations where there are no prospects of breastfeeding, F-100D (100 mL of F-100 diluted to 130 mL by adding water to decrease renal solute load) is used in place of F-100.

Step 9: Play and Stimulation

All children should receive sensory stimulation and structured play therapy for 15–30 minutes twice daily.

Step 10: Discharge and Follow-up

Mothers of children with SAM need to be educated, trained and encouraged to take care of the feeding, hygiene, stimulation, physical activity, supplements and signs of sickness in her child from the beginning of therapy. She should be confident of taking care of her child at home at the time of discharge. Follow-up vaccination and deworming also need to be assured. A child who has satisfactory weight gain (at least 5 g/kg/d) on catch up diet for 3 consecutive days and has recovered from medical complications may be discharged but should be followed up till his/her weight for length (or height) crosses -2 Z score.

In addition to above-mentioned ten steps, the child should receive appropriate treatment for other morbidities and any secondary causes.

KEY MESSAGES

- Children with severe acute malnutrition have profound disturbances of normal physiology, including electrolyte imbalances and altered fluid distribution.
- As a result of their reductive adaptive state, these children are prone to fluid and sodium overload and have reduced tolerance to rapid changes in circulating blood volume.
- WHO recommends a cautious approach to fluid management as overhydration is a common cause for high mortality in such children.
- Adherence to WHO recommended 10 steps decreases mortality significantly in these children.

REFERENCES

1. WHO. Updates on the Management of Severe Acute Malnutrition in Infants and Children. World Health Organization Guideline. 2013. Available from: *http://www.who.int/nutrition/publications/guidelines/updates_management_SAM_infantandchildren/en/index.html*. Accessed July 25, 2019.
2. WHO. Joint child malnutrition estimates—Levels and trends (2018 edition). WHO/UNICEF/WB Global Estimate 2018. Available from: *https://www.who.int/nutgrowthdb/estimates2017/en/*. Accessed July 25, 2019.
3. National Family Health Survey (NFHS-4). International Institute for Population Sciences. Mumbai, India. 2015-16.
4. Black RE, Cousens S, Johnson HL, *et al.* Global, regional, and national causes of child mortality in 2008: A systematic analysis. Lancet. 2010;375:1969-87.
5. WHO. Management of severe acute malnutrition in infants and children. Available from: *https://www.who.int/elena/titles/full_recommendations/sam_management/en/*. Accessed July 25, 2019.
6. Government of India. Facility-based care of children with severe acute malnutrition. New Delhi: MOHFW; 2011.
7. WHO. Updated guideline: Paediatric emergency triage, assessment and treatment. Geneva: World Health Organization; 2016.
8. Maitland K, Kiguli S, Opoka RO, *et al.* Mortality after fluid bolus in African children with severe infection. N Engl J Med. 2011; 364:2483-95.
9. Houston KA, Gibb JG, Maitland K. Intravenous rehydration of malnourished children with acute gastroenteritis and severe dehydration: A systematic review. Wellcome Open Res. 2017; 2:65.
10. Akech SO, Karisa J, Nakamya P, *et al.* Phase II trial of isotonic fluid resuscitation in Kenyan children with severe malnutrition and hypovolaemia. BMC Pediatr. 2010;10:71.
11. Alam NH, Islam S, Sattar S, *et al.* Safety of rapid intravenous rehydration and comparative efficacy of 3 oral rehydration solutions in the treatment of severely malnourished children with dehydrating cholera. J Pediatr Gastroenterol Nutr. 2009; 48:318-27.
12. Obonyo N, Brent B, Olupot-Olupot P, *et al.* Myocardial and haemodynamic responses to two fluid regimens in African children with severe malnutrition and hypovolaemic shock (AFRIM study). Crit Care. 2017;21:103.

CHAPTER 43

Malaria

Ritabrata Kundu, Aniruddha Ghosh

INTRODUCTION

Malaria, a vector-borne parasitic infectious disease, is a major health burden of third world countries like India. The total number of malaria cases as well as deaths due to malaria is following a decreasing trend with each passing year. In India, around 8.4 lacs of confirmed cases with 194 deaths were observed in 2017.[1]

EPIDEMIOLOGY AND ETIOLOGY

Malaria is caused by four species of the genus Plasmodium namely *P. vivax, P. falciparum, P. ovale* and *P. malariae*. A fifth species *P. knowlesi*, primarily an animal pathogen, has been reported to cause malaria in humans in south-eastern Asia, especially Borneo. In India, incidence of *P. falciparum* (62%) has surpassed that of *P. vivax* (37%) in the last year with a few cases of *P. ovale* reported from Odisha.[1] *P. malariae* is practically non-existent in India currently except for a few cases reported from Madhya Pradesh and Chhattisgarh.[2]

The problem became far more severe when *P. falciparum* acquired resistance to first line antimalarial drug chloroquine (CQ). CQ-resistant falciparum malaria, first reported from north-eastern states of India, gradually spread to other states also. Resistance to second-line antimalarial drugs sulfadoxine-pyrimethamine (SP) has also been reported from north-eastern states and some areas of West Bengal and Odisha.[3]

Chloroquine is still very much efficacious against *P. vivax* although handful cases of CQ-resistance have come into light.

PATHOGENESIS

Due to seasonal trend of malaria (increased incidence especially during or just after rainy season), the disease has unstable transmission dynamics in India. All the age groups are equally susceptible to the disease due to lack of long-lasting immunity.

During mosquito bite, sporozoites from mosquito get entry to human bloodstream and are picked up by the hepatocytes to produce merozoites. Unlike falciparum malaria, some sporozoites of vivax malaria instead of transforming into merozoites, remain dormant as hypnozoites for weeks to months and suddenly can become active causing relapse of vivax malaria.

Merozoites liberate into bloodstream after hepatocytes are ruptured and enter into red blood cells (RBC). Vivax shows preference for young RBCs but falciparum parasites attack all the RBCs with equal aggressiveness thus invading more RBCs at a time than vivax. During this erythrocytic schizogony phase, parasites pass through stages of early ring form, trophozoites, schizonts and finally merozoites. RBCs loaded with merozoites become swollen and deformed and rupture to release numerous merozoites, which again attack fresh RBCs to start new asexual cycle.[4]

Erythrocytic schizogony in vivax occurs in peripheral circulation but in falciparum takes place within capillaries of vital organs, i.e. spleen, liver, brain, etc. with only early ring forms sometimes found in peripheral blood. Parasitized RBCs in falciparum malaria becomes sticky thus demonstrating two important features—cytoadherence (adherence to endothelium of microvasculature) and rosetting (adherence to uninfected RBCs). This can block the forward flow of blood within venules and capillaries making the disease more sinister (cerebral malaria, algid malaria).[4]

During preying upon an infected host, female anopheline acquires male and female gametocytes (sexual forms) developed from some merozoites and through several steps forms and stores sporozoites within salivary glands.[4]

CLINICAL FEATURES

Initial presenting symptoms are nonspecific and almost same as any viral fever like influenza. Both the malaria species cause myalgia, headache, lethargy and vague abdominal colic. The classical cold, hot and sweating stages are seldom seen. *P. vivax* may present with periodic fever spikes with chills and rigor but presentation of *P. falciparum* is very irregular sometimes without any chills or rigor. With disease progression, spleen and liver gradually become palpable with ensuing anemia. Abdominal discomfort, diarrhea or constipation may accompany fever. Tachypnea may be there due to acidosis, anemia or dehydration. Children may have extreme irritability, lethargy and anorexia.[3]

COMPLICATIONS

Complicated or severe malaria is defined as symptomatic malaria with signs of severity or evidence of vital organ dysfunction.[3] Apart from occasional cerebral malaria or splenic rupture (spontaneous or traumatic), severe anemia and hypersplenism, severe malaria is rarely seen with vivax malaria and almost exclusively characteristic of falciparum malaria.

Complications are as follows:

- *Impaired consciousness in cerebral malaria*: Blantyre coma score >3 in children and Glasgow coma score <11 in adolescents.
- *Metabolic acidosis*: Base deficit of more than 8 mEq/L, if not available then plasma bicarbonate level below 15 mmol/L or venous plasma lactate ≥ 5 mmol/L.
- *Hypoglycemia*: Blood glucose level less than 40 mg/dL (2.2 mmol/L).
- *Severe anemia*: Hemoglobin ≤5 g/dL and hematocrit ≤15%.
- *Shock (Algid malaria) or circulatory collapse*: Compensated shock is defined as capillary refill time ≥ 3 seconds or temperature gradient on leg, but no hypotension. Decompensated shock is defined as systolic blood pressure below 70 mm Hg in children with evidence of impaired perfusion.
- *Pulmonary edema*: Infrequently observed but life threatening.
- *Abnormal bleeding or disseminated intravascular coagulation (DIC).*
- *Acute kidney injury*: Serum creatinine more than 3.0 mg/dL or urine output less than 0.5 mL/kg/hour despite adequate hydration. Due to lysis of RBCs often there is hemoglobinuria.
- *Jaundice*: Serum bilirubin exceeding 3 mg/dL or clinically evident icterus.
- *Hyperparasitemia*: *P. falciparum* parasitemia >10%.[5]

DIFFERENTIAL DIAGNOSIS

Differentials of uncomplicated malaria include all the common causes of febrile illness like influenza, dengue, enteric fever, and typhus. Cerebral malaria has to be differentiated from other etiologies of acute encephalitic syndrome (AES) like Japanese encephalitis, herpes encephalitis etc.[3]

APPROACH TO DIAGNOSIS

Diagnosis based only on clinical features should be strictly avoided as it has led to abuse of antimalarials and subsequently drug-resistance.[2,3] Only exception may be suspected case of cerebral malaria where delay in diagnosis can lead to fatal outcome where diagnostic facilities are not available.

Microscopy

Examining properly stained thick and thin smears with 100X oil immersion objective by a skilled microbiologist is still the gold standard to diagnose malaria. Blood sample should be collected without any unnecessary delay (irrespective of timing of fever spikes and especially before commencement of any antimalarial drug) if malaria is suspected. Blood smears are to be preferably prepared as soon as blood sample has been collected (within 2 hours if anticoagulants are used in the vial). Thick smears yield nearly 10 times more sensitive result to find out Plasmodium parasite than thin films, which are to be used for diagnosis of species. At least 100 fields are to be examined under microscope before providing a negative result and if clinical suspicion still persists, this slide can be reviewed for a minimum of 3 consecutive days.[3]

Rapid Diagnostic Tests (RDTs)

These are immunochromatographic tests (ICT) which utilize monoclonal antibodies to detect plasmodium specific antigens in blood samples. Target antigens currently used in RDTs are: Histidine rich protein II (HRP-II) for detecting young gametocytes and asexual stages of *P. falciparum*, parasite lactate dehydrogenase (pLDH) enzyme produced by all four species of malaria for detection of *P. vivax*, *P. falciparum* and other malaria species and certain new antigens like plasmodium aldolase, etc. World Health Organization (WHO) has set standards for RDTs as: sensitivity at least 95% (able to detect *P. falciparum* parasitemia as low as 200 parasites/μL) and a specificity of 95%. ICTs using HRP-II are found to be more sensitive in comparison with those using pLDH as antigens.[3,6,7]

The RDTs have several advantages like ease of interpretation, rapid result, low cost, no need of trained laboratory personnel, etc. but they also have several drawbacks: Firstly, they cannot differentiate between falciparum malaria and mixed infection. Secondly, they usually interpret other non-falciparum malaria cases as vivax malaria. Thirdly, low parasite load often give false-negative results with RDTs. Fourthly, response to treatment cannot be assessed based on RDTs. HRPII antigens persists for more than 4 weeks after successful therapy giving false-positive results. pLDH and aldolase levels decrease quickly after starting effective therapy but they may also persist in gametocytes after clearance of pathogenic asexual stages of the parasite. Hence, in all RDT-negative fever cases microscopy is to be done to exclude malaria.[3]

Therefore, in Indian scenario it holds its place only in certain conditions: health facilities in hard-to-reach and remote areas without any trained laboratory personnel to do a proper microscopy; need of a diagnosis at odd hours when facility of microscopy is not available; as a complementary diagnostic tool besides microscopy; failure to demonstrate parasites in peripheral blood due to sequestration in capillaries.

According to National Strategic Plan Malaria Elimination in India 2017-2022, both Microscopy and quality assured bivalent RDTs have been recommended for diagnosis of malaria diagnosis.[2] Other diagnostic modalities like polymerase chain reaction (PCR), molecular probes, serological test, etc. are only used for research and epidemiological purposes.

MANAGEMENT

Malaria parasite has been a notorious organism to acquire de novo mutations thus becoming resistant to antimalarial drugs. Adequate dosage and duration of antimalarial therapy is very crucial to fight malaria.[3] According to WHO, antimalarial drug combinations are now the recommended modality of treatment for *P. falciparum* infection.[5]

Artemisinin-based Combination Therapy

Antimalarial combination therapy (ACT) is simultaneous use of two or more individually effective schizonticidal drugs with separate modes of action and separate target biochemical stages of the parasite. Even if the parasite acquires resistance to one drug, it gets killed by the other partner drug thus decreasing chances of emergence of drug resistance. WHO has recommended artemisinin and its derivatives as the cornerstone of ACT due to following plus points: high parasiticidal action (decrease parasite load by 10,000 fold in every asexual cycle), low incidence of adverse effects, rapid elimination from blood thereby decreasing chances of developing drug-resistance by Plasmodium and gametocidal action of the drug leading to decreased gametocyte carriage state.[3]

The following ACTs are presently used in our country:

- Artesunate (AS) + Sulfadoxine-Pyrimethamine (SP)
- Artesunate + Mefloquine (MQ)
- Artemether + Lumefantrine - Only form available as oral preparation.[8,9]

These slowly eliminated partner drugs (SP, MQ, lumefantrine) make the ACT regimens shorter (3 days) ensuring better adherence. In these 3 days, artemisinin remain there during 2 asexual parasite life cycles decreasing the parasite load by approximately a factor of one hundred million (10^8).[4]

Treatment regimens have been decided keeping the drug resistance pattern in that particular geographic area. To combat the increasing rate of drug resistance, all falciparum cases are to be treated with ACT in government as well as private set-ups. Mixed infection by vivax and falciparum infections are to be treated with ACT plus a 14-day regimen of primaquine as in vivax malaria.[3,10,11]

Table 1: Treatment of uncomplicated *P. vivax* malaria[2]

		0 Hr	*6 Hr*	*24 Hr*	*48 Hr*	*Total base*
CQ base PLUS	Regimen 1	10 mg/kg	5 mg/kg	5 mg/kg	5 mg/kg	25 mg/kg
	Regimen 2	10 mg/kg	–	10 mg/kg	5 mg/kg	25 mg/kg
Primaquine	0.25 mg/kg once daily for 14 days to prevent relapse					

Treatment of uncomplicated P. vivax malaria

Recommended regimes are provided in **Table 1**.

- CQ is not to be given in empty stomach or at the height of temperature spikes.
- If patient vomits within 45 minutes of taking CQ, the dose is to be repeated after administering proper antiemetics (Domperidone/Ondansetron).
- Primaquine is to be given only after excluding G6PD deficiency.
- Patients with borderline G6PD deficiency 0.6–0.8 mg/kg once weekly dose of primaquine is given for 6 weeks.

Treatment of uncomplicated Plasmodium falciparum malaria[2]

- Artesunate 4 mg/kg orally once daily for 3 days plus Single administration of SP on day 1 (Sulfadoxine - 25 mg/kg and Pyrimethamine - 1.25 mg/kg)

OR

- Artesunate as above plus Mefloquine (15 mg/kg on day 2 and 10 mg/kg on day 3)

OR

- Coformulated tablets of 20 mg Artemether plus 120 mg Lumefantrine as six dose regimen (Oral twice daily regimen for 3 days):

Body weight	*At diagnosis*	*8–12 hours*	*Day 2*	*Day 3*
5–14 kg	1 tablet	1 tablet	1 tablet twice	1 tablet twice
15–24 kg	2 tablets	2 tablets	2 tablets twice	2 tablets twice
25–34 kg	3 tablets	3 tablets	3 tablets twice	3 tablets twice
35 kg and above	4 tablets	4 tablets	4 tablets twice	4 tablets twice

PLUS

A single dose of Primaquine (0.75 mg/kg) for gametocidal action

Points to remember:

- Artemether-lumefantrine is not recommended for infants with weight less than 5 kg.
- Lumefantrine monotherapy was never used so parasite could not develop resistance against it.
- Fatty foods (milk, etc.) increases oral absorption of lumefantrine.
- Artesunate-mefloquine combination is not promoted by Indian health planners as long-term safety and tolerability data regarding mefloquine at 25 mg/kg dosage is lacking and also it has cross-resistance with another very effective and frequently administered antimalarial drug - Quinine.
- All the three regimens mentioned above are recommended for all states of India except north-eastern ones. For north-eastern states, the regimen combining artesunate with SP is not recommended. Artemether-lumefantrine is the first choice in those states with artesunate-mefloquine as an alternative regimen. Although single dose primaquine is used in the same manner in all the states.

Recommended Treatment of Severe Malaria[5]

Severe life-threatening malaria is almost always caused by *P. falciparum*. High degree of clinical suspicion, prompt diagnosis and management are the keys to prevent fatal outcomes. It should be treated preferably in an intensive care unit so that apart from antimalarial therpy, management of other co-existing complications and good quality of supportive and nursing care can be provided to the patient (**Table 2**). Where delay in getting confirmatory laboratory results are contemplated, therapy should not be delayed like in cases of suspected cerebral malaria.

Intravenous quinine or ACT is the recommended choice of therapy irrespective of chloroquine-resistance status as per the National Strategic Plan Malaria Elimination in India 2017-2022. Artemisinin derivatives due to their potential to rapidly destroy the parasite and also lack of significant adverse effects are gaining popularity over quinine.[12] It may be converted to oral medication when patient's clinical condition permits. Where IV therapies

Table 2: Recommended treatment options for complicated and severe malaria

Quinine salt	• Loading dose: 20 mg/kg dissolved in 10 mL normal saline/kg by infusion over 4 hours • Maintenance dose: 10 mg/kg every 8 hours calculated from initiation of loading dose, until patient is able to swallow oral medicine. Subsequently quinine tablets 10 mg salt/kg 8 hourly to complete 7 day course of therapy (parenteral plus oral). • Once patient is able to swallow along with oral quinine one of the following drugs is to be started orally and continued for 7 days: Tetracycline (more than 8 years age) 4 mg/kg/dose 4 times daily OR Doxycycline (more than 8 years age) 3.5 mg/kg/dose once daily OR Clindamycin 10 mg/kg/dose twice daily
Artesunate	3 mg/kg (for <20 kg weight) and 2.4 mg/kg (for ≥20 kg) IV stat and then at 12 and 24 hours, then once a day. Once the patient can swallow complete the treatment by giving a course of • Artemether-lumefantrine combination in north-eastern states of India as in uncomplicated falciparum malaria • Artesunate plus SP in all states other than north-eastern states of India as in uncomplicated falciparum malaria
Artemether	3.2 mg/kg (loading dose) IM, followed by 1.6 mg/kg daily. Once patient can swallow oral medication, complete treatment by giving a course of • Artemether-lumefantrine combination in north-eastern states of India as in uncomplicated falciparum malaria • Artesunate plus SP in all states other than north-eastern states of India as in uncomplicated falciparum malaria

are not available and delay in referral is apprehended, crushed or liquid oral preparations can be administered via nasogastric tube.

Points to remember:

- Parenteral treatment should be at least continued for 24 hours irrespective of child's ability to take oral medications.
- Loading dose of quinine should not be given if patient quinine, quinidine or mefloquine within last 12 hours. Alternatively, loading dose can be given as 7 mg salt/kg IV infusion over 30 minutes, followed by 10 mg salt/kg dissolved in 10 mL isotonic fluid/kg by IV infusion over 24 hours.
- Quinine should always be given in slow infusion (infusion rate not exceeding 5 mg salt/kg/hour).
- Quinine if given in subcutaneous route can cause skin necrosis.
- If there is no clinical improvement after 48 hours of quinine therapy, the maintenance dose is to be reduced by one third to one half, i.e. 5–7 mg salt/kg.
- Mefloquine should be avoided in cerebral malaria due to inherent property to cause neuropsychiatric side effects.

Supportive Therapy

- Good quality nursing care, proper positioning, special attention to airways, eyes, mucosa and skin.
- For unconscious child, nasogastric feeding.
- Oxygen and respiratory supports as needed.
- Close monitoring of vital parameters like intake-output, heart rate, blood pressure, respiratory rate, oxygen saturation, level of consciousness.

TREATMENT OF COMPLICATIONS (TABLE 3)

Cerebral Malaria

Apart from prompt ACT therapy, management of airway, breathing, circulatory shock, control of convulsions with intravenous or rectal diazepam or intravenous lorazepam or midazolam, management of hypoglycemia are cornerstone of management. If GCS is less than 8 endotracheal intubation and mechanical ventilation are necessary. Intravenous 3% NaCl is the option to reduce increased intracranial tension leading to cerebral edema. Placing the patient in lateral position (recovery position) and insertion of nasogastric tube may be helpful to prevent aspiration. Exchange transfusion or RBC exchange transfusion has limited benefit. Other adjunctive treatment options like corticosteroids, mannitol and anti-TNF antibodies are also not recommended due to increased chances of mortality and morbidity.[13-16]

Hypoglycemia

In an unconscious patient with malaria glucose level should be monitored regularly and blood glucose level

Table 3: Complications of malaria and their management	
Convulsions	Benzodiazepines (diazepam/midazolam)
Hyperpyrexia	Tepid sponging, fanning, paracetamol
Severe anemia	Packed red blood cell transfusion
Lactic acidosis	Correct hypovolemia, shock, anemia and prompt management of any seizure
Hypoglycemia	IV 25% dextrose 2–4 mL/kg by bolus. Monitoring of blood glucose every 4–6 hour
Circulatory collapse (Algid malaria)	Adequate fluids, inotropes if required Exclusion of septic shock is essential

should be kept more than 70 mg/dL. If hypoglycemia is noted 2 mL/kg bolus of 25% dextrose or 1 mL/kg bolus of 50% dextrose is to be administered followed by hourly monitoring and appropriate glucose infusion rate should be maintained to prevent rebound hypoglycemia.[5,17,18]

Respiratory Distress

This may be due to metabolic acidosis, acute respiratory distress syndrome (ARDS), severe anemia or co-existing pneumonia. Treatment is according to etiology. Moist oxygen therapy should be guided by pulse oxymetry. ARDS in malaria should be treated just like non-malaria ARDS but permissive hypercapnia for management of ARDS is not recommended in cerebral malaria due to risk of worsening cerebral edema.[5,19-21] Luckily ARDS is less common in children than adults.

Shock

Fluid boluses may be detrimental and thus should be avoided to prevent rise in intracranial pressure and also worsening of cardiac function due to co-existing anemia. Slow correction with intravenous infusion of dextrose and normal saline with or without inotropes is the mainstay of treatment. Antibiotics should be promptly started after collection of appropriate cultures if co-existing sepsis is suspected.[5,22]

Severe Anemia

Threshold for blood transfusion in higher transmission areas is <5 g/dL (Hematocrit 15%) and in lower transmission areas it is taken as <7 g/dL (Hematocrit 20%).[23,24] Often timely transfusion is life-saving especially if hypoxia, acidotic breathing, coma due to cerebral malaria or hyperparasitemia is concurrently present. Packed red blood corpuscles (PRBC), if unavailable, then whole blood transfusion has been recommended.[5,25] Although the cut off values for above thresholds are debatable and do not have concrete evidences to support them.[26]

Acute Kidney Injury

It can be oliguric as well as as non-oliguric. Slow rehydration with 10 mL/kg of normal saline over 2 hours keeping an alert watch for fluid overload and pulmonary edema is recommended. Next line of management is intravenous turosemide. If none of these works, renal replacement therapy (RRT) in the form of hemofiltration or hemodialysis (if these are not feasible then peritoneal dialysis) should be started early in the disease process.[5,27] Indications for RRT are (i) oliguria or anuria; (ii) rapidly rising potassium level or >6.5 mEq/L; (iii) pulmonary edema resistant to diuretics; (iv) uncompensated metabolic acidosis (pH < 7.1); or (v) serum sodium level <110 mEq/L or >160 mEq/L.

Disseminated Intravascular Coagulation (DIC)

Spontaneous bleeding due to DIC in severe malaria should be treated with screened blood products like plasma and platelets. Heparin is reserved for DIC, acral ischemia and purpura fulminans like situations. Antiplatelet agents are to be avoided in severe malaria.[5,28]

PROGNOSIS

Poor prognostic factors are listed below:

- *Clinical*: Deep coma, documented active seizure, malarial papilledema retinopathy, multiorgan dysfunction, age <3 years.
- *Biochemical*: Acidosis, hypoglycemia (<40 mg/dL), decreased GFR, high serum lactate (>5 mmol/L), high CSF lactate, hyperparasitemia, coexistent HIV infection, increased PfHRP2 concentration, >20% of parasites in peripheral smear containing malaria pigment, >5% of neutrophils containing malaria pigment.[29]

Without treatment, cerebral malaria is almost universally fatal. Survivors may develop neurological sequelae like ataxia, poor vision including blindness, paresis. Cognitive problems, unmasking of seizure disorders etc. have also been reported.[5]

KEY MESSAGES

- Parasitological diagnosis is malaria diagnosis as it prevents unnecessary drug usage.
- Microscopy is still the gold standard of diagnosis, rapid diagnostic tests (RDTs) are reserved for areas without skilled microscopist.
- Complicated malaria prompt recognition as success of therapy decreases with time.
- For uncomplicated *P. vivax* malaria, chloroquine is the drug of choice.
- All cases of falciparum malaria should be treated with artemisinin combination therapy (ACT) irrespective of drug resistance status.
- All cases of complicated malaria should be treated with either IV artemisinin or quinine irrespective of species.
- IV artemisinin is superior to quinine for treatment of complicated malaria.
- Mosquito control is still most effective in malaria prevention as vaccine against malaria is not available.

REFERENCES

1. Country profile: India. World Malaria Report 2018. World Health Organisation. Available from: *https://www.who.int/malaria/publications/country-profiles/en/*. Accessed July 25, 2019.
2. National Strategic Plan for Malaria Elimination (2017-22). Directorate of National Vector Borne Disease Control Program. Directorate General of Health Services. New Delhi: Ministry of Health and Family Welfare, Govt. Of India; 2017. Available from: *http://www.indiaenvironmentportal.org.in/content/445149/national-strategic-plan-for-malaria-elimination-2017-22/* Accessed July 25, 2019.
3. Kundu R. Malaria. In: Gupta P, Menon PSN, Ramji S, Lodha R, editors. PC Textbook of Pediatrics, 2nd edition. New Delhi: Jaypee Brothers Medical Publishers; 2018. p. 1232-7.
4. White NJ. Malaria. In: Cook GC, Zumla A, editors. Manson's Tropical Diseases, 21st edition. London: Saunders; 2003. p. 1205-95.
5. World Health Organisation (WHO). Guidelines for the treatment of Malaria, 3rd edition. Geneva: World Health Organisation; 2015. p. 23-5.
6. Marx A, Pewsner D, Egger M, *et al.* Meta-analysis: Accuracy of rapid tests for malaria in travellers returning from endemic areas. Ann Intern Med. 2005;142(10):836-46.
7. Moody A. Rapid diagnostic tests for malaria parasites. Clin Microbiol Rev. 2002;15(1):66-78.
8. Mutabingwa TK, Anthony D, Heller A, *et al.* Amodiaquine alone, amodiaquine+sulfadoxine-pyrimethamine, amodiaquine+artesunate, and artemether-lumefantrine for outpatient treatment of malaria in Tanzanian children: A four-arm randomised effectiveness trial. Lancet. 2005;365(9469):1474-80.
9. Rediscovering wormwood: Qinghaosu for malaria. Lancet. 1992;339(8794):649-51.
10. Adjuik M, Babiker A, Garner P, *et al.* Artesunate combinations for treatment of malaria: Meta-analysis. Lancet. 2004;363(9402): 9-17.
11. Bassat Q. The use of artemether-lumefantrine for the treatment of uncomplicated *Plasmodium vivax* malaria. PLoS Negl Trop Dis. 2011;5(12):e1325.
12. Newton PN, Angus BJ, Chierakul W, *et al.* Randomised comparison of artesunate and quinine in the treatment of severe falciparum malaria. Clin Infect Dis. 2003;37:7-16.
13. Calvo-Cano A, Gomez-Junyent J, Lozano M, *et al.* The role of red blood cell exchange for severe imported malaria in the artesunate era: A retrospective cohort study in a referral centre. Malar J. 2016;15:216-22.
14. Tan KR, Wiegand RE, Arguin PM. Exchange transfusion for severe malaria: Evidence base and literature review. Clin Infect Dis. 2013;57:923-8.
15. Namutangula B, Ndeezi G, Byarugaba JS, *et al.* Mannitol as adjunct therapy for childhood cerebral malaria in Uganda: A randomized clinical trial. Malar J. 2007;6:138-43.
16. van Hensbroek MB, Palmer A, Onyiorah E, *et al.* The effect of a monoclonal antibody to tumor necrosis factor on survival from childhood cerebral malaria. J Infect Dis. 1996;174:1091-7.
17. White NJ, Miller KD, Marsh K, *et al.* Hypoglycemia in African children with severe malaria. Lancet. 1987;1:708-11.
18. Dekker E, Romijn JA, Waruiru C, *et al.* The relationship between glucose production and plasma glucose concentration in children with falciparum malaria. Trans R Soc Med Hygiene. 1996;90:654-7.
19. Taylor WR, Cañon V, White NJ. Pulmonary manifestations of malaria: recognition and management. Treat Respir Med. 2006;5:419-28.
20. Agarwal R, Nath A, Gupta D. Non-invasive ventilation in *Plasmodium vivax* related ALI/ARDS. Intern Med. 2007;46: 2007-11.
21. Price L, Planche T, Rayner C, *et al.* Acute respiratory distress syndrome in *Plasmodium vivax* malaria: Case report and review of the literature. Trans R Soc Trop Med Hyg. 2007;101:655-9.
22. Maitland K, Levin M, English M, *et al.* Severe *P. falciparum* malaria in Kenyan children. Q J Med. 2003;96:427-34.
23. WHO. Severe malaria. Trop Med Int Health. 2014;19 (Supplement 1):1-131.
24. White NJ. Anemia and malaria. Malar J. 2018;17(1):371.
25. Lakritz EM, Campbell CC, Ruebush TK 2nd, *et al.* Effect of blood transfusion on survival among children in a Kenyan hospital. Lancet. 1992;340:524-8.
26. Mpoya A, Kiguli S, Olupot-Olupot P, *et al.* Transfusion and Treatment of severe anaemia in African children (TRACT): A study protocol for a randomised controlled trial. Trials. 2015; 16:593.
27. Mishra SK, Das BS. Malaria and acute kidney injury. Semin Nephrol. 2008;28:395-408.
28. Angchaisukri P. Coagulopathy in malaria. Thromb Res. 2014; 133(1):5-9.
29. Marsh K, Forster D, Waruiru C, *et al.* Indicators of life-threatening malaria in African children. N Engl J Med. 1995; 332(21):1399-1404.

CHAPTER

44

Dengue Fever

SK Kabra, Rakesh Lodha

EPIDEMIOLOGY

Dengue infection has become endemic in most of the South-East Asian countries including India. A recent estimate suggests that every year about 390 million (95% CI 284–528 million) infections occur annually. However, clinically manifested dengue infections are estimated to be about 96 million (95% CI 67–136 million).[1] Dengue fever and severe dengue fever are caused by infection due to any of the four serotypes of dengue viruses (Den 1–4). *Aedes* mosquito transmits the infection. It is believed that dengue infection occurs periodically and one outbreak is predominantly caused by one type of dengue virus. Evolution of dengue infection over last one decade and report of all four strains of dengue virus in one season from Delhi suggests high endemicity of disease.[2,3]

PATHOPHYSIOLOGY

The major pathophysiologic changes include abnormal homeostasis, plasma leakage leading to hemoconcentration, thrombocytopenia and varying degrees of bleeding manifestations.

Precise pathophysiology of plasma leakage and its consequences is unclear. After infection; virus is taken by dendritic cells and after antigen processing, presents it to T cells, leading to immune activation and release of a cascade of cytokines (cytokine storm).[4] Initial studies suggest that in severe dengue there is reduced interferon-α levels and increased pro-inflammatory mediators such as IL-6, IL-8 and IL-10. Markers associated with higher chance of recovery include reduced levels of IL-8 and IL-10.[5] There is increased CD 8 cell population but interferon gamma (a protective cytokine) is not produced possibly due to T cell receptor signaling insufficiencies.[6]

The reasons for platelet deficiency in children with severe dengue infection are not known. Recent report suggests clearance of $CD14^{+}CD16^{+}$ monocyte-platelet complexes by body rather than direct destruction of platelets due to the dengue virus.[7]

CLINICAL MANIFESTATIONS

The clinical manifestations of dengue virus infection vary from asymptomatic to severe life-threatening illness in the form of severe dengue fever.

Dengue infection with undifferentiated symptoms

Children may have fever without localization, nonspecific symptoms of malaise, body aches and recover in 3–5 days.

Dengue without warning signs

Children may present with fever, headache, body aches, rashes, vomiting. Blood pressures and urine output are within normal limits. Majority recovers in 3–5 days time.

Dengue with warning signs

In this group, all children with suspected dengue with any of the following are included:

- Abdominal pain or tenderness, persistent vomiting
- Fluid accumulation in pleural cavity, abdomen (ascites) or subcutaneous tissues
- Mucosal bleeds

- Lethargy, restlessness or irritability, liver enlargement of >2 cm
- Progressive increase in hematocrit with concurrent decrease in platelet count.

Severe dengue

Children with suspected dengue and have any of the following are considered as having severe dengue:

- Severe plasma leakage
- Shock, delayed capillary refill or oliguria
- Fluid accumulation in serosal cavities with respiratory distress
- Severe bleeding manifestations
- Severe organ involvement: Liver failure, AST or ALT ≥1000 units, impaired consciousness, myocardial dysfunction.

Course of Dengue Fever

Symptomatic dengue fever can be described in following phases:

Febrile phase

Child presents with sudden onset of high-grade fever for period of 2–7 days. Children may have body aches, muscle pain, joint pains, headache, eye pain and throat pain. There may be facial flushing, skin rash/erythema, throat and conjunctival congestion. Tourniquet test may be positive in small number of cases and there may be minor hemorrhagic manifestations including petechiae, epistaxis or gum bleed. Tender hepatomegaly may develop by 2–5 days of fever and suggest child is at risk of developing severe disease. There is progressive decrease in total white cell count and platelet count. Majority of patients recover from this phase in 3–7 days. Small proportion may progress to critical phase. Risk factors for progression to severe dengue is not very well defined.[8]

Critical phase

Small proportion of children may enter in critical phase between 3 and 7 days of fever. It is characterized by defervescence, develop bleeding manifestations and shock. Capillary leakage may manifest as facial puffiness, edema, ascites and pleural effusion especially on the right side. Excessive leakage of fluid leads to hypovolemia and shock. Clinically child may have cold and clammy limbs, rapid thready pulse, low blood pressure with narrow pulse pressure (<20 mm Hg), poor tissue perfusion (delayed capillary refill time) and oliguria. Unusual findings include: severe hepatitis, encephalitis or myocarditis and/or severe bleeding without any obvious plasma leakage or shock. Clinical manifestations and outcome in immunocompromised hosts include more liver dysfunction, delayed recovery of platelets and possibly more plasma leak requiring higher fluid.[9] There is fall in platelet counts and increase in packed cell volume.

Recovery phase

Majority of children with supportive care start recovering in 24–48 hours of the critical phase. Extravasated fluid gets desorbed and diuresis start. Child shows recovery with improved appetite, general well-being and resolution of nausea and vomiting. Blood pressure improves; there may be transient hypertension and relative bradycardia. During recovery, patients may demonstrate marked erythema with extreme itching of the extremities, palms and soles. Some patients may have a skin rash suggestive of *"isles of white in a sea of red".* Total leukocyte counts improve in 3–4 days while platelet recovery may occur in 7–10 days.

DIFFERENTIAL DIAGNOSIS

Clinical features of dengue fever may overlap other conditions like influenza, malaria, enteric fever, leptospirosis, viral hepatitis and less commonly meningococcemia and rickettsial infections. Children with malaria, leptospirosis, flu and enteric fever may also occur during outbreak of dengue infection.

Other viral hemorrhagic fevers though not reported or uncommon in India such as Ebola, Marburg, Crimean Congo, Hanta virus, etc. may also resemble with dengue infection. Chikungunya infection is emerging disease in India and resembles that of dengue infection. All these can be differentiated from dengue infection by good history, examination, course of illness and lab investigations.

LABORATORY INVESTIGATIONS

Hematological Changes

Children with severe dengue infection show gradual increase in packed cell volume (PCV), decrease in platelet and leukocyte count with increase in lymphocyte population. Rising hematocrit or a single hematocrit value of more than 40% or retrospectively when peak hematocrit is more than 20% of the hematocrit at the time of recovery are suggestive of hemoconcentration due to widespread capillary leakage. A low WBC count in a child with febrile illness during the endemic season is a pointer towards possible dengue infection. However, malaria, flu, typhoid/paratyphoid, viral hepatitis and rickettsial infections may also present with low WBC count though the leukopenia tends to be more severe in dengue. The peripheral smear may show transformed lymphocytes. In severe illness with shock, there may be evidence of disseminated intravascular coagulation (DIC).

Biochemical Changes

Serum chemistry may show decrease in total protein and albumin, which is more marked in patients with shock. Levels of transaminases are usually raised. A higher increase in SGOT than SGPT suggests the possibility of dengue infection rather than viral hepatitis. In severe cases, there may be hyponatremia, and acidosis along with increase in blood urea nitrogen and creatinine. Activation of complement system leads to profound depression of C_3 and C_5 levels.

Imaging Studies

Skiagram of the chest or ultrasound examination may show varying degrees of pleural effusion, commonly on the right side and occasionally bilateral. Ultrasonography of abdomen may show ascites and enlarged gallbladder due to wall edema.[10] Abnormal electrocardiogram and myocardial dysfunction on echocardiogram has also been reported.[11] The mechanism of decreased cardiac output during toxic stage of DHF is complex. Decreased preload is accompanied by decreased left ventricular performance, and possibly a subnormal heart rate response in some patients.[12]

Virus Isolation and Molecular Diagnosis

Confirmation of diagnosis of dengue may be established by direct methods of isolation of virus by culture, genome detection by PCR and serologic diagnosis by detection of NS1 antigen, IgM and IgG antibodies.[13] Virus isolation is technically demanding, not universally available, expensive and hence of limited practical use. PCR which till now was mainly a research tool for dengue diagnosis and serotyping has now entered the commercial domain. Multiplex real time PCR kits targeting mainly dengue and chikungunya viruses but even leptospirosis, rickettsia, malaria, salmonella and West Nile virus are now available.[14] Cost however restricts the routine use of these PCR-based tests in clinical practice.

Serological Diagnosis

NS1 antigen is a highly conserved glycoprotein of dengue virus and secreted during the initial phase of illness. It disappears as the antibodies appear and its level declines as illness advances and in secondary dengue infections. The specificity of NS1 antigen is nearly 100% and sensitivity in the first 4 days of illness is 90% in primary dengue and 70% in secondary dengue infection.[15] It has emerged as an extremely important diagnostic tool for diagnosis of dengue in clinical practice.

Indirect methods for diagnosis of dengue infection based on antibody determination need careful interpretation.[16] Following primary dengue infection, 80% of patients will have detectable IgM antibodies by day 5 and 99% by day 10. IgM antibodies peak by day 14 and are undetectable by 2 to 3 months. Dengue-specific IgG antibodies rise later, peak to levels which are lower than IgM, decline slowly and remain detectable at low levels for life. Following secondary dengue infection, there is a rapid IgG response in the first 2–3 days, peaking to levels much higher than primary dengue infection. In secondary dengue infection, the IgM antibodies rise later, are blunted and may be absent in some patients. The drawbacks of antibody diagnosis include false negativity in early illness, false positivity due to a positive IgM from an earlier symptomatic/asymptomatic infection, cross reactivity with other flavivirus infections such as Japanese encephalitis, marked variability between kits and different cut offs in different endemic areas. ELISA based tests for serology is more sensitive and specific than the rapid immunochromatographic tests.

If serologic diagnosis of dengue is attempted, the best sensitivity is achieved with estimation of NS1 antigen, dengue-specific IgM and IgG all together in a single sample at the time of presentation.[17]

TREATMENT

Dengue Infection with Undifferentiated Symptoms and Dengue Fever without Warning Signs

Children need symptomatic treatment. Fever is treated with paracetamol. Salicylates and other nonsteroidal anti-inflammatory drugs (NSAIDs) should be avoided as these may predispose a child to mucosal bleeds. In an outbreak/epidemic setting all patients with suspected dengue fever need regular monitoring by a primary care physician for early detection of severe dengue fever. The primary care physician/healthcare worker should monitor the patient for clinical features of severe dengue along with hematocrit and platelet counts, if possible. Any patient developing cold extremities, restlessness, acute abdominal pain, decreased urine output, bleeding and hemoconcentration should be admitted in a hospital. Children with rising hematocrit and thrombocytopenia without clinical symptoms should also be hospitalized.

Dengue with Warning Signs

Children assessed to have any one of the warning signs, need hospitalization. In the hospital, all children should be given crystalloid (Ringer lactate/Normal saline) infusion at the rate of 7 mL/kg over one hour. After one hour, if hematocrit decreases and vital parameters improve, fluid infusion rate should be decreased to 5 mL/kg over next hour and to 3 mL/kg/hour for 24–48 hours. When the patient is stable as indicated by normal blood pressure, satisfactory oral intake and urine output, the child can be discharged (**Flowchart 1**).

If at one hour, the hematocrit is rising and vital parameters do not show improvement, fluid infusion rate is increased to 10 mL/kg over next hour. In case of no improvement fluid infusion rate is further increased to 15 mL/kg over the third hour. If no improvement is observed in vital parameters and hematocrit at end of 3 hours, colloids or plasma infusion (10 mL/kg) is administered. Once the hematocrit and vital parameters are stable, the infusion rate is gradually reduced and discontinued next 24–48 hours.

Severe Dengue

Children assessed to have severe dengue, need admission preferably in Pediatric Intensive Care Unit (PICU) if available. All such patients require infusion of crystalloids fluid 20 mL/kg over one hour or given as bolus if blood pressure is unrecordable. The bolus may be repeated twice if there is no improvement. If there is no improvement in vital parameters and hematocrit is rising, colloids 10 mL/kg are rapidly infused. If the hematocrit is falling without improvement in vital parameters, blood is transfused, presuming that lack of improvement is due to occult blood

Flowchart 1: Intravenous fluid infusion in dengue with warning signs

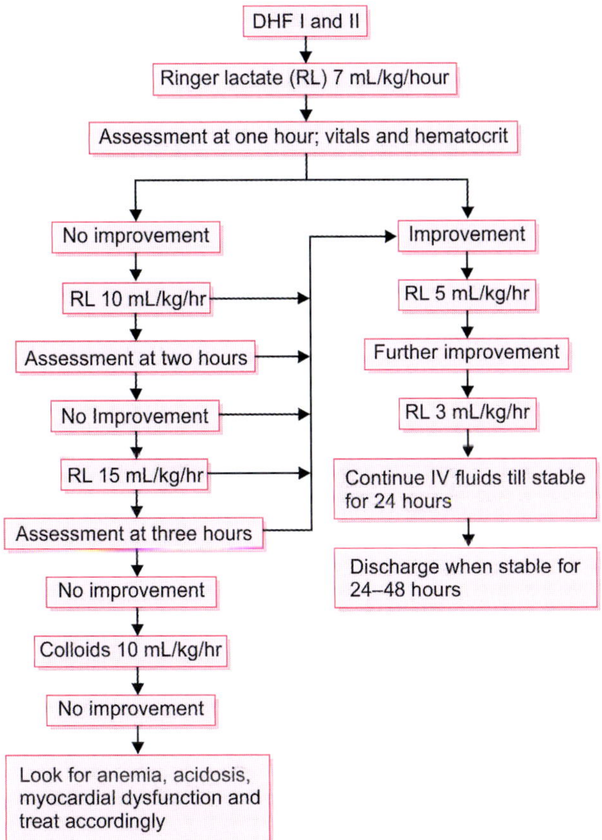

(DHF: dengue hemorrhagic fever)

loss (**Flowchart 2**). Once improvement starts then fluid infusion rate is gradually decreased. In addition to fluids, oxygen should be administered to all patients in shock.

Choice of fluids

There have been few studies that have evaluated the efficacy of different types of fluids in DHF/DSS. A randomized controlled trial comparing four different types of fluid in 230 children in Vietnam suggested that 0.9% saline is the resuscitation fluid of choice for the majority of patients with dengue shock syndrome.[18] Lactated Ringer's solution was not as effective as the other solutions, and allergic reactions occurred in five of the 56 children given 3% gelatin. Children given dextran 70 recovered more quickly, but they were not as ill as the children in the other treatment groups. With early aggressive fluid therapy, the mortality rate should be very low, even in severe dengue.

Flowchart 2: Treatment of severe dengue fever

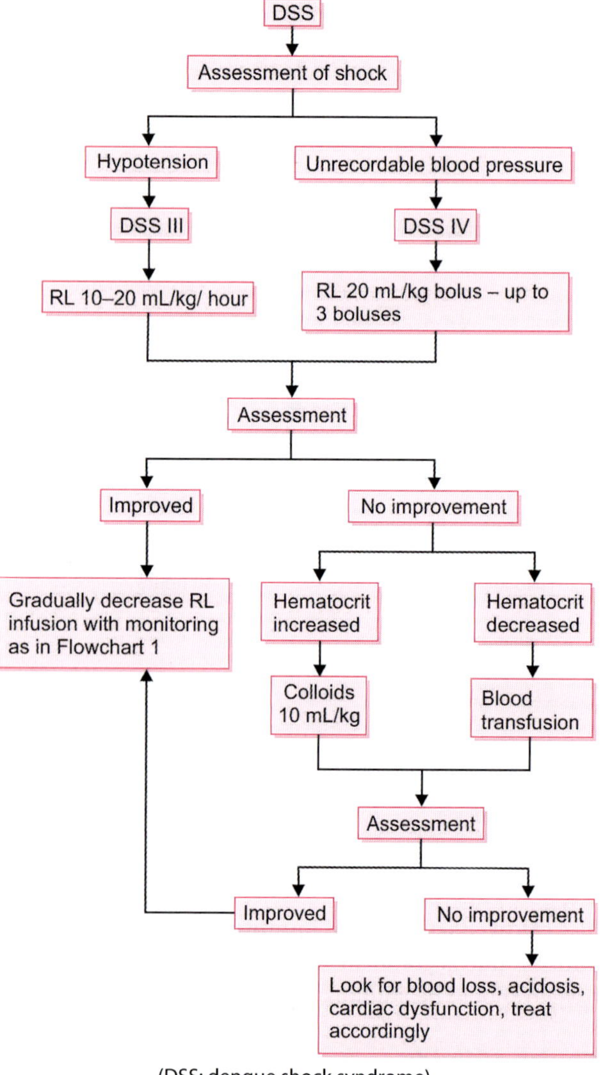

(DSS: dengue shock syndrome)

Wills *et al.* reported on a double-blind, randomized comparison of three fluids for initial resuscitation of Vietnamese children with dengue shock syndrome.[19] Authors concluded that initial resuscitation with Ringer's lactate is acceptable for children with moderately severe dengue shock syndrome. Six percent hydroxyethyl starch may be preferred in children with severe shock, the use of dextran is associated with various adverse reactions. However, a recent randomized controlled trial suggests no difference in outcome with different colloid solutions.[20] In view of non-availability of dextran solutions and no unequivocal support for particular colloid, it is suggested that when indicated, one can use any colloid solution till more studies are available. It is important to treat shock aggressively with fluid management and to avoid fluid overload, judicious use of furosemide infusion has been reported in one study.[21] However, patients with aggressive fluid therapy need very careful monitoring. In presence of clinical evidence of fluid overload, an intravenous dose of furosemide (1–2 mg/kg) may be given.

Management of bleeding

Platelet counts are unreliable to predict bleeding. In a small study in which children with severe thrombocytopenia were included, platelet infusion did not alter the outcome of patients.[22] A recently reported randomized controlled trial carried out in adult patients with dengue infection with thrombocytopenia (≤20 000 platelets per μL), without persistent mild bleeding or any severe bleeding, prophylactic platelet transfusion was not superior to supportive care in preventing bleeding; on the other hand administration of platelets was however associated with adverse events some of which were serious adverse events.[23]

- *Hemodynamically stable with mild mucosal bleeds* or few petechial spots may be managed *with* supportive care including rest, maintenance of hydration and monitoring. IM injections should be avoided. There is no role of prophylactic platelet rich plasma (PRP) infusions even with severe thrombocytopenia. Procedures predisposing to mucosal trauma such as NG tube insertion should be inserted with great care.
- *Hemodynamic instability with severe bleeding* should be treated with blood transfusion and monitoring. If disseminated intravascular coagulation (DIC) is considered, there may be role of fresh frozen plasma (FFP) and PRP and may be decided from patient to patient.

Management of fluid overload

Many children need excessive fluid infusion and may develop fluid overload. Fluid overload may also occur in patients with significant fluid leak. During recovery, the leaked out fluid will return back to the vascular compartment and may cause volume overload.

Fluid overload can be prevented by careful monitoring and discontinuation of IV fluids when the plasma leakage has stopped as suggested by stable blood pressure, pulse volume and peripheral perfusion; and decrease in hematocrit in the presence of a good pulse volume. Children admitted in hospital shows improvement in clinical condition such as defervescence for 24 to 48 hours, improved urine output.

- *Fluid overload with stable hemodynamic status and the patient is out of the critical phase*: In such patients intravenous fluids should be stopped but close monitoring continued. If necessary, oral or intravenous furosemide 0.1–0.5 mg/kg/dose once or twice daily, or a continuous infusion of furosemide 0.1 mg/kg/hour may be given. Serum potassium should be monitored and any hypokalemia should be corrected.
- *Fluid overload with stable hemodynamic status but patient is still in a critical phase*: The intravenous fluids should be reduced gradually. Diuretics during the plasma leakage phase should be avoided because they may lead to intravascular volume depletion. Patients who remain in shock with low or normal hematocrit levels but show signs of fluid overload may have occult hemorrhage. Further infusion of large volumes of intravenous fluids alone will lead to a poor outcome. Careful fresh whole blood transfusion should be given as soon as possible. If the patient remains in shock and the hematocrit is elevated, repeated small boluses of a colloid solution may be administered.

MONITORING

In view of the rapid and unpredictable course in dengue fever, close monitoring of the patient is crucial in the first few hours of illness. Heart rate, respiratory rate, blood pressure and pulse pressure should be measured every 30 minutes till the patient is stable and thereafter every 2–4 hours. Central venous pressure monitoring is desirable in all children who develop hypotension. Difficulties are often encountered in insertion of central lines in critically ill small children.

Laboratory monitoring includes hematocrit measurement every 2 hours for the first 6 hours or till stable. Absolute platelet counts may be carried out once a day till it shows a rising trend. Platelet counts are repeated and coagulation studies performed if there is uncontrolled bleeding. If insertion of a central line is not feasible, clinical and hematocrit monitoring every 30 minutes may guide the rate of fluid infusion. It is emphasized that infusion rates decrease rapidly in the first 6 hours following intervention in most uncomplicated cases of DSS and DHF.[24]

Criteria for discharge: Children should be kept in hospital for 24–48 hours after they are hemodynamically stable off intravenous fluid, accepting well orally, have good urine output and no evidence of fluid overload. It is desirable that platelet counts are more than 50,000/mm^3. However in outbreak situation, if a patient is well and does not have bleeding and platelets are showing rising trend; patients could be considered for discharge even with platelet counts of less than 50,000/mm^3.[3,8]

PROGNOSIS

If left untreated, the mortality in patients with DHF or DSS may be as high as 40–50%. Early recognition of illness, careful monitoring and appropriate fluid therapy alone has resulted in reduction in mortality to less than 1%.[25] Early recognition of shock is of paramount importance as the outcome in DSS depends on the duration of shock. If shock is identified when pulse pressure starts getting narrow and intravenous fluid are administered, the outcome is excellent. Recovery is fast and majority of the patients recover in 24–48 hours without any sequelae. The outcome may not be as good once patient develops cold extremities. The prognosis is grave in patients with prolonged shock and when blood pressure is not recordable.

KEY MESSAGES

- Dengue is an acute viral illness caused by four viruses 1 to 4; and spread by Aedes mosquito.
- Clinical presentation consists of a biphasic fever, myalgia, arthralgia, and hemorrhagic manifestations, lasting over 3–7 days. The most vulnerable stage is soon after defervescence (critical phase) characterized by increased capillary permeability.
- Increased capillary permeability and coagulopathy are major pathogenic abnormalities.
- Thrombocytopenia occurs both due to bone marrow suppression and immune-mediated destruction.
- Serological diagnosis is possible by detecting non-structural (NS) antigen 1 between 2 and 5 days, or fourfold rise in IgG antibodies after 7–10 days.
- Children with warning signs should be hospitalized. Those with severe shock, severe bleeding, and organ involvement need management in intensive care unit (ICU) setting.
- Fluid therapy is the mainstay of treatment. Crystalloid is the fluid of choice during resuscitation. Best guide to fluid therapy is hematocrit.

REFERENCES

1. Bhatt S, Gething PW, Brady OJ, *et.al.* The global distribution and burden of dengue. Nature. 2013;496:504-7.
2. Pandey A, Diddi K, Dar L, *et al.* The evolution of dengue over a decade in Delhi, India. J Clin Virol. 2007;40:87-8.
3. Bharaj P, Chahar HS, Pandey A, *et al.* Concurrent infections by all four dengue virus serotypes during an outbreak of dengue in 2006 in Delhi, India. Virol J. 2008;5:1.
4. Guglani L, Kabra SK. T cell immunopathogenesis of dengue virus infection. Dengue Bulletin. 2005;29:58-69.
5. Singla M, Kar M, Sethi T, *et al.* Immune response to dengue virus infection in pediatric patients in New Delhi, India—Association of Viremia, Inflammatory Mediators and Monocytes with Disease Severity. PLoS Negl Trop Dis. 2016;10: e0004497.
6. Chandele A, Sewatanon J, Gunisetty S, *et al.* Characterization of human CD8 T cell responses in dengue virus-infected patients from India. J Virol. 2016;90:11259-78.
7. Kar M, Singla M, Chandele A, *et al.* Dengue virus entry and replication does not lead to productive infection in platelets. Open Forum Infect Dis. 2017;4:ofx051
8. Anonymous. Dengue Guidelines for Diagnosis, Treatment, Prevention and Control. A joint publication of the World Health Organization (WHO) and the Special Programme for Research and Training in Tropical Diseases (TDR), 2009.
9. Singh A, Seth R, Singla M, *et al.* Clinical profile of dengue infection in immune-compromised children. Indian Pediatr. 2017;54:330-31.
10. Kabra SK, Jain Y, Pandey RM, *et al.* Dengue hemorrhagic fever in children in the 1996 Delhi epidemic. Trans R Society Trop Med Hyg. 1999;93:294-8.
11. Low GK, Looi SY, Yong MH, *et al.* Predictive and diagnostic test accuracy of ultrasonography in differentiating severe dengue from nonsevere dengue. J Vector Borne Dis. 2018;55: 79-88.
12. Kabra SK, Juneja R, Madhulika J, *et al.* Myocardial dysfunction in children with dengue hemorrhagic fever. Natl Med J India. 1998;11:59-61.
13. Khongphatthanayothin A, Suesaowalak M, Muangmingsook S, *et al.* Hemodynamic profiles of patients with dengue hemorrhagic fever during toxic stage: an echocardiographic study. Intensive Care Med. 2003;29:570-74.
14. Shu PY, Huang JH. Current advances in dengue diagnosis. Clin Diag Lab Immunol. 2004;11:642-50.
15. Simmons M, Myers T, Guevara C, *et al.* Development and validation of a quantitative, one-step, multiplex, real-time reverse transcriptase PCR assay for detection of dengue and chikungunya viruses. J Clin Microbiol. 2016;54:1766-73.
16. Datta S, Wattal C. Dengue NS 1 antigen. A useful tool for early diagnosis of dengue virus infection. Indian J Med Microbiol. 2010;28:107-10.
17. Mui Wang SM, Sekaran SD. Evaluation of a commercial SD dengue virus NS1 antigen capture enzyme-linked immunosorbent assay for early diagnosis of dengue virus infection. J Clin Microbiol. 2010;48:2793-97.
18. Ngo NT, Cao XT, Kneen R, *et al.* Acute management of dengue shock syndrome: A randomized double-blind comparison of 4 intravenous fluid regimens in the first hour. Clin Infect Dis. 2001;32:204-13.
19. Wills BA, Nguyen MD, Ha TL, *et al.* Comparison of three fluid solutions for resuscitation in dengue shock syndrome. N Engl J Med. 2005;353:877-89.
20. Kalayanarooj S. Choice of colloidal solutions in dengue hemorrhagic fever patients. J Med Assoc Thai. 2008;91 Suppl 3:S97-103.
21. Ranjit S, Kissoon N, Jayakumar I. Aggressive management of dengue shock syndrome may decrease mortality rate: A suggested protocol. Pediatr Crit Care Med. 2005;6:412-9.
22. Kabra SK, Jain Y, Pandey RM, *et al.* Dengue haemorrhagic fever in children in the 1996 Delhi epidemic. Trans R Soc Trop Med Hyg. 1999;93: 294-8.
23. Lye DC, Archuleta S, Syed-Omar SF, *et al.* Prophylactic platelet transfusion plus supportive care versus supportive care alone in adults with dengue and thrombocytopenia: A multicentre, open-label, randomised, superiority trial. Lancet. 2017;389(10079):1611-8.
24. Kabra SK, Verma IC, Arora NK, *et al.* Dengue hemorrhagic fever in children in Delhi. Bull WHO. 1992;70:105-8.
25. WHO publication. Dengue and Severe Dengue. Available from: *https://www.who.int/news-room/fact-sheets/detail/dengue-and-severe-dengue.* Accessed August 17, 2019.

CHAPTER

45

Fever without Focus

Bhavna Dhingra, Piyush Gupta

INTRODUCTION

Fever, defined as a rectal temperature of 38°C or higher is one of the commonest complaints and about one third of children presenting to the emergency are febrile.[1,2] It is known as *"Fever without focus"* when fever is the only presenting symptom and can be sub-categorized into *fever without localizing signs* (FWLS) and *fever of unknown origin (FUO).*

FEVER WITHOUT LOCALIZING SIGNS

Children presenting with history of acute onset of short duration fever (usually less than a week) as the only presenting complaint without any signs or symptoms localizing to any organ system are categorized as having fever without localizing signs. These represent about 20% of all children presenting with fever and pose a diagnostic dilemma in children less than 36 months of age. It has been estimated that approximately 1.4% children younger than 3 months of age report for evaluation of fever. These children have a higher risk of occult bacteremia and serious bacterial infections (SBI) (range 5–20%).[3,4] These children may require empirical antimicrobial therapy till the etiology is known or the cultures are reported to be negative. As the etiologies of this entity and risk of SBI are variable in different age groups, these children are usually subclassified into the following three categories:

1. Neonates (up to 1 month of age).
2. Infants, 1–3 months of age.
3. Infants, 3–36 months of age.

Children presenting with hyperpyrexia (>40°C); fever with petechiae; and immunocompromised patients with asplenia, sickle cell disease, complement deficiency states, agammaglobulinemia, hypogammaglobulinemia, congenital heart disease, malignancy, or AIDS represent the high-risk groups for bacteremia necessitating empirical antibiotics and aggressive management.

Fever without Localizing Sign in Neonates (Birth to 1 month of Age)

Rectal thermometry is the gold standard to record temperature in young infants, but is risky and is contraindicated in conditions like thrombocytopenia and necrotizing enterocolitis. Axillary temperature measurement should be done using a digital thermometer. Use of infrared, tympanic and temporal artery thermometers is not recommended in this age group.[5]

Etiology

Newborns lack diurnal temperature variation and have less variability of normal body temperature.[6] Neonatal fever without localizing signs is a challenge for the treating clinician. A normal physical examination in a febrile neonate cannot definitely rule out an SBI since signs of infection in this age group are few and that too are nonspecific. Immaturity of immune system, vaccine naivety and exposure to unique pathogens in the perinatal period makes them highly susceptible to develop serious bacterial infections (SBI).[6] It is difficult to differentiate between dehydration fever, a self-limited viral illness (e.g. enteroviral infections), and SBI. SBI ranges from occult bacteremia, pneumonia, meningitis, urinary tract infection, and enteritis, to osteomyelitis, and septic arthritis.

Haemophilus influenzae B and *Streptococcus pneumoniae* are the two most important causes of SBI in India, besides *Klebsiella*, *Staphylococcus aureus*, and *Escherichia coli*. *Listeria monocytogenes* and perinatally acquired herpes simplex virus (HSV) infection have also been implicated. Malaria should also be considered a strong possibility in endemic areas.

Fever in the Young Infant 1 to 3 Months of Age

A rectal temperature of more than 38°C (100.4°F) in conditions of normal ambient temperature and humidity should not be ascribed to overclothing (bundling) in young infants. Overclothing usually increases the skin temperature but does not increase the core (rectal temperature). A temperature of more than 38.5°C (101°F) should never be ascribed to overclothing, irrespective of the way the temperature has been recorded.

Etiology

Self-limited seasonal viral illnesses are the most common cause of fever without localizing signs in this age group. The possibility of SBI should always be entertained in any febrile child between 1 month and 3 months of age and the following conditions should be ruled out: otitis media, pneumonia, skin and soft tissue infections, omphalitis and urinary tract infections especially in uncircumcised boys and children with urinary tract anomalies.[7]

The most common implicated organisms are group B *Streptococcus*, *E. coli*, *S. aureus*, *S. pneumoniae*, *H. influenzae*, *Neisseria meningitidis* and enterococci. Pyelonephritis is the most common SBI and may be seen in well appearing as well as ill appearing children between 1 month and 3 months of age presenting with fever without localizing signs.[8,9]

Fever without Localizing Signs in 3 to 36 Months Old Children

Viral infections are responsible for majority of children having non-localizing fever in this age group. Serious bacterial infection can also occur due to *S. pneumoniae*, *Neisseria*, and *H. influenzae*. Important bacterial infections include otitis media, pneumonia, sinusitis, enteritis, urinary tract infection, osteomyelitis and meningitis. Pneumococcal bacteremia can resolve spontaneously in about one-third of cases or can lead to development of localized infections, e.g. meningitis, pneumonia, cellulitis, pericarditis, osteomyelitis or septic arthritis.

Children 3–36 months of age with temperature greater than 39°C and WBC counts greater than 20,000/mm^3 may have an occult pneumonia or urinary tract infection (UTI). Risk factors for UTI are female gender, uncircumcised boys and temperature greater than 39°C.

In children presenting with fever lasting for more than 5 days, a differential diagnosis of Kawasaki disease must be entertained.[6] In children with sickle cell anemia, due to splenic dysfunction, infections with capsulated organisms like *H. influenzae*, *S. pnuemoniae*, *E. coli* and *Salmonella* are frequent. Acute chest syndrome may be precipitated by any of these infections or *Chlamydia* or *Mycoplasma*. Parvovirus infection can lead to an aplastic crisis in these children.[6]

Clinical Features

Any afebrile newborn or young infant with history of documented fever at home should be treated as febrile. All febrile children in this age group should be hospitalized and after control of ambient environmental temperature and adequate hydration with increased frequency of breastfeeding, if the baby is still febrile—possibility of SBI should be entertained even in an apparently healthy neonate.

Febrile infants up to 3 months of age, at presentation may appear well or may present with diminished spontaneous activity, lethargy, convulsions, respiratory compromise (tachypnea, chest retraction and grunting), central cyanosis, diminished muscle tone, mottled cool extremities, irritability and/or weak sucking. Alteration of vital signs in these young children may be the only presenting feature of an SBI.[6]

Diagnosis of Kawasaki disease can be confirmed if fever is present along with any four of the following symptoms: non-exudative bilateral conjunctival injection, oropharyngeal mucous membrane changes (strawberry tongue and cracked lips), cervical lymphadenopathy ≥1.5 cm, extremity changes (palmar erythema, extremity swelling, periungual desquamation), and polymorphous moribilliform rash. Acute myocarditis, gallbladder hydrops and pulmonary involvement can also be present. Children less than 1 year of age may present with atypical features.[10]

Meningococcemia should be suspected in febrile children with a nonblanching petechial rash, which may progress to purpura fulminans. It may be complicated by pneumonia, otitis media, epiglottitis, uveitis, arthritis, pericarditis, myocardial dysfunction, stroke or adrenal hemorrhage.[11]

Approach to Diagnosis

A full sepsis evaluation is warranted in all febrile neonates, which includes complete blood counts with band form count, urine microscopy, urine culture, blood culture, chest X-ray, and peripheral smear for malarial parasite. Lumbar puncture and cerebrospinal fluid analysis (cell counts, glucose, protein, Gram stain and culture) should be undertaken in children with lethargy or refusal to breastfeeding.

Risk stratification for infants 1 to 3 months of age

Infants 1–3 months of age with fever who appear well and had been previously healthy, and have a normal physical examination, can be categorized as at low-risk or high-risk for serious bacterial infections by certain investigations.[12-14] **Table 1** lists the various criteria used for identifying children 1–3 months at low-risk of SBI.

Febrile children, 1–3 months of age who present with fever without localizing signs must be evaluated for sepsis by complete blood count, lumbar puncture, blood culture, urinalysis, urine culture and chest radiograph. Early ultrasound should be performed in male infants younger than three months and infants not responding to treatment.[6]

Risk factors for occult bacteremia in children between 3 and 36 months of age include rectal temperature >39°C, WBC counts >15,000/mm^3, raised ESR, and elevated C-reactive protein. Rectal temperature >40°C and WBC count > 25,000/mm^3 indicate a higher probability of serious bacterial infection.[15]

Increased C-reactive protein, sedimentation rate, and high WBC count in the first week of illness followed by thrombocytosis in the second week of illness, transaminitis and sterile pyuria help in confirmation of diagnosis of Kawasaki disease.

In children with known sickle cell anemia, temperature >40°C, poor perfusion, WBC counts >30,000 or <5000, platelet count < 1,00,000 per mm^3, Hb < 5 g/dL, infiltration of chest radiograph or history of pneumococcal sepsis raise the risk of bacteremia.

Gram stain and/or PCR of skin lesions or CSF are diagnostic of meningococcemia.

Management

In newborns, after obtaining relevant investigations, empirical antibiotic therapy should be initiated at the earliest with combination of ampicillin and cefotaxime or

Table 1: Low-risk criteria in 1–3 months old children with fever without localizing signs

	Philadelphia protocol	*Pittsburgh guidelines*	*Rochester criteria*	*Boston criteria*
General appearance	Well	Well	Well	Well
Physical examination	Normal	Normal	Normal	Normal
Complete blood count WBC/mm^3 I:T neutrophil ratio absolute band count	<15,000 <0.2	5,000–15,000 <1500/mm^3	5,000–15,000 <1500/mm^3	<20,000
Urine examination	<10 WBC/HPF No bacteria on Gram stain	9 WBC/mm^3 No bacteria on Gram stain	<10 WBC/HPF at 40X	Negative leukocyte esterase
Cerebrospinal fluid (If bloody tap)	<8 WBC/mm^3 No bacteria on Gram stain	5 WBC/mm^3 No bacteria on Gram stain WBC:RBC ≤ 1:500		< 10 WBCs/mm^3
Chest radiograph	No infiltrates	No infiltrates		
Stool examination	No RBC, few or no WBC	5 WBC/HPF with diarrhea	< 5 WBC/HPF if diarrhea	
				Caretaker contactable telephonically

(WBC: white blood cells; RBC: red blood cells; HPF: high power field; I:T: immature: total)

monotherapy with ceftriaxone (100 mg/kg per day) and modified later as per the reports of the sepsis screen and cultures. Acyclovir (20 mg/kg/dose IV 8 hourly for 14 to 21 days) may be added if HSV infection is suspected.[16]

Ill-appearing infants (1-3 months of age) require immediate hospitalization and prompt institution of empirical parenteral antimicrobial therapy. Ampicillin with either cefotaxime or ceftriaxone is an effective combination. Vancomycin should be included if possibility of meningitis with penicillin resistant *S. pneumoniae* is suspected. Antimicrobials can be modified as per the culture and sensitivity reports.[17,18]

In well-appearing infants, where a close follow-up within 24 hours can be ensured, a watchful observation without antibiotics may be planned and a sepsis screen obtained, although a lumbar puncture may be deferred. Prior to initiation of antibiotics in the event of clinical deterioration, a lumbar puncture should always be done.[17,18]

Management options for children between 3 and 36 months of age are detailed in **Flowchart 1**. Infants with moderate to high-risk factors should be treated with ceftriaxone (50–80 mg/kg/day in one or two divided doses IV or IM). In infants below 4 weeks of age, ampicillin

Flowchart 1: Management of fever without focus in young children

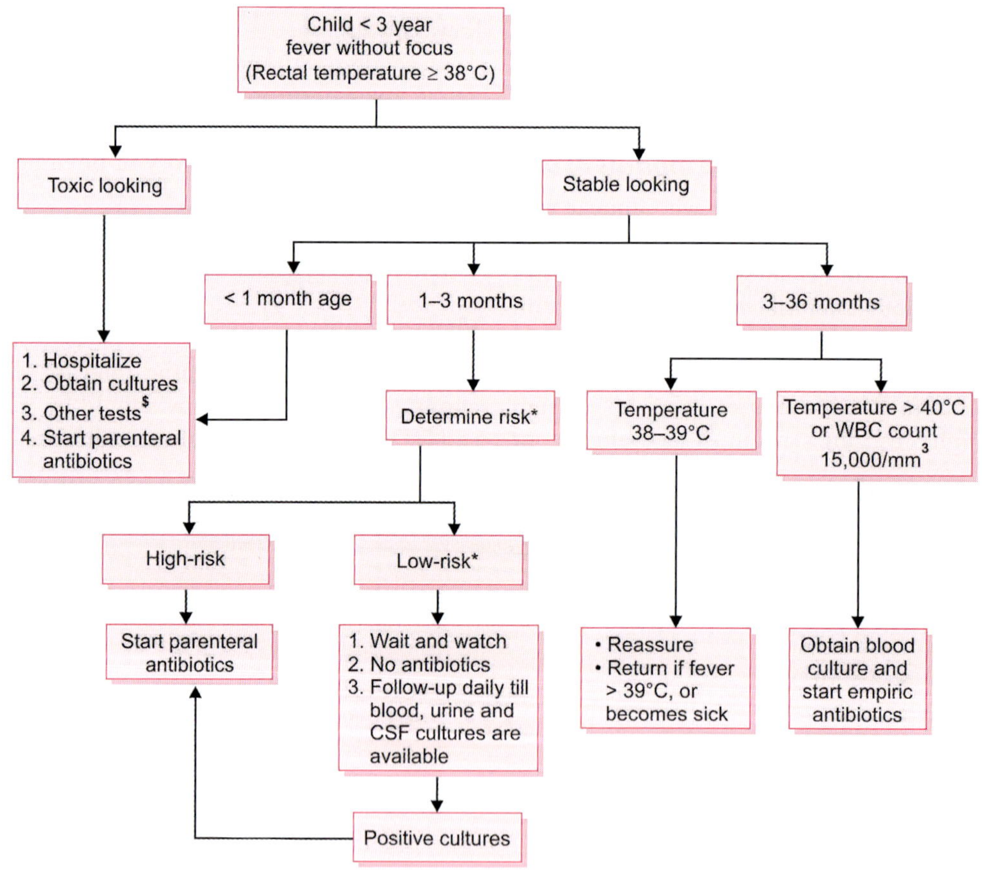

(*Reproduced from Gupta P. Textbook of Pediatrics. New Delhi: CBS; 2013*)

*Determine risk based on history, examination, and laboratory studies:

Low-risk: Normal history and physical examination; WBC 5,000–15,000/mm^3; band cell <1500/mm^3 urine pus cells <10/hpf; stool pus cells <5/hpf; normal chest radiograph; and CSF < 8 lymphocytes/mm^3.

$Other tests include WBC count; urine and stool microscopy; chest X-ray; CSF Gram stain.

Cultures include that of blood, urine, and CSF.

(50–100 mg/kg/day IM or IV two divided doses) should also be added to cover *Listeria monocytogenes* and enterococci, which are not sensitive to ceftriaxone.

Surgical intervention may be needed for drainage of abscesses, osteomyelitis, empyema, etc. Suspicion of Kawasaki disease warrants treatment with intravenous immunoglobulin (IVIG) at 2 g/kg along with aspirin (initially @80 mg/kg/day in four divided doses and reduced to 5 mg/kg/day after defervescence).[10]

Meningococcemia requires droplet isolation, aggressive antibiotic and fluid therapy. Steroids may be needed if adrenal hemorrhage is suspected. Chemoprophylaxis with rifampicin (10 mg/kg in 2 divided doses for 2 days) or ciprofloxacin 500 mg for adults, or ceftriaxone 125 mg IM for children <12 years or 250 mg for children >12 years is recommended for all contacts.[10]

FEVER (PYREXIA) OF UNKNOWN ORIGIN

Fever without an obvious cause, lasting for a period of more than 3 weeks after outpatient evaluation or after 7 days of detailed inpatient evaluation and investigation, is known as fever of unknown origin (FUO). Children presenting with FUO usually do not present as an emergency and empirical antimicrobial therapy is not warranted in majority of the cases.

The FUO has been categorized as: *Nosocomial* (or healthcare associated), *Neutropenic,* or HIV-*related*. The common causes of FUO can be grouped into Infections, Immune mediated disorders, Connective tissue disorders or Malignancies. In infants and young children, infections are the leading cause of FUO and the most commonly implicated infections are: Urinary tract infections (UTI), tuberculosis, infectious mononucleosis, osteomyelitis, deep seated abscesses, infective endocarditis, HIV, parasitic and fungal infections, etc.[6]

Juvenile inflammatory arthritis is the commonest connective tissue disorder presenting as prolonged fever in young children. Kawasaki disease should always be ruled out in young children presenting with FUO. Malignancies constitute up to 5% of such cases and leukemias are the commonest in this group.

Granulomatous and hypersensitivity disorders, certain familial and hereditary syndromes should also be considered in differential diagnosis. Collection of free blood, including intracranial hemmorhage, can present with fever without an obvious cause. Certain periodic syndromes like PFAPA (periodic fever, aphthous stomatitis, pharyngitis and adenitis) and drug fevers may also be implicated in the appropriate clinical setting. Factitious fevers should be considered if fever persists for more than 6 months despite complete workup and no obvious cause.

Detailed history including history of travel, recent immunization, animal bites or exposures, prior medications, contact with sick family members, etc. and a thorough physical examination to look for nonspecific and subtle signs are essential to establish a diagnosis in such cases. There is no algorithm that can be used to investigate such cases and the treating clinician must order investigations judiciously on the merit of each case and depending on their provisional diagnosis.

Empirical treatment with anti-inflammatory agents and antimicrobials should be avoided as they may alter the course of certain conditions and delay the establishment of diagnosis. Symptomatic therapy should be initiated and such cases should be investigated in detail.

KEY MESSAGES

- Children presenting with fever without localizing signs carry high chances of occult bacteremia and serious bacterial infection (SBI).
- Newborns or young infants with fever should be hospitalized and dehydration fever ruled out, before starting empirical therapy.
- Well appearing, 1–3 months old febrile children should be categorized into low-risk and high-risk categories, based on certain criteria.
- Empirical antibiotic therapy should be started in children at high-risk of serious bacterial infections/occult bacteremia.
- Children with FUO usually do not need empirical antimicrobials and/or anti-inflammatory agents.

REFERENCES

1. Chamberlain JM, Patel KM, Pollack MM. Association of emergency department care factors with admission and discharge decisions for pediatric patients. J Pediatr. 2006; 149:644-9.
2. Sands R, Shanmugavadivel D, Stephenson T, *et al.* Medical problems presenting to paediatric emergency departments: 10 years on. Emerg Med J. 2012;29:379-82.
3. Huppler AR, Eickhoff JC, Wald ER. Performance of low-risk criteria in the evaluation of young infants with fever: Review of the literature. Pediatrics. 2010;125:228-33.
4. Schwartz S, Raveh D, Toker O, *et al.* A week-by-week analysis of the low-risk criteria for serious bacterial infection in febrile neonates. Arch Dis Child. 2009;94:287-92.
5. Jain S, Cheng J, Alpem ER, *et al.* Management of febrile neonates in US Pediatric emergency departments. Pediatrics. 2014;133:187-95.

6. Claudius I, Baraff LJ. Pediatric emergencies associated with fever. Emerg Med Clin North Am. 2010;28:67-84,vii-viii.
7. Irwin AD, Drew RJ, Marshall P, *et al.* Etiology of childhood bacteremia and timely antibiotics administration in the emergency department. Pediatrics. 2015;135:635.
8. Greenhow TL, Hung YY, Pantell RH. Management and outcomes of previously healthy, full term, febrile infants ages 7 to 90 days. Pediatrics. 2016;138.
9. Aronson PL, Thurm C, Alpern ER, *et al.* Variation in the care of the febrile young infant < 90 days in US Pediatric emergency departments. Pediatrics. 2014;134:667-77.
10. Woodward AL, Sundel RP. Rheumatologic emergencies. In: Fleisher GR, Ludwig S, Henretig F, editors. Textbook of Pediatric Emergency Medicine, 5th edition. Philadelphia: Lippincott Williams & Williams; 2006. p. 1305-10.
11. Stephans DS, Greenwood B, Brantzaeg P. Epidemic meningitis, meningococcaemia, and *Neisseria meningitidis*. Lancet. 2007;369:2196-210.
12. Baskin MN, O'Fourke EJ, Fleisher GR. Outpatient treatment of febrile infants 28 to 89 days with intramuscular administration of ceftriaxone. J Pediatr. 1992;120:22-7.
13. Baker MD, Bell LM, Avner JR. Outpatient management without antibiotics of fever in selected infants. N Engl J Med. 1993;329:1437-41.
14. Jaskiewicz JA, McCarthy CA, Richardson AC, *et al.* Febrile infants at low risk for serious bacterial infections- an appraisal of the Rochester criteria and implications for management. Pediatrics. 1994;94:390-6.
15. Stoll ML, Rubin LG. Incidence of occult bacteremia among highly febrile young children in the era of the pneumococcal conjugate vaccine; a study from a children's hospital emergency department and urgent care center. Arch Pediatr Adolesc Med. 2004;158:671-5.
16. Steiner I, Kennedy PG, Pachner AR. The neurotropic herpes viruses: Herpes simplex and varicella-zoster. Lancet Neurol. 2007;6:1015-28.
17. Aronson PL. Evaluation of the febrile young infant: An update. Pediatr Emerg Med Pract. 2013;10:1-17.
18. Arora R, Mahajan P. Evaluation of child with fever without source: Review of literature and update. Pediatr Clin North Am. 2013;60:1049-62.
19. Singh J, Arrieta A. Management of meningococcemia. Indian J Pediatr. 2007;71:909-13.

CHAPTER

46

Fever with a Rash

Rachna Seth, Amitabh Singh

INTRODUCTION

Fever with rash is common among children and seen in both outpatient and emergency department. Most of them are benign viral exanthems without much clinical significance. The challenge lies in identifying conditions, which may be life-threatening or require specific treatment. There are a large number of infectious and noninfectious conditions presenting as exanthematous fevers. Many of them have a characteristic combination of clinical features. The rash is also morphologically different in different diseases. The identification of benign etiologies of fever with a rash also helps in allaying parental anxiety and avoids unnecessary laboratory investigations. It is also important to identify conditions, which require isolation to prevent spread of contagious infections. Viral exanthems are the most common cause of fever with rash in children. It is important to know the terminologies used for describing a skin rash to have a structured approach in making a differential diagnosis. The terminologies used are explained in **Table 1**.

EPIDEMIOLOGY[1-3]

- *Age*: The age of the child may help in narrowing the differential diagnosis. Viral exanthems like measles, roseola infantum, Epstein Barr virus occur more commonly in children below 3 years of age. Varicella

Table 1: Types and description of skin rash

Type of skin lesion	*Description*
Macule	Nonpalpable, circumscribed lesion that is flat and ≤ 1 cm in diameter
Papule	Palpable lesion that is solid, elevated, and ≤ 5 mm in diameter
Maculopapular	Confluent, erythematous rash made up of both macular and papular lesions
Purpura	Papular or macular nonblanching lesions that are due to extravasation of red blood cells, 1 to 2 mm lesions are called petechiae
Nodule	Deep-seated, roundish lesion ≥ 5 mm in diameter that can involve the epidermal, dermal, and/or subcutaneous tissue
Plaque	A palpable elevated lesion ≥ 5 mm in diameter
Vesicle	Distinct, elevated fluid filled skin lesion < 5 mm in diameter
Bulla	A vesicle ≥ 5 mm in diameter
Pustule	A vesicle containing pus
Ulcer	Loss of the epidermis and upper layer of the dermis
Eschar	Hard, black-color adherent necrotic skin with +/– overlying area of ulceration

and Rubella are common between 3 and 10 years of age. Parvovirus is common between 4 and 10 years of age. The incidence of scarlet fever is maximum between 2 and 10 years. Meningococcemia, which has characteristic rash is, one of the life-threatening condition which shows 2 peaks in age incidence (<5 years and 15–24 years). Kawasaki disease and staphylococcal scalded skin syndrome (SSSS) also occur more commonly in children less than 5 years. Rheumatological conditions (systemic lupus erythematosus, juvenile dermatomyositis) occur more commonly in older children (more than 6 years). Henoch Scholein purpura, another vasculitis disorder is more common between 2 and 8 years.

- *Season*: As underlying etiology is mostly infective, different etiologies show seasonal pattern because of the environmental condition which are important determinants for propagation of the offending organism. Measles epidemics occur in winter and early spring. Likewise Parvovirus B19 infections also occur mainly in winter and spring transmitted via respiratory droplets. The arbovirus transmitted by *Aedes aegypti* mosquito causes epidemics of dengue and chikungunya in the monsoon season. Herpes simplex infections are ubiquitous without any seasonal variation. Enteroviruses, known to cause numerous exanthems in children, occur round the year in tropical and subtropical areas. Leptospirosis is common in monsoon.
- *Geographical areas*: Some pathogens or their carrier are active only in certain climates and as a result, some of the diseases presenting as fever with rash are limited to geographical areas. Lassa virus, Ebola, yellow fever are mainly limited to Africa. Tropical climates give rise to a number of arbovirus infections. Rickettsial diseases occur worldwide. Measles and meningococcemia is less common in developed countries due to immunization coverage. Vibrio vulnificus and cutaneous larva migrans are common in coastal areas.
- *Incubation period*: A knowledge of incubation period is important when dealing with a child exposed to an individual with similar rash. The range of incubation period for common illness is shown in **Table 2**.
- *Exposure history*: Exposure to infected human secretion, close contact with a person infected with contagious disease, contact with animals, plant materials may provide a clue when evaluating a case of fever with rash.

Table 2: incubation period of common diseases presenting with fever and rash[4,5]

Disease/ Organism	*Incubation period*
Atypical measles	7 to 14 days
Cat scratch disease	7 to 14 days
Chancroid	1 to 35 days
Chickenpox	10 to 20 days
Chikungunya	3 to 7 days
Chlamydia psittaci	5 to 21 days
Coxsackie/echovirus	2 to 9 days
Cutaneous larva migrans	2 to 4 days
Dengue	3 to 14 days
Escherichia coli 0157:H7	3 to 8 days
Epstein-Barr virus (mononucleosis)	30 to 50 days
Hepatitis B	45 to 160 days
Hepatitis C	14 to 180 days
Herpes simplex (genital)	2 to 7 days
Human immunodeficiency virus (HIV)	28 to 180 days
Kawasaki disease	Unknown
Leishmaniasis	14 to 56 days
Lyme disease	3 to 30 days
Mycobacterium leprae	>1 year
Mycoplasma pneumoniae	7 to 28 days
Neisseria meningitidis	1 to 10 days
Parvovirus B19	7 to 21 days
Reiter's syndrome	7 to 14 days
Rheumatic fever	7 to 35 days
Rocky mountain spotted fever, *R. rickettsii*	2 to 14 days
Roseola infantum	5 to 15 days
Rubella	5 to 21 days
Rubeola	10 to 14 days
Salmonella typhi (enteric fever)	3 to 60 days
Staphylococcal toxic shock syndrome	2 days
Syphilis	9 to 90 days
Typhus: epidemic louse-borne, *R. prowazekii*	7 to 14 days
Typhus: scrub, *R. orientalis/R. tsutsugamushi*	6 to 21 days
Yersinia pestis	2 to 8 days
Zika virus	2 to 14 days

ETIOPATHOGENESIS

The list of underlying etiology for fever with rash consists of infective, immunological, rheumatological and other conditions.[3] Common causes are shown in **Table 3**.

The skin may be involved as systemic response to infection or by toxin-mediated disorders, including those

Table 3: Common causes of fever with rash in children

I. Infectious causes
Viral infections
• Measles • Rubella • Roseola infantum (human herpesvirus 6) • Parvovirus (fifth disease) • Epstein Bar virus • Enteroviruses • Adenovirus • HIV • Dengue virus • Chikungunya virus • Herpes simplex virus types 1 and 2 • Influenza A and B • Hepatitis B virus (Giannotti–Crosti Syndrome) • Lassa, Marburg, Ebola, Hantavirus (not seen in India)
Bacterial infections
• *Staphylococcus aureus* • Group A streptococcus • *Neisseria meningitidis* • *Listeria monocytogenes* • *Salmonella typhi* • *Yersinia pestis, Yersinia enterocolitica* • *Bartonela quintana* • *Borrelia* • *Leptospira* *Rickettsial infections (diseases)* • *R. prowazekkI* (Epidemic typhus) • *R. typhi vI* (Murine typhus) • *R. tsutsugamushi* (Scrub typhus) • *R. conorii* (Indian tick typhus) • *R. rickettsii* (Rocky mountain spotted fever) • *R. akari* (rickettsial pox)
II. Noninfectious causes
Collagen vascular diseases/Immune mediated conditions
• Systemic onset juvenile idiopathic arthritis • Systemic lupus erythematosus • Juvenile dermatomyositis • Kawasaki disease • Henoch Schonlein purpura • Polyarteritis nodosa • Wegener granulomatosis
III. Drug hypersensitivity rash
• Stevens-Johnson syndrome • Toxic epidermal necrolysis • Acute generalized exanthematous pustulosis • Drug reaction with eosinophilia and systemic symptoms (DRESS) • Leukocytoclastic vasculitis

associated with bacterial super antigen production or by inflammatory conditions, including vasculitides and rheumatologic diseases. The skin may be affected by (a) direct involvement by the infectious agent; (b) specific reaction to an infection; and (c) nonspecific reaction to an infection.

CLINICAL FEATURES

Fever and rash are common clinical constellation of myriad of etiologies. Some of the more common conditions are described here.[6,7]

Measles

This is an acute viral exanthematous illness with prodrome of malaise, fever, cough, running nose and conjunctivitis.[8] It has a brick red maculopapular rash which is blanching (**Fig. 1**). It starts from head and neck area and then spread centrifugally to trunk and extremities. It has a characteristic enanthem (Koplik spots) on buccal mucosa consisting of a red halo with bluish white central dot opposite the second molar, it has no or little pruritus. Rash appears at peak of fever usually on 3rd day. Fever and other symptoms resolve spontaneously after 48 hrs of appearance of rash. Fine desquamation usually starts from face and then to extremities and occurs over several days.

Chickenpox (Varicella)

It is characterized by prodrome of fever with a classical vesicular eruption on an erythematous base. The rash

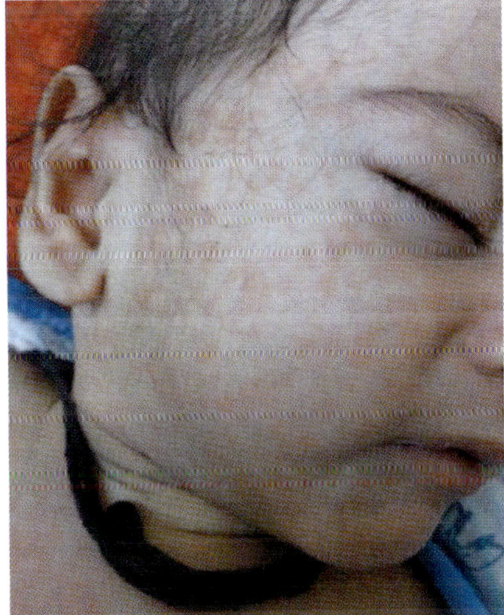

Fig. 1: Measles (*Courtesy*: Dr Neetu Bhari, Assistant Professor, Dermatology and Venereology, All India Institute of Medical Sciences, New Delhi)

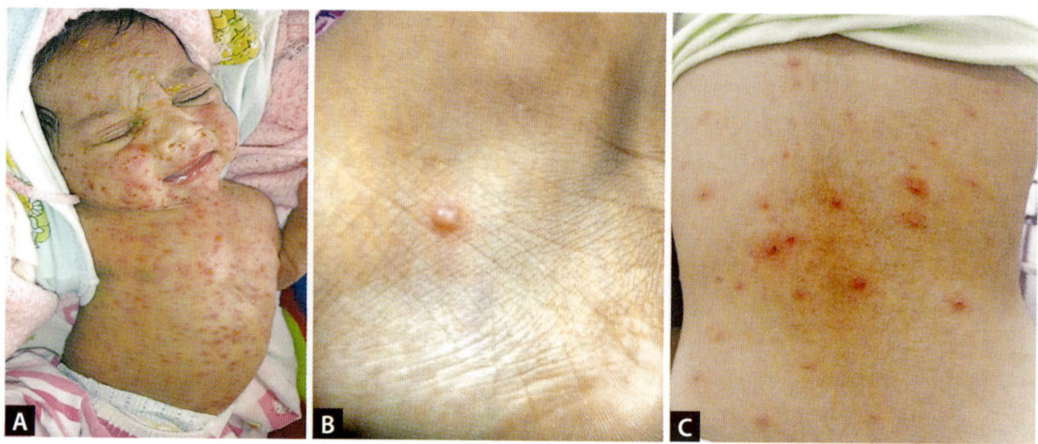

Figs. 2A to C: (A) Pleomorphic rash of varicella in a neonate; (B and C) Characteristic rash of varicella appearing in crop and are present in different stages from papules to vesicles to crusting in an older child (*Courtesy*: Dr Neetu Bhari, Assistant Professor, Dermatology and Venereology, All India Institute of Medical Sciences, New Delhi)

appears in crop and is present in different stages from papules to vesicles to crusting (**Figs. 2A to C**). There are pruritic papules, vesicles in various stages which appear in crops of 2–4 and then crusts.[9] The rash is distributed first on trunk and then involves face, extremities and it lasts for 7–10 days. The lesions may recur years later in dermatomal distribution (zoster, shingles) (**Fig. 3**). Recurrent lesions may be seen in immune compromised children.

Rubella

The rash mimics measles but the child does not appear sick. Presence of postauricular, posterior cervical or suboccipital adenopathy helps in making a diagnosis. Forchheimer spots, which are punctate soft palate macules are also helpful in diagnosis. The maculopapular rash starts on face and then involves peripheries, 1–4 days after a prodrome of mild systemic symptoms like low grade fever, cough and coryza.[8]

Parvovirus B19 Infection (Erythema Infectiosum)

Children usually develop a characteristic rash with a "slapped cheeks" appearance followed by an erythematous maculopapular rash that spreads from arms to trunk in a reticular pattern.[10] Rash may lag prodrome of headache, malaise, myalgia by 3–7 days; lasts 2–4 days and may recur 2–3 weeks later. Children are generally afebrile at time of appearance of rash. In patient with aplastic crisis associated with parvovirus, rash is usually absent. Pruritus may or may not be present.

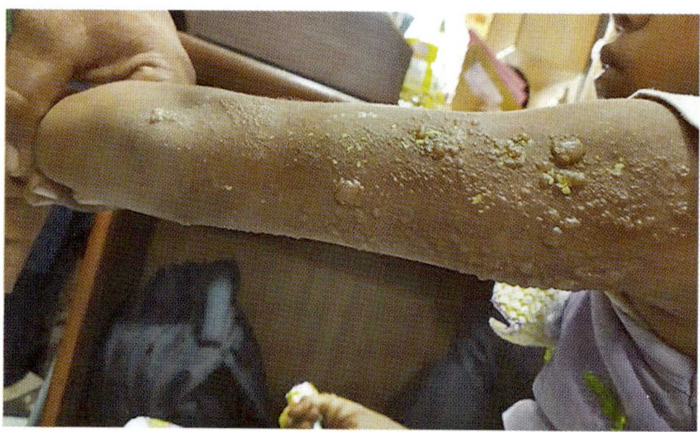

Fig. 3: Herpes zoster

Roseola Infantum (Sixth Disease; Exanthem Subitum)

This is an acute febrile illness caused by HHV 6 (younger children of 6 months–2 years) and HHV7 (older children) and is characterized by prodrome of irritability, high grade fever for 3–7 days with cervical, occipital adenopathy and non-toxic appearance.[11] Seizures are a known complication in young children. There is sudden-onset rash presenting as discrete macules on trunk and neck with defervescence lasting 1–2 days. There is sparing of the face. Rash may not be present in some children.

Enteroviruses (Coxsackievirus, Echovirus, and Others)

These infections present with variable prodrome of irritability, fever, sore throat, myalgias and headache in infants and young children. Hand-foot-mouth disease (HFMD)

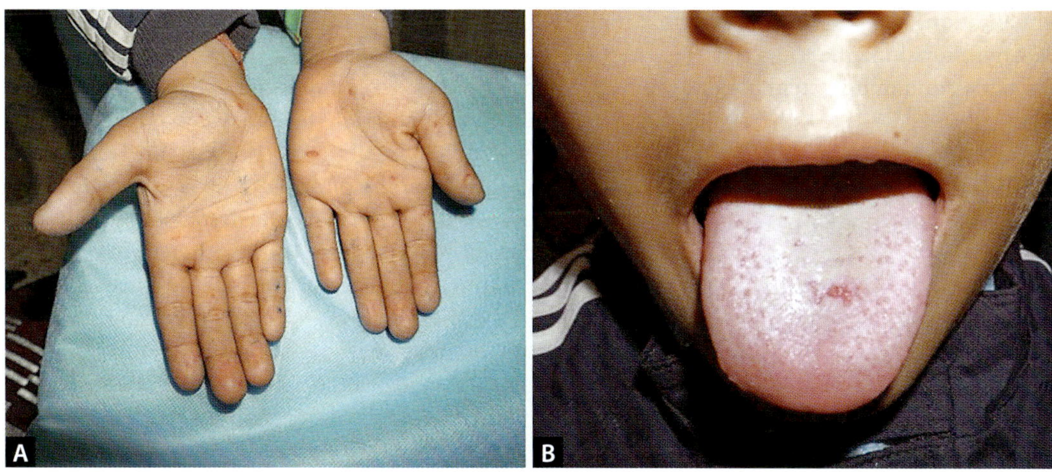

Figs. 4A and B: Hand foot mouth disease
(*Courtesy*: Dr Neetu Bhari, Assistant Professor, Dermatology and Venereology, All India Institute of Medical Sciences, New Delhi)

presents with vesicles in hand, foot, and mouth[12] (**Figs. 4A and B**). Other enteroviral infections may have fine non confluent, macular or maculopapular rash. Rarely petechial, urticarial, or vesicular rash may be present. The rash lasts for 3–7 days. HFMD outbreaks are common in play school and day cares. Children are contagious up to 2 weeks. Rash may appear with fever or after defervescence.

Infectious Mononucleosis

Illness caused by Epstein–Barr virus usually presents in older children and spreads by close contact (shed in saliva of infected children and adults). It is characterized by Fever, adenopathy, eyelid edema, sore throat, hepatosplenomegaly, malaise and atypical lymphocytosis.[13] The rash is maculopapular or morbilliform appearing on trunk and extremities and may be confluent, lasting 2–7 days. Children may have variable anemia and thrombocytopenia. The rash is typically aggravated by administration of ampicillin.

Scarlet Fever

This is an acute onset toxin mediated diffuse erythematous rash in setting of Group A streptococcal pharyngitis.[14] It has associated headache, abdominal pain, cervical lymphadenopathy. It is characterized by diffuse erythema with "sandpaper" feel, accentuation of erythema in flexural creases (Pastia lines); circumoral pallor and strawberry tongue. The rash lasts 2–7 days and ultimately desquamates. *Arcanobacterium haemolyticum* produces similar syndrome in adolescents.

Acute Rheumatic Fever

This is a Group A streptococcal pharyngitis related sequelae. The characteristic dermatological manifestation erythema marginatum (transient macular lesions with central clearing found on the extensor surface of the proximal extremities and trunk) is not discernible in Indian children due to their dark complexion.[15]

Staphylococcal Scalded Skin Syndrome

It is caused by *Staphylococcus aureus* producing exfoliative toxin. The rash is sudden onset, tender erythroderma which progresses to diffuse flaccid bullae. There is significant perioral, perinasal peeling which progresses to diffuse exfoliation (positive Nikolsky sign). There may be conjunctivitis and purulent rhinorrhea in the affected children.[16]

Toxic Shock Syndrome (TSS)

The offending organism is *S. aureus* producing toxic shock syndrome toxin-1 (TSST-1) and staphylococcal enterotoxins (SEs), Group A *Streptococcus* (SPEs). It is characterized by myalgias, fever, and gastrointestinal symptoms. It may be secondary to wound infection, trivial mucosal or respiratory infections or necrotizing fasciitis or myositis. The rash is diffuse sunburn-like erythroderma with late desquamation. Life-threatening systemic manifestations like hypotension, diarrhea, emesis, mental status changes, shock and multisystem organ dysfunction may be present.

Meningococcemia

Neisseria meningitidis infections can result in life threatening conditions. There is constellation of fever with rash, which presents with prodrome of fever, malaise, myalgia lasting 1–10 days. The rash is erythematous, non-confluent, discrete papules in early stages with presence of petechiae, purpura on trunk, extremities, palms and soles.[17]

Kawasaki Disease

It is a disease of unknown etiology, seen in younger children. It has standard diagnostic criteria with fever for more than 5 days, bilateral conjunctival injection, erythematous lips with fissuring, strawberry tongue, edema and erythema of hands or feet, cervical lymphadenopathy being important features. Periungual/generalized desquamation on follow-up is classical feature[18] (**Fig. 5**).

Mycoplasma Pneumoniae

Respiratory illness with mild erythematous maculopapular or vesicular rash is the presenting feature. It may be associated with erythema multiforme or Stevens-Johnson syndrome.

Dengue Fever and Chikungunya Fever

Another life-threatening exanthematous infection accompanied by fever is dengue fever. The arbovirus transmitted by *Aedes aegypti* mosquito causes explosive epidemics in the monsoon season in India. The disease occurs in all ages in both sexes and is clinically characterized by sudden onset of high grade fever associated with facial flushing, headache, myalgia, arthralgia, and abdominal pain. Within 48 hours of onset of fever, a transient generalized macular rash develops. Rash may be more typical during convalescence (**Fig. 6**). Another dengue-like illness is chikungunya fever, also transmitted by the same vector in the same season.[19] Chikungunya fever is characterized by high fever with rigors, intense joint pains, headache, myalgia, and rash. Chikungunya may have unusual skin manifestation in young children (**Fig. 7**).

Drug Rash

Antibiotics like penicillin, cephalosporin and sulfa drugs are the culprits in most of the allergic skin reactions to drugs. Skin lesions with high grade fever are indicator of severe drug reactions like one seen with systemic symptoms and eosinophilia in DRESS (**Fig. 8**), erythema multiforme, Stevens-Johnson syndrome (**Fig. 9**) and toxic epidermal necrolysis. These reactions develop 1–3 weeks after exposure to offending drug.

Erythema Nodosum

It is characterized by erythematous and painful nodules distributed over the extremities. It may be associated with viral infections. It is not diagnostic of any condition as etiology varies from viral (hepatitis B and C), bacterial (group A β-hemolytic *Streptococcus*, *Brucella* species, mycobacterial infections), fungal infection (*Candida*

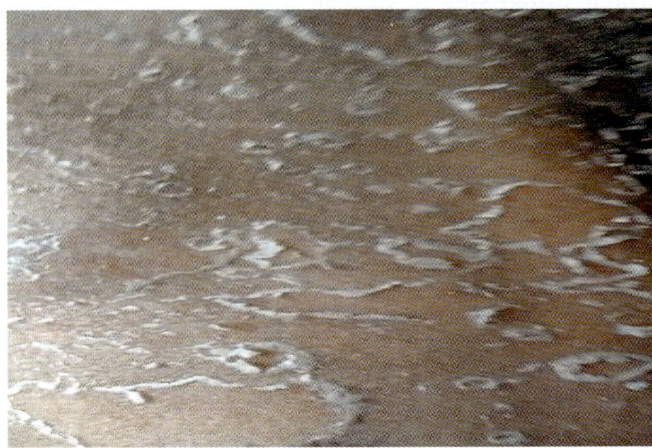

Fig. 5: Generalized desquamation of skin in a case of Kawasaki disease

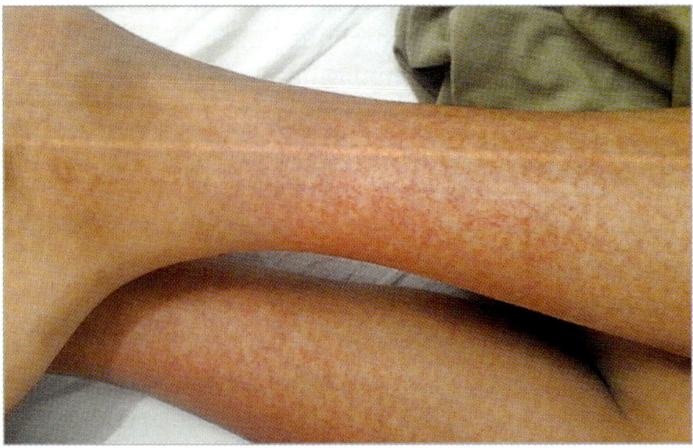

Fig. 6: Convalescent rash of dengue with characteristic "isle of white in sea of red appearance"

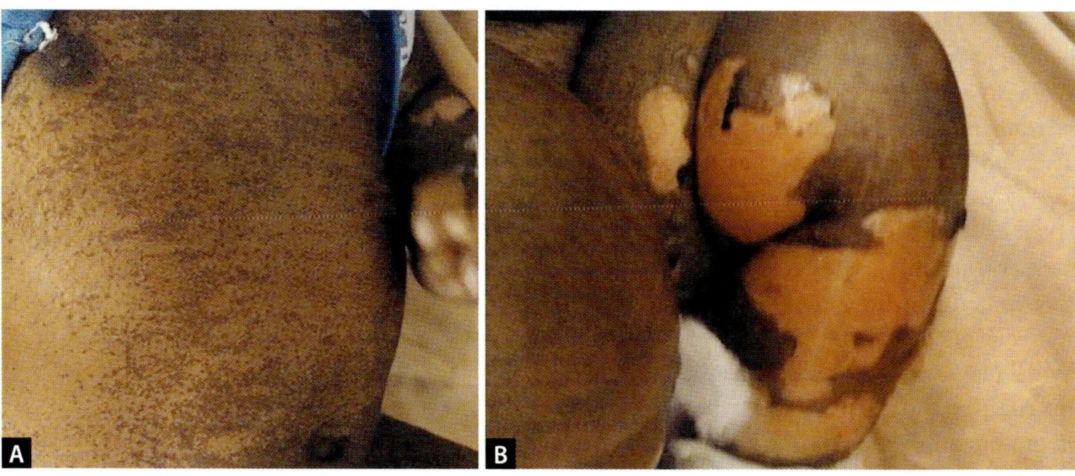

Figs. 7A and B: Skin manifestation of chikungunya in young children. (A) Hypermigmented, macular, coalescing skin lesions over trunk and limbs; (B) Burn-like peeling skin lesions over bilateral lower limbs

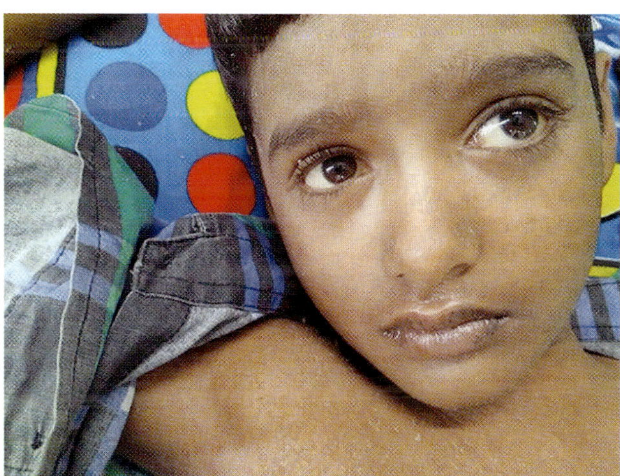

Fig. 8: DRESS syndrome in 11 years old, with generalized fine desquamation at time of diagnosis

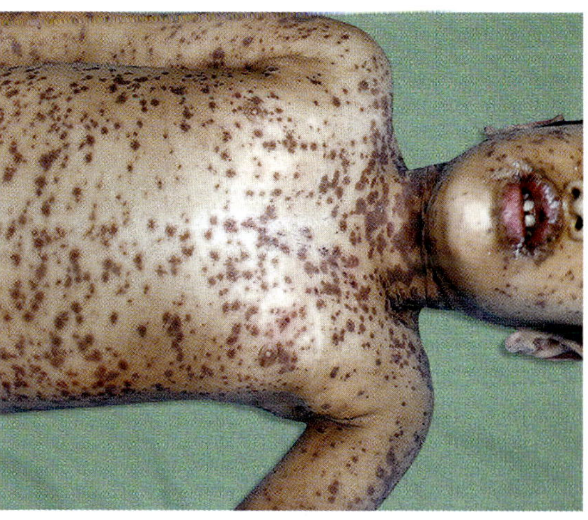

Fig. 9: Stevenson Johnson syndrome (*Courtesy*: Dr Neetu Bhari, Assistant Professor, Dermatology and Venereology, All India Institute of Medical Sciences, New Delhi)

species, *Histoplasma capsulatum, Cryptococcus neoformans*) or drug reactions (sulfonamides), and non-infectious causes [systemic lupus erythematosus (SLE), sarcoidosis, and inflammatory bowel disease].

DIFFERENTIATING FEATURES

Some of the findings present along with fever and rash also helps in narrowing the diagnosis:

a. Enanthem or *mucosal membrane lesions* are seen—measles, EBV, Kawasaki disease, scarlet fever and toxic shock syndrome.
b. *Palm/sole involvement* are characteristics of meningococcemia, dengue, drug rash, HFMD, measles, Kawasaki disease and erythema multiforme.
c. Presence of *joint symptoms* are seen in meningococcemia, acute rheumatic fever, Lyme disease, dengue, SLE, systemic onset juvenile idiopathic arthritis (JIA).
d. *Desquamation* is seen with Kawasaki disease, measles, scarlet fever, SSSS, SJS, and TSS.
e. *Cervical lymphadenopathy* is associated feature in Kawasaki disease, rubella, and scarlet fever. *Generalized lymphadenopathy* is seen in infectious mononucleosis,

systemic onset JIA, toxoplasmosis, SLE and localized lymphadenopathy in cat-scratch disease.

f. Meningeal involvement is common with infections by *Neisseria meningitidis*, enterovirus, *Leptospira*, Rickettsia and in Lyme disease.

g. *Pulmonary infiltrates* on imaging may be seen in complicated measles, *Mycoplasma pneumoniae* infections and varicella zoster.

h. *Characteristic rashes*: Some of the rashes are classical for underlying etiology (**Table 4**).

Differential diagnoses in a child presenting with fever and rash may be based on type of rash, associated localizing symptoms, presence of prodrome. The differential on basis of associated symptoms and presence of characteristic rash is explained already. The differential on appearance of rash is shown in **Table 5**.

COMPLICATIONS

The complications in cases presenting with fever and rash are due to widespread dissemination of underlying pathogen or due to the immune response. Some of

Table 4: Characteristic rashes which identify the underlying disease

	Characteristic rash	*Underlying disease*
1.	Erythema marginatum	Acute rheumatic fever (group A Streptococcus)
2.	Koplik spots	Measles
3.	Ecthyma gangrenosum	*P. aeruginosa, Vibrio vulnificus*
4.	Erythema migrans	Lyme disease
5.	Necrotic eschar	Aspergillosis, mucormycosis
6.	Erysipelas	Group A Streptococcus

Table 5: Differential diagnosis of fever based on appearance of rash[20]

Pathogen	*Maculopapular or Macular rash*	*Vesicles, bullae or pustules*	*Petechial/Purpuric*	*Diffuse erythroderma with desquamation*
Viral	Adenovirus Arbovirus Arbovirus- dengue, Chikungunya virus Coxsackie viruses A and B Epstein-Barr virus- primary infection Hepatitis B (Gianoticrosti syndrome) Human herpesvirus 6 (exanthem subitum) Human immunodeficiency virus (HIV) Measles (Rubeola) Parvovirus B19 (erythema infectiosum (fifth disease) Rubella (German measles)	Coxsackie viruses Echoviruses Herpes simplex Varicella (chickenpox) Varicella-zoster	Adenovirus Atypical measles Congenital cytomegalovirus Coxsackie A and B Dengue fever Epstein-Barr virus Enterovirust Hepatitis B HIV Rubella (congenital) Varicella (hemorrhagic) Yellow fever	
Bacterial	*Arcanobacterium haemolyticum* *Borrelia burgdorferi* (Lyme disease)	*Bacillus anthracis* *Listeria monocytogenes* *Mycoplasma pneumoniae*	*Borrelia* spp *Clostridium* spp *Infective endocarditis (many species)* *Haemophilus influenzae* type B *Neisseria gonorrhoeae* (disseminated gonococcal infection)	*Streptococcus* group A (scarlet fever, streptococcal toxic shock syndrome) *Stapylococcus aureus* (TSS, SSSS)

Contd...

Contd...

Pathogen	*Maculopapular or Macular Rash*	*Vesicles, bullae or pustules*	*Petechial/purpuric*	*Diffuse Erythroderma with desquamation*
	Borrelia spp (relapsing fever) *Brucella* spp (brucellosis) Group A streptococci-Rheumatic fever, scarlet fever, Erysipelas *Listeria monocytogenes* *Leptospira* spp (leptospirosis) *Mycoplasma pneumoniae* *Neisseria meningitidis* (meningococcemia) *Pseudomonas aeruginosa* *Salmonella typhi* (typhoid fever) Secondary syphilis	*Neisseria gonorrhoeae* *Neisseria meningitidis* *Pseudomonas aeruginosa* *Rickettsia akari* *Rickettsia rickettsii* *Staphylococcus aureus* (Toxic shock syndrome, staphylococcal scalded skin syndrome) Streptococcus group A (crusted impetigo)	*Neisseria meningitidis* (acute or chronic meningococcemia) *Pseudomonas aeruginosa* *Spirillum minor* *Staphylococcus aureus* (bacteremia) *Streptobacillus moniliformis* *Streptococcus group A* (streptococcal toxic shock syndrome, scarlet fever) *Streptococcus pneumoniae* (asplenic patient) *Yersinia pestis*	
Rickettsial/ Fungal/ Protozoal/ Parasitic	Early Rocky mountain spotted fever Scrub typhus Endemic typhus	*Histoplasma capsulatum* *Ricketssial pox*	*Rickettsia prowazekii* *Rickettsia rickettsia* Malaria	*Candida albicans* (erythroderma)
Others	Drug reaction Kawasaki disease Systemic onset JIA Hemophagocytic lymphohistiocytosis	Erythema multiforme bullosum Toxic epidermal necrolysis Stevens-Johnson syndrome	Immune thrombocytopenia Henoch Schonlein Purpura	Erythroderma Drug hypersensitivity Graft-versus-host reaction Kawasaki disease Stevens-Johnson syndrome Toxic epidermal necrolysis

the well-known complications with common illnesses presenting with fever and rash are shown in **Table 6**.

APPROACH TO MANAGEMENT

A careful history and examination will help a diligent clinician in narrowing the differentials.[21] The diagnostic approach to the patient with fever and rash should focus on the appearance of the rash in addition to other demographic and epidemiological history. The rash needs to be characterized by morphology and arrangement (e.g. annular, linear, serpiginous, dermatomal), distribution (e.g. isolated versus generalized, bilateral versus unilateral, symmetric, occurring on exposed areas), and evolution (centrifugal versus centripetal). In the same child, rashes have overlapping features, and several infectious agents can present with varied rash morphologies. Different infectious agents can also produce similar types of rashes. Presence of pathognomic rashes provide important clue to diagnosis. Characteristic prodromal symptoms may help differentiate viral and bacterial etiology. Generally, viral exanthems are benign and have nonspecific prodrome of respiratory symptoms. Bacterial etiologies may have more system specific findings and may have more toxic feature compared to viral.

Laboratory testing is usually not indicated in majority of fever with rash but when indicated they may include nonspecific routine investigation or etiology specific investigation. Majority of cases with fever and rash require supportive management. The details of treatment are given in **Table 7**.

Outcomes/Prognostic Factors

The list of causes of exanthematous fevers is exhaustive although most often the illness is benign and of viral etiology which improve spontaneously or with supportive management. In the life-threatening conditions, presenting with fever and rash, a stepwise algorithmic approach is helpful in reaching to a diagnosis.

Table 6: Complications associated with conditions presenting with fever and rash

Underlying disease/Etiology	*Known complications*
Measles	• Febrile seizures • Otitis media • Laryngotracheitis • Pneumonia • Encephalitis • Thrombocytopenia • Delayed- subacute sclerosing panencephalitis
Chickenpox (varicella)	• Staphylococcal or streptococcal skin infection • Arthritis • Cerebellar ataxia • Encephalitis • Thrombocytopenia • Reye syndrome (with aspirin) • Dissemination in immunocompromised—Myocarditis, nephritis, hepatitis, pneumonia
Rubella	• Arthritis • Thrombocytopenia • Encephalopathy • Intrauterine infection—fetal embryopathy
Parvovirus B19 infection (Erythema infectiosum)	• Arthritis • Aplastic crisis in patients with chronic hemolytic anemia (e.g. Sickle cell) • Vasculitis • Wegener granulomatosis
Roseola infantum (sixth disease; exanthem subitum)	• Single or recurrent febrile seizures • Encephalopathy • Disseminated infection (e.g. liver, CNS, lung) in immunosuppressed patients
Enterovirus	• Aseptic meningitis • Hepatitis • Myocarditis, paralysis usually in younger patients
Infectious mononucleosis	• Anemia, thrombocytopenia • Aplastic anemia • Hepatitis • Hemophagocytic lymphohistiocytosis (HLH) • Lymphoproliferative syndrome
Scarlet fever	• Peritonsillar abscess • Rheumatic fever • Glomerulonephritis
Acute rheumatic fever	• Rheumatic heart disease (RHD) • Jaccoud arthropathy
Staphylococcal scalded skin syndrome (SSSS)	• Shock
Toxic shock syndrome (TSS)	• Shock, multisystem organ dysfunction/failure
Meningococcemia	• Shock, meningitis, pericarditis, arthritis, endophthalmitis gangrene, disseminated intravascular coagulation
Kawasaki disease	• Coronary artery dilatation
Mycoplasma pneumoniae	• Hemolytic anemia • Stevens Johnson syndrome
Drug reaction with eosinophilia and systemic symptoms (DRESS)	• Hematological abnormality • Hepatitis • Involvement of kidney, heart and lung

Table 7: Treatment of underlying conditions presenting with fever and rash[20-23]

Underlying disease/Etiology	*Treatment*
Measles	• Supportive • Vitamin A deficiency contributes to delayed recovery and to the high rate of post-measles complications. The WHO recommends treatment with vitamin A in all patients with measles • Vitamin A for treatment of measles is administered once daily for two days at the following doses: – Infants <6 months of age: 50,000 IU – Infants 6 to 11 months of age: 100,000 IU – Children ≥12 months: 200,000 IU • Ribavarin has been used in trial setting for special situation like immunocompromised children
Chickenpox (varicella)	• Supportive (children<12 years of age) • In immunocompromised or at risk for complication • Children ≥1 year of age and adolescents-Acyclovir 1500 mg/m^2 per day in three divided doses **or** 30 mg/kg/day in three divided doses
Rubella	Supportive management
Parvovirus B19 infection (Erythema infectiosum)	• No supportive treatment required • Symptomatic therapy only for arthralgias, arthritis, or pruritus may be present
Roseola infantum (sixth disease; exanthem subitum)	No treatment warranted
Enterovirus (HFMD)	Supportive
Infectious mononucleosis	• Primary infection- supportive care • Acetaminophen or nonsteroidal anti-inflammatory for the treatment of fever, throat discomfort, and malaise. Adequate fluids and nutrition
Scarlet fever	• Oral penicillin or amoxicillin • Amoxicillin • Age 3 to 18 years: Oral: 50 mg/kg once daily **or** 25 mg/kg twice daily for 10 days
Acute rheumatic fever	Anti-inflammatory therapy, antibiotic therapy, and heart failure management
Staphylococcal scalded skin syndrome (SSSS)	• Prompt administration of intravenous penicillinase-resistant penicillin • Vancomycin in areas with a high prevalence of community-acquired methicillin-resistant *S. aureus* (CA-MRSA) • Supportive skin care - use of emollients, such as creams or ointments • Fluid and electrolyte replacement
Toxic shock syndrome (TSS)	• Empiric therapy • Vancomycin (children: 60 mg/kg per day IV in four divided doses) + • Clindamycin (children: 25 to 40 mg/kg IV per day in three divided doses) + • A combination drug containing a penicillin plus beta-lactamase inhibitor or A carbapenem • No controlled trials on role of IVIG therapy in staphylococcal TSS, use in TSS +/-
Meningococcemia	• Empiric therapy for patients with suspected (e.g. Gram stain with gram-negative diplococci) or culture-proven meningococcal infection consists of a third-generation cephalosporin
Kawasaki disease	IVIG (2 g/kg single infusion) with aspirin (30–100 mg/kg/day in 4 divided doses)
Mycoplasma pneumoniae	• Azithromycin 10 mg/kg in one dose (maximum dose 500 mg) on the first day and 5 mg/kg in one dose (maximum dose 250 mg) for the next four days, or • Clarithromycin 15 mg/kg per day in two divided doses (maximum daily dose 1 g) for 10 days, or • Erythromycin 30 to 40 mg/kg per day in four divided doses (maximum daily dose 2 g) for 10 days • Doxycycline 2 to 4 mg/kg per day in one or two divided doses (maximum daily dose 200 mg) for 10 days
Drug reaction with eosinophilia and systemic symptoms (DRESS)	Hematological abnormality, hepatitis, involvement of kidney, heart and lung

KEY MESSAGES

- Fever with rash is common among children and seen in both outpatient and emergency department.
- There are a large number of infectious and noninfectious conditions presenting as exanthematous fevers.
- Viral exanthems are the most common cause of fever with rash in children.
- Some conditions would require isolation to prevent spread of contagious infections.

REFERENCES

1. Valdez LM, Septimus EJ. Clinical approach to rash and fever. Infect Dis Pract. 1996;20:1.
2. Sarkar R, Mishra K, Garg VK. Fever with rash in a child in India. Indian J Dermatol Venereol Leprol. 2012;78:251e62.
3. Sumaya CV. Acute exanthematous disease. In: Pickering LK, DuPont HL, editors. Infectious Diseases of Children and Adults. A Step-by-Step Approach to Diagnosis and Treatment. Menlo Park, CA: Addison-Wesley; 1986. p. 167.
4. Nelson JSB, Stone MS. Update on selected viral exanthems. Curr Opin Pediatr. 2000;12:359-64.
5. Kang JH. Febrile illness with skin rashes. Infection and chemotherapy. 20151;47:155-66.
6. Biesbroeck L, Sidbury R. Viral exanthems: An update. Dermatol Ther. 2013;26:433-8.
7. Bolognia J, Schaffer JV, Duncan KO, *et al.* Fever and rash. In: Bolognia J, Schaffer JV, Duncan KO, editors. Dermatology Essentials. Oxford: Saunders/Elsevier; 2014. p. 28-38.
8. Fölster-Holst R, Kreth HW. Viral exanthems in childhood - infectious (direct) exanthems. Part 1: Classic exanthems. J Dtsch Dermatol Ges. 2009;7:309-16.
9. Dyer JA. Childhood viral exanthems. Pediatr Ann. 2007;36:21-9.
10. Anderson LJ. Role of parvovirus B19 in human disease. Pediatr Infect Dis J. 1987;6:711.
11. Cherry JD. Roseola infantum (exanthem subitum). In: Cherry JD, Harrison G, Kaplan SL, Steinbach WJ, Hotez PJ, editors. Feigin and Cherry's Textbook of Pediatric Infectious Diseases, 8th edition, Elsevier, Philadelphia. 2018. p. 559.
12. Messacar K, Modlin JF, Abzug MJ. Enteroviruses and parechoviruses. In: Long S, Prober C, Fischer M, editors. Principles and Practice of Pediatric Infectious Diseases. Philadelphia: Elsevier Saunders; 2017.
13. Morris MC, Edmunds WJ. The changing epidemiology of infectious mononucleosis? J Infect. 2002;45:107.
14. Stock I. Streptococcus pyogenes--much more than the aetiological agent of scarlet fever. Med Monatsschr Pharm. 2009;32:408-16.
15. Mc Donald M, Currie BJ, Carapetis JR. Acute rheumatic fever: A chink in the chain that links the heart to the throat? Lancet Infect Dis. 2004;4:240-5.
16. Manders SM. Toxin-mediated streptococcal and staphylococcal disease. J Am Acad Dermatol. 1998;39:383-98.
17. Sinclair D, Preziosi MP, Jacob John T, *et al.* The epidemiology of meningococcal disease in India. Trop Med Int Health. 2010;15:1421-35.
18. Singh S. Kawasaki Disease: A clinical dilemma. Indian Pediatr. 1999;36:871-5.
19. Krishnamoorthy K, Harichandrakumar KT, Krishna Kumari A, *et al.* Burden of chikungunya in India: Estimates of disability adjusted life years (DALY) lost in 2006 epidemic. J Vector Borne Dis. 2009;46:26-35.
20. Densmore EM, Lye PS. Fever and rash. In: Kliegman RM, Lye PS, Bordini BJ, Toth H, Basel D, editors. Nelson Pediatric Symptom-based Diagnosis. Elsevier; 2018. p. 726-45.
21. Sanders CV. Approach to the diagnosis of the patient with fever and rash. In: Sanders CV, Nesbitt LT Jr, editors. The Skin and Infection: A Color Atlas and Text. Baltimore: Williams and Wilkins; 1995. p. 296.
22. Mondiale de la Santé O, World Health Organization. Measles vaccines: WHO position paper–April 2017–Note de synthèse de l'OMS sur les vaccins contre la rougeole–avril 2017. Weekly Epidemiological Record= Relevé épidémiologique hebdomadaire. 2017;92:205-27.
23. Balfour HH Jr, Rotbart HA, Feldman S, et al. Acyclovir treatment of varicella in otherwise healthy adolescents. The Collaborative Acyclovir Varicella Study Group. J Pediatr. 1992;120(4 Pt 1): 627-33.

CHAPTER

47

Toxin Mediated Diseases

Jayashree M, Kavitha TK

High molecular weight toxins produced by some bacteria and fungi possess antigenic properties that result in impaired host immunity and direct host tissue damage.[1] These toxins mediated diseases produce multisystemic effects which require intensive care management in children. Common toxin mediated diseases include tetanus, diphtheria, botulism and toxic shock syndrome (**Table 1**).

TETANUS

Introduction

Tetanus is a non-communicable disease mediated by the tetanus toxin secreted by the spore forming *Clostridium tetani*. The disease is characterized by muscle hypertonia, spasms and autonomic instability. Improved vaccine coverage and availability of effective antitoxin has reduced incidence of disease and associated mortality worldwide. In India, nearly 5000 cases of tetanus were reported in 2017.

Etiopathogenesis

Clostridium tetani is a motile gram-positive obligate anaerobic bacillus whose spores are seen in soil or animal excreta. The usual portal of entry is a skin breach following minor trauma, surgical wound, fractures or through chronic infection sites like otitis media. Once inoculated into a suitable anaerobic environment, the spores germinate to produce vegetative forms which multiply inside the wound and produce exotoxins. Two plasmin mediated exotoxins are responsible for the pathogenesis; *tetanolysin* which damages tissues near the wound and *tetanospasmin* which causes neurotoxicity. Tetanospasmin, a two-peptide unit, after reaching neuromuscular junction traverses through axons by retrograde transport and reaches neuronal cell

Table 1: Common toxin mediated diseases and mechanism of host injury

Mechanism of toxin action	*Organism*	*Toxins*	*Disease*
Protease activity	*Clostridium tetani*	Tetanus toxins—tetanolysin, tetanospasmin Zn metalloproteases	Tetanus
	Clostridium botulinum	Neurotoxins A and B- Zn Metalloproteases	Botulism
Membrane damage	*Aeromonas hydrophila*	Aerolysis-pore former	Diarrhea
Inhibition of protein synthesis	*Corynebacterium diphtheria*	Diphtheria toxins ADP ribosyl transferase	Diphtheria
Activation of second messenger	*Clostridium difficile*	Toxin A-Glucosyl transferase	Diarrhea
Activation of immune response	*Staphylococcus aureus*	Toxic shock protein- Super antigens	Toxic shock syndrome (TSS)

body in spinal cord and brain stem. Inhibitory neurons in spinal cord are the most affected; tetanospasmin light chain decreases glycin and GABA release, thus resulting in unopposed antagonist muscle contractions and spasms. Simultaneous agonist and antagonist contraction results in characteristic muscle spasm and rigidity. Autonomic nerves including sympathetic chain, parasympathetic nucleus and motor nerves are also affected resulting in autonomic instability and muscle weakness.[2]

Clinical Features

The incubation period ranges from 7–10 days and may vary from one day to 2 months in some cases. Shorter onset time (the time between first symptom and first spasm) and shorter incubation period correlate with higher disease severity. Tetanus can present in four forms, generalized, localized, neonatal and cephalic.[3]

Generalized tetanus

Symptoms of generalized tetanus usually start with trismus (difficulty in jaw opening). Generalized spasms, rigidity, autonomic instability are other predominant symptoms which follow trismus. Initially spasms are precipitated by stimulation and subsequently become spontaneous. Excessive facial muscle spasms result in facial grimacing giving the typical risus sardonicus appearance. Spasms lead to opisthotonic posturing and airway compromise. Muscle spasms are severe in first week and improve gradually over 2 to 3 weeks, rigidity however may last longer. Autonomic instability begins after the onset of spasms and can last for 1–2 weeks. It is characterized by fluctuating BP records, arrhythmias, hyperpyrexia, ileus and even sudden cardiac deaths.[4]

Localized tetanus

Tetanus may occur only at the site of injury, like fingers or limbs. Partial immunity of the host against tetanus is a proposed mechanism. Generalized tetanus can develop later in some cases of localized tetanus.

Neonatal tetanus

Improper cord care practices in infants born to unimmunized mothers can result in neonatal tetanus. Initial symptoms are trismus, difficulty in sucking, excessive crying followed by varying degree of spasms and rigidity which develop later. Mortality is high and if child improves, spasms take 3–4 weeks to subside.

Cephalic tetanus

Chronic middle ear infections or head injury can predispose children to a localized form of tetanus called cephalic tetanus resulting in multiple cranial nerve palsies. Facial nerve palsy, followed by abducens, oculomotor and hypoglossal nerve palsies are usually seen. Generalized tetanus may follow these manifestations.

Grading of tetanus

Severity of tetanus is graded by various classification systems namely Philips, Dakar and Udwadia, but the commonly used one is the Ablett classification (**Table 2**).

Complications

Respiratory: Airway compromise is common in tetanus due to laryngeal, chest, diaphragm and abdominal muscle spasms. Mechanical ventilation related complications like pneumothorax or atelectasis may also be seen.

Table 2: Ablett classification for severity of tetanus

Grade		*Clinical features*
1	**Mild**	Mild to moderate trismus, generalised spasticity, no respiratory compromise, no spasms, little or no dysphagia.
2	**Moderate**	Moderate trismus, marked rigidity, mild to moderate but short spasms, moderate respiratory compromise with an increased respiratory rate (>30), mild dysphagia.
3	**Severe**	Severe trismus, generalised spasticity, reflex prolonged spasms, RR >40, apneic spells, severe dysphagia, tachycardia (heart rate >120)
4	**Very severe**	Grade III and violent autonomic disturbances involving the cardiovascular system. Severe hypertension and tachycardia alternating with relative hypotension and bradycardia, either of which may be persistent.

Source: Adapted from Ablett JJL. Analysis and main experience in 82 patients treated in the Leeds tetanus unit. In: Ellis M, editor. Symposium on Tetanus in Great Britain. Boston Spa, UK: National Lending Library, 1967.

Autonomic instability: The most common autonomic symptoms seen are bradycardia, tachycardia, arrhythmias, hyperpyrexia and profuse sweating. Sudden cardiac deaths have also been reported. Ileus and diarrhea can also occur as a part of autonomic instability.[5]

Rhabdomyolysis: Repeated muscle spasms can result in rhabdomyolysis and acute kidney injury.

CNS complications: Usually the consciousness remains unaffected in patients with tetanus. Seizures and encephalopathy are rare complications. Mononeuropathies involving laryngeal and phrenic nerve can also occur.

Diagnosis and Differential Diagnosis

Diagnosis of tetanus is clinical and the characteristic trismus, spasms, and rigidity in a child with clear consciousness clinches the diagnosis. Other diseases which may mimic tetanus include meningoencephalitis, drug induced dystonia, strychnine poisoning and trismus caused by peritonsillar or odontogenic abscesses.

Management

The goals of management are adequate source control, halting production of neurotoxins, neutralization of unbound toxin, spasm control and supportive care.

Source control

Probable source of infection has to be thoroughly debrided. Metronidazole (40 mg/kg/day) for 7 to 10 days is the drug of choice. Theoretically penicillin being a non-competitive inhibitor of GABA A receptors, has the potential to obtund post-synaptic inhibitory signals and increase the risk of convulsions. Additionally, it also carries a theoretical risk of potentiating the action of tetanospasmin. Although one study had shown survival benefit of metronidazole over crystalline penicillin, most RCTs have shown no difference between both antibiotics.[6] Alternative effective antibiotics against *Clostridium tetani* include macrolides, chloramphenicol and tetracyclines.[6]

Neutralization of toxins

Intrathecal tetanus immunoglobulin (TIG), 250 to1000 IU in addition to intramuscular TIG of 500 IU has been found to be helpful in reducing spasms, duration of hospital stay and mortality.[7]

Control of rigidity and spasms

Minimal stimulation, sedoanalgesia and neuromuscular blocking agents help in spasm control.

Benzodiazepines: GABA agonist property of benzodiazepines opposes the toxin action on inhibitory receptors and thereby helps prevent polysynaptic reflexes. Diazepam, midazolam and lorazepam are the commonly used benzodiazepines for spasm control. Of these, diazepam is preferred for spasm control owing to its pharmacological action of muscle re-laxation, sedation, and anxiolysis. It is started intravenously in doses of 0.1–0.2 mg/kg/dose and can be titrated 2–6 hourly to 1 mg/kg/hour based on clinical response. Doses as high as 40 mg/kg/day as infusion have been used in neonatal tetanus and shown to have improved mortality rate.[8] Once initial spasm control is achieved, diazepam can be shifted to enteral route through a feeding tube. Drug is usually continued in the same dose for 2–3 weeks followed by gradual tapering over next 2 weeks. Midazolam (0.1–0.3 mg/kg/hour) and lorazepam (0.15 mg/kg loading dose followed by 0.05–0.1 mg/kg/hour) are the other alternative drugs used for spasm control. There are no head to head comparison trials between diazepam and midazolam, although midazolam is short acting, has faster onset of action and causes lesser hypotension.

Neuromuscular blockers: Spasms not controlled by above measures may require neuromuscular blockade. Vecuronium or atracurium may be required in children with persistent muscle spasms. Better cardiovascular stability and less autonomic side effects makes vecuronium slightly better option than atracurium. Pancuronium may worsen autonomic instability through vagal blockade and inhibition of nor- epinephrine uptake by adrenergic nerves.

Other agents: Magnesium sulfate 50 mg/kg as intravenous infusion over 1 hour followed by 6 hourly repeated doses targeting a therapeutic magnesium level of 4-6 mEq/L (2-4 mmol/L) helps in muscle relaxation by virtue of its presynaptic neuromuscular blocking action. Use of intrathecal baclofen (GABA Agonist) and intravenous dantrolene (direct acting muscle relaxant) and propofol for spasm control have also been reported. High cost and variable pharmacological action of baclofen limit its usage in children.[9] Side effects of prolonged propofol use are lactic acidosis and bradycardia.

Control of autonomic instability

Morphine infusion (10–20 μg/kg/hour) acts by its central sympathetic inhibitory action. Additional sedative property helps to decrease autonomic symptoms like fluctuating heart rate and labile blood pressures. Magnesium sulfate helps in controlling autonomic instability by its central action. Other agents that can be used are clonidine, atropine and chlorpromazine. Labetalol (alpha and beta blocker) may also be used for high blood pressure but beta blocker like propanol in isolation has been reported to cause deleterious effects and hence not advocated in children.[10]

Supportive care

Airway protection and stabilization may be required in children with anticipated airway compromise. Intubation is indicated in all children presenting with generalized rigidity with or without frequent spasms, and those who need high dose benzodiazepines or neuromuscular agents for spasm control mandate intubation. Mechanical ventilation should be provided with adequate sedoanalgesia and gradual weaning may be started after second week of illness once spasms decrease in frequency and are less likely to progress. Tracheostomy may be considered in children on prolonged ventilation although no consensus regarding timing of tracheostomy is available in literature. Gastrointestinal hypomotility due to drugs or disease *per se* and risk of bedsores due to prolonged immobilization, are the other major concerns. Bedsore prevention, nutritional support and psychosocial support are important supportive management.

Prognosis

Mortality rate ranges from 10% to 50% in children. Shorter incubation period, shorter onset time and autonomic instability are poor predictors of outcome.[11]

Prevention

Adequate vaccination of children by three primary DPT vaccination at 6, 10, and 14 weeks followed by booster doses at 16–24 months and 5–6 years is recommended. Additional booster doses are recommended at 10 and 16 years. National immunization schedule recommends two doses of tetanus in pregnant mothers, first dose as early as possible and second 4 weeks after the first dose. Unimmunized children with contaminated wounds, should be immunized as per age and also receive TIG to prevent tetanus. A booster dose of tetanus is required in immunized children with contaminated wounds if 5 years have elapsed since last tetanus toxoid vaccination.

STAPHYLOCOCCAL TOXIC SHOCK SYNDROME

Introduction

Staphylococcal toxic shock syndrome (TSS) is caused by superantigen response to toxic shock protein-1 (TSST-1) produced by toxin producing strains of *Staphylococcus aureus* resulting in exuberant immune response and organ dysfunction. Toxic shock syndrome in early 80s was described in association with menstrual tampon use (menstrual TSS). TSS may be associated with staphylococcal infections elsewhere in body and without an obvious source (non-menstrual TSS). Nearly 50–80% of *Staphylococcus aureus* strains carry one or other super antigen gene. Toxic shock protein (Tst+) positive clonal complex (CC) 30 MSSA strain were associated with most cases of TSS in a UK study.[12]

Etiopathogenesis

Staphylococcal exotoxins (TSST-1), staphylococcal enterotoxins (SEs) or staphylococcal enterotoxin like toxins (SELs) are the major super antigens behind pathogenesis of TSS. Nearly 95% of menstrual TSS and 50% non-menstrual TSS is caused by TSST-1.[13] All these super antigens cause non-conventional activation of T cells resulting in cytokine storm. Super antigen directly gets attached with T cell receptor (TCR) and activates T cells and its clonal proliferation without help of antigen presenting cells (APC). Resultant cytokine storm releases IL-2, TNF-alpha, IL-6 and later on IL-12 and IFN-gamma.[14] Inability to mount antibody response against super antigens has also been attributed to development of TSS in hosts.

Clinical Features

TSS presents with high spiking fever, hypotension and progressive multiorgan dysfunction.

Foci of infection can vary from vaginal tampon, skin and superficial tissue infections or chronic rhinosinusitis. Initially fever, chills, myalgia, GI disturbances like diarrhea or vomiting may be present for 1–2 days prior to presentation to a healthcare facility. Child can present with features of warm shock with tachycardia, hypotension and altered sensorium. A macular erythrodermic rash is a usual characteristic clinical sign which appears within 24 hours. Children can progress to multiorgan failure within hours. Desquamation of palms and soles may ensue in first or second week. A history suggestive of probable staphylococcus infection may be present sometimes. CDC TSS clinical diagnostic criteria is given in **Table 3**.

Diagnosis and Differential Diagnosis

Diagnosis of TSS is based on clinical characteristics. Non-specific leucocytosis, thrombocytopenia, elevated transaminases, pyuria, proteinuria and altered renal function may be present. PCR based superantigen gene identification and low Anti TSST-1 antibody titres may corroborate the diagnosis. Flow cytometric evaluation of T cell subset to identify V beta positive T cell subset, proliferated by super antigen stimulation can be done.[13] Differential diagnosis includes viral exanthematous fever, scarlet fever, rickettsial infections, meningococcemia, and Kawasaki disease.

Complications

TSS leads to multiorgan dysfunction which include acute respiratory distress syndrome (ARDS), acute kidney injury (AKI), disseminated intravascular coagulopathy, hepatic dysfunction and myocardial damage.

Management

Management aims at supporting each and every organ dysfunction and control of bacterial proliferation and toxin production.

Source control and halting toxin production

Timely and adequate source control is paramount. Broad antistaphylococcal cover using cloxacillin, a bactericidal agent for MSSA, and vancomycin for MRSA has to be started based on community prevalence of MRSA. Intravenous clindamycin, a bacteriostatic lincosamide and protein synthesis inhibitor has been found to be useful in halting 90% toxin production and should be used in combination with bactericidal agents. It is postulated that clindamycin downregulates T cell response to super antigen through toll like receptor-2. Tigecycline and linezolid have also been

Table 3: CDC criteria for toxic shock syndrome (Other than streptococcal)

An illness with the following clinical manifestations:

- **Fever**—temperature ≥38.9°C (102°F)
- **Rash**—diffuse macular erythroderma
- **Desquamation**—1–2 weeks after onset of illness, particularly palms and soles
- **Hypotension**—Systolic blood pressure ≤90 mm Hg for adults or less than fifth percentile by age for children <16 years of age; orthostatic drop in diastolic blood pressure ≥15 mm Hg from lying to sitting, orthostatic syncope, or orthostatic dizziness
- **Multisystem involvement**—three or more of the following:
  - **Gastrointestinal**: Vomiting or diarrhea at onset of illness
  - **Muscular**: Severe myalgia or creatinine phosphokinase level at least twice the upper limit of normal for laboratory
  - **Mucous membrane**: Vaginal, oropharyngeal, or conjunctival hyperemia
  - **Renal**: Blood urea nitrogen or creatinine at least twice the upper limit of normal for laboratory or urinary sediment with pyuria (≥5 leukocytes per high-power field) in the absence of urinary tract infection
  - **Hepatic**: Total bilirubin, serum alanine aminotransferase (ALT), or serum aspartate aminotransferase (AST), at least twice the upper limit of normal for laboratory
  - **Hematologic**: platelets <100,000/cumm
  - **CNS**: disorientation or alterations in consciousness without focal neurologic signs when fever and hypotension are absent

Laboratory criteria

Negative results on the following tests, if obtained:

- Blood, throat, or CSF cultures (blood culture may be positive for *S. aureus*)
- Rise in titer to Rocky Mountain spotted fever, leptospirosis, or measles

Case classification

Probable: A case which meets laboratory criteria and four of five clinical criteria

Confirmed: A case which meets laboratory criteria and all five clinical criteria described above, including desquamation, unless the patient dies before desquamation occurs

Source: Adapted from Center for Disease Control and Prevention. Case definition; Toxic Shock Syndrome (Other Than Streptococcal TSS); CSTE position statement 10-ID-14 (page last reviewed and updated on January 17, 2014.

found to have effects on reduction of toxin production, hence may be used as alternative agents for MRSA infection with TSS.[13]

Immunomodulation

As defective immune response to super antigens has been demonstrated for TSS, intravenous immunoglobulin 1 g/kg over 48 hours may be used as an adjunctive therapy although major RCTs are lacking in this regard.[15] Postulated beneficial effects are toxin neutralization and *in vitro* studies have reported decreased leukocyte proliferation following super antigen stimulation with use of IVIG. Hence IVIG serves a dual role of immunosuppression and toxin neutralization. Studies suggest that staphylococcal TSS may require higher IVIG dose compared to streptococcal TSS.[16] Activated protein C has been used in few case reports.[17]

Supportive therapy

Adequate and timely organ support is very important in these children. Hemodynamic stabilization with fluids and vasoactive agents will be required as per patient's clinical status. Mechanical ventilation is indicated for shock and encephalopathy. Renal replacement therapy will be required in AKI. Child should be provided good nutritional support and measures to maintain electrolytes and blood glucose levels.

Outcome and Prognosis

Staphylococcal TSS mortality in children may vary from 3–5%.[18] Children with multiorgan dysfunction may require prolonged ICU stay.

STREPTOCOCCAL TOXIC SOCK SYNDROME

Introduction

Streptococcal TSS (STSS) is a potentially fatal disease caused by invasive infection with Group A beta hemolytic *Streptococcus* (GAS) characterized by shock and multiorgan failure. Nearly 8–14% of patients with invasive GAS infection have associated STSS.

Pathogenesis

GAS is a gram-positive coccus classified based on its surface protein M and T antigens. M protein confers virulence to the organism. STSS is usually caused by strains with M protein types 1 and 3. Streptococcal pyrogenic exotoxins A, B, C, and F causes super antigen response triggering massive T-cell proliferation and cytokine release resulting in TSS. M protein antibody and super antigen antibody titres were found to be less in patients with STSS compared to controls.

Clinical Features

Clinical features of STSS are usually abrupt, characterized by fever, pain and GI symptoms like vomiting or diarrhea which progress rapidly to shock and multiorgan dysfunction. Varicella infection and recent NSAIDs use predisposes children for TSS in some cases. TSS with necrotizing fasciitis, starts with extreme pain on the affected sites usually limbs or abdomen. Nearly 20% patients have influenza-like prodrome which include fever, nausea, vomiting, or diarrhea. Erythematous rash is rare (10%) in STSS as compared to staphylococcal TSS. Most patients will have confusion. Nearly 80% of patients may have obvious soft tissue infections and others may have respiratory tract infection as a focus. Clinical response to vasoactive drugs is not promising in TSS. Multiorgan dysfunction and requirement of RRT may ensue within 48–72 hours.[3]

Diagnosis

Diagnosis is based on clinical criteria (**Table 4**). Renal function derangement and hemoglobinuria may be seen. Leukocytosis and immature band forms are seen in peripheral smear. Metabolic derangements like hypocalcemia and altered liver function tests with hypoalbuminemia and elevated liver transaminases are seen commonly. TSS usually have bacteremia and blood culture positivity in nearly 60% of infections. Other fluids or infected tissue culture may be positive in 95% of cases.

Management

The goals of management include neutralization of toxins, source control and supportive care.

Source control: Antibacterial therapy with high dose penicillin and clindamycin is recommended. Clindamycin has better post antibiotic effect, reduces toxin production, helps in phagocytosis of *Streptococcus* by inhibition of M protein synthesis and decreases

Table 4: CDC case definition of streptococcal toxic shock syndrome

Clinical case definition

An illness with the following clinical manifestations*:

- Hypotension defined by a systolic blood pressure less than or equal to 90 mm Hg for adults or less than the fifth percentile by age for children aged less than 16 years
- Multi-organ involvement characterized by two or more of the following:
  - *Renal impairment*: Creatinine greater than or equal to 2 mg/dL (≥177 µmol/L) for adults or greater than or equal to twice the upper limit of normal for age. In patients with pre-existing renal disease, a greater than two-fold elevation over the baseline level
  - *Coagulopathy*: Platelets less than or equal to 100,000/mm^3 (≤ 100 × 10^6/L) or disseminated intravascular coagulation, defined by prolonged clotting times, low fibrinogen level, and the presence of fibrin degradation products
  - *Liver involvement*: Alanine aminotransferase, aspartate aminotransferase, or total bilirubin levels greater than or equal to twice the upper limit of normal for the patient's age. In patients with pre-existing liver disease, a greater than twofold increase over the baseline level
  - *Acute respiratory distress syndrome*: Defined by acute onset of diffuse pulmonary infiltrates and hypoxemia in the absence of cardiac failure or by evidence of diffuse capillary leak manifested by acute onset of generalized edema, or pleural or peritoneal effusions with hypoalbuminemia
  - A generalized erythematous macular rash that may desquamate
  - Soft-tissue necrosis, including necrotizing fasciitis or myositis, or gangrene.

**Clinical manifestations do not need to be detected within the first 48 hours of hospitalization or illness, as specified in the 1996 case definition. The specification of the 48-hour time constraint was for purposes of assessing whether the case was considered nosocomial, not whether it was a case or not.*

Laboratory criteria for diagnosis

- Isolation of group A *Streptococcus*

Probable: A case that meets the clinical case definition in the absence of another identified etiology for the illness and with isolation of group A streptococcus from a nonsterile site

Confirmed: A case that meets the clinical case definition with isolation of group A *Streptococcus* from a normally sterile site (e.g. blood or CSF, or less commonly, joint, pleural, or pericardial fluid)

Source: Adapted from Centers for Disease Control and Prevention. CSTE Position statement 09-1D-60 (page last reviewed and updated on January 17, 2014).

TNF production. Linezolid, daptomycin or tigecycline can also be used in resistant cases. Depending on the clinical presentation of necrotizing fasciitis, gram negative, anaerobic or anti-staphylococcal antibiotics should also to be considered before confirmation of specific etiological agent.

Toxin neutralization: Intravenous immunoglobulin (IVIG) reduces super antigen mediated T cell and decreases production of inflammatory tumor necrosis factor-α. Intravenous immunoglobulin 1 g/kg for 2 days should be given to neutralize toxins.[19]

Supportive care: Supportive care includes aggressive shock resuscitation, mechanical ventilation and renal replacement therapy.

Prognosis

TSS causes higher mortality in adults (30–70%) as compared to children (5–10%).[20]

DIPHTHERIA

Introduction

Diphtheria is an acute febrile illness caused by toxigenic strains of *Corynebacterium*, predominantly *Corynebacterium diphtheriae* and presents with a characteristic pseudomembrane in throat or non-healing skin infection. Bacterial toxins produced locally induce systemic signs and symptoms resulting in life threatening complications.[21] India continues to have high number of diphtheria cases contributing to 78% of global diphtheria cases. Resurgence has been reported from northern Kerala and Karnataka recently.[22,23] Diphtheria is associated with a significant mortality especially in the unimmunized group.

Pathogenesis

Transmission occurs through exposure to respiratory secretions and skin exudates and rarely through fomites.

Bacteriophage causes lysogenic conversion of diphtheria bacilli and helps in production of toxins. After colonization in the pharynx, bacilli rest in superficial layers of mucosa and produce toxins that cause local tissue necrosis resulting in pseudomembrane formation (necrotic tissue, fibrin, and neutrophils).[20] Toxin gets absorbed through blood leading to systemic complications like myocarditis and neuritis. Diphtheritic toxin contains 62 kDa peptide with two moieties, active moiety A and the binding segment B. Toxin moiety B helps in internalization of active moiety A by the cells. Cellular protein production is disrupted due to elongation factor 2 (EF 2) inhibition by active moiety.[3]

Clinical Features

The incubation period is 2–5 days but it can vary from 1–10 days.[24] Infection starts with low grade fever and sore throat. The pathognomonic greyish pseudomembrane which bleeds on touch appears within 24 hours over nasopharynx and can extend over palate, pharynx, uvula, and tracheobronchial mucosa. Unimmunized children tend to present more often with a fulminant course. Cervical lymphadenopathy and brawny edema give rise to the characteristic bull neck in severe disease. This along with the extensive membrane increases risk of upper airway obstruction leading to cough and stridor in 65–70% cases. Nearly 35–40% children may present with hoarseness and dysphagia. Extent of involvement in diphtheria is as follows: faucial (pharyngeal and palatal) 70%, pharyngo-laryngeal (25%), laryngeal (3–4%) or nasal (3–4%). Cutaneous diphtheria may present as non-healing ulcer and unilateral nasal discharge may be a presenting feature in nasal diphtheria.[3]

Complications

Airway compromise

Pseudomembrane formation and soft tissue edema results in airway compromise. Dislodgement of membrane into upper airways may result in sudden death. Early tracheostomy or intubation may be required in children with airway compromise.

Myocarditis

Diphtheritic myocarditis is a serious complication in diphtheria seen in nearly 10-20% and associated with high mortality (60–70%).[3] Indian studies have reported an incidence varying from 16–66%.[25,26] Myocarditis is usually a second week of illness complication but can be seen as early as first week in severe disease. Mild ECG changes like T inversion, ST depression, sinus tachycardia, ectopic beats and sinus bradycardia may be indicators of myocarditis. Severe conduction abnormalities like complete heart block can occur in nearly 50% of children followed by tachyarrhythmias like ventricular tachycardia, and atrial flutter. Studies have shown that higher aspartate amino transferase levels (AST), extensive pseudomembrane and delayed antitoxin administration are associated with increased risk of myocarditis.[27]

Neuropathy

Onset of neuropathy may vary from 3 weeks to 16 weeks of illness. Reported incidence varies from 3% to 40%.[28] Severity of infection and delayed antitoxin therapy predisposes to neuropathy. Cranial neuropathy along with peripheral motor neuropathy is a common finding (Cranial nerves III,IV, VI, VII, IX, and XII).[29] Neuropathy starts with proximal followed by distal weakness. Palatal paralysis occurs in second week followed by ocular palsies in third week and peripheral motor weakness in 3rd to 6th week of illness. Respiratory muscle involvement is described in up to 85% and limb muscle weakness up to 94% of cases; these cases require PICU care. The improvement in muscle power begins from respiratory muscle followed by palatal muscle and limb muscles.[30] Some studies suggest the contrary, palatal muscle recovery followed by other muscles recovery. Neuropathy resolves completely by 5–6 months and may take longer time up to 1 year in some individuals.

Renal failure and thrombocytopenia

Renal tubular cells are sensitive to diphtheritic toxins. Acute tubular necrosis and impaired renal perfusion can result in acute kidney injury. Rarely, thrombocytopenia may be seen in severe disease.

Diagnosis

Acute streptococcal pharyngitis, candidiasis, Vincent angina, infectious mononucleosis, and agranulocytosis should be considered in differential diagnosis. The characteristic bull neck and pseudomembrane in an unimmunized child helps clinch the diagnosis.

Diagnosis is confirmed by identification of the bacilli and tests for its toxigenicity. Gram stain shows the characteristic Chinese letter patterned club shaped bacilli with terminal swellings and Albert stain show green bacilli with blue metachromatic granules at the ends. Selective medium like tellurite blood agar, and a Loeffler slant are used for culture. *In vitro* toxicity may be demonstrated by the Elek test.[31] Polymerase chain reaction (PCR) to detect the toxin A subunit and enzyme immunoassay for toxin may also be used.

Management

Goals of management include initial stabilization, source control, toxin neutralization and treatment of close contacts.

Emergency room management

Assessment and stabilization of ABCs (Airway, breathing and circulation) is paramount. Emergent intubation or tracheostomy may be indicated as per the clinical need. Accessory muscle use may point towards immediate requirement of airway management. Tracheostomy is a better option than intubation in severe disease as it provides better airway visualization and conduit for tracheal toileting. Moreover, intubation carries risk of membrane dislodgement into lower airways. Cardiac monitoring to look for early myocarditis needs to be started. Immediate antitoxin administration after primary stabilization and appropriate cultures should be the main strategy to prevent complications.

Source control

Antibiotics prevent bacterial multiplication and toxin production. Crystalline penicillin 40,000 IU/kg 4–6 hourly IM/IV till toxicity subsides, followed by procaine penicillin 25–50,000 IU/kg IM once daily for a total of 10–14 days is recommended. Oral erythromycin 40–50 mg/kg/day (max dose 2 g/day) in four divided doses for 10–14 days is an alternative agent. Two negative cultures 24 hrs apart have to be obtained before stopping antibiotics.[3]

Toxin neutralization

Anti-diphtheritic serum (Diphtheritic antitoxin; DAT; ADS) has to be administered after a test dose for neutralization of unbound toxins. Dose of ADS varies with extent of involvement. Recommended dose is 20,000–40,000 units for faucial diphtheria, skin lesions or laryngeal diphtheria of 2 days duration, 40,000–60,000 units for nasopharyngeal disease, and 80,000–120,000 units for severe toxic state with bull-neck or severe disease of more than 2 days. Diphtheria antitoxin (DAT/ADS) has to be diluted in 250 mL of normal saline and given over 2–4 hours. A test dose by prick or scratch test with administration of 1:100 dilution drop of DAT or intradermal administration of 0.02 mL of 1:100 diluted DAT should be done prior to administration.[32]

Supportive therapy

Cardiac pacemaker and L-Carnitine supplementation has been tried in myocarditis with varying results. Systolic dysfunction secondary to conduction blocks and arrhythmias usually remains refractory to pharmacological management. Recent study from Vietnam reports survival benefit after pacemaker insertion in severe conduction defects after diphtheria.[33]

Mortality

Mortality varies between 5–10%. High case fatality rates are seen in children with myocarditis; recent outbreaks have reported mortality ranging from 21–30%.[34,35] Unimmunized children should get full vaccination and immunized children should receive booster once they recover.

Prevention

Contacts should receive oral erythromycin (40–50 mg/kg/day, maximum 2 g/day) in four divided doses for 7–10 days or IM benzathine penicillin (single dose of 0.6 mega units for patients <5 years of age and 1.2 mega units for those >5 years).

BOTULISM

Botulism is caused by a neurotoxin produced by *Clostridium botulinum*, an anaerobic spore forming gram-positive bacilli.

Pathogenesis

The organisms and its spores thrive in lakes, coastal areas, and digestive tract of fish and mammals. In a suitable environment these spores germinate, multiply and produce toxins. Toxins A, B, E, and, rarely, F cause human botulism. Different types of botulism described are infant botulism, food-borne botulism, wound botulism and two varieties associated with toxemia secondary to intestinal source and one associated with therapeutic botulinum toxin use. The toxin reaches body through a wound or mucosal surface. Toxins block the release of acetylcholine from nerve endings at neuromuscular junction, parasympathetic nerve endings, autonomic ganglia, and acetylcholine sympathetic nerve endings.[36]

Clinical Features

Infantile botulism

It is seen in children less than 6 months of age who ingest botulinum spores. Lack of normal intestinal flora in younger infants favor spore multiplication in intestine. Source of ingestion is usually unidentified, but at times it may reach body through soil or honey ingestion. Most cases are insidious in onset and constipation is a predominant symptom. Other symptoms include weakness, floppiness, poor feeding, constipation, lethargy or decreased activity, poor cry, irritability and respiratory distress. Sensorium is preserved and infection signs like fever are always absent. Infant will have normal sensorium, cranial nerve palsies and floppiness. Pupil reflex may become absent after repeated testing for 2–3 minutes.[37]

Food borne botulism

Gastrointestinal symptoms are abdominal pain, nausea, vomiting, and diarrhea that occur shortly after ingestion of toxin. Neurological symptoms occur 1–5 days after toxin ingestion and usually occur as early as 18–36 hours. Dry mouth, diplopia from cranial nerve paralysis, and dilated pupils are other common findings. Bulbar palsies are seen in later stages. Descending weakness with involvement of diaphragm followed by limb weakness can also be seen.

Diagnosis

Repetitive stimulation with 20–50 Hz in EMG may show staircase pattern. In food-borne botulism testing of botulinum toxin should be done in 10 mL of serum, stool samples, suspect foods in their original containers, and vomitus or gastric secretions.

Treatment

Human botulism immune globulin as a single dose of 50 mg/kg IV is given for infantile botulism. Supportive care should be provided for botulism. Recovery is almost complete with good supportive care and mechanical ventilation.

KEY MESSAGES

- Diseases mediated by toxins are characterized by multisystem involvement secondary to immune dysfunction and tissue damage.
- Diagnosis is usually based on specific clinical presentations.
- Main management strategies include adequate source control and neutralization of toxins by antiserum or by intravenous immunoglobulin.
- Supportive care includes airway management, mechanical ventilation and hemodynamic stabilization.
- Adequate immunization is important for prevention of diseases like tetanus and diphtheria.

REFERENCES

1. Schmitt CK, Meysick KC, Brien ADO. Bacterial toxins: Friends or foes? Emerg Infect Dis. 1999;5:224-34.
2. Cook TM, Protheroe RT, Handel JM. Tetanus: A review of the literature. Br J Anaesth. 2001;87:477-87.
3. Nichols D, Shaffner D, editors. Rogers' Textbook of Pediatric Intensive Care, 5th edition. Wolters Kluwer; 2015. p. 1550-68.
4. Poudel P, Budhathoki S, Manandhar S. Tetanus. Kathmandu Univ Med J. 2009;7:315-22.
5. Wasay M, Khealani BA, Talati N, *et al*. Autonomic nervous system dysfunction predicts poor prognosis in patients with mild to moderate tetanus. 2005;5(1):2.
6. Rodrigo C, Fernando D, Rajapakse S. Pharmacological management of tetanus: An evidence-based review. Crit Care. 2014;18:217.
7. Kabura L, Ilibagiza D, Menten J, *et al*. Intrathecal vs. intramuscular administration of human antitetanus immunoglobulin or equine tetanus antitoxin in the treatment of tetanus: A meta-analysis. Trop Med Int Heal. 2006;11:1075-81.
8. Khoo BH, Lee EL, Lam KL. Neonatal tetanus treated with high dosage diazepam. Arch Dis Child. 1978;53:737-9.
9. Rodrigo C, Fernando D, Rajapakse S. Pharmacological management of tetanus: An evidence-based review. Crit Care. 2014;18:217.
10. David N, editor. Rogers' Textbook of Pediatric Intensive Care, 5th edition. Wolters Kluwer; 2015.
11. Angurana K, Jayashree M, Bansal A, *et al*. Post-neonatal tetanus in a PICU of a developing economy: Intensive care needs, outcome and predictors of mortality. J Tropical Pediatr. 2017;64:15-23.
12. Sharma H, Smith D, Turner CE, *et al*. Clinical and molecular epidemiology of staphylococcal toxic shock syndrome in the United Kingdom. Emerg Infect Dis. 2018;24.
13. Silversides JA, Lappin E, Ferguson AJ. Staphylococcal toxic shock syndrome: Mechanisms and management. Curr Infect Dis Rep. 2010;12:392-400.

14. Schlievert PM. Use of intravenous immunoglobulin in the treatment of staphylococcal and streptococcal toxic shock syndromes and related illnesses. J Allergy Clin Immunol. 2001; 108:S107-10.
15. Kato K, Sakamoto T, Ito K. Gamma-globulin inhibits superantigen-induced lymphocyte proliferation and cytokine production. Allergol Int. 2007;56:439-44.
16. Darenberg J, Soderquist B, Henriques Normark B, *et al*. Differences in potency of intravenous polyspecific immunoglobulin G against streptococcal and staphylococcal superantigens: Implications for therapy of toxic shock syndrome. Clin Infect Dis. 2004;38:836-42.
17. Nasa P, Sehrawat D, Kansal S, *et al*. Use of recombinant human activated protein C in nonmenstrual staphylococcal toxic shock syndrome. Indian J Crit Care Med. 2010;14:147.
18. Chuang YY, Huang YC, Lin TY. Toxic shock syndrome in children. Pediatr Drugs. 2005;7:11-25.
19. Wilkins AL, Steer AC, Smeesters PR, *et al*. Toxic shock syndrome – the seven Rs of management and treatment. J Infect. 2017;74:S147-52.
20. Hadfield TL, McEvoy P, Polotsky Y, *et al*. The pathology of diphtheria. J Infect Dis. 2000;181:S116-20.
21. WHO. Disease surveillance and Burden. WHO. 2018.
22. Sangal L, Joshi S, Anandan S, *et al*. Resurgence of diphtheria in north Kerala, India, 2016: Laboratory supported case-based surveillance outcomes. Front Public Heal. 2017;5:218.
23. Murhekar M. Epidemiology of diphtheria in India, 1996–2016: Implications for prevention and control. Am J Trop Med Hyg. 2017;97:313-8.
24. Byard RW. Diphtheria – 'The strangling angel' of children. J Forensic Leg Med. 2013;20:65-8.
25. Havaldar PV, Sankpal MN, Doddannavar RP. Diphtheritic myocarditis: Clinical and laboratory parameters of prognosis and fatal outcome. Ann Trop Paediatr. 2000;20:209-15.
26. Jayashree M, Shruthi N, Singhi S. Predictors of outcome in patients with diphtheria receiving intensive care. Indian Pediatr. 2006;43:155-60.
27. Kneen R, Dung NM, Solomon T, *et al*. Clinical features and predictors of diphtheritic cardiomyopathy in Vietnamese children. Clin Infect Dis. 2004;39:1591-8.
28. Krumina A. Diphtheria with polyneuropathy in a closed community despite receiving recent booster vaccination. J Neurol Neurosurg Psychiatry. 2005;76:1555-7.
29. Piradov MA, Pirogov VN, Popova LM, *et al*. Diphtheritic polyneuropathy: Clinical analysis of severe forms. Arch Neurol. 2001;58:1438-42.
30. Kanwal SK, Yadav D, Chhapola V, *et al*. Post-diphtheritic neuropathy: A clinical study in paediatric intensive care unit of a developing country. Trop Doct. 2012;42:195-7.
31. Murphy JR. Corynebacterium diphtheriae. Medical Microbiology. 1996.
32. CDC, Ncird. Expanded Access Investigational New Drug (IND) Application Protocol: Use of Diphtheria Antitoxin (DAT) for Suspected Diphtheria Cases IND Sponsor: Centers for Disease Control and Prevention (CDC) Protocol CDC IRB # 4167 BB IND 11184. 2016.
33. Dung NM, Kneen R, Kiem N, *et al*. Treatment of severe diphtheritic myocarditis by temporary insertion of a cardiac pacemaker. Clin Infect Dis. 2002;35:1425-9.
34. Besa NC, Coldiron ME, Bakri a, *et al*. Diphtheria outbreak with high mortality in northeastern Nigeria. Epidemiol Infect. 2014; 142:797-802.
35. Saikia L, Nath R, Saikia NJ, *et al*. A diphtheria outbreak in Assam, India. Southeast Asian J Trop Med Public Health. 2010; 41:647-52.
36. Sobel J. Botulism. Clin Infect Dis. 2005;41:1167-73.
37. Cagan E, Peker E, Dogan M, *et al*. Infant botulism. Eurasian J Med. 2010;42:92-4.

CHAPTER

48

Rickettsial Infections

Atul Kulkarni, Ashutosh Yajurvedi

INTRODUCTION

Rickettsial infections holds considerable share of re-emerging infections which were often under diagnosed in past since its first documentation in India in 1930 from Kumaon region. Once thought to be diseases of rural population, these infections are increasingly reported from urban areas of India. Even though one of the easiest to treat infection early in course of the disease, but due to difficulty in diagnosis during this period, it becomes challenging to identify and treat the rickettsial infections.[1]

EPIDEMIOLOGY AND ETIOPATHOGENESIS

Rickettsial infections have been reported from multiples states and union territories of India including Delhi, Jammu Kashmir, Uttaranchal, Rajasthan, Maharashtra, Kerala, Karnataka, and Tamil Nadu. In India the most common reported rickettsial infection is scrub typhus followed by Indian tick typhus and murine typhus. The other types are less often reported.[1]

Tick, mite louse, flea are insect vectors as well as reservoirs of rickettsial infections while rodents, dogs, mice, cattle are mammalian reservoirs. Humans are accidental hosts. During bite of vector, there is regurgitation of the saliva through which transmission occurs.[2]

Classification of rickettsial infections is summarized in **Table 1**. Pathophysiology is detailed in **Flowchart 1**.

CLINICAL FEATURES

Incubation period is 2–14 days (may extend up to 28 days, with median of 7 days).

Table 1: Classification of rickettsial diseases

S.No	*Disease*	*Rickettsial agent*	*Insect vector*	*Mammalian reservoir*
I	**Typhus group**			
	a. Epidemic typhus	*R. prowazekii*	Louse	Humans
	b. Murine typhus	*R. typhi*	Flea	Rodent
II	**Scrub typhus**	*R. tsutsugamushi*	Mite	Rodent
III	**Spotted fever group***			
	a. Indian tick typhus	*R. conorii*	Tick	Dog/rodents
	b. Rocky mountain spotted fever	*R. rickettsii*	Tick	Dogs/rodents
IV	**Others**			
	a. Rickettsial pox	*R. akari*	Mite	Mice
	b. Q fever	*C. burnettii*	Nil	Cattle sheep goat
	c. Trench fever	*Rochalimaea quintana*	Louse	Humans
	d. Ehrlichioses	*Ehrlichia*	Tick	Deer/dog
	e. Anaplasmosis	Anaplasma phagocytophilum	Tick	Deer/dog

*More than 19 types of spotted fever varieties are described depending upon the geographical area where these are prevalent

Flowchart 1: Pathophysiology of rickettsial diseases

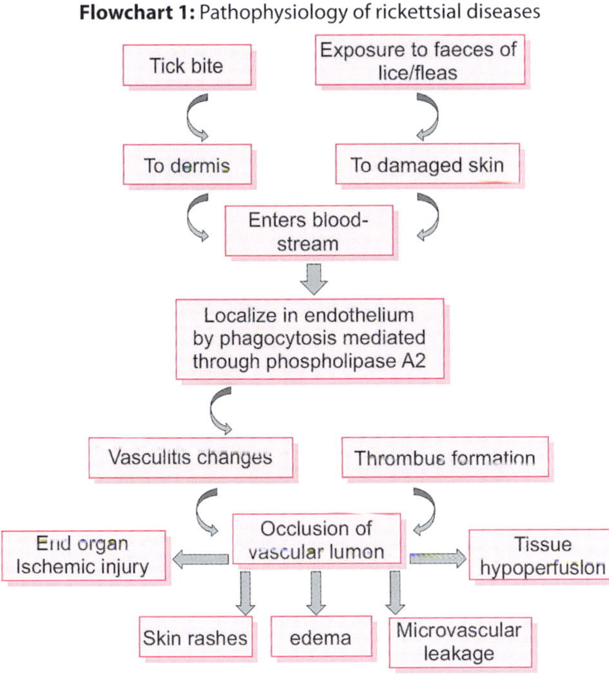

Acute febrile illness is the commonest presentation. Fever is usually high-grade sudden onset and often associated with anorexia, headache, myalgia and arthralgia. Very often there is history of visit to endemic area or contact with infected pets/animals. The triad of fever, headache and rash is observed in 44% of cases. Rash which is the hall mark of the disease, develops over the 3–5 days after onset of symptoms but may not be seen in all patients. Initially it begins as discrete, pink, blanching macular rash which progresses over days to become petechial (**Fig. 1**) hemorrhagic or gangrenous. Usually it spreads centripetally. Involvement of palms and soles is characteristic (**Fig. 2**). Rash in typhus group is atypical which spreads centrifugally and spares palms and soles.[2]

Eschar (**Fig. 3**) is pathognomonic of rickettsial disease which is more common in scrub typhus than spotted fever group. It represents the site of vector bite. These are crusty necrotic lesions with or without erythematous halo. These lesions are usually single painless non-pruritic and resemble cigarette burn. It is associated with regional lymphadenopathy, hence in cases with regional lymphadenopathy, one should actively search for eschar.[3]

Edema of hands and feet as well as periorbital puffiness or generalized edema can be observed. There can be hepatosplenomegaly.

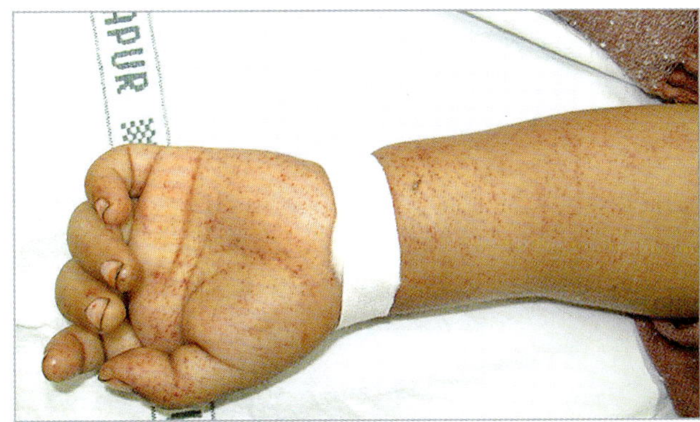

Fig. 1: Petechial rash

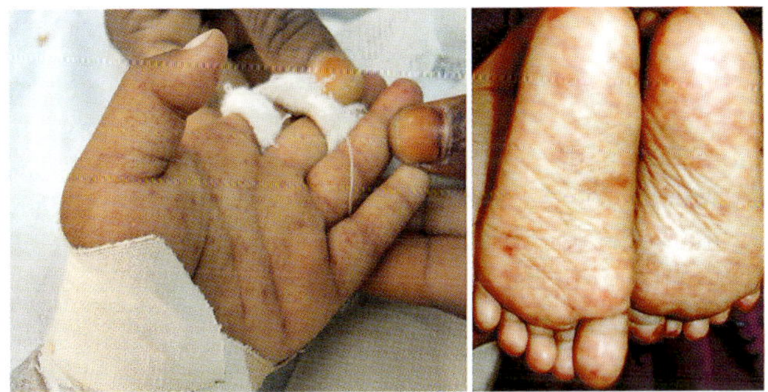

Fig. 2: Rash involving palms and soles

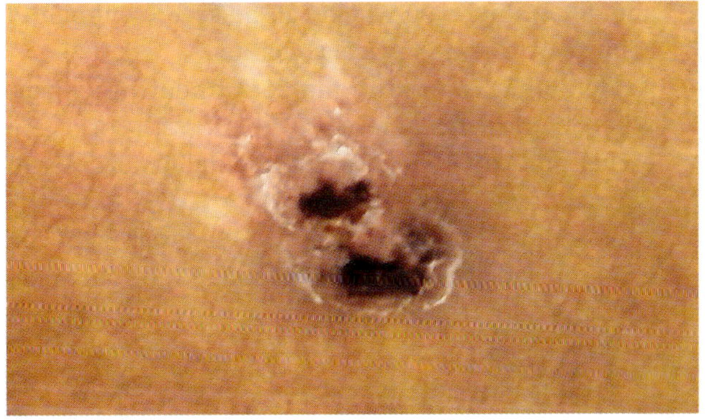

Fig. 3: Eschar

COMPLICATIONS

Complications are often seen after the first week of illness, commonly in untreated patients. These includes meningoencephalitis, pneumonitis, ARDS, hepatitis, AKI, myocarditis, septic shock, and DIC.[4]

- Meningoencephalitis is also one of most common and the lethal emergencies which may present as confusion, lethargy, progressing to stupor, delirium and coma. Seizures may also be the only manifestation

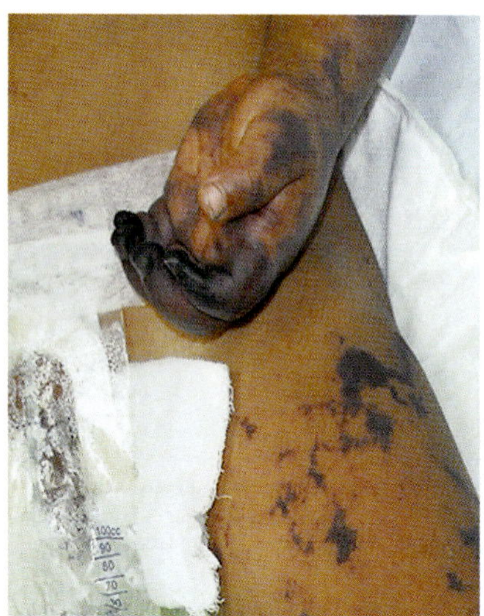

Fig. 4: Gangrene of digits

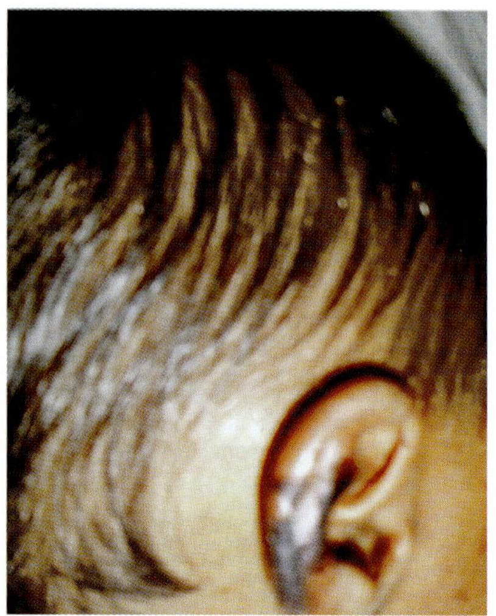

Fig. 5: Gangrene of ear lobe

of rickettsial encephalitis. Association of coma is marker of poor prognosis.[5,6]

- Pneumonitis can be a presenting complaint of scrub typhus. It presents with non-productive cough, breathlessness due to non-cardiogenic pulmonary edema sometimes culminating into dreadful ARDS.
- Hepatitis presents with nausea, vomiting, diarrhea and abdominal pain which can be severe enough to confuse with acute surgical abdomen.
- Acute kidney injury is a marker of poor prognosis. When febrile patient presents with AKI with coexisting eschar and compatible environmental history, scrub typhus should be ruled out.
- Other complications include DIC, hemophagocytic lymphohistiocytosis, purpura fulminanc and gangrene of digits (**Fig. 4**), ear lobes (**Fig. 5**), buttocks and scrotum. The gangrene of digits and ear lobe may progress to auto amputation.[3]

DIFFERENTIAL DIAGNOSIS

Rickettsial fever can mimic a great number of febrile illnesses. Most important of these are meningococcemia, measles and enteroviral exanthemas. Other diseases included in differential diagnosis are typhoid fever, secondary syphilis, leptospirosis, toxic shock syndrome, scarlet fever, rubella, Kawasaki disease, parvo-viral infection, idiopathic thrombocytopenic purpura (ITP), thrombotic thrombocytopenic purpura (TTP), hemolytic uremic syndrome, Henoch-Schönlein purpura, acute abdomen, aseptic meningitis, hepatitis, dengue fever, infectious mononucleosis, drug reactions, malaria, tularemia, anthrax and other causes of pyrexia of unknown origin.[7]

APPROACH TO DIAGNOSIS[7]

Rickettsial infections are diagnostic dilemmas due to non-specific clinical manifestations as well as lack of specific reliable laboratory tests in early phase of disease. Treatment in this period is inexpensive as well as it reduces complication rates. It is imperative to have high index of suspicion in endemic region in patient having compatible clinical scenario.

Rickettsial infection should be suspected in presence of fever and one or more of the following within 14 days of onset of illness: tick bite, ticks seen on clothes, visit to areas which are common habitats of vectors, contact with pet or stray dog infested with ticks, living in or travel to areas endemic for rickettsial diseases, and similar cases in family members or neighborhood. Case definitions are summarized in **Box 1**.

LABORATORY DIAGNOSIS

There is no widely available laboratory assay that provides rapid confirmation of early rickettsial fever.[7] Laboratory findings are usually non-specific. Total count may be normal or low with shift to left in early phase which in later course of illness have leucocytosis. There is anemia, thrombocytopenia, nonspecific features like hyponatremia, hypoproteinemia and raised transaminases. ESR and CRP are also elevated. CSF findings are usually normal but pleocytosis (<10–300 cells/μL) may be found

Box 1: Case definitions (ICMR 2015) for rickettsial diseases[1]

Suspected Case

Any undifferentiated fever without focus more than 5 days should be suspected as case of rickettsial infection. Presence of eschar suggests scrub typhus even if duration of fever is less than 5 days. Differential diagnosis of dengue, malaria, pneumonia, leptospirosis, enteric fever, meningococcaemia, measles, enteroviral exanthems and uncommon causes like toxic shock syndrome, rubella, parvoviral infection, ITP, TTP, HUS, and hepatitis should be considered.

Probable Case

Positive Weil Felix test with titres> 80- or four-fold rise in titres or Positive Elisa test with OD > 0.5 for IgM antibodies.

Confirmed Case

Positive Rickettsial DNA detection in blood or eschar, by PCR or Rising antibody titre in sera by Indirect Fluorescent Assay (IFA) / Indirect Immunoperoxidase Assay (IPA).

(ITP: immune thrombocytopenia; TTP; thrombotic thrombocytopenic purpura; HUS: hemolytic uremic syndrome)

especially in children with signs of encephalitis. There may be elevated CSF proteins (200 mg/dL).

Specific serological tests are expensive and may become positive only after first week of illness questioning the utility for the diagnosis of infections. The immunoperoxidase assay (IPA) and immunofluorescence assay (IFA) are considered serological gold standard. Molecular PCR based studies are not easily available.

Weil Felix Test

This test is economical and handy for laboratory diagnosis of rickettsial diseases in spite of having low specificity and sensitivity. The principle of this heterophile antibody testing is sharing of common antigens between rickettsia and *Proteus*. Depending on the agglutination with different non-motile strains of *Proteus*, specific rickettsial disease is suspected (**Table 2**). The local titers need to be defined for each geographical region. A titer of 1:80 is often suggestive of infection but high titers (1:320) and/or increasing titers have better positive predictive value and specificity. There are many reasons to question this test due to high cross reactivity leading to high false positivity.

Other Tests

Strain specific IgM ELISA testing has high sensitivity and specificity hence it is the choice of test. Detection of IgM antibodies confirms recent rickettsial infection. The cut off value taken is optical density of 0.5. Baseline titres for a particular geographical region need to be defined.

Table 2: Interpretation of Weil Felix test

	Weil Felix		
Disease	*OX 19*	*OX 2*	*OX K*
Epidemic typhus	+++	+	–
Endemic typhus	+++	+/–	–
Scrub typhus	–	–	+++
RMSF	++	++	–
Ricketssial pox	–	–	–
Q fever	–	–	–

(RMSF: Rocky mountain spotted fever)

Immunofluorescence assay (IFA) is considered gold standard test for the diagnosis of rickettsial infections. Because of prohibitive cost, meagre availability and test being technically demanding, the utility in clinical practice is limited. Usually titres start rising at 5–10 days of illness and reach its peak at 3–4 weeks. *Indirect Immunoperoxidase Assay (IPA)* gives equivalent results as IFA but this test also requires special instrument and experienced person for interpretation.

Polymerase chain reaction-based detection is useful for diagnosis in first week of illness even before the seroconversion. Rapid, reproducible, quantitative capability, and low risk of contamination are its advantages.

Approach to diagnosis is summarized in **Flowchart 2**.

TREATMENT

Severity and fatality of the disease increases with the delay in diagnosis and institution of the treatment. Treatment should never be delayed in cases where laboratory diagnosis is not yet confirmed and should not be stopped after negative test results as it does not rule out rickettsial infections. The empirical treatment of other differential diagnosis is also needed due to highly non-specific clinical features of rickettsial infection. For example, for a patient in whom meningococcal disease and tick borne rickettsial disease are being considered, administering antibacterial therapy to treat potential *Neisseria meningitidis* infection in addition to administering doxycycline to treat rickettsial agents is appropriate while awaiting additional diagnostic information.

Doxycycline

Doxycycline is the drug of the choice in all age groups. It can be used orally/intravenously in a dose of 2.2 mg/kg/dose BD (maximum dose 200 mg). The IV route is preferred

Flowchart 2: Approach to diagnosis and management of rickettsial infection

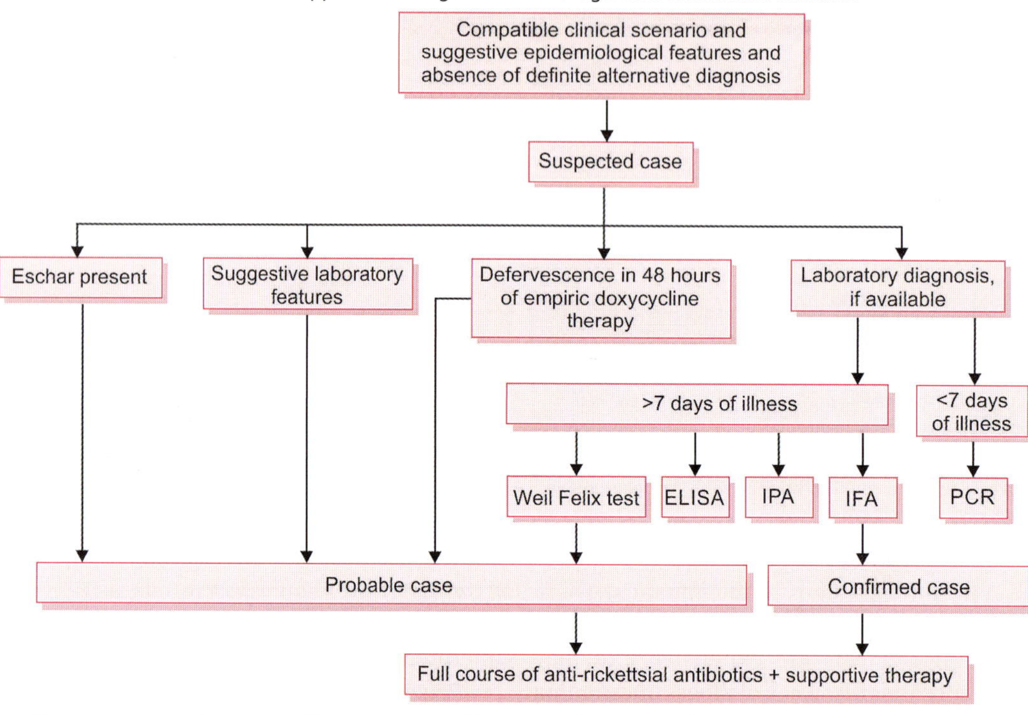

ELISA: enzyme-linked immunosorbent assay; IPA: immunoperoxidase assay; IFA: immunofluorescent assay; PCR: polymerase chain reaction)

in severely ill patients as well as in whom oral doxycycline cannot be given due to altered GI aspirates, persistent vomiting or comatose state.

Duration of the therapy is for 5–7 days or at least 3 days after subsidence of the fever whichever is longer. This strategy avoids the chances of recurrence of the disease.

Response to the treatment is dramatic and rapid defervescence occurs in 1–3 days and recovery within 7–10 days of starting of the therapy. Slower response may be seen if therapy is started late in the course of the illness or severely ill children with multiorgan failure. Failure of the response to treatment may suggest alternative diagnosis or rarely doxycycline resistance where alternate drugs can be tried.

Doxycycline in children

As per the recommendations from American Academy of Pediatrics and CDC, doxycycline is the drug of choice for tick-borne rickettsial infections. The concern about tooth staining and dental enamel hypoplasia is not seen with doxycycline as it used to be seen with older generation of tetracyclines. Doxycycline used at the dose and duration recommended for treatment of RMSF in children aged <8 years, even after multiple courses, did not result in tooth staining or enamel hypoplasia in a 2013 retrospective cohort study of 58 children who received doxycycline before the age of 8 years.

Pregnancy and lactation

Controlled studies to assess the safety of doxycycline use in pregnant women have not been conducted, and available data are primarily observational. An expert review on doxycycline use during pregnancy concluded that therapeutic doses were unlikely to pose a substantial teratogenic risk; however, the data were insufficient to conclude that no risk exists. Doxycycline has been used successfully to treat tick borne rickettsial diseases in pregnant women without adverse effects to the mother; however, follow-up to address adverse effects to the fetus was limited. Chloramphenicol is a potential alternative treatment for RMSF during pregnancy.

Doxycycline is excreted into breastmilk at low levels; however, the extent of absorption by nursing infants is unknown. Short-term use of doxycycline as recommended for the treatment of tick borne rickettsial disease is considered probably safe during lactation on the basis of available literature and expert opinion. Although doxycycline is not specifically addressed, tetracycline is listed by the American Academy of Pediatrics Committee on Drugs as "usually compatible with breastfeeding". Azithromycin can be used during pregnancy and lactation.

Treatment of Asymptomatic Persons Seropositive for Rickettsial Diseases

Regardless of previous treatment status, it is not recommended to treat asymptomatic seropositive asymptomatic patients, as there is persistence of rickettsial antibodies for months to years. This is also the reason that serological tests are not used for the monitoring of response to treatment.

Alternative Antibacterial Agents to Doxycycline

The alternate drugs can be used when the response to doxycycline is not seen as the reports of strains with resistance to doxycycline are on the rise. Tetracyclines including doxycycline are the only recommended drugs for the treatment of rickettsial infections. Chloramphenicol is alternate drug used for treatment of RMSF, but a CDC case series has shown higher risk of death with chloramphenicol than tetracyclines. Other effective drugs are macrolides (clarithromycin/azithromycin) and rifampicin. The use of rifampicin in India is not recommended. Many times, while awaiting laboratory reports or a specific diagnosis, broad spectrum antimicrobials like beta-lactams, aminoglycosides, fluoroquinolones and sulphonamides are used. But these agents are not active against the tick borne rickettsial infections. Even though fluoroquinolones show response in vitro, their use is associated with delayed response and longer hospital stay.

TREATMENT OF COMPLICATION

Meningoencephalitis

This is one of the complications with long term morbidity and high mortality. Apart from routine care like management of airway breathing and circulation, control of seizures with appropriate AEDs is required. Initially child should be loaded with lorazepam 0.05-0.1 mg (maximum 4 mg) IV/IM. The dose can be repeated after 10–15 mins. If seizures are still persisting, child should be loaded with anticonvulsants like phenytoin/fosphenytoin, levetiracetam. Child may sometimes go into refractory status epilepticus needing midazolam infusion. Child should be monitored for respiratory depression and can be electively intubated. Intubation and mechanical ventilation may also help to reduce raised ICP. Other measures like 3% Saline/mannitol, to reduce increased intracranial tension should be started. In a child with hyponatremia and hypotension 3% saline would be a better option. The role of steroids in encephalitis is controversial. While some authors recommend but the data supporting the use is lacking. Injection methyl prednisolone 30 mg/kg once a day for 3–5 days can be tried. Alternatively, dexamethasone can be used.

Pulmonary Edema

This is one of most frequently observed complication of rickettsial infection which can be because of disease severity itself or iatrogenically. The already damaged lung microvasculature may suffer further damage due to inadvertent fluid administration. Start with the supplemental oxygen therapy at the earliest sign of increased work of breathing. A tight fluid balance by monitoring input and output as well as restriction of fluids can be a strategy. With worsening of the respiratory status child may need noninvasive/invasive ventilation. For mechanical ventilation lung protective strategies in a form of smaller tidal volumes, optimum PEEP should be used. The child needs to be sedated and paralysed adequately to avoid asynchrony providing effective ventilation. Those requiring high pressure, can be shifted to HFOV. Adequate antibiotic covering organisms of community acquired pneumonia is warranted in addition to Doxycycline.

Myocarditis

This usually presents with tachycardia disproportionate to the temperature of the baby, low volume pulses and signs of failure. Cardiac involvement carries high mortality. There is no specific treatment available for this condition. It is treated symptomatically with restriction of fluids, inotropes. The role of steroids/intravenous immunoglobulin (IVIg) is controversial. IVIg 1 g/kg/day for 2 days or injection methyl prednisolone 30 mg/kg once daily may help.

Others

- Renal failure can be treated with fluid restriction or resuscitation depending on the type of AKI. Child may need diuretics, as well as peritoneal or hemodialysis.
- *Multiorgan failure and DIC*: This is one of the most dreaded complication of rickettsial fever. The child

Table 3: Summary of anti-rickettsial drugs

S. No.	*Name of drug*	*Dose, route and duration*	*Comments*
1.	Doxycycline	2.2 mg/kg/dose BD per oral or IV (Max 200 mg) 5 to 7 days or for at least 3 days until the patient is afebrile	• Drug of choice • Rapid defervesce within 48 hours • IV formulation for sick patients
2.	Tetracycline	25–50 mg/kg/dose every 6 hourly per oral (Max 2 g/day) 5 to 7 days or for at least 3 days until the patient is afebrile	• Rapid defervesce within 48 hours • IV formulation for sick patients
3.	Chloramphenicol	50–100 mg/kg/day every 6 hourly (Max 3 g/day) 5 to 7 days or for at least 3 days until the patient is afebrile	• Most common alternative for tetracycline • Most common adverse effect is agranulocytosis
4.	Azithromycin	10 mg/kg /day once daily (max 500 mg) 5 to 7 days or for at least 3 days until the patient is afebrile	• Preferred drug in pregnancy • Recommended when doxycycline resistant is present
5.	Clarithromycin	15 mg/kg /day bd 5 to 7 days or for at least 3 days until the patient is afebrile	
6.	Rifampicin	10 mg/kg Maximum is 300 mg 5 to 7 days or for at least 3 days until the patient is afebrile	• Doxycycline resistance cases • Shorter duration of fever with rifampicin in northern Thailand when compare with doxycycline
7.	Fluoroquinolones	Not recommended in pediatric age group	

may present with septic shock with bleeding. Child is treated like a septic shock with fluid boluses inotropes. Child is started with broad spectrum iv antibiotic to cover other infections mentioned in differential diagnosis. Child may need transfusion of various blood products like Packed cells, platelets or FFP depending on the blood picture and condition of the child. Other supportive measures like maintenance of electrolytes sugar fluid status should be provided as needed.

- Gangrene in earlobe, fingers, buttocks, scrotum can be managed with Low molecular weight heparin.

Recommended dosages, route and duration of the anti rickettsial agents are summarized in **Table 3**.

PROGNOSIS

Delayed treatment is invariably associated with irreversible vascular or end organ damage and long term sequalae or death. Those who survive without treatment, fever subsides within 2–3 weeks of illness. Younger age, male gender, shorter incubation period, absence of rash, comorbidities like diabetes, G6PD deficiency state, cardiac illness, and use of sulfonamides are poor prognostic factors.[7]

KEY MESSAGES

- Rickettsial infections are emerging infection with high mortality if not recognized early and treated.
- Basic cause of all manifestations is vasculitis with capillary leakage.
- Fever, rash, eschar, hepatosplenomegaly and edema are the common presenting symptoms.
- Suspect rickettsial infection in a case of non-specific acute febrile illness with possibility of vector exposure in light of supportive laboratory evidence.
- All the serological test should usually be carried out in second week of illness.
- Meningoencephalitis, myocarditis, renal failure and ARDS are fatal complications.
- Doxycycline is drug of choice in all age groups. Others options are tetracycline, chloramphenicol and azithromycin.

REFERENCES

1. DHR-ICMR. Guidelines for Diagnosis and Management of Rickettsial Diseases in India. ICMR; 2015, February.
2. Kulkarni A. Spotted fevers. PG Textbook of Pediatrics. New Delhi: Jaypee Brothers Medical Publishers; 2013. p. 1309-12.
3. Kulkarni A. Rickettsial infections. IAP Textbook of Infectious Diseases. New Delhi: Jaypee Brothers Medical Publishers; 2013. p. 376-85.
4. Reller ME, Dumler JS. Rickettsial infection. In: Kliegman RM, Bonita, Stanton, St. Geme J, Schor NF, editors. Nelson's Textbook of Paediatrics, 20th edition. Elsevier Health Sciences; 2015. p. 1497-511.
5. Baldwin K, Rathi N. Rickettsial disease. In: Robert L, Daniel T, William M, editors. International Neurology, 2nd edition. UK: Wiley Blackwell; 2016. p. 291-5.
6. Rathi N, Maheshwari M, Khandelwal R. Neurological manifestations of rickettsial infections in children. Pediatric Infectious Disease. 2016;7:64-6.
7. Rathi N, Kulkarni A, Yewale V. IAP guidelines on rickettsial diseases in children. Indian Pediatr. 2017;54(3):223-9.

CHAPTER

49

Post-exposure Prophylaxis

Abhay K Shah, Aashay A Shah

POST-EXPOSURE PROPHYLAXIS (PEP) FOR RABIES

Rabies, a zoonotic disease, is almost invariably fatal once clinical signs occur, as a result of acute progressive encephalitis. Rabies virus is rhabdovirus which infects several domestic and wild animals. It is secreted in the saliva of these animals and gets transmitted to humans through contact with infected animal's saliva in bites and scratches. Rabies occurs mainly in underserved populations, both rural and urban. Most cases occur in Africa and Asia, with approximately 40% of cases in children aged less than 15 years.[1] The important modes of transmission of rabies infection include (1) bite, (2) scratch, (3) lick on damaged skin and intact mucous membrane, (4) organ transplant, mainly cornea transplant, and (5) aerosol route.

The PEP is offered for preventing the development of clinical rabies after exposure has occurred, usually following the bite of an animal suspected of having rabies. In countries/ regions at risk of rabies, the circumstances of an animal bite or contact with a suspected rabid animal would warrant PEP. PEP comprises of local wound care and/or vaccines and/or immunoglobulin. With the availability of safe and effective modern tissue culture vaccines (MTCV), and the concept of sero-vaccination (immunoglobulin and vaccine - both), prevention of rabies is almost assured in post-exposure cases. Clinical categorization of the exposure as per WHO recommendation 2018 is a useful tool to treat an animal bite case **(Box 1)**.[2] **Table 1** summarizes the details of intervention for PEP in case of an animal bite.[2] PEP should be initiated promptly without any delay. There is no need to wait for any laboratory results or observe the dog.

Box 1: WHO rabies exposure categories

The WHO rabies exposure categories are:

Category I: Touching or feeding animals, licks on intact skin

Category II: Nibbling of uncovered skin, minor scratches or abrasions without bleeding

Category III: Single or multiple transdermal bites or scratches, contamination of mucous membrane or broken skin with saliva from animal licks, exposures due to direct contact with bats

Wound Care

Thorough cleansing of the wound with copious water and soap for minimum 10 minutes is the most vital step. This should be followed by irrigation with virucidal agent like 70% alcohol or povidine iodine. Majority of the wounds and exposures are of Category III. A total treatment procedure in category III cases is also very important medicolegally. The animal bite wound(s) is (are) not to be covered. RIG should be administered for severe Category III exposures. Any suturing of the wound(s) should be avoided. When the suturing is unavoidable for the purpose of hemostasis, it must be ensured that rabies immunoglobulin (RIG) has been administered in the wound(s) prior to suturing and that the suturing has been done loosely.

Passive Immunization

Rabies immunoglobulin (RIG)

There are 2 types of rabies immunoglobulin namely, (i) Human rabies immunoglobulin (HRIG) and (ii) Equine rabies immunoglobulin (ERIG). RIGs are specific rabies

Table 1: PEP for rabies following animal bite based on WHO categorization of patients

	Category I	*Category II*	*Category III*
Immunologically naive individuals of all age groups	Wash exposed skin surfaces. No PEP required	Wound washing and immediate vaccination 2-sites ID on days 0, 3 and 7 (2-2-2-0-0 regime) OR 1-site IM on days 0, 3, 7 and between day 14–28 OR 2-sites IM on days 0 and 1 site IM on days 7, 21 (2,1,1 regimen or 2-0-1-0-1 regimen) No RIG	Wound washing and immediate vaccination 2-sites ID on days 0, 3 and 7 (2-2-2-0-0 regime) OR 1-site IM on days 0, 3, 7 and between day 14–28 OR 2-sites IM on day 0 and 1 site IM on days 7, 21 (2,1,1 regimen or 2-0-1-0-1 regimen)* RIG recommended
Previously immunized individuals of all age groups	Wash exposed skin surfaces. No PEP required	Wound washing and immediate vaccination: 1-site ID on days 0 and 3 OR At 4-sites ID on day 0 OR At 1-site IM on days 0 and 3 RIG is not indicated	Wound washing and immediate vaccination: 1-site ID on days 0 and 3 OR At 4-sites ID on day 0 OR At 1-site IM on days 0 and 3 RIG is not indicated

*Except if complete PEP already received within 3 months

virus neutralizing antibodies that immediately neutralize rabies virus on contact. RIG gives a coating to the virus so that it cannot enter the nerve ending resulting in reduction or total obliteration of inoculated virus. RIG is mandatory for Category III patients and immunocompromised Category II patients, along with the vaccine.

Choice of RIG: Though HRIG represents the gold standard for passive immunization, its prohibitive cost and erratic supply are two important issues. ERIG is an acceptable alternative. The increased production of highly purified horse immunoglobulins (ERIG) should be promoted to provide an alternate and effective solution to the problems of supplies of HRIG. Studies have proved that the incidence of adverse reactions following RIG are as low as 2.4% and that of anaphylactic reaction is 0.2%.[3] Presently the purified ERIG preparation has been made available and is being produced by an Indian manufacturer. Central Research Institute, Kasauli, also produces a small quantity of anti-rabies serum (ARS). However, it is insufficient to meet the demands in a vast country like India.

Dose of RIG: The dose of HRIG is 20 IU per kg body weight and that of ERIG is 40 IU per kg body weight. In case of ERIG, skin test for sensitivity is essential but for HRIG no skin test is necessary. Maximum dose of ERIG and HRIG is 3000 IU and 1500 IU respectively.

As much as anatomically feasible the RIG should be infiltrated thoroughly into and around the wound. Intramuscular (IM) administration is now not advocated. If the administration of the RIG is delayed initially, it can be administered up to 7th day after the 1st dose of vaccine, i.e. along with 3rd dose of vaccine, but at a separate site. If the quantity of RIG is insufficient to infiltrate all the wounds it may be diluted with normal saline till sufficient quantity is available. RIG should not be given ≥8 days after the administration of anti-rabies vaccine since the antibody response to vaccine is presumed to have started. RIG is also not indicated in individuals who have completed pre-exposure/post-exposure prophylaxis in the past.

If a limited amount of RIG is available, RIG allocation should be prioritized for exposed patients based on the following criteria: Multiple bites, deep wounds, bites to highly innervated parts of the body (such as head, neck and hands), severe immunodeficiency, the biting animal is a confirmed or probable rabies case, and bites, scratches or exposures of mucous membranes caused by a bat. If RIG is not available, thorough, prompt wound washing, together with immediate administration of the first vaccine dose, followed by a complete course of rabies vaccine, is highly effective in preventing rabies. Vaccines should never be withheld, regardless of the availability of RIG.

Failure of RIG

Failure of RIG treatment may occur due to:[4]

- If RIGs are not used locally but administered only systemically.
- Insufficient quantity of RIG.
- Interval from the time of bite to RIG administration is unusually delayed, more than 7 days
- RIG and antirabies vaccine (ARV) given at the same site of injection.
- When infiltration of some wounds is not done especially where wounds are severe and extensive. It is better to dilute the RIG 2 to 3 folds with normal saline in this type of cases so that all wounds can be covered.
- RIG is administered alone without the use of vaccines.

Rabies monoclonal antibody (Rabies MAB)

The first monoclonal antibody product developed by recombinant DNA technology to replace the rabies immunoglobulin (RIG) component of rabies PEP[6] is now available across India. Rabishield® is manufactured by the Serum Institute of India, Pune, in partnership with Mass Biologics, of the University of Massachusetts Medical School in the US.

The extremely high cost and scarcity of HRIG is a huge problem in most canine rabies-endemic countries. ERIG is less scarce and much cheaper, but has been associated with very rare, but severe cases of anaphylactic shock. These issues will be taken care by Rabies MAB.

It has been tested *in vivo* and *in silico* against a large number of street rabies isolates and passed clinical trials in India showing that it is as effective as human RIG. It is described as more potent, requiring a lower dose (3.33 IU/kg body weight). It is available as 100 IU/2.5 mL and 250 IU/2.5 mL formulations.

PEP for Rabies in Immunocompromised

Would care and toileting are most important components as they may not mount desirable immune response. RIG is offered even in Category II patients who are immunocompromised. Rabies antibody estimation-10 days after the completion of course of vaccination-is recommended to assess whether an additional dose of vaccine is required.

Vaccination against Rabies

It is advisable to administer a potent modern tissue culture rabies vaccine (MTCV) following an approved schedule which results in production of systemic antibodies against rabies after a lag period of 7 to 14 days from the 1st dose of ARV. These antibodies are capable of neutralizing remaining virus particles. The use of MTCV is to be preferred to the brain tissue (nerve tissue) vaccines (NTV). Three types of MTCV are available in India. These are (i) Purified chick embryo cell vaccine (PCEC), (ii) Human diploid cell vaccine (HDCV), (iii) Purified vero cell vaccine (PVRV).

Schedules of vaccinations against rabies

The previously WHO-recommended *Essen protocol* which comprises of five IM injections on days 0, 3, 7, 14, 28/30 (6th dose on day 90 is administered in selected cases) is practiced in our country as we are in the highest endemic zone of rabies till today. But this protocol may not be as cost-, dose- or time-sparing, when compared to the WHO 2018 Protocol.[2]

WHO recommendations

- 1-site IM vaccine administration on days 0, 3, 7 and the fourth dose between days 14 to 28.
- Alternatively, on day 0 2 site IM vaccine can be administered, followed by 1 site IM vaccine on days 7 and 21

Criteria for intradermal (ID) use:[7] ID route is cost effective by 60–80% when used for a minimum 50 cases per day.[5] The dose of intradermal injection is 0.1 mL with both purified Vero cell rabies vaccine, and purified chick embryo rabies vaccine.

Management of Re-exposure Case

If a previously immunized person is bitten by a rabid dog within 3 months of completing a full course of PEP or PrEP, no new course of PEP is required.

For exposures occurring more than 3 months after a PEP or PrEP course, treat as PEP for previously immunized individuals; 1 site ID or IM vaccination at days 0 and 3, or a 4-site ID accelerated vaccination on day 0. RIG is not indicated **(Table 2)**.

Because rabies is a lethal disease there are no contra-indications for its PEP including infants, pregnancy, and

Table 2: Re-exposure recommendations for rabies

	Category I	*Category II*	*Category III*
Previously immunized individuals of all age-groups	Wash exposed skin surfaces. No PEP required	Wound washing and immediate vaccination 1 – site ID/IM on days 0 and 3* OR At 4 – sites ID on day 0# No RIG	Wound washing and immediate vaccination 1 – site ID/IM on days 0 and 3* OR At 4 – sites ID on day 0* RIG recommended

*The dose is either 1 single immunizing intramuscular (IM) dose (1 mL or 0.5 mL, depending on vaccine type) or one intradermal (ID) dose of 0.1 mL per site
#4 Injections of 0.1 mL equally distributed over left and right deltoids, thigh or suprascapular areas during a single visit

lactating mothers. Even if a person presents after several days/months/years after the bite, he/she should be managed in a similar manner as a person who has been bitten recently including using RIG (if indicated) as rabies may have a long incubation period.

POST-EXPOSURE PROPHYLAXIS FOR HEPATITIS B

Hepatitis B virus (HBV) is an important cause of chronic liver disease and often leads to hepatocellular carcinoma. In India, 2–4% of individuals are chronic carriers of HBV that place us in intermediate endemicity.[8] Infection with HBV may occur perinatally (vertical transmission), during early childhood (the so-called horizontal spread), through sexual contact or nosocomial. Horizontal transmission in children usually occurs by 5 years or before and is important cause of chronic HBV. The risk of infection in a child born to a hepatitis B positive mother ranges from 10% to 85% depending on the mother's hepatitis B e antigen (HBeAg) status. When HBV infection occurs at an younger there are higher chances of becoming chronic carriers. Those babies who are infected at birth, 90% of them will become chronic carriers and up to 25% of chronic carriers will succumb to chronic liver disease in adult life.[9]

HBV is concentrated most highly in blood, and is transmitted through percutaneous (i.e. puncture through the skin) or mucosal (i.e. direct contact with mucous membranes) exposure to infectious blood or body fluids and can be transmitted in the absence of visible blood and remains viable on environmental surfaces for at least seven days.[10] Semen and vaginal secretions are infectious, and HBV also can be detected in saliva, tears, and bile. Cerebrospinal fluid, synovial fluid, pleural fluid, peritoneal fluid, pericardial fluid, and amniotic fluid are also considered potentially infectious. Unless contaminated with blood, urine, feces, vomitus, sputum and sweat are not efficient transmissors of HBV. Hepatitis B surface antigen (HBsAg) found in breast milk is also unlikely to lead to transmission, and hence HBV infection is not a contraindication to breastfeeding.[10] When HBsAg in the serum persists for at least 6 months (chronic infection), it serves as a main reservoir for HBV transmission.[10] All HBsAg positive persons are infectious, but those with elevated HBV DNA or those with HBeAg are most infectious.[11] HBeAg is a marker of infectivity. Persons with occult HBV infection (i.e. those who test negative for HBsAg but have detectable HBV DNA) also might transmit infection.[11]

This underlies the importance of post-exposure prophylaxis (PEP) following exposure to HBV. Hepatitis B vaccine, and in certain circumstances, Hepatitis B immune globulin (HBIG) constitute the PEP regimen.

Hepatitis B Vaccine

Hepatitis B vaccines are available as monovalent formulations and in combination with other vaccines, including diphtheria-tetanus-pertussis (DTP), *Haemophilus influenzae* type B (HiB), and inactivated poliovirus (IPV). WHO recommends multiple options for HB vaccination schedule without requiring additional visits for immunization.[12] However "timely birth dose" is very crucial.

Hepatitis B vaccine, when administered as 0, 1 and 6 months schedule, provides the best immunogenicity. Ideal minimum interval between dose 1 and 2 is 4 weeks and between dose 2 and 3 is 8 weeks and final dose of the series should not be administered before age of 24 weeks. Several schedules for Hepatitis B vaccination (0, 1, and 6 months; at 6, 10, 14 weeks; at 0, 6, 10, and 14 weeks; at 2, 3, and 4 months; or 2, 4, and 6 months) have been studied, and almost all the studies showed adequate immunogenicity to prevent the disease. In various from India immunogenicity of Hepatitis B vaccine was also found in the range of 96–100% when using different schedules as 0, 6, 14 weeks and 0, 1, 2 months and 6, 10, 14 week.[13-15] Hence, the hepatitis B vaccine may be given using any of these schedules. However, considering the programmatic implications and logistic issues, Hepatitis B vaccine can be used in 6, 10, 14 weeks' schedule as combination vaccine.[16]

A substantial burden of chronic HBV infection persists because birth-dose coverage (estimated as 39% globally) is still low.[17] The WHO Position Paper 2017 recommends that a monovalent hepatitis B vaccine birth dose, ideally within 24 hours ("timely birth dose"), is a must. The birth dose of Hepatitis B vaccine is a critical safety net for infants born to infected mothers when the mother's results are not obtained, misinterpreted, falsely negative, transcribed or reported inaccurately, or not communicated to the infant care team.[18] The birth dose can reduce the perinatal transmission by 18–40%.[19] Delay in the administration of the first dose beyond the 7th day of life has been shown to be associated with higher rates of HBsAg acquisition in later childhood.

Hepatitis B Vaccination in High Risk Individuals

Hepatitis B vaccine should be offered to all health care professionals (HCP) who have a reasonable risk of being exposed to blood and body fluids. It is preferable that medical students and trainees be offered the vaccine, as exposure is more common during the training period. Hepatitis B vaccination should be routinely offered in high-risk setting that include health care workers, public safety workers, trainees working healthcare fields in schools of medicine, dentistry, nursing, laboratory technology, and other allied health professions. All HCP, who has had a direct patient contact or who drew/handled blood specimens from infected person should have post-vaccination testing for antibody to hepatitis B surface antigen (anti-HBs). Sero-conversion should be documented 1–2 months after the last dose of vaccine.

For immunocompetent HCP, periodic testing or periodic boosting is not needed. Persons with chronic liver disease including, those with hepatitis C virus infection, cirrhosis, fatty liver disease, alcoholic liver disease, autoimmune hepatitis, and an alanine aminotransferase (ALT) or aspartate aminotransferase (AST) level greater than twice the upper limit of normal are also high risk and should be administered Hepatitis B vaccine. Adults with risk factors for HBV infection should be administered Hepatitis B vaccine in a 0, 1, and 6 month schedule. An accelerated schedule may be offered alternately, where in dose 2 may be given at least 4 weeks after dose 1 and dose 3 at least 8 weeks after dose 2 and at least 16 weeks after dose 1.

Management of an Infant Born to Hepatitis B Positive Mother

All pregnant women should have HBs Ag screening. If them other is known to be HBsAg negative, hepatitis B vaccine can be given in the 0–6 weeks–6 months schedule or any other alternative suitable schedule. If the mother's HBsAg status is not known, it is important that hepatitis B vaccination should begin within a few hours of birth so that perinatal transmission can be prevented.

If the mother is HBsAg positive (and especially HBeAg positive), the baby should be given hepatitis B Immunoglobulin (HBIG) along with hepatitis B vaccine within 12 hours of birth, using two separate syringes and separate sites for injection. The dose of HBIG is 0.5 mL intramuscular. HBIG may be given up to 7 days of birth but the efficacy of HBIG after 48 hours is not known. Two more doses of hepatitis B vaccine at 1 month/6 weeks and 6 months are needed. If HBIG is not available or is unaffordable, hepatitis B vaccine may be given at 0,1 and 2 months with an additional dose between 9 and 12 months.

The efficacy of prophylaxis with both HBIG and hepatitis B vaccine is 85–95% and that with hepatitis B vaccine alone (1st dose at birth) is 70–75%. All infants born to HBsAg positive mothers should be tested for HBsAg and anti- HBsAg antibodies at the age of 9–15 months to identify carriers/non-responders.[20]

Hepatitis B Vaccination in Preterm Infants and Low Birth Weight Infants

Infants with birth weight less than 2000 g have a decreased response to hepatitis B vaccines administered before the age of one month. However, by the chronological age of one month, preterm babies irrespective of the initial birth weight and gestational age are likely to respond as adequately as full term infants.

PEP for Hepatitis B Infection in Healthcare Professional

Following a percutaneous or mucosal exposure to blood 3 factors need to be considered when deciding the

Table 3: PEP in healthcare professionals (HCP) after percutaneous or mucosal exposure*

Vaccination status of the exposed HCP	*HBs Ag status of source*		
	HBsAg positive	*HBsAg negative*	*HBsAg unknown*[#]
Unimmunized	HBIG (1 dose) and Hepatitis B vaccination series	Hepatitis B vaccination series	Hepatitis B vaccination series
Partially immunized	HBIG (1 dose) and complete vaccine series	No intervention	Complete Hepatitis B vaccination series
Response to vaccination series is unknown	Test exposed person for anti-HBs, if adequate: no treatment; if inadequate: HBIG (1 dose) and Hepatitis B vaccine booster dose	No intervention	Test exposed person for anti-HBs, if adequate: no treatment; if inadequate: vaccine booster dose
Known nonresponder to 3 dose series of vaccination	HBIG (1 dose) and start revaccination	No treatment; start revaccination for future protection	If known high-risk source, treat as if source were HBsAg positive
Known non-responder to initial and revaccination series	HBIG (2 doses); 2nd dose 1 month after 1st dose	No intervention	If known high-risk source, treat as if source were HBsAg positive

[#]If source is high risk, consider it as HBsAg positive source

*1. Persons known to have had HBV infection in the past or who are chronically infected do not require HBIG or vaccine
2. Hepatitis B immune globulin (0.06 mL/kg) administered IM.
3. Adequate response is anti-HB so fat least 10 mL U/mL after vaccination.
4. Revaccination: additional 3 dose series of hepatitis B vaccine administered after the primary series.
5. First dose as soon as possible after exposure and the second dose 1 month later.
6. Testing should be done as soon as possible after exposure.

nature of PEP. These include HBsAg status of the source, vaccination status of the exposed healthcare professional, and response to Hepatitis B vaccination in the healthcare professional **(Table 3)**.

POST-EXPOSURE PROPHYLAXIS FOR SUSPECTED HUMAN IMMUNODEFICIENCY VIRUS

Globally the number of HIV infected children in less than 15 years of age has increased from 1.6 to 2.5 million in 2009. But it is heartening to know that there has been decline in number of newly HIV infected cases since 2003 due to ever increasing access to prevention of parent to child transmission (PPTCT) services.[21] 90% of the children living with HIV are infected through mother-to-child transmission (MTCT) during pregnancy, around the time of birth or through breastfeeding. In the absence of any intervention, a substantial proportion of children born to women living with HIV infection will acquire the virus from their mother during pregnancy, labor, delivery and through breastfeeding;[21] the risk of transmission being 5–45%.[22] See **Box 2**. The use of antiretroviral (ARV) drugs for the prevention of parent-to-child transmission (PPTCT) of HIV has been shown to be effective for over a decade.

Box 2: Risk of HIV transmission in infant in relation to timing of maternal exposure in the absence of intervention[22]

Timing of HIV infection	*Percent of children at risk*
• During pregnancy	5–10%
• During labor and delivery	10–15%
• During breastfeeding	5–20%
• Overall risk without breastfeeding	15–25%
• Overall risk with breastfeeding to 6 months	20–35%
• Overall risk with breastfeeding to 18 to 24 months	30–45%

In addition to MTCT, other routes of transmission include transfusion with blood products from HIV-infected donor, injections with contaminated needles, sexual abuse or early sexual contact in children or adolescents. The mission of PMTCT services should be elimination of HIV of mother to child transmission.[23,24] It includes management of mother and her exposed infant.

Management of the HIV Positive Mother

The risk of perinatal HIV transmission can be reduced substantially by:

- Universal antenatal HIV screening

- All HIV-infected pregnant women should start Anti-retroviral therapy (ART) as soon as possible and continue ART throughout pregnancy, delivery, breast-feeding period and thereafter lifelong. Even if the pregnant women presents very late in pregnancy (including those who present after 36 weeks of gestation), ART should be initiated promptly.

Choice or anti-retroviral therapy: Pregnant women who are detected to be HIV infected during antenatal care should be initiated on ART (TDF+3TC+EFV) i.e. (TDF Tenofovir 300 mg, 3TC Lamivudine 300 mg, EFV Efavirenz 600 mg) regardless of clinical stage or CD4 count, provided there is no previous exposure to non-nucleoside reverse transcriptase inhibitors (NNRTIs) viz, Nevirapine (NVP) or Efavirenz (EVF).[23] HIV infected pregnant women who have had previous exposure to single dose Nevirapine (Sd NVP) or EFV, for PPTCT prophylaxis in prior pregnancies, an NNRTI-based ART regimen such as TDF+3TC+EFV may not be fully effective due to persistence of archived mutation to NNRTIs. Thus, these women will require a protease-inhibitor (PI) based ART regimen like TDF + 3TC + LPV/r (Lopinavir/ritonavir). The dose will be TDF (300 mg, OD) +3TC (300 mg, OD)+ LPV/r (200 mg/50 mg; 2 tablets BD).

Care of HIV-Exposed Infant/Child

a. *Immediate care at birth*: It is recommended to follow standard neonatal care guidelines including resuscitation guidelines and follow universal precautions. The cord should be clamped so on after birth and it should not be milked. The cord should be covered with a gloved hand and gauze before cutting to avoid blood splattering. Breastfeeding should be initiated within the first hour of birth, in accordance with the preferred and informed choice of the mother.
b. *Infant feeding*: Breastfeeding is the preferred choice in developing countries as it maximizes the chances of survival of the infant. Breastfeeding provides the infant with all the required nutrients and immunological factors. Mixed feeding, i.e. breast milk and replacement feeds combined increases the risk of transmission of HIV (as it increases mucosal abrasions) and should be avoided at all cost.[25] If child found to be HIV negative through Early Infant Diagnosis (EID), continue breast-feeding till 12 months. If found to be HIV positive through EID, continue breastfeeding till 2 years alongside appropriate ART. All children more than 6 months of age should be started on complementary feeding as per usual practice. Abrupt stopping of breast-feeding should NOT be done.

Anti-retroviral (ARV) prophylaxis

ARV prophylaxis to the infant must be given in accordance with the current National PPTCT Guidelines. For all exposed infants, oral Nevirapine (NVP) has to be given for 6 weeks regardless of whether the infant is exclusively breastfed or receives exclusive replacement feeding and these children have to be linked to the EID program **(Table 4)**. With effect from 1st January 2014, pregnant women who are found to be HIV positive are initiated on lifelong ART irrespective of CD4 count and WHO clinical Staging; their newborn (HIV exposed) babies are initiated on 6 weeks of Syrup Nevirapine immediately after birth so as to prevent transmission of HIV from mother to child and is extended to 12 weeks of Syrup Nevirapine if the duration of the ART of mother is less than 24 weeks.

Co-trimoxazole preventive therapy (CPT)

Oral co-trimoxazole is also given as prophylaxis for *Pneumocystis carinii* pneumonia, toxoplasmosis and other bacterial diseases for children below 5 years of age to reduce mortality and morbidity. CPT should be started from the age of 6 weeks till HIV is excluded. Once HIV is confirmed it should be continued till age of 5 years. The recommended dose is 5 mg/kg/day of trimethoprim (TMP) once daily.

Table 4: Dose and duration of Infant daily nevirapine prophylaxis[21]

Birth weight	*Dose of NVP (mg)*	*Dose of NVP (mL/kg)**
Birth weight < 2000 g	2 mg/kg once daily	0.2 mL/kg once daily
Birth weight 2000–2500 g	10 mg once daily	1 mL once daily
Birth weight >2500 g	15 mg once daily	1.5 mL once daily

*Considering the content of 10 mg Nevirapine in 1 mL suspension

HIV PEP for Occupational/Sexual Exposure

PEP must be started as soon as possible (ideally within 2 hours) to be effective—and always within 72 hours of a possible exposure.[26,27] PEP involves taking anti-HIV medicines every day for 28 days. PEP is not intended to replace regular use of other HIV prevention methods, such as consistent use of condoms during sex or pre-exposure prophylaxis (PrEP).[26] Important components are described below:

First aid

- Do not panic and ask for the help.
- Consult an expert physician for HIV exposure management.
- Clean the exposed area thoroughly.
- In case of an injury by needle or sharp instrument it is very important to immediately wash the wound and surrounding skin with water and soap, and rinse.
- Antiseptics and skin washes like bleach, chlorine, alcohol, betadine etc. are never to be used for wound care.
- Do not scrub.
- Do not squeeze or do not put injured finger in mouth.
- After a splash of blood or body fluids to unbroken skin: Wash the area immediately. Do not use antiseptic.
- *For the eye*:
  - Irrigate exposed eye immediately with water or normal saline.
  - Sit in a chair, tilt head back and ask a colleague to gently pour water or normal saline over the eye.
  - If wearing contact lens, leave them in place while irrigating, as they form a barrier over the eye and will help protect it.
  - Once the eye is cleaned, remove the contact lens and clean them in the normal manner. This will make them safe to wear again.
  - Do not use soap or disinfectant on the eye.
- *For mouth*: Spit fluid out immediately. Mouth should be thoroughly rinsed with saline or water and this should be repeated several times. Do not use soap or disinfectant in the mouth.

Establish the eligibility for PEP

This includes counseling, risk assessment, and testing of the source and exposed person.

- *Counseling*: Detailed and confidential counseling of the exposed person should be carried out about the risks and measures to be taken
- *Assessment of nature of exposure and risk of transmission*: The exposure can be mild, moderate and severe depending upon the type and amount of body fluid/ blood and portal entry. The risk of transmission depends on the amount of HIV transmitted (proportionate to the amount of contaminated fluid and the viral load). As an most urgent step, PEP should be started soon (within 72 hours as it is not effective if started after 72 hours), without waiting for the results of the source and the risk is to be evaluated soon. If it is found that risk is insignificant, PEP should be stopped.
- *Assessment of exposed person*: The exposed individual should be assessed for pre-existing HIV infection. Exposed individuals who are known or discovered to be HIV positive should not receive PEP. Such cases should be referred for clinical and laboratory assessment and if found eligible ART should be started. Counseling and detailed information on prevention of transmission are essential component of their management.

Counseling for PEP

- Exposed persons should receive appropriate information about PEP and the risk and benefits of PEP in order to provide informed consent. They should be clearly explained that PEP is not mandatory.
- Informed consent should be obtained before testing as per national HIV testing guidelines.
- Documentation of record is essential.

Regimens for PEP

There are two types of regimens: (1) Basic regimen which consists 2-drug combination (2) Expanded regimen having 3-drug combination. The decision to initiate the type of regimen depends on the type of exposure and HIV status of the source person.

Table 5 summarizes the regimens to be used in PEP for HIV. The 2-drug regimens could use AZT + 3TC, or d4T (Stavudine) + 3TC. 3-drug regimens need to be used after consulting experts. While NACO recommends 2 or 3 drug regimens, the international guidelines recommend

Table 5: Post-exposure prophylaxis (PEP) regimens for HIV

Exposure	*Status of source*		
	HIV+ and asymptomatic	*HIV+ and clinically symptomatic*	*HIV status unknown*
Mild	Consider 2-drug PEP	Start 2-drug PEP	Usually no PEP, or consider 2-drug PEP
Moderate	Start 2-drug PEP	Start 3-drug PEP	Usually no PEP, or consider 2-drug PEP
Severe	Start 3-drug PEP	Start 3-drug PEP	Usually no PEP, or consider 2-drug PEP

three drug regimes in all mucosal/percutaneous exposure irrespective of severity and host status.[25]

POST-EXPOSURE PROPHYLAXIS FOR DIPHTHERIA

Diphtheria is a serious bacterial infection which affects mucosa of nose and throat. It is an acute, toxin-mediated disease caused by the bacterium *Corynebacterium diphtheriae*. Human carriers are the reservoir for *C. diphtheriae* and are usually a symptomatic—Children act as transient carriers during diphtheria outbreaks.

Mode of Transmission

Most of the time person to person transmission occurs from the respiratory tract but rarely from skin lesions, fomites and contaminated articles. Transmission may occur as long as virulent bacilli are present in discharges and lesions. The time is variable, but without antibiotics, organisms usually persist 2 weeks or less and seldom more than 4 weeks. Chronic carriers may shed organisms for 6 months or more.[28] Effective antibiotic therapy promptly terminates shedding.

Prophylaxis

For close contacts like household contacts, a diphtheria booster (either Td or Tdap if no documentation of receipt of three-dose primary immunization series, or if last dose of vaccine was given more than five years ago), appropriate for age, should be given.

Chemoprophylaxis

All contacts should be treated with Benzathine penicillin G 600,000 units for persons younger than 6 years old and 1,200,000 units for those 6 years old and older, or a 7- to 10-day course of oral erythromycin 40 mg/kg/ day for children and 1 g/day for adults.[29] Contacts should be closely monitored and Diphtheria antitoxin should be started once signs of illness starts appearing. Identified carriers in the community should also receive antibiotics. Contacts of cutaneous diphtheria should be treated as described above; however, if the strain is shown to be nontoxigenic, investigation of contacts should be discontinued.

KEY MESSAGES

- Extensive flushing and meticulous wound care coupled with use of Rabies immunoglobulins or Rabies monoclonal antibodies and Anti rabies vaccine are the cornerstone of rabies prevention. Monoclonal antibodies provide cheaper and easily available alternative and must be infiltrated in to the wound only.
- The mainstay of Hepatitis B prevention is the timely use of Hepatitis B vaccine but in some case Hepatitis B immunoglobulins are to be used. This will go a long way for the prevention of chronic liver disease.
- PEP for HIV should be started as soon as possible within 72 hours of exposure and consists of use of Anti retrovirus agent daily for a period of 28 days. Perinatally exposed newborns are subjected to a 6 weeks course of a nevirapine as soon as possible after delivery Exclusive breastfeeding or exclusive replacement feeding on AFASS criteria should be offered.
- For close contacts of diphtheria, age appropriate booster dose of diphtheria containing vaccine along with 7 to 10 days course of oral penicillin or erythromycin is recommended.

REFERENCES

1. Tarantola A. Four thousand years of concepts relating to rabies in animals and humans, its prevention and its cure. Trop Med Infect Dis. 2017;2. pii: E5.
2. World Health Organization. Rabies vaccines: WHO Position Paper, April 2018 Recommendations. Vaccine. 2018;36:5500-3.
3. Goswami A. Safety and tolerance of equine rabies immunoglobulin in the Indian population. J Assoc Prev Control Rabies India. 2000;1:30-4.
4. Kundu R, Ramchandran P. Immunization against rabies. In: Thacker N, Shah NL, editors. Immunization in Clinical Practices, 2nd edition. New Delhi: Jaypee Brothers Medical Publishers; 2016. p. 235-43.
5. Bose A, Choudhury P. Rabies vaccines. In: Vashishtha V, Choudhury P, Bansal CP, Yewale VN, Agarwal R, editors. IAP Guidebook on Immunization 2013-2014. IAP National Publication House; 2013. p. 329-39.

6. Gogtay NJ, Munshi R, Ashwath Narayana DH, *et al.* Comparison of a novel human rabies monoclonal antibody to human rabies immunoglobulin for postexposure prophylaxis: A phase 2/3, randomized, single-blind, noninferiority, controlled study. Clin Infect Dis. 2018;66:387-95.
7. World Health Organization. WHO Guide for pre and post-exposure prophylaxis of rabies in humans. Available from: *https://www.who.int/rabies/PEP_prophylaxis_guidelines_June10.pdf.* Accessed August 17, 2019.
8. Acharya SK, Madan K, Dattagupta S, *et al.* Viral hepatitis in India. Natl Med J India. 2006;19:203-17.
9. Ott JJ, Stevens GA, Groeger J, *et al.* Global epidemiology of hepatitis B virus infection: New estimates of age-specific HBsAg seroprevalence and endemicity. Vaccine. 2012;30:2212-9.
10. Schillie S, Vellozzi C, Reingold A, *et al.* Prevention of hepatitis B virus infection in the United States: Recommendations of the advisory committee on immunization practices. MMWR Recomm Rep. 2018;67:1-31.
11. Centres for Disease Control and Prevention. Viral hepatitis—statistics and surveillance. Available from: *https://www.cdc.gov/hepatitis/statistics/.* Accessed August 17, 2019.
12. Expanded Programme on Immunization of the Department of Vaccines and Biologicals. Introduction of hepatitis B vaccine into childhood immunization services. Geneva: WHO; 2001. p. 48. Available from: *http://www.wpro.who.int/hepatitis/whovb0131.pdf.* Accessed August 17, 2019.
13. Mittal SK, Rao S, Kumar S, *et al.* Simultaneous administration of hepatitis B vaccine with other EPI vaccines. Indian J Pediatr. 1994;61:183-8.
14. Kumar TS, Abraham P, Raghuraman S, *et al.* Immunogenicity of indigenous recombinant hepatitis B vaccine in infants following 0, 1, 2 month vaccination schedule. Indian Pediatr. 2000;37:75-80.
15. Gomber S, Sharma R, Ramchandran VG, *et al.* Immunogenicity of Hepatitis B vaccine incorporated into Expanded Program of Immunization Schedule. Indian Pediatr. 2000;37:411-13.
16. Balasubramanian S, Shah A, Pemde HK, *et al.*; IAP Advisory Committee on Vaccines and Immunization Practices, 2018-19. Indian Academy of Pediatrics (IAP) Advisory Committee on Vaccines and Immunization Practices (ACVIP) Recommended Immunization Schedule (2018-19) and Update on Immunization for Children Aged 0 Through 18 Years. Indian Pediatr. 2018;55:1066-74.
17. World Health Organization. Hepatitis B vaccines: WHO position paper, July 2017-Recommendations. Vaccine. 2019;37:223-25.
18. American Academy of Pediatrics. American Academy of Pediatrics recommends that infants receive first Hepatitis B dose. Available from: *https://www.aap.org/en-us/about-the-aap/aap-press-room/Pages/AAP-Recommends-That-Infants-Receive-First-Hepatitis-B-Dose-Within-24-Hours-of-Birth.aspx.* Accessed August 17, 2019.
19. Kalra A, Kasi SG. Hepatitis B vaccine. In: Vashishtha V, Choudhury P, Bansal CP, Yewale VN, Agarwal R, editors. IAP Guidebook on Immunization 2013-2014. IAP National Publication House; 2013. p. 127-36.
20. Mast EE, Margolis HS, Fiore AE, *et al.*; Advisory Committee on Immunization Practices (ACIP). A comprehensive immunization strategy to eliminate transmission of hepatitis B virus infection in the United States: recommendations of the Advisory Committee on Immunization Practices (ACIP) part 1: immunization of infants, children, and adolescents. MMWR Recomm Rep. 2005;54(RR-16):1-31.
21. National AIDS Control Organization. Pediatric Antiretroviral Therapy Guidelines NACO 2013. Available from: *http://naco.gov.in/sites/default/files/Pediatric_14-03-2014.pdf.* Accessed August 17, 2019.
22. De Cock KM, Fowler MG, Mercier E, *et al.* Prevention of mother-to-child HIV transmission in resource-poor countries: translating research into policy and practice. JAMA. 2000; 283:1175-82.
23. WHO. Updated recommendations on first-line and second-line antiretroviral regimens and post-exposure prophylaxis and recommendations on early infant diagnosis of HIV Interim guidance. Available from: *https://www.who.int/hiv/pub/guidelines/ARV2018update/en/.* Accessed August 17, 2019.
24. WHO. Mother-to-child transmission of HIV. Available from: *https://www.who.int/hiv/topics/mtct/en/.* Accessed August 17, 2019.
25. Shah I, Karkera V. Antiretroviral therapy. In: Singhal T, Shah NK, Yewale V, Prabhu S, editors. Rational Antimicrobial Practice in Pediatrics (IAP Speciality Series), 3rd edition. New Delhi: Jaypee Brothers Medical Publishers; 2019. p. 384-98.
26. Preboth M. PHS guidelines for management of occupational exposure to HBV, HCV and HIV: Management of occupational blood exposures. Am Fam Physician. 2001;64:2012-4.
27. National AIDS Control Organization. Post Exposure Prophylaxis (PEP) - NACO Guidelines. Available from: *http://www.upsacs.in/pdf/GUIDELINES/PEP.pdf.* Accessed August 17, 2019.
28. Diphtheria: CDC pink book. Available from: *https://www.cdc.gov/vaccines/pubs/pinkbook/downloads/dip.pdf.* Accessed August 17, 2019.
29. Kulkarni P. Antimicrobial prophylaxis. In: Singhal T, Shah NK, Yewale V, Prabhu S, editors. Rational Antimicrobial Practice in Pediatrics (IAP Speciality Series), 3rd edition. New Delhi: Jaypee Brothers Medical Publishers; 2019. p. 343-54.

CHAPTER 50

Dermatological Emergencies

Atul Mohan Kochhar, Anuva Bansal

INTRODUCTION

Dermatological emergencies are life-threatening conditions attributed to the impairment in the structure and functioning of the cutaneous barrier. These conditions can be the outcome of syndromes ranging from benign transient skin diseases to potentially fatal systemic disorders. The prognosis of affected patients is serious and a prompt diagnosis in such cases is imperative. Various pediatric dermatological emergencies commonly present to a pediatric care facility and require a timely, multidisciplinary approach for their successful management. Since, several early cutaneous signs that initially seem benign, if neglected can result in fatal outcomes, pediatricians must be adequately sensitized to the early diagnosis and management of such cases.

EPIDEMIOLOGY

Dermatological conditions occurring in children and adolescents often first present to the pediatrician and constitute on an average 30% of all outpatient visits to a pediatrician.[1] Pediatric emergencies with cutaneous complaints is a wide spectrum and discerning these 'true dermatological emergencies' with a potential fatal outcome is crucial. Cutaneous dermatoses are responsible for around 4% of all pediatric emergencies with only 30% of these constituting true emergencies.[2,3]

In India, the incidence of dermatological emergencies has been reported by a few studies. One such study from a large tertiary care hospital reports that 103 such cases were seen over a year. The definition of pediatric dermatological conditions in this study included dermatological conditions in the children, which could be potentially severe or life-threatening; any case which was regarded as a dermatological emergency by the pediatrician but was not confirmed by the dermatologist was omitted. Objective scores have also been used for assessing severity of cutaneous disorders in children <18 years of age. **Table 1** summarizes the Nelson's severity index scoring system wherein patients are categorized as "very sick" when score was ≤7.[4]

Table 1: Nelson's severity index scoring system

Parameter	*0*	*1*	*2*
Respiratory effort	Labored/Absent	Some distress	No distress
Color	Cyanotic	Pale/Flushed/Mottled	Normal
Activity	Delirium/Stupor/ Coma	Lethargy	Normal
Temperature	<97.4 or >104°F	101.1–104°F	97.4–101°F
Play	Refuses to play	Decreased	Normal

Total score: 10 not sick; 8–9 moderately sick; ≤ 7 very sick

EPIDEMIOLOGY

Age-wise distribution of dermatological emergencies was described by a hospital-based Indian study as 15.5% neonates, 9.7% infants, 36.9% preschool and 37.2% school-going children.[1] The etiology of dermatological emergencies also tends to vary based on the age, and this shall be further elucidated in the next section.

PATHOPHYSIOLOGY

Dermatological emergencies result in what is known as "acute skin failure", a destruction of the structure and functioning of the skin. This loss of the normal skin barrier leads to fluid and electrolyte imbalance, metabolic abnormalities, altered thermoregulation, altered hemodynamics, altered immune function and disruption of the normal cutaneous homeostasis. This can culminate into acute renal failure, sepsis, high output cardiac failure, hypothermia, or hyperthermia, and a catabolic state resulting from an increased basal metabolic rate.[5] This has been depicted in **Flowchart 1**.

ETIOLOGY

The causes of dermatological emergencies in the pediatric age-group are many and various classification systems exist in order to provide a better understanding of these conditions. They have been variously classified as *primary and secondary*. Among the primary conditions, involvement of the skin is the major manifestation or cause whereas in the latter group, the cutaneous manifestations are secondary to underlying systemic involvement. The etiology may be categorized as *congenital and acquired* as well. *Age-wise* distribution of etiology has been described in **Box 1**. This is a practical approach, since the age-group based incidence of each etiology tends to vary due to age-related differences in anatomy and physiology. However, for the purpose of this discussion, we will elucidate the most common and practical classification based on the antecedent dermatological process as denoted in **Box 2**. Each of these causes will be discussed in greater detail in the following sections.

Box 1: Important causes of dermatological emergencies in various age-groups

Important causes of dermatological emergencies in various age-groups	
Neonatal period	Hereditary conditions: Ichthyosis, epidermolysis bullosa bacterial infections dermatological reactions associated with NICU seborrheic dermatosis
Post-neonatal period	Severe atopic dermatitis Infantile seborrheic dermatitis
Pre-school age	Infections
School going children (including adolescents)	Drug reactions

Flowchart 1: Pathophysiology and consequences of acute skin failure

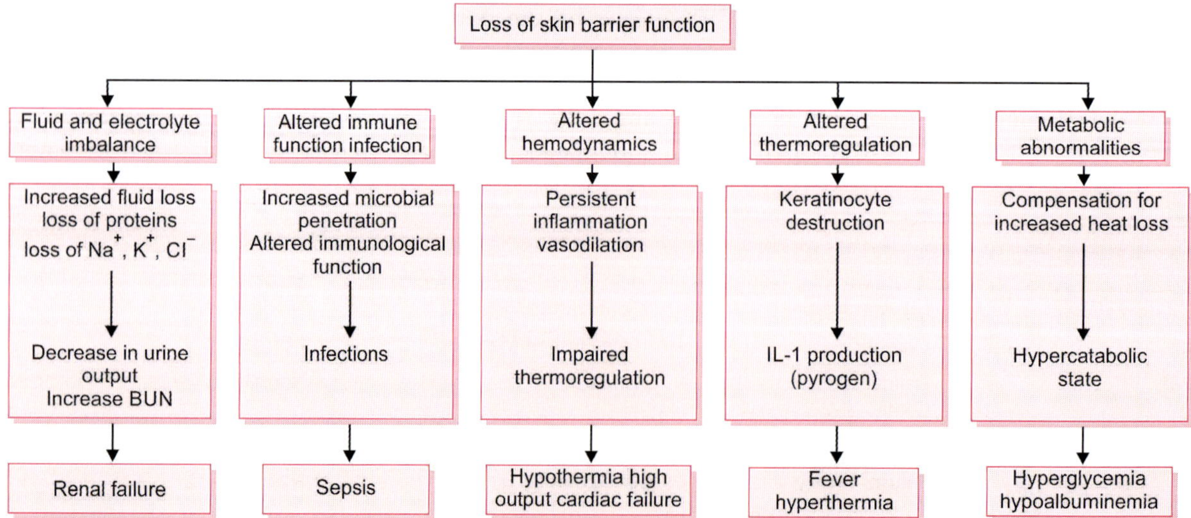

Box 2: Common causes of dermatological emergencies in the pediatric age-group

Causes of pediatric dermatological emergencies

1. Erythroderma (of various causes)
2. Urticaria and angioedema
3. Infections
4. Drug reactions
5. Metabolic conditions
6. Hereditary conditions
7. Miscellaneous

ERYTHRODERMA (EXFOLIATIVE DERMATITIS)

Definition

It is defined as redness and scaling involving greater than 90% of the body surface area and is a potentially life-threatening condition with a loss of the normal structure and function of the skin. It is the most common dermatological emergency and requires prompt diagnosis and management. It can be acute or chronic, and has a nonspecific disease pattern induced by various primary or secondary causes.

Etiology

The causes of erythroderma in children tend to differ from those in adults. According to a study done among neonates in a tertiary care center in Delhi, infections were the most common cause of erythroderma (40%), followed by ichthyosiform erythroderma (25%), atopic dermatitis (15%) and infantile seborrheic dermatitis (10%). Idiopathic erythroderma was reported in 10% of the cases.[6] In children, the most common causes of erythroderma were drugs (29%), psoriasis (18%), geno-dermatoses (18%), infections including staphylococcal scalded skin syndrome (18%), was reported from a tertiary care center in Delhi.

Clinical Features

The clinical features tend to vary (**Figs. 1 and 2**) and the child may present with the primary cutaneous lesions which tend to spread, or with a widespread erythema from the start (extends rapidly and becomes generalized in 12–48 hours). Scaling appears in 2–3 days, most commonly beginning in the flexures. The types of scales tend to vary based on the primary etiology and have been described below. Associated burning, itching and a tense, hot, palpably thickened skin is present in this stage (acute). Fever, lymphadenopathy, pedal edema, tachycardia, hepatomegaly may also be variably associated. With erythroderma becoming chronic, alopecia may set in along with nail dystrophy, ectropion and pigmentary changes. The important causes of childhood erythroderma, their clinical features and relevant investigations have been outlined in **Tables 2 and 3**.

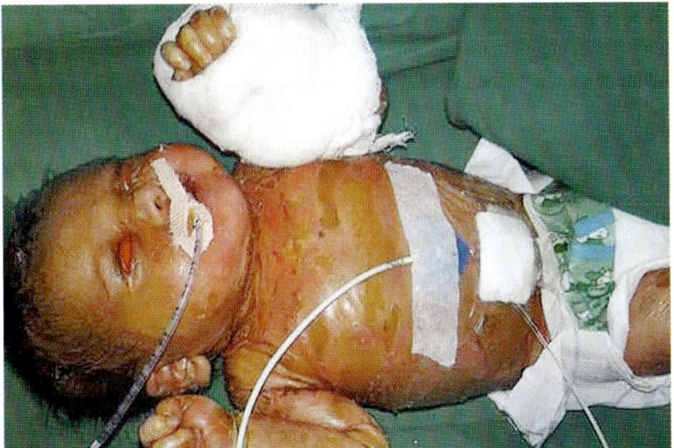

Fig. 1: Congenital ichthyosiform erythroderma. Neonate was born with a collodion membrane, ectropion and eclabium

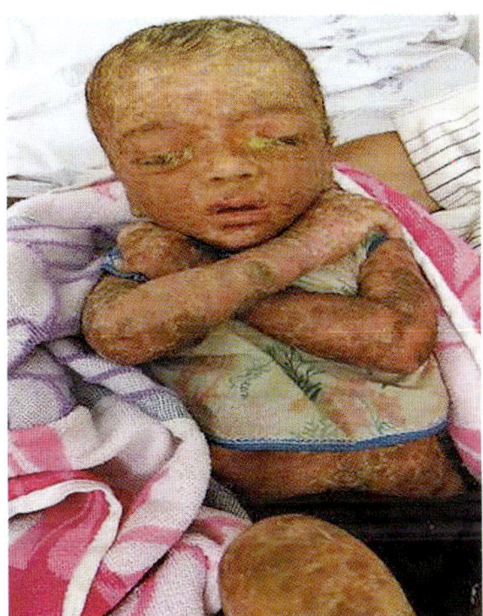

Fig. 2: Psoriatic erythroderma. Erythematous plaques with thick scales are seen all over the body, primarily the extensor surfaces. Involvement of the scalp is seen—a clue to the diagnosis

Complications

Erythroderma is characterized by a persistent inflammation of the skin, which can culminate into acute skin failure as outlined in **Flowchart 1**. It is thus a potentially life-threatening condition, which can lead to the following complications:

Table 2: Important etiologies of childhood erythroderma, clinical features and investigations

		Clinical features	*Investigations*
1.	**Infections and infestations**		
a.	Staphylococcal scaled skin syndrome (*Staphylococcus aureus*)	Most cases < 5 yrs Fever, skin tenderness, flexural and facial erythema which may coalesce into erythroderma; within 24 hours- large, flaccid, sterile bullae followed by erosions Positive Nikolsky sign	Microbiology - • Skin smears • Blood cultures
b.	Scarlet fever (*Streptococcus pyogenes* Group A)	Fever, chills, sore throat, sandpaper like rash on trunk and extremities, Pastia's lines (petechial streaks in the flexures), strawberry tongue, desquamation over palms and soles occurs later	Clinical diagnosis; Supportive serologies and isolation of group A streptococci from the pharynx.
c.	Congenital cutaneous candidiasis	Affected neonate presents with an erythematous maculopapular/ pustular or bullous lesion which may evolve into erythroderma; palmoplantar and periumbilical involvement, sparing of oral cavity and nappy area	*Full term babies*: 10% KOH mount – budding yeast cells *Pre-term LBW neonates*: Blood, urine and cerebrospinal fluid (CSF) cultures
2.	**Drug induced erythroderma** • Exfoliative rash • DRESS • SJS-TEN	History of sulfonamides, anti-epileptics, antimalarials, penicillin, isoniazid, thioacetazone, streptomycin, NSAIDs, topical tar, homeopathic and ayurvedic medicines, captopril, cimetidine and ampicillin Pruritus is prominent Nikolsky positive: SJS/TEN	Clinical diagnosis Temporal correlation Hemogram Peripheral eosinophilia Biopsy may show eosinophils +/- necrotic keratinocytes.
3.	**Ichthyosis**		
a.	Congenital ichthyosiform erythroderma (Fig. 1)	Collodion membrane at birth which is shed revealing erythroderma; ectropion, eclabium, palmoplantar keratoderma, alopecia	Clinical diagnosis Skin biopsy Electron microscopy Genetic analysis
b.	Harlequin ichthyosis	Neonates are born with truncal plates with fissuring; ectropion and eclabium are present. Around 10% of children develop auto-amputation of digits; infection; respiratory problems are the major cause of death in neonates. In those children who survive the critical phase -large lamellar scales with marked ichthyosiform erythroderma develops	
c.	Epidermolytic hyperkeratosis	Severe bullous lesions after birth, with widespread erosions, severe ichthyosiform erythroderma *Later-* hystrix-like hyperkeratoses and marked palmoplantar hyperkeratosis	
d.	Conradi-Hunermann's syndrome	Female neonates with ichthyosiform erythroderma; usually associated with hyperkeratosis and scaling following Blaschko's lines Extracutaneous features, which include frontal bossing, hearing loss, cataracts, punctate bone calcifications, mental retardation	
e.	Netherton syndrome	Ichthyosis linearis circumflexa- double edged scales; trichorrhexis in vaginata or bamboo hair and atopic diathesis, failure to thrive, chronic diarrhea	
4.	**Atopic dermatitis**	Onset below 2 years of age, history of atopy Pruritic, erythematous papules, plaques or vesicles *Infantile phase (2–18 months)* Face, extensors of elbows, knees in infants *Childhood phase (18–24 months)* Erythema, crusting, lichenification- elbow and knee flexures	Clinical diagnosis based on history and examination

Contd...

Contd...

		Clinical Features	*Investigations*
5.	**Infantile seborrheic dermatitis**	First few months of life Erythematous plaques with yellowish *greasy scales*- scalp (cradle cap), the napkin area and other intertriginous zones Generally transient, may progress to erythroderma	Clinical diagnosis
6.	**Immunodeficiency syndromes**		
a.	Omenn's syndrome	Lymphadenopathy, hepatosplenomegaly, elevated serum IgE and eosinophilia, failure to thrive; Pruritic eczematous lesions, nail dystrophy, alopecia	• Serum IgE • Peripheral eosinophilia • Skin biopsy: Hyperplasia, spongiosis, basal cell vacuolation, dermal inflammatory infiltrate
b.	Leiner disease	Most severe form of infantile seborrheic dermatitis with diarrhea and failure to thrive	Clinical diagnosis-More of a cutaneous phenotype for a number of underlying immunodeficiency disorders rather than a specific entity
7.	**Metabolic and nutritional disorders**		
a.	Multiple carboxylase deficiency	Starts in infancy with a facial/perioral eczematous rash; alopecia with loss of hair color; neurological involvement: convulsions, developmental delay, ataxia; metabolic acidosis, hyperammonemia, tachypnea	Diagnosis is suggested by urine organic acids analysis and confirmed by indirect holocarboxylase synthetase enzyme assay or DNA mutation analysis
b.	Essential fatty acid deficiency	Dry, scaly rash, hair loss, hair depigmentation, poor wound healing, growth restriction, infections	Elevated triene:tetraene ratio elevated liver function tests hyperlipidemia, thrombocytopenia altered platelet aggregation
c.	Protein malnutrition	Loss of subcutaneous fat, prematurely aged appearance, *flaky paint* dermatitis, brittle hair and nails, red-brown hair with *flag sign*	Clinical diagnosis Serum proteins, electrolytes serum iron, complete blood count
8.	**Inflammatory disorders**		
a.	Psoriasis (Fig. 2)	Erythematous scaly plaques which may generalize Pustules can also develop In neonates- psoriatic erythroderma presents as a recalcitrant diaper dermatitis which may become generalized	History of triggers- drugs, infections, stress Clinical diagnosis Pustules-Gram stain is sterile Histopathology for confirmation
b.	Pityriasis rubra pilaris	Follicular horny plugs on the knees, elbows, and dorsum of digits is characteristic. Islands of normal looking skin persist in the erythrodermic regions. Palmoplantar skin is thickened and has a typical orangish hue. The familial form has an autosomal dominant inheritance pattern	Clinical diagnosis Histopathology for confirmation
c.	Diffuse cutaneous mastocytosis	Presents in the neonatal period with diffuse skin thickening with a doughy consistency, bullae and erosions can develop; Systemic complications including diarrhea	History, examination for hepatosplenomegaly, CBC, DLC, LFT, Serum tryptase; Skin biopsy: mast cell infiltration – full thickness skin infiltration

- Secondary infections and septicemia
- Metabolic complications—hypoalbuminemia, hyperglycemia
- Hypothermia or hyperthermia
- Dehydration
- Electrolyte abnormalities—hypernatremia, hypokalemia.

Table 3: Work-up for a case of pediatric erythroderma

Investigations	*Etiology*
Gram stain, culture-skin swab, blood	SSSS, scarlet fever
KOH mount	Candidiasis
Complete hemogram, peripheral smear	Metabolic and nutritional disorders, diffuse cutaneous mastocytosis, infections
Lipid profile	Essential fatty acid deficiency
Hair mount	Ichthyosis – to see hair shaft abnormalities
Bone-marrow examination	Immunodeficiency syndromes, mastocytosis
Immunoglobulins and complement levels	Immunodeficiency syndromes
Plasma-amino acid levels	Protein energy malnutrition
Serum zinc and alkaline phosphatase levels	Acrodermatitis enteropathica
Biotinidase/ holocarboxylase synthetase levels	Multiple carboxylase deficiency
Genetic analysis	Ichthyosis
Skin biopsy	Serial skin biopsies may be needed for confirmation of primary etiology as the initial changes are common to all and are nonspecific
Ophthalmological evaluation	Ichthyosis

Management

The management of erythroderma, irrespective of the underlying cause consists of the following:[5-7]

1. Shift the patient in isolation in a warm-humid environment (30–32°C).
2. Withdraw all non-essential drugs.
3. Monitor the vitals—blood pressure, pulse rate, temperature, respiratory rate and input and output.
4. Administer IV fluids, correct electrolytes as needed.
5. Correct calorie and protein deficit—consider nasogastric tube feed or parenteral nutrition. An estimated energy intake of 120–130 kcal/kg/day is required to achieve a normal weight gain of 15 g/kg/day. The glucose infusion should provide 50–70% of energy requirement. The rest of the calorie is provided by lipids and the daily requirement of protein is 3–3.5 g/kg/day.[7]
6. Send an arterial or capillary blood gas analysis, serum electrolytes, hemogram, IgE.
7. Send cultures (blood, urine, skin swabs) if frank pus discharge is present or if suspecting infection; administer antibiotics accordingly.
8. Restore the cutaneous barrier—ensure barrier nursing, liberal use or bland emollients or paraffin gauze dressing is recommended.
9. After initial stabilization, a dermatology opinion must be taken to delineate the cause of the erythroderma and manage the patient accordingly (**Flowchart 2**).

Flowchart 2: Management of neonatal and childhood erythroderma

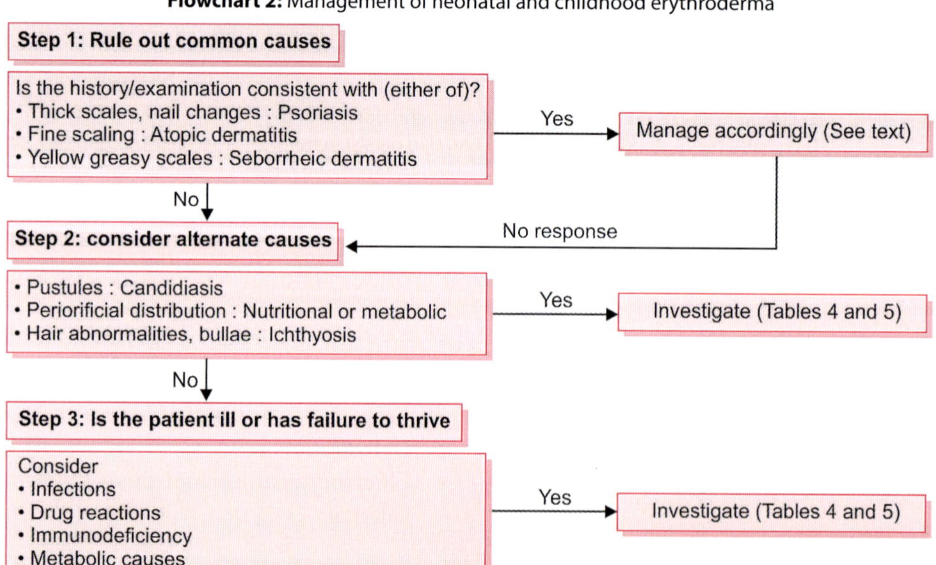

10. Further management will require a multidisciplinary team effort.

- A detailed history and examination are required to identify the cause.
- Common causes of erythroderma should be ruled out first and managed accordingly.
- Topical corticosteroids are required for the management of psoriasis and atopic dermatitis and are generally initiated after initial 1–2 weeks of conservative management.
- Appropriate investigations for the diagnosis of other causes must be sent as advised by the dermatologist.
- Specific systemic therapy is initiated once the primary cause has been identified.
- The efficacy of systemic retinoids in the treatment of ichthyosis except Netherton syndrome is well established. However, risk/benefit ratio is considered before using retinoids because of increased skin fragility and decreased barrier competence induced by them.[7]

Prognosis

Prognosis depends to a large extent on the primary etiology. Erythroderma secondary to drugs, seborrheic dermatitis, nutritional deficiencies and infections tends to have a good prognosis. Atopic dermatitis, psoriasis and pityriasis rubra pilaris tend to be chronic and recurrent with periodic flare-ups; and require specific and long-term systemic therapy. Ichthyotic erythroderma can be life-threatening at the onset and has a chronic course with a poor response to treatment. In a study on childhood erythroderma, the mortality was found to be around 16% and was attributed to both the primary cause as well as the complications.

URTICARIA AND ANGIOEDEMA

Definition

Urticaria is used to describe a condition characterized by the development of well-demarcated transient, pruritic, erythematous or pink dermal swellings known as '*wheals*', which occur as a result of dermal edema. These fade within hours with no residual changes. Urticaria can be acute (<6 weeks' duration) or chronic (>6 weeks' duration). It is also classified as spontaneous or idiopathic urticaria and inducible or physical/contact urticaria. Angioedema refers to a deeper swelling of the dermis, subcutaneous or submucosal tissue. These lesions are more painful than itchy, are ill-defined, with no skin discoloration and tend to persist for a longer duration than wheals. They can accompany wheals; however, when present alone it can be either mast cell mediated or bradykinin mediated.

Epidemiology

In children below 16 years of age, isolated urticaria is known to occur in around 85% cases, angioedema in 6% and both in around 9% cases. However, in children less than 3 years of age, angioedema is quite common and is seen in around 60% cases.

Etiology

Urticaria may occur at any age; although children often present with acute urticaria. Acute spontaneous urticaria can occur due to immediate hypersensitivity, allergy to food or drugs; however, in more than 50% cases the cause remains unknown.

In infants who are being exclusively breastfed, the main cause is cow's milk allergy, while in older children, infections especially viral and drugs are one of the most common causes of acute urticaria, and physical factors constitute an important cause of chronic urticaria in this age group.

In many cases, especially of chronic urticaria, the cause of the urticaria and/or angioedema remains unknown, however, in such cases triggering and contributing factors need to be identified and removed. **Table 4** illustrates the common causes of urticaria.

Clinical Features

Urticaria is characterized by wheals presenting as edematous lesions with a halo of erythema, and can vary in size from papules to larger lesions measuring several centimeters (**Fig. 3**). Lesions may coalesce to produce different patterns such as annular or oval. A bulla may develop at the center of lesion in rare cases. The lesions tend to resolve in a few hours leaving clinically normal skin, and cases with lesions persisting for >24 hours must be evaluated for urticarial vasculitis. In infants, lesions may become hemorrhagic and resemble erythema multiforme. Angioedema, edema of limbs and acrocyanosis may accompany these lesions.

Angioedema commonly affects the lips, tongue, oral cavity and pharynx. Involvement of the lips especially with an associated swelling/burning of tongue or buccal mucosa may be indicative of a food allergy. Laryngeal edema is uncommonly seen otherwise, and is a feature of hereditary angioedema.

Anaphylaxis is a rapidly developing dermatological emergency, which may start as palmoplantar itching, tingling of the soft palate followed by nausea, vomiting and wheezing. It may lead to hypotension, bronchospasm, and cardiac arrhythmias, thus warranting immediate attention. Urticaria and angioedema may also be associated.

Hereditary angioedema (HAE)

Recurrent episodes of angioedema characterized by swelling of the face, neck and extremities without urticaria, starting commonly in the adolescent age group, are suggestive of hereditary angioedema. It is more common in females, is autosomal dominant and is caused by a genetic deficiency of the inhibitor of complement 1 (C1 INH) as a result of the deletion or mutation of its gene present on chromosome.[11] Three subtypes have been recognized as outlined in **Table 5**. It is important to recognize that urticaria is not commonly seen associated with HAE. Moreover, the edema in these cases is painful and more persistent as compared to the other causes of angioedema. Patients may present with fatal airway obstruction or severe abdominal pain as a result of laryngeal and bowel edema respectively.

Table 4: Causes of urticaria in children

Type	*Causes*
Idiopathic	Multifactorial
Infections	Viral, e.g. upper respiratory tract infections, hepatitis B and C Bacterial, e.g. *Streptococcus pyogenes* Parasitic, e.g. *Anisakis simplex*
Food	Nuts, seeds, eggs, cow's milk, meat, fish, food color, preservatives
Drugs	Beta-lactams, aspirin, local anesthetics
Vaccines	Tetanus, measles, hemophilus b, hepatitis b
Stings	Bees, wasp venom
Others	Latex.
Physical	Cholinergic, cold, heat, pressure, solar, aquagenic, vibration
Systemic disease	SLE, Juvenile rheumatoid arthritis, mastocytosis
Metabolic	Autoinflammatory syndromes, TRAPS, Hyper-IgD syndrome

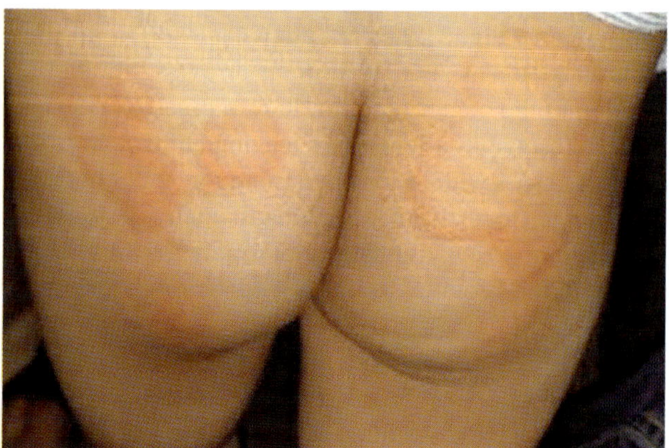

Fig. 3: Urticaria on the buttock region—A typical wheal is seen—edematous lesion a halo of erythema

Differential Diagnosis

Urticaria must be differentiated from few other conditions such as:

- Erythema multiforme—hemorrhagic lesions of urticaria in infants can resemble this
- Acute hemorrhagic edema
- Anaphylactoid Henoch Schönlein purpura
- Papular urticaria, insect bites
- Mastocytosis
- Annular erythema of infancy
- Urticarial vasculitis.

Differential diagnosis of angioedema includes:

- Acute hemorrhagic edema
- Contact dermatitis
- Erysipelas, cellulitis.

Management

In acute urticaria, the management starts with a detailed history aimed at identifying and removing any causative agent or trigger. In most cases, no additional work-up is required. In patients with chronic urticaria, after a detailed history and examination, few investigations are warranted such as hemogram, erythrocyte sedimentation rate, C-reactive protein, and liver function tests. Autoantibody testing may be needed including an antinuclear antibody test. In case of hypereosinophilia, stool microscopy may be needed to rule out parasitic infestation.

Table 5: Types of hereditary angioedema

Types of HAE	*Characteristics*
Type 1 HAE (85% cases)	• Gene deletion • Loss of protein to 40% of normal • Associated decreased C2 and C4
Type 2 HAE	• Gene mutation • Qualitative defect of C1 inhibitor
Type 3 HAE	• X-linked form • Described in adults

Acute and chronic urticaria both respond to treatment with antihistamines, which decrease the associated pruritus and wheals. General measures such as avoiding triggers—nuts, egg, meat, drugs, excessive heat, etc.; wearing loose fitting clothes; application of soothing lotions—calamine, menthol creams should be explained to every patient. The first line treatment in both cases is second generation antihistamines at usual doses (**Table 6**). Generally, treatment is required for up to a week in cases of acute urticaria and for several months in chronic urticaria. In case of no response or only partial relief even after two weeks of therapy, current recommendations **(Flowchart 3)** suggest increasing the dose of antihistamines to four times the usual doses.[8] If symptoms still persist, it is recommended to add anti-IgE monoclonal antibody—omalizumab (150 or 300 mg subcutaneous every 4 weeks, in adolescents >12 years of age). Another third line add on therapy is cyclosporine A and is recommended only for patients with severe disease refractory to any dose of antihistamine and omalizumab in combination due to its higher incidence of adverse events. Current recommendations suggest that there is low level of evidence for the efficacy of leukotriene antagonists such as Montelukast in the management of chronic spontaneous urticaria. For acute urticaria and acute exacerbations of CSU, a short course of oral corticosteroids, for maximum 10 days, may be helpful to reduce disease duration and activity.[8-10] In children with severe angioedema or anaphylactic shock, treatment with subcutaneous adrenaline (0.01 mg/kg), along with fluid replacement and appropriate resuscitation measures, is indicated. Corticosteroids are also infused during the treatment of anaphylactic shock. In cases of an acute attack of HAE, infusion of a purified inhibitor concentrate is the treatment of choice.

Table 6: Second-generation anti-histamines for trearing urticaria

Drug	*Adult dose*	*Pediatric dose and preparation*
Cetirizine	10 mg OD	Syrup: 5 mg/5 mL • 6 months to 2 years: 2.5 mg OD • 2 to 5 years: 2.5 mg OD-BD • 6 years or older: 5 to 10 mg OD
Levocetirizine	5 mg OD	Syrup: 2.5 mg/5 mL • 6 months to 5 years – 1.25 mg OD • 6 to 11 years – 2.5 mg OD • 12 years and older – 2.5 to 5 mg
Loratadine	10 mg OD	Syrup: 5 mg/5 mL • 2–5 years: 5 mg once daily • 6 years and over: usual adult doses
Desloratadine	5 mg OD	Syrup: 2.5 mg/5 mL • 6 months–6 yrs: 1.25 mg OD • 6 yrs–11 yrs: 2.5 mg OD
Fexofenadine	60 mg BD 180 mg OD	Syrup: 30 mg/5 mL 6–11 yrs: 30 mg BD

Flowchart 3: Management of urticaria

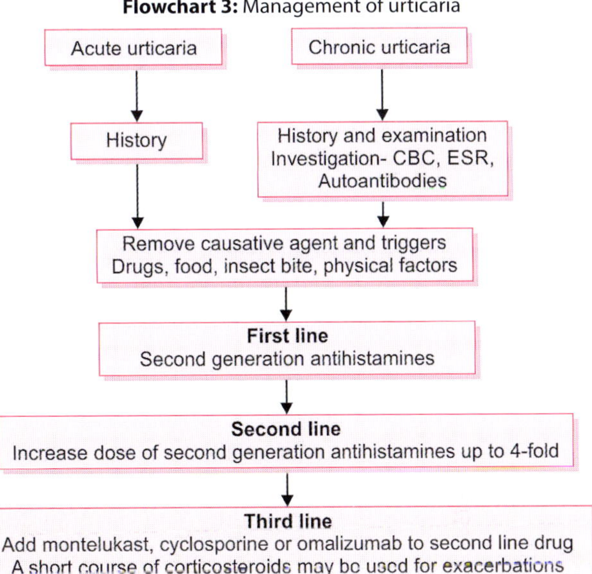

INFECTIONS PRESENTING AS CUTANEOUS EMERGENCIES

Some infections can present as a dermatological emergency. Most of these present as erythroderma and have been partially covered in the same section.

STAPHYLOCOCCAL SCALDED SKIN SYNDROME

Staphylococcal scalded skin syndrome (SSSS) is characterized by a generalized exanthem progressing to erythroderma, associated with cutaneous tenderness and widespread superficial blistering and denudation, caused by toxin producing *Staphylococcus aureus.*

Etiology

Staphylococcal exfoliative toxins are serine proteases that bind to the cell adhesion molecule desmoglein 1, which is expressed in the upper part of the epidermis, leading to epidermolysis between the stratum spinosum and granulosum. The risk factors, especially in adults include a compromised immune response and impaired toxin-neutralizing antibodies or renal insufficiency, which decreases the clearance of the toxin. Associated conjunctivitis, otitis media, nasopharyngeal infection, or a pyogenic skin infection may serve as staphylococcal foci from which the toxin is released and disseminated hematogenously.

Clinical Features

Most cases of SSSS occur in infants and children, and in those adults who have an underlying risk factor. It presents initially as an orange-red macular rash or uniform erythema associated with cutaneous tenderness. The rash spares the mucosal surfaces, and has a typical periorificial and flexural accentuation. Within 1–2 days the erythema and rash associated with a typical superficial tissue paper-like wrinkling, progresses to large flaccid bullae in flexural and periorificial regions. A positive Nikolsky sign can be elicited at this stage by stroking the skin resulting in a superficial blister. The epidermis is shed in large sheets, revealing a moist underlying erythematous base and may resemble burns. Fever may be associated, however the patient rarely looks toxic.

Investigations

Tzanck smear may show acantholytic cells. Cultures obtained from an intact blister are usually sterile. The diagnosis can be confirmed by a skin biopsy specimen, which can be expedited by frozen section processing which confirms the superficial level of cleavage. Histopathology shows acantholytic cells in the granular layer with shedding of the stratum corneum in the desquamative stage. Electrolyte abnormalities may be associated and require monitoring.

Differential Diagnosis

Generalized SSSS should be differentiated from toxic epidermal necrolysis (TEN). SSSS tends to occur in neonates and infants, never has mucosal erosions, is associated with acantholysis as seen on a Tzanck smear and epidermal separation is below the stratum granulosum. In contrast, TEN may occur in any age group, is preceded by a history of drug intake, has associated mucosal erosions, with no evidence of acantholysis and full-thickness epidermal necrosis and dermal-epidermal separation seen on histopathology.

Management

Patients with mild, localized disease may be discharged on oral antibiotics, however close follow-up is recommended. More severe cases benefit from admission to a burn unit when possible. Patients of SSSS require hospitalization and incubators to maintain temperature and humidity may be required for neonates. Vital monitoring, supportive skin care, management of potential fluid, and electrolyte abnormalities are essential and has been outlined in detail in the section on erythroderma. Management of skin involves the use of non-adherent dressings, including paraffin-impregnated gauze. Topical antibiotics such as mupirocin 2% ointment or fusidic acid 2% cream, should be applied twice daily to the affected areas, including the original focus of infection. Systemic antibiotic therapy is the keystone of management, and parenteral therapy is recommended. Nafcillin or Oxacillin is recommended for methicillin-sensitive *Staphylococcus aureus* (MSSA). Vancomycin should be administered if methicillin-resistant *Staphylococcus aureus* (MRSA) is suspected, especially in those with recent healthcare exposure or in areas with a high prevalence of MRSA. Furthermore, topical antibiotics alone are not effective, and even localized SSSS should be treated with systemic antibiotics.[11]

Prognosis

Resolution over 2–3 weeks is the usual outcome. The mortality in uncomplicated pediatric SSSS is very low (2%) and is not usually associated with sepsis.

TOXIC SHOCK SYNDROME

This is a serious life-threatening illness mediated by toxins produced by *Staphylococcus aureus* or *Streptococcus pyogenes* and is characterized by fever, erythema, epidermal denudation, circulatory shock and multiorgan failure.

Etiology

This syndrome was first reported to occur among menstruating women using highly absorbent tampons and the incidence decreased with the discontinuation of this particular type of tampon. The condition is common in the extremes of age as well as women of the reproductive age group. Underlying or preceding varicella, cellulitis, immunosuppression, malignancy constitute risk factors for varicella. Toxic shock syndrome (TSS) toxin 1 is produced by 80–90% of *S. aureus* isolates from affected cases and is able to stimulate T-lymphocyte proliferation in a non-antigen-specific manner resulting in fever, inflammation and shock. Rarely, it may be associated with infection caused by *Streptococcal pyogenes*. Non-menstrual TSS is associated with postsurgical wounds, burns, intravenous drug abuse, osteomyelitis, etc.

Clinical Features

It presents with acute onset of fever, sore-throat and myalgia. Diarrhea, vomiting and hypotension may also occur. The rash consists of a diffuse macular blanching erythema and scaling on the trunk, which spreads to extremities and is followed by palmoplantar desquamation. Multiorgan dysfunction may be associated deeming this condition to be potentially life threatening. Local signs of an infectious focus including pain, erythema and pus discharge may be present and careful wound examination is necessary in any case presenting with fever, hypotension and rash.

Investigations

All routine hematological and biochemical testing including liver function tests and kidney function tests is required to rule out any systemic involvement or multiorgan dysfunction. Cultures from skin swab, pus, throat, blood and cerebrospinal fluid may have to be sent and may come out to be positive for *Staphylococcus aureus*.

Differential Diagnosis

The differential diagnosis includes septic shock, staphylococcal exfoliative syndromes, viral hemorrhagic fever, Rocky mountain spotted fever, and Stevens-Johnson syndrome.

Treatment

Treatment is supportive and aimed eradicating *S. aureus*. Conventionally, beta lactamase resistant antibiotics such as nafcillin have been used, however, with the increasing frequency of methicillin resistant strains - a combination of vancomycin and clindamycin is preferred.

Intravenous immunoglobulins are used for severe or recalcitrant cases.

Prognosis

Mortality rate of TSS is around 5% in healthy individuals, however, recurrence may be seen.

SCARLET FEVER

This syndrome is caused by exotoxin producing group A *Streptococcus* and is characterized by a scarlatiniform rash, fever and pharyngitis, and most commonly occurs in early spring and winter.

Etiology

Scarlet fever is caused by group A *Streptococcus* which produces exotoxin that acts as a super antigen. Almost 10% of children who develop streptococcal pharyngitis go on to develop this syndrome.

Clinical Features

It begins 1–5 days after exposure with sudden onset pharyngitis, headache, vomiting, abdominal pain and fever. One to two days later the rash starts with the neck and trunk and spreads to the extremities, sparing the palms and soles. The rash is erythematous, with a sandpaper like texture. Around the skin folds, lines of confluent petechiae called Pastia's sign may be seen. The exanthem begins to fade 3–4 days after onset and a desquamation phase begins. Tonsillitis is commonly associated and a tender cervical lymphadenopathy is common. Tongue is typically red with prominent papillae known as the "strawberry tongue".

Differential Diagnosis

Kawasaki disease is an important differential and differs in that the course of fever is prolonged and cultures are negative.

Treatment

The treatment of scarlet fever includes antibiotics to eradicate *Streptococcus* and a localized nidus of infection like an abscess should be drained.

CONGENITAL CUTANEOUS CANDIDIASIS

This is a rare condition in newborn infants whose mother has an intrauterine *Candida* infection prior to delivery.

Etiology

Cutaneous candidiasis may be acquired in-utero and is known as congenital cutaneous candidiasis; and if acquired during passage through an infected birth canal it is known as neonatal candidiasis.

Clinical Features

Congenital infection presents as a generalized rash with macules, papules and/or pustules on an erythematous base, most commonly over back, extremities, skin folds, which tends to spread and may lead to erythroderma. It invariably involves the palms and soles, where pustular lesions are typically seen. The diaper area is usually spared and oral mucosa is uncommonly affected. The lesions resolve with desquamation in 1–2 weeks.

Differential Diagnosis

Congenital cutaneous candidiasis may resemble neonatal bacterial infections, transient neonatal pustulosis and congenital syphilis.

Investigations

The diagnosis can be confirmed by the demonstration of the yeast cells in a 10% potassium hydroxide mount or a positive culture of *Candida* species. Specimens should be examined for the presence of round or oval budding yeast cells of 2–4 μm in size.

Treatment

It responds well to topical antifungals such as nystatin or an azole except for those who are premature or low birthweight who typically require systemic therapy with agents such as fluconazole or amphotericin.

Prognosis

Full-term infants with congenital candidiasis generally follow a benign course and respond well to topical therapy. However, there is a potential for systemic involvement among premature and low birthweight infants.

DRUG REACTIONS

Drug reactions constitute a common dermatological emergency, and may present as erythroderma, and constitute one of the most common causes for the same, in children and adolescents. Drug reactions leading to erythroderma has been covered in a previous section.

Drug Reaction with Eosinophilia and Systemic Symptoms (DRESS)

It represents a rare but potentially fatal drug reaction. It is characterized by fever, maculopapular rash, lymphadenopathy and internal organ involvement. It commonly has a delayed onset, and presents almost 3 weeks after the initial drug exposure.

Etiology

DRESS is postulated to be a type IV hypersensitivity reaction to the bioactivated drug metabolite. Drugs most commonly implicated are aromatic anticonvulsants (phenytoin, carbamazepine, phenobarbital, oxcarbazepine) and lamotrigine. Other implicated agents include allopurinol, vancomycin, minocycline, sulfasalazine, aspirin, nevirapine and dapsone.

Clinical features

Symptoms begin up to 3 weeks after intake of the implicated drug. The syndrome begins with high grade fever (> 38.5°C), malaise, followed by the development of a polymorphous rash which starts rom the face and proceeds craniocaudally, which may be maculopapular or morbilliform and may show follicular accentuation. The rash can evolve into erythroderma in almost 40% cases. Vesicobullous lesions and targetoid lesions may also be seen. Cheilitis, conjunctivitis may also be seen in up to 50% cases. Facial edema and lymphadenopathy are common features. Systemic involvement may be delayed by up to a few weeks. Most children suffer from mild features. Hepatic dysfunction, acute kidney injury are the most commonly observed internal manifestations. Central nervous, respiratory and cardiac involvement can also occur. Hematological abnormalities are seen in more than 70% patients, and include peripheral leukocytosis ($>11\times10^9$/L), atypical lymphocytosis (>5%) and eosinophilia ($>1.5 \times 10^9$/L).

Complications: Fulminant liver failure is the most severe and life-threatening complication of DRESS. Others include a delayed onset interstitial nephritis, interstitial pneumonitis, autoimmune thyroid dysfunction and myocarditis have also been described.

Investigations

A temporal correlation with the drug intake, typical clinical features and investigations can be used to diagnose DRESS syndrome using the Regi SCAR criteria[12] mentioned in **Table 7**. Appropriate investigations for diagnosis and delineating extent of organ involvement include hemogram, LFT, KFT, peripheral smear, gamma-glutamyl transferase, alkaline phosphatase, serology for hepatitis A, B, C and mycoplasma and echocardiography. Cultures from various sites may be necessary to rule out sepsis.

Table 7: DRESS can be diagnosed using the regiSCAR DRESS scoring system	
Clinical features	*Score*
Extent of rash >50% body surface area	1 point
Rash suggestive of DRESS	1 point
Systemic involvement: • **Lymphadenopathy** – ≥2 sites, ≥1 cm. A maximum 1 point gained from lymphadenopathy • **Eosinophilia** – 10–19% of total white cell count = 1 point; ≥20% = 2 points – ≥20% = 2 points (if total leukocytes $<4 \times 10^9$/L, an eosinophil count of 0.7–1.5 $\times 10^9$/L will gain 1 point, an eosinophil count $\geq 1.5 \times 10^9$/L will score 2 points) • **Atypical lymphocytosis** – 1 point • **Organ involvement** – Liver: transaminases >2 × upper limit of normal (ULN) on two successive dates *or* bilirubin × 2 ULN on 2 successive days *or* aspartate aminotransferase (AST) – γ-glutamyl transferase (GGT) and alkaline phosphatase >2 × ULN on one occasion – Renal: creatinine 1.5 × patient's baseline – Cardiac: echocardiographic evidence of pericarditis. Maximum of 2 points gained from internal organ involvement – ≥3 of the following performed and negative: hepatitis A, B and C; *Mycoplasma/* chlamydia; antinuclear antibody; blood culture (performed ≤3 days after hospitalization)	Maximum 6 points
Relevant negative serological tests	1 point

Differential diagnosis

Differential diagnoses include bacterial and viral infections, which can be ruled out by sending cultures. Other differentials include: acute generalized exanthematous pustulosis (AGEP) which is characterized by flexural distribution of pustules, erythema multiforme-characterized by acral distribution of lesions and target lesions, Stevens Johnson syndrome and toxic epidermal necrolysis (SJS-TEN). Latency of onset of lesions in DRESS can help to differentiate it from these conditions.

Treatment

Identify and discontinuation of the culprit drug is of foremost importance. Rest of the management is similar to what has been discussed in the sections on erythroderma and SSSS. Isolation, barrier nursing, fluid and electrolyte correction, thermoregulation are essential. Care of the skin includes liberal emollient application, and topical corticosteroid in some cases. Specific management in the event of internal organ involvement and sepsis is required. A short course of systemic corticosteroids (oral prednisolone 1 mg/kg/day; tapering-off period varying from 1 to 3 months, or 1 g/day methyl prednisolone × 3 days)[13] may be needed for active disease and refractory or chronic cases may require treatment with agents such as cyclosporine. Other treatment options include intravenous immunoglobulin (IVIg) and plasmapheresis.

Stevens-Johnson Syndrome/ Toxic Epidermal Necrolysis

This entity constitutes a severe mucocutaneous reaction, most commonly to drugs and is characterized by epithelial sloughing. It can be frequently associated with systemic complications and can result in multiorgan failure and death, thus carrying an appreciable mortality rate. Severity of the process ranges from SJS to SJS-TEN overlap to the most severe variety, i.e. TEN.

Etiology

SJS/TEN is characterized by widespread skin and mucosal epithelial keratinocyte destruction, initiated in most cases by drug-induced cytotoxic T lymphocytes. Fas-Faslig and interaction, granzyme and perforins have all been implicated in causing keratinocyte apoptosis. Common drugs causing SJS/TEN have been enlisted in **Box 3**. Anti-epileptics, nonsteroidal anti-inflammatory drugs (NSAIDs) and antibiotics are the most commonly implicated groups. In almost 15% cases, where a culprit drug is not identified, infections, such as that caused by *Mycoplasma penumoniae* are common triggers. Moreover, certain individuals possess genetic susceptibility to the development of drug induced SJS/TEN. Strong genetic predisposition to the development of carbamazepine-induced SJS/TEN in individuals bearing HLA-B*1502 and an association of HLA-B*5801 with allopurinol-induced SJS/TEN is known.

Clinical features

Prodrome: The condition begins after a latent period of 7–10 days, after the initiation of the implicated drug with fever, malaise and upper respiratory tract symptoms, which constitutes the prodrome.

Cutaneous and mucosal involvement: The rash develops a few days later, starting with the face and chest **(Fig. 4)**, gradually spreading over the entire body, and may be accompanied by pruritus and/or pain. The earliest lesions are purpuric macules or atypical targets. Involvement of the palms and soles with target lesions (usually atypical) is often prominent. The lesions tend to increase in size and number over the next few days and coalesce leading to the production of vesicles, bullae and large areas of confluent erythema **(Fig. 5)**. Blistering and epidermal detachment ensues, producing large areas of denuded dermis **(Fig. 6)**. Detachable epidermis is demonstrated by a positive Nikolsky sign, in which gentle lateral pressure causes lesional epidermis to slide over the dermis. Erosive and hemorrhagic mucositis of the conjunctival, oral and genital mucosae is common. Painful mucosal erythema with subsequent blistering, ulceration of the oral cavity is seen, with adherent hemorrhagic crusts over the vermillion border of the lips and mucosal involvement may extend to the oropharynx, larynx, respiratory tract and esophagus. Around 25% of the patients may develop pulmonary complications, early in the disease. SJS/TEN is classified based on cutaneous lesions and the extent of maximal epidermal detachment[14] as shown in **Table 8**.

Box 3: Commonest drugs causing SJS/TEN

- Allopurinol
- Carbamazepine
- Lamotrigine
- Nevirapine
- Oxicam nonsteroidal anti-inflammatory drugs
- Phenobarbital
- Phenytoin
- Sulfamethoxazole
- Sulfasalazine

Differential diagnosis: The differential diagnoses include disorders that can present with vesico-bullous lesions, erosions and/or mucosal membrane involvement **(Table 9)**. Erythema multiforme major (EMM) closely resembles SJS, as both have less than 10% epidermal detachment and mucous membrane involvement. However, few key differences exist and have been described in **Table 10**.

Investigations

Investigations are needed to (a) support the diagnosis, (b) exclude other blistering disorders, and (c) identify systemic complications. These include hemogram, LFT, KFT, blood glucose, bicarbonate, erythrocyte sedimentation rate, amylase levels, C-reactive protein, coagulation studies,

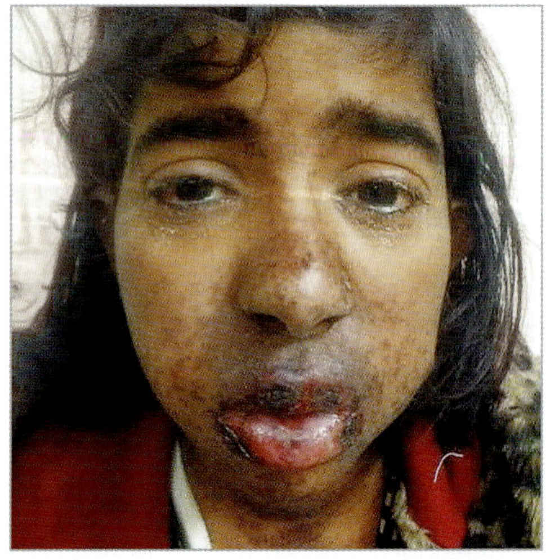

Fig. 4: Coalescent purpuric macules and hemorrhagic crusting in a case of Stevens-Johnson syndrome

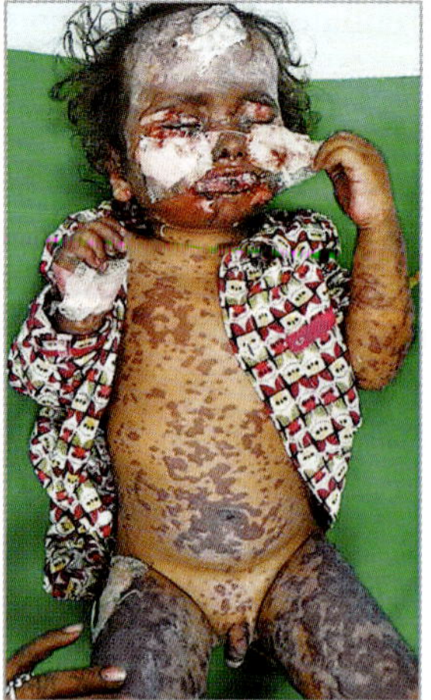

Fig. 5: Purpuric macules coalescing to form hemorrhagic bullae with predominant facial, truncal and proximal limb involvement in TEN. The body surface area involved is >30%

Mycoplasma serology and anti-nuclear antibody testing and chest X-ray. A biopsy from lesional skin should be sent for routine histopathology. A second biopsy taken from perilesional skin should be sent for direct immunofluorescence to exclude an immunobullous disorder. Swabs should be taken from affected skin and sent for culture. The extent of epidermal detachment should be recorded and the percentage of BSA involved should be estimated.

Complications

Acute complications: Epidermal detachment leads to the loss of the normal skin barrier leading to fluid and electrolyte imbalance, metabolic abnormalities, altered thermoregulation, hemodynamics, and immune function as well as the disruption of the normal cutaneous homeostasis. This is known as "acute skin failure" and has been described in detail in a previous section of the chapter (*see* **Flowchart 1**). Further anemia and leukopenia are common during the acute phase. The commonest life-threatening complication of acute SJS/TEN include septicemia, caused initially by *Staphylococcus aureus* and later by gram-negative rods from the digestive flora, especially *Pseudomonas aeruginosa*. This can frequently result in multiorgan dysfunction and death.

Late complications: These are long-term sequelae that can affect the survivor's quality of life and include: post-inflammatory dyspigmentation; onychomadesis (shedding of nails); telogen effluvium, corneal/conjunctival ulceration and scarring, dry eye, entropion, and gingival synechiae.

Long-term complications involving the systemic organs include: bronchiolitis obliterans, esophageal stricture, intestinal ulceration, vaginal adhesions. Finally,

Fig. 6: Superficial erosions and epidermal detachment is seen at sites of friction in TEN

Table 9: Differential diagnosis of SJS/TEN

Group of disorder		*Specific condition*
Drug reactions		• Erythema multiforme major • Acute bullous fixed drug eruption • Acute generalized exanthematous pustulosis
Immunobullous	*Intraepidermal*	• Pemphigus vulgaris • Paraneoplastic pemphigus
	Subepidermal	• Mucous membrane pemphigoid • Bullous pemphigoid • Bullous lupus erythematosus • Linear IgA bullous dermatosis
Infections		• SSSS • Erythema multiforme major

Table 10: Key differences between erythema multiforme major and Stevens Johnson syndrome

Parameters	*Erythema multiforme major*	*Stevens Johnson syndrome*
Lesions	Typical target lesions	Atypical targets
Distribution	Limbs and extremities	Trunk
Etiology	• Herpes simplex reactivation-common • Drugs-rare	• Drugs- common • Infection - rare

Table 8: Classification of severity in SJS/TEN[14]

Category	*Extent of epidermal detachment*	*Extent of purpura*
SJS	Epidermal detachment less than 10% BSA	Widespread purpuric macules or flat atypical targets
Overlap SJS-TEN	Detachment of 10–30% BSA	Widespread purpuric macules or flat atypical targets
TEN with spots	Detachment greater than 30% BSA	Widespread purpuric macules or flat atypical targets

the survivors of SJS/TEN suffer psychological sequelae, including post-traumatic stress disorder.

Management

The principals and pillars of management of SJS/TEN have been elaborated in **Table 11.**[12,15,16]

Prognosis: Score of ten (SCORTEN) **(Tables 12 and 13)** is a predictor of the severity of illness for SJS and TEN and is a useful parameter for predicting the mortality.[21] It is calculated on day 1, day 3 and day 5 of the illness. In general, the mortality of SJS is <5%, whereas around 30% of patients diagnosed with TEN die during the acute stage of the illness.

KEY MESSAGES

- Erythroderma, urticaria and angioedema, infections and drug reactions, are the most common dermatological emergencies.
- Erythroderma constitutes redness and scaling involving >90% of the body surface area and can be the end point of several conditions.
- Urticaria is used to describe a condition characterized by the development of well-demarcated transient, pruritic, erythematous or pink dermal swellings known as 'wheals', which occur as a result of dermal edema. Urticaria can be acute (<6 weeks duration) or chronic (>6 weeks). Angioedema refers to a deeper swelling of the dermis, subcutaneous or submucosal tissue.
- Infections presenting as a dermatological emergency include staphylococcal scalded skin syndrome, scarlet fever, and congenital cutaneous candidiasis.

Table 11: Management of SJS/TEN

Initial assessment	Evaluation and monitoring	• Detailed history and examination • Vital monitoring—temperature, pulse rate/ heart rate, blood pressure, input-output charting, oxygen saturation • Order baseline investigations—arterial blood gas analysis, hemogram, LFT, KFT, electrolytes, glucose, chest X-ray
Initiate primary management	Initial stabilization	• Establish peripheral venous access • Insert a nasogastric tube, if oral intake is affected • Urinary catheterization if significant urogenital involvement
Determination of causative drug	Detailed drug history–past 2 months Consider latent period of 7–10 days	• Discontinue all non-essential drugs
Care environment	If BSA>10%–Shift to ICU or burns unit	• Isolation • Barrier nursing • Ambient temperature—30–32°C • Humidity • Pressure relieving mattresses
Care team	Multidisciplinary approach	• Dermatologist • Intensive care specialist • Pediatrician/Physician • Ophthalmologist
Management of skin and topical therapy	Avoid shearing forces, trauma to prevent further loss of epidermis	• BP cuff, adhesive ECG leads to be used carefully • Proper patient positioning
	Restore the skin barrier	• Detached epidermis can be left *in situ- acts as biological dressing* • Blisters can be decompressed by fluid aspiration and the blister roof retained • Bland emollient—50% white soft paraffin with 50% liquid paraffin [white soft paraffin (WSP)] • Dressing • Paraffin gauze- preferred • Silicone dressings • Skin grafts
	Prevent secondary infection	• Barrier nursing • Skin swabs for cultures to be sent every 3rd day • Blood cultures—periodically • Cleansing using—weak antiseptic wash or warmed sterile water • Topical antibiotics—sloughy or crusted areas • Necrotic or infected epidermis that is fully detached may be removed

Contd...

Contd...

Local therapy for mucous membranes	Eyes • Lubrication • Prevention of synechiae formation • Prevention of infection	• Examination by ophthalmologist • Ocular lubricant—2 hourly (carboxy methylcellulose) • Ocular hygiene • Daily removal of pseudomembranes • Adhesiolysis using glass rod and lubricant gel daily • Broad spectrum antibiotic eye drops • Eye-pads/normal saline gauze to remove crusts
	Mouth • Hygiene • Analgesia	• Normal saline gauze to remove crusts • Topical emollient/antibiotic—framycetin cream • Antiseptic mouth wash—chlorhexidine • Choline—salicylate + lignocaine gel can be used half hour before feeds/meals
	Urogenital tract • Prevent infection • Prevent adhesions	• Hygiene • Emollient • Topical antibiotic cream • Topical corticosteroids—fluticasone propionate, betamethasone valerate 0.1% • Catheterization
Fluid, electrolytes and nutrition[15,17]	• Prevent fluid loss • Replace fluids • Prevent over-zealous fluid replacement • Enteral nutrition is preferred	• Establish peripheral intravenous access through non-lesional skin • Replace fluids (Ringer Lactate)– First 24 hours 2 mL × Body weight × BSA affected Half of this- first 8 hours Rest over 16 hours After 24 hours Use urine output to guide management With improvement in oral involvement- increase oral fluids • Nasogastric tube insertion • Energy requirements (in calories) for pediatric SJS/TEN patients is estimated by the following equation- **Daily requirement in calories =** **(Pre-injury weight [kg] × 9 24.6)** + **(Wound size [% of BSA] × 4.1)** + **940 calories**
Analgesia	NSAIDs are not recommended	Opiates are preferred for analgesia—Morphine
Supportive medication	• Gastric protection • Prevention of leukopenia and anemia	• Proton-pump inhibitors • Granulocyte-colony stimulating factor—treatment of severe neutropenia
Prevention and management of infection	• Send cultures frequently • Avoid unnecessary antibiotics • Monitor closely for signs of sepsis	• Swabs for bacterial and *Candida* culture should be taken from at least 3 sites particularly sloughy or crusted areas, throughout the acute phase • Antibiotics only if there are clinical signs of infection • Fever can be part of SJS/TEN- monitor other signs of sepsis – Confusion – Hypotension – Reduced urine output – Reduced oxygen saturation – Rise in CRP
Active therapy	• Early intervention during active stages • No randomized controlled trials available • Strength of recommendation- D[15]	• IVIg should be administered early, preferably within 48 h of onset of clinical disease at a total dose of 3 g/kg over a period of 3–5 days[18] • Systemic corticosteroids in the first 6 days—may decrease ocular complications[19] • Cyclosporine is given at 3–6 mg/kg for 1 week followed by a tapering course.[20]

Table 12: SCORTEN - Score of TEN

Prognostic factors	*Points*
Age >40 years	1
Heart rate >120/min	1
Cancer or hematological malignancy	1
>10% Body surface area	1
Serum urea >10 mmol/L	1
Bicarbonate <20 mmol/L	1
Serum glucose >14 mmol/L	1

Table 13: Mortality rates as determined by SCORTEN

SCORTEN	*Mortality rates*
0–1	3.2%
2	12.1%
3	35.8%
4	58.3%
>5	90%

- Drug reaction with eosinophilia and systemic symptoms (DRESS) is characterized by fever, maculopapular rash, lymphadenopathy and internal organ involvement. It commonly has a delayed onset, and presents almost 3 weeks after the initial drug exposure. Identify and discontinuation of the culprit drug is of foremost importance.
- Stevens-Johnson syndrome/toxic epidermal necrolysis constitutes a severe mucocutaneous reaction, most commonly to drugs such as antiepileptics, NSAIDs and antibiotics. Mucosal involvement is almost universal.
- Management of SJS-TEN includes discontinuation of culprit drug, vital monitoring, fluid, electrolyte and nutritional support, avoidance of infections and skin care. Skin care includes leaving the detached epidermis in situ, decompressing large bullae, application of bland emollient and dressing. Management of mucosal membranes includes hygiene, daily cleaning, emollient application prevention of adhesions and infection.

REFERENCES

1. Mathias RC, Jayaseelan E, Augustine M. Spectrum of pediatric dermatological emergencies at a tertiary care hospital in India: A descriptive study. Int J Dermatol. 2013;52:27-31.
2. Dolan OM, Bingham EA, Glasgow JF, *et al.* An audit of dermatology in a pediatric accident and emergency department. J Accid Emerg Med. 1994;11:158-61.
3. Auvin S, Imiela A, Catteau B, *et al.* Pediatric skin disorders encountered in an emergency hospital facility: A prospective study. Acta Derm Venereol. 2004;84:451-4.
4. Nelson KG. An index of severity for acute pediatric illness. Am J Public Health. 1980;70:804-7.
5. Inamadar AC, Palit A. Acute skin failure: Concept, causes, consequences and care. Indian J Dermatol Venereol Leprol. 2005;71:379-85.
6. Sarkar R. Neonatal and infantile erythroderma: 'The red baby'. Indian J Dermatol. 2006;51:178-81.
7. Ragunatha S, Inamadar AC. Neonatal dermatological emergencies. Indian J Dermatol Venereol Leprol. 2010;76: 328-40.
8. Zuberbier T, Aberer W, Asero R, *et al.* The EAACI/GA(2)LEN/EDF/WAO guideline for the definition, classification, diagnosis and management of urticaria. The 2017 revision and update. Allergy. 2018;73:1393-414.
9. Asero R, Tedeschi A. Usefulness of a short course of oral prednisone in antihistamine-resistant chronic urticaria: A retrospective analysis. J Investig Allergol Clin Immunol. 2010; 20:386-90.
10. Vena GA, Cassano N, Colombo D, *et al.* Cyclosporine in chronic idiopathic urticaria: A double-blind, randomized, placebo-controlled trial. J Am Acad Dermatol. 2006;55:705-9.
11. Ross A, Shoff HW. Staphylococcal Scalded Skin Syndrome. [Updated 2018 Oct 27]. In: StatPearls [Internet]. Treasure Island (FL): Stat Pearls Publishing; 2019 Jan. Available from: *https://www.ncbi.nlm.nih.gov/books/NBK448135/*. Accessed July 26, 2019.
12. Walsh S, Lee HY, Creamer D. Severe cutaneous adverse reactions to drugs. In: Griffiths C, Barker J, Bleiker T, Chalmers R, Creamer D, editors. Rook's Textbook of Dermatology, 9th edition. West Sussex: John Wiley & Sons; 2016. p. 1191-23.
13. Chiou CC, Yang LC, Hung SI, *et al.* Clinicopathological features and prognosis of drug rash with eosinophilia and systemic symptoms: A study of 30 cases in Taiwan. J Eur Acad Dermatol Venereol. 2008;22:1044-9.
14. Bastuji-Garin S, Rzany B, Stern RS, *et al.* Clinical classification of cases of toxic epidermal necrolysis, Stevens-Johnson syndrome, and erythema multiforme. Arch Dermatol. 1993; 129:92-6.
15. Creamer D, Walsh SA, Dziewulski P, *et al.* UK guidelines for the management of Stevens-Johnson syndrome/toxic epidermal necrolysis 2016. Br J Dermatol. 2016;174:1194-227.
16. Gupta LK, Martin AM, Agarwal N, *et al.* Guidelines for the management of Stevens- Johnson syndrome/toxic epidermal necrolysis: An Indian perspective. Indian J Dermatol Venereol Leprol. 2016;82:603-25.
17. Das S, Ramamoorthy R. Stevens-Johnson syndrome and toxic epidermal necrolysis in children. Indian J Paediatr Dermatol. 2018;19:9-14.
18. Ye LP, Zhang C, Zhu QX. The effect of intravenous immunoglobulin combined with corticosteroid on the progression of StevensJohnson syndrome and toxic epidermal necrolysis: A Meta-analysis. PLoS One. 2016;11:e0167120.
19. Araki Y, Sotozono C, Inatomi T, *et al.* Successful treatment of Stevens-Johnson syndrome with steroid pulse therapy at disease onset. Am J Ophthalmol. 2009;147:1004-11.
20. Law EH, Leung M. Corticosteroids in StevensJohnson syndrome/toxic epidermal necrolysis: Current evidence and implications for future research. Ann Pharmacother. 2015;49:335-42.
21. Bastuji-Garin S, Fouchard N, Bertochi M, *et al.* SCORTEN: A severity of illness score for toxic epidermal necrolysis. J Invest Dermatol. 2000;115:149-53.

CHAPTER

51

Gynecological Emergencies

Bindiya Gupta, Divya Chauhan

INTRODUCTION

The most common reasons for which a child may present to a gynecologist in the emergency room include abdominal/pelvic pain, vaginal bleeding, discharge and genital trauma. Timely and appropriate treatment is imperative for not only a successful outcome but also to prevent long-term morbidities and sequelae that may have an impact on future fertility and wellness. A very important aspect in adolescent medicine is psychological counseling to prevent unwanted pregnancy, knowledge on safe sexual practices, contraception and careful medicolegal approach to issues regarding sexual abuse. In this chapter, we will be dealing with common gynecological conditions seen in emergency department, their etiology, approach to diagnosis and management.

LOWER ABDOMINAL PAIN

Important gynecological causes for lower abdominal pain in children include ovarian/adnexal torsion, mullerian abnormalities, ectopic pregnancy and tubo-ovarian abscess and pelvic inflammatory disease. Besides gynecological causes, other differential diagnosis including appendicitis, diverticulitis, cystitis, renal stones etc. should always be considered.

OVARIAN/ADNEXAL TORSION

Introduction

Ovarian torsion is defined as complete or partial rotation of the ovarian vascular pedicle, thereby leading to impedance of blood supply to the ovary causing ischemia. When the fallopian tube twists along with the ovary, it is referred to as adnexal torsion. Early diagnosis is important to preserve the function of the ovaries. Surgery remains the mainstay of diagnosis and treatment.[1]

Epidemiology

Adnexal torsion is responsible for 2.7% to 7.4% of all gynecological emergencies in all age groups.[2] In children, the incidence is approximately 2%.[3] The mean age at presentation is 14.5 years and half of them are seen in Caucasians.[4] In a retrospective analysis of 5 years, Gupta, *et al.*[5] evaluated 94 benign and malignant ovarian masses in adolescent girls and reported that the most common presentation was pain abdomen (54%) and ovarian torsion was seen in 5%.

Ovarian torsion can occur both before or after menarche and one of the studies reported an incidence of as high as 67% in premenarchal girls.[6] It accounts for up to 30% of ovarian surgeries in children.[7] It is more common in benign ovarian cysts than malignancy.

Etiology and Pathogenesis

When ovarian torsion occurs, there is twisting of the adnexa around both the infundibulo-pelvic and the tubo-ovarian ligaments. Adnexal mass predisposes the ovary to torse on the axis of the infundibulo-pelvic and utero-ovarian ligaments. In fact, a finding of an adnexal mass of size ≥5 cm in size has a 83% sensitivity for predicting ovarian torsion.[8] Greater the size of the mass, more the risk of torsion until the mass becomes large enough to be fixed in the pelvis. In addition, fixed masses such as malignancies are less likely to undergo torsion. The incidence of malignancy in ovarian torsion is around 1.8%. In premenarchal girls up to 50% of torsed ovaries are normal.[9] Torsion is more common in the post-ovulatory period.[10] Ovarian torsion occurs in normal ovaries due to the longer utero-ovarian ligament in young age. The right ovary appears to torse more frequently than the left, possibly because the right utero-ovarian ligament is longer than the left and/or that the presence of the sigmoid colon in the left side may help to prevent torsion.[11] Prior ovarian torsion is also a risk factor and recurrent torsion occurs in 11% of cases.[12] Twisting of the infundibulo-pelvic ligament obstructs the lymphatic and venous outflow and arterial inflow leading to ovarian infarction. **Figure 1** shows the type of cysts in children.

Clinical Features

The child typically presents with acute onset of severe pelvic pain along with nausea and vomiting, seen in 70% cases. This occurs due to vagal reflex as a result of the pain. Rarely, fever may also be present. Low grade fever may be present in some patients with torsion. Most patients (70%) have pelvic and/or abdominal tenderness.[13] Tenderness may be localized to the side of the adnexal mass or may be diffuse. Palpable pelvic mass may or may not be present. Peritoneal signs, if present, should raise concern for adnexal necrosis. Failure to promptly diagnose torsion can lead to ovarian necrosis and loss of ovarian function; peritonitis may follow.

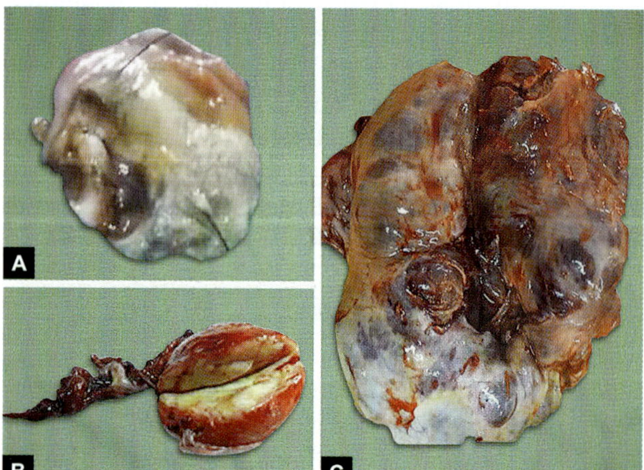

Figs. 1A to C: Ovarian cysts in adolescents. (A) Dermoid cyst after cystectomy; (B) Ovarian fibroma with torsion of fallopian tube; (C) Malignant germ cell tumor

Differential Diagnoses

The differential diagnoses of acute pelvic pain with an adnexal mass include ruptured ovarian cyst, tubo-ovarian abscess and ectopic pregnancy. Acute appendicitis can mimic adnexal torsion.

Laboratory Evaluation

There is no biochemical investigation for the diagnosis of adnexal torsion. Leukocytosis may be present. However, there is no correlation between leukocytosis and necrosis of ovarian tissue.

Imaging

Trans-abdominal ultrasonography with full bladder is the imaging modality of choice for patients with suspected ovarian torsion. Unilateral ovarian enlargement of more than 4 cm is common in adnexal torsion. Signs of ovarian ischemia such as increase in the size of the ovary, multiple small follicles and thickening of the interfollicular tissues may be seen. This occurs as a result of edema and vascular engorgement. Finally, the ovary may appear like an anechoic halo due to occlusion of arterial supply resulting in hemorrhage and infarction. Sometimes, no abnormality is seen on sonography. The sensitivity of ultrasound in diagnosing torsion is 40–75%.[14] Doppler may show a whirlpool sign of the twisted and coiled vessels, decreased or absent Doppler flow within the ovary. However, due to the dual blood supply of ovary, flow can be present even in the presence of torsion. Almost 60% of cases of torsion are missed by Doppler. However, its positive predictive value is 100%. Doppler cannot detect interruption of venous flow, which precedes arterial interruption. Therefore, a normal Doppler study cannot exclude the possibility of adnexal torsion. Other imaging modalities like CT scan or MRI may contribute as second line methods of imaging in case of inconclusive ultrasound. Out of the two, MRI is preferable as there is no radiation exposure.[15]

Shwartz, *et al.*[16] have developed a composite scoring system for premenarchal and menarchal girls based on three parameters: vomiting, total adenexal volume of the affected ovary and adenexal volume ratio (ratio of volume of affected ovary/unaffected ovary). Total score was 6; and if the score was < 2 there was least probability of torsion.

Management

Surgery provides the definitive diagnosis by direct visualization of the rotated adnexa. Laparoscopy is preferred unless malignancy is suspected. Ovarian conservation is of paramount importance. Despite the blue black appearance of ovary due to venous engorgement, arterial perfusion is still preserved for several days, preserving the physiological function of the ovary. Ovarian conservation rates are variable and range from 0% to 86% across several studies.[17,18] Hubner, *et al.*[19] showed that over time the rates of ovarian conservation have increased from 47.6% (1988–2002) to 85.6% (2004–2013). Studies have shown that the approach to surgery varies between the category of surgeons; pediatric gynecologists tend to perform ovarian conservation or detorsion 8–15 times more than pediatric surgeons.[20]

Ovarian detorsion

The torsed ovary should be untwisted and inspected for viability. Viable ovary should be conserved. It was hypothesized that untwisting the ovarian pedicle leads to release of thrombi causing pulmonary embolism. Studies have shown that there is no increase in the number of thromboembolic events after untwisting of adnexa, which used to be the concern with the conservative approach till recently.[21] After detorsion, ovarian cystectomy is done. In rare cases, when ovarian malignancy is suspected especially when the ovarian mass is more than 8 cm, frozen section analysis of adnexal masses should be performed and on confirmation, appropriate management should be followed. An ultrasound should be done after 3 months of ovarian detorsion to document follicles; however, it should be done sooner in case a neoplasm was suspected.

Oophorectomy or Salpingo-oophorectomy

Sometimes, salpingo-oophorectomy of the twisted adnexa has to be done if signs of necrosis are present or if clear signs of malignancy are evident.

Prevention

Ovarian torsion may recur. Recurrence is more in pre-menarcheal girls with normal ovaries and causes include long and lax utero-ovarian ligaments and long fallopian tube. Unilateral or bilateral oophoropexy following ovarian detorsion has been shown to prevent recurrence in a few studies.[22] The ovary is pexed to the peritoneum of the posterior wall of the abdomen maintaining the tubo-ovarian anatomic relationship using 3 anchoring vicryl 5-0 sutures. The argument against oophoropexy is that it alters the anatomy and interferes with the blood supply and function of the fallopian tube. It may be considered in cases of recurrent torsion, however there is lack of evidence to support this procedure during first surgery.

MULLERIAN ANOMALIES (OBSTRUCTIVE)

One of the differential diagnoses of acute abdomen with abdominal lump is obstructive mullerian abnormalities which include imperforate hymen, cervical or vaginal atresia, and transverse vaginal septum. There is a preceding history of primary amenorrhea and cyclical abdominal pain.[23] There may also be associated urinary retention (37–60%) or paralytic ileus (27%).[24,25] Urinary retention is due to urethral elongation and compression or due to irritation of nerves of the sacral plexus. The provisional diagnosis is made on basis of history and examination. A bluish bulge protruding at the introitus that increases on Valsalva maneuver indicates imperforate hymen. A per rectal examination is very useful in differentiating a hymenal obstruction from a lower transverse septum by measuring the distance of the bulge from the anal opening. The diagnosis is confirmed on ultrasound (transabdominal, endoluminal and transperineal) in 95% cases. MRI is more useful for complex anomalies, long cervicovaginal atresia and urogenital sinus syndrome.[26,27] Evaluation of the kidneys and spine need to be done using ultrasound and radiograph respectively.

Surgery is the mainstay of management. For imperforate hymen, a cruciate incision is performed on the hymen and hymenal edges are then attached to the vaginal epithelium. This prevents the narrowing and fibrosis. Lately, mini hymenotomy or annular hymenotomy followed by Foley's catheter drainage for 2 weeks is practiced in few centers with the aim of preservation of virginity. The intact hymenal tissue is spared circumferentially, at least 5 mm from the base. Sutures are put obliquely on the hymen to prevent refusion.[28,29] However, this may be associated with a high recurrence rate and more evidence is needed to introduce them in routine practice. Transverse septum excision is done for vaginal septum while complex obstructive anomalies require an abdominoperineal approach.

PELVIC INFLAMMATORY DISEASE AND TUBO-OVARIAN ABCESS (TO ABSCESS)

Another cause of acute onset abdominal pain is pelvic inflammatory disease (PID) with or without tubo-ovarian abscess. Pediatricians in the emergency department frequently diagnose PID in adolescents presenting in the emergency. In a questionnaire survey, 69% of pediatricians from the American Academy of Pediatrics had diagnosed PID, on average, once per month or more and 50% admitted them for treatment.[30]

Etiology

The most common organisms causing PID include sexually transmitted infections like *Neisseria gonorrhoea* and *Chlamydia trachomatis*. Other organisms include non-hemolytic *Streptococcus*, *Escherichia coli*, group B *Streptococcus*, coagulase negative *Staphylococcus*, *Bacteroides* species, etc.[31] Besides STIs, TO abscess has also been reported in virginal adolescents and various causes reported include Crohn's disease, labial agglutination due to lichen sclerosus, recurrent urinary tract infections and poor hygiene, and obesity. Organsisms isolated were *Escherichia coli*, alpha hemolytic *Streptococcus*, and *Pasteurella multocida*.[32-35] In Indian population, tuberculosis must always be ruled out.

Table 1: Diagnostic criteria for pelvic inflammatory disease (PID)

Minimum criteria

Cervical motion tenderness or uterine tenderness or adnexal tenderness

Additional criteria (to increase specificity and support diagnosis)

- Oral temperature >101°F (>38.3°C)
- Abnormal cervical or vaginal mucopurulent discharge
- Presence of abundant numbers of WBC on saline microscopy of vaginal secretions
- Elevated erythrocyte sedimentation rate
- Elevated C-reactive protein
- Laboratory documentation of cervical infection with *N. gonorrhoea* or *C. trachomatis*

The most specific criteria for diagnosing PID include the following:

- Endometrial biopsy with histopathologic evidence of endometritis;
- Transvaginal sonography or magnetic resonance imaging techniques showing thickened, fluid-filled tubes with or without free pelvic fluid or tubo-ovarian complex, or Doppler studies suggesting pelvic infection (e.g. tubal hyperemia)
- Laparoscopic abnormalities consistent with PID (TO masses, Fitz Hugh Curtis syndrome, pelvic congestion, salpingitis)

Clinical Presentation

Clinical presentation includes abdominal pain usually with fever and chills and vaginal discharge. Other associated complaints may be weight loss, diarrhea, dysuria, increased urinary frequency, dysmenorrhea, dyspareunia, and lump abdomen. On physical examination, patient is febrile, dehydrated, and abdominal examination may reveal tenderness, rigidity or guarding or lump abdomen. Some patients may also have features of septic shock. **Table 1** elucidates the diagnosis of PID according to the Center of Disease control (CDC) criteria, 2006.

Treatment

Adolescents with TO abscess warrant hospitalization while those presenting with acute PID alone should be hospitalized in case of pregnancy, non-compliance or non-response to outpatient therapy, high grade fever, nausea, or vomiting. CDC has given definite management guidelines for management of PID and some more commonly used are detailed below. Parenteral treatment is given for at least 48 hours till the patient shows clinical improvement. Once the condition stabilizes, oral treatment can be started. The recommended regimes by CDC are summarized in **Table 2**. Various other regimens using a combination of levofloxacin/ofloxacin, and metronidazole have also been described by CDC to improve response and compliance. Complete treatment should be ensured as to avoid the long-term sequelae of infertility, chronic pelvic pain, etc. Contraceptive counseling should also be done for all the adolescents.

Table 2: Treatment of pelvic inflammatory disease

Regimen A

Cefotetan 2 g IV every 12 hours OR cefoxitin 2 g IV every 6 hours PLUS doxycycline 100 mg orally or IV every 12 hours

In cases of tubo-ovarian abscess, anaerobic cover is added: Injection metronidazole 500 mg IV BD or Clindamycin 900 mg IV every 8 hours

Regimen B

Clindamycin 900 mg IV every 8 hours PLUS gentamicin loading dose IV or IM (2 mg/kg of body weight), followed by a maintenance dose (1.5 mg/kg) every 8 hours. Single daily dosing may be substituted

Once clinical improvement occurs, Cap doxycycline (100 mg twice a day) or clindamycin 450 mg orally four times a day should be given for 14 days

Prepubertal Bleeding

Prepubertal vaginal bleeding is rare and raises concern. Its evaluation requires comprehensive work-up to look for various causes which include:

- Vulvo-vaginitis
- Trauma
- Sexual assault
- Foreign body
- Urethral prolapse
- Precocious puberty
- Ovarian tumors
- Sarcoma botryoides.

Malignancy or abuse should be ruled out promptly. If a child is reluctant to undergo examination, or if the extent of injury or source of bleeding cannot be determined, examination under anesthesia and vaginoscopy is recommended. Vaginoscopy allows for clear visualization of the vagina and cervix without distorting hymenal anatomy. It also aids in diagnosis and removal of a foreign body and evaluation of mucosal damage caused.[36] In case vaginoscopy is not available, nasal speculum may be used to visualize the cervix and vagina.

Heavy menstrual bleeding

The term "abnormal uterine bleeding" (AUB) is used to collectively describe any abnormality in the volume, frequency and duration of menstruation. It encompasses absence of menses, irregular menses, heavy menstrual flow, and intermenstrual bleeding. When the duration of bleeding exceeds 7 days or blood loss exceeds 80 mL per menstrual cycle it is called heavy menstrual bleeding (HMB).[37] HMB is a common complaint due to which adolescents present in the gynecology emergency. It may be the first manifestation of a more serious underlying condition like coagulation defects, renal disease, etc. In all cases, pregnancy must be ruled out in case of missed periods.

Box 1: Causes of abnormal uterine bleeding

Structural causes

"PALM"

- Polyp (AUB-P)
- Adenomyosis (AUB-A)
- Leiomyoma (AUB-L)
- Malignancy and hyperplasia (AUB-M)

Non-structural causes

"COEIN"

- Coagulopathy (AUB-C)
- Ovulatory dysfunction (AUB-O)
- Endometrial (AUB-E)
- Iatrogenic (AUB-I)
- Not yet classified (AUB-N)

Epidemiology and Etiology

Prevalence of HMB in adolescents is between 12.1% and 37%.[38,39] The causes of AUB are described by the PALM-COIEN classification as shown in **Box 1**.[40]

Pathophysiology

In adolescent girls, the etiology of HMB is usually non-structural. It is often due to the immaturity of the hypothalamic-pituitary-ovarian axis, resulting in anovulatory cycles.[41] Anovulatory bleeding is typically associated with acyclical bleeding pattern. Although polycystic ovarian syndrome (PCOS) usually presents with oligomenorrhea, it can also present with HMB. The girls may be obese and have other signs of PCOS namely, acanthosis nigricans, hirsutism, and acne. Bleeding disorders such as von Willebrand disease, clotting factor deficiencies, immune thrombocytopenia, platelet function defects, and fibrinolytic pathway defects may also cause HMB in adolescents. In adolescents who present with first menses with very heavy flow, requiring blood transfusion or hospitalization, and patients with refractory excessive bleeding and anemia; presence of a bleeding disorder should always be ruled out. Bleeding abnormalities due to capillary fragility may be present in hereditary collagen disorders such as Ehlers-Danlos syndrome and benign joint hypermobility syndrome. A detailed drug history should also be elicited as antiplatelet drugs, anticoagulants, etc. can also cause abnormal coagulation leading to HMB. Structural causes like endometrial polyps and leiomyomas are rarely seen in adolescents. The approach to diagnosis is summarized in **Table 3**.

Management

When a patient presents with HMB to the emergency department, the first step is to assess the general condition including airway, breathing and hemodynamic status. Hemodynamically unstable patients should be resuscitated immediately. Intravenous access is obtained using a large bore cannula, crystalloids are started, emergency investigations including hemogram, coagulation studies are sent and sample is sent for grouping and cross match.

Table 3: Evaluation of an adolescent with heavy menstrual bleeding

History should be elicited regarding the following:

Bleeding pattern

Frequency of menses, regularity, duration of flow, volume of monthly blood loss, frequency of changing pads, effect on quality of life

Sexual history

Medical illness

- PCOS, hypothyroidism, hyperprolactinemia, hypothalamic or adrenal disorder
- Inherited bleeding disorders
- Connective tissue diseases
- Liver, renal or cardiovascular disease

Medications

- Anticoagulants/antiplatelet drugs, SSRIs and antipsychotics, hormone pills

Family history of bleeding/coagulation disorders

Physical examination includes assessment of acute blood loss, vital signs, pallor and assessment of medical stability. Other signs which should be noted are obesity, acanthosis nigricans, hirsutism, bruising and petechiae

Laboratory investigations

Blood should be sent for hemogram, liver function tests, kidney function tests, thyroid function tests, and coagulation studies

Ultrasonography pelvis (Transabdominal sonography) should be done to rule out any structural causes and polycystic ovaries

Blood transfusion should be done for severe anemia (Hb< 8 g/dL).

Drug therapy[42]

- *First-line medical treatment* for cessation of bleeding includes oral estrogen-progestin therapy (EPT) or progesterone-only hormones (when there are contra-indications to estrogen administration). In EPT, high dose combined oral contraceptive pills containing 50 µg ethinyl estradiol are used every 6 hours until the bleeding subsides, thereafter 8 hourly for 3 days, followed by 12 hourly for 3–7 days followed by 1 tablet daily thereafter. Once the patient is weaned to one pill per day and her anemia has resolved, she should be allowed to have a withdrawal bleed. For patients with a contraindication to EPT, progesterone-only treatments can be given as shown in **Table 4**. Progesterone pills are also tapered from a higher dose to a lower dosage schedule, i.e. TDS to BD and once daily dosing.
- *Estrogens only treatment*: Intravenous conjugated estrogen can be administered if available. 25 mg intravenous Premarin is given every 4 hours or till bleeding stops. This is followed by 2.5 mg Premarin three times a day × 7 d, then daily OCP × 3 weeks.[43]
- *Antifibrinolytic agents* are also a good option to arrest bleeding. These include tranexamic acid and aminocaproic acid in oral or intravenous form.
- *More invasive measures* need to be adopted following failed medical treatment. A few studies have reported that a 30 cc Foley balloon is an acceptable alternative for tamponade of uterus in adolescents. More invasive measures, such as endometrial ablation or hysterectomy, are reserved in case of a life-threatening emergency.[44]

Table 4: Medical therapy for acute heavy menstrual bleeding

Therapy	*Dose*	*Route*	*Initial frequency*
Conjugated estrogen	25 mg	IV	Every 4 to 6 hours
50 mg ethinyl estradiol combined pill	1 tablet	Oral	Every 6 hours
30–35 mg ethinyl estradiol combined pill	1 tablet	Oral	Every 6 hours
Medroxyprogesterone	10–20 mg (maximum 80 mg/d)	Oral	Every 6 to 12 hours
Norethindrone acetate	5–10 mg	Oral	Every 6 hours
Tranexamic acid	10 mg/kg	IV or oral	Every 6–8 hours
Aminocaproic acid	100–200 mg/kg (maximum 30 g/d)	IV or oral	Every 4 to 6 hours

Maintenance treatment

These include combination pills and progesterone-alone treatment, to be given in a cyclical fashion. Treatment of anemia is done using injectable or oral iron therapy.

GENITAL INJURIES

Introduction

Accidental injury in the genital area is an important reason for children attending gynecology emergency. Urogenital trauma should always raise suspicion of sexual assault and it should be ruled out on history and examination and if required medicolegal case should be made. As the genital tissues are unestrogenized in the prepubertal female and lack distensibility, even minor trauma can lead to extensive injury. Genital injuries often cause a lot of anxiety in both the child and parents, therefore gentle handling and adequate analgesia are important. In case of any doubt, clinician should not hesitate for examination under anesthesia, which often defines the true extent of injuries.

Etiology

Genital injuries in children and adolescents can be divided into 2 types namely sexual and accidental. Accidental genital injuries vary from abrasion to contusion, laceration and hematoma. They are further sub divided into 3 types based on mechanism of injury:[45]

1. Straddle injury
2. Non-straddle blunt injury
3. Penetrating trauma.

Straddle injury is the most frequent mechanism of injury among prepubertal children and occurs mostly during bicycle riding, fall and playing on monkey bars.[46] These injuries occur when a child straddles an object during fall and there is a blow to the genital area with the force of body weight. Injury occurs due to compression of soft tissues against the bony margins of pelvic outlet. Mostly straddle injuries involve the mons, clitoris and labia minora. Besides genital trauma other associated conditions like fractures, trauma to the bladder, bowel, and peritoneal cavity must also be ruled out.

Approach to Diagnosis

History should elicit the mechanism of injury, time, ability to pass urine and stools, and assessment for other injuries. Adequate analgesia/sedation should be given if the child is uncooperative and anxious or if the upper limit of the injury cannot be ascertained.

Examination is performed in supine frog-legged position. A nasal speculum can be used to examine the vagina.[47] Injury should be described in detail with description about urethral, anal and rectal involvement. Hematomas and lacerations in these regions are typically found. If there is a hematoma, it should be noted whether it is expanding or not. Obstruction of urethra and voiding difficulty may also occur in large hematomas of vulva.[48] Urethral injuries are uncommon but may occur. It is indicated by blood at the meatus and hematuria. It is important to ensure that the patient can urinate. Prolonged catheterization is required in urethral injuries. Less commonly, there may be penetrating injury in case the child falls on a stick, fence, posts, etc. they are more likely to be extensive.

Management

Severity of injury should be assessed. If the bleeding is minor or has stopped and the child has no difficulty in passing urine, then the injury is classified as minor. In such cases, salt water baths can give comfort. Topical anesthetic cream is locally applied to reduce pain. The child should avoid strenuous activity for 24 hours. Oral analgesics can be given for pain relief.[49]

Non-minor injuries include the following:

- On-going bleeding
- Laceration borders not visualized
- Labia minora tear
- Not able to void.

Such patients should be examined under anesthesia and repair should be done. Vulval hematoma should be drained and hemostais should be secured. Patient with voiding difficulty should be catheterized. A surgeon should be consulted in urethral, anal and rectal injuries. Ice packs should be used to reduce bleeding and swelling. Tetanus toxoid 0.5 mL intramuscularly should be given after reviewing immunization status. A broad-spectrum antibiotic cover with adequate analgesia should be given in the postoperative period.

SEXUAL ASSAULT

World Health Organization (WHO) defines child sexual abuse as "the involvement of a child in sexual activity that he or she does not fully comprehend, is unable to give informed consent to, or for which the child is not developmentally prepared and cannot give consent, or that violates the laws or social taboos of society".[50] These children normally present in emergency with injuries ranging from small lacerations to life threatening and grievous injuries like hemoperitoneum, colporrhexis, rectal and bladder injuries, pelvic hematoma, etc. There may be associated trauma to other areas also like abdomen, extremities, etc. The examination and treatment usually is performed under general anesthesia as children are not cooperative and when injuries inflicted are severe. Surgical treatment is given as per the extent of injuries.

The following guidelines describe the stepwise approach to be used for sexual violence survivor:[51]

- Initial resuscitation/first aid
- Informed consent for examination, evidence collection, police procedures

- Detailed history taking
- Medical examination
- Age estimation (physical/dental/radiological)—if requested by the investigating agency
- Evidence collection as per the protocol
- Documentation
- Packing, sealing and handing over the collected evidence to police
- Treatment of injuries
- Testing/prophylaxis for sexually transmitted infections (STIs), HIV, Hepatitis B and pregnancy
- Psychological support and counseling
- Referral for further help (shelter, legal support).

Treatment Guidelines

If clinical signs are suggestive of STIs start post-exposure prophylaxis. The preferred choice is azithromycin 1 g stat or doxycycline 100 mg BD for 7 days, with metronidazole 10 mg/kg/dose TDS for 7 days. Hepatitis B prophylaxis is given (0.06 mL/kg HB immunoglobulin anytime up to 72 hours after sexual act) and sample is also taken for testing for HBsAg. Tetanus toxoid is administered 0.5 mL IM in all cases. Post-exposure prophylaxis (PEP) for HIV should be given if a survivor reports within 72 hours of the assault. Before PEP is prescribed, HIV risk should be assessed.

Emergency contraception needs to be given if child has attained menarche and the preferred choice is one tablet of levonorgestrel 1.5 mg within 72 hours.

KEY MESSAGES

- Ovarian conservation is of paramount importance in children presenting with torsion as the arterial supply continues to be preserved despite extensive venous engorgement. Detorsion of the ovary followed by cystectomy is the primary surgery.
- Obstructive mullerian abnormalities are an important cause of acute onset pain; usually accompanied by history of primary amenorrhea and urinary retention. Surgery including hymenectomy or septum excision is the mainstay of management.
- Acute abdomen with history of fever may be due to PID or tubo-ovarian abscess. Management may require hospitalization and antibiotics are administered according to the CDC guidelines.
- In adolescent girls, the etiology of HMB is usually anovulatory and progestogens are the mainstay of management after ruling out structural causes and hematological conditions.
- Sexual assault should always be ruled out in adolescents presenting with genital injury. All cases should preferably be examined under anesthesia and appropriate guidelines should be followed in cases of sexual assault.

REFERENCES

1. Huang C, Hong MK, Ding DC. A review of ovary torsion. Ci Ji Yi Xue Za Zhi. 2017;29:143-7.
2. Hibbard LT. Adnexal torsion. Am J Obstet Gynecol. 1985;152:456-61.
3. Piper HG, Oltmann SS, Xu L, et al. Ovarian torsion diagnosis of inclusion mandates earlier intervention. J Pediatr Surg. 2012;47:2071-6.
4. Guthrie BD, Adler MD, Powell EC. Incidence and trends of pediatric ovarian torsion hospitalizations in the United States, 2000-2006. Pediatrics. 2010;125:532-8.
5. Gupta B, Guleria K, Suneja A, et al. Adolescent ovarian masses: A retrospective analysis. J Obstet Gynaecol. 2016;36:515-7.
6. Bertozzi M, Esposito C, Vella C, *et al.* Pediatric ovarian torsion and its recurrence: A multicenter study. J Pediatr Adolesc Gynecol. 2017;30:413-7.
7. Dasgupta R, Renaud E, Goldin AB, *et al.* Ovarian torsion in pediatric and adolescent patients: A systematic review. J Pediatr Surg. 2018;53:1387-91.
8. Oltmann SC, Fischer A, Barber R, *et al.* Cannot exclude torsion--a 15-year review. J Pediatr Surg. 2009;44:1212.
9. Panksy M, Abargil A, Dreazen E, *et al.* Conservative management of adnexal torsion in premenarchal girls. J Am Assoc Gynecol Laparosc. 2000;7:121-4.
10. Schultz LR, Newton WA Jr, Clatworthy HW Jr. Torsion of previously normal tube and ovary in children. N Engl J Med. 1963;268:343-6.
11. Huchon C, Fauconnier A. Adnexal torsion: A literature review. Eur J Obstet Gynecol Reprod Biol. 2010;150:8-12.
12. Tsafrir Z, Hasson J, Levin I, *et al.* Adnexal torsion: Cystectomy and ovarian fixation are equally important in preventing recurrence. Eur J Obstet Gynecol Reprod Biol. 2012;162:203.
13. Pena JE, Ufberg D, Cooney N, *et al.* Usefulness of doppler sonography in the diagnosis of ovarian torsion. Fertil Steril. 2000;73:1047-50.
14. Mashiach R, Melamed N, Gilad N, *et al.* Sonographic diagnosis of ovarian torsion: accuracy and predictive factors. J Ultrasound Med. 2011;30:1205-10.
15. Schuh AM, Klein EJ, Allred RJ, *et al.* Pediatric adnexal torsion: not just a postmenarchal problem. J Emerg Med. 2018;54:131-2.
16. Schwartz BI, Huppert JS, Chen C, *et al.* Creation of a composite score to predict adnexal torsion in children and adolescents. J Pediatr Adolesc Gynecol. 2018;31:132-7.
17. Tsafrir Z, Azem F, Hasson J, *et al.* Risk factors, symptoms, and treatment of ovarian torsion in children: The twelve-year experience of one center. J Minim Invasive Gynecol. 2012;19:29.
18. Kokoska ER, Keller MS, Weber TR. Acute ovarian torsion in children. Am J Surg. 2000;180:462.
19. Hubner N, Langer JC, Kives S, *et al.* Evolution in the management of pediatric and adolescent ovarian torsion as a result of quality improvement measures. J Pediatr Adolesc Gynecol. 2017;30:132-7.
20. Bristow RE, Nugent AC, Zahurak ML, *et al.* Impact of surgeon specialty on ovarian-conserving surgery in females with an adnexal mass. J Adolesc Health. 2006;39:411-6.

21. Houry D, Abbott JT. Ovarian torsion: A fifteen-year review. Ann Emerg Med. 2001;38:156.
22. Dolgin SE. Acute ovarian torsion in children. Am J Surg. 2002;183:95.
23. Nazir Z, Rizvi RM, Qureshi RN, *et al*. Congenital vaginal obstructions: Varied presentation and outcome. Pediatr Surg Int. 2006;22:749-53.
24. Chang JW, Yang LY, Wang HH, *et al*. Acute urinary retention as the presentation of imperforate hymen. J Chin Med Assoc. 2007;70:559-61.
25. Wang W, Chen MH, Yang W, *et al*. Imperforate hymen presenting with chronic constipation and lumbago: Report of one case. Acta Paediatr Taiwan. 2004;45:340-2.
26. Shaked O, Tepper R, Klein Z, *et al*. Hydrometrocolpos - diagnostic and therapeutic dilemmas. J Pediatr Adolesc Gynecol. 2008;21:317-21.
27. Hamed ST, Abdel Rahman RW, Desouky WR. An integrated imaging approach for diagnosis of cervico-vaginal outflow defects and associated genital anomalies. Egypt J Radiol Nucl Med. 2015;46:1249-6.
28. Cetin C, Soysal C, Khatib G, *et al*. Annular hymenotomy for imperforate hymen. J Obstet Gynaecol Res. 2016;42:1013-5.
29. Ali A, Cetin C, Nedim C, *et al*. Treatment of imperforate hymen by application of Foley catheter. Eur J Obstet Gynecol Reprod Biol. 2003;106:72-5.
30. Benaim J, Pulaski M, Coupey SM. Adolescent girls and pelvic inflammatory disease: Experience and practices of emergency department pediatricians. Arch Pediatr Adolesc Med. 1998;152:449-54.
31. Workowski KA, Bolan GA; Centers for Disease Control and Prevention. Sexually transmitted diseases treatment guidelines, 2015. MMWR Recomm Rep. 2015;64(RR-03):1-137.
32. Dogan E, Altunyurt S, Altindag T, *et al*. Tubo-ovarian abscess mimicking ovarian tumor in a sexually inactive girl. J Pediatr Adolesc Gynecol. 2004;17:351-2.
33. Teng FY, Cardone JT, Au AH. Pasteurella multocida tubo-ovarian abscess in a virgin. Obstet Gynecol. 1996;87(5 Pt 2):883.
34. Kim SH, Kim SH, Yang DM, *et al*. Unusual causes of tubo-ovarian abscess: CT and MR imaging findings. Radiographics. 2004;24:1575-89.
35. Hartmann KA, Lerand SJ, Jay MS. Tubo ovarian abscess in virginal adolescents: Exposure of the underlying etiology. J Pediatr Adolesc Gynecol. 2009;22:e13-6.
36. Dwiggins M, Gomez-Lobo V. Current review of prepubertal vaginal bleeding. Curr Opin Obstet Gynecol. 2017;29:322-7.
37. Hallberg L, Hogdahl A, Nilsson L, *et al*. Menstrual blood loss—a population study. Acta Obstet Gynaecol Scand.1966;45:320-51.
38. Friberg B, Ornö AK, Lindgren A, *et al*. Bleeding disorders among young women: A population-based prevalence study. Acta Obstet Gynecol Scand. 2006;85:200-6.
39. Barr F, Brabin L, Agbaje S, *et al*. Reducing iron deficiency anemia due to heavy menstrual blood loss in Nigerian rural adolescents. Public Health Nutr. 1998;1:249.
40. Munro MG, Critchley HO, Broder MS, *et al*. FIGO classification system (PALM-COEIN) for causes of abnormal uterine bleeding in nongravid women of reproductive age. Int J Gynaecol Obstet. 2011;113:3.
41. Committee on Practice Bulletins—Gynecology. Practice bulletin no. 128: Diagnosis of abnormal uterine bleeding in reproductive-aged women. Obstet Gynecol. 2012;120(1): 197-206.
42. James AH, Kouides PA, Abdul-Kadir R, *et al*. Evaluation and management of acute menorrhagia in women with and without underlying bleeding disorders: Consensus from an international expert panel. Eur J Obstet Gynecol Reprod Biol. 2011;158:124-34.
43. McWilliams GD, Hill MJ, Dietrich CS 3rd. Gynecologic emergencies. Surg Clin North Am. 2008;88:265-83.
44. Haamid F, Sass AE, Dietrich JE. Heavy menstrual bleeding in adolescents. J Pediatr Adolesc Gynecol. 2017;30:335.
45. Hwang HJ, Lim HW, Han YS, *et al*. Hematocolpos as a result of delayed treatment of acute straddle injury in an adolescent girl. Case Rep Obstet Gynecol. 2016;2016:1987690.
46. Casey JT, Bjurlin MA, Cheng EY. Pediatric genital injury: An analysis of the National Electronic Injury Surveillance System. Urology. 2013;82:1125-30.
47. Hertweck P, Yoost J. Common problems in pediatric and adolescent gynecology. Expert Review of Obstetrics & Gynecology. 2010;5:311-28.
48. Merritt DF. Genital trauma in children and adolescents. Clin Obstet Gynecol. 2008;51:237-48.
49. The Royal Children's Hospital Melbourne. Clinical Practice Guidelines: Straddle injuries. Available from: *https://www.rch.org.au/clinicalguide/guideline_index/Straddle_injuries/*. Accessed July 26, 2019
50. World Health Organization, Social Change and Mental Health, Violence and Injury Prevention, Report of the Consultation on Child Abuse Prevention. p. 13-7; Geneva: 29-31 March 1999.
51. Manual for Medical examination of sexual assault, CEHAT, 2010, reprinted 2012.

CHAPTER

52

Psychiatric Emergencies

Raman Deep, Rachna Bhargava

INTRODUCTION

In the recent decades there has been a steady increase in the number of visits for pediatric mental health problems in emergency departments (ED).[1] Another noteworthy point is that nearly half of adult psychiatric disorders begin before the age of 18 years.[2] Early detection in pediatric age groups may have far-reaching consequences in reducing psychiatric morbidity and improving treatment outcomes. As ED is often an entry point for children with mental health problems, improving the standard of care at this initial contact is likely to help in treatment retention and better outcomes. Pediatricians need to be aware of the short-term management of pediatric psychiatric emergencies.

Herein, we discuss the clinically oriented, pragmatic approach for evaluation and management of common psychiatric emergencies and crisis in children, along with relevant ethical and medicolegal considerations in the Indian context. The chapters aims to cover key general considerations followed by management of two common psychiatric presentations (aggression, suicidality). The psychological management of child sexual abuse and substance use which may be provided by a pediatrician in ED is also discussed.

EPIDEMIOLOGY

Nearly 5% of visits at pediatric EDs are related to mental health problems as per western data.[3,4] Systematic data from Indian EDs is not available. In a yet unpublished data from our centre, pediatric psychiatric emergencies comprised 9.7% of all age emergency referrals attended by specialist psychiatric emergency services (range: 8–17 years; 63% females), with the most common presentations being dissociative episodes, aggression and self-harm attempts.

There is considerable burden of pediatric mental and behavioral disorders in community based Indian studies from India. Between 10–12.5% of children (<16 years) suffer from a diagnosable psychiatric disorder, similar to western studies.[5,6] Between 4–16% of adolescents report suicidal ideation and nearly 0.4–5% have attempted suicide.[7] Suicides accounted for 25% of deaths in boys and 50-75% of deaths in girls aged 10–19 years in a rural community of over lakh population in south India.[8]

The prevalence of substance use among children and adolescents (10–17 years) was 1.3% for alcohol use, 1.17% for inhalant use, 0.9% for cannabis use and 1.8% for opioid use in a recent nation-wide survey.[9] Several psychosocial risk factors are present among substance using children.[10]

The prevalence estimates of child abuse were found to be 8–31% for girls and 3–17% for boys in a systematic review of 55 studies on child abuse from 24 countries.[11] An Indian study (12,447 children, including those in family, institutions, schools, work and street children) found that nearly half had experienced some form of sexual abuse and one-fifth had experienced severe forms of sexual abuse.[12]

CONCEPT AND OVERVIEW

A "psychiatric emergency" is any disturbance in thoughts, emotions or behavior for which an immediate therapeutic intervention is deemed to be necessary. Precise definition as to what qualifies as a psychiatric emergency varies, however, there is a broad consensus that it constitutes behaviors or conditions with a potential to rapidly eventuate to a catastrophic outcome and require an immediate intervention.[13]

Recent Mental Health Care Act (MHCA)[14] has defined emergency treatment in the context of mental disorders which emphasizes potential to harm self/others.

Broadly, psychiatric emergencies can arise as a result of:

1. *Complication/consequence of an underlying psychiatric disorder*: Pediatricians in ED may come across children with first episode of severe mental disorders (e.g. schizophrenia, first episode mania or major depression, etc.) (**Box 1**: Case A). Autism spectrum disorders, intellectual disability or attention deficit disorders may occasionally present to the ED due to behavioral issues. Conduct disorder may present with fights and injuries. Some presentations are related to a predisposed child's interaction with immediate environment (e.g. dissociative disorder after a change in school or conflicts at home).
2. *Medical condition, toxic exposure or drug adverse effects with brain involvement*: The behavioral symptoms can arise from systemic medical conditions or neurological disorders. Organic brain syndrome (delirium) may present with mental or behavioral symptoms, along with disturbances in consciousness and disorientation (**Box 1**: Case B). Certain drugs may cause neuropsychiatric adverse effects (e.g. steroids, antitubercular drugs, etc.).
3. *Psychosocial crisis or trauma*: Emergency visit for a child could also be triggered after exposure to a trauma or physical or sexual abuse, with consequent psychological or behavioral symptoms (**Box 1**: Case C). There may be familial crisis which can precipitate behavioral issues in children, with no specific diagnosis.

Box 1: Case vignettes

A. A 12-year-old boy was brought to emergency by his family members after he attacked the neighbor, accusing him to be a 'spy'. He then broke the television suspecting that it recorded their conversations. Over past week, he has been telling his parents that he felt that a 'chip' had been inserted in his brain and he can clearly hear some 'voices' commenting on him

B. A 10-year-old girl had fever, vomiting, lethargy and low appetite for past few days. Since morning, she was restless and slightly agitated. She was scared of 'an army of ants' crawling on her body. She misidentified her family members and could not recognize if she was in home or a hospital

C. A 14-year-old girl was brought to emergency after a sexual assault. She was tearful and in severe distress. She refused to talk to the medical team

Box 2: Challenges in management of psychiatric emergencies in pediatric EDs

- Non-availability of physical resources (e.g. safe rooms) and infrastructure
- Lack of specialized psychiatric referral/consultation services
- Lack of trained support staff
- Concerns about medicolegal aspects (e.g. Mental Health Care Act, 2017)
- Time-constraints and competing medical emergencies
- Lack of objective tests or markers for most psychiatric emergencies
- Diagnostic complexities (normal vs pathological mental states; developmental variations)
- Multitude of psychosocial and familial factors like stigma may complicate management

The pediatric EDs have various barriers to effective management of psychiatric emergencies, which need to be mentioned and addressed (**Box 2**).

PRIORITIES IN MANAGEMENT FOR PEDIATRIC PSYCHIATRIC EMERGENCY

Some aspects need to be taken care of on an immediate priority, while others can be taken up after the child is somewhat stable. Certain aspects need to be prioritized in the approach and management of a child presenting with mental and behavioral symptoms,[13,15,16] as follows:

Immediate goals

Immediate goals are to:

- Triage the patient
- Curtail risks associated with the condition
- Look for medical etiology, if any
- Stabilize the crisis through pharmacotherapy or psychological interventions, or both.

Triage

Initial evaluation in ED needs to be done in a prompt and focused manner. The triage of cases in emergency as urgent and non-urgent cases may help the pediatrician to prioritize the cases. Rosenn urgency classification system[15,17] is one of the systems used to classify the need and acuity for intervention, as follows:

- *Class I*: Potentially life-threatening emergencies (e.g. suicidal and homicidal behavior).

- *Class II*: States of heightened disturbance requiring urgent intervention (e.g. witnessing or being a victim of rape, kidnapping, death of a parent or sibling).
- *Class III*: Serious conditions requiring prompt but not immediate intervention (e.g. child not dangerous/ verbal anger outbursts, etc.).
- *Class IV*: Situations in which intervention is requested but not necessarily warranted (e.g. chronic antisocial behavior). An advice for out-patient treatment may be provided.

Safety Considerations

The foremost goal in case of psychiatric emergencies is to ensure the safety of the child in addition to the safety of other patients, doctors and staff.[1,16] Immediate environment of a child with class I psychiatric emergencies should be modified for safety. Specific sections on the management of aggression and suicidality deals with this aspect in more detail.

Need to Screen for Primary (or Comorbid) Medical or Physical Conditions

As a rule of thumb, clinical history and examination must be oriented towards ruling out physical disease in children with behavioral disturbances. A range of medical conditions, including seizures (especially temporal lobe seizures), infectious diseases, autoimmune encephalitis, head trauma, or hitherto undiagnosed chronic diseases e.g. Wilson's disease or genetic syndromes, can manifest with psychosis and behavioral dysregulation. Panic attacks may occur in certain cardiac and endocrine conditions.[15,16,18]

Importantly, if the child is already on prescribed psychiatric medication, care must be taken to rule out potentially severe and life-threatening adverse effects of that medication group. For example:

- Serotonin syndrome in a child on serotonergic antidepressants can present with headache, agitation, restlessness, sweating, diarrhea, tachycardia, myoclonus, increased reflexes, mental confusion, among others and can be a life-threatening condition.
- Neuroleptic malignant syndrome is characterized by fever, rigidity, autonomic dysregulation, altered mental state, along with a raised serum CPK level and a history of prescribed antipsychotic drugs.

Special attention must be paid to "red flags" which point more towards a medical/neurological causation with secondary psychiatric manifestations **(Box 3)**.

Box 3: "Red flags" for psychiatric symptoms secondary to a medical condition

- Disorientation to time, place and person
- Presence of visual, tactile or olfactory hallucinations (uncommon in primary psychiatric illnesses)
- Fluctuating or altered consciousness
- Memory impairments
- Recent fever
- Head trauma
- Abnormal vital signs
- Recent history suggestive of seizures
- Recent use of medications with neuropsychiatric adverse effects

A thorough general physical and neurological examination is indispensable. Complete hemogram and biochemical tests (liver and kidney function tests, electrolytes, blood sugar levels) must be done. Specialized tests such as thyroid function, serum vitamin B_{12}, lead or ceruloplasmin levels, ASO titres, EEG and neuroimaging may be planned, if indicated.

On the other hand, medical conditions may occasionally be over diagnosed in emergency settings. For instance, dissociative pseudo seizures may be treated as true seizures in busy emergencies with time constraints.[19]

PEDIATRIC PSYCHIATRIC ASSESSMENT IN ED

Interview and Approach

Psychiatric interview is a de facto tool to gather information, assess mental state and ascertain psychopathology (if any) by gathering information. Clinician must obtain thorough details of the events and symptoms leading up to patient's presentation in the emergency[20,21] which include:

- Reason for presentation
- History of present illness (or behavioral disturbances)
- Medical conditions (and medications, if any)
- Past psychiatric history and treatment response
- Substance abuse
- Developmental, educational and psychosocial aspects
- Family history
- Medical clearance including physical and neurological examination
- Mental state examination—which includes structured assessments of appearance, speech, affect, thought, perception, orientation, sustained attention, memory, intelligence, judgment and insight.

Certain considerations are important in the approach towards child psychiatric interview,[20-22] as discussed here.

- Approach to a child should be empathic while maintaining objectivity and goal-orientation.
- Effort must be made to interview child and parents together as well as separately. For very young children, parents may be interviewed first.
- Corroborative information is often needed from multiple sources.
- Evaluation must begin with open-ended questions like *What brings you here?*, *Can you tell me about the problem?*. Responses to open-ended questions provide information about problems, child's mental state and insight, and also conveys clinician's interest to listen.
- Closed-ended questions (i.e. those with yes/no answers) are used later to clarify finer details and/or rule out relevant negative history.
- Interaction with a child (including phrasing of the questions) should be as per age and cognitive development.
- Children younger than seven years of age have limited capacities to verbalize their feelings. It helps to engage them with play, drawing or stories as a means to assess their mental state.
- Concept of death and suicide changes with developmental stage. Young children may not understand death as something decisive, but more like sleeping and waking up.
- A child who refuses to talk should be given some time and space.
- Avoid direct confrontation with an adolescent in denial.

Age and Developmental Considerations

A clinician must be aware of certain age and developmental considerations which are relevant for any professional interaction with child, both in routine and emergency settings.

- *Developmental variation in clinical symptoms*: Symptom expression for mood or other psychiatric disorders can be different in childhood.[23,24] For instance, hopelessness and guilt are less frequent in young children with major depression, perhaps due to a less evolved cognitive structure and less capacity to articulate thoughts into words.
- *Symptoms may cut across multiple diagnoses*: Many children have behavioral problems that cannot be classified under a single diagnostic terminology. The spectrum of mental and behavioral symptoms present in a child or adolescent often cut across many diagnostic categories. Comorbidity is a rule rather than exception.
- *Normative transition vs pathological behaviors*: There are developmental periods in which distressing emotions or behavioral issues are expected, for example, the separation anxiety in children or rebelliousness in an adolescent, which may be difficult to differentiate from pathological behaviors.
- *Involvement of parents or guardians*: Parental involvement is crucial for a minor both from a clinical and legal perspective. India is also a collectivistic culture with interdependency, and involvement of family is crucial. In absence of parents, the legal guardianship must be ascertained at the time of presentation.
- *Privacy and confidentiality*: An adolescent may wish to retain privacy over certain aspects of his/her life such as psychoactive drug use, sexual encounters etc. It is pertinent to emphasize that privacy and confidentiality of the information would be strictly maintained even from a parent or caregiver, barring situations with risk of harm to self or others. Such exceptions for confidentiality in situations with high safety concerns have provision under Mental Health Care Act.[14]

LEGAL ASPECTS OF EMERGENCY TREATMENT

The Mental Health Care Act (MHCA) introduced in 2017[14] governs the mental health care and services for persons with mental illness in India, including admissions to mental health establishments. The act applies to any health establishment, including any general hospital or general nursing home, providing treatment and care for mental disorders.

Section 94 deals with "Emergency Treatment" which can be provided by a registered medical practitioner to person with mental illness, if it is immediately necessary to prevent:

1. Death or irreversible harm to the health of the person; or
2. The person inflicting serious harm to himself or to others; or
3. The person causing serious damage to property belonging to himself or to others where such behavior is believed to flow directly from the person's mental illness.

Emergency treatment shall be limited to maximum 72 hours or till person has been referred to mental health establishment, whichever is earliest. Consent of legal guardian must be taken for emergency treatment.[14,25]

Pediatricians must develop a close liaison with mental health establishments for making a referral, after the initial stabilization of the patient and after emergency treatment is over.

SPECIFIC PEDIATRIC PSYCHIATRIC EMERGENCIES

The general considerations in management as discussed in previous sub-sections must be kept in mind for any psychiatric emergency. Specific management of common psychiatric emergencies is discussed here.

Aggressive or Violent Child Patient

Aggression can be the final common pathway for severe mental illnesses, temperamental characteristics, medical conditions or emotional disturbances in response to environmental triggers.[13,15,26] One must always rule out a medical causation during evaluation of a seemingly agitated or aggressive patient.

Evaluation

Pediatric patients may be brought to emergency with specific threats to harm, overt physical aggression, or violent acts. Aggression may progress from verbal stage to psychomotor agitation to damage to property and physical aggression/violence. Psychiatric, medical and other conditions that may cause or contribute to aggressive behavior must be evaluated.[13,15,26] These include:

- Severe mental illness such as acute psychosis or manic episode
- Delirium (hyperactive type) due to medical conditions or toxic drug overdose
- Externalizing disorders (conduct disorders etc)
- Autism spectrum disorders
- Intellectual disability
- Alcohol or other substance intoxication
- Severe akathisia (adverse effect of anti-dopaminergic medications characterized by subjective and motor restlessness, inability to sit still and compelling urge to be in constant motion)
- Trait impulsivity and low frustration tolerance
- Familial conflicts or environmental stimuli in predisposed children.

Specific threats and their nature including any concrete plans must be enquired and ambiguous statements must be clarified. Special attention must be paid to access to weapons, past history of violence, substance use and known/suspected psychiatric disorders, all of which may increase the risk of violence.

While approaching an aggressive or violent child/adolescent, a pediatrician must follow some instruction[15,26,27] as listed below:

- Stay at safe distance (3–4 feet) at the time of patient interview. Standing across a table may provide a barrier. Do not turn your back towards patient
- Ensure that there is no access to breakable items or potentially dangerous objects
- Keep environmental stimulation to minimum in the vicinity of patient (less noise, no crowding, no bright lights, etc.)
- Maintain a non-threatening posture preferably with both hands open and visible to patient (especially for paranoid patients who may suspect hidden syringes or instruments in doctor's hand)
- Locate easy exit before hand
- Prepare staff to escalate the behavioral measures, including restraint or pharmacotherapy, if needed
- Introduce himself/herself and convey that she/he is there to keep the child safe
- Seek child's permission and observe willingness to initiate conversation
- Use a calm and even tone, no visible signs of impatience
- Clarify the reasons for aggression and understand the goals of child's behavior
- Assure that you shall try to address the child's concerns and elicit the concerns
- Be objective, non-judgmental.

Treatment

The overall goal of treatment is to:

- Provide a safe environment for the child (no access to breakable items, reduce environmental stimulation and other precautions discussed in the above sub-section).
- Provide adequate therapeutic interventions to calm the patient.
- Plan management in accordance to the underlying (medical/psychiatric) disorder.

A step-wise, hierarchical approach is advocated, contingent upon severity of the aggressive behavior.[15,28]

The least invasive means is preferred first (e.g. verbal strategies to calm the patient),[29] which can be escalated based on the observed response to more restrictive interventions. More restrictive measures include:

- Seclusion (in specially designed 'safe, padded' rooms);
- Physical restraint in children (using hands) and adolescents; and
- Chemical restraint (pharmacological treatment—oral or injectable).

Restraints may pose a threat to child's life, if not properly monitored. Several deaths have been attributed to the use of physical restraints, in response to which certain regulations were adopted to govern the use and monitoring of restraints[30] (**Box 4**).

Commonly used pharmacological agents, along with dose and routes, recommended for pediatric chemical restraint are shown in **Table 1**. The choice and route of medication depends upon the symptom severity and underlying diagnosis.[22,29,31,32] Very few children are included in research studies on aggression management in EDs and there are no high quality pediatric trials. Experts recommend that medications may be used for short-term pediatric chemical restraint with caution Antipsychotic use in very young children < 6 years must be avoided.[22,29,31,32]

Pediatric chemical restraint may result in myriad of adverse effects, including anti-psychotic induced dystonias (involving neck and limbs commonly), sinus tachycardia, QTc prolongation, orthostatic hypotension, paradoxical behavioral disinhibition (with benzodiazepines in younger children and those with developmental disabilities), respiratory depression, among others. Close monitoring is advisable while keeping in mind certain points[22,28,31,32] as below:

- Oral medication should be preferred if the child accepts the medication.
- Prefer intramuscular route for quick onset of action in severe aggression or violent patient.
- Intravenous route/IV haloperidol not preferred due to its association with QTc prolongation and ventricular arrhythmias.
- Atypical antipsychotics have safer adverse effect profile compared to typical drugs.
- For agitation associated with intellectual disability, or conduct disorders, Risperidone has more evidence base compared to other antipsychotics. Use of benzodiazepines may cause paradoxical excitation or disinhibition in this group of children.
- For drug-induced dystonias, administer PO/IM/IV Promethazine or Diphenhydramine immediately.

Box 4: Guidelines for physical restraints in children[15,28,30]

- Document the need and justification of restraint (never used for staff convenience or as punitive measure)
- Time limit (for restraint order renewal) of 1 hour (<9 years) and 2 hours (9–17 years); release it every 2 hours (and reapply, if required)
- Perform a visual check (constantly or every 15 min)
- Physical evaluation, vitals and behavior check (every 2 hours)
- Offer food, water, drinks, bathroom facilities, etc. (every 2 hours)
- Change position (every 2 hours)
- Physical restraint in children, with 5 staff (1 for each limb and one for patient's head) and same number must be available at time of reapplying it, if needed
- For physical restraint
  - Supine position preferred
  - Compulsory staff training
  - Take care that patient's nose, face or mouth is not covered
  - Avoid pressure on back, chest or neck
  - Elevate head end of bed, if possible

Table 1: Pharmacological agents for pediatric chemical restraint[22,29,31,32]

Medication	*Initial dose range[#] (mg/kg)*	*Route*	*Dose range[#]*	
			6–12 years age	*> 12 years age*
Haloperidol	0.025–0.075 mg/kg	PO, IM	0.5–2 mg	2–5 mg
Risperidone	0.025–0.05 mg/kg	PO (tablet, ODT, liquid)	0.25–0.5 mg	0.5–1 mg
Olanzapine	0.05–0.1 mg/kg	PO (tablet, ODT), IM	2.5 mg	5 mg
Lorazepam	0.05 mg/kg	PO, IM	1–2 mg	2–4 mg
Midazolam	0.05–0.15 mg/kg	PO, IM	1–2 mg	2–4 mg
Diphenhydramine	1 mg/kg	PO, IM	25–50 mg	50–100 mg

(PO: per-oral, ODT: oral disintegrating tablets, IM: intramuscular)
#precise doses should be determined individually based on several factors such as weight, age, medical conditions, diagnosis etc.

Diphenhydramine or promethazine may be given prophylactically in patients at high-risk for dystonia (for example, co-administration of haloperidol and promethazine).

- If a child/adolescent is already on an antipsychotic drug, administration of same medication at usual or increased dose is acceptable.
- Lowest effective dose to achieve the desired effect must be used.
- In case of non-response/sub-optimal to antipsychotic drug administration, repeat dose of same agent (or a benzodiazepine) may be given to an aggressive patient (after about 30 min of intramuscular route and an hour of oral medication, varies with drugs).

After the child/adolescent is somewhat calm and cooperative, a detailed mental state examination may be conducted to assess the emotional and cognitive state. Patient's explanation of the aggressive behavior may be explored. The goal at this stage is risk stratification for repeat aggression/violence.[28,29] If the patient has high risk for repeat aggression or has clear plans to harm others or continues to be agitated, then such patients must be referred for in-patient treatment/psychiatric hospitalization for further management. Stable patients must be referred for specialist out-patient psychiatric services.

Suicidal Behavior

Suicidal ideation is one of the frequent symptoms in severe mood disorders, including major depression, recurrent depression, bipolar depression etc. Suicidal attempts may occur in psychotic disorders in response to paranoid delusions or command hallucinations. The non-suicidal self-injurious behavior (where the intent is not to kill self) is more likely to be associated with maladaptive personality traits or temperament in response to environment. However, intent is not always too clear in ED and risk of inadvertent or accidental harm is present even in non-suicidal self-injury.

Screening

Children and adolescents with several risk factors must be specifically screened for suicidality as shown in **Box 5**.[33] Asking about the suicidal ideation or attempts does not increase suicide behaviors, and may lead to higher detection rates and early intervention.[31,34]

Box 5: Child/adolescent risk factors for suicidality screening

Certain risk factors in adolescents may warrant screening for suicidality, for example:

- Presence of a psychiatric diagnosis (history and/or evaluation)
- Depressive cognition
- Recent stressful life event or stressors
- Impulsivity as a trait
- Substance abuse
- Past history of suicide attempts
- Family history of completed suicide
- History of physical or sexual abuse
- Identification as lesbian, gay, bisexual, or transsexual adolescent

The Columbia Suicide Severity Rating Scale has been specifically studied in adolescents and youth presenting to ED with a psychiatric chief complaint.[35] The Ask Suicide-Screening Questions (ASQ) is a 4-item questionnaire which is both psychometrically sound and brief.[36]

Evaluation

Suicidality evaluation[15,22,26] must incorporate the following areas for determining the seriousness of immediate or future suicidal risk.

- Intent to die and expectation of outcome
- Suicidal ideations (frequency, intensity and associated distress)
- Suicidal plans (concrete plan to harm self, with some degree of preparation)
- Suicidal attempts (lethality of method, rescue measures, suicide note)
- Access to lethal means (e.g. firearms)
- Reasons for living etc.

Table 2 presents the various parameters which can be used as guide to ascertain the severity of suicidal behaviors. In assigning the risk level, it is the child's understanding and perceived lethality of the method which is more important than the method per se.[15,22,26]

Treatment

The safety of the child should be the paramount concern of the service provider. High risk precautions, as shown in **Box 6**, must be ensured and vigilance advised to parents or caregivers. Adolescents may make impulsive suicidal attempts, with little prior planning. Such attempts are often made using easily accessible methods in the vicinity, e.g. kitchen knives, shaving blades, firearms or even toilet

Table 2: Suicidal risk assessment: High vs low risk

Parameter	*High risk*	*Low risk*
Suicide attempt characteristics	Alone No rescue available Evidence of planning Lethal methods	In front of others Rescue available Impulsive Low lethality methods
Intent to die	High resolve/intent	Low, ambiguous
Psychopathology	Presence of syndromal psychiatric diagnosis with a cluster of symptoms (commonly, mood disregulation, severe hopelessness, expressed suicidality, ideas or delusion of guilt, etc.) Hopelessness is a strong predictor for suicidal attempts in future	No syndromal diagnosis
Communication	Poor, guarded, evasive	Open, clear
Family resources and support	Poor	Strong and consistent
Psychosocial stressors	Several	Minimal

Box 6: High-risk precautions for suicidality

- Constant monitoring, not to be left alone and unobserved
- Screen the belongings including clothing, bags, etc. for any potentially lethal items
- Keep the medications away from patient (for risk of overdose) under parental supervision
- Modifications for safe environment (e.g. removal of sharp instruments, cords, etc.)
- Parental education about "Means Restriction"

cleaners/'acids'.[22,37] Means restriction involves curtailing access to lethal means at homes and surroundings in at-risk population. All cases with high suicidal risk must be referred for admission psychiatric facility **(Box 7)**. Patients with low-grade attempts, low risk and high familial support and supervision can be advised to seek out-patient psychiatric consultation for further advice.[15,22,36]

Suicidality may occur in association with a wide range of conditions, and specific treatment shall depend on the diagnosis and its severity etc. Depressive disorders remain one of the common psychiatric diagnosis associated with suicidal risk.[38] **Box 8** shows the diagnostic criteria for depressive disorder in children and adolescents. Evidence suggests that a combination of antidepressant medication (SSRIs) and psychosocial interventions is effective for children with moderate to severe depressive disorder. Psychosocial interventions alone may be offered in those with mild depression. Certain points are worth a mention:[24,39]

- Two SSRIs have FDA approval for acute and maintenance treatment of major depression in children and

Box 7: Criteria for immediate referral for psychiatric admission

- Expressed suicidal ideation, high intent
- High lethality attempt (planned attempt, rescue measures not available, suicide note)
- Severe hopelessness (expresses no hope or 'can't see future')
- Known or suspected major psychiatric disorder (as per evaluation) e.g. Major depression with/without psychotic symptoms, psychosis, eating disorders, etc.
- Associated anxiety and agitation
- Inadequate family support systems
- Psychosocial stressors or conflicts

Box 8: DSM-5 diagnosis of depressive disorder in children and adolescents[38]

The diagnosis must be made after a thorough evaluation and interview by a trained professional. Criteria for are at least one major depressive episode in which there is:

- Minimum of 2- week duration
- 1 symptom out of (a) depressed mood (or irritable mood in children) or (b) a loss of interest or pleasure; and
- ≥ 4 symptoms of following:
  - Weight loss/weight gain (or failure to make expected weight gain in children), or an increase or decrease in appetite
  - Insomnia or hypersomnia
  - Psychomotor agitation or retardation
  - Fatigue or loss of energy
  - Feelings of worthlessness or excessive or inappropriate guilt
  - Diminished ability to think or concentrate or indecisiveness
  - Recurrent thoughts of death, recurrent suicidal ideation, suicide attempt, or suicide plan
- Impairment in functioning or clinically significant distress.
- Symptoms not attributable to other medical condition/s
- Specify: Single episode or Recurrent
- Severity: Mild, moderate, severe with/without psychotic features

adolescents: fluoxetine (>8 years old) and escitalopram (>12 years old).

- Drugs are initiated at lower doses (e.g. fluoxetine 10 mg/day and escitalopram 5 mg/day) with a gradual escalation.
- SSRIs often have an onset of action within 2–3 weeks, with an optimal response expected in 4–6 weeks or more. Overall benefits of use in depressed children outweigh the risks with careful monitoring and follow up with mental health professional.
- Short-term use of anxiolytic (e.g. Tablet Clonazepam 0.25 mg PRN/as needed) may help in co-existing anxiety, if any.

Conditions Requiring Mental Health Interventions in Emergency Department

Child sexual abuse

Children who have been abused commonly present to the emergency setting due to the acute nature of their injury, and are brought by law or social welfare agencies. Urgent evaluation is necessary in an emergency setting if the alleged abuse occurred within 72 to 96 hours (or in recent past), or if the child/adolescent has injuries or has significant psychological symptoms, including suicidal ideation.

There may also be an incidental detection of sexual abuse in a child who presents for an unrelated condition. Under the Protection of Children from Sexual Offences (POCSO) Act 2012,[40] it is mandatory for a doctor to report any case of child sexual abuse falling within the jurisdiction of a child welfare committee. If a person who has information of any abuse fails to report, they may face imprisonment up to six months or may be fined or both.

Screening and evaluation: History may be taken in a calm, quiet room with privacy considerations. Children often do not report about abuse or maltreatment due to fear of repercussions or fear of being blamed (especially as large majority of child abuse involves a close relative or known person). The child may feel trapped and helpless due to pressure of keeping it as secret and may fear that she/he may not be believed or supported by family due to stigma. It is important to look for various indicators which may raise clinical suspicion for child abuse as shown in **Box 9**.[41,42]

Evaluation includes clinical history and physical examination e.g. injury marks on inappropriate or unusual places on the body, and may include forensic evidence collection and/or screening for HIV and other sexually transmitted diseases and pregnancy screening.[43,44] **Box 10** summarizes some points that may be helpful in eliciting sensitive information during evaluation for child abuse.

Box 9: Clinical suspicion towards child abuse[41,42]

Clinical history

- Full or partial omission of trauma history
- Changes in reporting across the interview
- Inconsistencies between family members
- Inconsistencies between history and clinical findings
- Broken family structure or other risk factors (such as domestic violence, use of alcohol or drugs in family etc.)
- Unexplained decline in performance at school
- Sleep or appetite disturbances

Behavioral observations

- Child silent, withdrawn, evasive or takes a defensive position without reason
- Wearing season-inappropriate clothes to cover injured body parts in cases of physical abuse
- Dislikes even the 'good' physical contact (such as pat on the back or a gentle touch on the head)
- Subtle comments made by the child
- Self-destructive behaviors
- Regressive behaviors
- Inappropriate sexualized behaviors in a child
- May show apathy or poor self-esteem, or anger and impulsivity
- Depression, post-traumatic stress disorder, dissociative and somatoform symptoms

Box 10: Considerations during evaluation of child abuse[41,43,44]

- Interviews should not be conducted by multiple, different people (to avoid traumatizing the child further, and to maintain rapport and consistency)
- Interview should begun with neutral topics (school, play, interests, etc.) which would help the child in feeling comforatable and gradually specific questions should be introduced
- Ground rules for the interview should be established, including permission for the child to say that she/he doesn't know or permission to correct the interviewer, etc.
- Parents may be asked regarding the words the child or they use for genitals. The language usually gets structured between the ages of 4 and 6 years, but a younger child can also report sexual abuse
- Avoid the use of leading and suggestive questions (like he touched here, didn't he?)
- Examiner should avoid expressions of shock or disbelief, and may maintain flow of the conversations using statements such as "tell me more" or "then what happened?"
- End with assurance

Clinical assessment of a child with sexual abuse should include the following areas:

- Mental health and psychological trauma of child victim
- Risk factors of abuse to prevent recurrence (may require hospitalization if one of the close family members is suspected)
- Parental beliefs and support.

Documentation of identifying information with an accurate and detailed description of symptoms, injuries, verbatim statements, discrepancies, if any, between child and caregiver's account, etc. must be recorded without any interpretation. All such records must be treated with privacy and confidentiality.

Management: The psychological management of the child abuse in the emergency setting may be targeted at fulfilling four objectives:

- Safety and prevention of subsequent abuse
- Assessment of needs (emotional, social, and educational) and relief from acute distress
- Referral and liaison with mental health professionals for long term management
- Informing legal services (if already not done).

Psychological first aid is the first line of support recommended for children experiencing trauma. World Health Organization (WHO) guidelines and practice statements for management of child abuse emphasizes on a gender sensitive and child or adolescent centerd first-line approach.[43] Referral should be made to child mental health professional for more intensive interventions such as trauma-focused cognitive behavioral therapy. Children are assisted with emotional recognition and regulation, and attention to maladaptive ideas. Younger children may not appear distressed many times as they may not understand the implications of abuse.[11] It is important to address the issues of self-blame which if not handled adequately may trigger trauma and associated disturbances. Such feelings and reactions in families have been reported in Indian studies as well.[45,46]

Child and adolescent substance use

Screening and evaluation: Adolescent substance users are more likely to be heavy episodic users ("binge drinkers"), rather than daily dependent users. They are more likely to present with complications due to intoxication. for example, road traffic accidents etc. Pediatricians may tailor the substance use evaluation to suit immediate needs and priorities in emergency.

The 6-item CRAFFT and 8-item ASSIST are brief, valid screening tools for identifying hazardous and harmful substance users.[47,48]

Brief intervention: If the patient is still under intoxication of alcohol or drugs, one must monitor till the acute effects wears off. There is a limited role for any specific pharmacotherapy in non-dependent/non-regular users. The contact with healthcare professional may be used to enhance motivation to change trajectory of alcohol or drug use.

Brief intervention (BI) is an evidence-based intervention recommended in EDs for all adolescents who

- screen positive for hazardous or harmful use of alcohol or other substances
- are still in the early stages of use; and
- present with a medical complication and are unaware of the real or potential harms related to substance use.

BI is often described by using the acronym FRAMES as shown in **Box 11**.[49] It can be easily delivered by a physician, nurse, or paramedical personnel in a busy setting and usually takes 5-10 minutes.

Box 11: WHO-Brief interventions for hazardous or harmful alcohol use[49]

- **Feedback**: Provision of personally relevant information about his or her substance use. (e.g. hepatic derangements, or any other obvious harm in life)
- **Responsibility**: Help them to acknowledge that they alone are responsible for their own choices about their substance use
- **Advice**: Provide a clear advice to quit, in an objective and non-judgemental manner
- **Menu of options**: Discuss a range of treatment options, e.g. talking to the counselor, taking alternative hobbies, self-help resources, medication, etc. to help achieve the desired goal
- **Empathy**: Accepting, non-judgmental, non-critical approach
- **Self efficacy**: Enable the client to believe that goal is achievable and they have all the skills and potentials to achieve it

(WHO: World Health Organization)

KEY MESSAGES

- Pediatric ED is often the first contact for children with mental health problems.
- ED provide a unique opportunity for screening, evaluation and first-line treatment of psychiatric conditions among children.

- Aggression and suicidality are common presentations for which an urgent intervention is required.
- Psychological interventions are indicated in the context of child sexual abuse and adolescent substance use which may present to emergency.
- Safety concerns are paramount in a suicidal or aggressive child. Immediate environment should be suitably modified.
- Brief interventions using FRAMES approach are effective for hazardous or harmful adolescent substance use in emergency department.
- Referral must be made for psychiatric hospitalization in all high-risk cases, after the initial stabilization of the patient. Stable patients may be referred for out-patient psychiatric services.

Note: The word 'pediatric' or 'child' has generally been used in the chapter for age groups below 18 years of age, however the terms 'child' and 'adolescent' have been separately specified wherever age appropriate aspects were to be emphasized.

REFERENCES

1. Chun TH, Katz ER, Duffy SZ. Pediatric mental health emergencies and special health care needs. Pediatr Clin North Am. 2013;60:1185-201.
2. Kessler RC, Berglund P, Demler O, *et al.* Lifetime Prevalence and Age-of-Onset Distributions of DSM-IV Disorders in the National Comorbidity Survey Replication. Arch Gen Psychiatry. 2005;62;593-602.
3. Grupp-Phelan J, Harman JS, Kelleher KJ. Trends in mental health and chronic condition visits by children presenting for care at US emergency departments. Public Health Rep. 2007; 122:55.
4. Simon AE, Schoendorf KC. Emergency department visits for mental health conditions among US children, 2001-2011. Clin Pediatr (Phila). 2014;53:1359-66.
5. Sharan P, R Sagar. Need for national data on epidemiology of child and adolescent mental disorders. J Indian Ass Child Adolesc Mental Health. 2008;4:22-7.
6. Srinath S, Girimaji SC, Gururaj G, *et al.* Epidemiological study of child and adolescent psychiatric disorders in urban and rural areas of Bangalore, India. Indian J Med Res. 2005;122:67-79.
7. Mehta M, Pattanayak RD, Sagar R. Adolescent psychiatry: An overview of the Indian research. In: Malhotra S, Chakraborti S, editors. Developments in Psychiatry in India: Clinical, Research and Policy perspectives. New Delhi: Springer; 2014. p. 313-41.
8. Aaron R, Joseph A, Abraham S, *et al.* Suicides in young people in rural southern India. Lancet. 2004;363:1117-8.
9. Ambekar A, Agrawal A, Rao R, *et al.*; on behalf of the group of investigators for the National Survey on Extent and Pattern of Substance Use in India. Magnitude of Substance Use in India. 2019. Ministry of Social Justice and Empowerment, Government of India: New Delhi.
10. Dhawan A, Pattanayak RD, Chopra A, *et al.* Pattern and profile of children using substances in India: Insights and recommendations. 2017;30(4):324-9.
11. Barth J, Bermetz L, Heim E, *et al.* The current prevalence of child sexual abuse worldwide: A systematic review and meta-analysis. Intl J Public Health. 2013;58:469-83.
12. Kacker L, Varadan S, Kumar P. Study on Child Abuse: India 2007. Ministry of Women and Child Development, (supported by UNICEF, Save the Child and Prayas); Government of India; 2007.
13. Emergency Psychiatric Medicine. In: Sadock BJ, Sadock VA, editors. Kaplan & Sadock's Concise Textbook of Clinical Psychiatry, 3rd edition. Philadelphia, USA: Lippincott Williams and Wilkins; 2008. p. 434-44.
14. Mental Health Care Act 2017. The Gazette of India, April 7, 2017. Available from: *https://www.prsindia.org/uploads/media/Mental%20Health/Mental%20Healthcare%20Act,%202017.pdf.* Accessed July 26, 2019.
15. Pon N, Asan B, Anandan S, *et al.* Special considerations in pediatric psychiatric populations. Emerg Med Clin North Am. 2015;33:811-24.
16. Santillanes G, Gerson RS. Special considerations in the pediatric psychiatric population. Psychiatr Clin North Am. 2017;40:463-73.
17. Edelsohn GA, Braitman LE, Rabinovich H, *et al.* Predictors of urgency in a pediatric psychiatric emergency service. J Am Acad Child Adolesc Psychiatry. 2003;42:1197-202.
18. Alam A, Rachal J, Tucci VT, *et al.* Emergency Department Medical Clearance of Patients with Psychiatric or Behavioral Emergencies, Part 2: Special Psychiatric Populations and Considerations. Psychiatr Clin North Am. 2017;40:425-33.
19. Uldall P, Alving J, Hansen LK, *et al.* The misdiagnosis of epilepsy in children admitted to a tertiary epilepsy centre with paroxysmal events. Arch Dis Child. 2006;91:219-21.
20. Leckman JF, Taylor E. Clinical assessment and diagnostic formulation. In: Thapar A, Pine DS, editors. Rutter's Child and Adolescent psychiatry. West Sussex, UK: Wiley Blackwell; 2015. p. 407-18.
21. King RA, Schwab-stone ME, Peterson BJ, *et al.* Psychiatric examination of the infant, child and adolescent. In: Sadock BJ, Sadock VA, editors. Kaplan & Sadock's Comprehensive Textbook of Psychiatry, 7th edition. Philadelphia, USA: Lippincott Williams & Wilkins; 2000. p. 2558-86.
22. Chun TH, Katz ER, Duffy SJ, *et al.* Challenges of managing pediatric mental health crises in the emergency department. Child Adolesc Psychiatr Clin N Am. 2015;24:21-40.
23. Sagar R, Pattanayak RD, Mehta M. Clinical profile of pediatric mood disorders at a tertiary care centre. Indian Pediatr. 2012;49:21-3.
24. Pattanayak RD, Mehta M. Childhood and adolescent depression. In: U Nayar, editor. International Handbook on Mental Health of Children & Adolescents: Culture, Policy & Practices. New Delhi: Sage Publications India; 2012. p. 21-38.
25. Sharma E, Kommu JV. Mental Healthcare Act 2017, India: Child and adolescent perspectives. Indian J Psychiatry. 2019;61(Suppl 4):S756-62.

26. Margret CP, Hilt R. Evaluation and management of psychiatric emergencies in children. Pediatr Ann. 2018;47:e328-e333.
27. Richmond JS, Berlin JS, Fishkind AB, *et al.* Verbal De-escalation of the Agitated Patient: Consensus Statement of the American Association for Emergency Psychiatry Project BETA De-escalation Workgroup. West J Emerg Med. 2012;13:17-25.
28. Masters KJ, Bellonci C. Practice parameter for the prevention and management of aggressive behavior in child and adolescent psychiatric institutions, with special reference to seclusion and restraint. J Am Acad Child Adolesc Psychiatry. 2002;41:4S-25S.
29. Gerson R, Malas N, Mroczkowski MM. Crisis in the emergency department: The evaluation and management of acute agitation in children and adolescents. Child Adolesc Psychiatr Clin N Am. 2018;27:367-86.
30. Dorfman DH, Mehta SD. Restraint use for psychiatric patients in the pediatric emergency department. Pediatr Emerg Care. 2006;22:7-12.
31. Carubia B, Becker A, Levine BH. Child psychiatric emergencies: Updates on trends, clinical care, and practice challenges. Curr Psychiatry Rep. 2016;18:41.
32. Adimando AJ, Poncin YB, Baum CR. Pharmacologic management of the agitated pediatric patient. Pediatr Emerg Care. 2010;26:856-60.
33. Foley DL, Goldston DB, Costello EJ, *et al.* Proximal psychiatric risk factors for suicidality in youth: The Great Smoky Mountains study. Arch Gen Psychiatry. 2006;63:1017-24.
34. Wintersteen MB. Standardized screening for suicidal adolescents in primary care. Pediatrics. 2010;125:938-44.
35. Gipson PY, Agarwala P, Opperman MA, *et al.* Columbia-Suicide Severity Rating Scale: Predictive validity with adolescent psychiatric emergency patients. Pediatr Emerg Care. 2015;31:88-94.
36. Horowitz LM, Bridge JA, Teach SJ, *et al.* Ask Suicide- Screening Questions (ASQ): a brief instrument for the pediatric emergency department. Arch Pediatr Adolesc Med. 2012;166:1170-6.
37. Pattanayak RD, Kumar S, Khandelwal SK. Self-harm attempts with corrosive 'acid' among the patients referred to psychiatric emergency services: observations and implications. Natl Med J India. 2016;29:182-3.
38. American Psychiatric Association. Diagnostic and Statistical Manual. 5th edition. DSM-5; APA; 2013.
39. Brent D, Maalouf F. Depressive disorders in childhood and adolescence. In: Thapar A, Pine DS, editors. Rutter's Child and Adolescent psychiatry, 6th edition. West Sussex, UK: Wiley Blackwell; 2015. p. 874-92.
40. The Gazette of India. Protection of Children from Sexual Offences (POCSO) Act, 2012 Available from: *https://wcd.nic.in/sites/default/files/childprotection31072012.pdf.* Accessed July 26, 2019.
41. National Commission for Protection of Child Rights (NCPCR). A handbook on counseling for training and skill development of staff of Child Care Institutions. Available from: *http://ncpcr.gov.in/showfile.php?lang=1&level=2&&sublinkid=1227&lid=1473.* Accessed July 26, 2019.
42. Picherot G, Vabres N, Fleury J, *et al.* How do we recognize recent sexual abuse in children less than 10 years of age? What is the role of paediatric wards? Experience in a French paediatric hospital. In: Kalfoğlu EA, Faikoğlu R, editors. Sexual Abuse-Breaking the Silence, 1st edition. Croatia: Intech Open; 2012. p. 127-36.
43. World Health Organization. Responding to children and adolescents who have been sexually abused: WHO clinical guidelines; 2017. Available from: *https://apps.who.int/iris/bitstream/handle/10665/259270/9789241550147-eng.pdf;jsessionid=9D3D706AAC91F7789CC89E22E961C535?sequence=1.* Accessed July 26, 2019.
44. World Health Organization. Guidelines for medico-legal care of victims of sexual violence; 2003. Available from: *https://apps.who.int/iris/bitstream/handle/10665/42788 /924154628X.pdf;jsessionid = ACDB22AAA7396C6308 DDEA619DBE219F?sequence = 1.* Accessed July 26, 2019.
45. Sahay S. Compelled subjugation and forced silence: Sexually abused girls and their family members: A case of Western Madhya Pradesh (India). Int J Adolesc Youth. 2010;15,343-64.
46. Choudhary V, Satapathy S, Sagar R. Qualitative study on the impact of child sexual abuse: Perspectives of children, caregivers, and professionals in Indian context. J Child Sex Abus. 2019;28:489-510.
47. Harris SK, Knight JR Jr, Van Hook S, *et al.* Adolescent substance use screening in primary care: Validity of computer self-administered versus clinician-administered screening. Subst Abus. 2016;37:197-203.
48. Sue Henry-Edwards, Rachel Humeniuk, Robert Ali, *et al.* The Alcohol, Smoking and Substance Involvement Screening Test (ASSIST): Guidelines for Use in Primary Care (Draft Version 1.1 for Field Testing). Geneva: World Health Organization; 2003.
49. World Health Organisation. Babor TF, Higgins-Biddle JC. Brief intervention for hazardous and harmful drinking: A manual for use in primary care. Available from: *https://apps.who.int/iris/bitstream/handle/10665/67210/WHO_MSD_MSB_01.6b.pdf?sequence=1&isAllowed=y.* Accessed July 26, 2019.

CHAPTER

53

Emergencies in Pediatric Rheumatology

Narendra Kumar Bagri

The spectrum of pediatric rheumatic disorders is wide, and they can present with various organ or life-threatening emergencies. **Table 1** enlists the various rheumatic emergencies, commonly encountered in pediatric practice. This chapter shall focus on some of the life-threatening emergencies requiring immediate diagnosis and urgent interventions.

Table 1: List of common emergencies in pediatric rheumatology

Emergency	*Underlying common rheumatic disease*
Acute flare of pre-existing rheumatic illness	Lupus flare, flare in JIA especially sJIA
Macrophage activation syndrome	Any rheumatic disorder ; sJIA* in particular
Dislocation of atlantoaxial joint	JIA#
Hypertensive emergency	Takayasu arteritis, SLE^ , vasculitis
Gangrene, thrombus	APLA$, CAPS@ , vasculitis
Muscular paralysis	Juvenile dermatomyositis
Pulmonary hemorrhage or Pulmonary renal syndrome	Vasculitis like granulomatosis with polyangiitis
Renal failure	SLE, Vasculitis
Myocarditis	Kawasaki disease, SLE , dermatomyositis
Kawasaki disease shock syndrome, rupture of coronary aneurysm	Kawasaki disease
Intussusception, gastrointestinal bleed, bowel angina	Henoch Schonlein purpura, vasculitis, NSAID or steroid-induced gastrointestinal bleed
Seizures, transverse myelitis, neurological deficit, CNS vasculitis	SLE, vasculitis
Hypokalemic paralysis	Sjogren syndrome
Scleroderma renal crisis	Systemic sclerosis
Cardiac tamponade	sJIA, SLE
Congenital heart block	Neonatal lupus
Acute adrenal insufficiency	Due to steroid withdrawal in systemic rheumatic illness
Acute vision loss	Giant temporal arteritis

*sJIA: systemic onet juvenile idiopathic arthritis ,#JIA: juvenile idiopathic arthritis
^ SLE: systemic lupus erythematosus, $APLA: antiphospholipid antibody,@CAPS: catastrophic antiphospholipid syndrome

MACROPHAGE ACTIVATION SYNDROME

Macrophage activation syndrome (MAS) is a life-threatening rheumatic emergency resulting from an uncontrolled cytokine storm and can complicate broad spectrum of underlying rheumatic diseases. The most common rheumatic disorders, which can trigger MAS, is systemic onset juvenile idiopathic arthritis (sJIA), systemic lupus erythematosus (SLE), juvenile dermatomyositis (JDM) and Kawasaki disease (KD). It is most frequently encountered with sJIA with a prevalence of 10%. Herein, we will focus on the management guidelines of MAS in association with sJIA. However, the same may be extrapolated for MAS secondary to other rheumatic disorders.

Etiopathogenesis

The MAS results from the heightened activity of immune system, predominantly cytotoxic T-lymphocytes and macrophages, triggered by an underlying autoimmune disease or any infectious stimuli resulting in hypercytokinemia, predominantly involving IL-1, IL-6, IFN-γ, and TNF-α. The hypercytokinemia leads to various clinico-laboratory characteristics. The hyperferritinemia (>5,000–10,000 ng/mL) due to increased production of ferritin by macrophages is a highly sensitive marker for diagnosis of MAS. The increased activity of macrophages and hemophagocytosis leads to falling hemoglobin and cytopenias. The hemophagocytosis on bone marrow examination (**Figs. 1A to D**) is demonstrated in approximately 60% of patients with sJIA, is useful but not an essential criteria for diagnosis of MAS. Hemophagocytosis can also be demonstrated in lymph nodes, spleen or liver. Increased plasminogen activator secretion by macrophages results in hypofibrinogenemia and a resultant fall in ESR. The histiocytic infiltration of liver may lead to transaminitis. The increased levels of TNF-α reduces the activity of lipoprotein lipase and results in elevated serum triglycerides.

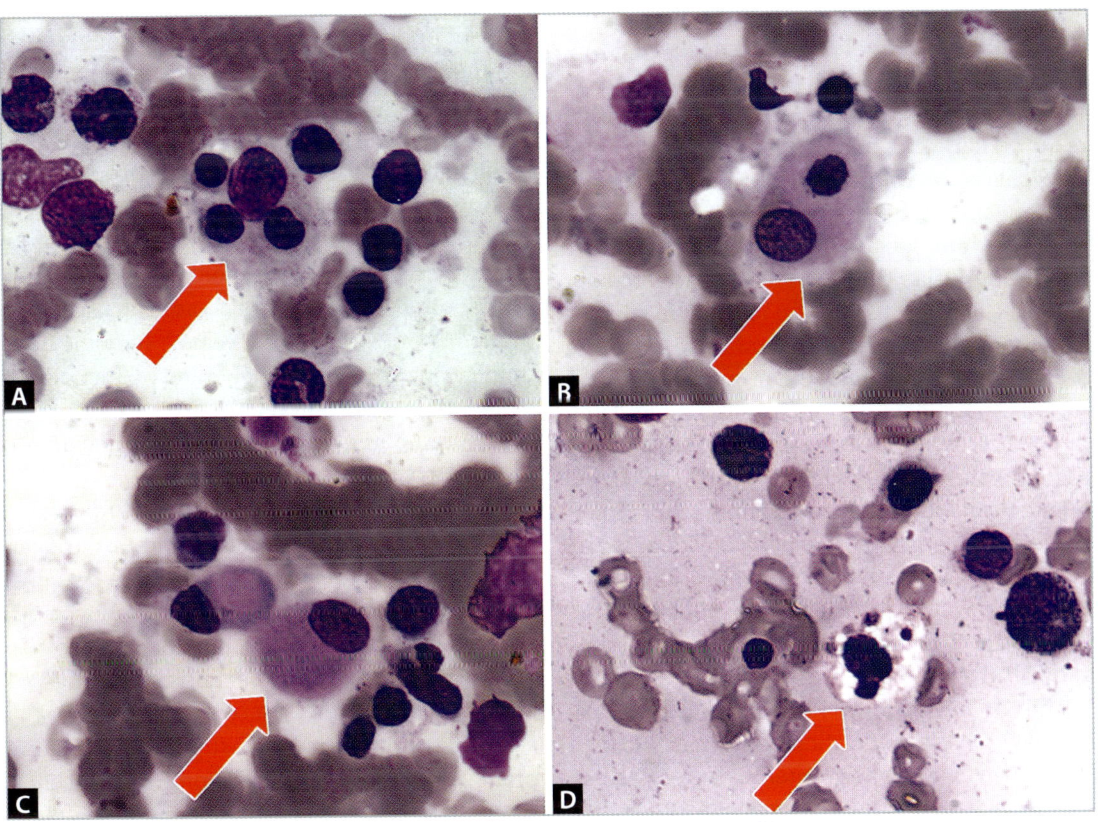

Figs. 1A to D: Giemsa Stain of bone marrow aspiration (ABCD: 10 × 100) showing multiple histiocytes with active hemophagocytosis in an 8-year boy with sJIA and MAS

Clinical and Laboratory Features

Recognizing MAS requires a high degree of suspicion and should be considered in any febrile child with underlying rheumatic disease. The typical pattern of fever in MAS change from an intermittent to a non-remitting fever in sJIA, and this change may help in differentiating MAS from the "underlying disease flare". MAS is a multisystem disorder and can have varied clinical features. CNS involvement in form of drowsiness, headache, altered behavior and seizures has been reported in approximately 30–35% patients. Hemorrhagic manifestations include petechial spots, mucosal bleeding, severe gastrointestinal bleeding, and disseminated intravascular coagulation. Unless promptly recognized, MAS can lead to multiple-organ involvement including cardiac, pulmonary, and renal failure. The reported mortality of MAS varies from 10–35% ; however, early recognition and prompt treatment can improve survival rates.[1]

The various laboratory parameters include falling total white cell count, low platelet counts, low fibrinogen and falling ESR. There is no single clinical and laboratory parameter, which can clinch the diagnosis of MAS. Kostik, *et al.*[2] demonstrated that a combination of >3 of the following laboratory variables were reliable indicators for an early diagnosis: declining platelet and white blood cell counts; decreased levels of albumin and fibrinogen; increased levels of ferritin, aspartate aminotransferase, and lactate dehydrogenase; and the presence of proteinuria. All these features accrue over time and hence a careful observation of trend of clinico-laboratory parameters remains pivotal for opportune diagnosis of MAS. Traditionally, the criteria developed by International Histiocytosis Society for diagnosing hemophagocytic lymphohistiocytosis (HLH) was being used for diagnosis of MAS,[3] however, this has low sensitivity and specificity owing to overlapping clinical and laboratory features (e.g. presence of hepatosplenomegaly and lymphadenopathy both in the sJIA and HLH diagnostic criteria). In an attempt to address this, recently, Pediatric Rheumatology International Trials Organization (PRINTO), have proposed a classification criteria (**Table 2**) for MAS in sJIA and found to have a sensitivity of 72% and a specificity of 97%.[4] Although originally designed for sJIA, these criteria may also help in early detection of MAS in other rheumatic disorders like SLE.[5]

Table 2: Pediatric rheumatology international trials organization (PRINTO) criteria for macrophage activation syndrome (MAS) in systemic onset juvenile idiopathic arthritis

A patient with systemic onset juvenile idiopathic arthritis with fever and serum ferritin > 684 ng/mL AND any two of the following:
- Platelet count ≤ 181 × 10^9/L
- Aspartate aminotransferase (>48 U/L)
- Triglycerides > 156 mg/dL
- Fibrinogen ≤ 360 mg/dL

Treatment

Currently, there are no validated evidence-based treatment guidelines on MAS in sJIA. Timely diagnosis and immediate therapeutic intervention is critical for successful outcome of this disorder. Intravenous methylprednisolone (IVMP) pulse therapy 30 mg/kg/day for 3–5 days, followed by oral prednisolone is the most widely used first line therapy. Oral steroids are initiated in a dose of 2 mg/kg/day and tapered after normalization of hematologic abnormalities. Doses of steroids are titrated as per the need of underlying disease. IVMP can be replaced with dexamethasone-palmitate (dose varying from 7.5 to 10 mg/day) in refractory cases or those with CNS involvement.[6]

Cyclosporine A, a T-cell blocking agent, has proven its efficacy in other histiocytic disorders, and has been reported to induce remission in the majority of cases. It is added as a combination therapy for rapid control and to limit the excessive use of steroids. The optimal duration of cyclosporine is unclear and it has been used for a variable duration from 3 months to 2 years.[6,7] It should be continued until normalization of all laboratory parameters, followed by tapering to prevent relapses. We usually consider oral cyclosporine in a dose of 2–7 mg/kg/day for a period of 3–6 months.

Intravenous immunoglobulin (IVIg) has also been used in treatment of refractory and EBV triggered MAS, and it used routinely as an adjunctive therapy to IVMP at some centers.[8] Given the relative safety and favorable adverse effect profile, it seems prudent to use IVIg as an adjunct to IVMP, especially in settings of serious underlying infection.

Along with the immunosuppressive therapy, appropriate antibiotics to cover the probable infectious trigger should also be initiated. **Box 1** summarizes the treatment approach for MAS in setting of sJIA.

Box 1: Treatment strategy for MAS

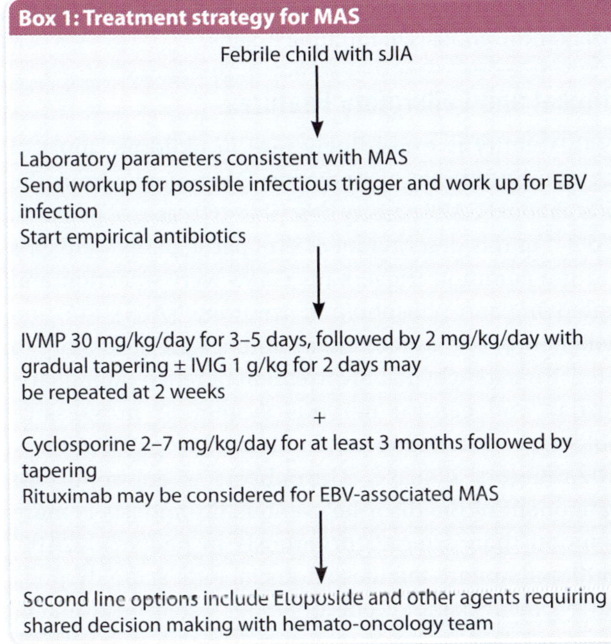

The MAS refractory to initial IVMP and cyclosporine is often challenging to manage. In refractory cases, additional use of etoposide, or shifting to HLH 2004 Protocol may be considered. However, this may be complicated with fatal myelosuppression and opportunistic infections. Biological agents like anti-IL-1 (anakinra) are increasingly used in the treatment of MAS in sJIA with successful results, however, these are not easily available in India. The anti-IL-6 receptor monoclonal antibody tocilizumab, which is available in India can trigger MAS and cannot be recommended for use in MAS. Rituximab, monoclonal antibody to CD 20 may be considered in EBV-triggered MAS. It may also be considered for MAS in underlying SLE. There are anecdotal reports of successful outcomes with the use of anti-thymocyte globulin (ATG) and cyclophosphamide in refractory MAS. Treatment of refractory MAS is often challenging and should be tailored judiciously in consultation with hemato-oncology team.

PULMONARY-RENAL SYNDROME

Several rheumatic conditions can present with multiorgan emergencies, one such life-threatening presentation is pulmonary renal syndrome (PRS) presenting with respiratory and renal failure as a result of underlying alveolar hemorrhage and rapidly progressive glomerulonephritis. The important rheumatic differentials for PRS include anti-neutrophil cytoplasmic antibody associated vasculitis (AAV), granulomatosis with polyangiitis and eosinophilic granulomatosis with polyangiitis, SLE or mixed connective tissue disease.[9,10] If unrecognized, PRS may lead to fatal pulmonary hemorrhage.

Clinical and Laboratory Features

These children may present with dyspnea, cough, hemoptysis, and hypoxemia. Renal impairment may manifest as hematuria or oligoanuria. The diagnosis of PRS secondary to rheumatic disorder rests on the presence of other clinical and serological markers of the underlying disease. The clinical features include constitutional symptoms like fever, arthralgia or arthritis, skin rash, oral or nasal ulceration, sinusitis, saddle nose, subglottic stenosis or ophthalmological symptoms.

Laboratory investigations suggestive of PRS in rheumatic illness include a falling hemoglobin level, leukocytosis, rising serum creatinine and urea levels, and presence of active urinary sediments. Demonstration of autoantibodies like antinuclear antibody (ANA) and anti-neutrophilic cytoplasmic antibody (ANCA) in the background of other clinical and laboratory features confirms the diagnosis of PRS secondary to rheumatic disorder. Anti-PR3 or anti-MPO specificity should be tested in the presence of ANCA. Chest X-ray may show presence of diffuse alveolar opacities secondary to hemorrhage (**Fig. 2**). Pulmonary function tests may show an increased diffusing capacity of the lungs for carbon monoxide (DLCO). Bronchoalveolar lavage may yield hemosiderin-laden macrophages due to intra-alveolar bleeding. Tissue diagnosis (lung or renal biopsy) may give specific clues to the underlying diagnosis.

Treatment

Once the presence of PRS is confirmed, presumptive immunosuppressive therapy should be instituted without undue delay. Initial therapy consists of high-dose intravenous methyl-prednisolone (IVMP) followed by oral prednisolone (1–2 mg/kg/day) which is tapered to 5 mg/day by the end of 6 months. In addition, the induction immunosuppressive regimen may incorporate intravenous cyclophosphamide 500 mg/m^2/month for 3 to 6 months. The RITUXIVAS trial; using rituximab at a dose of 375 mg/m^2/week, for 4 consecutive weeks, and

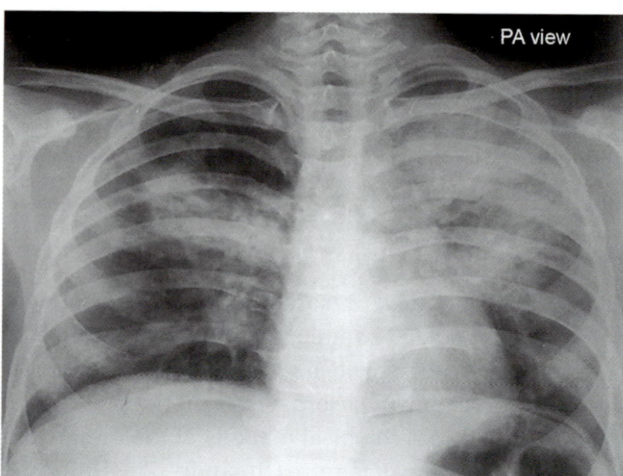

Fig. 2: X-ray chest of a 13-year old boy with ANCA-associated vasculitis showing patchy confluent alveolar opacities in left upper and right mid lung zones suggestive of pulmonary hemorrhage

intravenous cyclophosphamide at a dose of 15 mg/kg with the first and third rituximab infusions in AAV with renal disease has shown that rituximab is as effective as cyclophosphamide for remission induction.[11] Plasmapheresis may be considered as an adjunctive therapy for diffuse alveolar hemorrhage.[12] However, the final results of PEXIVAS assessing role of plasma exchange in addition to cyclophosphamide or rituximab in AAV are awaited.[13] The long-term management of SLE or ANCA associated vasculitis is beyond the scope of this chapter and readers should refer to treatment guidelines for detailed description.[14,15] Appropriate empirical antibiotics should be administered to control the underlying infection, which is often difficult to exclude in our settings.

CATASTROPHIC ANTI-PHOSPHOLIPID SYNDROME

Catastrophic anti-phospholipid syndrome (CAPS) is a rare but fatal rheumatic emergency with a case fatality rate of around 27–50%.[14,16] It may be primary phenomenon or can be associated with an underlying rheumatic disease like SLE.

Etiopathogenesis

Patients with CAPS have an underlying predisposition to thrombosis as a result of persistent anti-phospholipid antibodies. The precipitating trigger could be infection, flare of underlying rheumatic disease, surgery, trauma or malignancy. It involves multiple mechanisms like molecular mimicry, excessive cytokine storm, endothelial activation and/or complement activation leading to microvascular thrombosis in multiple organs.[14,16]

Clinical and Laboratory Features

As this entity is exceedingly rare in children, most of the manifestations of pediatric CAPS come from the International CAPS registry describing 60 cases of pediatric CAPS.[17] In this description, 67% of participants were girls and the common triggers for CAPS were infection and underlying anti-phospholipid syndrome (APS), SLE and malignancy. The predominant findings are secondary to extensive parenchymal involvement of renal, pulmonary, cardiac and central nervous system. A progressive multiorgan dysfunction sets in the backdrop of a primary inflammatory disease. Thrombosis is an important component of the disorder; venous thrombosis is more common than arterial thrombosis in pediatric CAPS. Cardiopulmonary manifestations include acute dyspnea and respiratory failure. Central nervous system involvement may manifest as cerebral venous sinus thrombosis, cerebral infarction, seizures, and encephalopathy. Renal and abdominal involvement can present with renal failure, proteinuria, and significant abdominal pain, which may be a manifestation of an intra-abdominal thrombotic event. Less common organ involvement includes the dermatological involvement presenting as livedo reticularis, purpura, and ulcers.[16] In the absence of a specific diagnostic clue, a high index of suspicion while evaluating patients with complex multisystem disease is warranted to diagnose CAPS. A diagnostic criteria (**Box 2**) for the CAPS have been proposed and subsequently validated.[18]

The other ancillary investigations include raised fibrin degradation products, thrombocytopenia (an important diagnostic clue), features suggestive of hemolytic anemia such as presence of schistocytes on peripheral blood smear, and evidence of organ infarction (e.g. renal or spleen) on imaging or biopsy with evidence of small-vessel thrombosis. A screening for underlying infection should also be done meticulously as infection is one of the most important triggers for CAPS.

Treatment

Early disease recognition with prompt initiation of aggressive therapy is pivotal for improving survival in children with CAPS. The Task Force on CAPS recommends anticoagulation and anti-inflammatory therapy, and

Box 2: Diagnostic criteria for catastrophic antiphospholipid syndrome (CAPS)

Definite CAPS; all four criteria should be met

1. Evidence of involvement of 3 or more organs, systems and/or tissues
2. Development of manifestations simultaneously or within 1 week
3. Laboratory confirmation of anti-phospholipid antibodies (lupus anticoagulant and/or anti-cardiolipin and/or anti-beta2-glycoprotein I antibodies in titers higher than 40 IU/L)
4. Exclusion of other diagnoses

Probable CAPS

All four criteria but only two organs, systems or tissues involved

All four criteria but laboratory confirmation at least 6 weeks apart is not available due to early death or no testing for APL prior to onset of CAPS

Presence of criteria 1, 2 and 4

Presence of criteria 1, 3 and 4, and the development of a third thromboembolic event despite anticoagulation treatment more than 1 week but less than 1 month after the second event

corticosteroids as the initial approach.[15-17] Appropriate treatment of inciting infectious agent must be started in all cases.

Anticoagulation

Acutely heparin is the preferred agent for initial 7–10 days owing to its rapid onset of action and additional anti-inflammatory properties. Weight-based dosing may not yield an equivalent anticoagulant effect in children; therefore, diligent monitoring and dose adjustments are required. The usual dose is 10–20 U/kg/hr titrated to aPTT control. Once the patient is stabilized, long-term anticoagulation has to be maintained with either oral warfarin or low-molecular-weight-heparin (LMWH). Oral anticoagulation with warfarin is generally used in our setting to target therapeutic INR (approximately 3).

Steroids

There is lack of evidence-based recommendations for the route, optimal dose and duration of steroids. Usual dose is intravenous methylprednisolone (30 mg/kg/day) for at least 3 to 5 days followed by tapering in conjunction with anticoagulation to muffle the systemic inflammation.

Other treatment options

Therapeutic plasma exchange (TPE) is the third most commonly used treatment modality in CAPS, especially, in the presence of microangiopathy. It effectively removes pathologic antibodies, immune complexes and cytokines. High-dose IVIG at doses of 0.4 g/kg/day for 4 to 5 days at slow infusion rates is used as a part of the "triple therapy" in CAPS and should be given after TPE for maximum benefit. Cyclophosphamide may be considered in CAPS secondary to SLE. Monoclonal antibodies like rituximab (anti CD-20) and eculizumab (a humanized monoclonal antibody against complement C5 that inhibits formation of C5a) has also been tried with success in anecdotal reports.[16]

INSTABILITY OF THE CERVICAL SPINE

Cervical spine involvement in juvenile idiopathic arthritis (JIA) ranges from 25% to 80% depending on the duration of disease and imaging modalities used for demonstrating cervical spine involvement.[19] In this context, atlanto-axial subluxation needs special attention due to associated risk of cervical myelopathy and even sudden death has been reported in patients with rheumatoid arthritis.[20] The prevalence of atlantoaxial subluxation in JIA is around 33% and diagnosed based on anterior atlantodental interval (AADI) seen on a lateral radiograph of cervical spine. AADI greater than 3 mm is suggestive of atlantoaxial dislocation. **Table 3** depicts Fielding and Hawkins classification for atlantoaxial dislocation is diagnosed on radiography and MRI.[21] **Figures 3A and B** demonstrate the imaging finding of AAD in juvenile idiopathic arthritis. They can present to emergency department with acute neck pain and restriction of neck movements.[22] Other manifestations include occipital headaches, aural or facial pain or tingling sensation of fingers due to C2 neural compression. Sensory and upper motor neuron signs are present in advanced cases with cord compression and cervical myelopathy.

Treatment

Emergency management of suspected atlantoaxial joint instability includes cervical immobilization using a cervical collar and a neurosurgical/orthopedic evaluation. The aim of management is to relieve pain and protect from neural damage. Surgical indications for axial spine fusion include AADI 8 mm on flexion/extension view, or AADI 5–8 mm with radiological evidence of cord impingement, and in all patients with neurological impairment.[19]

Table 3: Fielding and Hawkins classification of atlantoaxial subluxation

Type	Description	Anatomic considerations
I	Rotatory subluxation with no anterior displacement (AADI\3 mm)	Transverse ligament intact
II	Rotation about one intact facet with increase AADI 3–5 mm	Transverse ligament insufficient and unilateral capsular tear whilst the other acts as a pivot, alar ligaments intact
III	Bilateral anterior subluxation with AADI (5 mm)	Failure of the alar ligament, C1 facet locks over C2
IV	Complete posterior displacement of the atlas	A posteriorly displaced type II dens fracture

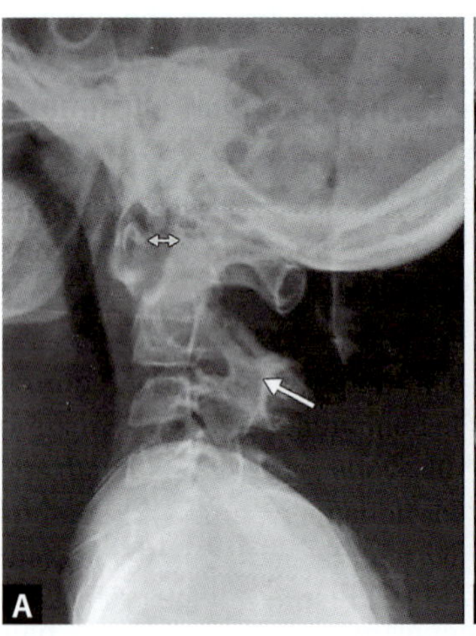

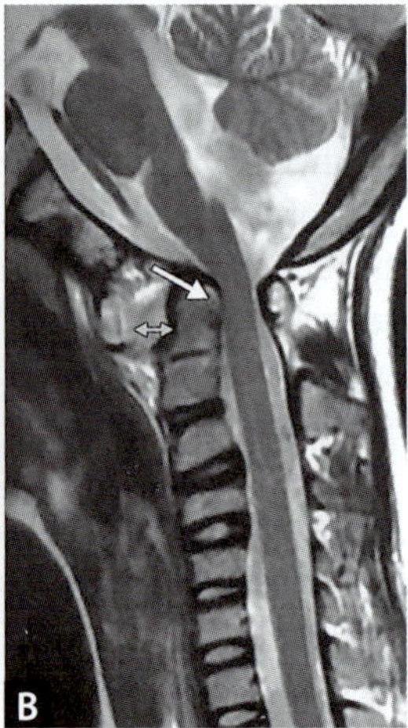

Figs. 3A and B: (A) X-ray cervical spine (lateral view) of 11-year-old boy with JIA showing increased atalanto-dens interval (double-head arrow) along with destruction of posterior cortex of anterior arch of atlas and incidental note of congenital fusion of posterior element of C3 and C4 vertebral bodies (white arrow); (B) T2 weighted MRI image showing inflammatory pannus with an increased atalanto-dens interval (double-head arrow) causing mild kink at the cervicomedullary junction (white arrow)

SEPTIC ARTHRITIS

Septic arthritis can present either in isolation, or as a monoarticular flare in child with underlying JIA. It is a joint threatening complication with long-term functional impairment. Any acutely presenting monoarticular arthritis should be promptly evaluated for septic arthritis. The most commonly affected joints are in the lower extremities: knees, hips, and ankles accounting for up to 80% of the cases.[23] The inflammatory cascade starts destroying the joint as early as within 8 hours of inoculation. The increasing intra-capsular pressure may lead to ischemia and avascular necrosis especially in joints like hip joint. The most common causative organisms include *Staphylococcus aureus*. The other agents include *Streptococcus pneumoniae, Haemophilus influenzae, Neisseria gonorrhoeae* and *Kingella kingae.*

Diagnosis is based on clinical examination coupled with laboratory studies, imaging, and arthrocentesis. Typical presentation includes acute onset joint pain, swelling and joint immobility associated with fever. Presence of redness over the involved joint, which is rather uncommon in JIA, should raise the suspicion of septic arthritis. The laboratory parameters include neutrophilic leukocytosis with raised ESR, CRP and blood cultures may be positive. Arthrocentesis may reveal opaque/turbid synovial fluid with total leukocyte count of greater than 50,000/mm^3 (>75% neutrophils) and low glucose (<40 mg/dL). Ultrasound is helpful in demonstrating joint effusion; absence of joint effusion usually rules out septic arthritis. Radiological changes of articular cartilage destruction, joint space narrowing and subchondral erosion usually become apparent after 7 to 10 days of infection **(Fig. 4)**. MRI of the involved joint is warranted if the clinical possibility is strong to delineate the exact site of involvement; joint cavity, osteomyelitis and muscle inflammation. The mainstay of treatment includes, pain management, arthrocentesis and prompt initiation of intravenous antibiotics.[23,24] Arthrocentesis (with closed needle aspiration) to remove bacteria, infected debris and relieve pressure in the joint cavity is safe, less invasive and associated with faster recovery compared to surgical drainage. However, open joint drainage may be considered for joints like hip and shoulder. The choice of empirical antibiotics is intravenous vancomycin (or clindamycin) and a third generation cephalosporin (ceftriaxone or cefotaxime). Shift to oral antibiotics may be considered once clinical response (absence of fever and improvement in joint mobility) and reduction in inflammatory markers is achieved to complete a total duration of 3–4 weeks of antibiotics. Early diagnosis and prompt treatment is essential for successful outcome and salvaging the joint.

NEONATAL LUPUS ERYTHEMATOUS

Neonatal lupus erythematous (NLE) results from transplacental passage of the maternal anti-SSA/Ro and anti- SSB/La antibodies and rarely anti-RNP antibodies

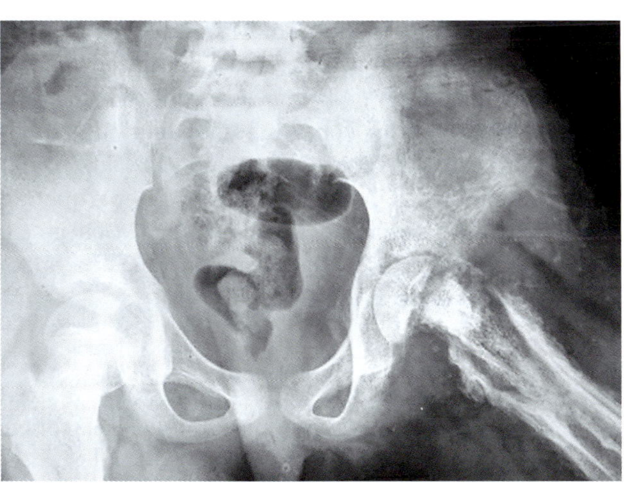

Fig. 4: X-ray pelvis with bilateral hip joints showing sequale of septic arthritis (reduced left hip joint space and irregular articular surfaces) with osteomyelitis of left femur

to the fetus. These antibodies may be found in mothers diagnosed with SLE, primary Sjogren's syndrome, antiphospholipid syndrome or other autoimmune disorders. The typical presentation of NLE includes the congenital heart block and transient skin rash, hepatic dysfunction and hematological abnormalities. The most feared complication is congenital heart block resulting bradycardia in the fetus or newborn. Congenital heart block carries 9–25% risk of fetal demise and a 5–13% risk of mortality through early childhood.[25] Hence, all mothers with anti-SSA/Ro and anti- SSB/La antibodies should be closely evaluated for fetal bradycardia using weekly fetal echocardiography after 16 weeks of gestation. Hydroxychloroquine should be initiated in all mothers and need of dexamethasone may be considered for heart block.[25] After birth, the need of pacemaker should be assessed in consultation with pediatric cardiologist.

BOWEL ANGINA IN HENOCH-SCHONLEIN PURPURA

Henoch Schonlein purpura (HSP) is one of the most common vasculitis of childhood involving small to medium vessels and is diagnosed in presence of palpable purpura (a mandatory criterion) along with least one of the following: (1) abdominal pain; (2) histopathology consistent with leukocytoclastic vasculitis with predominant IgA deposition; (3) arthritis or arthralgia; and (4) renal involvement (hematuria and/or proteinuria).

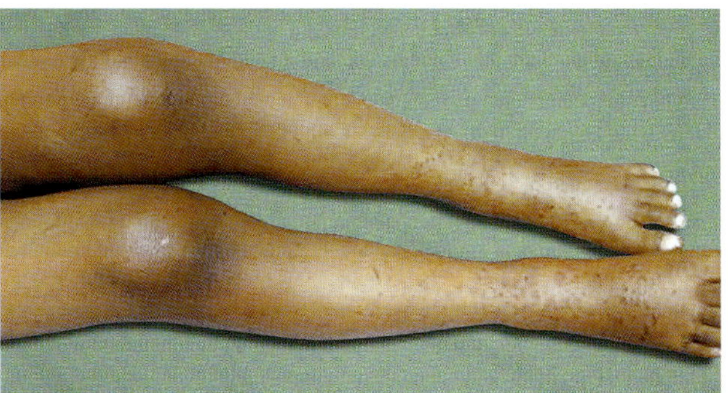

Fig. 5: Typical palpable purpura over bilateral lower limbs in an 8-year-old-boy with HSP

Children with HSP can present to emergency department with bowel angina, abdominal pain, associated with nausea, vomiting, or bleeding. The frequency of abdominal symptoms varies from 51–74%; and abdominal pain may be initial presentation in 12–19% of children with HSP. The periumbilical pain and epigastric pain worsening with meals from bowel angina, tender and distended abdomen may closely mimics acute abdomen and may result in unwarranted surgical exploration.[26] A meticulous clinical history and clinical examination can help the emergency care physician to explore the typical rash **(Fig. 5)** and unfolding the underlying cause of bowel angina. Ultrasound and CT scan show bowel wall thickening and intussusception. Treatment is usually supportive with nasogastric suction, parenteral nutrition, maintenance of hydration and pain control. Prednisolone (1 mg/kg/day for 2 weeks followed by weaning over next 2 weeks) may be advocated in severe gastrointestinal manifestation like gastrointestinal hemorrhage. However, there is lack of evidence in support of definite benefit of steroids over supportive care. In less than 5% of children, bowel edema and intramural hemorrhage resulting from vasculitis may lead to intussusception, massive gastrointestinal bleed, gangrene or perforation requiring surgical exploration.[26]

CORONARY ANEURYSMAL RUPTURE IN KAWASAKI DISEASE

Coronary artery aneurysms are the most common cause of long-term morbidity and mortality in children with Kawasaki disease (KD). The risk of coronary artery events, e.g. thrombosis, stenosis, myocardial ischemia related death increases with the size of coronary artery aneurysm and complicates approximately 48% of those with giant aneurysms, i.e. Z score >10, or absolute size >8 mm.[27] Children with giant aneurysms do not have symptoms unless myocardial ischemia develops secondary to severe coronary artery flow disturbances or thromboses and these symptoms are often nonspecific especially in infants; therefore, all children with KD with coronary aneurysms should be monitored periodically for aneurysmal dilatation and thrombosis. Rupture of a coronary artery aneurysm with subsequent myocardial ischemia and pericardial tamponade is extremely rare presentation and occurs during the acute illness in setting of a rapidly enlarging aneurysm. Timely diagnosis and management of KD to prevent these complications is the best strategy and regular ECHO screening and appropriate anticoagulation in consultation with cardiology team is the key to curtail such complications. Despite the rarity, an emergency care physician should be aware of these potentially life-threatening cardiac complications while attending a child with KD. The readers are referred to scientific statement of American Heart Association for an elaborate discussion on the management of KD.[28]

In addition to the aforementioned discussed emergencies rheumatic disorders can have various emergencies as tabulated in **Table 1** and readers should refer to concerned sections in the book for detailed description.

KEY MESSAGES

- Multisystem disorders with difficult cases without obvious diagnosis should be thoroughly evaluated for an underlying rheumatic disease as this may be their first presentation.
- Macrophage activation syndrome (MAS) is one of the most serious rheumatic emergencies and should be suspected in children with all underlying rheumatic disease especially sJIA and SLE.
- Appropriate immunosuppressive therapy when initiated early can be life saving in patients with MAS. However, empirical coverage of concomitant infections should also be initiated as underlying infection is difficult to exclude.
- Pain in cervical spine in setting of JIA should always be evaluated for atlantoaxial involvement.
- Any febrile child with monoarticular arthritis should be promptly evaluated for underlying septic arthritis to salvage the joint.

ACKNOWLEDGMENTS

Dr Pranay Tanwar, Associate Professor, Laboratory Oncology Unit, Dr BR Ambedkar Institute Rotary Cancer Hospital, All India Institute of Medical Sciences, New Delhi, for providing pictures and description of bone marrow slides of hemophagocytosis; Dr Manisha Jana, Associate Professor, Department of Radiodiagnosis, All India Institute of Medical Sciences, New Delhi, and Dr Neha Bagri, Assistant Professor, Department of Radiodiagnosis, Vardhman Mahavir Medical College and Safdarjung Hospital, New Delhi, for providing description of radiological images.

REFERENCES

1. Lerkvaleekul B, Vilaiyuk S. Macrophage activation syndrome: early diagnosis is key. Open Access Rheumatol. 2018;10: 117-28.
2. Kostik MM, Dubko MF, Masalova VV, *et al.* Identification of the best cutoff points and clinical signs specific for early recognition of macrophage activation syndrome in active systemic juvenile idiopathic arthritis. Semin Arthritis Rheum. 2015;44: 417-22.
3. Henter JI, Horne A, Aricó M, *et al.* HLH-2004: Diagnostic and therapeutic guidelines for hemophagocytic lymphohistiocytosis. Pediatr Blood Cancer. 2007;48:124-31.
4. Ravelli A, Minoia F, Davì S, *et al.* 2016 Classification criteria for macrophage activation syndrome complicating systemic juvenile idiopathic arthritis: A European League against Rheumatism/American College of Rheumatology/Paediatric Rheumatology International Trials Organisation Collaborative Initiative. Ann Rheum Dis. 2016;75:481-9.
5. Ahn SS, Yoo BW, Jung SM, *et al.* In-hospital mortality in febrile lupus patients based on 2016 EULAR/ACR/PRINTO classification criteria for macrophage activation syndrome. Semin Arthritis Rheum. 2017;47:216-21.
6. Boom V, Anton J, Lahdenne P, *et al.* Evidence-based diagnosis and treatment of macrophage activation syndrome in systemic juvenile idiopathic arthritis. Pediatr Rheumatol Online J. 2015;13:55.
7. Mouy R, Stephan JL, Pillet P, *et al.* Efficacy of cyclosporine A in the treatment of macrophage activation syndrome in juvenile arthritis: Report of five cases. J Pediatr. 1996;129: 750-4.
8. Carter SJ, Tattersall RS, Ramanan AV. Macrophage activation syndrome in adults: Recent advances in pathophysiology, diagnosis and treatment. Rheumatology. 2019;58:5-17.
9. Akikusa JD. Rheumatologic emergencies in newborns, children, and adolescents. Pediatr Clin North Am. 2012;59: 285-99.
10. West SC, Arulkumaran N, Ind PW, *et al.* Pulmonary-renal syndrome: A life threatening but treatable condition. Postgrad Med J. 2013;89:274-83.
11. Jones RB, Tervaert JWC, Hauser T, *et al.* Rituximab versus cyclophosphamide in ANCA-associated renal vasculitis. N Engl J Med. 2010;363:211-20.
12. Klemmer PJ, Chalermskulrat W, Reif MS, *et al.* Plasmapheresis therapy for diffuse alveolar hemorrhage in patients with small-vessel vasculitis. Am J Kidney Dis. 2003;42:1149-53.

13. University of Birmingham. PEXIVAS trial - Birmingham Clinical Trials Unit. Available from: *https://www.birmingham.ac.uk/research/activity/mds/trials/bctu/trials/renal/PEXIVAS/index.aspx*. Accessed July 26, 2019.
14. Groot N, de Graeff N, Avcin T, *et al.* European evidence-based recommendations for diagnosis and treatment of paediatric antiphospholipid syndrome: the SHARE initiative. Ann Rheum Dis. 2017;76:1637-41.
15. Groot N, de Graeff N, Avcin T, *et al.* European evidence-based recommendations for diagnosis and treatment of childhood-onset systemic lupus erythematosus: the SHARE initiative. Ann Rheum Dis. 2017;76:1788-96.
16. Go EJL, O'Neil KM. The catastrophic antiphospholipid syndrome in children. Curr Op Rheumatol. 2017;29:516-22.
17. Rodríguez-Pintó I, Moitinho M, Santacreu I, *et al.* Catastrophic antiphospholipid syndrome (CAPS): Descriptive analysis of 500 patients from the International CAPS Registry. Autoimmun Rev. 2016;15:1120-4.
18. Cervera R, Rodríguez-Pintó I, Colafrancesco S, *et al.* 14th International Congress on Antiphospholipid Antibodies Task Force Report on Catastrophic Antiphospholipid Syndrome. Autoimmun Rev. 2014;13:699-707.
19. Salem KM, Radhakrishnan A, Behrbalk E, *et al.* The surgical management of atlanto-axial subluxation in juvenile rheumatoid arthritis. Eur Spine J. 2016;25:2108-14.
20. Mikulowski P, Wollheim FA, Rotmil P, *et al.* Sudden death in rheumatoid arthritis with atlanto-axial dislocation. Acta Med Scand. 1975;198:445-51.
21. Fielding JW, Hawkins RJ. Atlanto-axial rotatory fixation. (Fixed rotatory subluxation of the atlanto-axial joint). J Bone Joint Surg Am. 1977;59:37-44.
22. Enazi AA, Morishita K, Cairns RA, *et al.* Early atlantoaxial subluxation in enthesitis-related arthritis. J Rheumatol. 2014;41:1190-1.
23. Montgomery NI, Epps HR. Pediatric septic arthritis. Orthopedic Clin North Am. 2017;48:209-16.
24. Gutiérrez-González LA. Rheumatologic emergencies. Clin Rheumatol. 2015;34:2011-9.
25. Clowse MEB, Eudy AM, Kiernan E, *et al.* The prevention, screening and treatment of congenital heart block from neonatal lupus: A survey of provider practices. Rheumatology (Oxford). 2018;57(suppl 5):v9-17.
26. Ebert EC. Gastrointestinal Manifestations of Henoch-Schonlein Purpura. Dig Dis Sci. 2008;53:2011-19.
27. Kato H, Sugimura T, Akagi T, *et al.* Long-term consequences of Kawasaki disease. A 10- to 21-year follow-up study of 594 patients. Circulation. 1996;94:1379-85.
28. McCrindle BW, Rowley AH, Newburger JW, *et al.* American Heart Association Rheumatic Fever, Endocarditis, and Kawasaki Disease Committee of the Council on Cardiovascular Disease in the Young; Council on Cardiovascular and Stroke Nursing; Council on Cardiovascular Surgery and Anesthesia; and Council on Epidemiology and Prevention. Diagnosis, Treatment, and Long-Term Management of Kawasaki Disease: A Scientific Statement for Health Professionals From the American Heart Association. Circulation. 2017;135:e927-e99.

Section Editor: Dheeraj Shah

CHAPTER 54

Burns

Arun Goel, Urmila Jhamb

INTRODUCTION

Injury due to burns is the second most important cause of trauma-related deaths in children, ranking only behind motor vehicular accidents. Although most burns in children are minor, and can be managed in the outpatient settings, significant number of children with serious burn injuries require hospitalization. In addition to the deaths caused by burns, a large number of survivors are left with various post-burn sequelae in the form of scars, contractures, amputations of limbs and loss of function leading to psychological consequences.[1] Although the basic principles of burn management in children are the same as for adults, there are key differences because of the unique physiology and psychology of a child.[2] Children account for almost 15% of all burn patients admitted to a large burn center.

EPIDEMIOLOGY AND ETIOLOGY

Although, as in adults, burns in children may be thermal, electrical, chemical or through exposure to radiation[3], the mode of getting injured and the frequency of getting affected from these agents differ. The vast majority of burns in children occur in their own home. The characteristics of the child and his environment are intertwined with the burn event, and suggest subgroups of children at risk for burn injury.[4] Worldwide published literature on pediatric burn injuries points out that children below the age of 4 years and boys are at increased risk. Infants and toddlers particularly suffer from scalds, in contrast to older children who mainly sustain flame burns.[5] An important factor leading to burns is overcrowding in a small house where a small room serves as a kitchen (with floor level cooking), a bedroom and even a bathroom. The victim is looked after by his/her siblings when the mother is away to work in order to make a living. Infants and small children are also the frequent victims when clusters of hundreds of '*jhuggis*' (shanties) catch fire, especially in hot summer months when they are either sleeping alone or unable to rescue themselves and get charred to death.

Toddlers, who have recently learned to creep or walk, actively explore and manipulate their physical environment. They usually suffer scalds by pulling down or knocking hot liquids onto themselves, and sometimes stumbling onto a fire. Immersion scalds are also common in a toddler. These burns occur when a child steps into a tub of hot water or stumbles into a container of hot milk or cooked food. Such cases have a higher morbidity and mortality as a larger body surface area is often involved.

Young children are fascinated by fire and if matchboxes are accessible, they are naturally curious to experiment. In this manner they may sustain flame burns which may be extensive and very serious. Fireworks during festivals are one such potential hazard. Although burns from firecrackers seldom cause deaths, they often cause serious injury to the eyes, face and hands. In winter season, it is a common practice amongst adults to collect wooden sticks, worn out tyres, *etc.,* and ignite them to keep warm. Small children often imitate adults and get burnt.

Electrical burns in children are generally caused by domestic voltage (220–250 V in India) electric currents.

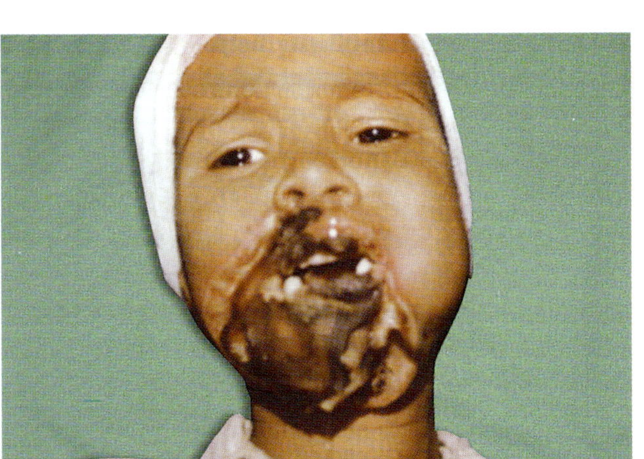

Fig. 1: Electric burn over the face in a child

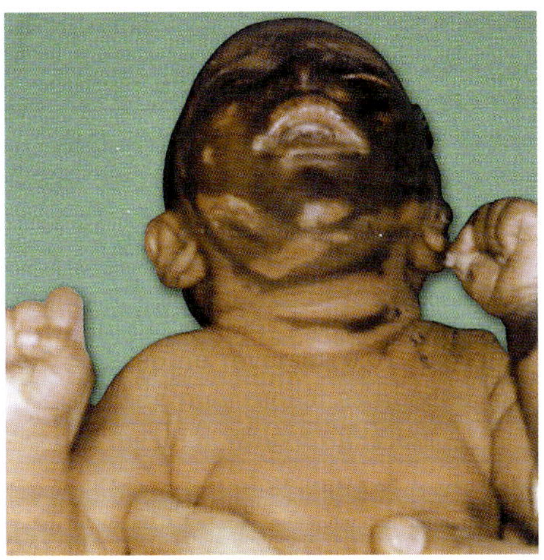

Fig. 2: Acid burn in an infant

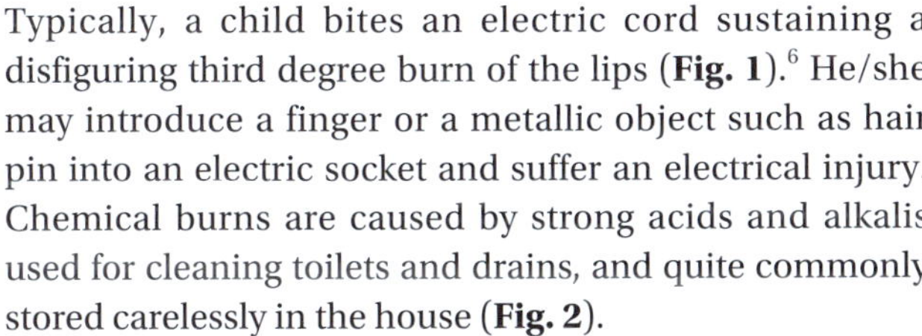

Typically, a child bites an electric cord sustaining a disfiguring third degree burn of the lips (**Fig. 1**).[6] He/she may introduce a finger or a metallic object such as hair pin into an electric socket and suffer an electrical injury. Chemical burns are caused by strong acids and alkalis used for cleaning toilets and drains, and quite commonly stored carelessly in the house (**Fig. 2**).

Almost all burn injuries in children are accidental, although a very small percentage can be attributed to homicide and child abuse.[7,8]

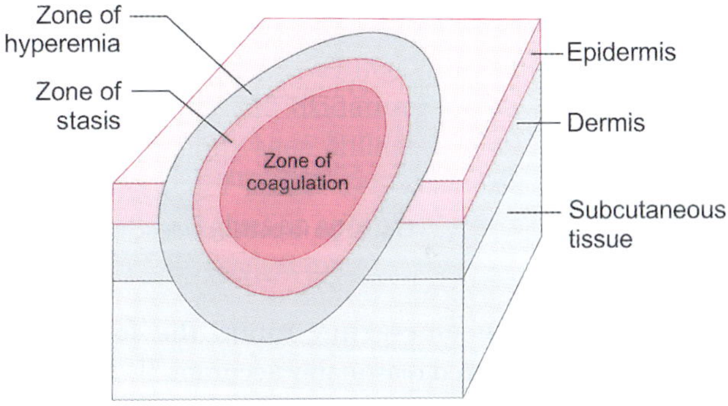

Fig. 3: Zones of burn injury

PATHOGENESIS/PATHOPHYSIOLOGY

A burn injury triggers various local and systemic pathophysiological alterations that increase in intensity with wound size and depth.[9]

Local Response

In addition to direct coagulation of skin, subcutaneous fat and other deeper tissues, the local response to a burn also includes microvascular vasoconstriction and thrombosis in peripheral unburnt tissues. This microvascular injury explains, in part, the common clinical observation that burns appear to deepen in the days after initial evaluation. This is an important consideration during the initial evaluation of children with extensive partial-thickness (second-degree) burns.

Zones of injury: Three zones of injury have been described in burnt skin[10] (**Fig. 3**). An inner *zone of coagulative necrosis* includes the tissue in most direct contact with the source and is irreversibly damaged, with no hope of recovery. The zone surrounding this is the *zone of stasis* that has some viable tissue. This intermediate zone is at risk for progression of the injury during resuscitation period unless adequate tissue perfusion is provided. The outermost zone is the *zone of hyperemia* characterized by inflammation and increased blood flow. The tissues here will invariably recover unless there is infection or prolonged hypoperfusion.

Burn size: An accurate estimate of the body surface area (BSA) burnt can be made by referring to detailed body surface area charts prepared by Lund and Browder.[11] This is because the surface area of head and lower limbs, as a proportion of total body surface area (TBSA), is variable, depending on the age (**Fig. 4**).

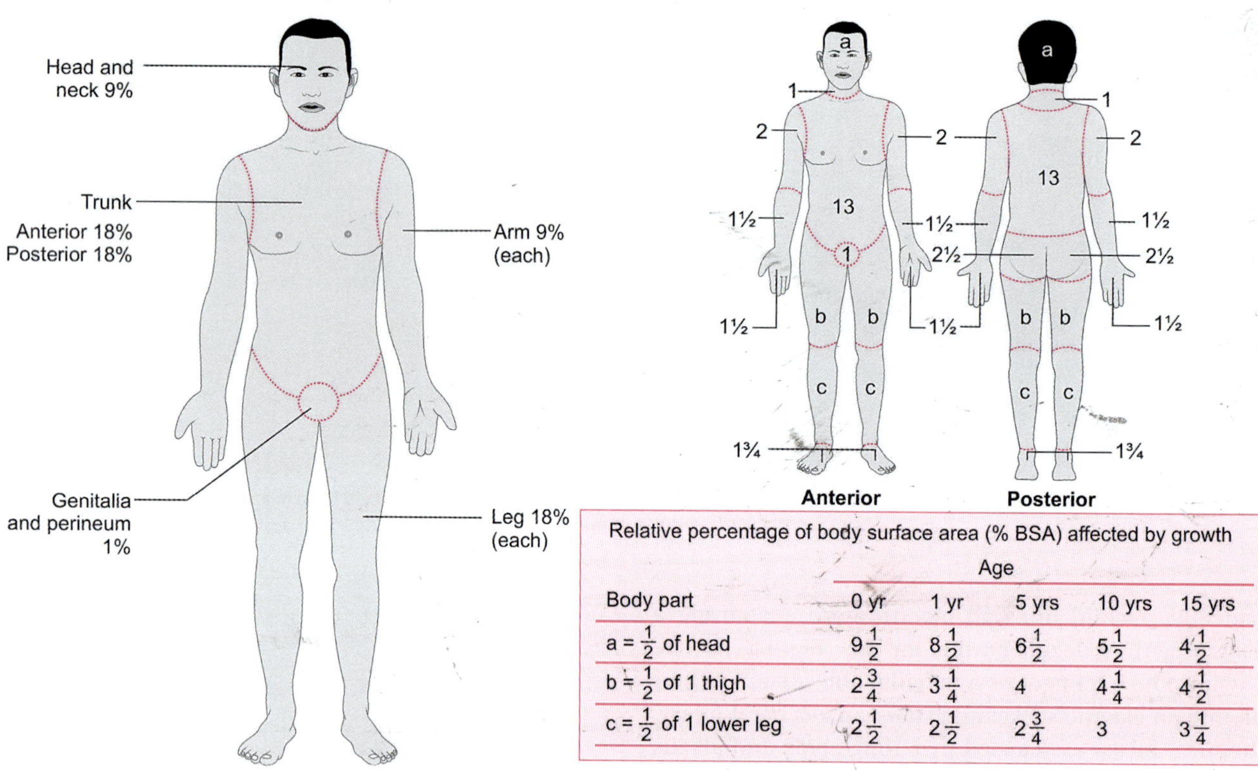

Relative percentage of body surface area (% BSA) affected by growth

Body part	Age				
	0 yr	1 yr	5 yrs	10 yrs	15 yrs
a = $\frac{1}{2}$ of head	$9\frac{1}{2}$	$8\frac{1}{2}$	$6\frac{1}{2}$	$5\frac{1}{2}$	$4\frac{1}{2}$
b = $\frac{1}{2}$ of 1 thigh	$2\frac{3}{4}$	$3\frac{1}{4}$	4	$4\frac{1}{4}$	$4\frac{1}{2}$
c = $\frac{1}{2}$ of 1 lower leg	$2\frac{1}{2}$	$2\frac{1}{2}$	$2\frac{3}{4}$	3	$3\frac{1}{4}$

Fig. 4: Lund and Browder chart for estimation of extent of burns at different ages

However, in an emergency room, the following formulae are considered reasonably accurate.

i. *Wallace's Rule of nine*:[12] In children over 15 years of age, extent of burnt area is estimated by this formula used for adults. According to this, the head and neck constitute 9% of TBSA, each upper extremity is 9%, each lower extremity is 18%, the anterior and posterior trunk are 18% each and the external genitalia is 1% (**Fig. 5**). This formula is not useful for children <15 years.
ii. *Rule of five*: Lynch and Blocker[13] developed a formula for estimating the extent of burns in children. This works very well in an infant where head and neck, anterior and posterior aspects of trunk are 20% each, and each limb constitutes 10%. For older children (age >1y), this is slightly modified. The head, posterior trunk and lower limbs are 15% each, anterior trunk is 20% and each upper limb is 10% (**Fig. 6**).
iii. *Rule of palm or hand*:[14] For all age groups, palmar surface of one's hand (from wrist to fingertip) with all the fingers and thumb by the side represents 1% of TBSA. This is useful for assessing scattered burnt areas.

Burn depth

A burn wound has been graded into degrees depending on the depth of skin involved.[3] *First degree burns* (e.g. sun burns) have only epidermal involvement, and are characterized by erythema, pain and swelling. There is no blister formation and it heals in 3-5 days without scarring. In *second degree burns*, dermis is also involved. They are further divided into superficial dermal (involvement up to papillary dermis) and deep dermal burns (involvement of whole of papillary and part of reticular dermis). As whole of skin is not burnt in first- and second-degree burn injuries, they are also known as partial thickness burns. The burnt area is pink, moist and edematous in appearance in superficial dermal burns. There is severe pain and hyperesthesia because of the exposure of nerve endings. Blisters may form if the overlying epidermis is intact. They heal spontaneously in about 10–20 days. Deep dermal burns appear waxy white in color and may take up to 5-6 weeks to heal. Also, there is a danger of their getting converted into a full thickness wound by infection and drying. Moreover, these wounds heal by hypertrophic scarring.

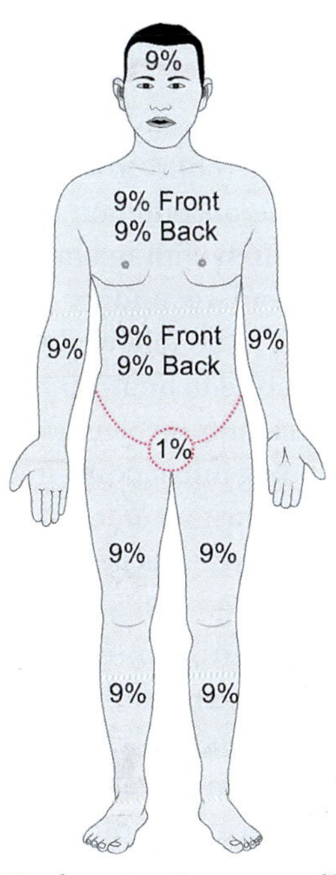

Fig. 5: Rule of nine for estimating extent of burns in adults

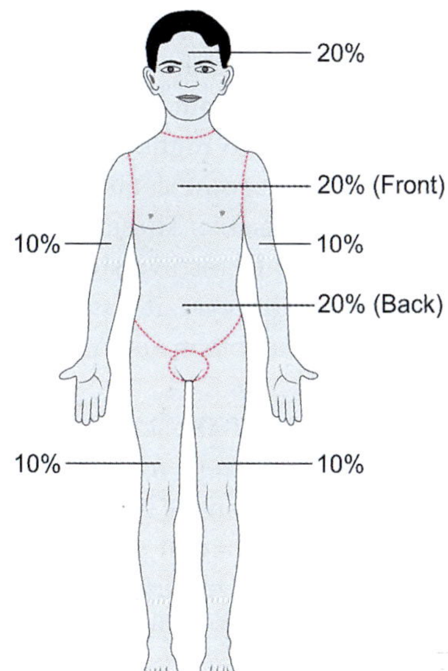

Fig. 6: Rule of five for estimating extent of burns in children

In *third degree* or full thickness burns, the entire thickness of the epidermis and dermis is involved. Young children have relatively thin skin, making burns more likely to be full thickness. The burnt skin is tough, dry, inelastic, translucent and parchment-like with thrombosed veins visible underneath and is called an eschar. These wounds are insensitive to pain as all the nerve endings are destroyed. The eschar generally separates in 3–5 weeks leaving a granulating, raw area, which undergoes wound contraction unless splinted and skin grafted. Sometimes a deeper subgroup of full thickness burns is referred to as *fourth degree* burns, which extend down to subcutaneous fat, muscle or bone and are caused by prolonged heat. The third- and fourth-degree burns require some sort of surgical intervention for their healing.

It is common to find different depths of burns in different areas or even the same area in a given patient. It must be remembered that the poor perfusion of the wound due to hypovolemia or anemia or infection of the wound may increase the depth of burn in later period.

Systemic Response

Following a burn injury, capillary permeability increases that leads to leakage of protein-rich plasma-like fluid into the extracellular space. In extensive burns (involving >30% TBSA), this phenomenon is not limited to the burnt area but occurs throughout the body. Several vasoactive mediators, including histamine, serotonin, kinins, arachidonic acid metabolites (thromboxane A_2 and leukotrienes) and fibrin degradation products, have been implicated for this response.[15] Capillary integrity gets restored within 24 hours of injury.

During the first 24–48 hours, a hypodynamic state with decreased cardiac output and metabolic rate is common. Subsequently, hypermetabolic physiology follows, with rising energy expenditure and cardiac output. This response is proportional to burn size, peaking at about twice the normal metabolic rate in children with burns involving more than half of the body surface. This later response has important nutritional implications, including enhanced gluconeogenesis, insulin resistance, and increased protein breakdown. The hypermetabolic response involves many pathways, two of which particularly seem to most profoundly affect outcomes after burn injury: (i) glucose metabolism with insulin resistance and hyperglycemia; and (ii) lipid metabolism with increased lipolysis. Hyperglycemia in patients with burns is associated with increased frequency of infections, sepsis, pneumonia, catabolism, hypermetabolism, and mortality.[16] Lipolysis and free fatty acids contribute to morbidity and mortality after burn injury through fatty infiltration of various organs. Fatty liver is very common after burn injury, and is associated with an increase in clinical morbidity and metabolic alterations. For a given body weight, children have higher energy needs than adults, and can quickly become catabolic; thus, an early nutritional support is advisable. These metabolic changes were previously thought to resolve shortly after wound closure was complete. However, it has been shown that burn-induced hypermetabolism seems to last for much longer.

The small diameter of the child's airway makes occlusion by edema more likely, mandating more liberal use of prophylactic intubation, as indicated for head and neck swelling in the presence of stridor or retractions. Children have a relatively large surface area to mass ratio, making them more susceptible to hypothermia.

CLINICAL FEATURES AND MANAGEMENT

First Aid

At the scene of the accident, the objectives are to extinguish the flames and to bring down the skin temperature to normal body temperature, in as short a time as possible. Damage due to heat is directly proportional to the temperature of the burning agent and the duration of contact. 'Pour water on burns' is the slogan to be taught to school children and the general public. This is true for all burns except electrical injuries where the victim has to be removed from the source of electricity first. All clothing and jewelry must be removed to prevent constriction and vascular compromise during the edema phase (first 24 hours) of burn injury. However, adherent synthetic clothing and tar may be left in place and cooled with water to be removed later by formal debridement. Tap water, instead of cold water or ice, should be used to bring down the temperature as it is easily available and has lesser chance of inducing hypothermia. Chemical burns require prolonged washing (half to one hour) with copious amounts of running tap water to dilute the chemical as much as possible. No household remedy or topical agent should be applied to the burnt site lest evaluation of depth of burns become difficult. Moreover, removal of this agent may be a painful. The burnt area should be covered with clean sheet to prevent contamination and hypothermia and the child should be transported to the medical facility at the earliest. The child should not be given anything orally on the way as vomiting may occur.

Hospital Management

Assessment of patient

With the arrival of the child to a clinician, one has to assess the child's general condition besides assessing the burn wound. In children with major burns, the standard protocol (primary and secondary surveys) as for any major trauma, needs to be followed meticulously. These children may be involved in house/building/bus on fire or other road traffic accidents involving mechanical injury as well as burns, including inhalational injury. Children with electrical burns with a history of fall from height also need to be assessed and managed as per trauma protocol.

Primary survey: Airway, breathing and circulation should be assessed and managed before assessing the exact extent of burn injury. Airway and breathing may be compromised due to inhalation injury as well as secondary to circulatory shock caused by burns. In presence of hoarseness, stridor or progressive facial or neck edema, intubation may be advisable. Intubation and ventilation is also required if respiratory failure occurs – PaO_2 <60 mm Hg or $PaCO_2$ >50 mm Hg with optimal conservative management. Endotracheal tube should be securely placed as edema can make re-intubation after unplanned extubation extremely difficult. If peripheral or central venous access is difficult, intraosseous access may be a good option.[9] If possible, intravenous or intraosseous access should be obtained in intact skin. Central venous catheter is avoided, especially in the early phase, as it is associated with high risk of infection.

Secondary survey: It includes a review of the mechanism of injury, a careful head to toe physical examination, and radiographs if required. All patients with burns should be registered as medicolegal cases. Child abuse or neglect should be considered when presentation for care is delayed or the reported injury mechanism is not consistent with the physical findings. Some wound patterns are particularly concerning, such as those including flexor sparing and wounds consistent with immersion or contact.[9]

A very brief history of the mechanism of burn and a quick look at the patient and burnt areas can tell the physician how to proceed. In patients with respiratory and/or circulatory compromise, appropriate intensive resuscitative measures are immediately instituted. As fluid loss into the interstitial space leading to decreased blood volume is the basic pathology occurring in a moderate to severely burnt patient, fluid replacement is the mainstay of treatment. All critical and moderate cases require immediate establishment of an intravenous access with a large bore cannula or even a venous cut down in long saphenous vein at the ankle.

Assessment of burn injury

The burn wound is evaluated for its extent in relation to the total body surface area, and the depth of skin burnt. This is important (i) to establish criteria for admission to a specialized burn care facility; (ii) to classify the wounds as minor, moderate or critical for the purpose of management; (iii) for calculating the initial fluid requirements during resuscitation; and (iv) to enable the clinician to prognosticate the parents regarding survival, expected time of healing, need for surgical interventions, rehabilitation and scarring.

Besides being a prognostic indicator, the depth of burn determines if the wound is going to heal on its own or else will require skin grafting for closure. Partial thickness burns, where whole of epidermis and only a part of dermal thickness is burnt, can heal by spontaneous epithelialization from the epithelial remnants in the sweat and sebaceous glands and hair follicles deeply placed in dermis. On the contrary, in a full thickness burn injury, when the whole of epidermis and dermis is burnt, skin grafting is invariably required to heal the wound. Those cases where subcutaneous fat, deep fascia and even muscle are burnt also come under this category.

Although, scalds are generally considered more superficial as compared to flame burns, they can also be full thickness burn injuries due to thin skin of a child. As the hair follicles do not extend deeper than dermis, it is an important marker for determining burn depth and potential for wound healing.

Assessment of the patient as a whole and his/her wounds allows the treating doctor to decide as to whether the child can be managed on an outpatient basis or needs admission to a hospital. It is convenient to categorize the burn patients as minor, moderate or critical **(Box 1)** for the purpose of establishing admission criteria. Patients with minor burns are managed on an outpatient basis. All other patients should be hospitalized, and the critically burnt patients are preferably admitted to a specialized burn care facility. Available data support the view that burns are most cost-effectively managed in dedicated burn centers rather than in general hospitals, with improved survival in higher volume centers.

Box 1: Categorization of patients with burns for triage and management

Critical burns
- Partial thickness burns >5% TBSA in infants and >15% TBSA in older children
- Full thickness burns >3% TBSA
- Burns of special sites like hands, face and perineum
- Burns with associated injury, inhalation injury or any pre-existing illness
- Electrical burns
- Chemical burns
- Burns with concomitant trauma (such as fractures)

Moderate burns
- Partial thickness burns 2–5% TBSA in infants and 10–15% TBSA in older children
- Full thickness burns1–3% TBSA

Minor burns

Partial thickness burns <2% TBSA in infants and <10% TBSA in older children

(TBSA: total body surface area)

Outpatient care of minor burn wounds

These patients do not require intravenous fluids. They are advised normal diet with increased intake of oral fluids. The wounds are to be dressed, and the child may be sent home with an advice to report back for change of dressing. Parents should be told about symptoms and signs of infection (fever, malaise, vomiting, undue/increased pain or foul smelling discharge), and told to return immediately if these are noted. Paracetamol is prescribed for pain control - for round-the-clock effect initially, and on as required basis, later. Prophylactic antibiotics are not routinely advised. Elevation of the burnt site above the heart level reduces edema and helps with pain control.

Management of hospitalized children

In patients admitted to a hospital, restoration of the blood volume is the single most important factor essential to the survival of a burnt patient in the initial period. Care must be taken to maintain temperature as hypothermia may occur. An assessment for associated injuries should also be made. In all major burns, baseline investigations like hemogram, blood glucose, serum electrolytes, blood urea nitrogen and creatinine, lactic acid and arterial blood gases should be done. Urinalysis is obtained to assess for myoglobin. For flame burns, a chest radiograph and blood carboxyhemoglobin levels are obtained.

Fluid and electrolyte therapy: Effective fluid therapy aims at restoring blood volume, maintaining acid-base and electrolyte balance, and preventing organ dysfunction. Intravenous fluid resuscitation is generally not required in children with burns <15% of the TBSA. These children can usually be managed with fluid administered orally at 150% of maintenance requirements while hydration status is monitored by physical examination and weighing diapers or measurement of urine output. With larger TBSA burns, several fluid regimens have been advocated but they all need to be modified in response to patient's vital parameters. Because capillaries are permeable to even larger molecules like albumin, it is generally agreed that the initial resuscitation should be with crystalloids. If colloids are used, they leak into interstitial space due to increased capillary permeability caused by the burn injury, and after the capillary permeability is restored, they increase the tissue edema. However, albumin or plasma may be administered after the first 24 hours to children with extensive burns. All formulae for fluid resuscitation have been devised for adult patients, and consequently they tend to under-estimate requirements in children who have a larger body surface area in relation to body weight. The most popular formula today is Parkland formula. According to this, in first 24 hours, Ringer's lactate solution is infused in a volume of 4 mL/kg body/TBSA% burn, in addition to the maintenance fluid requirement.[17] Half of the calculated requirement of fluids is transfused in first 8 hours, one-fourth in the second 8 hours, and the remaining one-fourth in the last 8 hours. The time periods are calculated from the time of burn and not the time of admission to the hospital. Infants are at risk of developing hypoglycemia because of limited glycogen stores, and hence require monitoring of blood glucose levels. For the next 24 hours, the fluid requirements are approximately halved, and resuscitation is followed-up with dextrose normal saline.

An indwelling urinary catheter is placed for monitoring hourly urine output, which is the single most important clinical parameter of adequacy of resuscitation[18] Average urine output must be maintained at around 1 mL/kg/hour to be considered adequate. Fluid overload can occur if urine output targets are set too high *i.e.* 2 mL/kg/hour.[19] Excess fluid induces 'fluid creep' that is associated with complications such as increased compartmental pressures (abdominal compartment syndrome, extremity compartment syndrome), Acute respiratory distress syndrome (ARDS), and pleural or pericardial effusions. It also causes conversion of burns to deeper wounds, blood stream infections, multiple organ failure and death.

Urinary catheter patency must be ensured before labeling a patient oliguric. Low urine output is treated by administering more fluids rather than by prescribing diuretics. However, a single dose of intravenous mannitol or furosemide may be required for persistent oliguria resistant to fluid therapy to rule out renal shut down. Other variables to judge the state of hydration and appropriateness of fluid and electrolyte therapy are pulse rate, blood pressure (difficult to measure with extremity burns), body weight, hematocrit, levels of blood urea and electrolytes, and urinary specific gravity. Despite success of various resuscitation approaches, optimal fluid requirement still remains a matter of debate. Whatever the approach, it is important to dynamically titrate fluids to the individual patient to prevent problems of over/under resuscitation.

In contact electrical burns, where there may be a lot of muscle damage, myoglobinuria may occur in addition to hemoglobinuria. To clear these pigments and prevent renal tubular blockade, intravenous mannitol is administered every 6–8 hours till the urine is clear. In patients with hemoglobinuria or myoglobinuria, the urine should be maintained at an alkaline pH by infusing sodium bicarbonate solution.

Blood transfusions are not required in the first 48 hours unless the child is severely anemic. It may be required later to maintain hematocrit of 30–35% and a hemoglobin level of more than 10 g/dL. Plasma or albumin has been traditionally added after 24 hours as it can minimize hypoproteinemia. This is significant when the burnt area exceeds 40% BSA. Albumin is given in a volume ranging from 0.3–0.5 mL/kg/TBSA% of burns, and the amount is to be subtracted from maintenance fluids. The rate of edema formation is maximal at 8 to 12 hours after injury.[20] Except for a transient loss of capillary integrity, non-burnt tissues soon regain the ability to sieve plasma proteins.

Although injured and burnt cells release potassium, hyperkalemia is noticed rarely. With adequate resuscitation, the excess potassium is effectively excreted. Additional potassium is only occasionally necessary during the diuretic phase. A close watch is maintained on serum electrolyte levels because rapid fluid and electrolyte shifts in burnt children can result in cerebral edema and convulsions. From second day onwards, the child is gradually started on liquid, semisolid and solid diet over a period of next 3–4 days with corresponding reduction in or complete omission of intravenous fluids. During this period, the patient should be watched for vomiting, paralytic ileus, abdominal distention, return of bowel sounds and activity, and passage of stools. As the capillary permeability is restored, urinary volumes far exceed the total of oral and intravenous intake due to return of fluid from the extracellular compartment into the intravascular compartment.

Pain relief: Pain relief and sedation must be preceded by correction of hypovolemia and hypoxia as they are the cause of restlessness in a burnt patient. Pentazocine and promethazine combination in appropriate doses are used intravenously (slowly) on "as and when required" basis. Dressing changes can be especially painful for which ketamine may be a useful drug. However, it needs the services of an anesthesiologist and specialized burn-care units.

Nutrition: An extensive burn is characterized by hypermetabolism, increased heat loss, accelerated tissue breakdown and erosion of body mass proportional to the extent of burns. Children are at a special risk because of higher basal metabolic requirements, increased body surface area in relation to bodyweight, decreased endogenous caloric reserves, and increased requirements for growth and development. Malnutrition and hypoproteinemia lead to lowered resistance and delay in wound healing. Hypermetabolism can be minimized by keeping the child in a warm environment (32°C) and by use of occlusive dressings to limit evaporative losses. Excessive evaporative water loss results in an expenditure of 0.5 kcal/g of water lost. Preventing hyperpyrexia and early treatment of sepsis also help in limiting metabolic requirements.

Burns involving >5% TBSA in infants and >15% TBSA in older children are universally accompanied by paralytic ileus because of hypovolemia and neuroendocrine changes. Therefore, the child should be kept nil per orally. If the stomach is already full, a nasogastric tube may be inserted for decompression, to prevent acute gastric dilatation. Oral intake is not restricted in children with less extensive burns. In fact, infants with <5% burns are encouraged to breastfeed. Many older children with less severe burns can also be completely managed by using oral rehydration solutions and milk.

Enteral route is preferred for nutritional support and is generally available. It preserves integrity of the gastrointestinal tract mucosa in addition to improving its blood flow and motility. Oral feeding should be started as soon as initial burn resuscitation is complete. In general, it is usually instituted by second to third post-burn day, and by the fifth day it is increased to meet the predicted calorie requirements. If the child is unable to take orally, a nasogastric tube may be placed, through which freshly prepared feeds at body temperature can be given as a drip. The feeds should have 1 kcal/mL and a low osmolality (300–700 mOsm/L) or else they may lead to osmotic diarrhea. Fat intake of <20% of overall caloric intake and vitamin A supplementation reduce the incidence of diarrhea in burn victims. Parenteral alimentation or supplements are necessary if the child is having vomiting, diarrhea or malabsorption.

There are many formulae to calculate daily caloric requirements in children, two of which are given below:

1. *Curreri's formula* 60 kcal/kg bodyweight + 35 kcal/%TBSA burnt [21]
2. *Carjaval's formula:* 2200 kcal/m^2 of burnt area + 1800 kcal/m^2 of BSA [22]

These formulae overestimate requirements by 20% and should be used as target levels only. Diets calculated in the above manner can lead to positive nitrogen balance and prevent weight loss. Along with calories, an adequate amount of protein is required. Higher protein intake (2 to 2.5 g/kg body weight per day) leads to better neutrophil function and improves resistance and survival. Dietary supplements of vitamins and trace elements, including zinc, copper, chromium and molybdenum, are also important for wound healing and should be given orally or in intravenous fluids.

Systemic antibiotics: A burn wound provides large, warm, moist and protein-rich medium for growth of microorganisms from endogenous and exogenous sources. The patient is also more susceptible to infection due to a depressed immune system. Consequently, sepsis is the leading cause of death from major burns. Routine use of prophylactic systemic antibiotics, however, is not recommended as it leads to rapid emergence of resistant strains.

Routine bacteriological monitoring of the burn wound is carried out with culture and sensitivity examination of swabs from the wound surface. Burn wound biopsies have been used to provide a quantitative estimation of the bacteria in the wound and infection is diagnosed when >10^5 bacteria are present per gram of tissue or there is invasion of subjacent healthy tissues. Local signs of burn wound sepsis include development of black or purple necrotic areas in the wound and hemorrhage in the sub-eschar fat. Bacteria generally isolated from the burn wound are *Pseudomonas, Klebsiella, Staph. aureus, E. coli, Strep. faecalis* and *Proteus* spp. Fungi and viruses are also being increasingly isolated. Septicemia in burns can also result by invasion of bacteria from the respiratory tract, indwelling cannula, urinary tract catheter, and sometimes from gastrointestinal tract. Whereas no clinical sign alone is diagnostic of septicemia, it is clinically suspected when there is a change in condition of the wound, presence of hyper- or hypothermia, deterioration in level of consciousness, tachypnea, tachycardia, abdominal distention, diarrhea and oliguria. Although infection is accompanied by fever and leukocytosis, burn wound sepsis may manifest with hypothermia and leukopenia.

Systemic antibiotics are the mainstay of treatment for wound infection. If the culture and sensitivity reports are available, the appropriate antibiotic treatment is directed towards the identified bacteria. Otherwise, antibiotics are started in broad-spectrum combinations (e.g. cephalosporin and aminoglycoside) empirically, pending culture reports. Antibiotics are started at the first sign of sepsis, in maximal therapeutic doses, and stopped only after seven days or so. The antibiotics useful in septicemia are penicillins (including amoxicillin with clavulanic acid and piperacillin), third generation cephalosporins (e.g. ceftazidime, cefotaxime, ceftriaxone), aminoglycosides (e.g. gentamicin, tobramycin, amikacin, netilmicin), quinolones (ciprofloxacin, ofloxacin) and carbapenems (meropenem, imipenem).

Other considerations: Tetanus toxoid injection should be administered for prophylaxis against tetanus along standard recommended lines. In children not properly immunized, passive protection should also be provided with 250 units of tetanus immunoglobulin. Children admitted to the hospital should be prescribed medicines for acid suppression (e.g. ranitidine, pantoprazole) for prophylaxis against gastroduodenal erosions and ulcerations (Curling ulcers).

Management of the burn wound

A burn wound is an area of coagulative necrosis with ischemia of the surrounding tissue from thrombosis of underlying microcirculation. The aim of local treatment is to prevent microbial colonization and proliferation, and allow a partial thickness burn to heal spontaneously or else prepare a full thickness burn for skin grafting. Bacterial growth can be prevented by a number of topical antimicrobial agents. In extensive burns, it is essential that the topical agent used should not only be a broad-spectrum agent but in order to prevent sepsis, it should also effectively penetrate the eschar for control of infection at that level. Because of impaired microcirculation, the systemic antibiotics cannot reach this level in sufficient concentration to limit bacterial growth.

Topical therapy: Silver sulfadiazine, available as 1% cream, is the most commonly used topical agent all over the world for major burns. It is a broad-spectrum agent, bactericidal to a wide range of bacteria known to colonize the burn wound, including *Pseudomonas.* It is applied as 5–10 mm thick layer and is painless. Transient leukopenia can occasionally result from its use. Mafenide (Sulfamylon) cream (11.1%) and silver nitrate solution (0.5%) are other topical agents used specifically in burns. Sulfamylon has a wide anti-bacterial spectrum and also penetrates the eschar readily. It is used as a substitute to silver sulfadiazine to control burn wound sepsis. However, its application is painful, and being carbonic anhydrase inhibitor, it can also lead to metabolic acidosis. Application of silver nitrate is tedious, and it penetrates the eschar rather poorly. It can also lead to methemoglobinemia and electrolyte disturbances by leaching cations into the wound. Presently, nano-crystalline forms of silver impregnated dressings are available in the market for application on the burn wounds.

A combination of neomycin, polymyxin and bacitracin (triple antibiotic cream), or povidone-iodine or framycetin containing ointments and creams are recommended in cases of minor burns only. Although, povidone-iodine can sometimes be used in extensive burns, its routine use in these cases can lead to iodine toxicity. In burn units, it is recommended that this agent be periodically alternated with silver sulfadiazine to prevent development of bacterial resistance with either agent.

Dressing technique: The burn wound is gently cleaned with dilute cetavlon and saline solutions and mopped dry. A topical chemotherapeutic agent is applied and covered with a single layer of non-stick paraffin gauze followed by multiple layers of absorbent gauze. Thereafter, Gamgee pads (thick cotton sandwiched between two layers of gauze) are applied and held in place with gentle compressive dressings. The dressings are changed daily in case of extensive burns. However, in minor or moderate burns, they may be changed after 2–4 days. Soakage of dressing, foul smell, and undue or increased pain and fever are indications for an earlier inspection of the wound.

Areas like face, perineum and buttocks cannot be dressed, and are kept exposed. After cleaning, the wound is left to dry. The exudate along with the superficial layer of burned skin forms a protective cover under which a partial thickness wound can heal. This technique can also be used if only one surface of the body is burnt. However, it is not practical to manage extensive burns by this method.

Burn wound excision: By conventional dressing techniques, a deep dermal burn heals generally in 3–6 weeks. It is highly prone to develop severe hypertrophic scarring. Check correctness of this statement. It is confusing regarding whether skin grafting has potential to prevent sepsis or exacerbate risk of sepsis.

A full thickness burn becomes fit for skin grafting after 3–4 weeks' time. Improvement in intensive care management has allowed burn surgeons to be positively aggressive towards a burn wound. This involves excising the dead skin, layer by layer, till viable dermis is reached in a case of deep dermal burn (tangential excision) or healthy and live tissues are reached in full thickness burns. The excised wound is preferably immediately split skin grafted to prevent its desiccation and further cell death. If enough autograft skin is not available, the excised wound is covered temporarily with a skin substitute to prevent plasma loss by exudation. Burn wound excision is done after the patient has been fully resuscitated but before significant bacterial proliferation has occurred. This is usually between 3rd and 7th day following the burn. This approach requires patient selection, an experienced team, sufficient operating time, adequate blood, donor sites for skin autograft and skin substitutes. Thus, this technique is generally practiced in specialized burn centers only. Circumferential full thickness burns are associated with a unique problem of compromising blood flow to underlying viable tissues due to edema and lack of elasticity of the burn wound (an eschar). Hence, they require escharotomies (incision through eschar) to release sub-eschar pressure. Fasciotomies of the various muscle compartments in upper and lower extremities is required, especially in electrical burns. Edema of the muscles under the tight deep fascia leads to ischemia, and even necrosis occurs along with compromise of arterial supply and venous drainage unless multiple fasciotomies are done to relieve all the muscle compartments.

Skin grafting: A full thickness burn will ultimately require autograft skin for permanent cover. Split skin grafts can be harvested from any part of the body with a manually operated Watson's modification of Humby Skin Grafting Knife with detachable and disposable blade or else with an electrical/power dermatome. The wound has to be adequately prepared to receive the graft. The donor area heals spontaneously from epithelial remnants in dermal appendages. Skin grafts can be applied as small stamps, strips or large sheets depending on the availability of the amount of graft. With the availability of skin graft mesher, a sheet of skin graft can be meshed and expanded several times to increase the size of graft when the donor area available is less than the area of recipient site. Presence of beta-hemolytic *Streptococci* is an absolute contraindication to skin grafting whereas *Pseudomonas* and *Staphylococcus* infections are relative contraindications. While Streptococcus does not allow the graft to stick to the wound, *Staphylococcus* starts eating away the graft after its initial "take".[23] Other bacteria when present in numbers less than 10^5 per gram of tissue allow satisfactory "take" of graft.

Skin substitutes: Many skin substitutes are available which can provide temporary and permanent wound coverage.[23-25] Because they adhere to the wound surface, they reduce pain and prevent exudative losses. They can also reduce bacterial proliferation and prepare a wound for autografting. If they are used to cover a partial thickness burn, they may aid the healing process. They are also valuable in providing temporary cover following excisional surgery when enough autograft is not available.

Biological skin substitutes like homografts (allografts), heterografts (xenografts) and amnion have traditionally had much appeal. Skin transplant from live donors (parents) or cadavers is being done occasionally. It must be remembered that they are all temporary as they get rejected as per principles of graft rejection. However, they do tide over the crisis for few days during which the child's condition improves. Their use involves a careful exclusion of hepatitis, syphilis and HIV infection. *Synthetic skin substitutes* like Epigard, Biobrane, Hydron and Opsite, though expensive, are appealing because of "off the shelf" availability. In laboratories, *Keratinocyte culture techniques* provide epidermal sheet of 1 m^2 in three weeks time, from a 1 cm^2 autograft. Although, it provides wound cover, it lacks skin texture because of the absence of a dermal layer. Burke and Yannas[26] developed a bilaminar, *biosynthetic substitute* to simulate skin. This "artificial skin" consists of an epidermal layer made from silastic and a dermal layer from bovine and shark collagen. It can be stored in 70% isopropyl alcohol. After removing the silastic sheet, autografts or cultured keratinocytes can be placed on the neodermis to complete the wound coverage.

Inhalational Injuries

Inhalation injury may also sometimes occur in burns patients. It is usually due to inhalation of toxic products of combustion, and not due to thermal injury as commonly thought. Clinical indicators of inhalation injury include face or neck burns, carbon deposits and acute inflammatory changes in the oropharynx, hoarseness of voice, or history of confinement in a burning environment.[2] Inhalation of smoke and toxic gases leads to pulmonary complications, including airway obstruction by bronchial casts, pulmonary edema, decreased pulmonary compliance and ventilation perfusion mismatch as well as systemic toxicity from carbon monoxide (CO) poisoning and cyanide toxicity.[27]

Carbon monoxide poisoning may lead to headache, coma and death. Diagnosis is mostly made by a history of burns in enclosed areas. Carboxyhemoglobin levels may be checked and more than 10% is consistent with significant inhalation injury. High flow O_2 may be administered by a non-rebreathing mask in cases of suspected CO poisoning.

The inflammatory reaction can lead to the formation of endobronchial casts and obstruction of the distal airways. Mucociliary clearance mechanisms are disrupted and the accumulation of necrotic debris and products of inflammation provide an environment conducive to infection. These patients often benefit from bronchoscopy to enhance pulmonary toilet and minimize the risk of pneumonia or, when pneumonia is present, facilitate its resolution. Although no data support the routine use of mucolytics in patients with inhalation injury, many experts recommend *N*-acetyl-cysteine (3–5 mL of a 20% solution nebulized 3–4 times a day) to help clear tenacious secretions.

Care of Healed Burn Wound

Once a burn wound has healed, either spontaneously or by skin grafting, it needs prolonged care. The patients usually complain a lot of itching, which is worse at night, in spontaneously healed areas and the donor sites of split skin grafts. Itching may be relieved by the use of oral antihistaminic drugs. There is also a tendency for hypertrophic scar formation in healed deep dermal burns. All the healed burn wounds and skin graft donor sites should be massaged with bland oils/cream (e.g. coconut oil) till the scar is mature (usually a period of a period of 9 months to one year). Pressure garments are prescribed to prevent as well as to treat already developed hypertrophic scar formation for a similar period. Exposure to sunlight (ultraviolet rays) should be strictly avoided till the healed wounds regain their normal pigmentation/coloration, generally a period of 3–4 months or more, to avoid hyperpigmentation. Last but not the least, the parents are counseled at every visit.

REHABILITATION

Physical therapy and occupational therapy consultation is required for all burn patients as soon as they are clinically stable. This is particularly important in patients with burns that extend over the joints. Range of motion and neutral positioning of joints needs to be stressed to prevent contracture formation.[2]

A burn injury is a traumatic experience for a child and the family, and requires long-term individualized psychological and emotional support. The child may exhibit signs of extreme anxiety as a result of the initial trauma, repeated exposure to painful procedures, possible separation from parents during procedures and long-term hospital stay. A burn injury not only leaves the scars on the skin but also on the mind. Returning to school and relating to their peers and teachers requires a major psychological adjustment on part of the child. The parents suffer not only monetary loss because of costly and lengthy treatment involving extended time away from work, but also psychologically because of the societal problems related with disfigurement and scars. They require a lot of emotional and psychological support.

PROGNOSTIC FACTORS

The likelihood of death is inversely related to age of child. Greater the extent and deeper the burn injury, higher is the mortality (**Fig. 7**). Flame burns are generally associated with higher mortality as compared to scalds. The risk of death rises sharply with concomitant inhalation injury. Management of extensive burns is extremely expensive and often prolonged. The poor socioeconomic status is certainly a contributing factor in increasing the morbidity and mortality.

PREVENTION

Often, the carelessness of adults is to be blamed for almost all cases of pediatric burns. Hence, the incidence of childhood burns can be greatly reduced only if a child is not left unattended/unobserved for even a very short period of time. Match boxes, lighters and inflammable materials must be kept out of reach of children. Kitchen burns in toddlers can be reduced either by excluding them from the kitchen or by avoiding easy access to pans, bright colored potter and by avoiding the use of tablecloth at mealtime. A child should not sit in one's lap while one drinks a hot beverage.

Firecrackers should be burst only under adult supervision. Minimize storage of flammable liquids, acids and other chemicals, and keep them away from areas where children play. The electrical sockets in the household must be at a higher level and out of reach of small children. Covers can be used on electrical outlets. The electrical appliances should be modified so as to be safe for children, e.g. use of hot blowers rather than heating rods during winters.

In addition, children should be taught about being careful of hot liquids, fire and electricity from a very young age (2-year onwards). Teach children to "stop, drop, and roll" if clothing is on fire. Schools, television and other media may help in spreading awareness at community level.

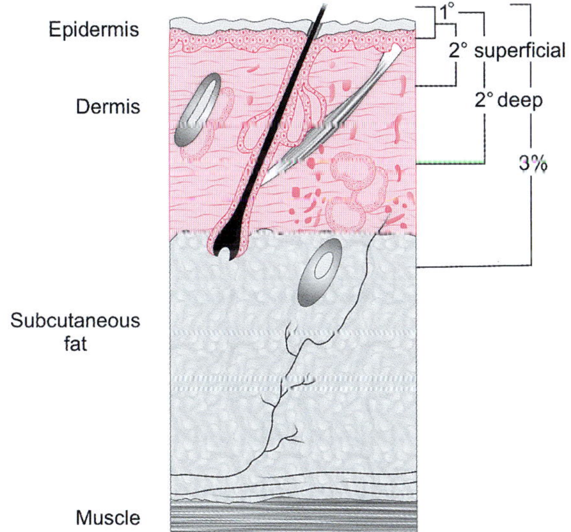

Fig. 7: A vertical section through skin to illustrate the basis of classification of depth of burns

KEY MESSAGES

- Burn injury is the second most important cause of trauma-related deaths in children and vast majority of burns occur in child's own home.
- Burn size is calculated by Rule of nine in children >15 years, and rule of five in children <15 years, or by detailed body surface area charts prepared by Lund and Browder.
- First aid includes extinguishing the flames and pouring tap water on the burn area and no topical application.
- Adequate fluid resuscitation with urine output monitoring is the most important aspect of burn management. Overhydration of patient is to be avoided.
- Routine use of prophylactic antibiotics is not recommended; wound is managed by proper dressings and if required skin grafting bacteriological monitoring of the burn wound should be carried out.

REFERENCES

1. Goel A. Post burn sequelae and their management. In: Sarabhai S, Tiwari VK, Goel A, Gupta LC, editors. Principles and Practice of Burn care, 1st edition. New Delhi; Jaypee Brothers Medical Publishers; 2010. p. 468-515.
2. Shah AR, Liao LF. Pediatric burn care: unique considerations in management. Clin Plastic Surg. 2017;44:603-10.
3. Cinat ME, Smith MM. Acute burn management In: Achauer and Sood's Burn Surgery Reconstruction and Rehabilitation. Edinburgh: Saunders Elsevier; 2006. p. 50-76.
4. Libber SM, Slayton DI. Childhood burns reconsidered: The child, the family and the burn injury. J Trauma. 1985;24:245-52.
5. Moehrlen T, Szucs T, Landolt MA, *et al.* Trauma mechanisms and injury patterns in pediatric burn patients. Burns. 2018,44.320-34.
6. Leake JE, Curtin JW. Electrical burns of the mouth in children. Clin Plast Surg. 1984,11.669-83.
7. Lenoski EF, Hunter KA. Specific patterns of inflicted burn injuries. J Trauma. 1977;17:842-6.
8. Wolf SE, Cancio LC, Pruitt BA. Epidemiological, Demographic and Outcome characteristics of Burn Injury In Herndon DN. Total burn care, 5th edition. Edinburgh; Saunders Elsevier; 2018. p. 14-27.
9. Sheridan RL. Burn care for children. Pediatr Rev. 2018;39:273-84.

10. Jackson DM. The diagnosis of depth of burning. Br J Surg. 1953;40:588-96.
11. Lund CC, Browder NC. The estimation of areas of burns. Surg Gynecol Obstet. 1944;79:352-8.
12. Knaysi GA, Crikelair GF, Cosman B. The rule of Nines: Its history and accuracy. Plast Reconstr Surg. 1968;41:560-3.
13. Lynch JB, Blocker V. The rule of five in estimation of extent of burn. In: Converse JM, editor. Reconstructive Plastic Surgery, 1st edition. Philadelphia: WB Saunders Co; 1964. p. 208.
14. Gore M. Initial evaluation and resuscitation of burn patient. In: Sarabhai S, Tiwari VK, Goel A, Gupta LC. Principles and Practice of Burn Care, 1st edition. New Delhi; Jaypee Brothers Medical Publishers; 2010. p. 101-26.
15. Wurzer P, Culnan D, Cancio LC, *et al.* Pathophysiology of burn shock and burn edema. In: Herndon DN. Total Burn Care, 5th edition. Edinburgh: Saunders Elsevier; 2018. p. 66-76.
16. Jeschke MG, Herndon DN. Burns in children: Standard and new treatments. Lancet. 2014;383(9923):1168-78.
17. Pediatric burn injury. In: Pierre L, Pringle EJ, editors. Pediatric Fundamental Critical Care Support, 3rd edition. 500 Midway Drive Mount Prospect, IL 60056 USA; Society of Critical Care Medicine; 2018. p. 421-46.
18. Fabri PJ. Monitoring of the burn patient. Clin Plast Surg. 1986; 13:21-7.
19. Pruit BA Jr. Protection from excessive resuscitation. "pushing the pendulum back". J Trauma. 2000;49:567-8.
20. Demling RH. The burn edema process: current concepts. J Burn Care Rehabil. 2005;26:207-27.
21. Curreri PW, Luterman A. Nutritional support of the burned patient. Surg Clin North Am. 1978;58:1151-6.
22. Hildreth M, Carjaval HF. Caloric requirements in burned children: A simple formula to estimate daily caloric requirements. J Burn Care Rehabil. 1982;3:78-80.
23. Bhandari PS, Goel A. Skin grafts and flaps in orthopedics. In: Jain AK. Turek's Orthopedics: Principles and their Applications, 7th edition. Wolters Kluwer; 2016. p. 1712-36.
24. Haddad AG, Giatsidis G, Orgill DP, *et al.* Skin substitutes and bioscaffolds. Clin Plast Surg. 2017;44:627-34.
25. Sheridan R. Closure of excised burn wound: Autografts, semi-permanent skin substitutes and permanent skin substitutes Clin Plast Surg. 2009;36:643-51.
26. Burke JF, Yannas IV, Quinby WC, *et al.* Successful use of a physiologically acceptable artificial skin in the treatment of extensive burn injury. Ann Surg. 1981;194:413-28.
27. Fidkowski KW, Fusaylov G, Sheridan RL, *et al.* Inhalation burn injury in children. Paediatr Anaesth. 2009;19(Suppl 1): 147-54.

CHAPTER

55

Drowning and Immersion Injuries

Lalitha Janakiraman, R Ganesh

INTRODUCTION

Drowning is a major but often neglected public health problem. Drowning is the 3rd leading cause of unintentional injury deaths worldwide accounting for 7% of all such deaths.[1] The most important steps to reduce the mortality due to drowning are prevention and timely initiation of cardiopulmonary resuscitation (CPR) at the site.

DEFINITION

According to World Congress of Drowning (WCOD), endorsed by WHO, drowning is the process of experiencing respiratory impairment from submersion (face and airway covered in water) or immersion (whole body including airway under water). The outcome can be fatal or non fatal while some non-fatal drowning events can result in significant neurological damage. The guidelines also state that the terms near-drowning, secondary drowning, wet/dry drowning should no longer be used.[2,3]

EPIDEMIOLOGY

Worldwide, an estimated 3,60,000 people died from drowning in the year 2015.[1] Majority of child deaths due to drowning occur in low- and middle-income countries. India and China have high drowning mortality rates, and together contribute to 43% of all drowning deaths worldwide.[4] In a study from Kerala in India, the prevalence of non-fatal drowning was 4% accounting to 270.6/1,00,000 persons/year.[5] Another study from Bihar reported that drowning deaths accounted for 7.2%, 12.5% and 5.8% of all deaths in children aged 1–4, 5–9 and 10–14 years, respectively.[6]

RISK FACTORS

The risk factors for drowning are as follows:

- *Gender*: Males have higher drowning rates than females because of increased exposure to water and riskier behavior.
- *Age*: The age distribution of drowning injury is bimodal. The first peak occurs in children below 5 years of age where they are inadequately supervised in or near bath tubs, swimming pools, garden ponds, and any other liquid-filled containers such as buckets and tubs. The second peak is seen in persons aged 15–25 years, and these episodes occur at ponds, rivers, lakes and sea.
- *Season*: Drowning is more frequently reported during the summer months and weekends.
- The other risk factors for drowning are use of liquor prior to swimming, under water swimming, pre-existing epilepsy and cardiac arrhythmias, travel on unsafe water transport (poorly manned/overcrowded boats and ferries), living in geographical areas that are prone for natural disasters like Tsunamis, lack of trained and adequate adult supervision, and overestimation of one's swimming capabilities.

PATHOPHYSIOLOGY

The sequence of events that follow during drowning is shown in **Flowchart 1**.

Flowchart 1: Sequential events following drowning

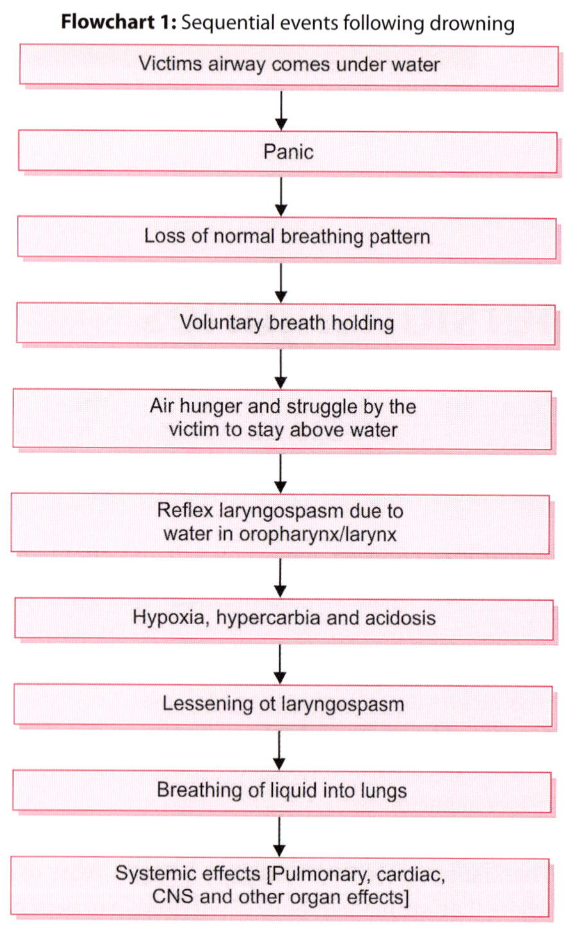

Pulmonary Effects

Functional residual capacity (FRC) is the only source of gas exchange at the pulmonary capillary level in the submerged state. Hypoxia, hypercarbia and acidosis hampers FRC. It has been reported that aspiration of liquid of 1-3 mL/kg body weight results in impairment of gas exchange.[7] Aspiration of liquid into the lungs washes away the pulmonary surfactant, and injures the alveoli and pulmonary capillaries resulting in increased membrane permeability, exudation of proteinaceous material into the alveoli, pulmonary edema, reduced lung compliance and increased airway resistance leading to Acute respiratory distress syndrome (ARDS). Also, the victim may aspirate mud, sewage or own gastric contents during the process of drowning, which might increase the risk of invasion by bacteria and fungi adding to the risk of morbidity and mortality.

Cardiovascular Effects

Severe cardiovascular instability is encountered following a drowning event that poses a threat to survival. Hypoxia results in ventilation perfusion mismatch leading to arrhythmias—ventricular tachycardia, fibrillation and asystole. Hypoxia also causes myocardial ischemia impairing the myocardial contractility. The presence of acidosis further impairs the myocardial contractility resulting in cardiogenic shock.

Central Nervous System Effects

Hypoxia results in neuronal damage, thereby leading to cerebral edema. The magnitude and severity of brain damage depends upon the duration of hypoxia, the degree of cerebral hypoperfusion, and the mechanism of secondary brain injury. The major determinant of long-term outcome in a drowning victim is the presence and degree of cerebral impairment.[8]

Acid Base and Electrolytes

Metabolic acidosis with or without respiratory acidosis is seen in a drowning victim. Electrolyte abnormalities such as hypernatremia, hypermagnesemia and hypercalcemia are seen in victims drowned in sea water.

Renal, Hepatic and Gastrointestinal Effects

Renal failure can be seen in victims of drowning, and that occurs due to hypoxia, renal tubular necrosis, hemoglobinuria or myoglobinuria. Liver dysfunction is manifested by elevation of serum bilirubin levels, elevated serum transaminase levels and impaired production of procoagulant factors. It can also lead to disseminated intravascular coagulation. Gastrointestinal injury is manifested as mucosal sloughing due to ischemia resulting in foul smelling bloody mucoid stools. This can result in bacterial translocation and perforation of the gastrointestinal tract.

Hypothermia and Diving Reflex

Apart from hypoxia, hypothermia is also responsible for many pathophysiological consequence of drowning. The most important effect of severe hypothermia is a decrease in energy utilization. Cerebral metabolism is depressed and oxygen consumption is reduced. Hypothermia also increases the blood viscosity by causing hemoconcentration. The oxy-hemoglobin dissociation curve shifts to the left. Hypothermia decreases white blood corpuscle (WBC) function increasing the risk of infection. It also decreases insulin production and impairs tissue glucose utilization resulting in hyperglycemia. Diving reflex acts as an oxygen conserving adaptation in response to submersion. It appears to be triggered by fear and cold stimulation. Cerebral blood flow is maintained while blood flow to gastrointestinal tract, skin and muscles is markedly reduced.[9]

MANAGEMENT OF DROWNING

The clinical outcome in a drowning victim is mainly determined by the duration of hypoxia. Hence, every attempt should be made to restore ventilation and circulation as early as possible. Therefore, the management of drowning victims are divided into three phases: Pre-hospital care (at the scene), Emergency care, and Pediatric intensive care.[10] The principles of management are listed in **Box 1**.

Pre-hospital Care

Cardiopulmonary resuscitation by the bystander improves the outcome of a drowning victim. Performing high quality chest compressions with delivery of rescue breaths restores circulation and ventilation. Heimlich maneuver and other postural drainage methods to remove water from the lungs are not advised. Less than 0.5% of drowning victims suffer from cervical spine injuries.[11] Hence, cervical spine immobilization is not routinely recommended unless there are signs of injury or the individual has attempted a shallow water diving/skiing/surfing. Removal of wet clothing and rewarming measures if an individual is hypothermic should begin at the scene itself, and should continue during transport. All patients of drowning— no matter how well they seem to appear— should be transported to the nearby hospital. During transport, oxygen must be administered, and measures of monitoring cardiac and respiratory parameters should be continued.

Box 1: Principles of management of children with drowning

At the scene
- Initial resuscitation
- Removal from water
- Assess ABC
- Begin CPR
- Remove debris from oropharynx
- Rescue breathing
- High quality chest compressions
- No Heimlich maneuver/other postural drainage methods to remove water from lungs
- Continue resuscitation till patient reaches emergency room

In the emergency room

Establish adequate oxygenation and ventilation
- Intubation if unable to protect airway
- Provide supplemental oxygen

Establish normal circulation
- Bolus IV fluids (NS)
- Vasopressor infusions for continued hypotension

Neurologic examination
- Determine GCS
- Consider therapeutic hypothermia (32–34°C) for 24–72 hours
- Control seizures -(Fosphenytoin)

Rewarming for hypothermia
- Removal of wet clothes
- Cover with warm blankets
- Give warmed humidified oxygen
- Use warmed fluids and ventilation with heated gas
- Consider peritoneal/bladder wash with warmed fluids

Metabolic
- Correction of dyselectrolytemias, hypo/hyperglycemia

Sepsis
- Apt treatment with appropriate antimicrobials

In the pediatric intensive care unit

Employ ventilator strategies for ARDS
- Limit ventilator peak pressures to 25 torr
- Limit tidal volume to 6–8 mL/kg
- Limit fraction of inspired O_2 to ≤ 0.6
- Optimal use of PEEP
- Consider the use of exogenous surfactant or
- ECMO for continued hypoxemia

Treat myocardial dysfunction
- Titrate vasoactive infusions to obtain normal cardiac output, adequate end organ perfusion

Employ brain protective strategies
- Avoid hyperthermia
- Treat clinical and subclinical seizures
- Frequent neurologic reassessments

Emergency Room Care

All resuscitative measures begun at the site of drowning should be continued. The need for hospitalization should be determined by the severity of drowning episode and clinical evaluation. Medicolegal formalities must be completed. All children with drowning should be observed in emergency room for at least 6 hours. Maintaining airway, monitoring breathing and circulation, assessment of disability, and analysis of exposure should be performed in all patients. The indications of intubation are deterioration of neurological function, not maintaining saturation >90% despite administering high-flow oxygen, or $PaCO_2$ >50 mm Hg. Maintaining optimal positive end-expiratory pressure (PEEP) is effective in reversing hypoxemia. Securing vascular access, drawing samples for blood gas analysis, complete blood counts, glucose, electrolytes, calcium, magnesium should be obtained, and appropriate intravenous fluids (Isotonic crystalloids 20 mL/kg over 15 minutes or colloids 10 mL/kg over 20 minutes) to be administered. A 12-lead electrocardiogram (ECG) and chest *X*-ray should be performed. Management of hypoglycemia and hypothermia should continue in emergency room and in ICU.

Intensive Care

Management of hypothermia

The management of hypothermia (core temperature <35°C) includes passive external rewarming by removing wet clothes and covering with warm blankets; active external rewarming with heated air blowers (avoiding direct blow); and active internal rewarming with warm intravenous fluids, heated humidified oxygen and pleuro/peritoneal/bladder lavage with warm fluids. Active rewarming efforts should be continued till core body temperature is 32–34°C.

Ventilation

The goal is to maintain oxygen saturation between 94% and 98%, PaO_2 between 70 and 100 mm Hg, and $PaCO_2$ around 40 mm Hg. Tidal volume is to be adjusted to 6–8 mL/kg, and optimal PEEP should be delivered. Exogenous surfactant administration may have a role; the role of corticosteroids is controversial. Recognition and apt treatment of secondary bacterial pneumonia with antimicrobials improves the outcome.

Neuroprotection

Intracranial pressure (ICP) should be monitored in ICU. Further brain injury can be prevented by apt recognition and treatment of hypo/hyperglycemia, treatment of seizures with non-sedating anticonvulsants, and raising head end of the bed to 30° after excluding cervical spine injuries. With optimal management, many children show neurologic improvement within first 24–72 hours.

Others

Apt recognition and treatment of complications such as electrolyte disturbances, shock, disseminated intravascular coagulation, and multiorgan dysfunction should be done in PICU.

PROGNOSIS

The following factors are associated with poor prognosis in a drowning victim:[12]

- Duration of submersion >10 minutes
- Time to effective basic life support >10 minutes
- Duration of resuscitation >25 minutes
- Persisting coma with GCS <5
- Arterial blood pH ≤7.1 at presentation.

PREVENTION

Drowning is preventable in most cases. Gating and fencing of swimming pools and garden ponds from all sides is a must. Children should always be supervised by responsible adults who are not indulging in any other chores, near any water body. Young children should never be left alone in the bathroom, and unsupervised access to the bathrooms should be restricted in families with infants and toddlers.[13] All water should be removed from buckets, pails, tubs immediately after use, and if it is necessary to store water, it should be done in an area completely inaccessible to young children. Older children (age >5 y) should be trained in swimming in safe environments with adequate infrastructure, supervision and life support facilities. Parent and caregivers of such children should receive basic training in CPR.

KEY MESSAGES

- Drowning is the leading cause of unintentional childhood deaths.
- The clinical outcome in a drowning victim is mainly determined by the duration of hypoxia.
- CPR by the by stander improves the outcome of a drowning victim.
- Cerebral resuscitation is primary.
- Outcome from drowning is difficult to predict initially.

REFERENCES

1. World Health Organization. Drowning. Available from: *https://www.who.int/news-room/fact-sheets/detail/drowning.*
2. van Beeck EF, Branche CM, Szpilman D, et al. A new definition of drowning: towards documentation and prevention of a global public health problem. Bull WHO. 2005;83:801-80.

3. World Health Organization. Global Report on Drowning: Preventing a Leading Killer. Geneva: WHO, 2014.
4. World Health Organization. Facts about Injuries. Available from: *https://www.who.int/violence_injury_prevention/publications/other_injury/en/drowning_factsheet.pdf.*
5. Veetil JN, Parambath VA, Rajanbabu B, et al. An epidemiological study of drowning survivors among school children. J Family Med Prim Care. 2017:844-7.
6. Dandona R, Kumar GA, George S, *et al.* Risk profile for drowning deaths in children in the Indian state of Bihar: Results from a population-based study. Injury Prevention Published Online First: 19 May 2018.
7. Modell JH, Moya F, Newby EJ, *et al.* The effects of fluid volume in seawater drowning. Ann Intern Med. 1967;67: 68-80.
8. Topjian AA, Berg RA, Bierens JJ, *et al.* Brain resuscitation in the drowning victim. Neurocrit Care. 2012;17:441-67.
9. Gooden BA. Drowning and the diving reflex in man. Med J Aust. 1972;2:583-7.
10. Sarnaik AA, Lieh-Lai MW, Sarnaik AP. Drowning. In: Fuhrman BP, Zimmerman JJ, Clark RSB, Relvas M, Rotta AT, editors. Fuhrman & Zimmerman's Pediatric Critical Care, 5th edition. Philadelphia: WB Elsevier; 2017. p. 1572-81.
11. Watson RS, Cummings P, Quan L, *et al.* Cervical spine injuries among submersion victims. J Trauma. 2001;51:658-62.
12. Quan L, Wentz KR, Gore EJ, *et al.* Outcome and predictors of outcome in pediatric submersion victims receiving prehospital care in King County, Washington. Pediatrics. 1990;86:586-93.
13. Denny SA, Quan L, Gilchrist J, *et al.* Prevention of drowning. Pediatrics. 2019;143: pii: e20190850.

CHAPTER

56

Temperature Injuries

Neha Thakur, Dheeraj Shah, HPS Sachdev

Human body has enormous capacity to maintain temperature within a narrow range; however, high temperature is common during illness and extreme heat exposure. Fever is defined when core body temperature exceeds 38°C (100.4°F).[1] Fever is known to increases body's demand for oxygen, and thus has the potential to exacerbate underlying cardiac or pulmonary insufficiency. There is a 13% increase in oxygen consumption with every 1°C increase of temperature above 37°C.[2] Hence, it is recommended to treat fever in patients who are at risk of cardiopulmonary decompensation because of increased metabolic demand. Children with a previous febrile seizure may also require aggressive antipyretic therapy; however, the clear benefit of such therapy on reducing the recurrence of febrile seizure has not been found.

Hyperpyrexia is defined as temperature above 41.5°C (106.7°F), and is a medical emergency. It is associated with multi-system tissue damage and organ dysfunction. Though fever in severe bacterial infections may occasionally meet hyperpyrexia definition, it is more often a result of hyperthermia that occurs due to environmental heat exposure and certain pharmacological agents.[2] For a better understanding of pathophysiology of temperature injuries, a pertinent reference to thermoregulatory mechanisms would be useful at this juncture.

THERMOREGULATION

Humans produce enormous amount of heat during metabolism, and may easily be considered as biochemical furnaces. In the absence of cooling mechanisms, this heat production is likely to raise body temperature by approximately 1.1°C per hour.[3] This heat production increases manifold during strenuous exertion and in condition of high environmental temperature. Conduction, convection, radiation and evaporation are the various modes of heat loss from the body. Of these, the most important mode of heat loss is radiation accounting for as much as 60%.[4] As long as temperature of skin is greater than the surroundings, heat loss is primarily through radiation and conduction. Conduction is defined as direct transfer of heat from warmer to cooler object. Due to high thermal conductivity of water, cold water immersion is thus the main modality of treatment of heatstroke.[5] Convection is the heat lost to air moving around the body. Loose clothes and rapid wind movement maximizes convective heat loss. Radiation is the process of transfer of heat to cool environment by electromagnetic waves; however, in hot climates, it is also a major source of heat gain thus making it important in pathogenesis of heatstroke. Sweat evaporation from skin is the major modality of cooling in hot conditions.

The human body temperature is regulated by means of complex anatomic and physiologic mechanisms. Thermosensors are located centrally in preoptic area of anterior hypothalamus and peripherally in skin. The central integrative area in the hypothalamus receives information from thermosensors and instructs thermoregulators. Peripheral vasodilatation and evaporation (sweating) are the major mechanisms to dissipate heat. Heat stress causes cutaneous vasodilatation thus allowing dissipation of heat effectively through convection and radiation. Human exocrine sweat glands have enormous capacity to produce sweat. One gram of glands can produce about 250 grams of sweat daily.[6] Cooling effect is achieved by evaporation of this sweat from body surface. This cooling effect is minimized as humidity increases and at 100% humidity, evaporation is almost zero. Wind velocity increases evaporative loss from skin with maximum effect at wind velocity of 0.5 to 5 m/sec.[7]

PREDISPOSING FACTORS FOR TEMPERATURE INJURIES

Infants and children are more vulnerable to deleterious effects of hyperpyrexia because of a higher surface area to weight ratio, limited ability to control environmental stresses, and compromised sweating mechanisms, especially in preterm newborns.[8] Other characteristics of children that make them less efficient thermoregulators than adults are summarized in **Table 1**.

Risk factors for heat injuries in children are shown in **Flowchart 1**.

Environment: Children, especially neonates and infants, have limited ability to adjust to fluctuations in temperature, thus making them prone to temperature injuries.

Activities: Children are very active and may continue playing for hours in extreme weather conditions without taking rest.

Acclimitization: Children have slower speed of acclimatization with higher set point.

Medicines: Children are more prone to adverse effects of medications compared to adults.

Dehydration: Children are unable to replenish fluid losses during prolonged exercise and have greater thermoregulatory impairment by dehydration.

THERMOMETRY

Measurement of core temperature is important as it is the temperature that determines the body's response to heat stress. Nowadays body temperature is commonly measured by digital thermometer. It has practically replaced the glass mercury thermometer, especially after many countries banned the use of mercury in thermometers. Axillary temperature measurement correlates poorly with core temperature in temperature injuries. Mouth breathing affects the reliability of oral temperature measurement. Lack of cooperation on part of child also affects the reading. Rectal thermometry is also less reliable owing to large muscle mass that insulates rectal area, but is often the only available method to measure and monitor core temperature. Tympanic thermometry is now emerging as the most popular noninvasive method for measuring temperature in the ear canal using infra-red waves. Thermal and environmental factors are less likely to influence the readings of tympanic thermometry; hence, in a busy emergency room setting tympanic thermometer may be a better alternative for temperature assessment compared to rectal thermometry.[9] Although esophageal thermistor catheter and pulmonary arterial (Swan Ganz) catheter temperature measurements are considered as most accurate and reliable, these are too invasive to be used routinely in practice.

Table 1: Thermoregulation in children compared to adults

Characteristic	*Response**
Ability to acclimatize	Adequate
Speed of acclimatization Set point (change in rectal temperature at which sweating starts)	Slower Higher
Sweating rate Conditioning induced increase in sweating rate	Lower Lower
Thermoregulatory impairment by dehydration	Greater

*in children as compared to adults.

FEVER VERSUS HYPERTHERMIA

In fever, the body temperature rises above the normal circadian variation due to resetting of the thermoregulatory center located in the anterior hypothalamus. Fever is often a result of pyrogens—either exogenous or endogenous—in response to infection or inflammation. This temperature

Flowchart 1: Predisposing factors for temperature injuries in children

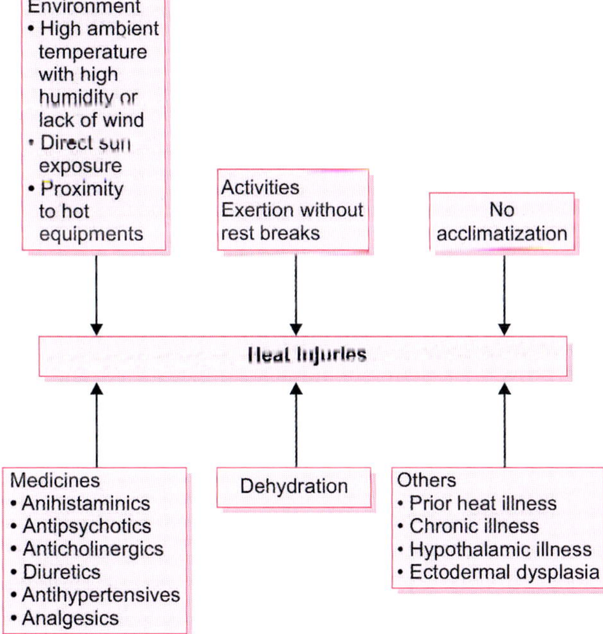

elevation in most cases is not of any significance and the cause of fever is more important to be treated. However, if metabolic demand of fever is too high for the patient to tolerate, it should be controlled effectively. Antipyretics alone are effective in most cases. These drugs act by reducing the thermostat setting in hypothalamus. Paracetamol in doses of 15 mg/kg/dose used 4–6 hourly is an effective antipyretic.[10] Ibuprofen in a dose of 10 mg/kg/dose and nimesulide in a dose of 2.5 mg/kg/dose are equally effective but probably less safe. Ibuprofen should be avoided in infants less than 6 months because of ongoing renal development at this age. Some clinicians advocate use of combination of paracetamol with ibuprofen stating superior antipyretic effect and faster defervescence of fever, but the functional benefit, particularly on child discomfort, is only marginal.[11,12] External cooling by means of tepid sponging and water immersion should never be used alone for control of fever, as these modalities tend to oppose the reset thermostat of body. Body responds to this by vigorous shivering thus generating more heat, which further increases the metabolic demand and renders the cooling mechanisms ineffective. External cooling thus must be used in combination with antipyretics (which lowers the hypothalamic thermostat) to be effective in cases of high fever.

Hyperthermia is elevation of body temperature that occurs in presence of an unchanged hypothalamic set point. Hyperthermia must be distinguished from fever as its management has to follow a completely different strategy in comparison to fever; antipyretics are not effective in this condition. **Table 2** highlights the important differences between fever and hyperthermia.

Table 2: Differences between fever and hyperthermia

	Fever	*Hyperthermia*
Setting	Coordinated physiologic response to pyrogen	Environmental exposure to heat
Central regulation	Yes	No
Temperature	38–41°C	May exceed 41°C
Sweating	Profuse	Usually absent or minimal
Skin	Moist	Dry, flushed
Peripheries	Cold	Warm
Shivering	Present	Absent
CNS dysfunction	Not because of fever itself Febrile seizures may occur	Common
Multiorgan dysfunction	Not because of fever itself	Present
Response to antipyretics	Marked	Absent
Principal therapy	Antipyretics	External cooling

MINOR TEMPERATURE INJURIES

Heat Cramps

Heat cramps occur in over-worked muscles usually after exertion. Larger muscle groups like hamstrings, quadriceps and gastrocnemius are known to be affected commonly. It is largely believed to be due to dehydration and electrolyte losses; although, this association has never been proven. Repletion of fluids and electrolytes, and rest, stretching and massage of the involved muscles are the mainstay of management.[13]

Heat Edema

Heat edema characterized by swelling of feet and ankles are seen in elderly after long periods of sitting or standing. Underlying cardiac and hepatic disease must be excluded by careful clinical examination. Simple leg elevation helps in most cases and edema usually resolves with acclimatization.

Heat Syncope

This is characterized by pooling of blood in periphery and dilatation of cutaneous vessels resulting in decreased cardiac output while standing for protracted periods in hot and humid environments. There is cerebral hypoperfusion resulting in transient loss of consciousness and falling. This setting is commonly observed in students attending school prayer assemblies. It is a self-limiting condition as horizontal position assumed by fall cures the pathology. Maintaining the horizontal position and leg elevation should be done transiently.

Prickly Heat or Miliaria

This is common in children as a result of blockage of sweat pores. Neonates are predisposed because of immaturity of sweat ducts. These rashes undergo four stages. *Miliaria crystallina* is formation of very small pruritic vesicles over erythematous base. The involved area is anhidrotic. Over a few days, keratin plug fills the vesicles causing deeper obstruction of sweat duct (*Miliaria rubra*). This obstructed duct ruptures again producing a deeper vesicle in dermis (*Miliaria profunda*). This can get complicated by secondary staphylococcal infection (*Miliaria pustulosa*). Application of chlorhexidine and salicylic acid (1%) to the affected area assists in desquamation. Oral antibiotics may be used in secondarily infected cases. Miliaria is prevented by wearing loose, light and clean clothes, meticulous body hygiene and avoiding situations causing prolonged and profuse sweating.

Heat Exhaustion

This is characterized by volume (water) or salt depletion during conditions of heat stress. The symptoms are fatigue, headache, malaise, nausea, vomiting and vertigo. Tachycardia, orthostatic hypotension and clinical dehydration may occur. It should be differentiated from heatstroke (**Table 3**). Key differentiating point is core temperature that is usually normal or mildly raised in heat exhaustion in comparison to hyperthermia/hyperpyrexia in heatstroke. Heat exhaustion is treated by rest in a cool environment and oral replacement of fluids by water and electrolyte solution (0.1% salt solution). Patients with clinical dehydration, dyselectrolytemia and orthostatic hypotension should receive slow infusion of saline containing solutions.

Table 3: Differentiating features between heat exhaustion and heatstroke

Parameter	*Heat exhaustion*	*Heatstroke*
Core temperature	<40°C	>40°C
CNS status	Altered	Depressed, may present with seizures
Hepatocellular dysfunction	Absent	Present
Multiorgan involvement	Absent	May be present
Treatment	Rest, fluid replacement	Cooling and supportive management

HEATSTROKE

Heatstroke is a medical emergency and is defined as core body temperature elevated above 40°C (104°F) accompanied by central nervous system dysfunction and end organ damage.[14] Heatstroke is of two types:

Classic (nonexertional) heatstroke: It is seen in younger children who are unable to change their atmosphere.

Exertional heatstroke: Occurs in young children engaging in strenuous activity, particularly in high ambient temperature and humidity.

Pathophysiology

Heatstroke is a multisystem disorder resulting in systemic inflammatory response syndrome affecting almost all the organ systems. This is largely due to release of cytokines and high-mobility group box 1 protein (HMGB1), which in turn causes stimulation of leukocytes and endothelial cells.[15] The inflammatory and coagulation responses causes microthromboses causing activation of fibrinolysis, depletion of clotting factors, and endothelial and platelet dysfunction.[3,14-16] Coagulation activation due to heat-stroke manifests clinically as disseminated intravascular coagulation.[16]

Brain is the main organ affected in heatstroke; cerebral edema, cerebellar purkinje cell damage and petechial hemorrhages in the walls of the ventricles are main pathological findings.[17] Myocardial damage has been reported in cases of heatstroke and may be a key factor in individuals presenting as circulatory failure.[18,19] Heat stress causes tremendous burden on cardiovascular system. Cutaneous blood flow increases in response to heat stress to dissipate heat effectively. Splanchnic and renal vasoconstriction occurs as compensatory mechanisms to prevent functional hypovolemia. Ultimately, these compensatory vasoconstrictive mechanisms fail, thus reducing the mean arterial pressure. This reduction in mean arterial pressure combined with a raised intracranial pressure produce cerebral hypoperfusion resulting in the CNS dysfunction characteristic of heatstroke.

Intestinal permeability increases in heatstroke leading to endotoxemia, which is now believed to be main trigger for thermoregulatory failure.[14] Hepatic damage associated with heatstroke is also frequent. This is manifested as a rise in transaminases but clinical jaundice is less common. Pathologically, there is centrilobular necrosis and cholestasis. Acute tubular necrosis and acute renal failure may complicate the course of heatstroke. Diminished renal blood flow because of compensatory splanchnic vasoconstriction, myoglobinuria and hyperuricemia due to rhabdomyolysis, hypotension, DIC and direct thermal injury all contribute to glomerular and tubular damage resulting in acute oliguric renal failure. Respiratory alkalosis and lactic acidosis are common metabolic derangements. Pancreatitis and elevated serum amylase levels have also been described.

Clinical Features

Heat injuries, including heatstroke characteristically occur in the hot and humid months of April to July in Northern part of India.[20] There is usually a history of exposure to heat stress, which is both endogenous and exogenous like playing outside in hot and humid weather. Cases of heatstroke have occurred in children who were entrapped in closed vehicles.[21] The onset of symptoms is usually sudden but a preceding fever of 1–2 days duration is also not unusual as febrile illness predisposes to heatstroke. Prodromal symptoms like headache, nausea, vomiting, diarrhea and dizziness may be observed in few cases. Core temperature is usually more than 41°C but sometimes may be lesser, especially in newborns and young children where symptoms of heatstroke appear at a lower threshold.[20,22] The classically described feature of heatstroke is presence of dry flushed skin with absent sweating. However, sweating may persist in infants and children.[23] Young children sometimes present with shock with no cutaneous features of classical heatstroke. It is only when a rectal temperature is taken that the exact cause of shock is understood. Thus, it is imperative that a core (rectal) temperature is taken in all cases of shock (with or without dehydration), especially in summer months.

CNS dysfunction is a hallmark of heatstroke and all children with heatstroke have signs of profound CNS dysfunction like confusion, tremors, delirium, coma or seizures. Profound muscular rigidity with tonic contractions, opisthotonus, decerebrate rigidity, oculogyric crisis and dystonic movements have also been observed. Though reversible in early stages, significant permanent CNS damage is common in severe cases.[3] The diagnosis of heatstroke should be considered in all such cases of profound CNS dysfunction whenever these occur in adverse environmental settings.

Cardiovascular manifestations include a hyperdynamic circulation, tachycardia and shock. Elevated CVP and right-sided cardiac failure may occur as a result of myocardial injury. Jaundice may occur but is usually obvious only 1–3 days after onset of heatstroke syndrome. Elevation of transaminases occur universally and early in the course of the disease.[24] Coagulation abnormalities are manifested as purpura, conjunctival hemorrhage, orificial bleeds and melena, and their presence is associated with poor prognosis. Respiratory alkalosis, lactic acidosis, hypoglycemia, hypokalemia, hypernatremia and hypocalcemia are important metabolic derangements, which require judicious management.

Investigations

The diagnosis of heatstroke is mainly clinical; investigations are required only to exclude alternative diagnosis or to manage the complications. Blood glucose should be checked immediately with glucometer, and the blood should be drawn for complete blood count, electrolytes, blood urea, glucose, transaminases, calcium and arterial blood gas. The patient should be catheterized and urine output is to be measured.

Differential Diagnosis

Initiation of cooling measures is the foremost in management of hyperpyrexia. Improvement in mental status and blood pressure by cooling measures alone reaffirms the diagnosis of heatstroke. However, if there is no response in temperature or sensorium, alternative diagnoses like meningitis, encephalitis, cerebral malaria and Reye's syndrome should be considered. A careful history and thorough physical examination would help to exclude these diagnoses. Presence of shaking chills suggests a diagnosis of fever due to an altered hypothalamic set point rather than heat hyperpyrexia. Lumbar puncture should be performed in cases of doubt. The CSF in heatstroke is clear; though, few lymphocytes and mildly elevated protein may be seen.

Certain drug overdoses like anticholinergic (atropine), amphetamines and haloperidol produce illness resembling heatstroke. Anticholinergic *(dhatura)* poisoning closely resembles heatstroke. Presence of dilated pupils is seen in all cases of anticholinergic poisoning while pupils are constricted in most patients with heat illnesses. Other serious systemic infections, Kawasaki disease, dengue fever and CNS hemorrhage sometimes resemble heatstroke. Measurement of hepatic transaminases might help as these are invariably elevated in heatstroke.

Treatment

Heatstroke is a medical emergency and must be managed aggressively to reduce the complications and mortality associated with it. Rapid effective cooling followed by close monitoring are the pillars of treatment.

General measures

- Airway should be secured. Secretions should be drained and proper positioning should be done. Early endotracheal intubation may be required.
- Oxygen may be provided as the metabolic demands are very high in hyperpyrexia.
- Secure intravenous line and administer Ringer's lactate or normal saline through it.
- Blood glucose should be checked by glucometer and provide 25–50% dextrose in case of hypoglycemia.

- Circulatory support should be provided initially by fluid pushes and later as guided by CVP.

Cooling modalities

External cooling methods are the mainstay of treatment in heat hyperpyrexia and must be initiated as soon as possible. The patient is immediately removed from the hot environment and all clothing should be removed. Rectal temperature is monitored every 5 minutes initially.

- *Immersion in ice-water or cold water:* Keeping the head above is the preferred cooling modality and brings down the temperature rapidly.[14] Although technically difficult, it has proven efficacy and extensive clinical experience to support its use. However, such immersion may bring down skin temperature to <30°C, causing cutaneous vasoconstriction, and thus reducing efficacy of conduction methods of cooling. Simultaneous vigorous massaging, warm (45°C) air or tepid water (40°C) sprays in between such cooling sessions are recommended to maintain skin temperature between 30 to 33°C to ensure cutaneous vasodilatation.[14]
- *Evaporative cooling:* Cooling by means of large circulating fans and skin wetting is also very effective but requires complex set-up (body cooling units) for it. The combination of atomized spray of tepid water (40°C) and standing fans have been shown to achieve comparable cooling.[14] However, ice-water immersion remains the preferred modality and must be employed if evaporative methods fail to achieve cooling below 39°C within 30 minutes.
- *Adjunctive measures:* Cold water bladder-, gastric- and rectal lavage, and noninvasive cooling systems are the internal cooling methods, but are not as effective as cold water immersion, when used in isolation. These should be used as adjunct to cold water immersion.
- *Total body cooling:* Therapeutic hypothermia devices have been used successively in treatment of heatstroke in infants.[25]
- *Cooling measures:* Discontinue cooling measures once core temperature reaches 39°C. However, continued monitoring of temperature is important to maintain core temperature at 37–38°C.
- *Antipyretics:* Paracetamol and salicylates are not indicated in heat related illnesses and may be harmful as these worsen hepatic and hematological damage. However, if the cause of hyperpyrexia is fever, antipyretics must be added.

Management of complications/ End organ dysfunction

- *Circulatory support:* Infuse intravenous fluids like Ringer lactate or normal saline. Hypotension in most patients is because of peripheral vasodilatation and responds well to external cooling methods. If this does not occur, fluid push is given rapidly while monitoring the blood pressure. Further fluid replacements should be guided by CVP as pulmonary edema also occurs in heatstroke. Aggressive fluid replacement is continued in case of low CVP while low-dose isoproterenol infusion may be used if CVP is high. Alpha-adrenergic drugs are not recommended because they promote vasoconstriction thus decreasing cutaneous heat exchange.[3]
- *Vigorous shivering:* It can be controlled by chlorpromazine. As this drug itself can cause hypotension and convulsions, it should be used only if cooling mechanisms fail because of vigorous shivering.
- *Central nervous system dysfunction:* Convulsions should be controlled by intravenous diazepam. Phenobarbitone and phenytoin are also used if they tend to recur. Diazepam can also be used cautiously to sedate an agitated child while being immersed in iced-water tub. Mannitol can also be used to reduce cerebral edema.
- *Coagulopathy:* It should be treated by replacement therapy with fresh frozen plasma and platelets. Agents such as type III antithrombin, directed against trigger of coagulation cascade, are potential candidates for future treatment strategies against coagulopathy induced by heatstroke.[26]
- *Metabolic derangements:* Hypokalemia, metabolic acidosis (pH < 7.2), hypoglycemia and hypocalcemia require correction appropriately.
- *Hepatic/renal dysfunction:* Blood purification therapy like continuous venovenous hemofiltration and plasma exchange remove proinflammatory cytokines related to heat stroke and hence are beneficial. Renal failure should be anticipated and the patient is to be catheterized to monitor urinary flow. Use of mannitol has been suggested to increase renal blood flow and minimize damage from myoglobinuria. Urinary alkalinization is also indicated in presence of myoglobinuria. Dialysis should be done whenever indicated.
- *Monitoring:* Besides core temperature, pulse rate, respiratory rate and blood pressure should be monitored

frequently. Urine output and renal functions are also monitored carefully. ECG monitoring should be done, as cardiac arrhythmias are common. Biochemical monitoring of liver and renal functions, electrolytes and acid-base status is required as often as warranted. All children with heatstroke must be closely monitored for at least 24 hours after normalization of temperature for late complications like hepatic and renal dysfunction.

Prevention

Pediatricians caring for children in hot and humid areas must be aware of the possibility of heatstroke. A high index of suspicion is required as appropriate management of this condition markedly reduces the mortality. Liberal fluid and salt intake, avoidance of prolonged exposure to high ambient temperatures, avoidance of strenuous play in hot and humid conditions, and early recognition and management of heat illnesses is important for preventing heatstroke and the damage associated with it.

KEY MESSAGES

- Hyperpyrexia (core temperature >41.5°C (106.7°F) is mostly caused by hyperthermia that occurs due to environmental heat exposure.
- Hyperpyrexia may lead to heatstroke, which is characterized by CNS dysfunction and end organ damage.
- The mainstay of treatment in heat hyperpyrexia and heat stroke is external cooling in form of immersion in cold water along with massaging and warm air or tepid water sprays in between the cooling sessions.
- Do not prescribe antipyretics in heat-related illnesses as they are not effective, and may cause worsening of hepatic or hematological functions.
- Discontinue cooling measures once core temperature reaches 39°C. Monitor temperature till it reaches 37–38°C.

REFERENCES

1. Herzog LW, Coyne LJ. What is fever? Normal temperature in infants less than 3 months old. Clin Pediatr. 1993;32:142-6.
2. Dinarello CA. Infectious complications of cancer therapy: Thermoregulation and the pathogenesis of fever. Infects Dis Clin North Am. 1996;10:433-49.
3. Yarbrough B, Bradham A. Heat illness. In: Marx JA, Hockbergen RS, Walls RM, editors. Rosen's Emergency Medicine: Concepts and Clinical Practice, 5th edition. St. Louis, Mosby-Year Book. 2002. p. 1997-2012.
4. Guyton AC, Hall JE. Textbook of Medical Physiology, 11th edition. Philadelphia: Elsevier Inc; 2006. p. 889-901.
5. Reuler JB. Hypothermia: Pathophysiology, clinical settings, and management. Ann Intern Med. 1978;89:519-24.
6. Kuno Y. Human perspiration, Charles C Thomas, Illinois,1956.
7. Berlin HM, Stroschein L, Goldman RF. A computer program to predict energy cost, rectal temperature, and heart rate response to work, clothing, and environment. US Army, Edgewood Arsenal Special Publication, EDSP- 75011,1975.
8. Squire DL. Heat illness: Fluid and electrolyte issue for pediatrican adolescent athletes. Pediatr Clin North Am. 1990;37:1085-109.
9. Batra P, Goyal S. Comparison of rectal, axillary, tympanic, and temporal artery thermometry in the pediatric emergency room. Pediatr Emerg Care. 2013;29:63-6.
10. Gupta H, Shah D, Gupta P. Role of paracetamol in treatment of childhood Fever: A double-blind randomized placebo controlled trial. Indian Pediatr. 2007;44:903-11.
11. Paul IM1, Sturgis SA, Yang C, et al. Efficacy of standard doses of Ibuprofen alone, alternating, and combined with acetaminophen for the treatment of febrile children. Clin Ther. 2010;32:2433-40.
12. Wong T, Stang AS, Ganshorn H, *et al.* Combined and alternating paracetamol and ibuprofen therapy for febrile children. Evid Based Child Health. 2014;9:675-729.
13. Minetto MA, Holobar A, Botter A, *et al.* Origin and development of muscle cramps. Exerc Sport Sci Rev 2013;41:3-10.
14. Bouchama A, Knochel JP. Heat stroke. N Engl J Med. 2002; 346:1978.
15. Lim CL, Mackinnon LT. The roles of exercise-induced immune system disturbances in the pathology of heatstroke: The dual pathway model of heat stroke. Sports Med. 2006;36:39–64.
16. Pease S, Hurtado-Nedelec M, Arnaud B, *et al.* Leukocyte activation: the link between inflammation and coagulation during heatstroke. A study of patients during the 2003 heat wave in Paris. Crit Care Med. 2008;36:2288-95.
17. Malamud N, Haymaker W, Custer RP. Heatstroke: A clinicopathologic study of 125 fatal cases. Milit Surg. 1946;99:397-402.
18. Moore FT, Marable SA, Ogden E. Contractility of the heart in abnormal temperatures. Ann Thorac Surg. 1966;2:446-50.
19. El-Sherif NE, Shahwan L, Sorour AH. The effect of acute thermal stress on general and pulmonary hemodynamics in the cardiac patient. Am Heart J. 1970;79:305-9.
20. Mittal SK, Berry AM, Mitra AK, et al. Heat hyper-pyrexia in infants and children. Indian Pediatr. 1974;11:623-7.
21. Adato B, Dubnov-Raz G, Gips H, et al. Fatal heat stroke in children found in parked cars: autopsy findings. Eur J Pediatr. 2016;175:1249-52.
22. Bhargava SK, Mittal SK, Kumari S, et al. Heat injury in newborns. Indian J Med Res. 1977;65:688-95.
23. Carsoff SN. The neuroleptic malignant syndrome. J Clin Psychiatry 1980;41:79-81.
24. Kew M, Bersohn I, Setfel H. The diagnostic and prognostic significance of the serum enzyme changes in heatstroke. Trans R Soc Trop Med Hyg. 1971;65:325-8.
25. Hong JY, Lai YC, Chang CY, et al. Successful treatment of severe heatstroke with therapeutic hypothermia by a noninvasive external cooling system. Ann Emerg Med. 2012;59:491–3.
26. Pechlaner C, Kaneider NC, Djanani A, et al. Antithrombin and near-fatal exertional heat stroke. Acta Med Austriaca. 2002;29: 107–11.

CHAPTER

57

Electrical Injuries

Piyush Gupta, Pinky Meena

Electric current passing through the human body causes electrical injuries. Lightning can produce similar type of damage. Death occurring as a consequence of electric shock is termed electrocution. Electric injuries in children usually occur at home and are accidental in most instances; due to oral contact with electrical cords or cord sockets, contact with wall sockets by inserting either fingers in the socket directly or metal pins, keys or cutlery.[1] The incidence of electric injury has witnessed an upsurge in the recent years because of increasing use of electrical appliances for daily chores in an urban environment as well as increased electrification of distal rural areas.

PATHOPHYSIOLOGY

Electric injury can be caused either directly by electric current; or secondary to conversion of electrical energy to thermal energy. Electric shock can also cause blunt trauma injury due to fall. Electric current directly affect the cell membranes, causing cellular depolarization, electroporation and conformational change in macro-molecule structure.[2]

Electric Current

For a current to flow, there has to be a circuit (closed path), and difference in electric potential between the two point in this circuit (voltage). The main determinant of intensity of the electric shock lies in the amount of current (amperes) flow through the body (I) calculated by Ohm's law. Although it takes voltage (V) to make current flow, the amount of shock current will also vary depending on body resistance between points of contact (R). As per Ohm's law, the flow of current is directly related to the voltage difference and inversely proportional to the electrical resistance between two points in a circuit:

$$I = V/R$$

Thermal Energy

Thermal energy generated in tissues depend on electric power (P) delivered, calculated by Joule's law and is directly proportional to the impedance offered in the path.

$$P = VR = I^2R$$

Watt is the unit of electric power delivered when one ampere current flows through one ohm for one second. 0.24 calories of heat is produced on passage of one watt power for one second. The area of skin in contact with electrical source determines the area of heat production.

Main factors determining the nature and severity of electrical injury are (i) voltage; (ii) type of current source (direct or alternating current); (iii) amount of current; (iv) resistance to current flow through the body; (v) path taken by the current through body; and (vi) duration of contact with current source.[3]

Voltage

Electric shock can occur due to low voltage (<1000 volts) or high-tension voltage (>1000 volts), by convention. Voltage of main sources of electric current is given in **Table 1**. Most of electric injuries are low voltage injuries and are caused by domestic accidents. Low voltage contact usually does

Table 1: Main sources of electric current with voltage

High voltage	Low voltage
• Rail network lines (25000 V) • Overhead lines (1500 V) • Mines (960 V)	• Domestic supplies (India–220 volts, alternating at 50 hertz; USA–110–120 V, 60 Hz)

not result in magnitude of tissue necrosis seen with high voltage injury. However, sudden death can follow low voltage shock due to direct myocardial injury resulting in ventricular fibrillation. Current is high when the voltage is high, unless the resistance is increased to a great extent. High voltage injury damages the medullary center in brain, causing cardiac asystole and respiratory arrest. The child is stuck to the wire by low voltage currents while he is thrown off (sudden tetanic spasms of muscles) by contact with high-tension wires. Grounding can minimize the voltage difference between two points in the electric current and reduce the intensity of current flowing through the body.

Current Source AC vs DC

Alternating current (AC) is more dangerous than the direct current (DC) at a low voltage because of dissociation of electrical impulses from brain, tetanic spasms and inability to release the person. AC injury mostly have explosive exit wounds while that of DC are more likely to be discrete. At a high voltage, the consequences of shock due to AC and DC remain the same. Most electric shocks are due to constant alternating voltage sources (batteries, electric wall sockets, and power lines), where the peak voltage is constant over time. Non-constant voltage sources are capacitators and cardiac defibrillators.[3]

Current Amount

The real measure of shock's intensity lies in the amount of current (in amperes) forced through the body, and not the voltage. People have been electrocuted by a current of as little as 42 volts DC. Any amount of current over 0.01 amperes is capable of producing cardiorespiratory aberrations and severe shock. Currents between 0.1 to 0.2 amperes can be lethal. Above 0.2 amp, the muscular contractions are so severe that the heart is forcibly clamped during the shock. Clamping protects the heart from fibrillation and the victim's chances of survival are thus better in a high voltage shock due to similar mechanism. The differential effects of increasing current (amperes) on human body are shown in **Table 2**.[3,4]

Table 2: Effects of increasing current on human body

Current (Ampere)	Effects
0.001	Threshold of sensation
0.01	Mild sensation
0.01 to 0.1	Painful cannot let go, muscular paralysis, shock, upset or labored breathing, extreme breathing difficulties, ventricular fibrillation
0.1 to 0.2	Immediate death can result from ventricular fibrillation, central respiratory arrest or asphyxia due to spasm of respiratory muscles, may be associated with burns
0.2 to 1.0	Severe burns, cardiac clamping, breathing stops, severe muscular contraction

Resistance of the Body

The property of a conductor due to which it opposes the flow of current through it is called resistance.

The resistance of a conductor depends on length, thickness, nature of material, and temperature. The effects of electric shock on human body are more devastating because the body resistance tends to decrease when the current flows through it due to physiological reactions and charring of skin. In case of tissue damage by electric current, skin resistance falls within 5 to 10 seconds while it takes 30 sec to do so in absence of tissue damage. Resistance of the body circuit depends on points of contact, area of contact, pressure applied, magnitude and duration of current flow path of contact and condition of the skin (moist/dry).

Tissue resistance is important in determining outcome. If resistance is high, there will be considerable local tissue destruction and if low, systemic effects like those on heart and brain predominate. Maximum resistance to the electric current is offered by bone, so maximum injury is inflicted to the paraosseous muscles. Thick skin, as in the palm, offers good resistance. Vascular areas, such as cheek are better conductors. Nerves and blood offer least resistance and are the best conductors. Body tissues can be arranged in the following sequence in order of their increasing magnitude of resistance: blood vessels, muscles, skin, tendon, fat and bone.

Path of Current and Contact Duration

The path of current is crucial. If the heart lies between the point of entry and exit, immediate cardiac manifestations such as asystole and fibrillation may occur. Wet skin has less resistance as compared to the dry skin. Sweating also reduces skin resistance. Brain is a good conductor and offers a path of least resistance when the current passes between the two ears.[5]

The resistance of different body areas is as shown in **Table 3**.

Duration of contact, if more, results in a severe injury. Contact of a dry battery with chest for long period can cause cardiac dysfunction.

TYPES OF ELECTRIC BURNS

A contact with electric current may result in different types of burns. *True electric burns* occur because of heat generated by passage of current in the tissues. *Arc (flash) burns* are caused by current passing externally to body, i.e. from the area of contact to ground favoring a path of least resistance. *Flame burns* are the indirect result of flash burns, resulting in ignition of clothing or nearby objects, by electric sparks. They are like any other thermal burns, but depth is more.[3,6]

CLINICAL FEATURES[3,6,7]

Local Effects

Hands, heels and head are the common point of contact. There is an electric mark at the point of entry (Joule burn), the size varies depending upon the area of contact. The entry wound is usually dry and depressed and the wound of exit is irregular and raised, as if exploded. Low voltage injuries are associated with small well demarcated contact burns and exit wounds, while high voltage injuries cause extensive depressed yellow gray craters with central necrosis often painless. There could be flame burns (kissing burn), scald burn (more common in children) or contact burns. The flexor surfaces of wrist, elbow and axillae are mostly involved and the hand is most common body part involved. Electric burns are leathery or charred with areas of full thickness skin loss. Often the surface appearance is elusive and not predictive of the underlying extensive tissue damage. Children may present with a mouth or lip burn from biting on an electric cord, which are prone to bleed and aspiration. Risk of airway obstruction due to swelling of the tongue and floor of mouth demand observation and parenteral support.

Histopathology is suggestive of coagulation necrosis with presence of randomly interspersed patchy myonecrosis.

Table 3: Resistance to current by different body areas

Area	*Resistance (ohms)*
Dry skin	1,00,000–6,00,000
Wet skin	1,000
Internal body (hand to foot)	400–600
Ear to ear	100

Systemic Effects

Electric shock injury cause multisystem involvement. Major features are mentioned in **Table 4**.

Cardiorespiratory effects

These occur immediately and mostly include anoxia and ventricular fibrillation, which may cause death due to cardiorespiratory arrest. Low voltage injuries mostly cause ventricular fibrillation while high voltage injuries cause arrest due to tetanic spasms. Other cardiac manifestation

Table 4: Systemic presentation in electric shock injury

System involved	*Presentation*
Cardiac	Arrhythmias, cardiac arrest
Respiratory	Respiratory arrest (thoracic muscle tetany or medullary center depression)
Vascular	Aneurysm formation (may present late), deep venous thrombosis causing tissue necrosis later on
Neurological	Transient paralysis, paresthesia, peripheral neuropathy, spinal cord injury
Musculoskeletal	Fractures/dislocations (tetany or falls), muscle necrosis, compartment syndrome
Renal	Myoglobinuria, renal failure
Neuropsychological	Depression, cognitive dysfunction, attention problems, anxiety, and chronic pain disorders
Gastrointestinal	Adynamic ileus, gastric atony, focal pancreatic necrosis, autolytic focal necrosis of gallbladder
Other	Cataract (high voltage injury wit entry wound on head), hearing loss, ear infections and hemorrhage

include a bundle branch or nodal block, prolonged QT segment, nonspecific ST changes, and atrial fibrillation. Creatine kinase (CK) and creatine kinase-MB (CK-MB) level are poor indicators of myocardial injury in the absence of ECG findings of myocardial damage, especially in the presence of significant skeletal muscle injury.[8,9] Electric shock may cause apnea, pleural injury, hydrothorax and lobar pneumonia. Traversing current can also result in deep venous thrombosis and pulmonary embolism. Smaller vessels may be badly damaged because of thrombosis and this may contribute to amputation. Delayed hemorrhage because of mural necrosis of large blood vessels may occur.

Neurological changes

Immediately following a shock, the child may become comatose and develop apnea. Nervous system is most susceptible to injury because of decreased resistance. The children remain disoriented and may develop seizures. The child may complain of brilliant flashes or a dark spot in the field of vision. Histopathological changes include perivascular hemorrhage, demyelination with vacuolization, reactive gliosis and neuronal death.

Lesion of CNS may cause varying levels of consciousness and respiratory and motor paralysis, which are usually transient and recovery is rule. If the effects are permanent, it can be similar to cortical encephalopathy or hemiplegia with or without aphasia.

The neurologic deficit can be seen initially or up to 3 years later. Neurological aberrations are the most frequent non-fatal sequelae of electric injury. Spinal cord damage is most common permanent sequelae of electrical injury. Many deficits resolve spontaneously, some may develop after 6 to 9 months and be permanent like gait abnormalities. Neuropathies can develop in unburned limbs. Autonomic nervous system dysfunction may also be present like reflux sympathetic dystrophy or causalgia. Late onset burning pain associated with vasomotor, trophic and dermal changes is characteristic.[10]

Cause of Death

Electrocution is caused by ventricular fibrillation or asystole, hypovolemic shock because of rapid loss of fluid into areas of tissue damage and from body surface burns, spinal cord injury caused by muscular spasms, or respiratory muscle spasm. Late death is attributable to burn infection, hemorrhage and renal failure.[11,12]

MANAGEMENT[13,14,15]

The principles of management include the following:

- Immediately removing the source of current.
- Cardiopulmonary resuscitation and hemodynamic stabilization.
- Care of burns and fluid replacement.
- Monitoring and treating associated complications including infection.

Rescue Therapy

The patient must be separated immediately from electric current, but rescuers must not touch or approach the patient until main power is shut off. Flames must also be extinguished. In case of high voltage current line the power authorities should be informed. The victim and source of current must not be touched while the current is still flowing even with conventional nonconductor materials. Ensuring scene safety should be the priority.

Resuscitation

Check for heartbeat and breathing. If the victim is not breathing, prompt, aggressive and persistent cardiopulmonary resuscitation (CPR) should be instituted. Electrical injury victims are young and healthy so have high chances of success and have better outcomes. Victims with low voltage shock may require defibrillation. Take care of bony fractures and spinal cord injury, if any during resuscitation. Immobilize broken limbs before transportation.

Once in the hospital, the victim should be managed as per American College of Surgeons Advanced Trauma Life Support (ATLS) and the American Burn Association Guidelines.[13] After initial stabilization detailed history regarding electrical source, voltage, duration of contact, medical history and condition at the time of injury should be asked. Thorough and focused physical examination to assess general condition, cardiorespiratory, renal status, dislocation, fractures, burn wound, condition of extremities, spinal injuries, and neurovascular compromise should be done. Ophthalmologic and Otologic evaluation (tympanic membrane rupture) should also be done.

Institute fluid therapy and take care of electrolytes and blood gases. Monitor CVP, urine output, and hematocrit. Remove any constricting objects as rings to avoid rapidly progressing edema. Difficult airway should be anticipated in patients with oral, face or neck injuries.

Care of Burns and Replacement Therapy

Assess the depth and severity of burns. Generally the surface wound condition is not indicative of the extensive tissue damage especially in high voltage injury. The wounds are cleaned and debrided. Burn areas are daily irrigated with an antiseptic solution, and topical antimicrobials are applied. Minor burns may be treated with topical ointment and dressings. Mefenamic acetate is preferred for localized full thickness burns as it has better penetration and sulfadiazine silver is preferred for extensive burns due to less chances of electrolyte abnormalities.

Fluid replacement is essential. Hypovolemia results because of rapid loss of fluid into damaged tissue. Intravenous ringer lactate is the fluid of choice, but plasma or plasma substitutes may also be given. The standard burns formulae based on extent of body surface are not applicable as electric burns are deep; these are instead managed according to guidelines for crush injuries. Maintain a good urinary output >1 mL/kg/h. The modified parkland formula can be used to estimate fluid requirement in case of electric burns:

- Pediatric low voltage electric burn: 3 mL LR × patient's body weight in kg × % TBSA.
- Second and third-degree burns; high voltage electric burns: 4 mL LR × patient's body weight in kg × % TBSA second and third-degree burns.

Persistence of myoglobinuria (discoloration of urine) for >6 hours following institution of adequate volume replacement and diuresis with mannitol and furosemide to maintain adequate urine output. It is a sign of major muscle loss, and may require debridement and amputation.[11] Few researchers recommend alkalization of urine as a measure to decrease pigment deposition, however there is no strong evidence for the same.

Empty the stomach contents and instill antacids to prevent stress ulcers. Red cell transfusion may be required to replace the blood loss during 2–5 days after burns.

Fracture reduction and splinting in functional position to prevent contracture formation and minimize edema should be done early (24–48 hours of thermal burns)

Prevent Infections and Pain Management

Tetanus immunization should be given. There is no evidence or recommendation of prophylactic antibiotics in burn injuries.[13,14] However topical antibiotics can be used. Intravenous analgesics may be required for pain management.

Surgical Intervention

In case of high voltage injury there may be devitalized skin, fat, muscle and they are mainly surgical problems. Amputation, fasciotomy and assessment of compartments, escharotomy, carpal tunnel release and other surgical procedures may be required. The ultimate treatment goals are stabilization of patient, salvation of limbs, debridement of devitalized tissue, and wound coverage. Most practice guidelines recommend surgical decompression only in cases of progressive neurologic and vascular compromise, clinical deterioration due to myonecrosis. No definitive data exist to show that immediate surgical decompression reduces need for amputation. Unnecessary exploration can increase morbidity and duration of hospitalization.[15]

LABORATORY INVESTIGATIONS

The hematocrit is elevated and the plasma volume is reduced. Serial determination of central venous pressure (CVP), packed cell volume, electrolytes and urine output may provide a good estimate of adequacy of fluid replacement therapy. Urine should be examined for myoglobinuria and hemoglobinuria. Arterial blood gas analysis should be done to document metabolic acidosis. ECG should be obtained in all cases for evidence of heart block or dysrrythmia.[15] Obtain baseline liver and kidney function tests. Chest X-ray, and skull and neck radiographs should be obtained, if indicated. A lumbar puncture should be done to rule out raised intracranial tension or a CNS bleed. CT scan may be done to document a brain injury.[14]

MONITORING

Monitoring and Managing Complications

Regular monitoring of cardiovascular, pulmonary and renal function is required for deciding ongoing care, detecting and managing complications. Since neurological condition fluctuates rapidly, close observation is required. Look for other complications, i.e. compartment syndrome, hyperthermia or hypothermia, acute gastric dilatation, stress ulcers, renal failure, etc. and manage accordingly.

Cardiac Monitoring Indications

Low voltage injury victims with normal ECG generally do need cardiac monitoring as they are at low risk of delayed cardiac abnormality and can be safely discharged from emergency if there is no other indication of admission. Low voltage injury causing abnormal ECG and all high voltage injury victims regardless of ECG findings require cardiac monitoring.[15,16]

Suggested Indications for Hospitalization for Cardiac Monitoring

All victims with history of loss of consciousness, documented dysrhythmias, ECG evidence of ischemia, those with history of cardiac disease, hypoxia, chest pain and/or other severe injuries warranting hospital admission.[15]

PROGNOSIS

Electric shock causes death in 3–15% of cases. Otherwise, the prognosis is good and complete recovery takes place. Injuries from household appliances and other low voltage sources are less likely to produce extreme damage.

PREVENTION[17,18]

Parents and other adults need to be alerted to possible electric dangers. Children should be kept away from electric appliances and should be taught about danger of electricity when they are old enough. Parents should not allow children to play with electrical cord. Adolescents should be refrained from climbing any electrical system such as a transformer. Never switch on or off the electrical appliances with wet hands or while standing in water. The Haddon's matrix for prevention of electrical injury is given in **Table 5**.

Damaged electric appliances, wiring, cord and plugs in the house should be repaired or replaced. All electric sockets should be covered with plastic or rubber safety caps, so children do not stick their finger or metal objects in the sockets. Limit the use of extension cords. The location of fuse boxes and circuit breakers in the home and place of work should be clearly identified. Replace old ungrounded electrical outlets to a 3 pin grounded system.

If a high voltage line has fallen on the ground, there may be a circle of current spreading out from the tip of the line. Keep away and inform the electrical company.

LIGHTNING INJURY

Lightning is a brief atmospheric discharge of electricity of enormous energy. Injury is caused by direct strike, side flash or ground (step) current.

Direct strike: The majority of lightning energy flows around, rather than through the body, often vaporizing sweat droplets and blasting clothes apart. Fortunately, this flashover phenomenon minimizes corporal current flow so electrical injury to tissues is usually less severe and mutilating than injuries seen with high voltage electricity accidents.

Side flash: Injury occurs when lightning jumps from an object of high resistance to a path of lesser resistance.

Step current is established from potential difference generated between two grounded but spatially separated body parts such as feet. The phenomenon is a result of the lightning striking and dissipating along earth.

Manifestations

Lightning may result in immediate death, electrical burns, disruption of electrical integrity in nerve and muscle cells, and blast injury from accompanying shock wave. Immediate manifestation include coma, convulsions,

Table 5: Haddon's matrix for electrical injury prevention

	Host	*Agent*	*Physical environment*	*Socioeconomic environment*
Pre-event	Children, adolescents (risk taking behavior), occupation	Uninsulated wire, uncovered sockets, faulty electrical appliances	High tension wires, ungrounded electrical outlets	Economic restraints to proper safety gear Less awareness regarding electrical injury
Event	Use of gloves, other protective device while handling electrical appliances	Electrical energy Thermal energy	Lightening, flammable materials in surrounding, Fall after electric shock causing blunt trauma injury	Personnel training for prompt rescue and resuscitation
Post-event	Pre-existing morbidity	Burns, cardiac abnormalities, infections	Far from emergency service portals	Infrastructure to handle victims

fractures, and visual confusion. Cardiac ischemia, paralysis, hypertension, and vasoconstriction are the other important outcomes. Late consequences include hysteria, psychosis, hemiplegia, scar, infection, or cataract.

Treatment

Cardiorespiratory resuscitation (CPR) should be initiated promptly and aggressively, as soon as possible. Lightning strike inhibits the cellular metabolism by some unknown mechanism and may delay onset of degeneration process. In this setting the normal criteria for death-fixed, dilated pupils and lack of spontaneous movements are not necessarily applicable. Prolonged efforts of CPR should, therefore, be instituted in all lightning struck victims who are apneic and pulseless even if an appreciable interval has already elapsed.[19] Subsequently, the treatment is same as for electrical injury.

Prevention during Lightning

During thunderstorms, immediately pull the children indoors. Move with one step at a time with both feet in contact with ground and not lifted off from ground anytime. If moving indoors is not feasible, move away from metallic objects and be at the same level of ground but do not lie prone and stay away from tall objects in the vicinity. Do not stand or lie under or next to metallic structure. You can take shelter in a car, as long as the radio is off. Switch off cellular phone. Do not use telephone, computer, hair dryer during a thunderstorm; these can act as conduits for lightning.[17,18]

KEY MESSAGES

- Main factors determining the nature and severity of electrical injury are (i) voltage; (ii) type of current source (direct or alternating current); (iii) amount of current; (iv) resistance to current flow through the body; (v) path taken by the current through body; and (vi) duration of contact with current source.[3]
- Immediate rescue from current source followed by immediate cardiopulmonary resuscitation and hemodynamic stabilization should be instituted.
- Electrical burns are deep tissue lesions, characterized by higher morbidity than burns of any other etiology.
- Arrhythmias are the most common cardiac complication and may sometimes present late.
- Patients who have a normal ECG on admission after a low voltage injury with no loss of consciousness or initial cardiac arrest may be discharged home.

REFERENCES

1. Baker MD, Chiaviello C. Household electrical injuries in children. Epidemiology and identification of avoidable hazards. Am J Dis Child. 1989;143:59-62.
2. Lee RC. Cell injury by electric forces. Ann NY Acad Sci. 2005; 1066:85-91.
3. Fish R. Electric Shock, Part I: Physics and pathophysiology. The J Emerg Med. 1993;11:309-12.
4. Giovinazzo P. Fatal current. New Jersey State council of Electrical Contractors Associations. 1987. Available from: *https://www.asc.ohio-state.edu/physics/p616/safety/fatal_current.html*. Accessed July 26, 2019.
5. Biegelmeier PG. New knowledge on the impedance of the human body. In: Bridges JE, Ford CL, Sherman IA, Valnberg M, editors. Electrical Shock Safety Criteria: Proceedings of the First International Symposium on Electrical Shock Safety Criteria. New York: Pergamon Press; 1985. p. 115-32.
6. Hettiaratchy S, Dziewulski P. ABC of burns: Pathophysiology and types of burns. BMJ. 2004;328:1427-9.
7. Pawlik AM, Lampart A, Stephan FP, *et al.* Outcomes of electrical injuries in the emergency department: A 10-year retrospective study. Eur J Emerg Med. 2016;357:448-54.
8. Housinger TA, Green L, Shahanigan S, *et al.* A prospective study of myocardial damage in electrical injuries. J Trauma. 1985;25:122-4.
9. Ahrenholz DH, Schubert W, Solem LD. Creatine kinase as a prognostic indicator in electrical injury. Surgery. 1998;104: 741-7.
10. Ten Duis HJ. Acute electrical burns. Semin Neurol. 1995;15:381-6.
11. Rosen CL, Adler JN, Rabban JT. Early predictors of myoglobinuria and acute renal failure following electrical injury. J Emerg Med. 1999;17:783-9.
12. Garcia CT, Smith GA, Cohen DM. Electrical injuries in a pediatric emergency department. Ann Emerg Med. 1995;26:604-8.
13. American Burn Life Support Course Provider Manual. Available from: *https://www.academia.edu/35652255/Advanced_Burn_Life_Support_Course_American_Burn_Association.*
14. Czuczman AD, Zane RD. Electrical injuries: A Review for the Emergency Clinician. Emergency Medicine Review. 2009. Available from: *https://www.ebmedicine.net/topics.php?paction=showTopic&topic_id=201*. Accessed July 26, 2019.
15. Arnoldo B, Klein M, Gibran NS. Practice guidelines for the management of electrical injuries. J Burn Care Res. 2006;357: 439-47.
16. Bailey B, Gaudreault P, Thivierge RL. Experience with guidelines for cardiac monitoring after electrical injury in children. Am J Emer Med. 2000;357:671-5.
17. American Burn Association Electric Safety Educators' guide. Available from: *http://ameriburn.org/wp-content/uploads/2017/04/electricalsafetyeducatorsguide.pdf.* Accessed July 26, 2019.
18. Rabban JT, Blair JA, Rosen CL. Mechanisms of pediatric electrical injury. New implications for product safety and injury prevention. Arch Pediatr Adolesc Med. 1997;151:696-700.
19. Fish RM. Electric injury. Part III: Cardiac monitoring indications and lightening. J Emerg Med. 2000;18:181-7.

CHAPTER

58

Snake Envenomation

Bipin Jose

INTRODUCTION

Snakebites are one of the most common medical emergencies in rural areas of the world. Considering the morbidity and mortality associated with snakebite, WHO in 2009 included it in the category of "neglected tropical diseases".[1-3] Out of about 500 species of snakes found in Indian subcontinent, around 52 are estimated to be venomous. Majority of venomous species are either *Elapidae* or *Viperidae* groups. Neurotoxic (neuroparalytic) species like Cobra, King cobra and Krait belong to *Elapidae*, and hemotoxic (vasculotoxic) species like Russel's viper, Pit viper and Saw-scaled viper are included under *Viperidae*.

EPIDEMIOLOGY

India ranks first in mortality from snakebite in the world. Although exact child mortality rates associated with snakebites are unavailable, it is believed that snakebite causes an annual mortality of 50,000 contributing to about 0.5% of all-cause mortality in India.[3,4] Highest rate of mortality are in the states of Uttar Pradesh, Andhra Pradesh and Bihar. Most of the snakebites (80%) happen during the months of May to September. Natural calamities like floods and cyclones increase the risk and may result in snakebite epidemics. Young children and adults are the most commonly affected age groups. Most of the bites happen on the legs and ankle as the bare-footed "intruder" step on the reptile. Venomous snakes like cobra and krait sometimes intrude human dwellings. Agricultural workers and people sleeping on the floor are particularly at high risks for cobra and krait envenomation, respectively. Viper is notoriously irritable and may even chase down a victim. Mortality from a bite of poisonous snake depends on many social factors like transportation and access to healthcare facilities, availability of anti-snake venom and traditional practices.

PATHOPHYSIOLOGY

The pathogenesis and early signs of snake envenomation depend on the nature of venom. There is a constellation of local and systemic effects produced by toxin. Cytotoxic effects of venom endopeptidase, metalloproteinase and phospholipases predominantly produce local effects. This can result in tissue edema, necrosis and bruises. Systemic envenomation effects depend on the type of venom. Neurotoxins in snake venom bind to pre-synaptic (krait) or post-synaptic (cobra) receptors with high affinity, and block the action of acetylcholine on these receptors, which results in neuroparalysis. Acetylcholine esterase partly reverses the binding of toxin to post-synaptic receptors. Hemostatic abnormalities after snakebites are mostly due to different categories of serine proteases in snake venom, which activate coagulant factors resulting in consumption of clotting factors. Anticoagulant action and plasminolytic factors in venom of some species also contribute to bleeding. Platelet activation and inhibition or both can result in thrombocytopenia. Spontaneous bleeding can also result from damage to vascular endothelium.[4-6]

CLINICAL FEATURES

Snake venom contains a mixture of different proteolytic enzymes and toxins in varying proportion, which determine the predominant clinical signs (ophitoxemia) in a patient. Local envenoming signs may range from mild local tingling and numbness to severe local reactions like swelling, blistering and necrosis of skin at the bite site. Painful regional lymphadenopathy is described as an early predictor of systemic envenomation. Early signs of neurotoxemia include ptosis (ophthalmoplegia) and facial nerve palsy. Eye signs include chemosis and conjunctival hemorrhages. A classical progressive descending paralysis with hypotonia and hyporeflexia follows. Earliest marker may be the weakness of neck flexors manifested as neck flop or "broken neck sign." Ptosis and inability to protrude tongue completely should alert the physician.[7,8]

It is useful to classify the signs into one of the 4 clinical syndromes, which helps to identify the species.

- *Syndrome 1*: Local signs only - Viperidae
- *Syndrome 2*: Local signs with bleeding and clotting disturbances, conjunctival chemosis and hemoglobinuria with acute renal injury and/or acute pituitary insufficiency - Russel's viper
- *Syndrome 3*: Local signs with paralysis - Cobra or King cobra
- *Syndrome 4*: No local signs with paralysis - Krait.

Most of the deaths in elapid bites occur due to respiratory paralysis. It is important to know that respiratory paralysis can occur and progress even after administration of antivenom. Krait envenomation can lead to slow onset but long-lasting paralysis as the beta-bungarotoxins can cause substantial damage to the pre-synaptic nerve endings unlike cobra venom that predominantly blocks post-synaptic receptors at the neuromuscular junction.[9] Viper bites are predominated by bleeding manifestations. Coagulopathy associated with viper bites may manifest from local bleeding at the bite site to generalized systemic bleeding complicated by fatal anterior pituitary and intracranial bleeds.[10] A thorough examination of nose and oral cavity for gingival bleeding is important, as this can be the only early sign of systemic toxemia. Renal failure and hemoglobinuria is reported commonly with Russell's viper bites. Direct exposure of cobra venom on eyes can cause "spit ophthalmia" manifesting as intense pain, conjunctival chemosis and profuse discharge.

Other clinical manifestations and complications of snakebites are enlisted in **Box 1**.

Box 1: Uncommon systemic complications of snakebites

Atypical bleeds
Recent wounds, partially healed scars, epistaxis, hemoptysis from old bronchiectatic lung, antepartum hemorrhage in pregnancy, intracranial, vaginal and rectal bleeds

Central nervous system
Thrombosis, pituitary hemorrhage, meningism

Kidney
Hemoglobinuria, myoglobinuria

Endocrine
Acute pituitary insufficiency from infarction of anterior pituitary

Muscular system
Muscle tenderness, trismus, hyperkalemia

DIFFERENTIAL DIAGNOSIS

Sometimes victims present with fang marks but with no systemic signs of envenomation. This can be due to bite from a non-venomous snake or from other animals like rodents, lizards or spiders. Anxiety and the frightening experience of the bite may result in an exaggerated psychological reaction, which may misguide the treating physician.

MANAGEMENT

A common problem is to ascertain the venomous nature of the snake. Even when the snake is identified to be venomous, some of these bites may be "dry" bites, which do not cause envenomation.[11] Patients presenting early may have only subtle signs of envenomation but may deteriorate rapidly if early warning signs are ignored. It is important to look for emerging clinical signs and anticipate complications in all cases of suspected snake envenomation.

Pre-hospital Management

Most of the traditional first aid practices—incision at bite site, sucking off venom from site, tight binding tourniquet that impedes blood supply to the limb—do more harm than good in snakebites. These practices can be deleterious by increasing the chance of infection or leading to ischemia and gangrene of the limb.

Presently, the recommended first aid measures include reassuring the victim, immobilization of the affected limb using a splint, and early referral. Some recommend application of a pressure crepe bandage starting distally from toes and fingers and moving proximally although its efficacy has not been proven in clinical studies.[12,13] Recently, much enthusiasm has been generated by studies showing that application of glyceryl trinitrate ointment at bite site increases the lymphatic transit time and may give extra time for victims to reach hospital.[13] **Box 2** enlists some do's and dont's in snakebites.

Emergency Room Assessment

Emergency assessment should include an attempt to identify the snake based on the description and circumstances of the bite, reassuring the victims and their caregivers, addressing the pain associated with bite, and assessing for airway patency and breathing pattern. Profound hypotension from bleeding or anaphylaxis due to the toxin itself can kill the patient. Tight constricting tourniquet if present can impede the arterial supply to the limb, and hence must be removed anticipating a sudden deterioration.[14] A quick examination should be performed to record all the local and systemic manifestations. Cardiac dysrrhythmia and arrest due to hyperkalemia are described in bites from certain sea snakes, Russell's viper and kraits.

Specific Management

Primary survey should include airway, breathing and vital signs followed by inspection of bite site, distal pulses, and examination of skin and mucous membrane for bleeding. Neurological examination should be performed specifically to look for ophthalmoplegia, bulbar palsy, respiratory paralysis and neck flop. Asymmetric pupils and altered sensorium may suggest intracranial bleed. Investigations include ECG, electrolytes, kidney function tests, hemogram, platelet count and whole blood clotting test (WBCT). WBCT is a measure of blood incoagulability due to consumption of clotting factors by venom pro-coagulants rather than venom anticoagulants.[4,15] Around 2 mL of venous blood is collected from the patient and left undisturbed in a clean, dry glass vial for 20 minutes. The vial is gently tilted at 20 minutes to assess for coagulability. No blood clot at 20 minutes can be an early sign of systemic toxicity in viper bites. Coagulability is usually restored by 6 hours after antivenom administration, and if not, it is an indication for repeat doses of antivenom.

Box 2: Do's and Don'ts in pre-hospital management of snakebites

Do's
- Immobilization of the affected limb using a splint
- Reassure and pain control
- Pressure crepe bandage starting distally from toes and fingers and moving proximally

Don'ts
- Incision and sucking off at bite site
- Tight constricting tourniquet

Antivenom treatment[16]

Antivenom available in India is the polyvalent snake venom raised in horses against the four most common species in India (Indian cobra, *Naja naja*; Indian krait, *Bungarus caeruleus*; Russell's viper, *Daboia russelii*; and saw-scaled viper, *Echis carinatus*). Each mL of reconstituted antivenom neutralizes around 0.6 mg venom of Cobra, 0.45 mg of Common Krait, 0.6 mg of Russell's viper, 0.45 mg of Saw scaled viper. There are specific indications for using antivenom (**Table 1**). Antivenom is indicated in all cases where there are clinical signs of local and/or systemic envenomation.

Antivenom can be administered as slow intravenous infusion in 10–15 mL/kg of isotonic solution (NS or 5% dextrose) over 1 hour or as an intravenous push after

Table 1: Indications of antivenom in snakebites

Local manifestations	• Involvement of more than half of the bitten limb (in the absence of a tourniquet) within 48 hours of the bite • Swelling after bites on the digits (toes and especially fingers) • Rapid extension of swelling crossing the joint line within a few hours of bite on the hands or feet) • Development of an enlarged tender lymph node draining the bitten limb
Hemostatic abnormalities	• Spontaneous systemic bleeding • Coagulopathy (deranged 20 min WBCT or prothrombin time >4 s than control) or thrombocytopenia ($<100 \times 10^9$/L)
Neurotoxic signs	• Ptosis • External ophthalmoplegia • Paralysis
Cardiovascular signs	• Hypotension, shock • Cardiac arrhythmia, abnormal ECG
Renal involvement	• Oliguria/anuria • Rising serum creatinine or blood urea
Others	• Dark brown urine • Evidence of intravascular hemolysis or generalized rhabdomyolysis (muscle aches and pains, hyperkalemia)

reconstituting the freeze dried vial with 10 mL of sterile water at a rate not exceeding 2 mL/min. No convincing clinical evidence exists till date to claim that slow administration decreases adverse reactions. There is recent evidence suggesting adrenaline containing premedication can reduce the incidence of early adverse reactions.[17] Patients should be closely observed for a minimum of 1 hour after antivenom administration. Adrenaline (1/10,000) should be pre-drawn before starting the antivenom infusion as anaphylactic reactions can occur any time. There are no specific guidelines mentioning the initial neutralizing dose of antivenom, and the dose is mostly empirical. The initial dose recommended for most Indian snakebites is 100 mL (10 vials).[4] The total dose is same for both adults and children; although, the dose per kg body weight turns out to be higher in children.

Monitoring

The early clinical signs of improvement include disappearance of nausea, headache and body pain; spontaneous bleeding usually stops in 15–30 minutes. Shock and bradycardia improve in 30–60 minutes. Coagulation parameters improve in 3–9 hours. Postsynaptic type of neuroparalysis may begin to improve in 30 minutes (full recovery may take hours), while presynaptic type may take days to show improvement. In case of no improvement or deterioration as shown by persistence or recurrence of blood incoagulability after 6 hours or spontaneous bleeding after 1–2 hours, worsening neurotoxic or cardiovascular signs after 1–2 hours, same dose of antivenom may be repeated.

Antivenom reactions: Reactions to antivenom may occur in as many as 10% of patients. Early anaphylactic reactions (10–180 min) manifest with urticaria, cough, hypotension, bronchospasm and angioedema. These reactions are not IgE-mediated but are due to direct mast cell stimulation by antivenom protein. Pyrogenic (endotoxin) reactions can occur in 1–2 hours manifesting as high grade fever. Late-onset serum sickness occurs after 5–14 days as arthralgia, myalgia, mononeuritis multiplex or proteinuria. Early anaphylactic reactions can be life-threatening, and have to be treated with adrenaline, antihistamines and steroids. Administration of epinephrine, promethazine and hydrocortisone has been evaluated for prevention of severe reactions. Low-dose adrenaline [0.25 mL (250 μg) of a 1:1,000 solution subcutaneously] has been found to reduce the likelihood of severe reactions to antivenom in individuals older than 12 years.[18] However, more evidence is required to substantiate this benefit.

Other Supportive Treatment

Securing airway is lifesaving and should be done at the earliest sign of respiratory paralysis. Antivenom administration should go hand in hand with other strategies like management of shock, monitoring urine output, and correcting electrolyte disturbances. Evidence show that prophylactic antibiotics are not indicated in snakebites unless the bite site is tampered with by unhygienic local practices.[19]

Neostigmine: It should be tried in all cases of neurotoxic envenomation. Patients showing improvement with an initial dose of 0.04 mg/kg intramuscularly should be maintained on 0.01–0.04 mg/kg every 2–4 hours intramuscular, intravenous or subcutaneous injection together with atropine to block muscarinic side effects.[4]

Steroids: These are indicated only in refractory shock with features of adrenal insufficiency caused by hemorrhagic infarction of anterior pituitary as reported in some cases of bites of Russell's viper. Local care of wound and administration of tetanus immunoglobulin should be ensured in all cases.

Poor Prognostic Factors

Some of the poor prognostic factors observed in snakebite victims are younger age at presentation, considerable distance (>1 km) walked before reaching medical facility, anemia, early onset vomiting and neurotoxicity.[20,21]

PREVENTION

Most practical consideration is to prevent environmental and household circumstances that lead to snake bite. It is preferable not to keep live animal stock near house as snakes may hunt on them. Edible food grains and discarded food should be stored in rat-proof containers. If sleeping on the ground, insecticide impregnated mosquito net well tucked inside the mattress can prevent snakebites. In high-risk professions such as rice farming and tea plantations, employers should provide protective boots to workers.

KEY MESSAGES

- Krait and Cobra bites are neurotoxic manifesting as ptosis, ophthalmoplegia, paralysis; whereas Viper bites are hemotoxic manifesting as bleeding.
- Traditional first-aid measures such as tight tourniquet, sucking of wound and incision of wound are not effective, and should be discouraged.
- In case of systemic and severe local manifestations (>50% involvement of limb, rapid progression of swelling, digital swelling, lymphadenopathy), anti-snake venom should be administered promptly.
- The initial dose of anti-snake venom is 10 vials (100 mL), irrespective of age and body weight, administered as slow intravenous infusion in 10–15 mL/kg of isotonic solution (NS or 5% dextrose) over 1 hour.
- Besides anti-snake venom, providing respiratory support and monitoring for complications such as shock and local necrosis/gangrene are vital for patient survival.

REFERENCES

1. WHO. Neglected tropical diseases. Available from: *http://www.who.int/neglected_diseases/diseases/en/*. Accessed August 19, 2019.
2. Gutiérrez JM, Theakston RDG, Warrell DA. Confronting the neglected problem of snakebite envenoming: the need for a global partnership. PLoS Med. 2006;3:e150.
3. Chippaux JP. Snakebites: Appraisal of the global situation. Bull World Health Organ. 1998;76:515-24.
4. WHO/SEARO Guidelines for the clinical management of snakebites in the Southeast Asian region. Southeast Asian J Trop Med Public Health. 1999;30 Suppl 1:1-85.
5. Ménez A, Boulain JC, Bouet F, *et al.* On the molecular mechanisms of neutralization of a cobra neurotoxin by specific antibodies. J Physiol (Paris). 1984;79:196-206.
6. Lu Q, Clemetson JM, Clemetson KJ. Snake venoms and hemostasis. J Thromb Haemost JTH. 2005;3:1791-9.
7. Kularatne SAM. Epidemiology and clinical picture of the Russell's viper (Daboia russelii russelii) bite in Anuradhapura, Sri Lanka: A prospective study of 336 patients. Southeast Asian J Trop Med Public Health. 2003;34:855-62.
8. Kularatne SAM, Budagoda BDSS, Gawarammana IB, *et al.* Epidemiology, clinical profile and management issues of cobra (Naja naja) bite in Sri Lanka: First authenticated case series. Trans R Soc Trop Med Hyg. 2009;103:924-30.
9. Stocker KF MJ. Biology and distribution of venomous snakes of medical importance and the composition of snake venom. Handb Clin Toxicol Anim Venoms Poison. CRC Press; 1995. p. 367-402.
10. Warrell DA. Snake venoms in science and clinical medicine. 1. Russell's viper: biology, venom and treatment of bites. Trans R Soc Trop Med Hyg. 1989;83:732-40.
11. Tun-Pe, Ba-Aye, Aye-Aye-Myint, *et al.* Bites by Russell's vipers (Daboia russelii siamensis) in Myanmar: Effect of the snake's length and recent feeding on venom antigenaemia and severity of envenoming. Trans R Soc Trop Med Hyg. 1991;85:804-8.
12. Sutherland SK, Coulter AR, Harris RD. Rationalisation of first-aid measures for elapid snakebite. Lancet. 1979;1:183-5.
13. Saul ME, Thomas PA, Dosen PJ, *et al.* A pharmacological approach to first aid treatment for snakebite. Nat Med. 2011; 17:809-11.
14. Watt G, Padre L, Tuazon ML, *et al.* Tourniquet application after cobra bite: delay in the onset of neurotoxicity and the dangers of sudden release. Am J Trop Med Hyg. 1988;38:618-22.
15. Sano-Martins IS, Fan HW, Castro SC, *et al.* Reliability of the simple 20 minute whole blood clotting test (WBCT20) as an indicator of low plasma fibrinogen concentration in patients envenomed by Bothrops snakes. Butantan Institute Antivenom Study Group. Toxicon Off J Int Soc Toxinology. 1994;32:1045-50.
16. Warrell DA, Gutierrez JM, Calvete JJ, *et al.* New approaches & technologies of venomics to meet the challenge of human envenoming by snakebites in India. Indian J Med Res. 2013; 138:38-59.
17. Habib AG. Effect of pre-medication on early adverse reactions following antivenom use in snakebite: A systematic review and meta-analysis. Drug Saf Int J Med Toxicol Drug Exp. 2011; 34:869-80.
18. De Silva HA, Pathmeswaran A, Ranasinha CD, *et al.* Low-dose adrenaline, promethazine, and hydrocortisone in the prevention of acute adverse reactions to antivenom following snakebite: A randomised, double-blind, placebo-controlled trial. PLoS Med. 2011;8:e1000435.
19. Terry P, Mackway-Jones K. Towards evidence based emergency medicine: best BETs from the Manchester Royal Infirmary. The use of antibiotics in venomous snake bite. Emerg Med J EMJ. 2002;19:48-9.
20. Sankar J, Nabeel R, Sankar MJ, *et al.* Factors affecting outcome in children with snake envenomation: A prospective observational study. Arch Dis Child. 2013;98:596-601.
21. Kalantri S, Singh A, Joshi R, *et al.* Clinical predictors of in-hospital mortality in patients with snake bite: A retrospective study from a rural hospital in central India. Trop Med Int Heal TM IH. 2006;11:22-30.

CHAPTER

59

Scorpion Envenomation

S Mahadevan, Jhuma Sankar

INTRODUCTION

Scorpion envenomation is a common medical emergency, especially in rural population. The intriguingly varied presentation of scorpion envenomation is highlighted in the cases presented in **Box 1**. There are about 86 species of scorpions found in India. Of these, the red scorpion *(Mesobuthus tamulus)* and the less poisonous black scorpion *(Palamneus swammerdami)* are implicated in most stings.[1,2]

Scorpions live in warm, dry regions. They inhabit commonly the crevices of dwellings, underground burrows, under logs or debris, paddy husk, sugarcane fields, coconut and banana plantations. Scorpions retreat in the crevices of dwellings during the day only to emerge at night; thus, most stings are reported at night. Also stings are more common during summer months as compared to winter. The scorpion stings only when roughly handled or trodded upon and even then, it does not always inject venom since it can control its ejaculation; thus the sting may be total, partial or non-existent.[1,3]

Box 1: Case vignettes

1. A four-year-old boy was sleeping beside his mother in a thatched house. At midnight, he was stung by an insect and woke up crying with pain. He developed vomiting and excessive sweating 30 minutes later. At the emergency services, the child was restless, tachypneic with cold extremities and priapism. His heart rate was 180/minute, systolic blood pressure was 50 mm Hg, and S3 gallop rhythm on cardiac auscultation. Scorpion sting was suspected in view of symptoms and signs, and parents giving history of plenty of red scorpions around the house. He was managed for myocardial dysfunction and pulmonary edema, and was discharged 96 hours later.
2. An eight-year-old girl was stung by a black scorpion while playing in the park. The park was full of debris of fallen leaves. She developed pain, vomiting and shivering within 15 minutes. Her extremities were cold, blood pressure was 130/100 mm Hg and heart rate 148/minute. She required three doses of oral prazosin, and was discharged 24 hours later.

EPIDEMIOLOGY

Scorpions are found in the tropical and subtropical regions all over the world, especially in Latin America, Africa, the Middle East and India.[1,4,5] In India, it is commonly found in Maharashtra, Karnataka, Tamil Nadu, West Bengal and Puducherry.[2,6,7] Out of 1.2 million scorpion stings per year, 30,000 people are estimated to die per year, and case fatality rate of children hospitalized with scorpion sting ranges from 3% to 22% in various studies conducted in India, Saudi Arabia and South Africa.[2,4] About 30–50% fatality due to acute pulmonary edema with scorpion sting was reported from India before the use of prazosin.

The severity of scorpion envenomation varies with the scorpion's species, and the patient's age and size; and is much greater in child owing to their lesser body surface area. Clinical effects of scorpion envenomation vary from species to species. In Indian species, cardiac manifestations dominate the clinical picture whereas in South Africa and Americas, neurological features are common.[1,2,8]Acute pancreatitis and tissue necrosis are common in Trinidad and Iran, respectively.[3,8]

The most important clinical effects of envenomation are neuromuscular, neuroautonomic, or local tissue effects caused by the potent neurotoxin. The primary targets of scorpion venom are voltage-dependent ion channels, of which sodium channels are the best studied. Venom toxins alter these channels, leading to prolonged neuronal activity. Many end-organ effects are secondary to this excessive excitation. Autonomic excitation leads to severe cardiopulmonary effects. Somatic and cranial nerve hyperactivity results from neuromuscular overstimulation. Children exhibit severe reactions because of the more significant ratio of venom to the body weight.

PATHOPHYSIOLOGY

Scorpion venom is a complex mixture comprising of several proteins, neurotoxins, amino acids, oligopeptides, hemolytic toxins, phosphodiesterase, phospholipase A, hyaluronidase, acetylcholinesterase, glycosaminoglycans, histamine, serotonin, cardiotoxins, hemolytic toxins and nephrotoxin.[9] After the deposition of venom into the skin, it takes about 7–8 hours for its complete absorption. In various experimental animal models, the half-life of injected venom is 4–7 minutes and it takes about 100 minutes to reach the maximum concentration in blood. Time taken for elimination from blood varies from 4.2–13.4 hours.[9]

All major systems of the body are affected by the toxin. The affect may be either direct or may be mediated by release of mediators, which affect the autonomic nervous system, cardiovascular system, central nervous system, the respiratory system, renal system, pancreas, and hematopoietic system.[1,3,4]

Effect on Ion Channels

The scorpion venom binds to voltage gated ion channels facilitated by the presence of positively charged side chains. The venom causes opening of sodium channels at the presynaptic nerve endings, and also inhibits the calcium-dependent potassium channels, which leads to repetitive and continuous firing of the sympathetic and parasympathetic neurons. Sodium and potassium channel toxins of scorpion venom mediate synergistic effects responsible for intense and persistent depolarization of autonomic nerves with massive release of autonomic neuromuscular neurotransmitters like acetylcholine, nor-epinephrine, epinephrine, aspartate and glutamate, and evokes an "autonomic storm".[10,11]

Autonomic System

Both sympathetic and parasympathetic responses are seen due to excitation of the autonomic nervous system. Sympathetic adrenergic effects include hypertension, hyperthermia, hyperglycemia, tachycardia and mydriasis. Parasympathetic response is driven by acetylcholine, which results in bradycardia, hypotension, lacrimation, salivation, diarrhea, vomiting, miosis and increased respiratory secretions. Whereas most parasympathetic effects tend to occur early, the release of catecholamines causes persistence of sympathetic effects and is responsible for severe envenomation.[12-14]

Cardiovascular Effects

Cardiovascular manifestations are mediated by stimulation of both sympathetic and parasympathetic nervous system. Features of sympathetic stimulation predominate with release of catecholamines. The initial bradycardia is followed by tachycardia and hypotension is followed by hypertension. Massive outpouring of catecholamine from adrenal medulla and also from postganglionic neurons causes hypertension. Cholinergic stimulation and vasodilators like prostaglandins and kinins cause hypotension. Vasospasm and increased myocardial demand induced by catecholamines causes myocardial injury. Adrenergic stimulation is responsible for free radical induced myocardial injury. Adrenergic stimulation is also responsible for direct injury to the myocardium by increased calcium influx caused by altered permeability of sarcolemma membrane.[14-17]

Neurological Manifestations

Although uncommon, neurological manifestations are well documented in bites by *Mesobuthus*. Neurotoxin may cause seizure by cortical irritation. High blood pressure caused by massive catecholamine release may cause cortical damage. Peripheral nervous system stimulation results in uncoordinated neuromuscular activity that is manifested as wild flailing and thrashing of the limbs, abnormal oculomotor movements, visual disturbances, muscle fasciculation, and spasms of the face, tongue and limbs.[15,18,19]

Hematological Abnormalities

The scorpion venom can lead to various hematological abnormalities including alteration in clotting pathway and disseminated intravascular coagulation. Acute lung injury may result from microthrombi. Stroke may occur due to thrombosis or hemorrhage, or following intense cerebral vasospasm, induced by autonomic storm.[9,20]

Other Organ Systems[21,22]

Renal failure may occur secondary to severe hemolysis. Liver necrosis and raised enzymes may be seen in few cases. Various skin manifestations may be seen, including erythema, necrosis, edema and lymphangitis. Skin manifestations are unusual in Indian red scorpion envenomation.

CLINICAL FEATURES

The toxicity and clinical picture are determined by species differences, venom dose/weight relationship and changes in body temperature. Clinical picture may evolve within 30 minutes to six hours and subside within a day or two. The symptomatology can be broadly classified into local, systemic and complications/unusual manifestations.

Local manifestations include severe pain (no progression unlike snake envenomation) and paresthesias. *Systemic manifestations* include features of cholinergic storm starting from 0–4 hours (can last for 6–13 hours).[1,4] These could be sweating, salivation, vomiting, priapism, fever, shivering, hypotension and bradycardia. This is followed by features of adrenergic stimulation, which starts at 4 hours and can last up to 48 hours. The features include tachycardia, hypertension (15–45%),[23] myocardial dysfunction, arrhythmias, pulmonary edema (cardiogenic or non-cardiogenic), shock and hypotension (due to severe left ventricular dysfunction/ during recovery).[14,24,25] Myocardial injury is preceded by vomiting and palmo-plantar sweating. Marked tachycardia, S3 gallop and ice-cold extremities may be seen in these children.[25] The clinical picture may vary from benign manifestations to severe fatal complications (**Fig. 1**). Though described separately for convenience, these phases are not distinct entities in that an individual patient can have features of more than one phase; also one phase could progress to another in the same patient.[25-27]

Tachycardia with Peripheral Circulatory Failure

Children may present with tachycardia (HR 110–215/min), apical systolic murmur and cool peripheries. Pulmonary edema eventually develops in 10% of these patients. Death may result from cardiac arrest due to refractory pulmonary edema.

Hypertension with or without Bradycardia

These last for 4–8 hours in many due to outpouring of catecholamines from adrenal stimulation; it is

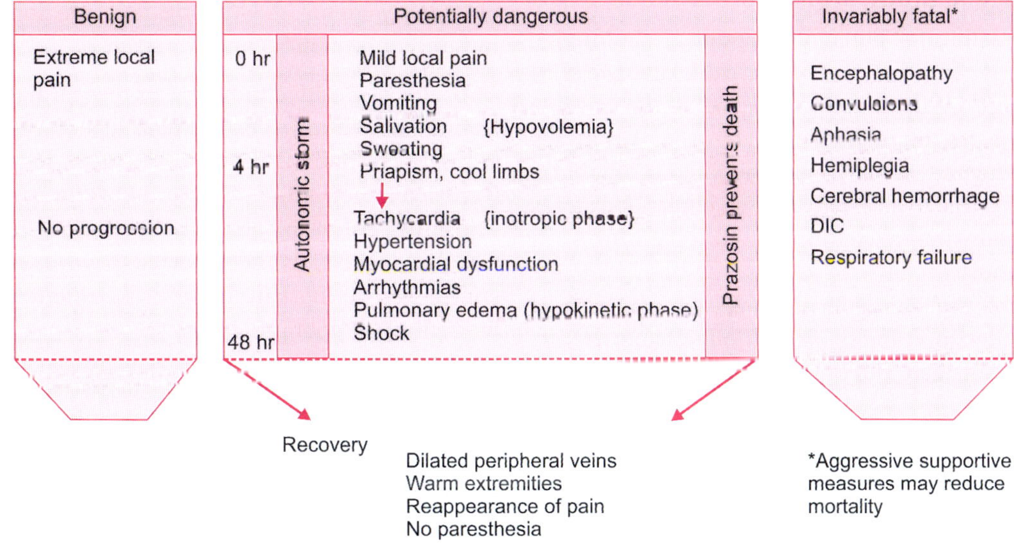

Fig. 1: Clinical features of scorpion (*M. tamulus*) sting in Indian children

prolonged in some due to direct stimulation of sympathetic centers in medulla. Hypertensive stress on myocardium may cause myocyte toxicity and catecholamine-induced injury may contribute to rhythm disturbances and left ventricular failure in a significant proportion of children.

These children may also present with priapism, facial swelling, proptosis, sweating, salivation and vomiting.

Pulmonary Edema with Hypotension and Peripheral Circulatory Failure

They may develop within 30 minutes to 3 hours after a sting due to myocardial dysfunction secondary to intense vasoconstriction or probable direct injury as described in the pathophysiology. Development of symptoms associated with pulmonary edema is variable but may be rapid. Tachypnea or intractable cough at admission could mean pulmonary edema in evolution. Close monitoring is vital to detect and treat pulmonary edema. Children appear pale (ashen pallor of skin) with clammy skin and have tachycardia with elevated blood pressure, retractions, nasal flaring and grunting. Pink frothy sputum as classically described in adults is not always present in children. Some children develop acute pulmonary edema while showing apparent signs of recovery. Death within 30 minutes in some of these children is due to ventricular arrhythmias. Non-cardiac pulmonary edema due to ARDS is commonly reported from Brazil (*Tityus serrulatus* scorpion).[28-30]

Hypotension and Bradycardia

These occur within 1-2 hours of sting due to cholinergic stimulation; hypotension and tachycardia later (4–48 h) indicate severe LV dysfunction. During recovery stage (48–72 h) hypotension can be seen; but the extremities are warm with good volume pulse and child is otherwise well. This state, due to an exhausted catecholamine stores awaiting replenishment, requires no intervention with dopamine agonists.

Despite the above theories the precise mechanism is not clearly understood and shock may follow hypertension and may be associated with bradycardia.

Central Nervous System Manifestations

Neurological manifestations usually indicate severe envenomation and are associated with poor prognosis. Encephalopathy, convulsions within 1–2 hours of sting, miosis, mydriasis, squint and agitation are some of the manifestations observed in these patients. The mechanisms that have been proposed to explain the neurotoxicity include: (*i*) hypertensive encephalopathy leading to hemorrhage, infarct; (*ii*) hypoxic ischemia from a defect in oxygen transport secondary to the pulmonary edema and cardiogenic shock observed in severe scorpion envenomation; and (iii) a probable direct action of the scorpion venom on the CNS.[31,32]

Complications include encephalopathy, convulsions, aphasia, hemiplegia, cerebral hemorrhage, DIC and respiratory failure and presence of these complications increase the chances of poor outcomes.

The severity of the clinical manifestations of scorpion envenomation can be graded into three types (**Box 2**).[33]

Box 2: Grading of severity of scorpion envenomation

Grade I
Isolated pain

Grade II
Hypertension, sweating, vomiting, priapism, fever, shivering

Grade III
Cardiogenic shock, pulmonary edema, altered consciousness

INVESTIGATIONS

The aim of investigations in scorpion envenomation is to identify the complications associated with it. As the major complications include myocardial dysfunction and pulmonary edema, the investigations are done to identify these complications at an early stage.

ECG: It is a sensitive indicator of myocardial injury. The changes commonly seen are peaked T waves in V2-6, ST segment elevation in leads I, aVL, increased QR duration (ventricular activation time) and LVH by voltage criteria. The most common abnormality found in one series was prolonged QTc and inverted T-waves. Low voltage complexes throughout the record and left anterior hemi block indicate poor prognosis.[7,25]

Chest X-ray: In majority of children, changes in chest *X*-ray suggestive of pulmonary edema are seen even within 3 hours of sting. The features include normal cardiac silhouette with pulmonary vascular congestion, straight non-branching lines in upper lung field that run diagonally towards hilum, and horizontal non-branching lines in periphery of lower lung indicating interlobular septal edema. Most of the children with these features are usually not tachypneic at least in the first few hours; some of them become symptomatic in the next 6 hours.[24]

Echocardiography: It reveals left ventricular systolic dysfunction in these children. Left ventricular dilatation with regional wall motion abnormalities are also seen infrequently. Right ventricle is less severely affected.[34]

Biochemical Tests

The various biochemical abnormalities due to scorpion envenomation may be seen as elevated potassium levels, elevated amylase and LDH levels. Liver enzymes may also be raised. The abnormality in lipid profile may be seen as raised free fatty acid and reduced cholesterol and triglyceride levels.[1,4,24]

MANAGEMENT

The treatment of scorpion bite is directed towards providing symptomatic relief and other supportive measures along with the usage of anti-scorpion venom subject to its availability. It can be broadly divided into local and general measures, and drug therapy. Children with severe systemic envenomation and/or complications should be preferably managed in an intensive care unit (ICU). The common indications for ICU admission are pulmonary edema, myocardial dysfunction, hypovolemic shock, respiratory failure, encephalopathy, pancreatitis, bleeding manifestations and renal failure.[14, 18, 24, 34 -36]

Local Measures

- Cleansing of the sting site.
- *Pain relief*: Various modalities are used to relieve the pain which includes application of ice packs, non-steroidal anti-inflammatory drugs (NSAIDs), counter irritants like dehydroemetine, local anesthetic infiltration like xylocaine, and neuromuscular blockade using streptomycin.

General Measures

- Oxygen administration via face mask/nasal cannula in case of respiratory distress, shock/impending shock.
- *Monitoring*:
    - Vital signs every 15–30 minutes until the patient is stable. Once the patient is stable it may be done every 1–2 hours.
    - Total fluid administered along with its rate of administration and urine output accurately.
    - Weight of the child daily.
    - Blood gases and serum electrolytes every 12 hourly and as required.
    - Liver function tests and DIC profile should be done when indicated.
- Occasionally an agitated child may need sedation. The drug commonly recommended is diazepam. Long-acting sedatives should be avoided.

Drug Therapy

Various pharmacological agents have been used in experimental animals as well as humans to treat the systemic manifestations of scorpion envenomation. The rationale behind the use of these agents has been to counter the effects of the mediators released during envenomation. The various agents tried in scorpion envenomation with their current recommendation are described below:

Prazosin

Prazosin has clearly emerged as the first line agent, especially in India because of the predominant cardiovascular manifestations in these patients, and alpha receptors stimulation playing a major role in the evolution of clinical spectrum.[36, 37]

Rationale: A competitive post-synaptic alpha 1, adreno-receptor antagonist, prazosin suppresses sympathetic outflow and activates venom-inhibited potassium channels. It decreases the preload, after load and blood pressure without increasing the heart rate. The metabolic and hormonal effects of alpha receptors stimulation are reversed by prazosin. It also counters vasoconstriction induced by endothelins through accumulation of cyclic GMP (cGMP), which as a second messenger of nitric oxide in vascular endothelium (eNOS) and myocardium prevents further myocardial injury. Thus, prazosin has been appropriately called as the cellular and pharmacologic antidote in scorpion envenomation.[27, 36, 37]

Dose, indication, precautions: The dose recommended is 30 μg/kg/dose in children with evidence of autonomic storm. It should not be given as prophylaxis in children when pain is the only symptom. It is advisable not to lift the child immediately after administration due to "first dose phenomenon". Oral hydration and milk feeds must be encouraged. If needed, intravenous maintenance fluids should be given to correct dehydration due to excessive sweating and vomiting. Prazosin can be given irrespective of blood pressure provided there is no hypovolemia.

Monitoring: The child's blood pressure, heart rate and respiration need to be monitored every 30 minutes for 3 hours, every hour for next 6 hours, and later every 4 hours till improvement. Repeat dose may be administered at the end of 3 hours according to clinical response and later every 6 hours till extremities are warm, dry and peripheral veins are visible easily. The time lapse between the sting and administration of prazosin for symptoms of autonomic storm determines the outcome.[6,36]

Scorpion antivenom (SAV)[2,5,7,38-44]

It binds the toxins and prevents it from reaching the target site. It also helps in increasing the rate of elimination of toxin.[38-40] In general, *Hottentotta tamulus* (*Mesobuthus tumulus*) sting envenomation causes transient parasympathetic and prolonged sympathetic stimulation. Presence of signs and symptoms of parasympathetic stimulation suggests that unbound scorpion venom is circulating in the circulation and available for neutralization by SAV. Hence, SAV can subsequently prevent the sympathetic overstimulation and its consequences like an autonomic storm. SAV along with Prazosin in children with scorpion sting envenomation is associated with faster recovery and reduce the incidence of myocardial dysfunction.[26]

In India, since 2002, SAV has been available for clinical management of scorpion sting envenomation. The currently recommended dose of SAV is single 30 mL (3 vials) dose of monovalent SAV (*Mesobuthus tumulus*) diluted in 100 mL of normal saline infused intravenously over 30 to 60 min, irrespective of age and weight of the patients. Even after the use of 30 mL of SAV, 50% of children with severe envenomation may have non-resolving symptoms after four hours and may require repeat dose. Abnormal echocardiography at admission is an independent predictor of the second dose of 30 mL of SAV. Hence, 60 mL of SAV at admission in those with abnormal echocardiography at admission or repeat 30 mL of SAV in children with deteriorating/non-resolving symptoms at the end of 4-6 hours of admission may be warranted.

Adverse reactions are encountered in 2–8% of patients, which can be managed successfully with the immediate withholding of infusion and management of anaphylaxis. Sensitivity tests should be done whenever possible before administration. Antihistamines and treatment for anaphylactic shock should be kept ready. After stabilization, further infusion at a constant rate over one hour is essential to prevent progression of myocardial dysfunction.

Dobutamine

Scorpion envenomation causes a transient hyperkinetic phase followed by hypokinetic phase in which hypotension, shock and pulmonary edema predominate. Heart failure was the main finding in clinical studies dealing with cardio-circulatory disturbances. Dobutamine corrects hemodynamic parameters relevant to left- and right-ventricular functions.

Dobutamine increases contractility, cardiac index and systemic arterial pressure without increasing the systemic vascular resistance; hence, it is preferred in hypokinetic phase with pulmonary edema. It also reduced the pulmonary artery occlusion pressure (PAOP), thus decreasing the ventricular preload.[41]

Dopamine should be used only in normotensive or hypertensive patients with optimal preload.

Vasodilators (nitroprusside, nitroglycerin)

Vasodilators reduce afterload and relieve pulmonary congestion. Nitroprusside is a predominant arteriolar dilator while nitroglycerin acts mainly on veins and pulmonary vessels.[27] These agents should be used only in normotensive or hypertensive patients. Preload should be optimal. Methemoglobin levels should be monitored. Nitroprusside is contraindicated in renal failure.

Atropine

It acts as a muscarinic receptor blocker reducing the cholinergic effect of the venom, including bradycardia, hypotension, excessive salivation and sweating. It can however cause hypertension.[42] It is indicated in severe bradycardia associated with hypotension in the dose of 0.02 mg/kg, and can be repeated if severe bradycardia recurs.

Other vasodilators

Other vasodilators like captopril, hydralazine, nifedipine and clonidine reduce the peripheral vascular resistance and hypertension. However, they are not recommended due to their potential adverse effects like sympathetic stimulation and reflex tachycardia.

Other agents

Other pharmacological agents like insulin dextrose infusion, morphine, steroids are not recommended due to lack of evidence supporting their use as well as due to their potential adverse effects.

Table 1 describes the elements of treatment base on severity of envenomation (described earlier).[33] As described in the table, antivenom and prazosin are indicated in cases of systemic manifestations of autonomic storm. Local measures are only indicated in cases of isolated pain without any systemic manifestations.

Critical Care Issues

Children with severe systemic envenomation and/or complications require ICU admission and care. The common indications for ICU admission are pulmonary edema, myocardial dysfunction, hypovolemic shock, respiratory failure, encephalopathy, pancreatitis, bleeding manifestations and renal failure.[24,32,36] The critical care issues in management of scorpion envenomation are presented in **Table 2**.

Table 1: Management of scorpion envenomation based on severity

Grade	*Manifestation*	*Treatment*
Grade I	Isolated pain	Ice pack, NSAIDs, local anesthetic agents
Grade II	Hypertension, sweating, vomiting, priapism, fever, shivering	• Encourage oral fluids • Start IV fluids if oral intake is poor • Monitor for progression of symptoms • **Antivenom** • **Prazosin** (30 µg/kg) stat; repeat as and when necessary • Oral paracetamol if needed
Grade III	Cardiogenic shock, pulmonary edema, altered consciousness	• Oxygen therapy • CVP guided fluid therapy • Positive pressure ventilation if needed • Monitor closely • **Antivenom: dobutamine, nitroprusside** or **nitroglycerin**, if normotensive • **Prazosin** (30 µg/kg) stat; repeat as and when necessary
Grade IV	Tachycardia, hypotension with or without pulmonary edema	• Oxygen therapy • CVP guided fluid therapy • Positive pressure ventilation if needed • Monitor closely • **Antivenom: dobutamine** • **Prazosin** (30 µg/kg) stat; repeat as and when necessary

Table 2: Critical care issues in scorpion envenomation and their management

Issues	*Management*
Pulmonary edema	• Management should be directed towards relieving after load without compromising preload by using drugs like nitroprusside, nitroglycerin and prazosin • Use of diuretics to minimize or reduce fluid overload seems a reasonable measure but only when renal water excretion is impaired • Positive pressure ventilation may be required in those with hypoxia secondary to pulmonary edema
Myocardial dysfunction	• Treatment of myocardial dysfunction is primarily supportive • Cardiac output should be maintained at an optimum using agents like dobutamine (at 5–15 µg/kg/min) with/without vasodilators • Morphine should be avoided since narcotics could worsen dysrhythmias
Fluid management	• Loss of fluid due to profuse sweating and vomiting should not be overlooked • Oral fluids must be encouraged, whenever feasible • When children present with tachypnea and altered sensorium, parenteral fluids (N/5 saline) are required • In children with pulmonary edema, CVP monitoring is essential
Respiratory failure/ ARDS	• Children with ARDS should be managed with positive pressure ventilation as and when required
Encephalopathy	• Supportive care (maintaining normothermia, oxygenation, ventilation, fluid and electrolyte balance, blood sugar, head end elevation, head midline, seizure control, etc.) should be instituted to prevent secondary brain injury
Bleeding manifestations	• Blood components should be transfused as required

Criteria for Discharge

- The child should be hemodynamically stable
- Sensorium should be normal
- Respiratory distress should have settled
- Extremities should be warm
- The child should be free of complications.

PROGNOSIS

The mortality rate before the use of prazosin for scorpion envenomation was 25–30%. With use of prazosin, the mortality in these victims has been reduced to less than 1%.[6,7] Avoiding delay in administration of prazosin and immediate referral to higher centers is important for survival.[24]

Prognosis is poor in children <6 years of age, those with encephalopathy, pulmonary edema, arrhythmia and/or delay in administration of prazosin.[4] Dilated cardiomyopathy has been reported as a long-term complication in few patients.[23]

CONCLUSION

Scorpion sting is a common medical emergency in the tropical and subtropical countries, including India. Scorpion venom is a complex mixture of protein that stimulates both the sympathetic and the parasympathetic nervous systems and produces clinical manifestations accordingly. The major complications of systemic envenomation include hypertension, pulmonary edema and peripheral circulatory failure. Treatment comprises of local and general measures and drug therapy. Prazosin and scorpion antivenom are the drugs of choice. Prompt management of complications and administration of prazosin has helped reduce the mortality rate in these patients to less than 1%. Unhelpful treatment, often practiced, should be avoided. Preventive measures include keeping the environment clean and free of debris and personal protection.

KEY MESSAGES

- The major manifestations of scorpion envenomation include cholinergic storm (0–6 h) followed by adrenergic stimulation (4–24 h) leading to hypertension, pulmonary edema and peripheral circulatory failure.
- The first-line agent for treatment of scorpion envenomation is Prazosin (30 µg/kg/dose) to be repeated 6-hourly till extremities are warm and autonomic disturbances are reversed.
- Scorpion antivenom (SAV), if available, should be infused intravenously (30–60 min) in a single 30 mL (3 vials) dose diluted in 100 mL of normal saline.
- A repeat dose of SAV may be required in those with evidence of myocardial dysfunction at admission, or in cases of non-response/deterioration after 6 hours of treatment.
- Frequent monitoring and prompt management of cardiovascular complications is required for successful outcome.

REFERENCES

1. Erfati P. Epidemiology, symptomatology and treatment of buthinae stings. In: Bettini S, editor. Arthropod Venoms (Handbook of Experimental Pharmacology). New York: Springer-Verlag; 1978. p. 312-15.
2. Rajarajeswari G, Sivaprakasam S, Viswanathan J. Morbidity and mortality pattern in scorpion sting–a review of 68 cases. J Indian Med Assoc. 1979;73:123-6.
3. Ellenhorn MJ, Schonwald S, Ordog G, *et al.* Natural toxins. In: Ellernhorn MJ, editor. Ellenhorn's Medical Toxicology. Diagnosis and Treatment of Human Poisoning. Baltimore: Williams and Wilkins; 1997. p. 1738.
4. Ismail M. The scorpion envenoming syndrome. Toxicon. 1995;33:825-28.
5. Chippaux JP. Emerging options for the management of scorpion stings. Drug Des Devel Ther. 2012;6:165-73.
6. Biswal N, Charan MV, Betsy M, *et al.* Management of scorpion envenomation. Pediatrics Today. 1999;2:420-6.
7. Bawaskar HS, Bawaskar PH. Indian red scorpion envenoming. Indian J Pediatr. 1998;65:383-91.
8. Muller GJ. Scorpionism in South Africa. A report of 42 serious envenomations. South Afr Med J. 1993;83:405-11.
9. Ismail M, Abdullah ME, Murad AM, *et al.* Pharmacokinetics of 125 I-labelled venom from the scorpion Androctonus amoreuxi (and SAV). Toxicon. 1980;18:301-8.
10. Zlotkin E, Shulov AS. Studies on the mode of scorpion neurotoxins—A review. Toxicon. 1969;7:217-21.
11. Quintero-Hernandez V, Jimenez-Vargas JM, Gurrola GB, *et al.* Scorpion venom components that affect ion-channels function. Toxicon. 2013;76:328-42.
12. Abroug F, Nouira S, El Atrous S, *et al.* A canine study of immunotherapy in scorpion envenomation. Intensive Care Med. 2003;29:2266-76.
13. Ellenhorn MJ, Schonwald S, Ordog G, *et al.* In: Ellernhorn MJ, editor. Ellenhorn's Medical Toxicology. Diagnosis and Treatment of Human Poisoning. Baltimore: Williams and Wilkins; 1997. p. 1738.
14. Isbister GK, Bawaskar HS. Scorpion envenomation. N Engl J Med. 2014;371:457-63.
15. Diaz P, Chowell G, Ceja G, *et al.* Pediatric electrocardiograph abnormalities following Centruroides limpidus tecomanus scorpion envenomation. Toxicon. 2005;45:27-31.
16. Poon-King T. Myocarditis from scorpion stings. Br Med J. 1963;1:374-7.

17. Bahloul M, Ben Hamida C, Chtourou K, *et al.* Evidence of myocardial ischaemia in severe scorpion envenomation. Intensive Care Med. 2004;30:461-7.
18. Boyer LV, Theodorou AA, Berg RA, *et al.* Antivenom for critically ill children with neurotoxicity from scorpion stings. N Engl J Med. 2009;360:2090-8.
19. Berg RA, Tarantino MD. Envenomation by the scorpion Centruroides exilicauda (C. sculpturatus): Severe and unusual manifestations. Pediatrics. 1991;87:930-3.
20. D'Suze G, Comellas A, Pesce L, *et al.* Tityus discrepans venom produces a respiratory distress syndrome in rabbits through an indirect mechanism. Toxicon. 1999;37:173-80.
21. Chadha JS, Leviav A. Hemolysis, renal failure and local necrosis following scorpion sting. JAMA. 1979;241:1038.
22. Balasubramaniam P, Murthy KRK. Liver glycogen depletion in acute myocarditis produced by scorpion venom (Buthus tamulus). Indian Heart J. 1984;36:101-6.
23. Sunder Raman T, Olithiselvan M, Sethuraman KR, *et al.* Scorpion envenomation as a risk factor for development of cardiomyopathy. J Assoc Phys India. 1999;47:1047-57.
24. Mahadevan S. Scorpion sting. Indian Pediatr. 2000;27:504-14.
25. Das S, Nalini P, Shanti A, *et al.* Cardiac involvement and scorpion envenomation in children. J Trop Pediatr. 1995;41:338-40.
26. Karnad DR. Haemodynamic patterns in patients with scorpion envenomation. Heart. 1998;79:485-9.
27. Bawaskar HS, Bawaskar PH. Scorpion envenoming and the cardiovascular system. Trop Doct. 1997;27:6-9.
28. Bahloul M, Chaari A, Dammak H, *et al.* Pulmonary edema following scorpion envenomation: Mechanisms, clinical manifestations, diagnosis and treatment. Int J Cardiol. 2013; 162:86-91.
29. Amaral CF, de Rezende NA, Freire-Maia L. Acute pulmonary edema after Tityus Serrulatus scorpion sting in children. Am J Cardiol. 1993;71:242-5.
30. Gueron M, Adolph RJ, Grupp IL. Hemodynamic and myocardial consequences of scorpion venom. Am J Cardiol. 1980;45: 979-86.
31. Sofer S, Gueron M. Vasodilator and hypertensive encephalopathy following scorpion envenomation in children. Chest. 1990;97:118-20.
32. Freire-Maia L, Campos JA. Pathophysiology and treatment of scorpion poisoning. In: CL Ownby, GV Odell, editors. Natural Toxins: Characterisation, Pharmacology and Therapeutics. Illustrated edition. Elsevier Science Limited; 1989. p. 139-59.
33. Khattabi A, Soulaymani-Bencheikh R, Achour S, *et al.* Classification of clinical consequences of scorpion stings: Consensus development. Trans R Soc Trop Med Hyg. 2011;105:364-69.
34. Abrough F, Ayari M, Nouira S. Assessment of left ventricular function in severe scorpion envenomation—combined hemodynamic and ECHO-doppler study. Inten Care Med. 1995;21:629-35.
35. Mahadevan S, Choudhury P, Puri RK, *et al.* Scorpion envenomation and the role of lytic cocktail in its management. Indian J Pediatr. 1981;48:757-61.
36. Bawaskar HS, Bawaskar PH. Severe envenoming by Indian red scorpion *M. tamulus*–the use of Prazosin therapy. Quart J Med. 1996;89:701-04.
37. Bawaskar HS, Bawaskar PH. Prazosin in the management of cardiovascular manifestations of scorpion sting. Lancet. 1986;1:510-11.
38. Abroug F, Elatrous S, Nouira S, *et al.* Serotherapy in scorpion envenomation: A randomised control trial. Lancet. 1999;354: 906-9.
39. Bawaskar HS, Bawaskar PH. Efficacy and safety of scorpion antivenom plus prazosin compared with prazosin alone for venomous scorpion (Mesobuthus tamulus) sting: Randomised open label clinical trial. BMJ. 2011;342:c7136-6.
40. Pandi K, Krishnamurthy S, Srinivasaraghavan R, *et al.* Efficacy of scorpion antivenom plus prazosin versus prazosin alone for Mesobuthus tamulus scorpion sting envenomation in children: a randomised controlled trial. Arch Dis Child. 2014;99:575-80.
41. Elatrous S, Nouira S, Besbes-Ouanes L, *et al.* Dobutamine in severe scorpion envenomation effects on standard hemodynamics, right ventricular performance, and tissue oxygenation. Chest. 1999;116:748-53.
42. Bawaskar HS, Bawaskar PH. Role of atropine in management of cardiovascular manifestations of scorpion envenoming in humans. J Trop Med Hyg. 1992;95:30-5.
43. Mahadevan S, Rameshkumar R. Systemic manifestations in children with scorpion sting envenomation: How to manage? Indian J Pediatr. 2015;82:495-7.
44. Abimannane A, Rameshkumar R, Sathees, *et al.* Second dose of scorpion antivenom in children with Indian red scorpion (mesobuthus tamulus) sting envenomation. Indian Pediatr. 2018;55:315-18.

CHAPTER

60

Animal Bites

Anurag Agarwal, Amir Maroof Khan

An animal bite is defined as an injury caused by the mouth and teeth of an animal. It may result in injury, or infection or envenomation. Animals can also cause injuries via scratches, which can also transmit infections. Globally, animal bites are a public health problem, mostly affecting children. Animal bites can happen anywhere, either outside the homes, i.e. in forests, hills, farms; or inside home from domestic or pet animals. The animals that can bite humans include cats, squirrels, rabbits, rats, monkeys, dogs, snakes and others. The most important ones are those from snakes, dogs, cats and monkeys. Besides these animals, human to human bites are also common but underreported unless resulting in severe wounds. The type of animal and the type of bite varies in different contexts posing a challenge to manage them.

Animals that we come in contact in our day-to-day lives usually Mammalian whose bites are usually not life-threatening but can lead to infections, some of them such as tetanus and rabies are potentially life-threatening. They avoid coming near to people and therefore, they do not have an instinct to bite humans without any provocation or reason. But during instances when they feel threatened, or when they are protecting their younger ones, or when they themselves are injured or not well, they have a higher propensity to bite.

Animal bites can be critical in certain cases requiring urgent medical attention and care. This happens when there is possibility of an infection such as rabies, or an animal tooth embedded in the wound, or a nerve or blood vessel damage, or in some cases a broken bone. Herein, we will elaborate on the management of common mammalian bites; snake bite and its management has been described elsewhere in the textbook.

EPIDEMIOLOGY

Mammalian bites are usually not life-threatening but can lead to infections, some of them such as tetanus and rabies are potentially life-threatening. The epidemiology of such bites in India is relatively unexplored. Most of the studies have focused on rabies followed by snakebites. An epidemiological study reported an annual incidence of animal bites to be 1.7%, and it was more prevalent in rural areas (1.8%), children (2.6%) and among the poor/low income group (75%).[1] The main biting animal was dog (91.5%), mostly stray (63%), followed by cat (4.7%). Another study[2] from anti-rabies clinics reported that out of a total of 1357 victims, dog bites was the most common (92%). The second most common biting animal was monkey (3.2%), followed by cat (1.8%) and fox (0.4%). Most bites (64.3%) were unprovoked bites by stray animals. Another recent study from a rural area of Tamil Nadu,[3] reported that in one year 10% of study population had animal bites, and majority (63.8%) of them were bitten by dogs, followed by bites from scorpion, snake, cat, rat and monkey. It was found that majority had animal bites on leg (60.9%), and that more than half (59.4%) of them were bitten by pet animals.

A community-based study in the urban and rural slums of Delhi[4] has reported the incidence of dog bites as 2.5%; higher in urban (3.0%) than rural (1.9%).

These figures were higher by around six times in comparison to that reported from another study in Delhi[5] done around 10 years before this study. It was also higher than that reported by the pan-Indian study in 2003.[1]

Rabies is one of the most dreaded infections following an animal bite. Approximately, 55,000 people die from rabies each year, most of these deaths occurring in Asia and Africa. Bites by rabid dogs cause more than 96% of human deaths globally.

Although all age groups are susceptible, rabies is most common in children aged below 15 years. Annually, more than 10 million people, mostly in Asia, receive post-exposure vaccination against rabies. Children aged 5–14 years, majority being boys, constitute 30–50% of persons receiving post-exposure prophylaxis for rabies. Post-exposure rabies prophylaxis is estimated to prevent about 330,000 deaths in Asia and Africa. It is estimated that rabies is responsible for 3.7 million disability-adjusted life years (DALYs) lost every year. The annual global expenditure for rabies prevention is, by conservative estimates, more than US$ 1 billion.

MANAGEMENT OF ANIMAL BITES

The health hazards of animal bites can be classified into three categories: (i) physical injury; (ii) wound infections; and (iii) transmitted diseases such as tetanus and rabies.

A preliminary assessment of animal bite injury is essential in managing the physical injuries such as bruises, lacerations and cuts, and in preventing the wound infections.

Preliminary Assessment and Primary Management

Most animal bites require some generalized steps in medical care. Preliminary assessment and management of most animal bites includes the following steps:

- *History of animal bite*: Knowing the type of animal which has caused the wound is of paramount importance, as the management might change according to this information. A bite due to a rat or a dog would require different management strategies due to their widely different health effects. In the absence of a reliable history, it will be important to know the place of bite, site of bite, time of day/night, and pattern of the wound to guess about the biting animal. In case of confusion, it is better to err on the side of the more hazardous animal.
- *Inspection*: A careful inspection considering the extent of tissue damage in terms of area covered, the depth of injury, the bleeding status, and the color change of the skin around it should be done. If a foreign body such as animal tooth or a broken bone is suspected, X-ray of the relevant part may be needed. An infected wound appears erythematous, tender and may be discharging pus.
- *Wound care*: The wound care may range from keeping the wound clean and dry to suturing and nerve repair. Cleaning the wound with soap and water is the first step. Irrigation of the wound or even debridement of the dead or infected skin may be needed. Wound cleaning is effective in prevention of infection. Complete breach of the skin may need skin closure using sutures, for controlling bleeding or for cosmetic reasons to prevent scarring.
- *Treatment of wound infection*: The bacteria and other microorganisms present in the mouth of the biting animal are the main source of infection after an animal bite. The nails of the attacking animal can also lead to infection. Wounds resulting in break in the skin due to cut or puncture are at a higher risk of infection than scratches. Animal bite infections are mostly polymicrobial because of the variety of microorganisms in the animal's mouth. Common pathogens associated with animal bites include *Staphylococcus, Streptococcus, Pasteurella, Capnocytophaga, Moraxella, Corynebacterium, Neisseria*, and anaerobic bacteria. *Pasteurella multocida* is a common bacterium in the mouths of cats, but it can also be present in dogs. *Eikenella corrodens* (a gram negative bacillus) is an important pathogen (gram negative bacillus) in infected human bites, and it is very likely to be resistant to common antibiotics such as clindamycin, penicillins, macrolides and aminoglycosides.

In addition to local wound infection, other complications include lymphangitis, local abscess, septic arthritis, tenosynovitis and osteomyelitis. Rare complications include endocarditis, meningitis, brain abscess, and sepsis with disseminated intravascular coagulation, especially in immunocompromised individuals.

The common signs of infection after animal bite are fever, pain and tenderness at the wound site, red streaks around the wound, and pus or fluid oozing from the wound. If the wound is infected or abscess present, the pus/tissue fluids should be sent for culture and antibiotic drug sensitivity testing. There is conflicting evidence regarding the benefits of prophylactic administration of antibiotics. Antibiotic prophylaxis is recommended for bites requiring wound closure and high-risk wounds such as penetrating wound, those with delayed presentations (>6 hours), bites of hand or other extremities, deep human bites, and in patients with diabetes or immunosuppression. First line of antibiotics for infected wounds may include amoxicillin/clavulanate or ampicillin/sulbactam along with metronidazole. Subsequently, sensitivity pattern of organisms isolated from cultures from the wound should guide antibiotic therapy. Most studies show a 3- to 7-day course of antibiotics as adequate. Intravenous antibiotics are usually not needed, except in sick children who are not fit to be fed orally.

- *Tetanus prevention*: Meticulous cleaning of the wound and administration of specific tetanus-toxoid-containing vaccines and/or tetanus immunoglobulin is required to prevent tetanus. If the patient gives a reliable and or documented history of a tetanus vaccination in the last ten years, only a booster dose of tetanus is recommended. If the patient has received tetanus toxoid vaccine more than 10 years ago or has not received any vaccination, tetanus immunoglobulin is recommended as soon as possible. Tetanus toxoid (0.5 mL) is administered intramuscularly in the anterolateral aspect of mid-thigh for children aged less than 2 years, and in the lower deltoid for children aged more than 2 years.
- *Rabies prevention*: Bites from dogs, cats, cattle (cows, buffaloes, camels), horses, sheep, goats, mules and wild animals like monkeys, mongoose, bats, coyotes, foxes, raccoons, bears, skunks can transmit rabies. Rodents and squirrels have not been reported to transmit rabies, except one case with insufficient evidence, where squirrel was reported to cause rabies.[6] In India, bats also have not yet been reported to be transmitting rabies.

Washing the site with copious amount of water and soap/detergent for about 15 minutes reduces the risk of developing rabies by about 50%. Even if the patient has reported late, wound toilet should be done as the virus can persist and multiply at the site for a long time. After washing and drying of the wound, chemical disinfectants (e.g. povidone iodine, cetrimide) can be applied in recommended dilutions. Suturing of the wound should be avoided as it further creates entry points for the virus to enter the body. But in case of severe bleeding, suturing may be unavoidable, and minimum stay sutures after administration of rabies immunoglobulin should be applied.[7] Bite wounds are categorized as per the World Health Organization's guidelines, and it determines the post-exposure prophylaxis (**Table 1**).

Vaccine for post-exposure prophylaxis of rabies can be given either by intramuscular route or by intradermal route. The preferred route of anti-rabies vaccine is intradermal as it is cost-saving and equally efficacious as intramuscular route. For intramuscular route, 5-dose regimen prescribes 1 dose (1 mL or 0.5 mL depending upon the type of vaccine) to be injected into the deltoid muscle (or anterolateral thigh in children aged <2 years) on each of days 0, 3, 7, 14 and 28. For intradermal administration 2-site schedule (Thai Red Cross regimen 2-2-2-0-2) with 0.1 mL given over each deltoid on days 0, 3, 7, 28. The doses of vaccines are age independent. Pregnancy and lactation are not a contraindication to post-exposure prophylaxis.[8] Immunocompromised individuals, patients on immunosuppressant drugs or steroids, those with HIV/AIDS, and those on chloroquine should receive the vaccine by the IM route. Change of brand of vaccine or the route of vaccination is not advisable, but in cases when it is unavoidable, it can be accepted as an alternative rather than discontinuing the schedule.[9] In cases of bite wound with complete breach of skin, passive immunity by administration of Rabies Immunoglobulin (RIG), also

Table 1: Category of animal bites and management – post-exposure prophylaxis

Category I	Touching or feeding animals, animal licks on intact skin (no exposure)	None
Category II	Nibbling of uncovered skin, minor scratches or abrasions without bleeding (exposure). The integrity of the dermis is intact	Wound cleaning, Administer Antirabies Vaccine (ARV) immediately
Category III	Single or multiple transdermal bites or scratches, contamination of mucous membrane or broken skin with saliva from animal licks, exposures due to direct contact with bats (not in India) (severe exposure). Any ooze of serum or blood from the bite or scratch site	Wound cleaning Administer Rabies Immunoglobulin (RIG) immediately Administer ARVs immediately

called as Anti-Rabies Serum (ARS) is recommended. It should be administered as soon as possible, and not later than seven days after initiation of anti-rabies vaccine. In the case of immunocompromised individuals, RIG should be administered even in the case of category II bites. The dose for Equine Rabies Immunoglobulin (ERIG) is 40 IU/kg body weight and for Human Rabies Immunoglobulins (HRIG) is 20 IU/kg body weight. The anti-rabies serum should always be brought to room temperature (20–25°C) before use. Sensitivity testing for ERIG as per the manufacturer's guidelines should be performed before administration. However, WHO does not recommend routine sensitivity testing before ERIG administration, but advises that its administration should be done in settings that allow management of anaphylactic reaction. Pregnancy and lactation are not a contraindication for administration of RIGs.[8] The calculated amount of RIGs should be administered at the site of the wound. If the amount is insufficient to cover infiltration of the wound, it can be diluted with normal saline to 2 or 3 times so that the infiltration of the wound is covered. RIGs should be administered at the site only, as much as possible. In cases where after complete coverage of the wound, some amount is remaining, then it should be administered intramuscularly at a site distant from the site where the vaccine is to be administered. Preferably vaccine should be given after half an hour of serum administration. This period can be gainfully utilized to observe the patient for any reactions of the serum.

A novel product in the form of rabies monoclonal antibody (RMAB) is now available in the Indian market. Sensitivity testing is not required. It is used in a dose 3.33 IU/kg body weight. Rest of the instructions for use remain the same.[10]

Booster doses are not recommended as a routine practice to everyone who has received a full course of primary immunization against rabies. Periodic booster injections are recommended only for people whose occupation puts them at continuous or frequent risk of rabies exposure. If the Virus Neutralizing Antibody (VNA) level is less than 0.5 IU/mL, boosters on days 0 and 3 are recommended.

Pre-exposure immunization is recommended for anyone at increased risk of exposure to rabies virus, such as laboratory staff, veterinarians, animal handlers, wildlife officers with frequent exposure to potentially infected animals, as well as visitors to areas with high risk of rabies. Both the intramuscular route and the intradermal route schedule, days 0, 7, and 28, the vaccine is administered. The dose is 1 mL (or 0.5 mL depending on the type of vaccine) for intramuscular route and is 0.1 mL for intradermal route schedule.

If the animal bite exposed patient gives a reliable or documented history of having received a full course of anti-rabies vaccination schedule, 2 intramuscular or intradermal doses of such a vaccine administered on days 0 and 3 are enough for booster dose. RIG is not necessary in such cases.

The World Health Organization in 2018 update, has recommended a new PEP regimen known as the Institut Pasteur du Cambodge (IPC) regimen (11): 2-site (0.1 mL per site) intradermally on days 0, 3 and 7; and The Essen regimen: 1-site (1 vial per site) intramuscular on days 0, 3, 7 and 14/28, unrestricted for all populations. These guidelines have not yet been accepted by the Government of India. More evidence from Indian context is needed regarding this new regimen.

CONCLUSION

Animal bites are a public health problem. There is scarcity of epidemiological data regarding animal bites from India. Physical trauma, polymicrobial infections, and prevention of tetanus and rabies need to be taken care of in animal bite cases. Wound toilet and infection control are a priority in most animal bite cases. Rabies, being an almost 100% fatal disease, need to be managed by post-exposure prophylaxis following a bite of an animal which can potentially transmit rabies.

KEY MESSAGES

- Management of all bites should be as per the type of the animal and the severity of the bite.
- Thorough washing of the wound must always be done to prevent infections.
- Most animal bites lead to polymicrobial infections.
- Tetanus prophylaxis is a key component in animal bite management and should be given as per the guidelines
- Rabies is an almost 100% fatal infection after bites of warm-blooded animals such as dogs, cats, monkeys, and cattle.
- Both rabies immunoglobulin (RIG) and anti-rabies vaccine (ARV) should be considered as per the category of animal bite.
- High risk individuals should receive Pre-exposure prophylaxis for rabies.
- Pregnancy and lactation are not a contraindication for either RIG or ARV.
- ARV dose is independent of body weight, whereas RIG dose is dependent on body weight.

REFERENCES

1. Sudarshan MK, Madhusudana SN, Mahendra BJ, *et al.* Assessing the burden of human rabies in India: Results of a national multi-center epidemiological survey. Int J Infect Dis. 2007;11:29-35.
2. Ichhpujani RL, Mala C, Veena M, *et al.* Epidemiology of animal bites and rabies cases in India. A multicentric study. J Commun Dis. 2008;40:27-36.
3. Sangeetha S, Sujatha K, William RF. An epidemiological study of animal bites among rural population in Tamil Nadu, India. J Community Med Public Health. 2016;3:1413-8.
4. Sharma S, Agarwal A, Khan AM, *et al.* Prevalence of dog bites in rural and urban slums of Delhi: A community-based study. Ann Med Health Sci Res. 2016;6(2):115-9.
5. Lai P, Rawat A, Sagar A, *et al.* Prevalence of dog-bites in Delhi: Knowledge and practices of residents regarding prevention and control of rabies. Health Popul Perspect Issues. 2005;28:50-7.
6. Kumari PL, Mohanan KR, Kailas L, *et al.* A case of rabies after squirrel bite. Indian J Pediatr. 2014;81:198.
7. Consortium Against Rabies. Delhi. Maroof KA, Agarwal A, editors. Guidelines for Human Rabies: Managing animal bites for Consortium Against Rabies. 2013.13.
8. National Centre for Disease Control. National Guidelines on Rabies Prophylaxis. 2015. National Rabies Control Programme. India. National Centre for Disease Control, Ministry of Health and Family Welfare, Delhi, India.
9. Ravish HS, Sudarshan MK, Madhusudana SN, *et al.* Assessing safety and immunogenicity of post-exposure prophylaxis following interchangeability of rabies vaccines in humans. Hum Vaccin Immunother. 2014;10:1354-8.
10. Gogtay NJ, Munshi R, Ashwath Narayana DH, *et al.* Comparison of a novel human rabies monoclonal antibody to human rabies immunoglobulin for postexposure prophylaxis: A phase 2/3, randomized, single-blind, noninferiority, controlled study. Clin Infect Dis. 2018;66:387-95.

Section Editor: Rakesh Lodha

CHAPTER 61

Management of a Poisoned Child

Suresh Gupta, Bharat Choudhary

Poisoning in children is one of the common complaints in emergency, which ranges from ingestion of nontoxic household substances to lethal drugs. Incidence of poisoning in children is common in toddlers' age group which has tendency to put everything in mouth and also in adolescent age group because of high suicidal tendency. Poisoning in child differ from adult as the incident is unnoticed by the parent most of the time so the exact amount and type of substance ingested is difficult to know and also because of small body weight, little amount of ingestion becomes toxic to them.

The field of toxicology (the science of poisons) is broad and multidisciplinary. Emergency toxicology is the application of toxicological knowledge with a limited data to formulate the most effective management plan. Any substance can behave as poison if taken in excess amount. To provide the details of all possible poisons is therefore impossible for practical purposes. This chapter aims at formulating a general approach to a poisoned child. A poisoned child should be approached like a polytrauma case where a *primary survey* aims at supporting vital functions and *secondary survey* (called detoxification phase) is aimed at evaluation, decontamination, and neutralization with continued supportive care. The basic elements of the medical management of poisoning are:

1. Support vital functions.
2. Identify agent (when possible).
3. Remove, neutralize or reverse toxic effects of poison.
4. Hasten recovery.
5. Treat damaged or poisoned organs or systems and prevent further damage whenever possible.

INITIAL MANAGEMENT

When a patient has been poisoned, the immediate priority must be to maintain life. The general approach to evaluation and support of airways and cardiorespiratory function remains same as taught in pediatric advanced life support course (PALS). In a poisoned child, some points deserve special attention. Special care should be given to any impaired airway protective reflexes. Children with poisoning tend to vomit more or undergo gastric lavage, which puts them at increased risk of aspiration. So, these children may require early endotracheal intubation, if neurologically depressed. Comatose poisoned patients can suddenly develop respiratory failure and arrest. Respiratory support should be provided at the earliest evidence of respiratory insufficiency as evident on arterial blood gas study. An intravenous access should be obtained at the beginning.

During the initial evaluation and support of vital functions, a member of the emergency team should make every effort to identify the poison. A constellation of signs and symptoms consistent with ingestion or exposure to a toxin is called **toxidrome**. It is important to recognize various toxidromes when an acutely ill patient does not have any obvious history of poisoning. For some of these toxidromes'[1] life-saving therapies are available (**Table 1**).

At the completion of initial management, the patient should have been assessed for airway, breathing, circulation, and neurological status. Appropriate resuscitative measures should have been instituted by this time. The critical evaluation of respiratory status

Table 1: Toxidromes for which life-saving therapies are available	
Toxidromes	*Therapy*
• *Opioid:* Miosis, central nervous system, depression, respiratory depression	Intravenous naloxone
• *Cholinergic:* (caused by organophosphates and carbamates) SLUDGE syndrome (salivation, lacrimation, urination, defecation, garlic odor, emesis with pin-point pupils)	Atropine and pralidoxime
• *Cyclical antidepressant toxidrome:* Altered sensorium, seizure, wide QRS complexes, arrhythmias	Sodium bicarbonate
• *Hypoglycemia:* It should be suspected in any child with altered sensorium or seizures, (occurs due to oral hypoglycemics, beta-blockers, salicylates and ethanol) glucose	Intravenous 25% glucose

is essential in any comatose child. A therapeutic trial of oxygen, glucose and naloxone[2] may be tried in an unconscious child if required. The anticonvulsant or antiarrhythmic drugs should have been used wherever indicated. A thought process for the decontamination options should have begun by now.

EVALUATION

The evaluation of a poisoned patient involves an interpretation of history, physical examination and investigations. Following is the outline of the questions that must be kept in mind.

History

Parents or caregiver should be inquired about exact substance and amount ingested. It is often very helpful if empty canister or blister back is brought, as many time parents are not aware about the substance. Exact amount will help in calculation of dose whether the particular substance is ingested in toxic dose or not. The time spent after ingestion helps in taking decision of decontamination, as children who are brought within 1-2 hours of ingestion, gastric lavage and charcoal administration can help in limiting absorption unless it is contraindicated. It is also important to ask for home management for the poisoning, most of the time, which include induction of vomiting, which might be more harmful.

In the condition where child was brought with history of altered sensorium where ingestion of any substance was not noted, inquiring about family history of any chronic disorder or another member in family on medications such as antiepileptic or diabetes controlling drugs becomes important.

Emergency physician should also ask about the onset of symptoms following ingestion and the order of onset of symptoms. If more than one children are affected, then whether the symptoms are similar in nature or not.

Identification of multiple ingestions, underlying medical problems, and maintenance medications may significantly alter these findings, and must be included in the history.

Physical Examination

Each substance produces a particular set of symptoms based on their pharmacodynamics and kinetics, constellation of this signs and symptoms is known as **Toxidrome.**[1,2] Identification of these toxidromes is useful in improving the diagnosis and specific management. Certain agents produce peculiar odor when ingested, recognition of the same also points out towards the ingested substance. Clinical features of various poisonings and toxidromes are listed in **Tables 2 and 3**.

Table 2: Clinical manifestations of poisoning	
Pulse	
Bradycardia	Organophosphates, cyanide, digoxin, narcotics, carbon monoxide, clonidine, beta-blockers, calcium channel blockers
Tachycardia	Amphetamines, sympathomimetic, atropinics, tricyclic antidepressants, theophylline, salicylates, phencyclidine, alcohol, cocaine
Respiration Slow depressed	Sedative—hypnotics, alcohol, barbiturates (late), narcotics
Tachypnea	Amphetamines, salicylates, barbiturates (early), methanol, carbon monoxide
Blood pressure Hypotension	Narcotics, nitrates, nitrites, cyanide, carbon monoxide, phenothiazines, tricyclic antidepressants, barbiturates, iron theophylline, clonidine, , beta-blockers, calcium channel blockers
Hypertension	Amphetamines, sympathomimetics [especially phenylpropanolamine in over-the-counter (OTC) cold remedies], phencyclidine, MAO inhibitors, antihistamines, atropinics, clonidine, cocaine
Temperature Hypothermia	Ethanol, barbiturates, sedative—hypnotics, narcotics, phenothiazines, antidepressants, clonidine, carbamazepine

Contd...

Contd…

Hyperpyrexia	Atropinics, quinine, salicylates, amphetamines, phenothiazines, tricyclic antidepressants, MAO inhibitors, theophylline, cocaine
Neuromuscular Coma	Narcotics, sedative—hypnotics, anticholinergics (Antihistamines, antidepressants, phenothiazines, atropinics), alcohol, anticonvulsants, carbon monoxide, salicylates, oganophosphate insecticides, clonidine
Delirium/ Psychosis	Alcohol, phenothiazines, drugs of abuse (phencyclidine, LSD, mescaline, marijuana. cocaine, heroin, methaqualone), sympathomimetics and anticholinergics (including prescription and OTC cold remedies), steroids, heavy metals
Convulsions	Alcohol, amphetamines, cocaine, phenothiazines, antidepressants, antihistamines, camphor, boric acid, organophosphates, isoniazid, salicylates, lindane, lidocaine, phencyclidine
Ataxia	Alcohol, barbiturates, carbon monoxide, diphenylhydantoin, heavy metals, organic solvents, sedative/hypnotics, hydrocarbons
Paralysis	Botulism, heavy metals, tick paralysis, shellfish poisoning
Eyes Miosis	Narcotics, organophosphates, plants (Mushrooms of muscarinic type), ethanol, barbiturates, phenothiazines, clonidine

Contd…

Contd…

Mydriasis	Amphetamines, atropinics, barbiturates (if comatose), cocaine methanol, glutethimide, LSD marijuana, phencyclidine, antihistamines, antidepressants
Nystagmus	Diphenylhydantoin, sedative—hypnotics, carbamazepine, glutethimide, phencyclidine, barbiturates, ethanol
Skin Jaundice	Carbon tetrachloride, acetaminophen, naphthalene, phenothiazines, plants (Mushrooms, fava beans), heavy metals iron, phosphorous, arsenic)
Cyanosis	Methemoglobinemia due to aniline dyes, nitrites, benzocaine, phenacetin, nitrobenzene, phenazopyridine
Pinkness to redness	Atropinics, antihistamines, alcohol, carbon monoxide, cyanide, boric acid
Smell Acetone	Acetone, isopropyl alcohol, phenol and salicylates
Alcohol	Ethanol (Alcoholic beverages)
Bitter almond	Cyanide
Garlic	Organophosphates, heavy metal (Arsenic, phosphorous and thallium)
Hydrocarbons	Hydrocarbons (gasoline, turpentine, etc.)

Table 3: Toxidrome (constellation of signs/symptoms due to poisonings)

Poison syndrome	*Symptoms and signs*	*Possible toxins*
Cholinergic syndrome	Tachypnea, bradycardia or tachycardia, salivation, bronchorrhea, bronchospasm pulmonary edema, urinary frequency, diarrhea, lacrimation, confusion to drowsiness to coma, convulsions, muscle fasciculations, weakness to paralysis, miosis, blurry vision, , sweating, garlic odor,	Organophosphates Drugs for myasthenia
Anticholinergic activity	Fever, tachycardia, hypertension, cardiac arrhythmia, delirium, psychosis convulsion, coma, mydriasis, flushed dry skin	Atropine, antihistamines, antidepressants (TCA), antispasmodics, antiparkinson drugs, mushroom poisoning
Increased sympathetic activity	• Fever, tachycardia, hypertension, mydriasis, sweating, hyperactive to delirious, tremor, myoclonus, psychosis, convulsions, bradycardia, bradypnea, hypotension, hypothermia, euphoria to coma, hyporeflexia, pin-point pupils • Hypothermia, hypotension, bradypnea, confusion to coma, ataxia, nystagmus, miosis or mydriasis, vesicles, bullae • Postural hypotension, hypothermia, tachycardia, tachypnea, extrapyramidal syndrome (ataxia, torticollis, back arching, oculogyric crisis, trismus, tongue protrusion or heaviness), miosis (majority of cases) • Tachycardia, hypotension, cardiac arrhythmias, tachypnea, agitation, convulsions, vomiting	Amphetamines, cocaine Decongestant preparations Ecstasy, theophylline, narcotics, clonidine, barbiturates salicylates, phenothiazines Theophylline
Methhemoglobinemia	Cyanosis resistant to oxygen therapy	Chlorates, alanine dyes, nitrates, nitrobenzene, sulfonamides
Renal failure	Oliguria or anuria, hematuria myoglobinuria	Oxalates, carbon tetrachloride Methanol, ethanol mushrooms

Table 4: Investigations for a poisoned child [4,5]

Lab test	*Implication*	*Poisoning*
Blood sugar	Hypoglycemia	Beta blockers, Insulin, oral hypoglycemic agents, quinine, salicylates
	Hyperglycemia	Albuterol, theophylline, epinephrine, caffeine, Iron, calcium channel blocker
Blood gas	High anion gap metabolic acidosis	Methanol, Iron, isoniazid, salicylates, metformin
Electrolytes	Hypocalcemia, hypokalemia	Ethylene glycol, oxalate, fluoride Beta agonist, diuretics Cardiac glycosides
Serum osmolality	Increased	Methanol, ethanol, acetone, mannitol
Urinalysis	For rhabdomyolysis, myoglobinuria	
Electrocardiogram	Tachyarrhythmias	Sympathomimetic, anticholinergics
	Bradyarrhythmias	Beta blockers, calcium channel blockers, cardiac glycosides, cholinergic
	QRS and QT prolongation	Antidepressants, antihistaminic, antiarrhythmic
Toxicology screen	Qualitative/ Quantitative	Indicated when uncertain poisoning, comatose child, child abuse
X-ray	Radio-opacity in abdomen	Iron Pills, chloral hydrate, salicylates

Vital Signs and Initial Patient Assessment

Although the history of drug ingestion or toxin exposure is important, many clinical decisions are based on the patient's physical examination. A thorough evaluation can confirm the suspected diagnosis and detect the unexpected, as well as follow the response to therapeutic interventions.[3] All physical assessment must begin with an analysis of the vital signs. The abbreviation WNL (**w**ithin **n**ormal **l**imit) is not acceptable information as normal means different things to different people. Frequently WNL means, "**W**e **N**ever **L**ooked".

Laboratory Evaluation

Laboratory evaluation in a child with unknown ingestion is done with aim to detect the effect of poisoning as well to find out the probable agent. **Table 4** enlists the investigations that may help in initial management.

REMOVE, NEUTRALIZE OR REVERSE EFFECTS

While the patient is being stabilized, the decision process for removal of toxin from body should be taken. This may involve gastrointestinal decontamination, hastening the excretion of toxin, and use of appropriate antidote.

Gastrointestinal Decontamination

Gastrointestinal decontamination methods involve clearing of the ingested poison from the gastrointestinal tract to remove the unabsorbed substance. There are various techniques, which include use of agents which induces vomiting, gastric lavage, charcoal administration and whole bowel irrigation.[6,7] Indication of each method varies from poison to poison and depends upon arrival of the victim after ingestion of poison.

Syrup of ipecac (SOI)

Syrup of ipecac has been used to induce vomiting and decrease the absorption of ingested poison, but the risk of aspiration of vomitus is higher than the benefit, so its use is not recommended now days.

Gastric lavage

Gastric lavage involves clearing the stomach with neutral solution. It involves insertion of large bore orogastric tube through which normal saline is pushed in the aliquots of 15 mL/kg and aspirated again till the affluent becomes clear.

It is important to note that this procedure involves the risk of aspiration therefore should be done carefully and to be avoided in those victims who have poor sensorium or whose airway is not maintained. In those conditions, there are higher chances of risk of aspiration then the benefit from it. It is also preferred to be done when victim is brought to the emergency within 1–2 hours of ingestion or substance with delays gastric emptying.[8]

Contraindications to gastric lavage include corrosive poisoning (acid as well as alkali) and hydrocarbon ingestion. Gastric lavage in corrosive poisoning may lead to esophageal perforation from a misplaced tube whereas gastric lavage in hydrocarbon ingestion increases the risk of pulmonary aspiration of oropharyngeal/gastric contents.

Activated charcoal (AC)

Activated charcoal is highly absorptive material because of high absorptive surface area. It has the capacity to absorb majority of toxins when ingested orally. Usual dose is 1–2 g/kg. it is usually available in tablet form of 250 g–500 mg. Tablets are crushed and given in slurry form with soft drink.

It is effective when given within 1–2 hours of ingestion of the poison. Caution should be taken for those victims who has altered sensorium or at risk of poor airway, in those patients it can be given after securing airway with intubation to prevent the aspiration.

There are few substances in which multiple dose charcoal is effective like carbamazepine, phenytoin, digoxin, barbiturates, phenylbutazone, dapsone, methotrexate, salicylates and amitriptyline. It is not effective in poisonings due to caustics, hydrocarbon, heavy metals, iron, methanol, and ethylene glycol.[9]

Whole bowel irrigation (WBI)

Whole bowel irrigation includes flushing the whole gastrointestinal tract to remove the ingested toxin per rectally. It is usually done with polyethylene glycol (PEG) which is non-absorbable solution that is commonly used to preparing the bowel before surgery. WBI is specifically indicated for heavy metals or substances with extended release formulation, cocaine or heroin body stuffers.[10]

The dose of PEG for WBI used is 25–40 mL/kg/h either orally or through nasogastric tube till rectal effluent become clear. In condition of bowel obstruction, perforation or ileus WBI is contraindicated.[11]

Hastening Elimination of Toxin

Diuresis and alkalinization

Forced diuresis is an overused and probably ineffective treatment for most poisonings.[12] There is virtually no role for diuresis in the management of acutely poisoned patient. However, urinary pH manipulation may increase the excretion of weak acids or bases by maintaining the drug/toxin in its ionic state within the renal tubules, thereby preventing its reabsorption into the circulation. Maintaining an adequate output of alkaline urine is useful to enhance the excretion of salicylates and phenobarbitone. The urinary pH should be maintained between 7 and 8. Attempts should be made to avoid systemic alkalosis. The serum pH should not go beyond 7.5.

Hemodialysis

It is not a widely used tool in toxicology, but it can be effective in certain selected poisonings. The dialysis is effective for those toxin which are of low molecular weight (<500 RMM), has low protein binding and small volume of distribution. Examples include salicylates, ethylene glycol, methanol, lithium, theophylline, vancomycin and isopropranolol poisonings. Peritoneal dialysis is rarely useful. [13]

Hemoperfusion

Hemoperfusion over a charcoal or resin column may be an effective treatment in certain poisonings. It was used to remove substance with high molecular weight, those could not be removed through dialysis, but it now less commonly used because of availaibilty of high flux dialysis membranes.[14]

Specific Antidote Therapy

Unfortunately, there are very few poisonings in which a specific antidote is useful to reverse the toxicity. For this reason, meticulous attention must be given to the techniques for gastrointestinal decontamination or enhanced elimination. A timely supportive care alone may result in a good outcome. **Table 5** lists the antidotes which are used for patients presenting with acute ingestion of particular toxins.

SUPPORTIVE CARE

An important rule in toxicology is to "treat the patient, not the poison". There are few agents for which a specific antidote dramatically reduces the patient's symptoms. More often, supportive care with meticulous attention to vital functions, is all that is needed to ensure a good outcome.

The ABCs should always take to priority with adequate support for a clear airway, breathing and circulation throughout the management. The supportive measures needed depend on the clinical status of the child. For hypotension, the use of Trendelenburg position, intravenous fluid or pressor agent (e.g. dopamine or norepinephrine) may be indicated. For hypertension, administration of agents appropriate for the severity of the hypertension may be necessary. Appropriate antiarrhythmic therapy may be needed for the treatment of drug-induced cardiac arrhythmias. Seizures deserve special attention because toxin-induced seizures may be difficult to control. Benzodiazepines are preferred for

Table 5: Antidote therapy for poisonings[15–17]

Toxins	*Antidotes*	*Pediatric doses*
Acetaminophen	N-acetylcysteine	Loading dose: 140 mg orally; Maintenance doses: 70 mg/kg/every, 4 hours for 17 doses orally Intravenous (IV) administration: 150 mg/kg over 1 hour (loading dose); 50 mg/kg IV over 4 hours; 100 mg/kg IV over 16 hours
Anticholinergics	Physostigmine salicylate	0.02 mg/kg slow IV infusion over 3–5 minutes titrated to effect
Arsenic	Succimer (DMSA) British anti-Lewisite (BAL) (dimercaprol) only if unable to tolerate oral succimer	10 mg/kg/orally 3 times a day 3–5 mg/kg intramuscular every 4–6 hours
Benzodiazepines	Flumazenil	0.01 mg/kg IV bolus titrated to effect or total dose of 1–3 mg
β blockers	Glucagon	0.15 mg/kg IV bolus, then 0.1 mg/kg/h IV infusion titrated to effect
Calcium channel blockers	Calcium chloride 10% & Calcium gluconate	Calcium chloride- 20–30 mg/kg Calcium gluconate- 100–200 mg/kg IV
	Glucagon	0.15 mg/kg IV bolus followed by 0.1 mg/kg/h IV infusion titrated to effect
Carbamates	Atropine	0.02 mg/kg mg/kg max 0.5 mg/dose IV bolus, repeat doses titrated to effect
Cyanide	Cyanide antidote kit: Sodium nitrite 3% Sodium thiosulfate and or hydroxocobalamine	Hydroxocobalamin: 70 mg/kg IV (maximum 5 grams) Sodium thiosulfate: 400 mg/kg IV (maximum 12.5 grams) Sodium nitrite: 6 mg/kg by slow IV infusion (maximum 300 mg, only give if not contraindicated and hydroxocobalamin is not available)
Digoxin	Digoxin immune Antibody fragment	Empiric dosing: 10–20 vials IV bolus for life-threatening toxicity
Ethylene glycol, Methanol	Ethanol 10%	Loading dose 10 mL/kg IV or orally followed by maintenance dose 1–2 mL/kg/h IV infusion or orally
	Fomepizole	15 mg/kg IV bolus, followed by 10 mg/kg 12 hrly- 4 doses repeat doses may be necessary
Iron	Deferoxamine	5–15 mg/kg/h IV infusion titrate to effect
Isoniazid	Pyridoxine	1 g per gram ingested or empiric dosing 75 mg/kg IV bolus up to 5 g
Lead	Succimer (DMSA) if Patient is able to tolerate oral medication	10 mg/kg orally 3 times a day, repeat doses are common
	BAL (dimercaprol) (only for lead encephalopathy)	3–5 mg/kg IM or 50–75 mg/m^2
	Calcium disodium EDTA	20–30 mg/kg diluted in 250 mL IV infusion over 12–24 hours (start 4 hours after BAL administration)
Methemoglobinemia	Methylene blue	1–2 mg/kg slow IV infusion, repeat doses as needed
Opioids	Naloxone hydrochloride	0.4–2 mg IV titrated to effect
Organophosphates	Atropine	0.1 mg/kg IV bolus, repeat dose titrated to effect
	Pralidoxime	20–40 mg/kg slow IV infusion followed by 5–10 mg/kg/h continuous infusion or 20 mg/kg every 4 hours
Salicylates	Sodium bicarbonate	150 mEq + 40 mEq KCl in one liter of D5 w infused to maintain urine output at 1–2 mL/kg/h and a urine pH approximately 7.5
Tricyclic antidepressants	Sodium bicarbonate	1–2 mEq (kg IV bolus, titrate repeat boluses, do not exceed arterial pH 7.55)
Warfarin, Superwarfarins	Fresh frozen plasma Vitamin K1	Fresh frozen plasma for life-threatening hemorrhage 0.6 mg/kg/slow IV infusion, subcutaneously or orally

Table 6: Non-toxic substances

- *Pharmaceuticals*: Antacids, antibiotics, contraceptives, corticosteroids, laxatives, mineral oil, vitamins (without iron), zinc oxide
- *Cosmetics*: Baby products, cologne, deodorants, eye makeup, hand lotion, hair products, hydrogen peroxide (household, 3%), lipstick, perfumes
- *Soaps and detergents*: Suntan lotion, soap, bath foam, bubble bath, fabric softener, hand and dish washing soap, laundry detergent, shampoo
- *Household products*: Artificial sweeteners, lubricating oil, ballpoint pen ink, bath oil, matches, candles, crayons, dehumidifying packets, deodorizers, silica gel, household bleach, shaving cream, shoe polish, thermometers (mercury), water colors
- *Miscellaneous*: Chalk, cigarettes, clay, glues and paste, greases, pencil lead, paint (without lead)

control of seizures due to poisoning. If a specific antidote is available to counteract a toxin-induced seizure, it should be given.[18] For example—isoniazid-induced seizures are difficult to control without the administration of pyridoxine.

THE STABLE ACCIDENTAL POISONED PATIENTS

The approach to the stable accidental poisoning patient includes all the components as for any other poisoned patient like history, physical examination, clinical investigation (as needed) and management. The point that needs to be stressed is that many of the accidental poisonings are trivial. These children do not require any gastrointestinal decontamination, investigation or treatment. A few hours observation may be all that is needed. Many of the household products are non toxic, which do not necessitate any kind of treatment (**Table 6**). These children can be safely sent home after providing anticipatory poison prevention guidance.

KEY MESSAGES

- Children with poisoning tend to vomit more or undergo gastric lavage, which puts them at increased risk of aspiration. So these children may require early endotracheal intubation, if neurologically depressed.
- A constellation of signs and symptoms consistent with ingestion or exposure to a toxin is called toxidrome. It is important to recognize various toxidromes.
- Syrup of ipecac has been used to induce vomiting and decrease the absorption of ingested poison, but the risk of aspiration of vomitus is higher than the benefit, so its use is not recommended now days.
- Gastric lavage in corrosive poisoning may lead to esophageal perforation from a misplaced tube whereas gastric lavage in hydrocarbon ingestion increases the risk of pulmonary aspiration of oropharyngeal/gastric contents.
- There is virtually no role for diuresis in the management of acutely poisoned patient. However, urinary pH manipulation may increase the excretion of weak acids or bases.
- An important rule in toxicology is to "treat the patient, not the poison". There are few agents for which a specific antidote dramatically reduces the patient's symptoms.

REFERENCES

1. Mofenson HC, Caraccio TR. Toxidromes. Compr Ther. 1985;11:46-52.
2. Mofenson HC, Greensher J. The unknown poison. Pediatrics. 1974;54:336-42.
3. Hoffinan JR, Schrigr Luo JS. The empiric uses of naloxone in patients with altered mental status—A reappraisal. Ann Emerg Med. 1991;20:246-52.
4. Osterloh JD. Utility and reliability of emergency toxicological testing. Emerg Med Clin North Am. 1990;8:693-723.
5. Mahoney JD, Gross PL, Stern TA, *et al.* Quantitative serum toxic screening in the management of suspected drug overdose. Am J Emerg Med. 1990;8:16-22.
6. Rogers GC, Matyunas NJ. Gastrointestinal decontamination for acute poisoning. Pediatr Clin North Am. 1986;33:261-85.
7. Bryant S, Singer J. Management of toxic exposure in children. Emerg Med Clin North Am. 2003;21:101.
8. Kulig K, Bar-Or D, Cantrill SV, *et al.* Management of acutely poisoned patients without gastric emptying. Ann Emerg Med. 1985;14:62-7.
9. Levy G. Gastrointestinal clearance of drugs with activated charcoal. N Engl J Med. 1982;307:676-8.
10. Tenebein M, Cohen S, Sitar DS. Whole bowel irrigation as a decontamination procedure after acute drug overdose. Arch Intern Med. 1987;147:905-7.
11. Albertson TE, Derlet RW, Foulke GE, *et al.* Superiority of activated charcoal alone compared with ipecac and activated charcoal in the treatment of acute toxic ingestions. Ann Emerg Med. 1989;18:56-9.
12. Prescott LF, Balali-Mood M, Critchley J, *et al.* Diuresis or urinary alkalinization for salicylate poisoning? Br Med J. 1982;285: 1383-6.
13. Pond SM. Extracorporeal techniques in the treatment of poisoned patients. Med J Aust. 1991;154:617-22.
14. Higgins RM, Hearing S, Goldsmith DJ, *et al.* Severe theophylline poisoning: Charcoal, hemoperfusion or hemodialysis? Postgrad Med J. 1995;71:224-6.
15. Poisodex, Engelwood, CO: Micromedex. Inc., 1998;95.
16. Sivilotti ML. Flumazenil, naloxone and the 'coma cocktail'. Br J Clin Pharmacol. 2016;81:428.
17. Sutter ME, Gerona RR, Davis MT, *et al.* Fatal fentanyl: One pill can kill. Acad Emerg Med. 2017;24:106.
18. Shannon M. Ingestion of toxic substances by children. N Engl J Med. 2000;342:186.

CHAPTER

62

Plant Related Poisonings

Baljeet Maini, Parveen Kumar Antil

INTRODUCTION

Plants are common causes of poisoning in children in India, especially in rural areas. According to one study, plants accounted for 1.7% of all poisons exposures.[1] Most exposures are accidental in children.[2] Poisonous plants encountered in India include nearly 10 species but serious common poisonings are due to only a few of them like datura, wild mushroom, etc.[3] Suicidal and homicidal use of plants is also reported. More recently, litchi encephalopathy has been described from India's litchi producing regions of eastern Uttar Pradesh and Bihar. **Table 1** highlights main plant related poisonings in India.

General Management Principles

Toxic plants contain numerous chemical components including toxic alkaloids, glycosides, terpenes, proteins, lectins, etc.[4] Determination of the specific plant ingested helps guide in management. Whenever possible, samples of the plant, including, flower, leaves, stem, and root should be obtained. Consultation with a medical toxicologist and botanist is advised when attempting plant identification whenever feasible and required. Symptomatic patients can be classified according to presenting features to guide therapy and identify the type of plant ingested.

Role of advanced studies: Although specific plant toxins can be identified using techniques such as thin layer chromatography, high-performance liquid chromatography, mass spectrophotometry, and ultraviolet absorption, these analytic methods are neither routinely available in most hospital laboratories nor timely aid in management.[5]

DATURA POISONING

Datura stramonium is one of the most poisonous plants in India found in most of the states. The whole plant especially the foliage, and seeds contain anticholinergic tropane alkaloid.[6,7] Seeds contain highest amount of atropine (0.1 mg per seed). Intoxication occurs by ingesting the seeds, drinking the brewed tea, or from the "milk" of stem and leaves. Intentional use of Datura plants for recreational use is increasing especially among youths.[7] Accidental cases are also seen from use of Datura seeds by quacks for treatment of various ailments.

Pathophysiology

Datura species contain alkaloids that can cause anticholinergic effects centrally and peripherally. The chief sites of action of these alkaloids are cholinergic muscarinic receptors. These are the post ganglionic receptors of the parasympathetic nervous system as well as sympathetic system supplying sweat glands and smooth muscle tissues. Central nervous system (CNS) muscarinic receptors are located in the spinal cord, extrapyramidal system, reticular activating system, vestibular system and cerebral cortex. Nicotinic receptors are much less sensitive to anticholinergic action of belladonna alkaloids and do not play significant role in Datura poisoning.

Clinical Features

The typical representation of anticholinergic intoxication is well known:

- Red as a beet (flushing)
- Dry as a bone (anhidrosis)

Table 1: Plants causing poisoning and their pathophysiologic principles

Systemic manifestation	*Plants causing poisoning*
Cardiotoxic plants (cardiac glycoside)	Neerium (oleander), Cerbera odollam (suicide tree)
Neurotoxin plant	Datura, calotropis
Hepatotoxic	Mushroom
Miscellaneous toxic plant and plant products	Arecanut, parthenium, ricinus (castor), litchi fruit

- Hot as a hare (anhidrotic hyperthermia)
- Blind as a bat (nonreactive mydriasis)
- Mad as a hatter (delirium; hallucinations), and
- Full as a flask (urinary retention).[8]

Other clinical features not included above are tachycardia, which is the earliest and most reliable sign of anticholinergic toxicity and decreased or absent bowel sounds.

Treatment

Initial treatments of the poisoned patient begin with assessment and stabilization of the airway, breathing, and circulation with rapid intravenous access, oxygen if required along with vital monitoring. Agitation and seizures initially should be treated with benzodiazepines. Hyperthermia should be treated with evaporative cooling in moderate to severe cases.

Decontamination

Although systemic anticholinergic toxicity has been reported from cutaneous and ocular absorption, most anticholinergic toxicity results from ingestion.[9,10] If the patient's mental status is intact and ingestion of an anticholinergic agent is likely, activated charcoal (AC) (1 g/kg; maximum 50 g) should be administered. Activated charcoal should not be given in patients with depressed conscious level; however, tracheal intubation is done first as patient in such state not able to protect the airway. Gastric lavage is seldom needed, and induced emesis should be avoided.

Antidote therapy with physostigmine

Most patients with anticholinergic toxicity do well with supportive care alone, but some may benefit from antidote therapy with physostigmine.[10] Physostigmine is indicated when patients have manifestations of both central and peripheral anticholinergic toxicity with (moderate to severe agitation/delirium) as it crosses the blood brain barrier. Physostigmine should **not** be given if a condition other than a purely anticholinergic poisoning is suspected. Once physostigmine blocks acetylcholinesterase, the concentration of acetylcholine at muscarinic receptors increases, and overcomes anticholinergic blockade. The atropine, cardiac monitor and resuscitative equipment should be available at the bedside before physostigmine is given. In children, the recommended dose of physostigmine is 0.02 mg/kg by slow IV push over 5 minutes, up to a maximum of 0.5 mg per dose in pediatric patients. Rapid administration may result in cholinergic symptoms or seizures. Additional, smaller doses may be repeated after 20 to 30 minutes if agitated delirium recurs.[11] Physostigmine appears to be superior to benzodiazepines in the management of agitation and delirium due to anticholinergic toxicity. Patients treated with physostigmine have shorter recovery times and less complications. Although patients with very minor anticholinergic toxicity may respond well to small doses of benzodiazepines, those with moderate to severe agitation will likely respond better to physostigmine.[12] Treatment with physostigmine can elucidate the diagnosis of anticholinergic poisoning in some cases. If physostigmine leads to dramatic clinical improvement, further workup is often unnecessary.

WILD MUSHROOM POISONING

Mushroom is used as food but some species are poisonous. Around 100 species of mushrooms in India are known to be poisonous to humans.[13] In poisonous fungi, common varieties are *Amanita phalloides* and *Amanita muscaria*. *A. muscaria* contains an alkaloid muscarine, the action of which resembles stimulation of parasympathetic postganglionic nerves. *A. phalloides* has polypeptides, which are heat stable, insoluble in water and are powerful protein synthesis inhibitors. Muscarine stimulates postganglionic cholinergic fibers.[14]

Symptoms

In some cases, irritant symptoms may be present, while in others neurotic or a combination of both. The irritant symptoms are delayed for 6 to 12 hours. There is constriction of the throat, burning pain in the stomach with nausea, vomiting and diarrhea followed by cyanosis, weak pulse, labored respirations, convulsions, eventually collapse and death. The neural symptoms are giddiness, headache, delirium, diplopia, constriction of pupils,

Table 2: Clinical phases of mushroom poisoning

Phases	Symptoms and signs	
Stage 1	Lag phase 0–24 h	Asymptomatic
Stage 2	Gastrointestinal phase 6–24 h	Nausea, vomiting, crampy abdominal pain, and severe secretory diarrhea
Stage 3	Apparent convalescence 24–72 h	Asymptomatic, worsening of hepatic and renal function indices
Stage 4	Acute liver failure 4–9 days	Renal and hepatic failure → multiorgan failure → death

cramps, twitching of the limbs, convulsions, salivation, bradycardia and coma. Sometimes renal and hepatic toxicity occurs between 3 and 6 days. **Fatal dose**: Two to 3 mushrooms. **Fatal period**: Usually 2 hours. **Table 2** describes phases of mushroom poisoning.

Management

The main treatment in mushroom poisoning is supportive care. However, for some mushroom poisonings there are specific antidotes. It is needed in cases of cholinergic excess, seizures, methemoglobinemia and delayed gastroenteritis. After initial assessment and support of airway, breathing, and circulation as needed, the clinician should anticipate and aggressively manage fluid losses caused by vomiting and diarrhea, intravenous fluids should be given based upon clinical assessment of losses and evidence of dehydration. Hypoglycemia should be treated, for hyperammonemia, lactulose may be administered, Vitamin K replacement and infusions of fresh frozen plasma are indicated for significant coagulopathy. Management of other common comorbidities includes acute renal failure, sepsis, metabolic disturbances, hepatic encephalopathy, and cerebral edema depending upon the complications noted in course.

Gastrointestinal decontamination: Patients who are alert and present for care within one hour of a potentially toxic mushroom ingestion should receive activated charcoal (AC) [dose in less than 2 yr (1-2 g/kg orally up to 15 g and more than 2 yr (1 g/kg orally up to 50-100 g)].

Elimination: In addition to a single dose of AC, patients who ingest amatoxin-containing mushrooms should receive mushroom derived active compound (MDAC) to decrease the enterohepatic circulation of amatoxin. The dose is 0.5 g/kg (maximum dose up to 50 g) every 4 hours.

Penicillin G: High-dose IV penicillin G may inhibits toxin uptake by organic anion transporting polypeptides (OATP) thereby preventing cellular toxicity. Recommended dosing varies from 400,000 units/kg per day and can be given as a continuous intravenous infusion.[15]

OLEANDER AND SUICIDE TREE POISONING

Two main plants causing cardiac toxicity in India are Kaner (local name) (*Nerium oleander/indicum*) and suicide tree *(Cerbera odollam)*. *Nerium* sp. is an ornamental shrub, with flowers in various colors (pink, red, white, peach, yellow).[16] The oleander is most prevalent, alluring flowers make it a particular hazard.[17] All parts of this plant contain cardiac glycosides and even on burning, smoke produced is toxic, as heat does not inactivate the glycosides. Human poisoning with the fruit kernels of plant *Cerbera odollam* ("suicide tree") is common in the state of Kerala where it accounts for 10% of all fatal poisoning cases.[18]

Clinical Features

Initial symptoms from oleander and *Cerbera odollam* poisoning are gastrointestinal in nature and appear within 4 hours of ingestion. The most serious side effects of oleander poisoning are cardiac abnormalities, including various ventricular dysrhythmias, tachyarrhythmias, bradycardia, and heart block.[19] Electrocardiography often reveals an increased PR interval, QRS-T interval decreased and flattening or inversion of T wave. It is thought that these clinical manifestations are the result of both increased vagal tone and also direct cardiac glycoside toxicity.[20] ECG changes noted with *Odollam* poisoning, are sinus arrhythmias, notably sinus pauses. Further emergence of ECG changes is seen in course of treatment.[21]

Management

The treatment consists of hemodynamic support and administering atropine for severe bradycardia, controlling dysrhythmias by lidocaine, installing a temporary venous pacemaker; and administering digoxin-specific Fab antibody fragments.[22]

LITCHI ENCEPHALOPATHY

This is a recently described entity which until recently was an enigma in litchi producing regions of India (Bihar). This condition is due to chemicals hypoglycin A and methylene cyclopropyl glycine (MCPG) in unripe and ripe litchi fruit (*Litchi sinensis*).[23] Children consuming them in significant amounts in absence of evening meal are chiefly affected. These chemicals block the gluconeogenesis and β-oxidation of fatty acids, leading onto acute complications. Patients present in acute state of altered sensorium, vomiting and seizures. Delayed presentation to hospital increases the mortality. Acute presentation of a child with altered sensorium/seizures in summer season in Litchi producing areas should always prompt this entity as a possibility.

Management

This condition is treated entirely with supportive management. Children respond variably due to variable times of presentation to hospitals. Prompt correction of blood sugar levels along with other supportive treatment is lifesaving.

KEY MESSAGES

- Serious plant poisoning is seen in setting of suicidal ingestion or intentional recreational use in adolescent age group.
- Identify the plant and part of plant ingested as far as feasible.
- Asymptomatic individuals with plant ingestions that are unlikely to be toxic may be observed without any testing.
- Differential diagnosis should always be kept in every seriously ill case of suspected plant poisoning.
- Knowledge of local plants of wild type as well as household plants is beneficial in treating plant related poisonings.
- Schools should be involved in disseminating awareness of local poisonous plants among children to decrease unintentional cases of plant-related poisonings.

REFERENCES

1. Manzar N, Saad SM, Manzar B, *et al.* The study of etiological and demographic characteristics of acute household accidental poisoning in children--a consecutive case series study from Pakistan. BMC Pediatr. 2010;10:28.
2. Lamminpää A, Kinos M. Plant poisonings in children. Hum Exp Toxicol. 1996;15:245-49.
3. Pillay VV. Modern Medical Toxicology, 4th edition. New Delhi, India: Jaypee Brothers Medical Publishers; 2013. p. 10-28.
4. Palmer M, Betz JM. Plants. In: Nelson LS, Lewin NA, Howland MA, Hoffman RS, Goldfrank LR, Flomenbaum NE, editors. Goldfrank's Toxicologic Emergencies, 9th edition. McGraw-Hill: New York; 2011. p. 1537.
5. Smolinske SC, Daubert GP, Spoerke DG. Poisonous plants. In: Shannon MW, Borron SW, Burns MJ, editors. Haddad and Winchester's Clinical Management of Poisoning and Drug Overdose, 4th edition. Saunders Elsevier, Philadelphia. 2007. p. 473.
6. Krenzelok EP. Aspects of Datura poisoning and treatment. Clin Toxicol. 2010;48:104-10.
7. Vearrier D, Greenberg MI. Anticholinergic delirium following Datura stramonium ingestion: Implications for the Internet age. J Emerg Trauma Shock. 2010;3:303.
8. Richmond M, Seger D. Central anticholinergic syndrome in a child: A case report. J Emerg Med. 1985;3:453-56.
9. Reilly JF Jr, Weisse ME. Topically induced diphenhydramine toxicity. J Emerg Med. 1990;8:59-61.
10. Thompson HS. Cornpicker's pupil: Jimson weed mydriasis. J Iowa Med Soc. 1971;61:475-7.
11. Rosenbaum C, Bird SB. Timing and frequency of physostigmine redosing for antimuscarinic toxicity. J Med Toxicol. 2010;6: 386-92.
12. Pentel P, Peterson CD. A systole complicating physostigmine treatment of tricyclic antidepressant overdose. Ann Emerg Med. 1980;9:588-90.
13. Purkayastha RP, Chandra A. Manual of Indian Edible Mushrooms. New Delhi: Today and Tomorrows Printers and Publishers; 1985. p. 192-4.
14. Karlson-Stiber C, Persson H. Cytotoxic fungi—an overview. Toxicon. 2003;42:339-49.
15. Nakajima N, Ueda M, Higashi N, et al. Erythromelalgia associated with Clitocybe acromelalga intoxication. Clin Toxicol (Phila). 2013;51:451-4.
16. Frohne DP, Fander HJ. A Colour Atlas of poisonous plants. London: Wolfe Publishing Ltd; 1984. p. 190.
17. Ansford AJ, Morris H. Fatal oleander poisoning. Med J Aust. 1981;1:360-1.
18. Gaillard Y, Krishnamoorthy A, Bevalot F. Cerbera odollam: A 'suicide tree' and cause of death in the state of Kerala, India. J Ethnopharmacol. 2004;95:123-6.
19. Behcet AI, Yarbil P, Dogan M, et al. A case of non-fatal oleander poisoning. BMJ Case Reports. 2010.
20. Osterloh J, Herold S, Pond S. Oleander interference in the digoxin radioimmunoassay in a fatal ingestion. JAMA. 1982;247:1596-7.
21. Monon MS, Kumar P, Jayachandran CI. Clinical profile and management of poisoning with suicide tree: An observational study. Heart Views. 2016;17:136-9.
22. Shumaik GM, Wu AW, Ping AC. Oleander poisoning: Treatment with digoxin-specific Fab antibody fragments. Ann Emerg Med. 1988;17:732-5.
23. Shrivastava A, Kumar A, Thomas JD, *et al.* Association of acute toxic encephalopathy with litchi consumption in an outbreak in Muzaffarpur, India, 2014: A case-control study. Lancet Glob Health. 2017;5:e458-66.

CHAPTER

63

Drug Overdose

Rajniti Prasad, Utpal Kant Singh

63.1 ACETAMINOPHEN POISONING

INTRODUCTION

Acetaminophen (paracetamol) is the most widely used antipyretic and analgesic, which is also used in combination with other medications in hundreds of formulations. Its therapeutic safety in children has been directly related to absence of significant cumulative kinetics. In USA, it is the leading cause of drug overdose.[1] Free over the counter availability and careless use of acetaminophen is responsible for drug overdosage. In adolescents, acetaminophen ingestion may be suicidal. Following ingestion of sufficient acetaminophen to produce potentially toxic blood level, an adolescent is six times more likely to develop evidence of hepatotoxicity than in a child under age of 6 years.[2,3] Adolescents are two times more likely to develop potentially toxic blood levels.

PATHOPHYSIOLOGY

The prime target organ of acetaminophen toxicity is the liver. In addition to hepatotoxicity, renal tubular damage and hypoglycemic coma may occur due to toxic action of active intermediate metabolites. Acetaminophen is rapidly absorbed after therapeutic dose and produces peak plasma level in about 90 min. In overdose, this absorption may be delayed for 4 hours. The volume of distribution and half-life of acetaminophen with normal liver function are 1 L/kg and 1 to 3 hours respectively. The drug is primarily metabolized in liver with less than 2% being excreted unchanged in urine.[4]

In children, between 9 and 12 years of age, acetaminophen is primarily metabolized in the liver to the sulfate or glucuronide conjugates, which are metabolically inert. The remaining 2–4% is metabolized through cytochrome P450 mixed functions oxidase system, which conjugates it with glutathione to produce mercaptopuric acid, a non-toxic product. The lower incidence of toxicity in young children may be related to lesser metabolism via P450.[5]

With acetaminophen overdose, when hepatic stores of glutathione are depleted to less than 70% of normal, highly reactive intermediate toxic metabolites bind with hepatic macromolecules and cause hepatic necrosis.[6] Hepatic enzyme induction by barbiturates, narcotics, hydantoin and histamines may increase the formation of reactive metabolites, predisposing the patient to hepatic damage even if a minor overdose of acetaminophen is ingested.[7] Co-ingestion of ethanol and acetaminophen is cytoprotective in both adults and children, probably as a result of competition at P450 site but ethanol is not recommended as therapy.[8] Therapeutic accumulation to plasma levels of 40 μg/dL, which is still lower that required for hepatotoxicity, may occur if the highest recommended dose of 15 mg/kg is given every 4 hours for extended period, child abuse or intentional overdose must be considered in children who develop high plasma levels at therapeutic overdose.[9]

CLINICAL FEATURES

Children with overdose of acetaminophen usually present with features of hepatic cell damage, renal tubular necrosis and hypoglycemic coma. Following four stages of toxicity are described if left untreated.[10]

Stage I

Lasts for first 24 hours after ingestion. Average time of onset of symptoms is 6 hours after ingestion; children usually become symptomatic by 14 hours. Children present with anorexia, nausea, vomiting, malaise, pallor, and diaphoresis; children less than 6 years of age rarely show diaphoresis but present with early vomiting. Laboratory investigations such as ALT, AST, serum bilirubin and prothrombin time are normal.

Stage II

Lasts for next 24 hours after stage I. It is characterized by resolution of symptoms of stage I with upper right quadrant abdominal pain and tenderness. Mild hepatomegaly and jaundice may be present. Laboratory investigations show elevated serum bilirubin, AST, ALT and prothrombin time. Some children may develop oliguria.

Stage III

This stage is seen 48–96 hours after ingestion. Maximum liver functions abnormalities are seen during this period. Hepatotoxicity due to acetaminophen is characterized by elevated transaminases, increased serum bilirubin and prolonged prothrombin time.

Plasma AST level in excess of 1000 IU/L, prolongation of prothrombin time and serum bilirubin more than 4 mg/dL on third to fifth day after ingestion are indicators of severe toxicity.[11] Acute renal failure may also occur in some patients. Anorexia, nausea, vomiting and malaise may reappear during this stage. Less than 1% of patients develop fulminant hepatotoxicity and eventually die of hepatic failure, if left untreated. Liver biopsy in this stage reveals centrilobular necrosis of hepatocytes with sparing of periportal area.

Stage IV

This is the stage of resolution and extends from 4–14 days. It is characterized by resolution of hepatic dysfunction although AST may remain elevated for few more days. Patients who had hepatotoxicity, usually revealed no sequelae either clinically or on liver biopsy, 3–12 months later.

Biochemical and hematological abnormalities in acetaminophen poisoning are shown in **Table 1**.

Table 1: Biochemical and hematological abnormalities in acetaminophen poisoning
Biochemical
• ↑ ALT/AST • ↑ Bilirubin • ↓ Blood glucose • ↓ Lactate • ↑ Amylase • ↑ Creatinine • ↓ Phosphate
Hematological
• Thrombocytopenia • ↑ Prothrombin time • ↓ Clotting factors II, V, VII

DIAGNOSIS

1. History of ingestion
2. Clinical features
3. Laboratory investigations
   a. Plasma level of acetaminophen to assess the severity of hepatotoxicity: Serum concentrations greater than 200, 100 and 50 µg/mL at 4, 8 and 12 hours after ingestion respectively or any concentration above the values depicted on the Rumack Mathew nomogram indicates a potential risk of hepatotoxicity.[2]
   b. Plasma AST level greater than 1000 IU/L.
   c. Bilirubin more than 4 mg/dL.
   d. Prolonged prothrombin time.

MANAGEMENT

Assessment

In children with acetaminophen overdose, efforts should be made to determine the amount of drugs and co-ingestants, if any. Acetaminophen alone will not produce any alteration in the sensorium in first 24 hours and usually will not produce such an alteration unless patient develops hepatic encephalopathy. If a patient comes with a significant change in sensorium, some other agents should be considered in addition to or instead of acetaminophen. Care of airways, breathing and circulation should be done properly. A sample of blood should be drawn and sent for laboratory investigations including serum acetaminophen level.

General Measures

When a child presents within 4 hours, gastrointestinal decontamination should be done. Emesis should be induced with syrup of ipecac to get rid of remaining acetaminophen. Gastric lavage must be done with normal saline. Activated charcoal is effective in adsorbing acetaminophen. At physiological pH, adsorption is rapid and pH independent.[12] The dose of activated charcoal is 10 times the ingested dose of acetaminophen.[13] For maximal effect, activated charcoal should be administered within 30 minutes of ingestion. However, activated charcoal effectively adsorbs both methionine and N-acetylcysteine, concurrent administration of both would markedly diminish their antidotal effectiveness.[14]

Specific Measures

N-acetylcysteine

It is the specific antidote and drug of choice for prevention of hepatotoxicity. Other drugs like methionine, cysteamine are available but are not popular due to their side effect. Oral or intravenous N-acetylcysteine mitigates acetaminophen induced hepatorenal damage, if given within 10 hours. In vivo, N-acetylcysteine increases hepatic glutathione and other protective amino acids in blood.[15] The beneficial effects of N-acetylcysteine include increase in hepatic blood flow, glutathione store, and free radical scavenging and alteration of cytokine production.[16]

The oral dosage schedule of N-acetylcysteine is 140 mg/kg as loading dose followed by 70 mg/kg body weight 4 hourly for 17 doses.[17] If the patient vomits within an hour of administration of dose, it should be repeated. For intravenous route, usual dose is 300 mg/kg given over 21 hours. The optimal route and duration of administration of N-acetylcysteine are controversial. On basis of selected post-hoc analysis, oral route were found superior to intravenous route in children who presented after 15 hours. A shorter hospital stay, patient convenience, and concerns over the reduction in bioavailability of oral N-acetylcysteine by charcoal and vomiting make intravenous N-acetylcysteine preferable for most patients.[18] Prior charcoal administration does not reduce the efficacy of N-acetylcysteine and may provide additional hepatoprotective benefit. However, some workers have suggested increment of loading dose by 40% or from 140 mg/kg to 235 mg/kg body weight.[19]

As unpleasant odor and frequent vomiting is associated with its use, N-acetylcysteine may be diluted to a final concentration of 5%(w/v) and to mask the unpleasant flavor, citrus fruit juices or carbonated beverages may be added. For intravenous preparations, loading dose of 150 mg/kg should be given with 3 mL/kg of 5% dextrose over 15 min; followed by 50 mg/kg dose in 7 mL/kg 5% dextrose over 4 hours and the third dose of 100 mg/kg in 14 mL/kg 5% dextrose over 16 hours. Adverse reactions such as angioedema, bronchospasm, flushing, hypotension, hypokalemia, nausea/vomiting, rashes, tachycardia and respiratory distress have been reported in about 10% of patients.[15] Oral therapy with N-acetylcysteine or methionine is contraindicated in coma and children with recurrent vomiting. Vitals and SpO_2 should must be monitored regularly in children with fulminant hepatic failure.[16]

Methionine

It acts by replenishing cellular glutathione stores and generation of cysteine and/or glutathione. Methionine is more effective when given orally than IV. The initial dose is 2.5 g then 2.5 g 4 hourly to a total of 10 g over 12 hours.[14]

Ethyl pyruvate

It has been reported to have beneficial effect as anti-inflammatory and antioxidant therapy after acetaminophen intoxication in experimental animals. In addition, ethyl pyruvate also exerts as anti-apoptotic, increases heme-oxygenase-1 enzyme, and stimulates Krebs cycle. The dose is 0.01 to 100 mg/kg intravenously. It causes increase in lung and kidney NF-kB activation, which is associated with higher mortality.[20]

During treatment, laboratory investigations should be repeated. If the liver function tests become abnormal, proper measures should be taken. Once hepatic failure occurs, use of N-acetylcysteine is contraindicated[15] and patient should be managed along conventional line with lactulose, vit-K, 20% mannitol and appropriate IV fluids. Renal function should be evaluated periodically and necessary measures should be taken, if deterioration occurs. Forced alkaline diuresis is of no therapeutic value. Hemodialysis or charcoal hemoperfusion enhances elimination of acetaminophen but not the toxic metabolites.

PROGNOSIS

The poor prognostic factors in established paracetamol induced hepatic failure are pH below 7.3, serum creatinine above 300 μmol/L and prothrombin time above 100 secs in grade III to IV encephalopathy. However, factor VIII to factor V ratio above 30 is the best poor prognostic indicator.[16]

KEY MESSAGES

- The prime target organ of acetaminophen toxicity is the liver. In addition to hepatotoxicity, renal tubular damage and hypoglycemic coma may occur due to toxic action of active intermediate metabolites.
- When a child presents within 4 hours, gastrointestinal decontamination should be done.
- N-acetylcysteine is the specific antidote and drug of choice for prevention of hepatotoxicity.
- The poor prognostic factors in established paracetamol induced hepatic failure are pH below 7.3, serum creatinine above 300 μmol/L and prothrombin time above 100 secs.

REFERENCES

1. Clark J. Acetaminophen poisoning and the use of intravenous N-acetylcysteine. Air Med J. 2001;20:7-16.
2. Rumack BH, Mathew H. Acetaminophen poisoning and toxicity. Pediatrics. 1975;55:870-1.
3. Peterson RG, Rumack BH. Age as variable in acetaminophen overdose. Arch Intern Med. 1981;141:390-3.
4. Rumack BH. Acetaminophen overdose in young children. Am J Dis Child. 1984;138:428-433.
5. Lich Lai MW, Sarnaik AP, Newton JE. Metabolism and pharmacokinetics of acetaminophen in severely poisoned young child. J Pediatr. 1984;105:125-8.
6. Mitchell JR, Thorgeirsson SS, Potter NZ. Acetaminophen induced hepatic injury. Clin Pharmacol Ther. 1974;16:676.
7. Miller RP, Robert RJ, Fisher LJ. Acetaminophen elimination kinetics in neonates, children and adults. Clin Pharmacol Ther. 1976;19:284-94.
8. Rumack BH. Acetaminophen overdosage in young children, treatment and effects of alcohol and additional ingestions in 417 cases. Am J Dis Child. 1984;138:428-33.
9. Nahata MC, Powel DA, Durell DE. Acetaminophen accumulation in a pediatric patient after repeated therapeutic doses. Eur J Clin Pharmacol. 1984;27:57-9.
10. Rumack BH, Peterson RC, Koch GG. Acetaminophen overdose: 662 cases with evaluation of oral acetylcysteine treatment. Arch intern Med. 1981;141:380-5.
11. James O, Lesna M, Roberts SH. Liver damage after paracetamol overdosage: comparison of liver function tests, fasting serum bile acids and liver histology. Lancet. 1975;2:579-81.
12. Riper W, Piperno E, Mosher AH, *et al.* Pathophysiology of acute acetaminophen toxicity: Implication for management. Pediatrics. 1978;62:880-9.
13. Buckley NA, Whyte IM, O'Connell DL, *et al.* Activated charcoal reduces the need for N-acetylcysteine treatment after acetaminophen overdose. J Toxicol Clin Toxicol. 1998;37: 753-7.
14. Klein-Schwartz W, Oderda GM. Adsorption of oral antidotes for acetaminophen poisoning (methionine or N-acetylcysteine) by activated charcoal. Clin Toxicol. 1981;18:283-90.
15. Flanagan RJ, Meredith TJ. Use of N-acetylcysteine in clinical toxicology. Am J Med. 1991;91:131-9.
16. Jones AL. Mechanism of action and value of N-acetylcysteine in the treatment of early and late acetaminophen poisoning: A critical review. J Toxicol Clin Toxicol. 1998;36:277-85.
17. Smilkstein MJ, Knapp GL, Kuling KW, *et al.* Efficacy of oral N-acetylcysteine in the treatment of acetaminophen overdose. Analysis of national multicenter study (1976 to 1985). N Engl J Med. 1988;319:1557-62.
18. Buckley NA, Whyte IM, O' Connell DL, *et al.* Oral or intravenous N-acetylcysteine: which is the treatment of choice for acetaminophen (paracetamol) poisoning? J Toxicol Clin Toxicol. 1991;37:759-67.
19. Chamberlain JM, Gorman RL, Oderda GM, *et al.* Use of activated charcoal in a simulated poisoning with acetaminophen: A new loading dose for N-acetylcysteine? Ann Emerg Med. 1993;22:1398-402.
20. Yang R, Zou X, Koskinen ML, *et al.* Ethyl pyruvate reduces liver injury at early phase but impairs regeneration at late phase in acetaminophen overdose. Crit Care. 2012;16:R9.

63.2 IRON INTOXICATION

INTRODUCTION

Iron is an essential micronutrient but overdose after accidental ingestion is common and may lead to death in children.[1,2] The exact incidence of iron overdose in children and associated mortality in India is not known. Accidental iron poisoning in children is common because of the following:

- Iron preparations are freely available over-the-counter in developing countries and easily available in home.
- Lack of awareness that iron can be dangerous.
- Various chewable tablets of iron are often in attractive shape with fruit flavors and candies available in market.

PATHOPHYSIOLOGY

Iron is normally absorbed from duodenum and jejunum in ferrous form and gets oxidized into ferric form. In blood, it is transported with transferrin protein and utilized in synthesis of hemoglobin, myoglobin, catalase, cytochrome oxidase. It is stored in liver and bone marrow as ferritin or hemosiderin.

In acute overdose, iron is absorbed by a passive first order process.[3] Ascorbic acid, valine, histidine, succinate, pyruvic acid, and citric acid rich diet increases absorption of iron. Furthermore, iron toxicity is also influenced by serum copper, phosphorus and vitamin E levels, and associated diseases such as primary hemochromatosis, thalassemia, liver diseases that in turn enhance toxicity.

- Large amount of accidentally ingested iron gets deposited in liver and heart and causes cell damage. With acute iron poisoning, deposition of large amount of iron in liver results in free radical production, which causes lipid peroxidation and destruction of hepatic mitochondria, thus hepatotoxicity.[3,4] Various mechanisms of iron toxicity have been suggested: It exerts a direct corrosive effect on gastrointestinal tract leading to hemorrhagic necrosis and cause nausea, vomiting, diarrhea and abdominal pain. The ferrous form remains stable in acid pH and cause direct irritation of gastric mucosa whereas in duodenum, it gets converted into insoluble iron complexes causing further mucosal damage.
- Free iron crosses cellular membranes and inhibits electron transport system of mitochondria, thus favors anaerobic metabolism. Increased lactic acid production from anaerobic metabolism results in metabolic acidosis.[4]
- Reduction-oxidation reactions of excess iron may lead to excessive production of free radicals in the body, which cause damage to cells of various organs by peroxidation of lipids and proteins. The pulmonary damage manifests as ARDS, respiratory failure and acidosis.
  - $Fe^{++} + H_2O_2 \rightarrow Fe^{+++} + OH^- + OH^\cdot$

  Free iron causes damage to vascular endothelium, post-arteriolar dilatation and increased capillary permeability, which leads to venous pooling, decreased blood volume and reduced cardiac output.[3,4]
- Excess free iron leads to functional, reversible and concentration dependent impairment of coagulation within first few hours, probably because of susceptibility of serine proteases to non-transferrin bound ferric ion.[5]

Box 1: Pathological changes in iron poisoning

- Esophagus: Ulceration, edema, hemorrhage
- Stomach: *Early* – Ulceration, venous thrombosis, gastritis, necrosis, perforation; *Late* – Stricture/obstruction
- Liver: Swelling, hemorrhagic periportal necrosis, iron deposition in Kupffer or parenchymal cells
- Lung: Vascular congestion, edema, atelectasis
- Heart: Fatty degeneration of cardiac muscles
- Kidneys: Fatty degeneration of renal tubules
- Pancreas: Hemorrhagic necrosis.

Pathological Changes

Iron overdose exerts its primary effects on GI tract, liver and cardiovascular system (**Box 1**). The lowest reported lethal dose for children is 600 mg. However, iron ingestion less than 20 mg/kg body weight though considered subtoxic will rarely produce mild symptoms, 20–60 mg/kg body weight is considered potentially serious, and more than 60 mg/kg body weight, potentially lethal.

CLINICAL FEATURES

The clinical features of iron overdose are classically divided in five stages but may not be observed in all patients.[6]

Stage I (Gastrointestinal)

This usually appears 30–120 minutes after ingestion of iron. The clinical manifestations during this phase, i.e. nausea, vomiting, bloody diarrhea, abdominal pain and hematemesis are the result of local necrosis and hemorrhage at the site of contact. Sometimes pallor or cyanosis, lassitude, drowsiness, hyperventilation due to acidosis and severe hypotension or cardiovascular collapse may occur.

Stage II (Stage of Apparent Recovery)

It is a poorly defined stage during which child appears better. In this stage, iron accumulation continues in mitochondria and various organs. The careful observations reveal ongoing problems, which manifest as hyperventilation, oliguria, poor tissue perfusion, and vague gastrointestinal symptoms.

Stage III (Stage of Circulatory Failure)

Stage III is characterized by shock, which is usually multifactorial. Gastrointestinal fluid or blood loss, increased capillary permeability, postarteriolar and venous dilatation are the principal contributing factors.

Coexisting metabolic acidosis and coagulopathy further aggravate circulatory failure. Clinical features in this stage include tachycardia, pallor, hypotension, oliguria, altered sensorium and metabolic acidosis. Acute tubular necrosis, pulmonary hemorrhage and pancreatic necrosis may occur in severe cases.

Stage IV (Stage of Hepatic Necrosis)

It is usually seen 2–4 days after ingestion, is rarely encountered and is characterized by severe hepatic necrosis with elevation of AST, ALT, prothrombin time and serum bilirubin.

Stage V (Stage of Gastric Scarring)

This stage is usually seen 2–4 weeks after ingestion and patients present with features of gastric outlet or intestinal obstruction due to scarring from its corrosive effects. *Yersinia enterocolitica* sepsis is an infrequent complication.

Other clinical features include anorexia, diarrhea, hypothermia, shock, metabolic acidosis and death. As a result of iron storage disease, the liver becomes cirrhotic and incidence of hepatoma, primary cancer of liver increases several folds. Also, when siderosis becomes severe in young people, myocardial disease is a common cause of death. Impotence may occur in young male and amenorrhea may occur in adolescent girls. Both sexual related problems are due to iron loading in the anterior pituitary.[7]

MANAGEMENT

When a child presents with acute iron intoxication, the clinician is faced with two important management issues. Does the child warrant intervention? If yes, how exactly should she/he manage the patient? These issues are addressed in the algorithm shown in **Flowchart 1**. Every attempt must be made to calculate the elemental iron dose ingested.

Laboratory Investigation

Serum iron-total and free, and total iron binding capacity should be carried out to aid in the diagnosis and delivery of supportive care. Free serum iron is the best way to determine the potential for toxicity.

a. If free serum iron is less than 50 µg/dL – toxicity unlikely.
b. If free serum iron is 50 µg/dL or more – toxicity manifests.
c. Total serum iron 350 µg/dL or more – toxicity evident.

Flowchart 1: Algorithm for management of Iron overdose

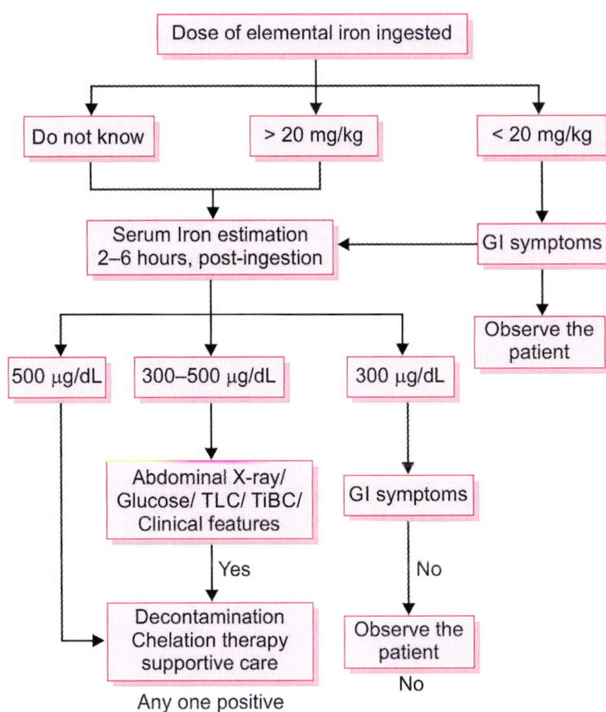

A hematocrit, total leukocyte counts, arterial blood gases and electrolytes, serum glucose and a plain X-ray of the abdomen comprise the minimal essential laboratory workup in iron poisoning. The presence of radiopaque shadow in radiograph, total leukocyte counts greater than 15,000/ mm^3, metabolic acidosis and increased anion gap in ABG and blood glucose more than 150 mg/dL warrants urgent interventions. Individual cases of severe poisoning may require monitoring of coagulation profile and serum calcium. Transaminase determinations are useful only after 24 hours to indicate possible hepatic damage.

Treatment

When a child presents in emergency with iron poisoning, the following measures should be promptly started after care of airway, breathing and circulation.

Decontamination

This should be done as rapidly as possible. In conscious patients, who has presented to emergency within 30 to 60 minutes and tablets are visible in abdominal radiograph, emesis may be induced with ipecac syrup. Gastric lavage with wide bore tube should be done in all cases irrespective of previous vomiting either spontaneous or induced. Following lavage, 100 mL of milk of magnesia[8] or 50–100 mL of 5% sodium bicarbonate solution may be left within the stomach.[9] They form complex iron to prevent further absorption and also decrease the corrosive effects on a denuded gastric mucosa.[8,9] Oral desferrioxamine should not be given as it enhances iron absorption from GI tract as observed in experimental animals.[6]

Whole bowel irrigation using polyethylene glycol solution should be used as an alternative to emesis, lavage and cathartics, particularly if large numbers of tablets are visible in abdominal radiograph beyond stomach.[10] Activated charcoal should not be administered as it does not adsorb iron. Following lavage, abdominal radiograph should be done to look for presence of remaining tablets.

In some children, bezoars of iron tablets in abdominal radiograph is an indication of surgical removal of the tablets (gastrotomy).[11] Endoscopy is sometimes useful to break-up clumps of tablets in the stomach.

Definitive therapy

The definitive therapy of iron poisoning is chelating agent desferrioxamine. Desferrioxamine binds with iron in plasma resulting in excretion of ferrioxamine complex via urine which is typically Vinrose (pink) in color.[6,10,12] At sub-cellular level, i.e. mitochondria, it chelates free iron.

Indications of chelation therapy:[12,13]

1. Clinical manifestation like lethargy, hypotonia, tachypnea and tachycardia.
2. If free serum iron more than 50 μg/dL or total serum iron more than 350 μg/dL.
3. Abdominal radiograph showing large mass of remaining tablets.
4. Total leukocyte count more than 15,000/mm^3.

Routes and dosage of desferrioxamine

For acute cases, continuous intravenous infusion is preferred while in less severe cases it can be given intramuscularly. The dose of desferrioxamine is 15 mg/kg/hour for intravenous infusion and 50 mg/kg (maximum 1 g per dose) given every 4 hours by intramuscular route. Total dose of desferrioxamine should not exceed 6.0 g IV or IM For practical purposes, it is useful to remember that 1 g of desferrioxamine chelates about 90 mg of elemental iron. It is available as white powder in injectable form (500 mg/vial). It is diluted by adding 5 mL of distilled water to produce 10% solution. It is further diluted with normal saline or 5% DNS and administered as a continuous infusion. The clinical improvement can be observed in 1–2 hours.

The effectiveness of chelation therapy is judged by passage of pink or port wine urine. The duration of continuous infusion remains a debatable issue. Pink or vinrose color urine indicates high iron load and treatment should be continued till urine is clear for 24 hours. Occasionally urine color may not change despite serum iron level of more than 500 μg/dL.[6,13] Therapy is continued till the urine color becomes normal or serum iron falls to less than 300 μg/dL. In severe poisoning, additional 12–24 hours chelation therapy is recommended.[14] Recently, urinary iron to creatinine ratio have been suggested as an objective criterion for cessation of desferrioxamine therapy.[15]

Adverse reactions include hypersensitivity reactions and anaphylaxis. In higher dose, hypotension may occur due to histamine release. Pulmonary edema and ARDS have been reported in patients receiving desferrioxamine infusion for more than 65 hours. Long-term use may cause optic neuritis, hearing loss and cataracts.[16]

Other oral chelating agents available are Deferiprone and Deferasirox. The dose of deferiprone is 25 mg/kg 8 hourly. It is more effective in reducing cardiac iron and has a half-life of 3 hours. Deferasirox has a half-life of 16 hours. The initial dose is 20 mg/kg with gradual escalation to 30 mg/kg once a day. Oral deferiprone is effective in acute iron overdose in rats and human being.[17]

Supportive therapy

Care of airway, breathing and circulation is important in patients with altered sensorium. Shock must be treated with IV fluid and ionotropic support with frequent monitoring of CVP as per standard hospital protocol. Blood transfusion may be required. Persistent acidosis should be corrected with sodium bicarbonate. Liver and renal failure should be managed as per hospital standard protocols. Dyselectrolytemia and hyperglycemia associated with stage III and IV should be managed appropriately. *Yersinia enterocolitica* or *Listeria monocytogenes* septicemia may occur either due to free iron induced mucosal damage or desferrioxamine induced growth.[18]

Other measures

Hemodialysis is only indicated in patients who developed acute kidney injury (removal of ferrioxamine).[19] Exchange transfusion along with desferrioxamine is indicated only in cases where serum iron levels exceeds 1000 μg/dL and there is no response to routine treatment. It may increase clearance of free irons to as much as 30-fold as compared to desferrioxamine alone.[6,20] Charcoal hemoperfusion is not useful as charcoal has poor affinity for iron. Experimental modalities of therapy include IV administration of liposomal encapsulated desferrioxamine.[21]and high molecular weight derivatives of desferrioxamine, i.e. desferrioxamine covalently attached to high molecular weight carbohydrates such as dextran and hydroxyethyl starch.[22]

PROGNOSIS

The prognosis of iron overdose is usually good with conservative treatment and chelation therapy but presence of shock and hypotension indicate poor prognosis. Untreated children with shock have almost 100% mortality compared to 10% among those receiving chelation.[4]

PREVENTION

Education of parents, restriction on over the counter prescription of iron, safe and child resistant packaging, unit-dose packaged product in original containers, storage of product beyond reach to children and conspicuous warning about dangers are important steps of prevention. Simultaneously, additional resources should be directed towards the identification, testing and marketing of improved antidotes.[1]

KEY MESSAGES

- Large amount of accidentally ingested iron gets deposited in liver and heart and causes cell damage.
- The lowest reported lethal dose for children is 600 mg. However, iron ingestion less than 20 mg/kg body weight though considered sub-toxic will rarely produce mild symptoms, 20–60 mg/kg body weight is considered potentially serious, and more than 60 mg/kg body weight, potentially lethal.
- Iron poisoning is characterized by 5 stages: gastrointestinal, apparent recovery, circulatory failure, hepatic necrosis, and gastric scarring.
- Treatment consists of decontamination and chelation with desferrioxamine.
- Untreated children with shock have almost 100% mortality compared to 10% among those receiving chelation.

REFERENCES

1. Litovitz T, Manoguerra AS. Comparison of pediatric poisoning hazards. An analysis of 3.8 million exposure incidents. Pediatrics. 1992;89:999-1106.
2. HHH News. U.S. Department of Health and Human services, Food and Drug Administration. Jan 15, 1997; p. 97-3.
3. Singh UK, Layland FC, Suman S, *et al.* Iron poisoning. In: Poisoning in Children, 2nd edition. New Delhi: Jaypee Publishers Ltd.; 2001. p. 40-6.
4. Eisen TF, Lacouture PG, Lovejoy FFH. Iron. In: Haddad LM, Winchester JF, editors. Clinical Management of Poisoning and Drug Overdose, 2nd edition. Philadelphia: WB Saunders Co.; 1990. p. 101-7.
5. Rosenmund, Haecberli A, Straub PW. Blood coagulation and acute iron toxicity, reversible iron-induced inactivation of serine protease in vitro. J Lab Clin Med. 1984;103:324-533.
6. Banner Jr W, Tong TG. Iron poisoning. Pediatr Clin North Am. 1986;33:393-409.
7. Riederer P, Youdim M. Iron in Central Nervous System Disorders. New York: Springer-Verlag. 1993.
8. Corby DG, Mc Cullen AH, Chadwick EW, *et al.* Effects of orally administered magnesium hydroxide in experimental iron intoxication. J Toxicol Clin Toxicol. 1986;23:489-99.
9. Bachrach L, Correa A, Levin R, *et al.* Iron poisoning: complications of hypertonic phosphate lavage therapy. J Pediatr. 1979;94:147-9.
10. Tenenbein M. Whole bowel irrigation in iron poisoning. J Pediatr. 1987;111:145-52.
11. Venturelli J, Kwee Y, Morris N, *et al.* Gastrotomy in the management of acute iron poisoning. J Pediatr. 1982;100:768-9.
12. Proud Foot A. Management of acute iron poisoning. Med Toxicol. 1986;1:83-100.
13. Klein Schwartz W, Oderda GM, Gorman RL, *et al.* Assessment of management guidelines in acute iron ingestion. Clin Pediatr. 1990;29:316-21.
14. Freeman DA, Manoguerra AS. Absence of urinary colour change in a severely iron-poisoned child treated with desferrioxamine. Vet Hum Toxicol. 1981;23:351.
15. Yatscoff RW, Wayne EA, Tenenbein M. An objective criterion for the cessation of desferrioxamine therapy in the acutely iron poisoned patient. J Toxicol Clin Toxicol. 1991;29:1-10.
16. Shannon M. Desferrioxamine in acute iron poisoning. Lancet. 1992;339:1601.
17. Berkovitch M, Livne A. Lushkov G, *et al.* The efficacy of oral deferiprone in acute iron poisoning. Am J Emerg Med. 200;18:36-40.
18. Melby K, S Slørdahl, T J Gutteberg, *et al.* Septicemia due to yersinia enterocolitica after oral overdose of iron. BMJ. 1982; 285:467-8.
19. Richardson JR, Sugerman DL, Hulet WH. Extraction of iron by chelation with desferrioxamine and hemodialysis. Clin Res. 1967; 15:368.
20. Movassaghi N, Purugganan GG, Leikin S. Comparison of exchange transfusion with desferrioxamine in treatment of acute iron poisoning. J Pediatr. 1969;75:604-8.
21. Tabak A, Hoffer E. Depletion of serum iron levels in rats by intravenous administration of liposome-encapsulated desferrioxamine. Acta Hematol. 1994;91:111-3.
22. Mahoney JR, Hallaway PE, Hedlund BE, *et al.* Acute iron poisoning: Rescue with macromolecular chelators. J Clin Invest. 1989;84:1362-6.

63.3 CYCLIC ANTIDEPRESSANTS

INTRODUCTION

Cyclic antidepressants are used in treatment of depressive disorders, in management of chronic pain syndromes, and in childhood nocturnal enuresis. Children account for approximately 20% of tricyclic intoxications either due to overdose of the drug prescribed or accidental ingestion of drugs at home. Amitryptiline and imipramine are the two most commonly prescribed and hence most commonly implicated in intoxications.[1]

PATHOPHYSIOLOGY

Tricyclic antidepressants are rapidly absorbed from gastrointestinal tract and undergo a major first pass metabolism in liver. They are highly lipid soluble and are rapidly distributed to body tissues such as myocardium.

Only a small amount of the absorbed drug remains in the blood, of which 85–95% is bound to plasma proteins. Extensive binding to tissues and plasma proteins explain the ineffectiveness of forced diuresis and dialysis techniques in the removal of these drugs. They are eliminated (expect amoxapine) mainly by hepatic metabolism and minimally by renal excretion. In the liver, they are metabolized by monodemethylation producing active metabolites, desipramine, and nortriptyline. Subsequently, following ring hydroxylation and demethylation, these metabolites undergo an enterohepatic circulation and a final stage of glucuronidation before being excreted by kidney. The elimination of amoxapine is primarily renal.

Cyclic antidepressants, particularly tricyclics are structurally similar to phenothiazines and have similar anticholinergic, adrenergic and alpha-blocking properties. They block neuronal reuptake of norepinephrine, serotonin or dopamine and cause drowsiness and impair concentration and thought process even in therapeutic doses. They also block H_1 receptor, which explains its sedative and antihistaminic properties. Peripheral anticholinergic effects include mydriasis, dry mucous membrane, tachycardia, urinary retention and decreased intestinal peristalsis while the central effects include confusion, agitation, hallucination, myoclonus, choreoathetosis and seizures. Trazodone inhibits the neuronal reuptake of serotonin and has anti-serotonergic and alpha-adrenergic blocking properties.[2] The average lethal dose is 30 mg/kg but as little as 8 mg/kg may be fatal.

CLINICAL MANIFESTATIONS

Wide ranges of clinical manifestations are seen in children intoxicated with cyclic antidepressants.[3,4] Initial manifestations, usually anticholinergic, include tachycardia, mydriasis and dryness of mucous membranes, urinary retention, hallucinations and flushing. Fever may occur as a drug effect but should raise the possibility of aspiration pneumonia particularly in comatose patient. Hypothermia may also occur occasionally.

The central nervous system toxicity is prominent feature of tricyclic toxicity and includes alteration in mental status, depression, lethargy and hallucination. Myoclonus and choreoathetosis occur variably. Seizures occur in up to 20% of patients typically in first 12 hours and may progress to status epilepticus. Seizures are more frequent with amoxapine and maprotiline overdosage. Coma may occur which rarely lasts for more than 48 hours, persistence beyond this period should suggest the ingestion of additional drugs or development of complications.

Common cardiovascular manifestations of cyclic antidepressant overdose and intoxication are arrhythmias-supraventricular tachycardia, premature atrial, and ventricular fibrillation. Various conduction disturbances such as right bundle branch block (RBBB) and left bundle branch block (LBBB), various degrees of A-V block including complete heart block are usually associated with seizures, coma, respiratory depression and arterial hypotension. Electrocardiographic changes include widening of QRS complex, prolongation of QT interval with flattening or inversion of T-wave, ST-segment depression and evidence of RBBB, LBBB and complete heart block.

A withdrawal syndrome occurs in neonates born to mothers who have been taking tricyclics. The features of withdrawal syndrome are tachypnea, irritability and restlessness, which may last for first month of life. Amoxapine causes a higher incidence of seizures and coma. Exposures to tetracyclics are associated with higher incidence of cardiovascular effects as compared to tricyclics. Bicyclics are like tetracyclics but it causes less cholinergic toxicity.

DIAGNOSIS

1. History of ingestion of antidepressant.
2. Suggestive clinical signs and symptoms.
3. Measurement of blood levels of the drug and arterial blood gases to detect acidosis and hypoxemia.
4. *Physostigmine test*: Administration of IV physostigmine in the obtunded or comatose patient causes arousal in patient with antidepressant intoxication. The sensitivity of the test is greater than 90%, the specificity however is not known. Adverse effects due to IV physostigmine are anticholinergic syndrome, seizures, bradyarrhythmias and asystole. This test in tricyclic overdoses is both reproducible and sensitive. The results of test appear to have minimal impact on management and no beneficial effect on outcome.[5]
5. Leukocytosis, increased transaminases and hyponatremia.

MANAGEMENT

Standard conservative life support measures should be employed in all patients. Emesis should be avoided in symptomatic children because of danger of aspiration. Emesis is only indicated in asymptomatic children. Gastric lavage should be done immediately after ingestion to remove the unabsorbed drugs from stomach. It is followed by administration of activated charcoal, 50–100 g in adolescents and 15–30 g in younger children. Activated charcoal 10–20 g may be given repeatedly every 2–6 hours in symptomatic children. A single dose of cathartic such as sorbitol, magnesium or sodium sulfate should be administrated. Unfortunately, no method exists to hasten the process of metabolism or excretion of tricyclics and tetracyclics. Forced diuresis, peritoneal dialysis, hemodialysis and charcoal hemoperfusion are usually ineffective because of large volume distribution.[6]

Sodium Bicarbonate Therapy

The aim of sodium bicarbonate therapy is to raise sodium concentration and arterial pH. It also shortens QT interval, narrows QRS complexes and increases myocardial contractility, thus often suppress ventricular arrhythmias and reverse hypotension. These can be achieved by administering 1–2 mEq/kg bolus infusion of sodium bicarbonate until arterial pH is ≥ 7.45 and is followed by continuous infusion as a solution of 150 mEq/L of 5% dextrose to maintain alkalosis.[7] Thus, it helps in correction of hyponatremia and reduces cardiotoxicity.

Respiratory depression: Intubation and mechanical ventilation are indicated in the presence of respiratory depression. Arterial blood gases should be monitored.

Choreoathetosis and myoclonus: They generally do not require treatment. Rarely myoclonus is so severe that it may produce rhabdomyolysis. Physostigmine is effective in controlling both the choreoathetosis and myoclonus but should be used only to prevent secondary complications. Physostigmine is given slowly as 0.5 mg test dose in children and may be repeated every 20 minutes (maximum dose: 20 mg). Atropine must be available to reverse any toxic effects of physostigmine.[5]

Seizure Management

A single seizure does not require specific treatment but repetitive or continuous seizure activity must be controlled rapidly to avoid secondary complication particularly systemic acidosis, with resultant increase in free drug and rhabdomyolysis. IV lorazepam or diazepam is the drug of choice and controls most of the seizures. The dose of lorazepam is 0.1 mg/kg to a maximum of 4 mg and diazepam is 0.1–0.3 mg/kg to a maximum of 10 mg in children. If seizures are not controlled with diazepam, phenytoin may be used an alternative but has disadvantage of long half life and the potential for causing hypotension, bradycardia and conduction defects. Barbiturates should not be used because they may further depress respiration and exacerbate hypotension.

Status epilepticus is usually refractory to conventional anticonvulsants (lorazepam, diazepam, phenytoin, barbiturates) as well as physostigmine.

Arrhythmia Management

The following is generally accepted modality for the treatment of arrhythmias. Sinus tachycardia generally requires no treatment. Sodium bicarbonate[7] is administered first to achieve a pH of 7.45–7.55. Phenytoin is given if electrocardiogram shows widened QRS (more than 0.12 seconds) and prolongation of QT interval. The dose of phenytoin is 15 mg/kg, IV up to a maximum of 1 g and the rate of administration should not exceed more than 0.5 mg/kg/min. In children with ventricular arrhythmias, the acidosis is corrected first with sodium bicarbonate or mechanical hyperventilation then lidocaine is administered at a loading dose of 1 mg/kg/dose and appropriate maintenance dose thereafter. Bretylium should not be used in hypotensive patients or in those with fixed cardiac output.[8,9] In adolescents, propranolol may be used in a dose of 1.0-mg IV every 2 to 5 minutes until a response is seen. In younger children, the dose of propranolol is 1 mg/kg IV up to a maximum of 1 mg. Physostigmine used only rarely, is administered in the dose of 0.5 mg IV over 2 to 3 minutes and repeated two to three times. Physostigmine and propranolol are most useful in supraventricular arrhythmias. Second or third degree A-V block, bradyarrhythmias should be treated with alkalization, isoproterenol and cardiac pacing, physostigmine and phenytoin being contraindicated in these setting. Antiarrhythmic drugs, which are contraindicated in arrhythmias induced by antidepressants, are quinidine, procainamide and disopyramide.[8,9]

Since antidepressants have high protein biding and large volume of distribution, plasmapheresis[10] and charcoal hemoperfusion[11] are reported to be effective modality in treatment of antidepressant overdose.

Hypertension and Hypotension

Hypertension is usually self-limited and requires no treatment. It usually responds to physostigmine. Hypotension should be initially managed with cautious crystalloid fluid administration and monitoring of central venous pressure. Alkalinization may also be effective. Hypotension sometimes responds to norepinephrine. Physostigmine may be effective and should be used if other measures fail. Severe hypotension may require intra-aortic balloon. Digitalis should be avoided.

All patients with antidepressant overdosage should be closely monitored for at least 24 hours or until their mental status has returned to baseline and conduction defects (excluding QTc prolongation) and arrhythmias are absent. Only completely asymptomatic children should be discharged after 6 hours.

KEY MESSAGES

- Amitriptyline and imipramine are the two most commonly prescribed and hence most commonly implicated in intoxications.
- Initial manifestations, usually anticholinergic, include tachycardia, mydriasis and dryness of mucous membranes, urinary retention, hallucinations and flushing.
- CNS toxicity is prominent feature of tricyclic toxicity and includes alteration in mental status, depression, lethargy and hallucination. Myoclonus and choreoathetosis occur variably. Seizures occur in up to 20% of patients.
- Common cardiovascular manifestations include supraventricular tachycardia, premature atrial, and ventricular fibrillation.
- Sodium bicarbonate therapy shortens QT interval, narrows QRS complexes and increases myocardial contractility, thus often suppress ventricular arrhythmias and reverse hypotension. These can be achieved by administering 1–2 mEq/kg bolus infusion of sodium bicarbonate until arterial pH is ≥7.45 and is followed by continuous infusion as a solution of 150 mEq/L of 5% dextrose to maintain alkalosis. Thus, it helps in correction of hyponatremia and reduces cardiotoxicity.

REFERENCES

1. Nelson JC, Spyker DA. Morbidity and mortality associated with medications used in the treatment of depression: An analysis of cases reported to U.S. Poison Control Centers, 2000-2014. Am J Psychiatry. 2017;174:438-50.
2. Crome P, Newman B. Fatal tricyclic antidepressant poisoning. J Roy Soc Med. 1979;72:649-53.
3. Clement A, Raney JJ, Wasserman GS, *et al.* Chronic amitriptyline overdose in a child. Clin Toxicol (Phila). 2012;50:431-4.
4. Olgun H, Yildirim ZK, Karacan M, *et al.* Clinical, electrocardiographic, and laboratory findings in children with amitriptyline intoxication. Pediatr Emerg Care. 2009;25:170-3.
5. Aquilonium SM, Hedstrand U. The use of physostigmine as an antidote in tricyclic antidepressant intoxication. Acta Anaesth Scand. 1978;22:40-5.
6. Miller J. Managing antidepression overdoses. Emerg Med Serv. 2004;33:113-9.
7. Bradberry SM, Thanacoody HK, Watt BE, *et al.* Management of the cardiovascular complications of tricyclic antidepressant poisoning: role of sodium bicarbonate. Toxicol Rev. 2005;24:195-204.
8. Foianini A, Joseph Wiegand T, Benowitz N. What is the role of lidocaine or phenytoin in tricyclic antidepressant-induced cardiotoxicity? Clin Toxicol. 2010;48:325-30.
9. Sarisoy O, Babaoglu K, Tugay S, *et al.* Efficacy of magnesium sulfate for treatment of ventricular tachycardia in amitriptyline intoxication. Pediatr Emerg Care. 2007;23:646-8.
10. Kolsal E, Tekin IO, Piskin E, *et al.* Treatment of severe amitriptyline intoxication with plasmapheresis. J Clin Apher. 2009;24:21-4.
11. Bek K, Ozkaya O, Mutlu B, *et al.* Charcoal haemoperfusion in amitriptyline poisoning: Experience in 20 children. Nephrology. 2008;13:193-7.

63.4 BARBITURATE INTOXICATION

INTRODUCTION

Barbiturates are used as hypnotic, sedative, anti-convulsant, and short-term anesthetic agents. Poisoning in children is usually accidental from over dosage. An uncommon type of accidental poisoning, "involuntary suicide" or "barbiturate automatism", occurs in children who are taking usual dose of barbiturate. The doses may be repeated several times in succession due to mental confusion produced by the drug ultimately resulting in fatal overdosage.[1] Easy availability of these drugs make it a common agent used for suicides. Based on duration of action, barbiturates are classified into four groups (**Table 1**).

PATHOPHYSIOLOGY

Barbiturates act on GABA-A receptors by increasing the opening time of chloride channel, and increase the affinity of receptor for GABA. Thus, it decreases the excitability of all cells of central nervous systems. Reticular formation of thalamus and midbrain are particularly affected. Large doses depress respiratory and vasomotor centers. The renal function may be impaired secondary to fall in blood pressure. Barbiturates stimulate the production of ADH by neurohypophysis and thus, prevent diuresis. The basal metabolism and intestinal motility are reduced.[1,2]

Table 1: Classification of barbiturates based on duration of action

Type	*Drugs*	*Half life*	*Fatal dose*
a. Long acting	Phenobarbitone Barbitone sodium Barbitone Methyl phenobarbitone	8–12 hrs	3–4 g
b. Intermediate acting	Allobarbitone Amylobarbitone Aprobarbitone Butobarbitone Pentobarbitone	4–8 hrs	2–3 g
c. Short acting	Cyclobarbitone Hexobarbitone Quinalbarbitone Quinal with amylobarbitone	2–4 hrs	1–2 g
d. Ultra-short acting	Pentothal sodium Hexabarbital sodium Kemittal sodium Thiamylal sodium	For anesthetic purpose	1 g

Barbiturates are rapidly absorbed from gastrointestinal tract and subcutaneous tissues. Then they are stored in liver for a short time and later evenly distributed in body fluids. In general, the long acting ones are excreted in urine while the short acting stable compounds are detoxified in the liver.[2]

Fatal period: Usually ranges from 1 day to 2 days.

CLINICAL FEATURES

The clinical features depend upon the amount and type of drug ingested and the time elapsed since ingestion. In general, larger doses of long acting preparations are required to produce the depth of unconsciousness comparable to that produced by short acting compound.[3,4]

Mild Poisoning

The patient is drowsy and can be readily aroused by shaking or calling name. There may be confusion, impairment of judgments, emotional liability, disorientation, slurred speech, nystagmus and ataxia. The reflex activity, blood pressure and respiration are not affected.

Moderate Poisoning

The patient is usually in coma and can be aroused only by vigorous stimuli. Reflexes, except corneal and pharyngeal ones, are depressed or absent. Respiration is shallow.

Severe Poisoning

The patient is in deep coma. Respiration is slow and shallow and may be Cheyne-Stokes type in character. Cyanosis and pulmonary edema may be present. There is marked hypotension due to direct action of barbiturates on cardiac and smooth muscles of blood vessels. In presence of severe anoxia, rigidity of limbs, exaggerated reflexes, ankle clonus and decerebrate rigidity are present. Involuntary movements in the form of tremor and spasm may occur. Pupils are contracted or even unequal. Skin lesions such as patches of erythema and blisters may occur. In 6–8% cases, bullous lesions occur on the pressure areas but are also found on the hand and feet. Fixed drug eruptions and exfoliative dermatitis may occur. There may be jaundice and hypothermia. Urine output could be severely reduced due to a number of factors such as hypotension, anoxia and toxic action of barbiturates on renal tubular cells.

The cause of death is usually respiratory failure. If recovery occurs, headache, dizziness somnolence, diplopia, ptosis, ataxia and hypotension may be present for several days.[4]

DIAGNOSIS

The diagnosis is based on history, clinical features and circumstantial evidences like presence of tablets or capsules in gastric contents. The poisoning resembles glutethimide intoxication except that pupils are fixed and child has conversion reactions.

Differential Diagnosis

The differential diagnosis should include intoxication by other substances with sedative effects, such as benzodiazepines, anticonvulsants (carbamazepine), alcohols (ethanol, ethylene glycol, methanol), opioids, carbon monoxide, and gamma-hydroxybutyric acid (GHB- a known date rape drug).

INVESTIGATIONS

1. *Serum barbiturate level*: If the serum level of long acting and intermediate acting barbiturates are more than 10 mg/dL and 33 mg/dL respectively they reflect a severe degree of intoxication.
2. *EEG*: The electroencephalogram provides useful evidence of poisoning.
   a. *Mild intoxication*: The normal activity is replaced by fast activity in the range of 20–30 Hz, which appears first in frontal regions and spreads to parietal and occipital regions as toxicity increases.
   b. *Severe intoxication*: The fast waves become less regular and are interspersed with 3 to 5 Hz slow wave activities.

In extreme overdosage, all electrical activity ceases and EEG records show a flat line. CBC, RFT, LFT and ABG should be done in all cases.

TREATMENT

Children with mild to moderate intoxication require no vigorous treatment. Emesis is contraindicated in children with altered sensorium. Gastric lavage should be done, if the drug has been ingested within 4–6 hours. The patient is then watched for signs of impending coma, the presence of which necessitates treatment for severe intoxication.

After gastric lavage, activated charcoal should be administered for adsorption of remaining drug in GI tract. The dose of activated charcoal is 1 g/kg/dose via nasogastric tube in infants; 1–2 g/kg/dose (25–50 g/dose) in children and 5–10 times the estimated weight of drug/chemical ingested in adolescents and may be repeated q4-6 hr. Multiple doses of charcoal may interrupt enterohepatic recirculation as intestinal mucosa serves as a dialysis membrane for reverse-absorption of drug from intestinal villous capillary blood back into the intestine.[2,5]

Elimination of Absorbed Drug

The aim is to decrease the duration of ventilatory support, combat hypotension, and decrease morbidity/mortality. Forced alkaline diuresis using sodium bicarbonate is very effective because of high water solubility and low hepatobiliary excretion of phenobarbiturates. The dose of sodium bicarbonate is 1 mEq/kg intravenously followed by a constant infusion to maintain a urine pH of greater than 7.5 and arterial pH of less than 7.50. The urine output should be 2 mL/kg/hr or more. Adverse effects are hypokalemia, hypocalcemia, fluid overload and metabolic alkalosis. Extracorporeal elimination is rarely recommended.[5]

Intravenous lipid emulsion (ILE) decreases serum drug concentration and thus toxicity. However, its role is limited in management of phenobarbiturate overload.

Severe Intoxication

Severe intoxication constitutes emergency. The aim of treatment is to maintain adequate perfusion and pulmonary gas exchange and prevent complications after care of airways, breathing and circulation. If ventilation is inadequate, mechanical ventilation should be started. Shock should be managed with intravenous crystalloid, plasma or whole blood. Norepinephrine infusion increases cardiac output and blood pressure; the dose of norepinephrine is 0.05–0.1 μg/kg/min infusion to a maximum of 1 μg/kg/min. Continuous monitoring of rectal temperature and urine output is mandatory.[6]

Hemodialysis and charcoal hemoperfusion are useful in removing the drug from circulation. If the child remains in coma for more than 24 hours, prophylactic antibiotics should be given to prevent secondary bacterial infections like hypostatic pneumonia.

On recovery, some children suffer a short period of psychosis. They may become hyperactive or agitated and sustain injuries from falls. Continued supervision by a nurse or an attendant is essential. Clonazepam may be used to control agitation.

KEY MESSAGES

- CNS symptoms are predominant. Severe poisoning causes coma. Cyanosis and pulmonary edema may be present.
- There is marked hypotension. Involuntary movements in the form of tremor and spasm may occur. Pupils are contracted.
- Serum level of long acting and intermediate acting barbiturates more than 10 mg/dL and 33 mg/dL, respectively reflect severe intoxication.
- Children with mild to moderate intoxication require no vigorous treatment. Emesis is contraindicated in children with altered sensorium.
- Forced alkaline diuresis using sodium bicarbonate is very effective because of high water solubility and low hepatobiliary excretion of phenobarbiturates.
- Hemodialysis and charcoal hemoperfusion are useful in removing the drug from circulation.

REFERENCES

1. Aronson JK. Barbiturates. In: Aronson JK, editor. Meyler's Side Effects of Drugs, 16th edition. Waltham, MA: Elsevier; 2016. p. 819-26.
2. Gussow L, Carlson A. Sedative hypnotics. In: Walls RM, Hockberger RS, Gausche-Hill M, editors. Rosen's Emergency Medicine: Concepts and Clinical Practice, 9th edition. Philadelphia, PA: Elsevier; 2018. p. 159.
3. Birnbaumer D. Poisonings and ingestions. In: Bongard ES, Sue Dy, editors. Current Critical Care Diagnosis and Treatment. London: Appleton and Lange; 1994. p. 686-715.
4. Henderson LW, Merrill JP. Treatment of barbiturate intoxication. Ann Intern Med. 1966;64:876.
5. Roberts DM, Buckley NA. Enhanced elimination in acute barbiturate poisoning—a systematic review. Clin Toxicol (Phila). 2011;49:2-12.
6. Ducluzeau R, Genty A. Severe acute intoxication by barbiturates, tranquilizers, tricyclics, paracetamol, salicylates. Diagnosis, treatment. Rev Prat. 2001;51:557-64.

63.5 BENZODIAZEPINES

INTRODUCTION

Benzodiazepines are used in the treatment of insomnia, anxiety, seizure disorders, and as muscle relaxants and preanesthetic medication. It is one of the common drugs of abuse. Benzodiazepine overdoses are commonly observed in emergency. The overdose is usually accidental in children but may be intentional in adolescents. Its co-ingestion with alcohol may cause profoundly depressed levels of consciousness.[1]

PATHOPHYSIOLOGY

Ingested benzodiazepines are rapidly absorbed from gastrointestinal tract. In the serum, more than 70% of the drug is protein bound. The free fraction crosses the blood-brain barrier and acts on benzodiazepine receptors and thereby, enhances activity of the inhibitory neurotransmitter GABA. The clinical effect is directly related to drug concentration in the central nervous system. The increased GABA release causes sleep and inhibition of excitement.[1]

CLINICAL FEATURES

The main effect of benzodiazepines is on the central nervous system and clinical features include depression, blurred vision, confusion, drowsiness, and unresponsiveness or coma. On examination, patients may have decreased respiratory rate, hypotension, slurred speech, ataxia, hallucination, altered sensorium, coma and decreased oxygen saturation. There is a risk of aspiration, respiratory failure, anoxic brain damage, rhabdomyolysis and death. It may cause A-V block.[2]

History of ingestion and suggestive clinical features should prompt suspicion. Benzodiazepines can be easily identified in routine urine toxicologic screens.

TREATMENT

Majority of children with benzodiazepine overdose improve with conservative management. The care of airways, breathing and circulation should be taken on priority. Such patients should be preferably be managed in ICU with frequent monitoring of vitals and SpO_2. Endotracheal intubation is indicated in patients with GCS score 8 or less, and those who cannot maintain airway and breathing on their own. Significant cardiovascular instability may warrant central venous access in order to provide medications, fluids, and invasive monitoring.

Activated charcoal is administered if patients reaches emergency within one hour of ingestion. The dose may repeated if patients has ingested sustained release preparations. Electrolyte abnormalities must be corrected judiciously. Dialysis is not useful because of its large volume of distribution and high protein binding.

Flumazenil, a competitive antagonist of the GABA receptor, is the specific antidote for benzodiazepine overdose. However, use of flumazenil is associated with significant adverse effects, such as seizures and benzodiazepine withdrawal syndrome. Flumazenil also decreases seizure threshold by blocking the binding of GABA receptor.[3,4] The dose of flumazenil is 0.002–0.02 mg/kg IV over 1 min and may be repeated if required. If there is no response after 5 minutes of receiving a total dose of 5 mg, the sedation is not due to benzodiazepines.[5]

KEY MESSAGES

- The main effect of benzodiazepines is on the central nervous system and clinical features include depression, blurred vision, confusion, drowsiness, and unresponsiveness or coma.
- Patients may have decreased respiratory rate, hypotension, slurred speech, ataxia, hallucination, altered sensorium, coma and decreased oxygen saturation.
- Majority of children with benzodiazepine overdose improve with conservative management.
- Flumazenil, a competitive antagonist of the GABA receptor, is the specific antidote for benzodiazepine overdose.
- The dose of flumazenil is 0.002–0.02 mg/kg IV over 1 min and may be repeated if required.

REFERENCES

1. Buckley NA, Dawson AH, Whyte IM. Relative toxicity of benzodiazepines in overdose. BMJ. 1995;310:219-21.
2. Arroyo Plasencia AM, Ballentine LM, Mowry JB, *et al.* Benzodiazepine-associated atrioventricular block. Am J Ther. 2012;19:e48-52.
3. Spivey WH, Roberts JR, Derlet RW. A clinical trial of escalating doses of flumazenil for reversal of suspected benzodiazepine overdose in the emergency department. Ann Emerg Med. 1993;22:1813-21.
4. Weinbroum AA, Flaishon R, Sorkine P, *et al.* A risk-benefit assessment of flumazenil in the management of benzodiazepine overdose. Drug Safe. 1997;17:181-96.
5. Kreshak AA, Tomaszewski CA, Clark RF, *et al.* Flumazenil administration in poisoned pediatric patients. Pediatr Emerg Care. 2012;28:448-50.

63.6 DIGITALIS

INTRODUCTION

The incidence and severity of digitalis toxicity have declined substantially in past three decades due to development of alternative drugs for treatment of supraventricular arrhythmias, increased understanding of digoxin pharmacokinetics and recognition of important interactions.

Digitalis poisoning occurs most frequently due to overdosage during chronic maintenance therapy, accidental ingestion and rarely due to ingestion of crude digitalis from the dried leaf of the Foxglove plant digitalis purpura.

PATHOPHYSIOLOGY

Digitalis acts by inhibiting the enzyme sodium-potassium ATPase, leading to increase intracellular Na^+ and Ca^{++} and decreased K^+. Digitalis is absorbed from GI tract and serum levels does not correspond to pharmacologic effects for up to 8 hours.[1]

Digoxin is 25–30% protein bound in plasma and has a large volume of distribution of 5 to 6 L/kg of body weight. It is localized in skeletal muscle, liver and heart. Elimination is primarily by the kidney (85%) in unchanged form and the remainder is metabolized by the liver. The half-life ranges between 36 and 45 hours. The mean therapeutic concentration ranges from 0.6 to 2.5 nmol (0.5–2.0 mg/mL).

CLINICAL FEATURES

The clinical features are divided into two categories, extra-cardiac and cardiac.[2]

Extracardiac: Anorexia, nausea, vomiting, abdominal pain, fatigue, malaise, dizziness, confusion, delirium, hallucinations, scotomata and altered color perception (yellow vision).

Cardiac: Cardiac manifestations include sinus arrhythmias, sinus bradycardia and variable type of A-V block. Supraventricular tachycardia, bigeminy, ventricular tachycardia and fibrillation may occur. The presence of supraventricular tachycardia and A-V block is highly suggestive of digitalis toxicity. Clinical toxicity occurs with serum digoxin levels greater than 3.8 to 6.4 nmol/L (3–5 ng/mL) and levels as high as 64 to 77 nmol/L have been observed.

INVESTIGATION

- ECG changes in children with overdose include depression of ST segment with inverse check mark configuration, flattening or inversion of T-wave, shortening of Q-T interval, extrasystoles, bigeminal rhythm either unifocal or multifocal, multifocal ventricular tachycardia, ventricular fibrillation, first degree heart block (common) second and third degree heart block.
- Serum digoxin level.

MANAGEMENT

Gastric lavage should be done if digoxin is ingested within one hour. Gastrointestinal decontamination should be done as soon as possible followed by administration of activated charcoal, which reduces absorption from GI tract and also enhance elimination. Emesis should be avoided as it stimulates vagus nerve and further worsen bradycardia.

Potassium, magnesium and calcium abnormalities should be corrected. Potassium is contraindicated, if higher degree of A-V block is present. Temporary cardiac pacing may be needed in second and third degree heart block in children with refractory hypotension that fails to respond to atropine and isoprenaline. Magnesium sulfate as well as phenytoin (1 mg/kg over 5 min to a maximum of 10 mg/kg IV) and lidocaine (1 mg bolus followed by 0.03 µg/kg/min) may be useful in treatment of ventricular arrhythmias induced by digitalis.

Digoxin-specific antibody fragments (Fab) prepared from IgG produced in sheep has been available commercially since 1986 (Digibind, Ovine). Antibody therapy is quite valuable because of risk of life with severe toxicity and limited clinical benefit from conventional treatment. The antibody fragments rapidly bind intravascular and interstitial digoxin. Their low molecular weight (50-KDa) permits rapid diffusion into interstitial space where binding of free digoxin sets up a concentration gradient leading to egress of tissue stores of the glycoside. An initial clinical response can usually be expected within 20–40 minutes and complete reversal of toxicity within about 4 hours. If the renal function is normal, the digoxin bound to Fab is excreted with a half-life of approx 16-hour.[3,4] Fab antibody fragments lack complement fixing activity. Allergic reactions have been reported in less than 1% of patient treated with Fab. The usual dose is 6–8 mg/kg intravenously with isotonic saline over 30–60 minutes as bolus. 40 mg of digoxin specific Fab can neutralize approximately 0.6 mg of digoxin.[3,4]

Forced diuresis, hemoperfusion and hemodialysis have very little role to play in the management of digitalis toxicity.

KEY MESSAGES

- Cardiac manifestations of digitalis toxicity include sinus arrhythmias, sinus bradycardia and variable type of A-V block. Supraventricular tachycardia, bigeminy, ventricular tachycardia and fibrillation may occur.
- Digoxin-specific antibody fragments (Fab) prepared from IgG produced in sheep rapidly bind intravascular and interstitial digoxin.
- An initial clinical response can usually be expected within 20–40 minutes and complete reversal of toxicity within about 4 hours.

REFERENCES

1. Mégarbane B, Aslani AA, Deye N, *et al.* Pharmacokinetic/pharmacodynamic modeling of cardiac toxicity in human acute overdoses: Utility and limitations. Expert Opin Drug Metab Toxicol. 2008;4:569-79.
2. Bara V. Digoxin overdose: Clinical features and management. Emerg Nurse. 2001;9:16-21.
3. Milani L, Bizzaro N, Sanson A. The monitoring of plasma digoxin levels during acute digitalis poisoning treated with Fab anti-digoxin fragments. G Ital Cardiol. 1992;22:97-101.
4. Woolf AD, Wenger TL, Smith TW, *et al.* Results of multicenter studies of digoxin-specific antibody fragments in managing digitalis intoxication in the pediatric population. Am J Emerg Med. 1991;9(2 Suppl 1):16-20.

63.7 SALICYLATE INTOXICATION

INTRODUCTION

Salicylate poisoning is one of the common forms of poisoning in children. It may result from overdosage in an already sick child, accidental ingestion or deliberate self-poisoning, and use of oil of wintergreen, salicylate powder, or ointment on broken skin. In neonates and infants, salicylate intoxication may occur inadvertently through placental transfer, breast milk or by application of teething gels to gums.

PATHOPHYSIOLOGY

The primary effects of salicylate intoxication includes direct stimulation of the central nervous system, the respiratory center, and uncoupling of oxidative phosphorylation.

There is inhibition of Krebs cycle enzymes, stimulation of gluconeogenesis, and increased tissue glycolysis. Lipid metabolism is stimulated while there is inhibition of amino acid metabolism and interference with hemostatic mechanism.[1]

The respiratory stimulation caused by salicylate intoxication is characterized by increase in both the depth and rate of respiration which results in increased exhalation of CO_2 and decreased pCO_2 leading to alkalosis and a compensatory increase in renal excretion of bicarbonate. Thus, early in the course, there is respiratory alkalosis followed by metabolic acidosis. Inhibition of Kreb cycle enzyme results in accumulation of pyruvic, lactic acids, amino acids and aminoaciduria. These changes results in metabolic acidosis. Children under 4 years may develop poisoning due to prolonged therapy; hence, initial phase of respiratory alkalosis is less prominent whereas metabolic acidosis is readily detected.[1,2]

Fluid and electrolyte imbalance is frequently associated with salicylate intoxication and results from increased metabolism and heat production leading to increase cutaneous insensible loss, organic aciduria accompanied by increased excretion of sodium, potassium and water, gastrointestinal loss due to emesis, increased pulmonary insensible loss due to increased respiratory rate. In severe intoxication, the child may lose 4–6 L/m^2 of fluid.

Table 1: Clinical manifestations of salicylate intoxication

Gastrointestinal	Nausea, vomiting, epigastric pain, hematemesis, melena due to irritation of gastric mucosa
Respiratory	Tachypnea and hyperpnea initially followed by acidotic breathing (direct stimulation of respiratory center)
CNS	Headache, vertigo, lethargy, drowsiness, excitement, talkativeness, mental confusion, convulsion and coma. The mental changes are termed as "salicylate Jag"
Cardiovascular	Tachycardia due to direct paralysis of vasomotor center
Vision and hearing	Tinnitus, deafness and blurring of vision
Renal	Oliguria or anuria
Fluid and electrolyte disturbances	Dehydration, hyper or hyponatremia are common due to profuse sweating, vomiting and over breathing
Coagulation system	Bleeding tendency due to decreased platelet aggregation and defective prothrombin synthesis

Normally, Vitamin K is converted to vitamin 2,3-epoxide and then reconverted to Vit-K, by reductase enzyme, which is inhibited competitively by warfarin and salicylate. Thus, results in deficiency of Vit-K1 dependent factors II, VIII, IX and X as Vit-K1 is essential for post-transational Y-carboxylation of glutamyl residues.

Fatal dose is 200 mg/kg body weight (less than 100 mg/kg body weight is usually safe). And fatal period is 1–3 hours of ingestion but the fatal period varies from a few minutes to several hours.

CLINICAL FEATURES

Young children are more severely affected. A mixed acid-base disturbance occurs with respiratory alkalosis followed by metabolic acidosis. It can affect all the systems of the body. The face is red and swollen. There is profuse sweating. The temperature is either subnormal or raised (due to increased metabolism). Paresthesia and muscle weakness may occur. The salient clinical manifestations are mentioned in **Table 1**. Complications include acute drug induced hepatitis, Reye syndrome, cerebral edema, acute renal failure. GI bleeding, severe cardiovascular collapse and respiratory failure.

LABORATORY INVESTIGATIONS

The blood salicylate level is one of the best indicator of severity of the intoxication (**Table 2**).[3]

Serial salicylate levels estimation at 4 to 6 hours interval should be done. There may be hypoglycemia, or hyperglycemia, hyponatremia or hypernatremia, hypokalemia, elevated pyruvate and lactate, acidemia, hypoprothrombinemia, abnormal liver and renal functions.

TREATMENT

The basic principles of poisoning management are applied with salicylate intoxication, which include stabilization of airway, restoration of circulation, removal of drug from the body and correction of acidosis and the related complications. Gastric emptying is done by using syrup of

Table 2: Blood salicylate levels in different severity of poisoning

Blood salicylate level (at 6 hours)	*Severity of poisoning*
<50 mg/dL	Mild
50–100 mg/dL	Moderate
>100 mg/dL	Severe

Table 3: Guidelines of fluid therapy in salicylate intoxication

	Rate of administration mL/kg/hour	*Duration*	*Na^+*	*K^+*	*Cl^-*	*HCO_3^-*	*Dextrose*
Initial hydration	10–15	1–2 hours	75	0	50	25	5–10%
Subsequent hydration	4–8	3–8 hours Until salicylate level therapeutic	*40	35	50	*20	5–10%
Maintenance	2–3	As per necessity	25	20	25	20	5%

** In refractory metabolic acidosis, these constituents should be increased by addition of 15 mEq/L $NaHCO_3$. If pH is <7.15, give an additional 1–2 mEq/kg $NaHCO_3$ every 1–2 hours. Usual fluid loss approximates 200–300 mL/kg. Suggested minimum urine flow 5–10 mL/kg/hour.*

ipecac as an emetic. If emesis is not successful, then gastric lavage is done and at the end of lavage, activated charcoal along with cathartic is left in the stomach.[4]

Since there is no specific antidote available for salicylates, supportive therapy plays a vital role in the management of salicylate intoxication. The primary objective is correction of metabolic imbalances and enhancement of drug elimination. Fluid therapy in a patient of salicylate intoxication is crucial, the guidelines of fluid therapy is given in **Table 3**. If the above solution is not available then 0.25% normal saline with appropriate addition of sodium bicarbonate can be used. Fluid administration must be monitored carefully to avoid pulmonary edema or fluid retention. Shock is treated with 5% albumin or plasma in a dose of 10 mL/kg. Since neuroglycopenia may occur even in the presence of normal blood glucose, glucose administration is essential.

For elimination of absorbed salicylates, forced alkaline diuresis should be done with sodium bicarbonate (1-2 mEq/kg) over 1-2 hours to maintain urinary pH 8.0 or more. This enhances urinary excretion and decreases serum level of salicylates. Unfortunately, this urine pH is very difficult to achieve with sodium bicarbonate unless it is combined with acetazolamide. Close monitoring of fluid and electrolyte status must be maintained during forced diuresis.[5]

Seizures should be controlled with phenobarbitone (5 mg/kg) or diazepam (0.2 mg/kg/dose). Hypocalcemic tetany is treated by 10% solution of calcium gluconate and prolonged prothrombin time by parenteral administration of Vitamin K. Naloxone should be given parenterally if there is history of associated opioid ingestion. If the patient develops respiratory failure, supportive ventilation may help.

Indications for Hemodialysis or Hemoperfusion

1. Clinical features:
   i. Renal failure
   ii. Persistent CNS manifestations
   iii. Non-cardiogenic pulmonary edema
   iv. Progressive deterioration of patient.
2. Unresponsive acidosis (pH<7.1).
3. *Blood salicylate level*: Initial level 90 mg/dL and 100 mg at 6 hours after ingestion.

Hemodialysis is preferred over hemoperfusion or peritoneal dialysis, if facilities are available.

The unfavorable prognostic indicators of salicylate intoxication are prolonged seizures, severe respiratory acidosis, hypoglycemia and life-threatening bleeding.[6]

KEY MESSAGES

- Young children are more severely affected. A mixed acid-base disturbance occurs with respiratory alkalosis followed by metabolic acidosis.
- The blood salicylate level is one of the best indicator of severity of the intoxication.
- The basic principles of management of salicylate intoxication include stabilization of airway, restoration of circulation, removal of drug from the body and correction of acidosis and the related complications.
- Hemodialysis/hemoperfusion is indicated in severe manifestations, unresponsive acidosis and blood salicylate level >100 mg at 6 h after ingestion.

REFERENCES

1. Temple AR. Acute and chronic effects of aspirin toxicity and treatment. Arch Int Med. 1981;141:364-69.
2. Anderson RJ, Potts DE, Gabow PA, *et al.* Unrecognized adult salicylate intoxication. Ann Intern Med. 1976;85:745.
3. Done AK. Salicylate intoxication. Significance of measurements of salicylate in blood in cases of acute ingestion. Pediatr. 1960;26:800-07.
4. Done AK, Temple AR. Treatment of salicylate poisoning. Med Treat. 1971;8:528-51.
5. Lawson AA, Proudfoot AT, Brown SS, *et al.* Forced diuresis in the treatment of acute salicylate poisoning in adults. QJ Med. 1969;38:31-48.
6. Shively RM, Hoffman RS, Manini AF. Acute salicylate poisoning: risk factors for severe outcome. Clin Toxicol (Phila). 2017;55:175-80.

CHAPTER

64

Insecticide and Pesticide Poisonings

Amit Kumar Satapathy, Joseph John

INTRODUCTION

Any substance used to control pests including insecticides, herbicides, rodenticides and fungicides are called pesticides. These are chemicals which are mostly used in agriculture for improving productivity. The primary route of human exposure is through ingestion—intentionally (suicidal) or unintentionally (accidental) or by the ingestion of its residue in our diet. Exposure of children to these pesticides can be in the following settings:

- *Non-agricultural*: Pesticides are also used at home or in the workplace for control of pests, which creates additional exposure routes through inhalation, dermal absorption and ingestion, particularly if food is handled after touching surfaces contaminated with pesticides.
- *Agricultural*: This is seen amongst agricultural workers and their families in the fields/plantations, more so in developing countries where child labour in not uncommon.

Pesticides have been used extensively over last century to increase agricultural production and for preservation of crops. It is used both in the public and private domain. Though the benefit of pesticide use is significant but its overuse and misuse can lead to toxicity too. Morbidity and mortality secondary to intentional or accidental exposure/ingestion is reported worldwide and across all age groups. The incidence of pesticide poisoning is high in developing countries as it is used widely, more so in rural areas in view of dependency on agriculture as a means of livelihood. According to the WHO around 30% people are estimated to have pesticidal poisoning annually and more than 90% of these belong to developing countries.[1] This data is probably under estimated as a majority of cases are not reported.

Children are more vulnerable to pesticide poisoning in view of developmental and physiological factors. Children having frequent hand mouth activity, predisposes them to more accidental ingestion than adults. The exploratory behavior of children, playing on the ground and putting objects into their mouth, increases their risk of dermal, inhalation and oral exposure to residues on surfaces or in the air as it settles.[2,3] Exposure is more likely unintentional in those less than 6 years of age and intentional in older children. A list of various categories of pesticides that children are exposed is mentioned in the **Table 1**.[4]

Organophosphates (OP) and carbamates were introduced as "safer" alternatives as compared to organochlorines due to its early "decay and disappearance" from the environment. The pyrethroids are an additional class of non-persistent insecticide chemicals that interfere with sodium channels; these are often a component of residential pest (insect) control products. Newer insecticides include the neonicotinoids and the ryanoids which have more to be learnt about their action.

SOURCE OF EXPOSURE

Food remains the most important source of pesticide poisoning as demonstrated in few studies, where consuming organic food has led to decrease in urinary excretion of metabolites of pesticides.[5]

Table 1: Categories of pesticides and major classes[4]

Categories	*Major classes*	*Examples*
Insecticide	Organophosphates Carbamates Pyrethroids/Pyrethrin Organochlorines Neonicotinoids N-Phenylpyrazoles	Malathion, Methyl parathion, acephate Aldicarb, Carbaryl, Methomyl, Propoxur Cypermethrin, Fenvalerate, Permethrin Lindane Imidacloprid Fipronil
Herbicide	Phosphonates Chlorophenoxy herbicide Dipyridyl herbicide Nonselective	Glyphosate 2,4-D, Mecoprop Diquat, Paraquat Sodium chlorate
Rodenticide	Anticoagulants Convulsants Metabolic poison Inorganic compounds	Warfarin, Brodifacoum Strychnine Sodium fluroacetate Aluminium phosphide
Fungicide	Thiocarbamates Triazoles Strobilurins	Metam-sodium Fluconazole, Myclobutanil, Triadimefon Pyraclostrobin, Picoxystrobin
Fumigants	Halogenated organic Organic Inorganic	Methyl bromide, Chloropicrin Carbon disulfide, Hydrogen cyanide, Naphthalene phosphine
Miscellaneous	Arsenicals Pyridine	Lead arsenate, chromated Copper Arsenate, Arsenic Trioxide 4 - aminopyridine

Proximity of pesticide treated agricultural areas or contact with household members working with pesticides are the other source of exposure in children either through ingestion or transdermal route. While playing, children may be exposed to insecticides and rodenticides in the household due to its unsafe storage. This risk of contact with pesticides is high in developing countries, especially in rural areas.[6] Child labor, those engaged in agricultural fields are the other major reason of exposure of children with these poisons.

CLINICAL MANIFESTATIONS

The clinical manifestation of pesticide poisoning varies with the amount/dose/type of agent and duration of exposure. It can be an acute poisoning with immediate symptoms or a chronic poisoning due to exposure to a low dose or not a very potent agent over a long period of time. Describing the clinical features and management of each type of pesticide is beyond the scope of this chapter, but we are including a few of the common pesticides that are encountered in the Indian scenario. As per the data published in the various studies from India, the common pesticide poisonings seen are mentioned in **Table 2.**[7,8]

Table 2: Common pesticide poisonings in India

Type of poison	*AIIMS, New Delhi[7]*
Household	
• Rodenticide	17.1%
• Pyrethrin	26.2%
• Organophosphate	6.3%
• Carbamate	4.9%
• Others	4.9%
Agriculture	
• Organophosphate	9.0%
• Aluminum phosphide	9.3%
• Organochlorine	9.3%
• Carbamate	0.2%
• Pyrethrin	3.9%
• Herbicide	3.2%
• Others	1.7%
	South India[8]
• Organophosphorus	60.6%
• Organochlorine	20.7%
• Pyrethrin	5.7%
• Others	9.9%

Organophosphates, pyrethrin and pyrethroid poisoning followed by organochlorine are amongst the most commonly seen poisonings in children in India.

ORGANOPHOSPHATE AND CARBAMATE POISONING

Approximately 3 million people are exposed to OP or carbamates worldwide each year with about a 10% fatality. OP and carbamate are commonly used pesticides in household and agriculture fields worldwide. The incidence of poisoning due to both the pesticides is high as per the study published by the National Poison Cell, AIIMS, New Delhi.[7] The commonly used products are parathion and chlorpyrifos. The other chemical compositions available in Indian market are methyl parathion, malathion, acephate, etc. An OP variant like malathion has a lower acute toxicity as compared to others and is even used as a medication for treatment of lice too. On the other hand there are highly potent OP variants like tabun, sarin, soman which were developed for use in the event of a war. Inhalational, ingestion and cutaneous exposure are the predominant sources of exposure in adults. In children, accidental ingestion and cutaneous exposure through parents remain to be commonest source of exposure. Though OP and carbamates are structurally distinct, their clinical manifestations and management follow similar lines.

Clinical Features

Organophosphate and carbamates act by binding with acetylcholinesterase enzyme which is responsible for metabolism of acetylcholine, making it non-functional. Inhibition of the enzyme leads to accumulation of acetylcholine at synapses, neuromuscular junction and other end organs causing continuous stimulation. OP usually binds irreversibly with acetylcholinesterase whereas the carbamate binding is reversible. Hence, symptoms due to exposure to similar doses of acute OP poisoning are more severe and catastrophic than carbamate poisoning.

The clinical features in acute poisoning are due to a cholinergic crisis primarily involving the neuromuscular junction, autonomic nervous system and central nervous system. The muscarinic and nicotinic signs are what are manifest. The muscarinic signs can be remembered by using the DUMBBBELS mnemonic—**D**efecation, **U**rination, **M**iosis, **B**ronchorrhea, **B**ronchospasm, **B**radycardia, **E**mesis, **L**acrimation, **S**alivation. The nicotinic effects are fasciculations, muscular weakness and paralysis. Diaphoresis is due to stimulation of post-ganglionic muscarinic receptors. Though bradycardia is a common cardiovascular manifestation, but tachycardia too may be observed in the initial phase due to nicotinic receptor stimulation. Rarely cardiac arrhythmias, heart block, prolonged QTc interval may be seen and myocardial ischemia too has been reported. There can be muscle weakness and respiratory involvement too. The serious CNS signs like lethargy, seizures, central respiratory depression, stupor and coma are due to nicotinic and muscarinic receptor stimulation and are not uncommon in children.[9-11]

Evaluation

The diagnosis is based on clinical grounds with history of exposure and suggestive clinical features. Laboratory confirmation or severity assessment can be done by measuring the red blood cell acetylcholinesterase and plasma acetylcholinesterase levels which are reduced both in OP and carbamate poisoning. Red blood cell cholinesterase levels though are more specific for acute poisoning than its plasma levels. Most hospitals though do not have access to both these tests, reiterating the importance of a clinical diagnosis. If available, these tests can guide the effectiveness of oxime therapy in the management of the patient. Measuring the ingredients of the poison in plasma is not recommended as it undergoes metabolism rapidly in the liver.

Management

The ABCD approach is followed here. Early control of **A**irway and **B**reathing is usually required in this condition. This is due to either

- Depressed mentation, or
- Evolving respiratory failure due to central respiratory depression and nicotinic receptor stimulation induced diaphragmatic weakness, and
- Airway flooding due to excessive secretions.

Circulation—bradycardia and hypotension are more commonly seen as compared to tachycardia and hypertension which are rare manifestations due to sympathetic nervous system overstimulation. Skin **D**econtamination is an important and mandatory part of therapy to decrease the continuing exposure to the poison. For this the child's clothes are removed and fresh clothes used.[12] Gastric decontamination remains controversial. The American Academy of Clinical Toxicology and the

European Association of Poisons Centres recommends use of activated charcoal within the first hour of acute poisoning and its use beyond that is ineffective. Gastric decontamination with activated charcoal at 1 g/kg up to a maximum of 50 grams is used **BUT** is contraindicated if airway is not protected. Similarly, induced vomiting is contraindicated. Seizure should be treated with antiepileptics if needed.

Atropine can be used as a non-specific antidote in both OP and carbamate poisoning. It is helpful in recovery of the muscarinic effect but ineffective for the CNS symptoms. It is given at a dose 0.05 to 0.1 mg/kg per dose and can be repeated every 3–5 mins interval and with doubling of the dose till respiratory secretions and bronchoconstriction are controlled.[13]

Though atropine decreases the symptoms, there is need for a cholinesterase reactivating agent. Pralidoxime (2-PAM) and similar other oximes help in the same. This helps in taking care of both nicotinic and muscarinic symptoms. A word of caution though needs to be mentioned here that Pralidoxime should be administered following atropine as there may be a transient worsening of symptoms due to Oxime induced acetyl cholinesterase inhibition.

Pralidoxime is the specific antidote to reverse acetylcholinesterase inhibitor complex. It is usually used in cases with OP poisoning as the inhibition of enzyme complex is irreversible unlike carbamate poisoning where inhibition is reversible. A loading dose of 25–30 mg/kg of pralidoxime over 30 minutes followed by repetitive administration or a continuous infusion of >8 mg/kg/hr (usual dose 10–20 mg/kg/hr) is administered until muscle weakness and fasciculations resolve.[14]

There are two conditions that need to be mentioned here.

Intermediate syndrome: is a neurologic syndrome seen after 24 hrs to 96 hrs of exposure to OP. It is characterized by weakness of the flexors of the neck and proximal muscles, respiratory failure, depressed DTR's and cranial nerve abnormalities. This is seen mostly following OP poisoning and rarely, following carbamate poisoning. With good supportive care most patients recover completely.[15]

OPIDN – **O**rganophosphorus **I**nduced **D**elayed **N**europathy – This occurs 1 to 3 weeks after exposure to the OP agent. Carbamates are rarely associated with this condition. Patients complain of the transient painful glove stocking paresthesia with symmetrical motor polyneuropathy leading to a flaccid paralysis of both lower limbs to begin with and ascends to involve the upper limbs also. There is usually no sensory involvement.[15]

Prognosis

The outcomes depend on the dose, route, type of OP, time from exposure to initiation of therapy, complications and quality of care received which would decide the outcome. There is some preliminary data that suggests that a Glasgow Coma Scale of less than 13 may predict poorer outcomes.

PYRETHRIN AND PYRETHROID INSECTICIDES

Pyrethrin and pyrethroids are usually used as insecticides for pest control measure in urban areas and agricultural fields. Pyrethrin is a plant extract which rapidly degrades whereas pyrethroids are the synthetic derivative of pyrethrin which are more stable and long lasting. Pyrethrin and pyrethroids act by inhibiting the sodium channels at cell membrane causing hyperpolarization, resulting in prolonged excitation. Thus, the clinical features are predominant secondary to excessive neuronal excitation. Nausea, vomiting, headache, paresthesia, dizziness and anorexia are the initial manifestation of acute toxicity whereas CNS depression, blurred vision, excessive salivation, seizure, lethargy, coma, respiratory failure is seen in severe toxicity. Many of the clinical features mimics OP poisoning due to the chemical ingredient of pyrethroids which contain cholinesterase.[16,17]

Management

Pyrethrin and pyrethroid poisoning are diagnosed by clinical features and history of exposure. Unlike OP and carbamate poisoning, there is no specific laboratory test to diagnose acute intoxication.

Management of pyrethroid poisoning is mostly supportive. There is no specific antidote for it. Paresthesia usually resolve by 24 hrs. Vitamin E, oils and creams have shown some benefit in resolving cutaneous paresthesia. Gastrointestinal decontamination, respiratory failure and seizure should be managed. Though many of the features resemble OP toxicity, atropine should be used judiciously in pyrethroid poisoning unlike OP. Hence, it is imperative to distinguish pyrethroid poisoning from OP toxicity.

ORGANOCHLORINE POISONING

The organochlorines were one of the first insecticides synthesized and included compounds like dichlorodiphenyltrichloroethane (DDT), chlordane, methoxychlor, lindane, hexachlorocyclohexane and dieldrin. Due to low cost and easy availability, organochlorine pesticides are widely used. India now is the only country in the world where these are still being manufactured. DDT was used widely in many countries in its fight against malaria for achieving good vector control. Though its use has been banned in most countries now, unfortunately, its exposure continues as these chemicals persist in the environment for very long periods. There is little that individuals can do to alter their own exposure. The toxicity is due to inhibition of sodium and calcium channels in neuronal cell membrane. The clinical features include paresthesia, ataxia, tremor, hyperreflexia, altered mental status and seizures. The treatment of organochlorine toxicity is mostly supportive. Gastric and skin decontamination should be done immediately. No specific antidote is available for organochlorine poisoning.[18]

ALUMINUM PHOSPHIDE POISONING

Aluminium phosphide (ALP) is a cheap and highly effective pesticide used in agricultural fields in most parts of India as it is free from toxic residue and does not affect seed viability. Accidental ingestion is the common source of exposure in pediatric age group. ALP liberates phosphine gas, when it comes in contact with gastric hydrochloric acid or the moisture in the air causing widespread cellular hypoxia by inhibiting the mitochondrial cytochrome oxidase C and generating oxygen free radicals. The symptoms start almost instantaneously and involve almost all systems primarily the cardiovascular system leading to palpitation, a thready pulse, tachycardia and marked hypotension with signs of cardiac failure and ECG changes of ischemia. This does not mean that the other systems are spared. The gastrointestinal symptoms include vomiting, abdominal pain, loose stools. Drowsiness, delirium and coma are the typical CNS manifestations seen in severe cases of ALP poisoning. Dyspnea, cyanosis and pulmonary edema followed by respiratory failure are the respiratory complications.

Management

Diagnosis

Diagnosis of ALP poisoning is based on history and clinical features as mentioned above. The smell of the breath in ALP toxicity has a characteristic garlic odor. Phosphine positivity on silver nitrate impregnated paper on gastric aspirate or a breath sample helps in confirming the diagnosis of ALP poisoning. Gas chromatography is the most sensitive and specific test used for detecting phosphine in postmortem samples.

Treatment

Prompt and adequate cardiovascular support is important and core in the management to attain adequate tissue perfusion, oxygenation and physiologic metabolic milieu compatible with life until the tissue poison levels are reduced and spontaneous circulation is restored. In most of the studies, poor prognostic factors were presence of acidosis and shock. The overall outcome improved in the last decade due to better and advanced intensive care management.

Management should be initiated as soon as diagnosis of ALP poisoning is considered based on history and clinical features. There is no known specific antidote, hence the management remains primarily supportive. Early arrival to the emergency department, establishing the diagnosis, early resuscitation, decreasing the continuing exposure to the ALP by decontamination of skin and eye must be carried out immediately as phosphine is absorbed through skin. Gastric lavage with potassium permanganate (1:10,000), or coconut oil, followed by activated charcoal is recommended. Intensive monitoring and supportive therapy may result in good outcome. Antacids and proton pump inhibitors are used to relieve gastric symptoms. The most important step of successful treatment is management of shock by fluid resuscitation and judicious use of inotropes. Endotracheal intubation and need for mechanical ventilation depends on the severity of respiratory involvement. Intravenous sodium bicarbonate is used to correct mild to moderate metabolic acidosis whereas presence of severe metabolic acidosis and renal failure are indication for hemodialysis in ALP poisoning. Intravenous magnesium sulfate injection has beneficial effect in acute ALP poisoning reducing mortality and hence, is being used routinely.[19]

KEY MESSAGES

- Accidental (unintentional) exposure is most common mode of exposure in children with poisoning.
- Detailed history and clinical evaluation are key to diagnosis. Investigations has limited role except for a few poisonings like OP poisoning.
- Organophosphate and carbamate poisonings are commonly seen in rural India as they are used widely in agricultural fields.
- Gastric lavage and skin decontamination are essential wherever indicated.
- The clinical features of OP poisoning are due to cholinergic crisis which presents as: **D**efecation, **U**rination, **M**iosis, **B**ronchorrhea, **B**ronchospasm, **B**radycardia, **E**mesis, **L**acrimation, **S**alivation (**DUMBBBELS**)
- Pralidoxime is used as specific antidote in cases with OP poisoning while Atropine can be used as a non-specific antidote in both OP and Carbamate poisoning.
- Management is mostly supportive in most of the acute poisoning except for OP/Carbamate poisoning.

REFERENCES

1. World Health Organization (WHO). Principles for Evaluating Health Risks in Children Associated with Exposure to Chemicals. Geneva: Switzerland; 2006.
2. Freeman NCG, Hore P, Black K, *et al*. Contributions of children's activities to pesticide hand loadings following residential pesticide application. J Expo Anal Environ Epidemiol. 2005; 15: 81-8.
3. Freeman NC, Jimenez M, Reed KJ, *et al*. Quantitative analysis of children's microactivity patterns: The Minnesota Children's Pesticide Exposure Study. J Expo Anal Environ Epidemiol. 2001;11:501-9.
4. Council on Environmental Health. Pesticide Exposure in Children. Pediatrics. 2012;130:e1757-e63.
5. Riederer AM, Bartell SM, Barr DB, *et al*. Diet and nondiet predictors of urinary 3-phenoxybenzoic acid in NHANES 1999–2002. Environ Health Perspect. 2008;116:1015-22.
6. Gunnell D, Eddleston M. Suicide by intentional ingestion of pesticides: A continuing tragedy in developing countries. Int J Epidemiol. 2003;32:902-9.
7. Peshin SS, Srivastava A, Halder A, *et al*. Pesticide poisoning trend analysis of 13 years: A retrospective study based on telephone calls at National Poison Information Centre at All India Institute of Medical sciences, New Delhi. J Forensic Leg Med. 2014;22:57-61.
8. Ram P, Kanchan T, Unnikrishnan B. Pattern of acute poisonings in children below 15 years - a study from Mangalore, South India. J Forensic Legal Med. 2014;25:26-9.
9. Lifshitz M, Shahak E, Sofer S. Carbamate and organophosphate poisoning in young children. Pediatr Emerg Care. 1999;15: 102-03.
10. Zwiener RJ, Ginsburg CM. Organophosphate and carbamate poisoning in infants and children. Pediatrics. 1988;81:121-6.
11. Sofer S, Tal A, Shahak E. Carbamate and organophosphate poisoning in early childhood. Pediatr Emerg Care. 1989;5: 222-25.
12. Geller RJ, Singleton KL, Tarantino ML, *et al*. Centers for Disease Control and Prevention (CDC). Nosocomial poisoning associated with emergency department treatment of organophosphate toxicity - Georgia, 2000. MMRW Morb Mortal Wkly Rep. 2001;49:1156-8.
13. Reigart JR, Roberts JR. Recognition and Management of Pesticide Poisoning, 6th edition. Washington, DC: U.S. Environmental Protection Agency (EPA); 2013. p. 41-55.
14. Schexnayder S, James LP, Kearns GL, *et al*. The pharmacokinetics of continuous infusion pralidoxime in children with organophosphate poisoning. J Toxicol Clin Toxicol. 1998;36: 549-55.
15. Sidell FR. Clinical effects of organophosphorus cholinesterase inhibitors. J Appl Toxicol. 1994;14:111-3.
16. Ray DE, Forshaw PJ. Pyrethroid insecticides: Poisoning syndromes, synergies, and therapy. J Toxicol Clin Toxicol. 2000; 38:95-101.
17. Ray DE, Fry JR. A reassessment of the neurotoxicity of pyrethroid insecticides. Pharmacol Ther. 2006;111:174-93.
18. Jayaraj R, Megha P, Sreedev P. Organochlorine pesticides, their toxic effects on living organisms and their fate in the environment. Interdiscip Toxicol. 2016;9:90-100.
19. Bajpai SR. Aluminum phosphide poisoning: management and prevention. J Indian Acad Forensic Med. 2010;32:352-4.

CHAPTER

65

Hydrocarbon Poisoning

Indumathy Santhanam, Sharada Sathish Kumar

INTRODUCTION

Hydrocarbon (HC) ingestions account for approximately 5% of all accidental poisonings and 25% of all fatal ingestions in the under-five age group.[1] Emergency department visits due to hydrocarbon exposure occur in four ways. In children less than 5 years, ingestion is accidental. The latter causes aspiration induced pulmonary toxicity. This mode of presentation is the commonest. Substance abuse due to recreational inhalation by adolescents, accidental inhalation or dermal exposure in rural settings is other less common modes of presentation. Massive oral ingestion of HCs due to a suicide attempt has also been reported.[2]

Since hydrocarbon solvents are often volatile, exposure by inhalation is a common hazard. Inhalational exposure can occur in gasoline stations, while painting a room or while applying or removing fingernail polish. The inherent solubility of hydrocarbons in lipids predisposes to dermal absorption when skin is exposed.

A recent study from south India reported that amongst non-drug related poisoning in children, hydrocarbon poisoning accounted for approximately 50% of cases.[3] HC poisoning is a major public health concern in rural areas due to the easy accessibility to kerosene. The latter is the most important fuel used for cooking or lighting lamps. Its accidental ingestion can often lead to pulmonary aspiration and acute respiratory distress syndrome (ARDS), leading to death. More recently, substance abuse by inhalation has also been resulted in similar complications.

ETIOLOGY

The commonly encountered HC are a mixture of compounds, obtained by distilling petroleum products. These products are used for multiple common household products such as paints, thinners, furniture polish, lamp oils, and lubricants.

PATHOPHYSIOLOGY

A hydrocarbon is an organic compound made up primarily of carbon and hydrogen atoms, typically ranging from 1 to 60 carbon atoms in length. The two basic types of hydrocarbon molecules, aliphatic (straight or branched chains) and cyclic (closed ring), have their own subclasses.

Most commonly available hydrocarbons exist as solvents. They are composed of a mixture of hydrocarbons emanating from a common petroleum distillation fraction. Belonging to a class of chemicals known as xenobiotics, they are used to dissolve and provide a vehicle for delivery of other xenobiotics. Examples of commonly used solvents are: Limonene (lemon oil), menthol (mint oil), pinene (turpentine) and camphor.

Hydrocarbons are variably absorbed into human systems by ingestion, inhalation, or dermal routes. When inhaled, the solvent crosses the alveolar membrane by passive diffusion. The absorbed dose is determined by the air concentration, duration of exposure, minute ventilation, and the blood-to-air partition coefficient **(Table 1)**. Hydrocarbons that are highly soluble in blood and tissues are readily absorbed, and blood concentrations rise rapidly following inhalation exposure.

Table 1: Hydrocarbons are classified based on viscosity

Hydrocarbons	*Commonly used as*	*Viscosity (units)*
Aliphatic		
Petrol	Motor vehicle fuel	30
Kerosene	Heating fuel	35
Turpentine	Paint thinner	33
Aromatic		
Toluene	Spray paint thinner	28
Xylene	Paint thinner	28
Halogenated		
Methylene chloride	Solvent, propellant	27
Carbon tetrachloride	Solvent, Refrigerant	30

CLINICAL FEATURES

Respiratory Effects

Clinical manifestation depends on the physical properties of the ingested hydrocarbon, volume ingested whether vomiting had occurred. Physical properties that predispose to aspiration are viscosity, surface tension, and volatility. Hydrocarbons with low viscosities (<60 SUS; e.g. turpentine, gasoline, naphtha) **(Table 1)** and low surface tension have an increased risk of aspiration. HC, with high volatility tend to vaporize, displace oxygen, leading to transient hypoxia.[4]

Pulmonary toxicity manifests with tachypnea, respiratory distress, crackles, bronchospasm leading to wheeze and hypoxemia. More severe toxic effects can cause hemoptysis and acute respiratory distress syndrome (hemorrhagic or non-hemorrhagic). Cyanosis, secondary to ventilation-perfusion mismatch or methemoglobinemia have noted in toxicity due to aniline, nitrobenzene, or nitrite-containing hydrocarbons.

Cardiac Effects

Hydrocarbons increase the risk of cardiac toxicity due to their potential to sensitize the myocardium. The resultant arrhythmias can worsen prognosis. Halogenated and aromatic compounds have been most frequently associated with inducing arrhythmias. Arrhythmias ranging from atrial fibrillation, ventricular tachycardias, junctional rhythms, ventricular fibrillation, and cardiac arrest have been described. This has been termed the "sudden sniffing death syndrome". Prolongation of the QT interval leads to the development of *torsade de pointes*.

CNS Depression

Inhaled hydrocarbon vapor depresses consciousness. Acute central nervous system (CNS) toxicity from occupational overexposure or recreational abuse parallels the effect of administering an inhaled general anesthetic.

Gastrointestinal Irritant

Hydrocarbons are also GI mucosal irritants leading to nausea and vomiting. The latter, increases the risk of aspiration induced pulmonary toxicity.

MANAGEMENT

History

Identification of the specific type, route, and amount of hydrocarbon exposure is essential to plan effective management. On arrival, obtain the following information: Whether ingestion was accidental or intentional? Nature of exposure: Inhalational or ingestion? How much was consumed? What was the type of hydrocarbon ingested? When did exposure or ingestion occur? An approach to hydrocarbon poisoning is summarized in **Flowchart 1**.

Decontamination

This is essential to prevent further absorption. During decontamination, care is taken to avoid contamination of the healthcare providers. Protection of rescuers with personal protective equipment and rescue protocols is crucial especially where the victim is unresponsive. The caregivers should also be aware that some hydrocarbons are highly flammable posing risk of fire.

Flowchart 1: Approach to hydrocarbon poisoning

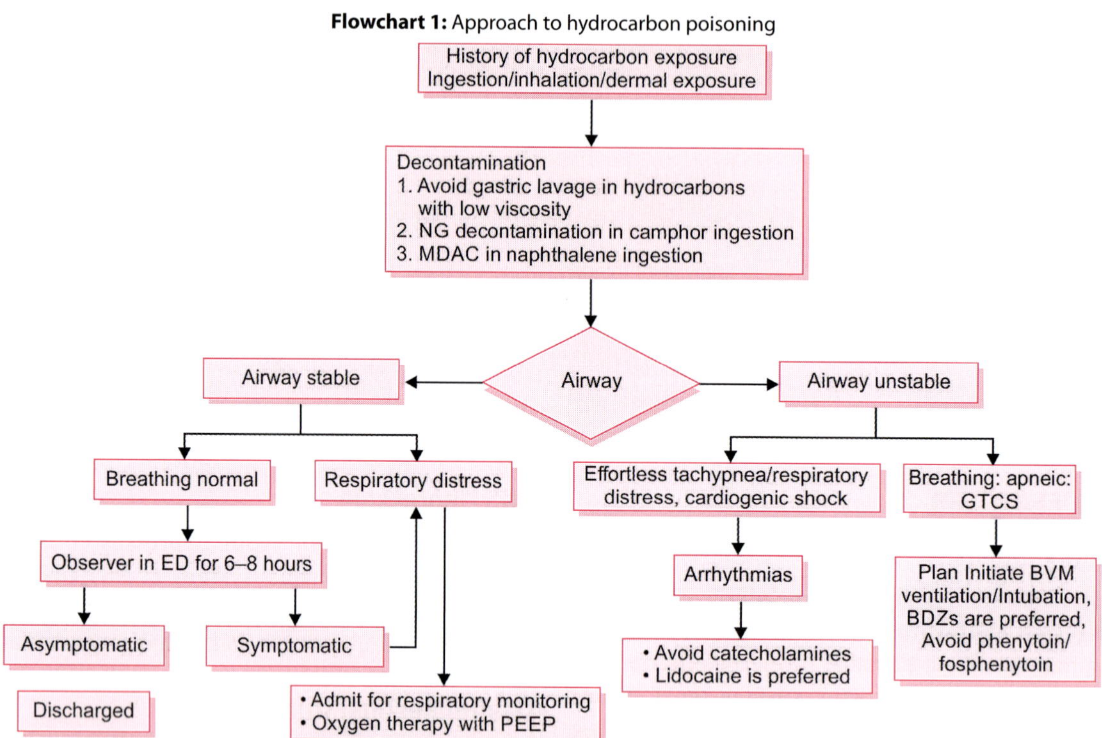

(GTCS: generalized tonic clonic seizures; NG: nasogastric; MDAC: multi-dose activated charcoal; ED: emergency department; BDZs: benzodiazepines; PEEP: positive end-expiratory pressure)

Exposed clothing should be removed and safely discarded as further absorption or inhalation of hydrocarbons from grossly contaminated clothing can worsen systemic toxicity. Decontamination of the skin should have a high priority in massive hydrocarbon exposures, particularly those exposures involving highly toxic hydrocarbons. Early decontamination with soap and water may be adequate. Water alone, may be ineffective in decontaminating most hydrocarbons.

Activated charcoal (AC) has limited ability to decrease gastrointestinal absorption of hydrocarbons and may distend the stomach and predispose patients to vomiting and aspiration. AC, do not bind HC and has been found to increase risk of HC aspiration. Hence, AC has been specifically contraindicated and can use can worsen prognosis in Hydrocarbon poisoning.

Antibiotics and steroids also play no role in the management of hydrocarbon toxicity.

Management in the Emergency Department

Patients with severe hydrocarbon toxicity develop respiratory distress associated with a large ventilation-perfusion mismatch resulting in hypoxia.

Provide oxygen

Noninvasive ventilation to provide high levels of positive end-expiratory pressure (PEEP) is beneficial. Early intubation is planned if there is no response.

Correct shock if identified

Small volumes may be needed, unless complicated by persistent vomiting. Monitor for arrhythmias, because of hypokalemia and acidosis. Clinically cardiac dysfunction can also result in hypotension and cardiogenic shock. Avoid catecholamines for ventricular fibrillation. Lidocaine is the preferred drug.

Manage seizures

Development of seizures warrant the use of benzodiazepines. Phenytoin is avoided due to its potential cardiotoxic effects.

Monitoring

Patients who are asymptomatic and have normal chest radiographs, and remain normal during 6 hours of observation can be discharged.

Children with history of hydrocarbon ingestion should be monitored in the emergency department for 6–8 hrs and a chest radiograph should be obtained at the end of the observation period. Spontaneous or induced emesis and gastric lavage have led to aspiration pneumonitis. Children who are symptomatic require admission to the hospital for cardio-respiratory monitoring and supportive care. Approximately 90% of hospitalized children have a benign clinical course.

Patients who are asymptomatic but have radiographic evidence of pneumonitis; or who have initial respiratory symptoms but quickly become asymptomatic during medical evaluation, need to be hospitalized.

CAMPHOR POISONING

Camphor (2-bormanone, 2-camphonone), a cyclic ketone of the terpene group camphor is synthesized from a derivative of turpentine oil. Camphor is a commonly used ingredient found in many non-prescription remedies for cold symptoms and in muscle liniments. Ingestion is the most common route of exposure, resulting in significant camphor toxicity.[5]

Camphor is a highly lipophilic compound that is rapidly absorbed from the gastrointestinal tract and can be detected in the blood within 15 to 20 minutes following ingestion. The presence of food in the stomach may delay the absorption of camphor. A significant amount of camphor can be absorbed through normal skin. Dermal absorption of camphor is slow but can produce systemic toxicity up to 72 hours following exposure.

Clinical Effects

Exposure to camphor can often be detected by its characteristic odor. Camphor ingestion results in oropharyngeal irritation, nausea, vomiting, and abdominal pain. Generalized tonic–clonic seizures may occur within 1 to 2 hours of ingestion. The onset of systemic toxicity, particularly CNS toxicity, can occur as early as 5 minutes after ingestion. Some patients may develop status epilepticus. Delayed seizures, occurring up to 9 hours following ingestion and up to 72 hours following dermal exposure, are reported.

Diagnostic testing: No specific diagnostic test is available or indicated when managing patients with camphor toxicity. Camphor and its metabolites can be identified in blood and urine.

Management

Camphor is rapidly absorbed in the gastrointestinal tract due to its high lipophilic property. Thus, the benefit of gastrointestinal (GI) decontamination rapidly diminishes with time following acute ingestion. If lavage is deemed necessary following recent ingestion of a camphor-containing solution, nasogastric suctioning and lavage are preferable to orogastric lavage. The utility of activated charcoal in acute camphor ingestion is unknown. There is no antidote for camphor. Most patients survive with supportive care. Although the management of camphor induced seizures is not well studied, the first line therapy for camphor induced seizures is a benzodiazepine. Repeat doses of benzodiazepines may be needed to control seizures.

NAPHTHALENE

Naphthalene ($C_{10}H_8$), an aromatic bicyclic hydrocarbon, is commonly found in products such as moth repellents.

Pharmacology

Naphthalene is a white, flaky crystalline solid with a noxious odor. Naphthalene toxicity is reported following ingestion, dermal application, and inhalation. Naphthalene is initially metabolized to an unstable epoxide intermediate, 1,2-naphthalene oxide. Naphthalene 1,2-oxide can react with cellular components such as DNA and protein to form covalent adducts or can get spontaneously converted to 1-naphthol and 2-naphthol, which undergo glucuronidation or sulfation to form conjugates that are subsequently eliminated in urine. Glutathione-S-transferase and glutathione play an important role in detoxification of 1,2-naphthalene oxide by converting the reactive epoxide to nonreactive mercapturic acid metabolites.[6]

Reactive hepatic metabolites, 1-naphthol, 1,2-naphthoquinone, and 1.4-naphthoquinone, are cytotoxins which deplete intracellular glutathione stores and generate reactive oxygen species. They are responsible for the oxidative stress leading to naphthalene-induced hemolysis and methemoglobinemia.

Clinical Features

Naphthalene-induced hemolysis and methemoglobinemia result when physiologic compensatory mechanisms to oxidative stress are overwhelmed. Hemolysis and methemoglobinemia can occur in children with either normal or deficient glucose-6-phosphate dehydrogenase (G6PD) activity. Children, with G6PD deficiency are at greater risk of hemolysis due to their decreased glutathione stores. Infants have an increased risk of methemoglobinemia, since fetal hemoglobin is more susceptible to the formation of methemoglobin and also because nicotinamide adenine dinucleotide phosphate (NADPH) methemoglobin reductase activity is less well developed, impairing the reduction of methemoglobin to hemoglobin.

Hemolysis and methemoglobinemia can become clinically evident, as early as 24 to 48 hours post-exposure. However, it has been noted more typically on the third day post-exposure, since time is necessary for the hepatic metabolism of naphthalene. Anemia secondary to hemolysis manifests between 3 and 5 days post-exposure. Both acute and chronic exposures to naphthalene result in similar toxicity. Renal failure is reported as a complication of naphthalene-induced hemolysis and hemoglobinuria.

Diagnostic Testing

No specific diagnostic testing is indicated. Naphthalene-induced hemolysis is similar to hemolysis from other causes. Reticulocytosis and elevation of the unconjugated bilirubin are noted. Serum haptoglobin falls because the haptoglobin–hemoglobin complex is cleared by the kidneys. Lactate dehydrogenase is elevated. Hemoglobinuria is usually present. It should be differentiated from myoglobinuria. Serum creatine phosphokinase is elevated in patients with rhabdomyolysis and myoglobinuria. Examination of a peripheral blood smear can suggest hemolysis before a patient develops clinical or laboratory evidence of anemia. The percentage of methemoglobin can rapidly be determined using a co-oximeter.

Management

Even one naphthalene containing mothball can be hazardous to young children. Administration of activated charcoal, 1 g/kg, followed by repeat doses of activated charcoal 0.5 g/kg and/or whole-bowel irrigation with polyethylene glycol electrolyte lavage solution are indicated for children with significant ingestions of naphthalene.

TURPENTINE OIL POISONING

Turpentine is an oleoresin solvent—a mixture of pine oils and resins distilled from the tree genus Pinus. Pine oil is also distilled from the same trees but does not include any resins. Turpentine is used as a degreaser and paint thinner. Pine oil and turpentine are volatile hydrocarbon compounds with low viscosity. Aspiration and inhalational injury are common when low-viscosity hydrocarbons are ingested or inhaled. Although, acutely toxic, once the victim improves, there is no evidence of permanent damage due to hydrocarbon toxicity.

KEY MESSAGES

Do's

- Early decontamination of skin with soap and water is a priority.
- Avoid gastric lavage in kerosene poisoning.
- Nasogastric suctioning and lavage are preferable to orogastric lavage in camphor poisoning.
- Benzodiazepines are preferred antiepileptic in camphor poisoning.
- Multi-dose activated charcoal are indicated in naphthalene ingestions but contraindicated in other hydrocarbon ingestion.

Don'ts

- Spontaneous or induced emesis and gastric lavage.
- Administration of antibiotics and steroids.
- Catecholamines for arrhythmia resuscitation.

REFERENCES

1. Sarker AK, Ghosh S, Barik K. A study of accidental poisoning (in children) in a rural medical college hospital of West Bengal. Indian J Public Health. 2005;34:159-62.
2. Tormoehlen LM, Tekulve KJ, Nañagas KA. Hydrocarbon toxicity: A review. Clin Toxicol (Phila). 2014;52:479-89.
3. Thomas M, Zach MS, Atkinson SD. Profile of hospital admissions following acute poisoning-experiences from a major teaching hospital in south India. Adverse Drug React Toxicol Rev. 2000; 19:313-7.
4. Makrygianni EA, Palamidou F, Kaditis AG. Respiratory complications following hydrocarbon aspiration in children. Pediatr Pulmonol. 2016;51:560-9.
5. Narayan S, Singh N. Camphor poisoning-An unusual cause of seizure. Med J Armed Forces India. 2012;68:252-3.
6. Chauhan V, Sharma R, Sharma K, *et al*. Naphthalene poisoning manifesting as hemoglobinuria. Toxicol Int. 2014;21:314-5.

CHAPTER

66

Heavy Metal Poisoning

Javed Ismail, Jhuma Sankar

INTRODUCTION

Our environment comprises many chemicals, which we use in our daily life. When human body is exposed to higher than tolerable quantities, these chemicals are dangerous. Heavy metal exposure is a cause of growing concern in our era of industrialization with increased exposure to chemicals. Lead, arsenic, mercury, cadmium are 4 heavy metals listed among the World Health Organization (WHO) list of 10 major chemicals of concern.[1]

Heavy metals are those with specific gravity more than 4 or those with atomic weight more than that of sodium. Many of these are found in miniscule quantities in our body and have physiological roles like co-factor for enzymes, as a part of proteins (iron in hemoglobin, myoglobin) or as a part of enzymes (zinc, selenium, chromium). Some of these are being used solely or as a mixture in treatment of some diseases (for example, gold in rheumatoid arthritis, aluminum in antacids, or iron, zinc, selenium in food supplements).[2] As in any toxicological exposure, management revolves around decreasing absorption, treatment of toxic manifestations, increasing excretion and monitoring for recovery of organ functions.[2] In this chapter, we shall discuss 4 common heavy metal exposures (lead, mercury, arsenic and cadmium), their modes of exposure, mechanism of toxicity, clinical manifestations and management principles.

LEAD

It is one of the most studied environmental heavy metal toxin. Human exposure to lead has increased dramatically over past two centuries with industrial revolution, burning fossil fuels, use of lead-based paints and from mining industries.[3,4]

Chemical Forms

Lead is a bluish-white lustrous metal. It exists in four isotopic forms in nature. Because of its non-corrosive and non-biodegradable nature, it accumulates in the environment with its continuous use.

Main Sources of Exposure

Exposure to lead can occur through inhalation, ingestion or direct skin contact.

- Inhalation of smoke generated by burning lead containing materials. Leaded petrol was an important source of exposure, which was banned by India in March 2000.
- Ingestion of lead contaminated water, dust and food, peeling paints, recently renovated houses are other important sources.
- Children are vulnerable to lead poisoning because of their curiosity and age appropriate non nutritive hand to mouth behavior. It results in swallowing and ingestion of lead containing objects and soil or dust.
- Lead can readily cross placenta resulting in in-utero lead poisoning.

Pathophysiology

After absorption, lead is disseminated throughout the body. More than 90% of lead is stored in the bones, where it can reside for decades. In body, it circulates bound to red blood cells. A very small fraction is found in plasma. When red blood cells become saturated with lead, the plasma levels begin to increase. The plasma lead portion gets distributed to various organs and tissues and is responsible for lead toxicity. This being a slow process, takes months to years before clinical toxicity occurs.

Various pathophysiological mechanisms described are:

- It binds to various enzymes especially sulfhydryl groups containing enzymes, diminishing their function. Two major enzymes involved in heme synthesis are susceptible to lead inhibitory effects.
- Lead has a higher affinity for calcium dependent process, thereby, inhibits calcium uptake, disrupts intra and intercellular signaling and disrupts mitochondrial function.
- It interferes with the neurotransmitter functions at presynaptic level by inhibiting calcium dependent protein-kinase C, which is required for brain function.
- During the infancy and childhood, it inhibits formation of interneuron connections and hence results in an abnormal tertiary brain structure which is an irreversible damage.

Clinical Features and Complications

The appearance of clinical symptoms varies among various individuals and as lead exposure increases, the range and severity of symptoms also increases. Children are more vulnerable to lead poisoning because they absorb lead 4–5 times as much as adults.[3,4]

Neurologic: Nervous system is most vulnerable to lead toxicity in children. Symptoms include headache, lethargy, seizures, papilledema, coma and death. Poor scholastic performance and behavioral changes like hyperactivity are reported in school-age children. Adolescents may present aggressive, violent behaviors.[2] Cognitive and behavioral effects are irreversible and permanent correlating with blood lead levels (BLL) done serially or at 2 years of age. Peripheral neuropathy and foot drop has been seen in older patients. Lead encephalopathy can occur in children with BLL more than 100 µg/dL. Prenatal lead exposure has also been implicated in cognitive and behavioral disorders.

Renal: Renal tubular dysfunction is seen at levels more than 100 µg/dL. Laboratory evaluation may reveal glycosuria, phosphaturia or Fanconi's syndrome. Tubulointerstitial fibrosis, glomerulosclerosis and chronic renal failure may occur with chronic toxicity.

Gastrointestinal: Gastrointestinal symptoms include anorexia, abdominal pain, vomiting and constipation. These symptoms are usually seen at BLL more than 20 µg/dL.

Hematologic: Anemia occurs as lead interferes with activity of essential enzymes like delta-aminolevulinic acid dehydratase and ferrochelatase involved in heme biosynthesis. A decrease in the activity of ferrochelatase results in an increase of the substrate erythrocyte protoporphyrin in the red blood cells. Acute lead poisoning results in hemolytic anemia by disrupting red cell membrane. Chronic lead poisoning induces anemia by diminishing red cell survival as well as heme biosynthesis.

Others: Chronic exposure results in accumulation in bones resulting in demineralization and rachitic deformities in children. Hearing defects, growth retardation, delay in puberty, are proportionately worse with levels of lead exposure.

Diagnosis

There is no known safe blood lead concentration. Centers for Disease Control and Prevention have set the standard elevated BLL for children to be 5 µg/dL and for adults at 10 µg/dL of the whole blood.[3]

Management

Prevention of exposure remains the key in sustaining a low lead levels. Treatment of iron deficiency and food fortification with iron has been found to decrease blood lead levels in children.

Chelation therapy

Chelation therapy is lifesaving in children with lead poisoning. Guidelines for chelation are based on BLL. Children with BLL of 40–70 µg/dL can be treated with single agent, whereas those with levels > 70 µg/dL require two agents. DMSA and Calcium disodium edetate are the preferred agents (**Table 1**). Other agents, which can be used, are BAL and D-Penicillamine. For children with encephalopathy a combination of calcium disodium edetate and BAL is used. These chelating agents reduce the circulating lead levels and do not reverse the

Table 1: Chelating agents

Drug	Dose	Route	Indication	Side effects
Dimercaprol (BAL)	3 mg/kg (max 150 mg) 4 hourly for 2 days followed by twice daily for 10 days (for inorganic mercury toxicity – 5 mg/kg on first day followed by 2.5 mg/kg every 12 hourly for 10 days)	Intramuscular	Acute arsenic toxicity Inorganic mercury toxicity	Pain at injection site, nausea, abdominal pain, feeling of constriction of chest, sweating, tachycardia, hypertension, hemolysis in G6PD deficient
Calcium disodium edetate	1000–1500 mg/m²/day divided every 12 hourly for 5 days	Intravenous infusion or intramuscular	Lead toxicity	Proteinuria, pyuria, rising blood urea nitrogen, creatinine
Dimercapto-1-propane sulfonic acid (DMPS)	10 mg/kg/dose thrice daily for 3 days	Oral, intravenous	Acute and chronic mercury toxicity	Nausea, vomiting, fatigue, rash, pruritus
2,3 Dimercaptosuccinic acid (DMSA)	350 mg/m² or 10 mg/kg every 8 hourly for 5 days, then 12 hourly for 14 days	Oral	Acute lead toxicity Cadmium toxicity Chronic arsenic toxicity	Nausea, vomiting, diarrhea, anorexia, transaminitis, transient hemolysis, reversible neutropenia
Penicillamine	5–7.5 mg/kg every 8–12 hourly for 4–12 weeks	Oral	Low grade mercury poisoning Lead toxicity	Leukopenia, thrombocytopenia, proteinuria, fever, rash, transaminitis

neurological impairment. Eventually, the lead levels rise despite preventing further exposure, probably originating from bone reservoir. Repeat chelation may be indicated if the BLL surge beyond 45 µg/dL after a treatment gap of 3 days.

MERCURY

Three chemical forms of mercury are elemental, organic and inorganic. At room temperature, it exists in elemental form as a silvery white liquid metal. Inorganic forms are being used as a mixture in ayurvedic products, traditional skin lightening creams, pesticides, fungicides, button batteries and as preservatives in medicines (thiomersal). Organic forms (methylmercury) exist in environment polluted with mercury and enter the human body via ingestion of contaminated food items especially seafood. It accumulates through the food chain and are found in high quantities in predator fish like shark, tuna, sword fish and other seafood like mussels and crayfish.[2,5]

Historically, mercury poisoning with its clinical effects was described in Japan (1959, called as minimata disease) due to ingestion of fish contaminated with methylmercury. Other instance was from Iraq (1970) where mass toxicity occurred due to ingestion of grains contaminated with mercury fungicides.

Common Modes of Toxicity

1. Acute household exposure in children can occur with inhalation of mercury vapors from broken fluorescent light bulbs and broken thermometers. Skin contact of this metal can also result in minimal absorption. Elemental mercury is poorly absorbed through the gut whereas its vapors are absorbed readily through the lungs. Ingestion of inorganic compounds can result in symptoms of acute toxicity.
2. Chronic exposure commonly occurs with ingestion of contaminated seafood or ingestion of traditional ayurvedic medicines, dental amalgams. Maximum permissible levels of mercury in drinking water is 2 parts per billion parts of water and for seafood 1 ppm.

Pathophysiology

Elemental mercury is absorbed rapidly through the lungs and is distributed all over the body especially to the central nervous system due to its lipid solubility. However, enteral absorption is poor (< 0.1%). In tissues, it is oxidized to form a cytotoxic divalent compound by hydrogen peroxidase-catalase pathway. Once oxidized, its ability to cross the tissue barriers is restricted and hence elimination is impeded. Elemental form is excreted through kidneys, gut and respiratory tract.

Inorganic forms are absorbed poorly (10%) through the gut and hence toxicity is less with this form. Whereas the organic form (methyl mercury) is rapidly absorbed through gut and is distributed throughout the body and crosses the blood brain barrier. It binds with cysteine to form a complex and is transported across the tissues through carrier proteins. Half-life in human ranges from 44 to 80 days.

Mercury or its compounds in the environment are methylated by soil microbes to form methylmercury. Enteral absorption of this form is high (90%). It has high affinity for sulfhydryl groups and binds with reduced glutathione and avidly binds to metallothionein in kidneys and if accumulated in large quantities can cause acute renal failure.[5]

Clinical Features

Acute exposure

Exposure to mercury vapors are toxic and can present with malaise, fever, headache, respiratory symptoms like cough, dyspnea, headache, visual disturbances. In severe cases, these symptoms may progress on to respiratory failure due to necrotizing bronchiolitis and interstitial pneumonitis. Neurological disturbances like tremors, movement disorders, excessive sensitivity may develop later.

Acute ingestion of inorganic compounds can present with gastrointestinal symptoms like nausea, severe abdominal pain, hematochezia, hematemesis. In severe cases, it can progress to result in myocardial infarction, arrhythmias and renal failure. Ingestion of large quantities can result in death due to myocardial infarction.

Chronic exposure

Prolonged inhalation of small quantities of mercuric vapors (elemental form), ingestion of inorganic compounds or contaminated seafood (organic) is the common mode of chronic toxicity.

Clinical manifestations include a triad of fine tremors, neuropsychiatric symptoms and gingivostomatitis. Symptoms begin with malaise, headaches, lack of concentration, hair loss, excessive salivation and gingivitis. If prolonged, neurological symptoms like tremors, movement disorders, ataxia, incoordination and behavioral disturbances like delirium, insomnia, memory loss. Renal manifestations like proteinuria, hematuria and nephrotic syndrome have been described.

Pink disease or acrodynia occurs as dermatological hypersensitivity to mercury in children. Clinical presentation includes reddish pink exanthems, pain, desquamation and edema of hands and feet with neurological symptoms like paresthesia. Other features like anorexia, tremors, insomnia, excessive sweating, photophobia and proximal weakness can occur.

Laboratory Testing

Urinary mercury levels estimated in 24-hour sample is the preferred method for all forms except organic compound exposure (methylmercury). It is useful in measuring the total body burden of elemental and inorganic mercury especially in occupational exposure. Peak levels are attained about 2–3 weeks of exposure. Treatment is warranted for urinary levels >150 μg/L.[6] For organic compound poisoning, blood and hair mercury levels can be estimated. Blood levels have a half-life of only 3 days and hence, have limited value if estimated beyond this time. Blood levels of >35 μg/L is an indication for chelation.[6] Renal injury can be detected by microalbuminuria.

Management

Chelation therapy: Dimercapto-1-propane sulfonic acid (DMPS) and dimercaptosuccinic acid (DMSA) are preferred chelating agents for both acute and chronic mercury toxicity. They both bind inorganic mercuric compounds and are effectively excreted. However, they do not chelate from the central nervous system and effectiveness in reversing symptoms is not clear.

Prevention

Chronic dietary intake of mercurial compounds can be prevented by avoiding seafood grown from contaminated waters. The United States Environmental Protection Agency recommends avoiding fish with mercury more than 0.66 μg/g. Inhalation of mercury vapors can be prevented by avoiding exposure to broken fluorescent bulbs or elemental mercury from broken thermometers.

ARSENIC

Arsenic is abundantly available toxic metal in the natural earth's crust. The chemical forms available are elemental arsenic, arsine gas, inorganic arsenic salts and organic arsenic. Among these, arsine gas is the most toxic.

Chemical Characteristics

- Elemental arsenic is insoluble in water, hence not absorbed and non-toxic.
- Arsine gas—colorless, non-irritant gas emitted when arsenic compounds are treated with acid. Inhalation of even small quantities like 25–50 ppm can result in death in 30 minutes and quantities up to 150 ppm can cause immediate death.
- Inorganic form is found in—pesticides, dyes, homeopathic medicines, household medications. It is well absorbed through skin, mucosal membranes and eliminated predominantly by kidneys. The trivalent form (arsenic trioxide) is lipid soluble and hence more toxic. Exposure to about 2 mg/kg in a child can be fatal.
- Organic compounds are poorly absorbed through gut, are less soluble and less toxic.

Main Sources of Exposure

- Natural resources—rocks, soil, well water. Humans are exposed to an average of 20 µg/day from food and water.[6] According to WHO guidelines, drinking water should not contain more than 10 µg/L of arsenic.[7] Epidemiological studies in West Bengal, Uttar Pradesh, Bihar, Jharkhand and Assam have revealed higher levels in drinking water and high prevalence of skin manifestation of arsenic poisoning.
- Parental smoking.
- Industrial sources—burning of fossil fuels, as a byproduct in smelting of copper, lead, zinc, as a component in wood preservatives, and pesticide manufacture.

Pathophysiology

After exposure to arsine gas, absorbed metal binds to hemoglobin and is oxidized to arsenic dihydride and elemental arsenic, which results in cell membrane instability and massive hemolysis. Arsenic trioxide (inorganic form) binds to sulfhydryl groups and causes uncoupling of oxidative phosphorylation by being substituted for phosphate in glycolytic pathway and decreases adenosine triphosphate production by inhibiting enzymes like pyruvate dehydrogenase and alpha-ketoglutarate complex. It also induces reactive oxygen species and oxidative stress, which in turn triggers apoptosis and cell death. Arsenic is methylated and mainly excreted by kidneys with a half-life of 2.5 days. High concentrations are reached in bone and keratinized tissues like hair, nails and skin.[7]

Clinical Features

Acute toxicity

Gastrointestinal manifestations are common and begin within 30 minutes after oral consumption of arsenic compounds often presenting with dysphagia, garlic taste and severe thirst. Abdominal pain, vomiting, bloody or rice water diarrhea are also common. Inhalation of arsine gas results in malaise, gastrointestinal side effects, massive hemolysis presenting as hemoglobinuria, jaundice, pallor, renal failure. Cardiac arrhythmias like torsade de pointes, ventricular fibrillation are common. Severe muscle cramps, neurological manifestations like delirium, seizures, encephalopathy, coma and death can occur. Exposure to low doses presents with maculopapular eruption in the intertriginous areas along with other manifestations. Patients who recover from the acute illness may develop peripheral neuropathy, hematuria, proteinuria after days to weeks of exposure.

Chronic toxicity

It usually occurs in areas with high concentrations of arsenic in drinking water. Clinical manifestations usually appear after 5 to 20 years of exposure. Common manifestations are as follows:

- Garlic odor on breath
- Muscle weakness, tenderness on examination
- Generalized fatigue
- Excessive perspiration
- Sensorimotor polyneuropathy—paresthesia of hands and foot
- Hyperpigmentation (rain drop shaped discolored spots, diffuse dark brown spots, diffuse darkening of skin), keratosis especially of palms and soles
- Mees lines on the nails (transverse white striae)
- Intellectual disabilities
- Gangrene of foot
- Laboratory features of bone marrow suppression
- Cancers of lung, bladder and skin in adults.

Prenatal arsenic exposure can lead on to spontaneous abortion, stillbirth, increased risk of pneumonia and diarrhea in infancy.

Management

In patients with acute toxicity, stabilize airway, breathing and circulation. Gastric lavage should be performed if the patient presents within initial few hours of exposure. In those with clinical signs of acute toxicity, chelation therapy should be initiated. Those exposed to arsine gas need close monitoring for evidence of hemolysis. Patients with circulatory failure may require fluids, blood transfusion, vasoactive medications and mechanical ventilation for stabilization.

Chelating agents are dimercaprol or dimercaptosuccinic acid (DMSA) or d-penicillamine. In acute toxicity, dimercaprol is most preferred while DMSA is preferred in chronic toxicity.[8] Monitoring in the intensive care unit is indicated in patients with hemodynamic compromise, neurological symptoms, respiratory failure, severe hemolysis and those with multiple organ dysfunction syndrome.

Laboratory tests: Arsenic concentration should be estimated with 24-hour urine sample and any level more than 50 μg/L suggests toxicity and is an indication for chelation therapy.[2] Other organ function tests including liver function test, renal function test, total leukocyte counts, platelet counts, urine protein, urine hemoglobin tests can be done based on clinical presentation. Estimation of arsenic levels in hair, nails and skin can be done in patients with chronic toxicity.

CADMIUM

Sources of Exposure

- Animal foods—fish, oysters, mussels from polluted water bodies
- Rice, wheat grown in contaminated soil
- Tobacco smoke
- Industrial dust—copper or zinc smelting factories, batteries, paints, plastics, coal mining, etc.

Pathophysiology

Cadmium is a highly toxic heavy metal. It is absorbed in the body after ingestion or inhalation of cadmium containing compounds. Intestinal absorption increases in children during calcium, zinc and or iron deficiency states. After absorption, it binds with metallothionein and the circulating free metal determines the toxicity. Cadmium generates a metabolic stress and affects mitochondrial respiration, oxidative phosphorylation and increases production of reactive oxygen species. At higher concentrations, it affects cell proliferation, halts metabolism and induces apoptosis. In acute exposure, it can affect the kidneys with damage to proximal tubules resulting in acute tubular necrosis. With chronic exposure, cadmium gets deposited in bones, causing demineralization and skeletal deformities. It also gets concentrated in kidneys and causes cortical damage and chronic kidney disease. Along with lead exposure, it can act synergistically resulting in neurodevelopmental disabilities and high risk of proteinuria, renal failure in children.

Clinical Features

Acute tubular injury and necrosis is the predominant manifestation of acute toxicity. Ingestion of cadmium of about 70 mg/kg may prove fatal.[9] Chronic cadmium exposure is much commoner and it affects the bones, kidney and neurodevelopment. Bone involvement clinically manifests as osteomalacia in severe cases (also called as Itai-Itai disease in adults, first described in Japan). It can result in renal damage presenting early with features of proximal tubular dysfunction like polyuria along with aminoaciduria, sub-nephrotic proteinuria, glucosuria, phosphaturia and hypercalciuria. In long-term, these patients may evolve into chronic kidney disease. Neurodevelopmental disabilities like hyperactivity, cognitive dysfunction, behavioral changes have been described with chronic toxicity and in those with in utero cadmium exposure. Immune dysfunction especially of T cell lineage is increasingly described. Inhalation of cadmium vapors can manifest with signs of lung inflammation and may evolve into emphysema. Cadmium is carcinogenic and has been associated with liver, bladder, gastric and hematopoietic malignancies in adults.

Laboratory Evaluation

Cadmium can be detected in blood and urine. Elevated blood levels indicate acute exposure while elevated urinary levels indicate high cadmium load in the body suggesting chronic exposure. Urinary cadmium concentration of more than 0.5 µg/g of creatinine correlates with renal injury.[10] Blood cadmium levels can be detected if it is above 0.3 µg/L. It can also be estimated in nails, hair and saliva. Accurate testing of total body load of cadmium requires urine provocation testing.

Management

Chelating agent—DMSA and its monosters are effective in cadmium toxicity. Commonly used DMSA monoesters are—monoisoamyl DMSA, monomethyl DMSA, monocyclohexyl DMSA. They bind both the circulating and the intracellular forms and so is more effective form of chelation. A combination of DMSA and its monoester can also be used. N-acetyl cysteine decreases heavy metal induced hepatic and renal oxidant stress and has been recommended as an adjuvant therapy. Zinc and magnesium are protective by decreasing reactive oxygen species and lipid peroxidation, can be used in reversing cadmium induced renal toxicity. BAL binds with cadmium form a complex (BAL-cadmium complex), which is more nephrotoxic, increases liver and kidney cadmium levels, may result in poor outcomes. Hence, BAL is not used in cadmium intoxication.

In severe cases with renal failure, hemodialysis may be needed as a supportive measure. Plasma exchange in younger children or plasmapheresis has been used in patients with high levels of cadmium as a measure to remove the protein-bound heavy metals.

CONCLUSION

Environmental heavy metal poisoning is common and preventable cause of morbidities in children. Preventive measures include regular screening of drinking water, soil, air to assess the exposure to these metals, legislative measures to ban the use of these chemicals in household products, relocating of factories in the non-residential areas and creating public awareness about the problem. The acuity of exposure, duration, route, type of compound, clinical manifestations and organ systems involved should guide the diagnosis and treatment of heavy metal toxicity.

KEY MESSAGES

- Lead, arsenic, mercury and cadmium are 4 heavy metals listed among the WHO list of 10 major chemicals of concern.
- Lead exposure in children has decreased with use of unleaded petroleum products. Chronic lead exposure can result in multisystem involvement and a blood lead level of >40 µg/dL requires chelation.
- Garlic odor on breath, muscle weakness, tenderness on examination, generalized fatigue, excessive perspiration, sensorimotor polyneuropathy, hyperpigmentation, keratosis of palms and soles and Mees lines on the nails are classical manifestations of chronic arsenic toxicity.
- A triad of fine tremors, neuropsychiatric symptoms and gingivostomatitis indicates chronic mercury toxicity.
- Acute tubular injury and necrosis is the predominant manifestation of acute cadmium toxicity.

REFERENCES

1. WHO. Ten chemicals of major public health concern. Available from: http://*www.who.int/ipcs/assessment/public_health/chemicals_phc/en/*. Accessed July 26, 2019.
2. Mahajan PV. Heavy metal intoxication. In: Kliegman R, Behrman RE, Nelson WE, editors. Nelson Textbook of Pediatrics, 20th edition. Philadelphia, PA: Elsevier; 2016.
3. Chandran L, Cataldo R. Lead poisoning: Basics and new developments. Pediatrics in Review. 2010;31:399-406.
4. Advisory Committee on Childhood Lead Poisoning Prevention (ACCLPP). Recommendations for blood lead screening of young children enrolled in medicaid: targeting a group at high risk. MMWR Recomm Rep. 2000;49:1-13.
5. Bhan A, Sarkar NN. Mercury in the Environment: Effect on Health and Reproduction. Reviews on Environmental Health. 2005. Available from: https://*www.degruyter.com/view/j/reveh.2005.20.1/reveh.2005.20.1.39/reveh.2005.20.1.39.xml*. Accessed July 26, 2019.
6. Roychowdhury T. Groundwater arsenic contamination in one of the 107 arsenic-affected blocks in West Bengal, India: Status, distribution, health effects and factors responsible for arsenic poisoning. Int J Hyg Environ Health. 2010;213:414-27.
7. World Health Organization. Guidelines for drinking-water quality. 2017.
8. Stephanopoulos DE, Willman DA, Shevlin D, *et al.* Treatment and toxicokinetics of acute pediatric arsenic ingestion: Danger of arsenic insecticides in children. Pediatric Critical Care Medicine. 2002;3:74-80.
9. Rafati-Rahimzadeh M, Rafati-Rahimzadeh M, Kazemi S, *et al.* Cadmium toxicity and treatment: An update. Caspian Journal of Internal Medicine. 2017. Available from: *http://caspjim.com/article-1-798-en.html*. Accessed July 26, 2019.
10. Bernhoft RA. Cadmium toxicity and treatment. Sci World J. 2013;2013:1-7.

CHAPTER

67

Corrosive Poisoning

Ujjal Poddar, Jayendra Seetharaman

INTRODUCTION

Corrosive ingestion is common in developing countries as there is no legislation to reduce the concentration to <10% and non-existence of child-proof packing as in developed countries. It is common in younger children (<6 years) due to their natural curiosity to explore and often deceived by the container (acids are often kept in cola's bottle). On the contrary, corrosive ingestion in adolescent age group is often suicidal. In a recent meta-analysis[1] of 64 studies comprised of 11,345 cases of corrosive ingestion in children, the mean age of corrosive ingestion was 2.78 ± 2.02 years with boys were slightly more than girls (58% vs. 42%). The types of ingested corrosive by children vary from country to country. In most developed world, alkali ingestion is more common than acid ingestion,[2,3] whereas in India multiple studies have shown that acid ingestion is more common than alkali, as acid is cheap and easily available toilet cleaner used in rural India.[4,5]

TYPES OF CORROSIVES

Common caustic agents include strong acids and alkali, concentrated weak acids and alkali, oxidizers and alkylating agents. The sources are usually from common household liquids such as toilet cleaner (hydrochloric acid), drain cleaner (sodium hydroxide), bleach (sodium hypochlorite), car batteries (sulfuric acid), rust removers (hydrogen fluoride) etc.[2,3,6] Aqua regia or Goldsmith liquid is a combination of hydrochloric acid and nitric acid in 3:1 ratio, used by Goldsmith as a solvent for gold, is also a common source.[7] Paraquat commonly used pesticide in North India is said to have corrosive action.

PATHOGENESIS

The severity of corrosive ingestion depends on whether the substance is acid or alkali, liquid or solid, diluted or concentrated, pH of the agent, presence or absence of food in the stomach and quantity of agent ingested. The mechanism of injury produced by acid and alkali is different. Acids cause coagulative necrosis of the mucosa.[8] This causes hydrogen (H^+) ions to desiccate in epithelial cells leads to eschar formation on the esophagus. This eschar prevents further penetration of the acid into deeper tissue and thus prevents deeper injury. The process also causes edema, erythema, mucosal sloughing and ulceration. On the contrary, alkali ingestion causes liquefactive necrosis that leads to deeper injury. This process includes protein dissolution, collagen destruction, fat saponification, cell membrane emulsification, submucosal vascular thrombosis and cell death. Acid ingestion usually causes gastric injury as the acids acts longer time in gastric mucosa, but alkali causes more of esophageal injury with transmural involvement.[9] Both alkali and acid injury heal with fibrosis and stricture formation. Time sequence of various pathogenetic events which happen after corrosive ingestion is given in **Table 1**.

CLINICAL FEATURES

The clinical manifestations are shown in **Table 2**. The clinical presentations depend on the timing of corrosive ingestion and the time at which the patient presents to the physician. Many a time patient presents to the tertiary care center with manifestations which are different from what was there at the time of ingestion. Patients may

Table 1: Pathogenesis: time frame of events following corrosive ingestion	
Pathology	*Timing*
Necrosis	Within seconds to minutes
Ulceration and perforation	24–72 hours
Fibrosis	2–3 weeks
Stricture	Weeks to years
Carcinoma	Years to decade

present with symptoms or without any symptoms as well. It has been shown that there is no correlation of presence or absence of symptoms and the severity of esophageal burn. This is important to note that the severity of oral injury does not accurately predict the severity of esophageal injury.[10] In a study of 473 children with corrosive ingestion, Dogan *et al.*,[11] showed that 61% without any oral burn had esophageal lesion. Similarly, there is no correlation between symptoms and severity of esophageal injury. In a study of 378 children with acute corrosive ingestion, Gaudreault *et al.*,[12] showed that 82% children with symptoms did not have any esophageal burn on endoscopy whereas 12% children without any symptoms had severe esophageal burn. Most severe complications like perforation can occur as early as in first 48 hours and as late as 14 days because of progression of tissue injury by free radical damage, ulceration and sloughing. Hence, it is warranted to observe these children for this complication. In a study of 162 children, Betalli P *et al.*,[13] have shown that the presence of three or more symptoms such as oral burns, dyspnea, vomiting, drooling, dysphagia, hematemesis and shock are important predictors of severe esophageal injury (Odds ratio: 11.97 [95% CI: 3.49–42.04], p = 0.001).

INVESTIGATIONS

X-ray

A simple chest X-ray suggest mediastinitis in case of esophageal perforation and abdominal erect X-ray suggest air under diaphragm in case of gastric perforation. These complications are expected in corrosive ingestion in significant volume and concentration, in case of symptomatic children immediately after taking corrosives. The findings are confirmed by water soluble contrast study showing leak from the perforated area or by CT scan.

CT Chest

The efficacy of CT in diagnosing depth of injury and predilection of strictures is better than X-ray and fluoroscopy. In a retrospective analysis of more than 300 CT scan in corrosive injury, a simplified radiological classification was proposed in adults (**Table 3**). The same can be extrapolated in children, although it has not yet been validated in children.[14]

Table 2: Clinical manifestations of corrosive ingestion[10]	
Gastrointestinal (GI) manifestations	Drooling, oral pain, dysphagia, odynophagia, retrosternal or abdominal pain, vomiting Examination may show ulceration in oral cavity, features of mediastinitis and GI perforation
Respiratory manifestations	Cough, choking, stridor, hoarseness of voice, wheezing, aspiration pneumonitis
Other systems	Burns in eyes and skin, renal, hepatic failure and disseminated intravascular coagulation (DIC)

Table 3: CT scan grading of corrosive injury[14]		
CT grades	*CT finding*	*Corresponding endoscopic finding*
Grade 1	Normal esophagus	0–2a
Grade 2	Wall edema, surrounding soft tissue inflammation and increased postcontrast wall enhancement	2b–3a
Grade 3	Absence of postcontrast wall enhancement suggestive of transmural necrosis	3b

Laboratory Investigations

Investigations to look for metabolic acidosis, disseminated intravascular coagulation, super-added infection, electrolyte disturbances and multiple organ dysfunctions are to be checked in children who are sick and as pre-operative measures when surgery is indicated.

Endoscopy

Endoscopy helps in assessing the extent and severity of mucosal injury. Endoscopic grading of injury helps in planning management and predicts outcome. Endoscopic evaluation is to be done by a trained endoscopist and should be done as early as possible and preferably within 48–72 hours post ingestion as the risk of perforation goes up after that due to sloughing of mucosa and ongoing necrosis. On the contrary, only a few centers prefer to do endoscopy once a mature necrosis sets in but is not routinely practiced.

Principle of endoscopy consists of procedure under deep sedation without intubation, in case of stridor and hoarseness of voice, laryngeal involvement has to be suspected and airway has to be protected and needs pre-emptive intubation to prevent airway compromise during the procedure. During the procedure, air should be insufflated less to prevent perforation in case of severe injuries, need gentle maneuvering and in case of excessive mucosal injury scope need not be negotiated. The main purpose of endoscopy is to assess the severity of mucosal injury. The grading mucosal injury is given by Zargar *et al.* and is shown in **Table 4**.[15] Although esophagus is commonly involved (**Figs. 1A to D**), stomach can also get injured especially in suicidal ingestion (**Figs. 2A to C**).

- Grade 1, 2A have better prognosis and can be started on oral feeds and may be discharged early.
- Grade 2B and 3 have the risk of stricture formation and definitive sequalae.[16] Endoscopic classification helps to identify patients who are at risk of complication and provides crucial information which helps in deciding management and to predict the outcome.[17]

MANAGEMENT

General Measures

Do's and don'ts of acute corrosive management is given in **Table 5**.[18] Management of caustic injury starts with

Table 4: Endoscopic grading of corrosive injury[15]

Grade of injury	*Endoscopic findings*
0	Normal appearance
1	Edematous and hyperemic mucosa
2A	Superficial injury—friability, hemorrhagic areas, erosions with whitish exudates and membranes, superficial ulceration
2B	Grade 2A with deep discrete ulcers or circumferential involvement
3A	Scattered and small areas of necrosis
3B	Extensive areas of necrosis

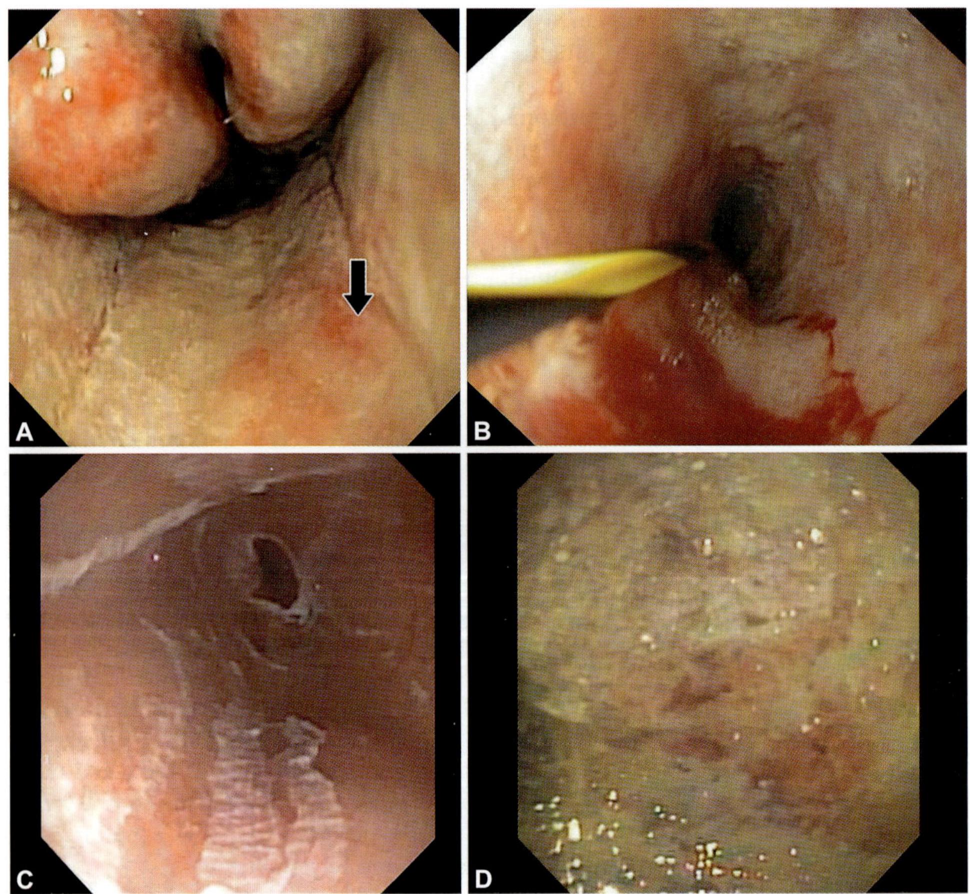

Figs. 1A to D: (A) Upper gastrointestinal endoscopy in a 14-year-old boy showing hyperemia, edema, exudates and superficial ulcers (arrow) in esophagus (grade 2A injury); (B) In a 10-year-old boy showing circumferential hyperemia, edema and friability (grade 2A injury) with guidewire in situ; (C) In a 4-year-old girl showing hyperemia, edema and membrane in esophagus (grade 2A); (D) Endoscopic view of the stomach of the same patient showing circumferential involvement with ulcers (grade 3A injury)

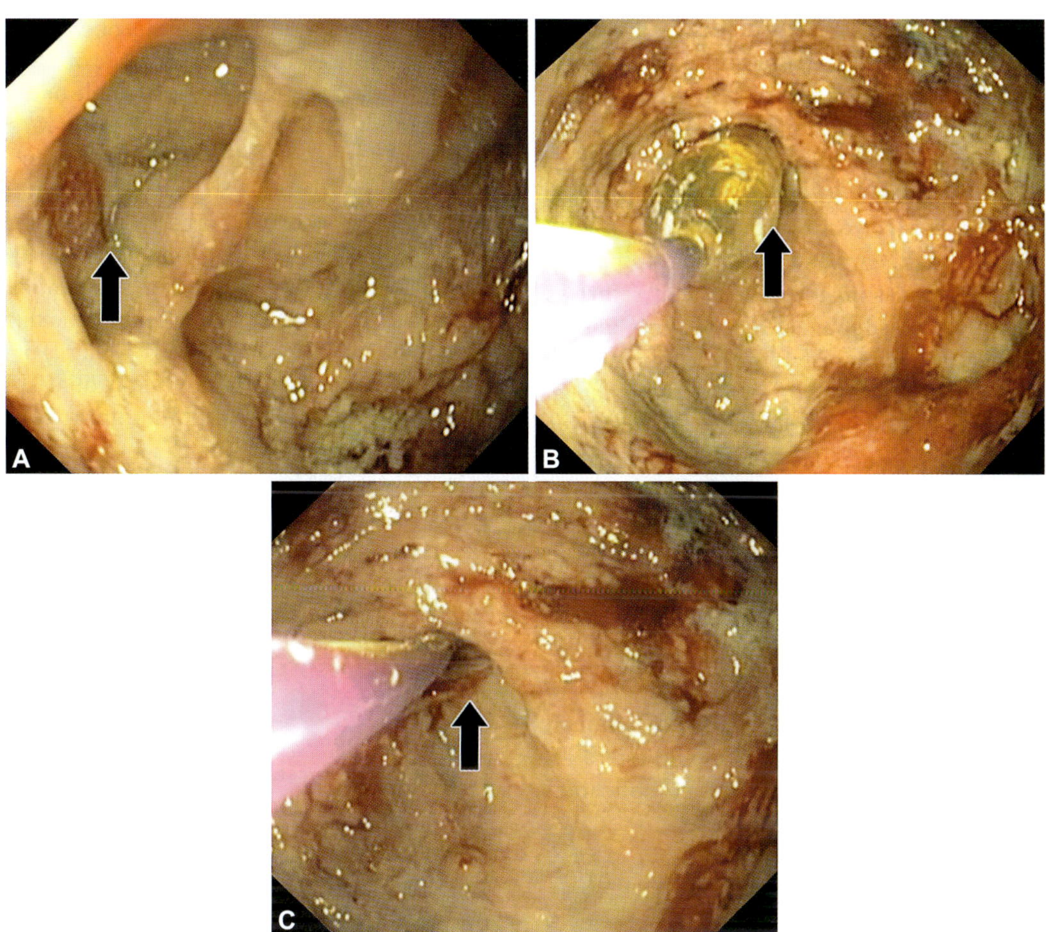

Figs. 2A to C: Upper gastrointestinal endoscopy in a 14-year-old girl showing (A) Distorted antrum with pyloric stenosis (arrow); (B) Balloon dilatation of pyloric stricture (arrow); (C) Opened up pylorus following dilatation (arrow)

immediate resuscitation (ABC: airway, breathing and circulation) in severe cases. In cases with tachypnea, stridor and respiratory distress, elective intubation should be done as airway maintenance. If X-ray chest and abdomen show features of perforation, child should be immediately taken up for surgery. After hemodynamic and airway stabilization, diagnostic endoscopy should be performed if perforation is ruled out. As there is poor correlation of symptoms with oral and esophageal burn, endoscopy should be done in all patients with corrosive ingestion. Endoscopic grading also helps to decide management. However, in Indian setting where pediatric endoscopy is not readily available, especially in primary care level, asymptomatic patient with no oral burn and questionable history of ingestion can be observed without endoscopy and can be discharged if patient can swallow liquid. On the contrary, if there is strong history of ingestion and patient having oral burn with or without symptoms, upper gastrointestinal endoscopy (UGI endoscopy) should be done to look for extent and severity of injury in esophagus and stomach. During endoscopy a naso-gastric or naso-jejunal tube may be placed under endoscopic visualization, if there is

Table 5: Do's and Don'ts in the management of corrosive ingestion

Do's
• ABC: Airway and hemodynamic stabilization • X-ray chest & abdomen: to look for perforation/aspiration • Examination of oral cavity • Endoscopy: within 24 to 48 hrs
Don'ts
• No gastric lavage • No induction of vomiting • No neutralizing agents (alkali for acid or vice-a-versa)

grade 2b or more injury. Naso-enteric tube helps in enteral feeding and also maintains a track for future dilatation as the risk of stricture development is high in this subset of patients.[19,20] Neutralizing agents such as weak acids and weak bases should not be used, as they aggravate injury by causing exothermic reaction. Similarly, gastric lavage is contraindicated in acute corrosive injury.

Although it is a routine practice to start Proton pump Inhibitor (PPI) at admission to prevent acid reflux as it might aggravate the esophageal injury, there are no studies that support PPI administration except for a small prospective study showing improvement of esophageal injury after 72 hours of omeprazole infusion.[21] In cases with symptomatic injury, sucralfate can be given for relief of symptoms as it provides physical barrier in the ulcers from corrosive injury and also hastens mucosal healing.

Antibiotics are not routinely used for Grade 1 and grade 2 injury, and their role in grade 3 injury is also controversial. Antibiotics have a definite role in perforation and if steroids are administered for airway edema.[22]

There is controversy about use of systemic steroids to prevent stricture formation in corrosive ingestion. Though there was some case series in favor of using early steroids, the controversy was set to the rest after the publication of a randomized controlled trial by Anderson KD et al.,[23] which has clearly shown that steroids (given for 3 weeks) do not decrease the risk of stricture formation. However, in a recent randomized trial from Turkey with high dose methyl prednisolone (1 g/1.73 m^2 for 3 day) in children with grade IIb injury has shown that stricture development was less in those children who received steroids (11% vs. 30%, p = 0.04).[24] Since there is high risk of developing infective complications in high grade esophageal burn, routine use of steroids in this subset of patients is not currently recommended. Steroids play an important role in reducing airway edema in cases with stridor. Intralesional steroids as an adjunct of endoscopic dilatation (triamcinolone 40 mg/session) has shown to improve outcome of dilatation.[25-27] Similarly, topical application of mitomycin C, a chemotherapeutic agent, as an adjunct to endoscopic dilatation, showed some encouraging results in small studies.[28]

Management of Strictures

Overall risk of stricture development is just 5% but the risk increases to >50% in grade IIb and grade III injury.[29] Stricture formation in esophagus gives rise to dysphagia whereas the stricture formation in antrum and pylorus of stomach produces symptoms of gastric outlet obstruction (**Figs. 3A and B**). Stricture can occur at any part of esophagus, can be long (>5 mm) or short (<5 mm), single or multiple with varying grades of severity (**Fig. 4**). It is not recommended to do endoscopy in children within 3 weeks (barring first 48–72 hours) after corrosive ingestion due to risk of perforation. After 4–6 weeks of corrosive ingestion, contrast study (barium swallow and meal) should be done to have a road map before initiating endoscopic dilatation in cases with dysphagia (**Figs. 2A to C**). Endoscopic dilatation can be done either with bougie (Savary Gilliard) or by balloon dilatation. Long strictures are better dilated by bougie. Dilatation is done till symptoms improve and lumen opened as per age-based cut off (11 mm in <5 years and 15 mm in >5 years).[5] The interval between dilatations varies

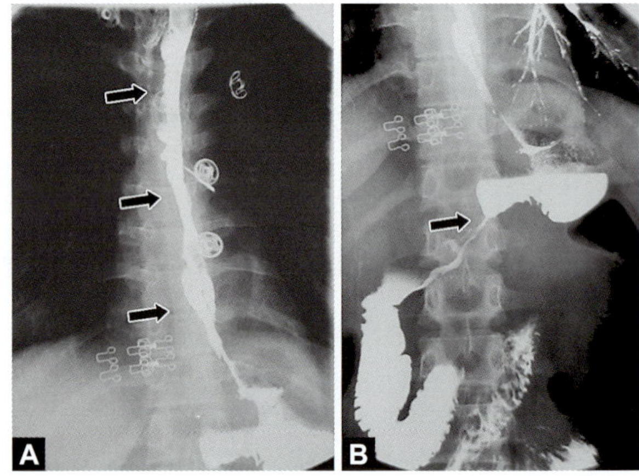

Figs. 3A and B: Barium swallow and meal of a 16-year-old girl showing. (A) Long, tight stricture in esophagus (arrows); (B) Contracted stomach with pyloric stenosis (arrow)

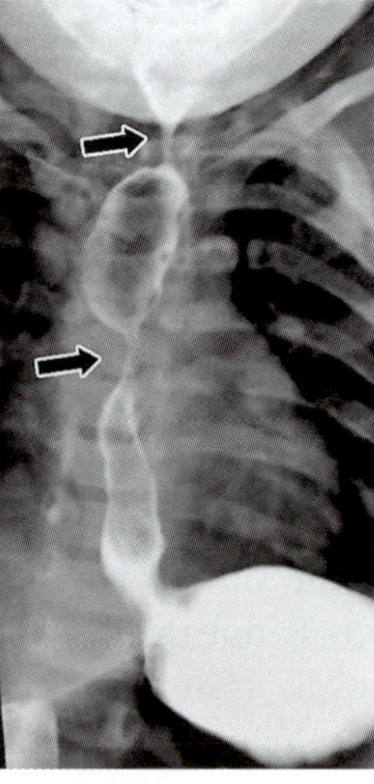

Fig. 4: Barium swallow of a 2-year-old girl showing multiple, short segment esophageal strictures (arrows).

from 1 to 3 week and usually 3–4 sessions are considered sufficient for optimal results, However, the number of dilatation sessions is most of the time unpredictable.[30]

KEY MESSAGES

- Please do not attempt gastric lavage and restrain from making an effort to neutralize acid/alkali.
- Early management includes immediate resuscitation in severe cases (ABC: airway, breathing, circulation) followed by detailed clinical examination and X-ray to rule out perforation.
- Examine the oral cavity but absence of oral burn does not rule out esophageal injury.
- Early endoscopy (within 24–48 hrs of ingestion) is the key step in assessment of mucosal injury and predication of morbidity.
- Patients with superficial injury may be started with oral feeding and can be sent home early; whereas patients with deep injury need endoscopically inserted nasogastric/nasojejunal tube or surgical feeding jejunostomy to maintain nutrition.
- There is no role of prophylactic antibiotics, proton pump inhibitor and steroids.

REFERENCES

1. Rafeey M, Ghojazadeh M, Sheikhi S, *et al.* Caustic ingestion in children: A systematic review and meta-analysis. J Caring Sci. 2016;5:251-65.
2. Yeom HJ, Shim KN, Kim SE, *et al.* Clinical characteristics and predisposing factors for complication of caustic injury of the upper digestive tract. Korean J Med. 2006;70:371-7.
3. Yoon KW, Park MH, Park GS, *et al.* A clinical study on the upper gastrointestinal tract injury caused by corrosive agent. Korean J Gastrointest Endosc. 2001;23:82-7.
4. Poddar U, Thapa BR. Benign esophageal strictures in infants and children: Results of Savary-Gilliard bougie dilation in 107 Indian children. Gastrointest Endosc. 2001;54:480-4.
5. Broor SL, Lahoti D, Bose PP, *et al.* Benign esophageal strictures in children and adolescents: Etiology, clinical profile and results of endoscopic dilatation. Gastroint Endosc. 1996;43: 474-7.
6. Schaffer SB, Hebert AF. Caustic ingestion. J La State Med Soc. 2000;152:590-6.
7. Lakshmi CP, Vijayahari R, Kate V, *et al.* A hospital-based epidemiological study of corrosive alimentary injuries with particular reference to the Indian experience. Natl Med J India. 2013;26:31-6.
8. Contini S, Scarpignato C. Caustic injury of the upper gastrointestinal tract: A comprehensive review. World J Gastroenterol. 2013;19:3918-30.
9. Millar AJ, Cox SG. Caustic injury of the esophagus. Pediatr Surg Int. 2015;31:111-21.
10. Previtera C, Giusti F, Guglielmi M. Predictive value of visible lesions (cheeks, lips, oropharynx) in suspected caustic ingestion: May endoscopy reasonably be omitted in completely negative pediatric patients? Pediatr Emerg Care. 1990;6:176-8.
11. Dogan Y, Erkan T, Cokugras FC, *et al.* Caustic gastroesophageal lesions in childhood: An analysis of 473 cases. Clin Pediatr (Phila). 2006;45:435-8.
12. Gaudreault P, Parent M, McGuigan MA, *et al.* Predictability of esophageal injury from signs and symptoms: A study of caustic ingestion in 378 children. Pediatrics. 1983;71:767-70.
13. Betalli P, Falchetti D, Giuliani S, *et al.* Caustic ingestion in children: Is endoscopy always indicated? The results of an Italian multicenter observational study. Gastrointest Endosc. 2008;68:434-9.
14. Ryu HH, Jeung KW, Lee BK, *et al.* Caustic injury: Can CT grading system enable prediction of esophageal stricture? Clin Toxicol (Phila). 2010;48:137-42.
15. Zargar SA, Kochhar R, Nagi B, *et al.* Ingestion of corrosive acids. Spectrum of injury to upper gastrointestinal tract and natural history. Gastroenterology. 1989;97:702-7.
16. Havanond C. Is there a difference between the management of grade 2b and 3 corrosive gastric injuries? J Med Assoc Thai. 2002;85:340-4.
17. Zargar SA, Kochhar R, Mehta S, *et al.* The role of fiberoptic endoscopy in the management of corrosive ingestion and modified endoscopic classification of burns. Gastrointest Endosc. 1991;37:165-9.
18. Kay M, Wyllie R. Caustic ingestion in children. Curr Opin Pediatr. 2009;21:651-4.
19. Ramasamy K, Gumaste VV. Corrosive ingestion in adults. J Clin Gastroenterol. 2003;37:119-24.
20. Krey H. On the treatment of corrosive lesions in the oesophagus; an experimental study. Acta Otolaryngol Suppl. 1952;102:1-49.
21. Cakal B, Akbal E, Köklü S, *et al.* Acute therapy with intravenous omeprazole on caustic esophageal injury: a prospective case series. Dis Esophagus. 2013;26:22-6.
22. Salzman M, O'Malley RN. Updates on the evaluation and management of caustic exposures. Emerg Med Clin North Am. 2007;25:459-76.
23. Anderson KD, Rouse TM, Randolph JG. A controlled trial of corticosteroids in children with corrosive injury of esophagus. N Engl J Med. 1990;323:637-40.
24. Usta M, Erkan T, Cokugras FC, *et al.* High doses of methylprednisolone in the management of caustic esophageal burns. Pediatrics. 2014;133;e1518-24.
25. Gandhi RP, Cooper A, Barlow BA. Successful management of esophageal strictures without resection or replacement. J Pediatr Surg. 1989;24:745-50.
26. Zein NN, Greseth JM, Perrault J. Endoscopic intralesional steroid injection in the management of refractory esophageal strictures. Gastrointest Endosc. 1995;41:596-8.
27. Kochhar R, Poornachandra KS. Intralesional steroid injection therapy in the management of resistant gastrointestinal strictures. World J Gastrointest Endosc. 2010;2:61-8.
28. Berger M, Ure B, Lacher M. Mitomycin C in the therapy of recurrent esophageal strictures: hype or hope? Eur J Pediatr Surg. 2012;22:109-16.
29. Bautista Casasnovas A, Estevez Martinez E, Varcela Cives R, et al. A retrospective analysis of ingestion of caustic substances by children. Ten-year statistics in Galicia. Eur J Pediatr. 1997;156:410-4.
30. Contini S, Scarpignato C, Rossi A, *et al.* Features and management of esophageal corrosive lesions in children in Sierra Leone: lessons learned from 175 consecutive patients. J Pediatr Surg. 2011;46:1739-45.

CHAPTER 68

Neonatal Emergencies in Delivery Room

Swathi Chacham, Madhuradhar Chegondi, Rachna Pasi, Siddarth Ramji

INTRODUCTION

Neonatal survival depends on the successful transition from fetal to neonatal life soon after birth, which involves major cardiopulmonary adaptation. A shift from parallel placental circulation to a highly complex neonatal circulation must occur very swiftly and systematically for a safe and smooth transition to extrauterine environment. Initiation of effective gas exchange coupled with functional closure of fetal circulatory pathways is vital for effective fetal to neonatal transition. Although majority of the term neonates make the transition without assistance, it is estimated that 5–10% neonates require some assistance to initiate breathing and 1:10 require advanced resuscitative measures.[1] World Health Organization estimates that about 3–5% of babies are depressed at birth and in need of resuscitation. Failure to provide appropriate support to a newborn who is depressed at birth can result in mortality and long-term disability. It is important to understand that not all emergencies are predictable before birth of a neonate. Thus, every birth must be considered as a potential emergency and adequate resources, both trained personnel and equipment, must be available in the delivery room.

EPIDEMIOLOGY AND ETIOLOGY

The most frequent emergencies encountered in the delivery room are a neonate who fails to initiate breathing, has respiratory distress soon after birth, is in shock or has major malformations.

- *Failure to initiate or sustain breathing*: The most common emergency in the delivery room is a neonate who fails to breathe or sustain respiration after birth. The burden of such babies is estimated to be about 5% of all live births. **Table 1** provides a list of conditions that contribute to the neonate's failure to initiate or sustain breathing at birth.
- *Respiratory distress*: The most common reasons are either airway obstruction; or parenchymal disorders of the lung due to developmental anomalies (e.g. pulmonary hypoplasia), prematurity (i.e. hyaline membrane disease) or acquired (e.g. meconium aspiration syndrome or congenital pneumonia). The common causes of respiratory distress in the delivery room are given in **Table 2**.
- *Shock*: Shock in the delivery room is not common but can be due to severe intrapartum asphyxia, acute blood loss due placental abruption or placental previa, accidental cord rupture, or due to pneumothorax.
- *Major congenital malformations*: These include conditions such as congenital diaphragmatic hernia, gastroschisis, open neural tube defects, obstructive uropathy.[2] These conditions would need initiating supportive care in the delivery room before they are shifted to an appropriate facility for advanced care.
- *Other causes*: These include birth trauma (fractures and nerve palsies), severe anemia (due to feto-maternal hemorrhage) or convulsions. These are rare and dealt with elsewhere in this book.

PATHOGENESIS

Ashyxia can occur as a result of impaired gas exchange across the placenta either antepartum or intrapartum (**Table 1**). As a result of impaired oxygenation, the fetus attempts to oxygenate itself by initiating breathing efforts

Table 1: Common causes for failure to initiate/sustain breathing at birth

Timing of risk factor	*Maternal*	*Placenta and umbilical cord*	*Fetal*
Antepartum	• Pregnancy induced hypertension/preeclampsia • Maternal diabetes • Maternal chorioamnionitis • Severe maternal disease (renal, pulmonary, cardiac, neurological, etc.) • Mother > 35 yrs • Premature rupture of membranes • Maternal substance abuse	• Antepartum hemorrhage (due to abruption of placentae, placenta previa) • Cord compression or nuchal cord	• Feto-maternal hemorrhage • Hydrops fetalis • Fetal growth restriction • Multiple gestation
Intrapartum	• Administration of drugs to mother such as morphine, barbiturates, tranquilizers in 2nd stage of labor (narcotics within 4 hrs of delivery) • General anesthesia • Precipitous labor • Prolonged rupture of membrane • Obstructed labor	• Intrapartum hemorrhage (Abruption/placenta previa) • Cord prolapse, Nuchal cord, cord compression	• Multiple gestation • Macrosomia • Fetal growth restriction • Abnormal fetal presentation (breech, transverse) • Major malformations

Table 2: Causes of respiratory distress in delivery room

Category	*Etiology*
Developmental	• Congenital airway obstruction (choanal atresia, laryngeal atresia, tracheal webs or atresia, Pierre Robin anomaly) • Congenital diaphragmatic hernia (CDH) • Pulmonary hypoplasia (e.g. secondary to severe renal anomaly) • Congenital cyst adenomatoid malformation (CCAM) • Cardiac anomaly (e.g. Ebstein anomaly)
Prematurity or Transitional	• Hyaline membrane disease • Transient tachypnea of newborn
Acquired	• Meconium aspiration syndrome (MAS) • Congenital pneumonia • Hydrops fetalis • Pneumothorax

and if the placental oxygenation is not established stops these breathing efforts - the phase of primary apnea. Continued hypoxia results in attempts to establish breathing again (which are less sustained and irregular) followed by apnea - the phase of secondary apnea. This phase may be preceded by increase in fetal heart rate and as metabolic acidosis sets in, there is fetal bradycardia followed by hypotension due to myocardial pump failure.[3] With prolonged asphyxia, there is loss of cerebral autoregulation and CO_2 responsiveness resulting in reduced cerebral perfusion and consequent hypoxic-ischemic injury to the brain.

The delay in initiating breathing contributes to inadequate increase in arterial paO_2, resulting in persistence of pulmonary vasoconstriction, and delayed clearance of fluid from the lungs. This manifests as transient tachypnea of newborn. In addition, if the fetus had passed meconium in utero, the gasping efforts of the fetus during hypoxia can result in aspiration of meconium manifesting after birth as meconium aspiration syndrome.

CLINICAL FEATURES

Noninitiation or Lack of Sustained Breathing Efforts

This is identified at birth when the baby is apneic (no breathing) or has gasping respiratory efforts. These babies are also usually hypotonic and show little body movements. They are usually cyanosed, but if the cause of apnea is acute blood loss, they may be pale. Note must also be made of whether the baby is preterm, and if the amniotic fluid was meconium stained.

- The heart rate of all such babies must be assessed by auscultating over the left side of the chest. One can multiply the number of beats in 6 seconds by 10 to provide a quick estimate of the beats per minute. The heart rate should be more than 100 bpm. However, auscultation may be un reliable, prone to errors, especially if the asphyxia is prolonged. Current evidence suggests that heart rate may be better assessed by use of a 3-lead ECG connected to a monitor than auscultation of the heartbeat.[4] Where feasible, this may be a more reliable and accurate method of assessing infant's heart rate during resuscitation in the delivery room. *Auscultation for the heartbeat may also help*

Table 3: APGAR scoring

Sign	*Score*		
	0	**1**	**2**
Color	Blue, pale	Pink body, blue extremities	All pink
Heart rate	Absent	< 100 bpm	>100 bpm
Breathing	Absent	Slow, Irregular	Good crying
Reflex irritability	No response	Grimace	Cough, sneeze
Muscle tone	Limp	Some flexion of extremities	Active motion

Table 4: Target preductal oxygen saturation levels

Time after birth	*Oxygen saturation*
1 min	60–65%
2 min	65–70%
3 min	70–75%
4 min	75–80%
5 min	80–85%
10 min	85–95%

detect a congenital diaphragmatic hernia, which may be suspected if heart sounds are not heard on the left but better on the right side of the chest.

- The use of the APGAR score (**Table 3**) at 1 minute can also assist in assessing the severity of the asphyxial state and, subsequent assessments at 5 and 10 minutes can help the physician in evaluating the baby's response to treatment. An APGAR score >7 at 1min or more is more reassuring.

Respiratory Distress

If the baby is breathing, but has difficulty breathing as evidenced by grunting, severe chest indrawing or a respiratory rate > 60/minute, it indicates the baby is having respiratory distress. The baby may be cyanosed or if a pulse oximeter probe is attached to the baby, the oxygen saturation values may be below the target pre-ductal oxygen saturation levels (**Table 4**).

The causes of respiratory distress as listed in **Table 2** must be sought for by appropriate clinical history and examination. As illustrations, in a preterm baby it may indicate hyaline membrane disease; maternal chorioamnionitis or prolonged rupture of membranes may indicate congenital pneumonia; meconium stained amniotic fluid may indicate meconium aspiration syndrome; absence of breath sounds and heart sounds better heard on right than left may suggest a congenital diaphragmatic hernia or a pneumothorax (if baby had been provided positive pressure ventilation at birth for noninitiation of breathing); birth by cesarean section or noninitiation of breathing at birth may indicate transient tachypnea of the newborn. A small mandible may suggest Pierre Robin anomaly and breathing with mouth open may suggest choanal atresia, which can be confirmed by inability to pass a suction catheter through the nostrils into the oral cavity.

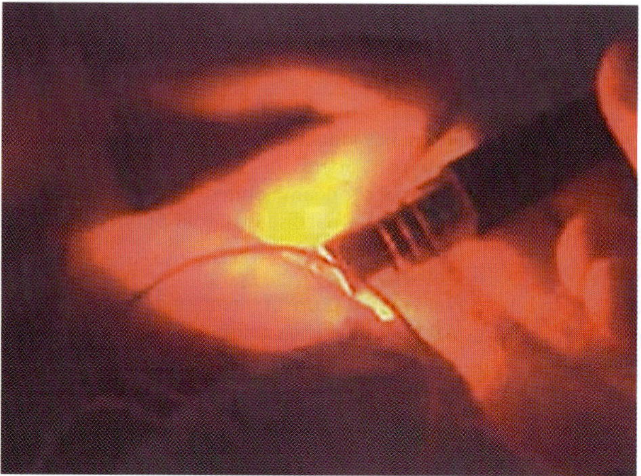

Fig. 1: Brilliant transillumination of chest in a neonate with pneumothorax

Shock

Babies in shock usually would have poor respiratory efforts, would be limp and have poor palpable pulses. History of acute bleeding such as severe vaginal bleeding in the mother or accidental rupture of the cord during delivery, would provide clues to a hypovolemic shock. In a baby born apneic, limp and has bradycardia in spite of adequate assisted ventilation support, the cause of shock could be myocardial injury due to prolonged intrapartum asphyxia, or pneumothorax, especially if the baby went into shock after initiating assisted ventilation. Transillumination (**Fig. 1**) of the chest wall in the delivery room can help diagnose pneumothorax. It is important to identify the etiology of shock in the delivery room since each of them have different treatment modalities.

Congenital Malformations

Central nervous system (CNS) malformations can present with abnormal facies, absent scalp vault (anencephaly), large head (hydrocephalus) swelling over spine (meningomyelocele). Cardiac malformations can present with cyanosis, respiratory distress, heart failure, hepatomegaly, murmur and cardiogenic shock. Airway abnormalities can present with grunt, stridor, cyanosis, respiratory distress, scaphoid abdomen (CDH), and drooling of saliva (TEF).

Birth Injuries

In babies who are macrosomic, those who have been delivered by breech extraction or assisted instrumental deliveries, should be examined for evidence of birth trauma. Inability to move the upper limbs or an asymmetric Moro reflex may indicate either Erb's or Klumpke's paralysis. Abnormal contour of the limbs and decreased movement could indicate fractures of the long bones. Paradoxical breathing could indicate a diaphragmatic paralysis (phrenic nerve palsy). There could be soft injuries such as bruising due to difficult deliveries or use of forceps; or cuts due to accidental injury during cesarean birth.

MANAGEMENT

As it is difficult to predict which neonate requires resuscitation and respiratory support in the absence of antenatal risk factors, each delivery should be attended by at least one person who has optimum training and skill in newborn resuscitation. Also, it is necessary to have extra personnel with expertise in advanced resuscitative skills for high risk deliveries. Successful outcome of neonatal resuscitation depends on a team approach. Ideally, a team leader should be identified, who can anticipate and implement the plan of resuscitation, possess effective communication skills, and is able to delegate a specific task to each team member. Before each newborn delivery, availability and functional status of resuscitation equipment needs to be checked and ensured.

Management of Baby Who Has Not Initiated Breathing at Birth

Preparation: Preparation for neonatal resuscitation starts with evaluation of each pregnancy for risk factors that can predispose to a baby not initiating breathing at birth (**Table 1**). The newborn corner should have all the equipment and supplies required for the management of such babies (**Table 5**).

Initial steps: Once the baby has been identified as not breathing and in need of resuscitation, the umbilical cord must be cut and baby separated and placed under a preheated radiant warmer in the newborn corner. **Flowchart 1** provides the neonatal resuscitation guidelines adapted for India from the International Liaison Committee on Resuscitation (ILCOR) 2015 guidelines.[4] The baby must be positioned with neck slightly extended by placing a shoulder roll. A gentle thorough suction of the mouth, oropharynx followed by that of nose should be done with a mucus extractor (or any other suction device available). Deep pharyngeal suction should be avoided, as it can result in vagal stimulation and can lead to apnea and bradycardia. *Routine suction is not recommended in vigorous neonates.* If the infant is still not breathing, then tactile stimulus by flicking the soles or rubbing the back may be carried out to initiate breathing.

Assessment of baby: After providing initial steps, the baby's breathing and heart rate should be assessed.

Table 5: Equipment required for neonatal resuscitation

A. For providing warmth - Radiant warmer - Plastic wraps, blankets, caps - Pre warmed linen **B. For suction and airway maintenance** - Mucus extractor - Suction machines/central wall mounted suction facility - Suction catheters 5F, 6F, 8F, 10F, 12F - Shoulder roll - Oropharyngeal airway (size 0,00 or 30, 40 mm lengths)	**C. For positive pressure and ventilation** - Self-inflating bag (250 mL 500 mL)/T piece resuscitator - Face masks for term and preterm (size 0, 1) - Oxygen source - Compressed air source - Oxygen blender (with flows up to 10 L/min) - Pulse oximeter with probe - Cardiac monitors/electrodes (optional) - Clock with seconds hand **D. For intubation** - Laryngoscope with straight blades # 0 and 1 - Endotracheal tubes—2.5, 3.0, 3.5 and 4.0 mm internal diameter - Extra batteries - Stethoscope - Laryngeal mask airway (desirable) - Scissors and tape for securing endotracheal tube	**E. Medications** - Epinephrine (1:1000) - Fluid for volume expansion—0.9% saline or Ringer's Lactate - Dextrose (10%) **F. Supplies** - Umbilical catheterization tray with 3.5F and 5F catheters - Syringes (1.0, 3.0, 5.0, 10.0, and 20.0 mL), needles (18 to 25G), T-connectors, and stopcocks - 10% dextrose for hypoglycemia after resuscitation - Food grade plastic wrap (for preterm babies)

Box 1: Routine essential care after birth

- Examine the baby for malformations/birth injury
- Place an identity label on baby
- Give Inj. Vitamin K $_1$ mg IM (0.5 mg for preterm)
- Weigh the baby
- Place baby between mother's breast to start skin-to-skin care
- Initiate breastfeeding

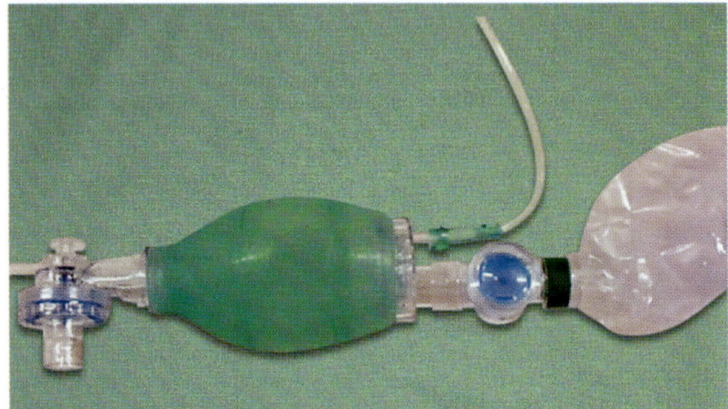

Fig. 2: Self-inflating bag with oxygen tubing and reservoir
Source: Reprinted with permission from National Neonatology Forum (NNF), India

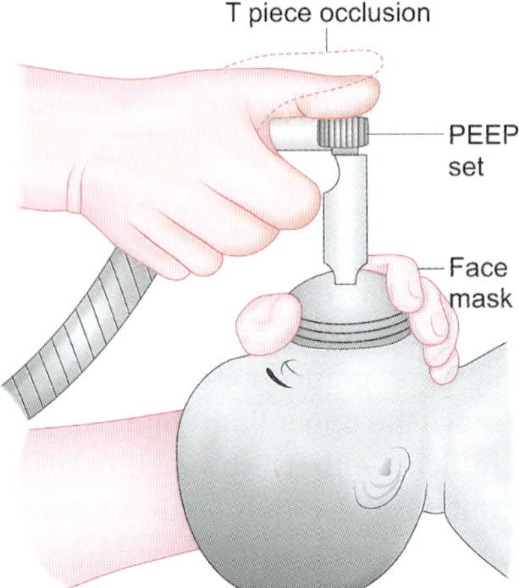

Fig. 3: T-piece resuscitator
(PEEP: positive end-expiratory pressure)
Source: Reprinted with permission from National Neonatology Forum (NNF), India

- *Baby has good breathing efforts and the heart rate is more than 100 beats/min.* Provide routine essential care as described in **Box 1**.
- *Baby has poor breathing efforts/is apneic or has a heart rate less than 100 beats/min.* Positive pressure ventilation (PPV) with bag and mask (**Fig. 2**) or T-piece resuscitator (**Fig. 3**) must be initiated. The team must also connect a pulse oximeter to the right wrist of the baby to assess level of oxygenation.

Positive pressure ventilation: PPV should be provided at a rate of about 40 breaths/min. In term babies, PPV should be initiated with 21% oxygen and then titrated based on oximetry readings. In preterm babies too it is advisable to initiate PPV with room air and then subsequently titrate with pulse oximetry readings. Current recommendations do not recommend use of oxygen concentrations greater than 65% even in preterm babies. The oxygen concentration should be titrated to maintain target oxygen saturations outlined in **Table 4**. The baby should be assessed for effectiveness of PPV after 30 seconds of the procedure.

- *Effective ventilation* is indicated by increase in heart rate, appearance of spontaneous breathing efforts, improvement in color and muscle tone. PPV can be stopped when baby has good spontaneous breathing efforts and has a heart rate greater than 100 beats/min.
- *Baby is not improving*, i.e. no spontaneous breathing or no rise in heart rate, then the following actions should be considered based on the assessment of the baby:
  - *If the heart rate is more than 60 beats/min but less than 100 beats/min.* Continue PPV as long as the baby is improving and reassess every 30–40 sec.
  - *If the baby's heart rate is below 60 beats/min despite 30 sec of effective PPV.* Continue PPV, increase oxygen supplementation to 100% and consider initiating chest compressions.

Chest compressions: Chest compressions would need at least two healthcare personnel as chest compression has to be coordinated with ventilation. The baby should preferably be intubated (**Fig. 4**) before commencing chest compressions. For every PPV breath that is provided, three chest compressions should be provided (1:3 ratio). Chest compression should be continued for at least 1 min before the baby is reassessed. Chest compressions are best administered using the two-thumb technique as it has been shown to result in higher blood pressure and coronary perfusion pressure, and results in less fatigue for the health-care provider. Chest compressions are discontinued when heart rate goes above 60 beats/min. However, if the heart-rate remains less than 60 beats/min, one must consider use of medications.

Drug therapy: *Epinephrine* is indicated when the heart rate does not go above 60 beats/min after PPV and chest compressions. It is administered intravenously in a dose of 0.1–0.3 mL/kg of a 1:10,000 solution.

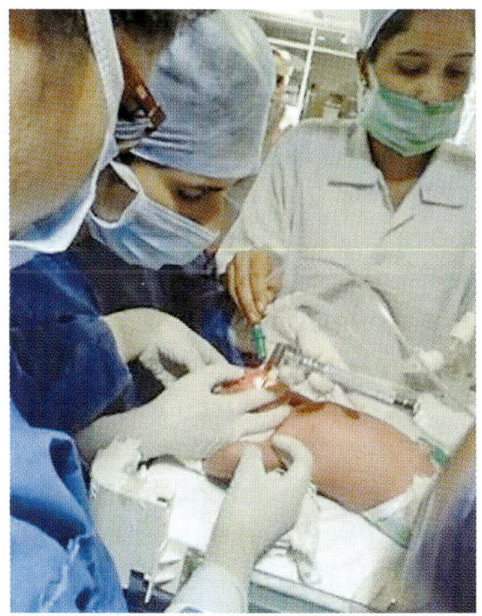

Fig. 4: Endotracheal intubation

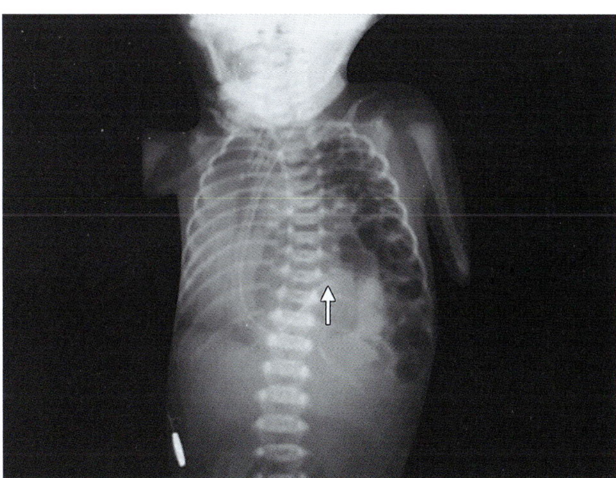

Fig. 5: Congenital diaphragmatic hernia (left side)

Naloxone (dose 0.1 mg/kg) administration should be considered when there is maternal opiate exposure about 4 hours before the delivery and results in respiratory depression in the baby.[5] Give *flumazenil* (dose 200 µg/kg) for benzodiazepine associated respiratory depression. Magnesium sulfate toxicity in the baby presents as generalized hypotonia and areflexia along with respiratory depression and a dose of intravenous calcium gluconate (2 mL/kg) can be given over 5–10 minutes.

Resuscitation of preterm babies: Babies who are born preterm need additional strategies to stabilize them in the delivery room soon after birth. Drying the baby and placing the baby under the radiant warmer may not be sufficient to prevent heat loss in babies born before 32 weeks gestation. It is currently recommended that these newborn infants, rather than being dried, should be covered or wrapped up to their neck in polythene plastic immediately after birth and the head covered with a cap.

Discontinuation of resuscitation: If there is no heart rate despite of all the resuscitative steps outlined above, resuscitation efforts may be discontinued. Further when very low birth weight and gestation, or severe congenital anomalies are unlikely to survive or are likely to have unacceptable high morbidity if they survive, resuscitation may be withheld.

Management of Baby Who Has Respiratory Distress

- A baby with respiratory distress must have a pulse oximeter probe connected to the right wrist of the baby to assess level of oxygenation. If the baby's oxygen saturation is below the target level as indicated in **Table 4**, supplemental oxygen either by nasal prongs or head box should be provided.
- *In a preterm baby who has grunting and/or chest retractions*, continuous positive end expiratory pressure (CPAP) should be initiated in the delivery room itself. CPAP may be initiated with a CPAP pressure of 5 cm H_2O and an FiO_2 of 0.5. The oxygenation may be titrated based on pulse oximetry readings and targeted to be between 87% and 93%. A 5F or 6F orogastric tube must be inserted to prevent gastric distention.
- *If CDH is suspected*, bag and mask ventilation should be avoided and the baby must be intubated and provided PPV. CDH can be confirmed on a chest skiagram (**Fig. 5**).
- *If the baby has a choanal atresia*, an oropharyngeal airway should be inserted.
- *If the baby has Pierre Robin anomaly*, the baby should be placed prone to allow the tongue to fall forward to clear the airway for breathing. If this does not help, a 2.5 mm ID endotracheal tube may be inserted through one of the nostril with the tip deep in the nasopharynx (behind the tongue and above the laryngeal inlet).
- *If pleural effusion is suspected (as in baby with hydrops fetalis or chylothorax)* fluid needs to be aspirated from the pleural cavity. An 18G or 20G percutaneous intracath can be used to drain the fluid. The needle should be inserted at the fourth intercostal space in the anterior axillary line on the side on which fluid collection is suspected. Once the needle enters the pleural space, the needle is removed from the intracath and connected to a 3-way stopcock connected to a 10 or 20 mL syringe. An X-ray chest should be done after

the procedure to ascertain the amount of residual fluid and the expansion of the lung.

- *If a pneumothorax is suspected*: The same can be screened for by transillumination of the chest. A bright source of light is held against the side of chest where pneumothorax is suspected. The ipsilateral side to the pneumothorax will appear brighter than the contralateral side. In preterm, one has to be cautious while interpreting the observations, since the thin chest wall in these babies may cause both sides to be equally bright. A chest skiagram would be confirmatory of a pneumothorax (**Fig. 6**). If it is causing significant respiratory distress or is affecting lung expansion during PPV, the air should be drained as mentioned for pleural effusion. If even after draining the air, the baby continues to have severe respiratory distress or SpO_2 is not improving, a thoracostomy tube would have to be inserted for continuous drainage of the air from the pleural cavity.
- All babies with respiratory distress should be shifted to the neonatal intensive care unit as soon as the baby is stabilized in the delivery room.

Management of Shock in Delivery Room

- A neonate in shock should first be stabilized by providing effective respiratory support which may include intubation and positive pressure ventilation (as described for managing babies who have not initiated breathing after birth).
- *Umbilical venous cannulation*: There is a need to have a secure vascular access to manage neonates with shock for administration of medication and fluids. In all such babies, an umbilical venous cannulation must be done using a 3.5F or 5F umbilical cannula, and secured adequately to prevent any accidental dislocation.

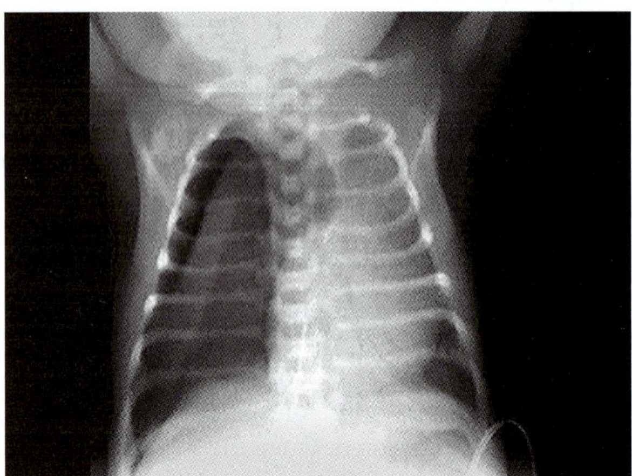

Fig. 6: Right side pneumothorax

- *History of maternal antepartum/intrapartum hemorrhage or accidental rupture of umbilical cord*: When hypovolemia is the likely cause of shock, the immediate treatment includes infusion of crystalloids for volume expansion - normal saline or Ringer's lactate. The fluid in a dose of 10 mL/kg loaded in a 20 mL syringe should be infused over about 10 minutes. A repeat dose may be considered if the baby does not show improvement in signs of shock.[6]
- *Fetal anemia (Rhesus isoimmunization)*: If a fetus with severe anemia is anticipated, O Rh-negative packed red blood cells, cross-matched with the mother should be arranged before the delivery. If not arranged before delivery, one may request for O Rh-negative uncross matched blood from the blood bank on emergency basis.
- *Vasopressors*: Use of vasopressor is infrequent in the delivery room and vasopressor therapy should be considered if inadequate response is seen despite two fluid boluses of 10 mL/kg. Dopamine, dobutamine and epinephrine are frequently used vasopressors.[6]

Management of Babies with Major Congenital Malformations

Certain airway anomalies can create an emergency in the delivery room. Upper airway anomalies including choanal atresia, laryngeal web, laryngeal stenosis, bilateral vocal cord palsy, tracheal stenosis, and tracheomalacia can present with significant respiratory distress. Other airway anomalies like cystic hygroma, hemangioma, lymphangioma, macroglossia, Pierre Robin sequence and Treacher Collins syndrome can cause difficulty in resuscitation **(Flowchart 1)**. In a neonate with suspected airway anomaly, if the baby is having spontaneous breathing, consider placing airway adjuncts such as nasopharyngeal airway to maintain airway patency. If the baby is in significant respiratory distress, start PPV with bag and mask ventilation (BMV) while preparing for endotracheal intubation. Emergent tracheostomy is indicated if BMV is ineffective and difficult to intubate the baby. BMV role is limited in babies with congenital diaphragmatic hernia (CDH) and requires immediate endotracheal intubation.

In neonates with *gastroschisis* avoid direct trauma and ischemic injury to the eviscerated organs. The eviscerated

Flowchart 1: Neonatal resuscitation algorithm

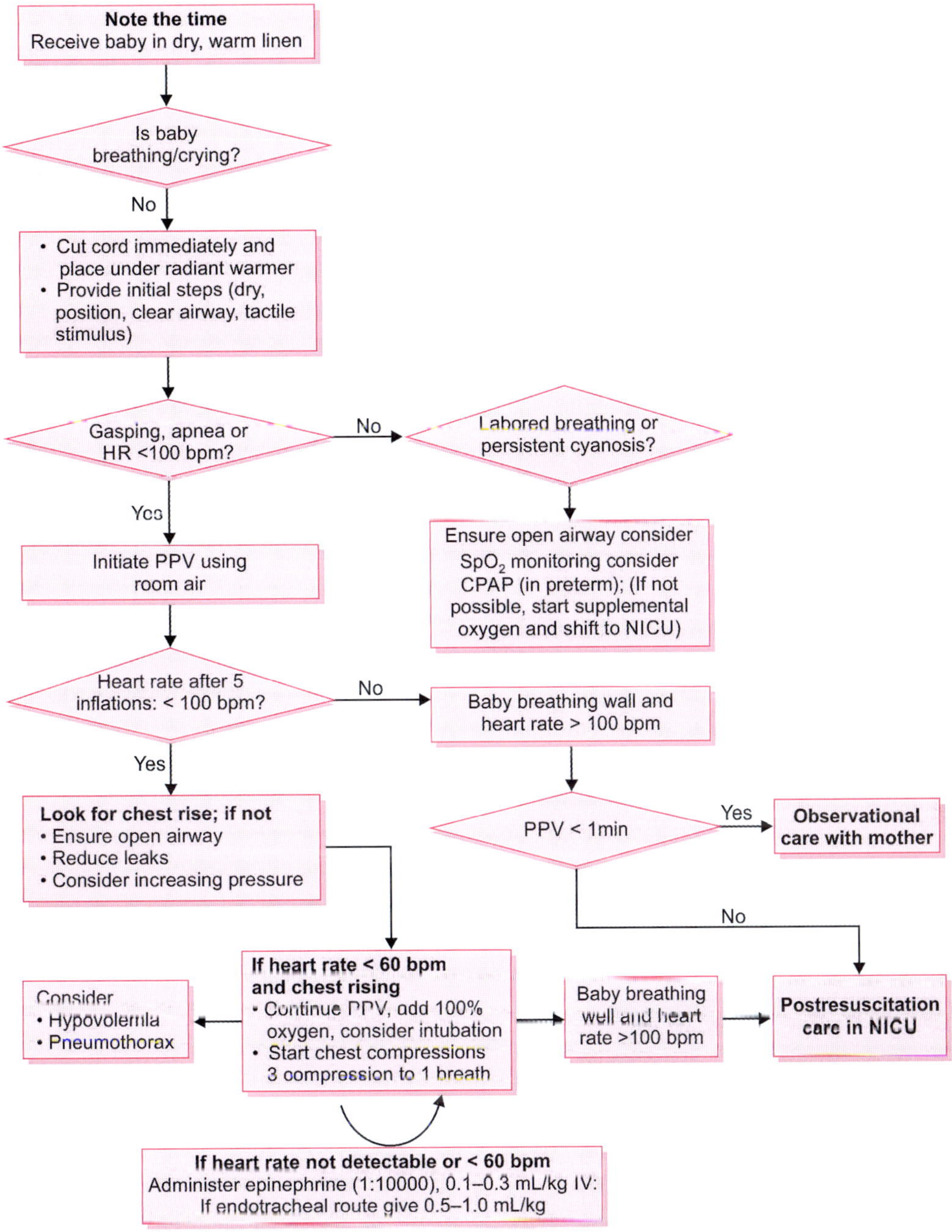

Note the time
Receive baby in dry, warm linen

↓

Is baby breathing/crying?

No ↓

- Cut cord immediately and place under radiant warmer
- Provide initial steps (dry, position, clear airway, tactile stimulus)

↓

Gasping, apnea or HR <100 bpm?

- No → Labored breathing or persistent cyanosis? → Ensure open airway consider SpO_2 monitoring consider CPAP (in preterm); (If not possible, start supplemental oxygen and shift to NICU)
- Yes ↓

Initiate PPV using room air

↓

Heart rate after 5 inflations: < 100 bpm?

- No → Baby breathing wall and heart rate > 100 bpm → PPV < 1min
  - Yes → **Observational care with mother**
  - No → **Postresuscitation care in NICU**
- Yes ↓

Look for chest rise; if not
- Ensure open airway
- Reduce leaks
- Consider increasing pressure

↓

If heart rate < 60 bpm and chest rising
- Continue PPV, add 100% oxygen, consider intubation
- Start chest compressions 3 compression to 1 breath

← Consider
- Hypovolemia
- Pneumothorax

→ Baby breathing well and heart rate >100 bpm → **Postresuscitation care in NICU**

↻ **If heart rate not detectable or < 60 bpm**
Administer epinephrine (1:10000), 0.1–0.3 mL/kg IV: If endotracheal route give 0.5–1.0 mL/kg

(PPV: positive pressure ventilation; CPAP: continuous positive airway pressure; NICU: neonatal intensive care unit; bpm: beats per minute)

gut should be immediately covered by a cling film to prevent fluid and heat loss. The baby should be nursed supine to prevent drag on the mesentery. Intravenous access should be established immediately and fluid bolus given in the delivery room. In neonate with a *large omphalocele*, the neonate should be nursed supine and the sac supported on both sides to prevent rupture. In neonates with open neural tube defects to prevent the rupture of the membranes and exposure of neural tissue, keep the baby in prone position or to the sideways. Also, apply sterile saline soaked gauze on the defect and then wrap with a plastic cover (avoid examining with a latex glove) and consider empiric antibiotic therapy to prevent infection.

Management of Birth Injuries

- *Fractures*: In case of fractures of the long bones, it should be splinted to reduce pain due to movement and handling till such time investigations and definitive treatment are initiated. Fractures can be confirmed by a skiagram (**Fig. 7**).
- *Nerve injuries*: Nerve injuries detected in the delivery room do not require active management. However, the parents and family must be informed of the injury and the subsequent proposed plan of management.
- *Laceration or cuts*: Most would need only local dressing of the wound. Deep cuts may need suturing, which should be preferably done by a trained healthcare provider after the baby is shifted from the delivery room.

OUTCOME

Outcomes of neonatal emergencies are dependent on how efficiently and effectively they are managed. A well-coordinated team if it can provide effective and timely resuscitation in asphyxiated babies can prevent mortality and improve long-term outcomes. Respiratory distress also would need effective ventilatory support to minimize hypoxia and prompt identification of the underlying cause.

PREVENTION

Early identification of high-risk pregnancies, timely referral of complicated pregnancies to the tertiary care centers equipped with optimum facilities for the care of sick newborn can prevent majority of the delivery room emergencies. Air leaks can be prevented by judicious use of positive pressure ventilation, avoiding high peak inspiratory pressure and PEEP.[7] Timely performance of C-section in at risk deliveries (obstructed labor, face presentation, abnormal position, transverse lie, large babies) can prevent birth trauma to a major extent. Also careful delivery of macrosomic babies can prevent bony injuries like clavicular fracture and also Erb's palsy.

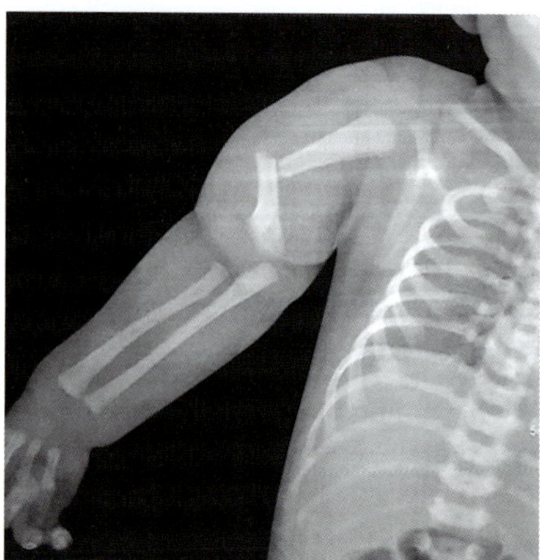

Fig. 7: Fracture humerus

KEY MESSAGES

- Although, majority of the neonates have a smooth adaptation to extrauterine life, about 10% of neonates require some assistance to initiate breathing.
- Each delivery should be attended by at least one person who has optimum training and skilled in newborn resuscitation.
- In term babies resuscitation should be initiated with 21% oxygen and in preterm babies less than 35 weeks of gestation, resuscitate with 21–30% oxygen preferably with oxygen saturation monitoring.
- Effective positive pressure ventilation is the key foundation for neonatal resuscitation.
- Respiratory distress and its etiology must be promptly identified and managed with CPAP (in preterm) and if needed intubation and PPV.
- Shock in the neonates will need umbilical vascular access and fluid boluses.
- Major life-threating malformations must be identified and provided prompt supportive care.

REFERENCES

1. Sankar MJ, Neogi SB, Sharma J, *et al.* State of newborn health in India. J Perinatol. 2016;36:S3-S8.
2. Bhide P, Kar A. A national estimate of the birth prevalence of congenital anomalies in India: Systematic review and meta-analysis. BMC Pediatr. 2018;18(1):175.
3. Weiner GM, editor. Textbook of Neonatal Resuscitation, 7th edition. American Academy of Pediatrics and American Heart Association: Illinois; 2016.
4. Wyckoff MH, Aziz K, Escobedo MB, *et al.* Part 13: Neonatal Resuscitation: 2015 American Heart Association Guidelines Update for Cardiopulmonary Resuscitation and Emergency Cardiovascular Care. Circulation. 2015;132: S543-60.
5. Moe-Byrne T, Brown JVE, McGuire W. Naloxone for opioid-exposed newborn infants. Cochrane Database Syst Rev. 2018;10:CD003483.
6. Wynn JL, Wong HR. Pathophysiology and treatment of septic shock in neonates. Clin Perinatol. 2010;37(2):439-79.
7. Ramesh Bhat Y, Ramdas V. Predisposing factors, incidence and mortality of pneumothorax in neonates. Minerva Pediatr. 2013;65(4):383-8.

CHAPTER

69

Approach to a Sick Newborn

Siddarth Ramji

INTRODUCTION

Neonatal mortality continues to be the major contributor to deaths among under-five children. A large proportion of these deaths occur in low and middle income countries (LMIC), which contributed to 98% of the 2.6 million neonatal deaths worldwide in 2016.[1] Most deaths amongst sick infants brought to hospitals occur within the first 24 hours. Many of these deaths can be prevented if very sick infants are identified soon after they arrive at the hospital and appropriate treatment is started immediately. The recent UNICEF-WHO joint report indicates that of the 2.5 million newborns who died in 2017, some died because they received poor quality care and some because they received no care at all.[2] A survey of district and teaching hospitals from 7 developing countries revealed that two-thirds of the hospitals lacked an adequate setting for priority screening (or triage).[3] This was evidenced by poor initial patient assessment and delay in treatment. Most emergency treatment areas were poorly organized and lacked essential supplies (families being required to buy essential drugs before they could be administered). It was also observed that most personnel had inadequate knowledge and skill for managing these children. There is thus a need for initial triage, emergency care, assessment and monitoring if mortality amongst sick newborn infants is to be reduced.

EPIDEMIOLOGY

A recent household survey from Bangladesh[4] reported that about 31% of neonates <28 days reported an illness and a third of them had more than one symptom. Two-third reported to have had fever, 28.1% had difficult or fast breathing, 27.8% had low temperature, 13.4% reported poor feeding and 10.4% had chest in-drawing. Ijaz *et al.*[5] in a recent study from a Karachi hospital reported that 29.8% of emergency visits were neonates <28 days, with 22.5% being preterm babies and 25% being low birth weight. The most common presenting symptom was a respiratory problem (30.5%), followed by fever (16.2%), poor feeding (14.1%), diarrhea (12.8%), jaundice (11.6%), and convulsions (5.9%). Neonates under 10 days of age have a relatively high risk of serious illness with about 10–33% needing hospitalization.[6] This early presentation has been further compounded by the early discharge of neonates from hospitals.

CLINICAL FEATURES

Every infant on arrival at the hospital should be assessed for symptoms and signs that are indicative of serious illness and adverse outcome, and thus form the criteria for immediate hospitalization of these infants. There have been several studies that have evaluated the sensitivity and specificity of clinical signs in predicting serious illness and the need for hospitalization. In a study by Singhi *et al.*[7] in sick young infants less than 2 months old, decreased activity, abnormal cry, presence of pallor, fast breathing, decreased consolability and consciousness level had a sensitivity of >90% and a negative predictive value of >95% for prediction of an adverse outcome. Altered consciousness level followed by poor feeding and color were the most important predictors of outcome. In an attempt to identify the simplest symptoms and signs for use as a triaging procedure in young infants for identifying those in need of hospital intervention, Hewson *et al.*[8] observed that the presence of any one of the following markers: drowsiness, significant chest retraction, generalized pallor, history of poor feeding or decreased activity, had a sensitivity of 91% and a specificity of 72%. Another recent study has also affirmed that drowsiness, breathing difficulty, pallor and fever identified 82% of babies deemed to be subsequently seriously ill.[9]

Emergency Triage Assessment and Treatment

Table 1 provides the list of symptoms or signs when present alone or together, suggests serious illness and the immediate need for hospitalization. These signs therefore could be used for emergency triage assessment and treatment. Tamburlini *et al.*[10] evaluated a simplified algorithm for emergency triage assessment and treatment (ETAT). The ETAT assessment algorithm had a group who had an emergency condition needing immediate treatment (the signs included in this group were severe respiratory distress, shock, coma and convulsions). The other group were those with priority signs requiring hospitalization but not emergency treatment (the signs included were non-severe respiratory distress, severe pallor, lethargy, irritability, severe wasting or edema). It was observed that about 3% infants attending the emergency room had signs of an emergency condition and they constituted 37% of all in-patient admissions. There were 17% infants who had priority signs and this group made up about 48% of all in-patient admissions. When this algorithm was administered by nurses in infants < 1 month of age, it had a sensitivity of 82.2% and specificity of 89.2% in identifying those in need of emergency treatment and those needing priority assessment.

Table 1: Clinical symptoms/signs suggesting serious illness

- Drowsiness/coma
- Convulsions
- Shock
- Breathing difficulty (apnea, gasping, fast breathing > 60/ min, severe chest retractions)
- Decreased feeding, decreased activity
- Severe jaundice (palms and soles stained)
- Severe pallor
- Bleeding

Emergency Triage

All infants must be initially assessed for signs needing emergency care. These signs include:

- Gasping breathing or apnea
- Severe respiratory distress
- Central cyanosis/ SpO_2 <85%
- Shock (poor perfusion indicated by cool peripheries with capillary refill longer than 3 seconds and weak, fast pulse). Blood pressures may be normal is some of these neonates.
- Coma (these infants are unconscious and do not respond to stimuli)
- Convulsions
- Bleeding.

Presence of these signs requires immediate emergency treatment. **Flowchart 1** gives the outline on how to carry out an emergency assessment and treatment.

Flowchart 1: Emergency assessment and treatment

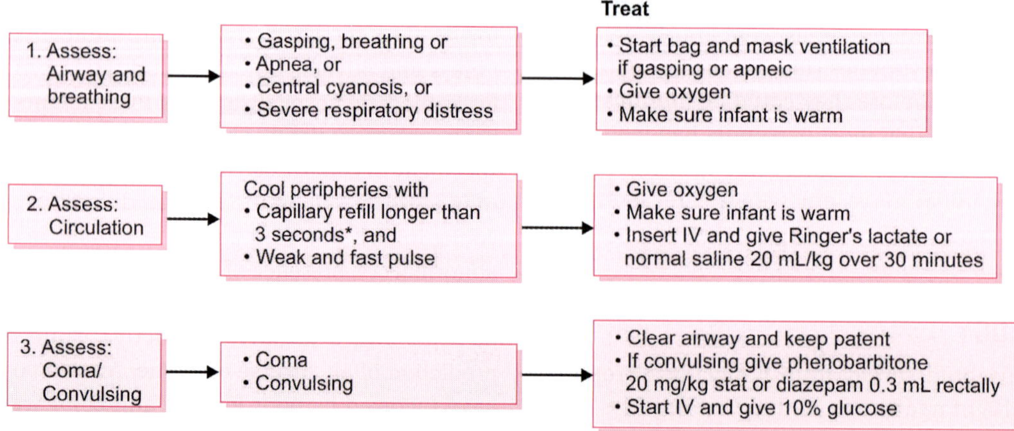

** Capillary refill is assessed over the sternum*

BREASTFEEDING PROBLEMS PRESENTING IN THE EMERGENCY ROOM

Early discharge of newborns from the hospital by 48 hours often results in mothers bringing in their newborns with breastfeeding problems to the emergency room.[11] Any difficulty mentioned by the mother is important. Breastfeeding difficulties mentioned by the mother may include her infant feeds too frequently, not frequently, she does not have enough milk, her nipples are sore, she has flat or everted nipples, or infant does not want to take to the breast. The other common complaints with which they present include excessive crying by the baby (often due to colic) and failure to thrive. If a mother says that the infant is not able to feed, assess breastfeeding or watch her try to feed the infant with a cup to see what she means by this. An infant who is not able to feed may have a serious infection or other life-threatening problem and needs immediate hospitalization. Most often the problem of insufficient milk is more a "maternal perception" than a reality. It requires careful assessment of breastfeeding (**Table 2**). Observe the baby's attachment, position and sucking at the breast. Most often these problems are related to faulty feeding techniques, insufficient feeding frequency and inadequate emptying of both breasts during feeding.

Table 2: Assessment of an infant's breastfeeding

Ask: • Has the infant breastfed in the previous hour?	If the infant has not fed in the previous hour, ask the mother to put her infant to the breast. Observe her breastfeed for 4 minutes If the infant was fed during the last hour, ask the mother if she can wait and tell you when the infant is willing to feed again • Is the infant able to attach? Classify as: *No attachment at all, Not well attached, Good attachment* To check attachment, Look for: – *Chin touching breast* – *Mouth wide open* – *Lower lip turned outward* – *More areola visible above than below the mouth* (All of these signs should be present if the attachment is good) • Is the infant suckling effectively (that is, slow deep sucks, sometimes pausing)? Classify as: *Not suckling at all, Not suckling effectively, Suckling effectively* • Clear a blocked nose if it interferes with breastfeeding • Look for ulcers or white patches in the mouth (thrush)

Rarely, it can also be due to a blocked nose or oral thrush. These problems are seen both in term and preterm babies but are probably more common amongst low birth weight babies who are born at home or babies who have been discharged from hospital prior to 72 hours after birth. Careful assessment and counseling in the emergency room can solve most of these problems. The rest may require hospitalization.

DIFFERENTIAL DIAGNOSIS

After the initial assessment has been completed, consider the various conditions that could cause the infant's illness. The detailed history of the neonate's illness, the mother's antepartum and intrapartum course and family history are necessary to arrive at the likely cause of the neonate's illness.

The most common presenting acute problems in a young infant presenting in the emergency room usually are:

- *Unconsciousness, lethargy* or *convulsions*
- *Respiratory distress*
- *Diarrhea or blood in stools*: In the neonate, blood in stools in the first 5 days could be due to hemorrhagic disease of the newborn which is due to vitamin K deficiency, and after 7 days it could be due to surgical conditions such as necrotizing enterocolitis.

The common conditions presenting with an alteration in sensorium, activity or convulsions are listed in **Table 3**. The most common conditions in the first week of life include birth asphyxia/trauma, kernicterus, hypoglycemia, intracranial hemorrhage and infections (especially sepsis and meningitis). After the first week, infections dominate the conditions causing these signs.

Table 4 provides a brief differential diagnosis to infants presenting with respiratory distress. The most common conditions in the first week include respiratory distress syndrome, pneumonia and sepsis. After the first week, infections (especially pneumonia) are the predominant cause.

Infection

Infections can present with a range of clinical features – minor to very serious signs such as shock. While fever is an important sign of infection, it is an uncommon presentation in preterm infants with sepsis. Every ill neonate should be considered to be septic, unless proven otherwise.

Table 3: Differential diagnosis of infant presenting with lethargy, unconsciousness or convulsion

Diagnosis or underlying cause	*Supporting information*
Birth asphyxia/ Hypoxic ischemic encephalopathy	• Onset in first 3 days of life • Delayed cry at birth • Need for PPV in delivery room
Birth trauma	• Abnormal/difficult labor • Instrumental delivery
Intracranial hemorrhage	• Onset in first 3 days in low birth weight or preterm infant
Hemolytic disease of newborn/ Kernicterus	• Onset in first 3 days • Jaundice • Pallor
Hypoglycemia	• Onset in first 3 days • Low birth weight baby • Serious bacterial infection
Inborn error of metabolism	• Previously well neonate • Onset of illness after feeding initiated • Family history of unexplained sibling deaths in newborn period • Family history of consanguinity
Neonatal tetanus	• Onset at day 3–14 days • Irritability • Difficulty in breastfeeding • Trismus • Convulsions
Meningitis	• Lethargy • Apneic episodes • Convulsions • High-pitched cry • Bulging fontanelle
Sepsis	• Fever or hypothermia • Shock • Seriously ill with no apparent cause

Congenital Heart Disease

The congenital heart diseases (CHDs) that generally present in the neonatal period include left sided obstructive lesions (e.g. hypoplastic left heart syndrome, coarctation of aorta), right sided obstructive lesions (e.g. tricuspid atresia, tetralogy of Fallot) and mixed lesions with increased pulmonary blood flow (e.g. transposition of great arteries). *CHD should be suspected in any neonate who was previously healthy and presents with respiratory distress and/or shock.*[6]

Table 4: Differential diagnosis of infant with respiratory distress

Diagnosis or underlying information	*Supporting information*
Respiratory distress syndrome (hyaline membrane disease)	• Preterm birth • Onset within 1 hour of birth • Lower chest in-drawing • Grunting • Fast breathing
Sepsis/Pneumonia	• Lethargy • Hyper or hypothermia • Difficulty in breastfeeding • Difficult breathing
Congenital cardiac disease	• Difficult breathing • Difficulty in breastfeeding • Cyanosis • Shock • Hepatomegaly • Gallop rhythm • Cardiomegaly
Meningitis	• Lethargy • Apneic episodes • Convulsions • High-pitched cry • Bulging fontanelle
Neonatal tetanus	• Onset at day 3–14 days • Irritability • Difficulty in breastfeeding • Trismus • Convulsions

Gastrointestinal Emergencies

Vomiting (particularly bilious) and abdominal distension are important indicators of a gastrointestinal emergency which could include necrotizing enterocolitis, volvulus or intestinal obstruction at any level. *Bilious vomiting should be considered a surgical emergency unless proved otherwise.*

Inborn Error of Metabolism (IEM)

The clinical presentations of IEM are nonspecific and could overlap with that of neonatal sepsis. IEM should be suspected especially in a well neonate who becomes ill after a symptom free period and rapidly deteriorates with no apparent cause or where there is a family history of an unexplained sibling death or developmental delay.[12]

Mnemonic

Kim *et al.*[13] have proposed a mnemonic that could be a valuable aid to determine the etiology in a sick neonate presenting to the emergency department—"NEO SECRETS"

- N: i**N**born errors if metabolism
- E: **E**lectrolyte abnormalities
- O: **O**verdose (toxins, drugs)
- S: **S**eizures
- E: **E**nteric emergencies
- C: **C**ardiac emergencies
- R: **R**ecipes (additives, herbs)
- E: **E**ndocrine emergencies
- T: **T**rauma
- S: **S**epsis

MANAGEMENT

If any of the emergency triage signs are present, initiate treatment, call for help into the emergency room and take blood samples for laboratory investigations (glucose, hemoglobin, blood group, smear). Treatment that must be urgently initiated in the emergency room is outlined in **Flowchart 1**.

Initial Stabilization

Positive pressure ventilation (PPV)

In infants with *gasping respiration or apnea (not breathing even when stimulated)*, immediate positive pressure ventilation with bag and mask/T-piece resuscitator, must be initiated to establish and maintain adequate ventilation. If the oxygen saturations are <85% on pulse oximetry (SpO_2) after 1 minute of PPV consider giving supplemental oxygen using a blender to maintain the SpO_2 between 85–93%. If the infant does not establish adequate spontaneous respiration, it would be necessary to intubate the infant and continue assisted ventilation till the infant is stabilized and can be transferred to an intensive care facility.

Oxygen therapy

In infants with *cyanosis, severe respiratory distress and shock*, supplemental oxygen therapy must be initiated with a facemask, head box or nasal cannula. Care must be taken to ensure that the oxygen is humidified and warmed. If oxygen is being bubbled through a bottle of warm water, care must be taken to ensure that the water is frequently changed with warm water. If oxygen is being administered by head box, the minimum oxygen flow in the head box needs to be at least 2–3 L/min to prevent accumulation of exhaled carbon dioxide. With a head box, oxygen concentration delivered can be up to 80–90%. When oxygen is administered by a nasal cannula, a flow rate of 0.5 L/min provides about 25% oxygen, while 2 L/min can deliver up to 40% oxygen. Provide sufficient oxygen till the baby becomes pink or if a pulse oximeter is available, to raise the oxygen saturation up to 88–95%.

Clear airway

In infants who are *comatose or those who are convulsing*, it is important that the airways are kept patent. This is achieved by suctioning out secretions and appropriately positioning the infant with slight neck extension (facilitated by placing a one-inch thick shoulder roll). Placing the baby in a lateral position can also help by preventing obstruction due to falling back of tongue or pooling of secretions.

Bleeding

If visible bleeding is present stop it, if possible (if bleeding from umbilical cord, reclamp/retie the cord; if from a cut or male circumcision, press the bleeding site with sterile compress).

Establish vascular access and provide fluids

Once ventilation and oxygenation have been stabilized, it is important that a vascular access is established. If a peripheral venous access cannot be established, the possibility of umbilical venous cannulation or intraosseous route must be considered.

- *Shock present*: If the baby is in shock, then 20 mL/kg of Ringer's lactate or normal saline should be infused over 20–30 minutes. If there is no response to volume expansion and there is an obvious cause for hypovolemia such as diarrhea, persistent vomiting or bleeding, further volume administration can be attempted (up to 2 more doses of volume expansion with 10 mL/kg over 20–30 minutes). If shock persists in spite of adequate volume expansion, ionotrope administration with dopamine or dobutamine must be considered.
- *Shock due to bleeding*: If the shock is not improving in spite of volume replacement, then arrange and administer blood transfusion. In an emergency type O, Rh negative blood can be used for transfusion.

- *No shock*: If there is no perfusion problem, fluids must be initiated with 10% dextrose with a volume appropriate for the infant's age as provided below:
  - Day 1—60 mL/kg/d
  - Day 2—80 mL/kg/d
  - Day 3—100 mL/kg/d
  - Day 4—110 mL/kg/d
  - Day 5—120 mL/kg/d

  After day 2, if baby well hydrated and passing urine, electrolytes-glucose infusion can be initiated.

Prostaglandin E1

In critically sick neonates where ductus dependent cardiac lesions are suspected, it is recommended that prostaglandin E1 infusion IV in a dose of 0.05–0.1 μg/kg/min is initiated even before confirmation by echocardiography. Improvement in 15 minutes will invariably confirm the ductus dependent cardiac lesion as the cause of the critical illness.

Maintain warmth/Rewarming

Record the baby's temperature on arrival and assess for hypothermia (<36°C) or fever (temperature >38°C). Hypothermia may be a sign of cold environment or a sign of serious systemic infection in the infant. It is essential to rewarm a baby who is hypothermic as soon as possible.

- Rewarming can be achieved by placing a baby under a thermostatically controlled radiant warmer or heated mattress set at 36.5° to 37°C.
- Before rewarming, the infant's cold clothing should be removed and replaced with pre-warmed clothes and a cap/bonnet.
- If the baby does not need interventions for breathing, shock or convulsions, rewarming can be done by placing the baby in skin-to-skin contact on the mother or caregiver's chest (Kangaroo Mother Care).
- The infant's temperature should be monitored every half-hour till it returns to normal.

Control of convulsions

The initial control of convulsions requires an immediate check of the blood sugar. If that is not possible or blood sugar <40 mg/dL, administer 2–4 mL/kg of 10% glucose IV (200–400 mg/kg) as a bolus, thereafter they would need a sustained infusion of glucose at the rate of 4–6 mg/kg/min.

Hypocalcemia: If hypocalcemia is present, then 2 mL/kg of 10% calcium gluconate should be given as a slow infusion and subsequently continued as oral supplementation.

Anticonvulsant therapy: If blood sugar is normal or convulsions are not controlled with bolus glucose or calcium, then phenobarbitone at a dose of 20 mg/kg can be infused slowly over 20 minutes for seizure control. If there is no control, the drug can be repeated in a dose of 10 mg/kg. If there is no response another anticonvulsant such as phenytoin can be used in dose of 10 mg/kg or diazepam (dose 0.3 mg/kg IV or rectally) can be used.

Neonatal tetanus: If neonatal tetanus is suspected then diazepam is the drug of choice and may be required in dose of 5 mg/kg every 6 hours.

Vitamin K_1

In all sick newborns 1mg of Vitamin K_1 must be given intramuscularly or IV (if an IV access has been established), even if the infant is not bleeding.

Antibiotics

In a sick neonate, it must be assumed that all are septic, unless proved otherwise. Keeping this dictum, it would be advisable to initiate the first dose of antibiotic therapy in all sick neonates in the emergency room. The choice of antibiotic would be determined by the institution's existing protocol.

Nasogastric decompression

In all neonates with vomiting and/or abdominal distension, a nasogastric tube must be placed *in-situ* for gastric decompression.

Laboratory Investigations

The investigations that may be useful in the emergency room management are summarized here.

- *Blood sugar* should be done in all sick newborns because it may be the cause of some of the emergency signs such as convulsions or lethargy or may be an associated feature in any sick newborn. Treatment of hypoglycemia is important because of its association with poor long-term outcome especially in symptomatic newborns.
- *Serum calcium*: In neonates with seizures particularly when blood glucose values are normal.

- *Bacterial infection* is suspected as a cause of illness. Then the helpful laboratory investigations are:
  - *Blood examination* of the peripheral blood smear may be useful if increased number of immature polymorphs (> 20%) are seen along with leukopenia or leukocytosis. One can also assess the adequacy of platelets by detecting platelet clumps on peripheral smear. A total leukocyte count, micro-ESR and C-reactive protein may be useful in deciding on a positive sepsis screen.
  - *Lumbar puncture* for CSF examination and culture should be carried out if meningitis is suspected.
  - *Blood culture* should be taken in all cases before antibiotics are started.
- *Chest skiagram* is required especially in infants with respiratory distress. This may help in diagnosing hyaline membrane disease, pneumonia, air-leaks, some congenital heart diseases (estimate cardiac size, contour and pulmonary markings) or other congenital defects such a diaphragmatic hernia. It will also be useful in gastrointestinal emergencies such as NNEC and intestinal obstruction.
- *Hematocrit/hemoglobin* to diagnose anemia especially in infants with pallor.
- *Prothrombin time (PT) and partial thromboplastin time (PTT)* for those with clinical bleeding.
- *Blood grouping* for those in need of blood transfusion or exchange transfusion.
- *Serum bilirubin* in severely jaundiced newborns, because it helps in deciding the need for exchange transfusion or phototherapy.
- *Serum electrolytes*: This is particularly important when one is suspecting hypernatremic dehydration in the neonate.
- *Arterial blood gas analysis* can be useful in critically sick newborns if the facilities are available. It helps in assessing the extent of metabolic and respiratory acidosis. This would optimize further treatment of these infants especially to decide need for ventilatory support, initial management of IEMs.

PREVENTING DELAY IN EMERGENCY ROOM CARE

Delay in initiation of emergency room care of sick newborns increases their risk of mortality and long-term disability. In a study on the quality of emergency care of sick newborns, Mallick *et al.*[14] observed that following quality improvement initiatives the proportion of neonates who received emergency care with 30 minutes of arriving in triage area rose from 20% (pre-intervention) to 76% (post-intervention) and the mean (SD) time for initiation of treatment decreased from 80.8 (20.9) min to 19.8 (5.6) min post-intervention. Hospital mortality also decreased from 33% to 15% post-intervention.

All sick newborns presenting in the emergency room must be immediately assessed using a triage system to help identify those in need of emergency treatment, assessment and hospitalization. Investigations and diagnosis should be delayed till the infant is stabilized. This approach can prevent delay in institution of therapy and save many lives and prevent disability

KEY MESSAGES

- Neonates presenting in the first week of life often are critically ill and would need hospitalization.
- Emergency rooms must be well equipped to triage and initiate emergency treatment to sick newborns.
- Neonates presenting with altered consciousness, lethargy, respiratory distress, cyanosis, convulsions, shock, feeding difficulties, severe jaundice or bleeding have emergency signs and must be immediately managed.
- Sepsis, inborn errors of metabolism, cardiac, gastrointestinal and endocrine causes are most frequent reasons for presentation in the emergency room.
- Initial stabilization should address breathing, airway patency, oxygenation, maintaining blood pressure and hydration and controlling convulsions.
- All sick neonates should also receive vitamin K1 and first dose of antibiotic in the emergency room.
- Delays in initiating management of sick newborns in the emergency room increases the risk of death and long-term disability.

REFERENCES

1. UNICEF. Levels and trends in child mortality: Report; 2017. p. 2017.
2. Survive and thrive: transforming care for every small and sick newborn. Key findings. Geneva: World Health Organization; 2018 (WHO/FWC/MCA/18.11).
3. Nolan T, Angos P, Cunha AJ, *et al.* Quality of hospital care for seriously ill children in less developed countries. Lancet. 2001;357:106-10.
4. Chowdhury SK, Billah SM, Arifeen SE, *et al.* Care-seeking practices for sick neonates: Findings from cross-sectional survey in 14 rural sub-districts of Bangladesh. PLoS ONE 2018;13:e0204902.
5. Ijaz N, Strehlow M, Wang NE, *et al.* Epidemiology of patients presenting to a pediatric emergency department in Karachi, Pakistan. BMC Emergency Medicine. 2018;18:22.

6. Peréz AM, Martínez S, Corrales AY. A Practical Approach to Emergencies in the Neonatal Period. J Neonatal Biol. 2016;5:213.
7. Singhi S, Chaudhuri M. Functional and behavioral responses as marker of illness and outcome in infants under 2 months. Indian Pediatr. 1995;32:763-71.
8. Hewson PH, Gollan RA. A simple hospital triaging system for infants with acute illness. J Pediatr Child Health. 1995;31:29-32.
9. Hewson P, Poulakis Z, Jarman F, *et al*. Clinical markers of serious illness in young infants: a multicentric follow-up study. J Pediatr Child Health. 2000;36:221-5.
10. Tamburlini G, Di Mario S, Maggi S, *et al*. Evaluation of guidelines for emergency triage assessment and treatment in developing countries. Arch Dis Child. 1999;81:478-82.
11. Newman J. Breastfeeding problems presenting to the emergency department: Diagnosis and management. Pediatr Emerg Care. 1989;5:198-201.
12. Saudubray JM, Desguerre I, Sedel F, *et al*. A clinical approach to inherited metabolic diseases. In: Saudubray JM, Baumgartner, John Walter, editors. Inborn Metabolic Diseases: Diagnosis and Treatment. 6th edition. Berlin: Springer-Verlag; 2016. p. 6-10.
13. Kim UO, Brousseau DC, Konduri GG. Evaluation and management of the critically ill neonate in the emergency department. Clin Ped Emer Med. 2008;9:140-148C.
14. Mallick A, Banerjee M, Mondal B, *et al*. A quality improvement initiative for early initiation of emergency Management for sick neonates. Indian Pediatr. 2018;55:768-72.

CHAPTER

70

Respiratory Failure in Newborn

Rhishikesh P Thakre, Nandkishor S Kabra

INTRODUCTION

The unique physiology of the newborn not only predisposes them to a higher risk of respiratory morbidity but is also responsible for their rapid progression to respiratory failure needing ventilatory support. Respiratory distress and respiratory failure are the most common causes of morbidity and mortality in newborn infants, accounting for almost a third of all NICU admissions.[1-7] Early recognition of respiratory distress and its underlying etiology are critical not only for initiating appropriate supportive care but also specific (and in some cases definitive) treatments. The assessment of both etiology and severity often need laboratory support. The implications for early diagnosis and referral cannot be more explicit for facilities without the supportive aids for diagnosis and management.

EPIDEMIOLOGY AND ETIOLOGY

Respiratory conditions are the most common reason for admission to a neonatal intensive care unit in both term and preterm infants. An Indian study showed that 6.7% of all births were complicated by a respiratory disorder.[8] Respiratory distress in newborns is often due to lung and airway pathologies. In a preterm newborn, the most common cause of respiratory distress is respiratory distress syndrome - RDS (previously called as hyaline membrane disease - HMD). In a full term newborn, common causes of respiratory distress includes transient tachypnea of newborn (TTNB) and meconium aspiration syndrome (MAS). Congenital anomalies, cardiac, neurological, metabolic, hematologic and infectious etiologies also may cause respiratory distress in newborn.[1-2] **Table 1** summarizes the etiologies of neonatal respiratory distress.

Table 1: Causes of respiratory distress in newborn

Preterm newborn	*Full term newborn*	*Congenital anomalies and surgical conditions*	*Non-respiratory conditions*
Respiratory distress syndrome Pneumothorax Pneumonia Pulmonary hemorrhage Aspiration pneumonia Pleural effusion including chylothorax Chronic lung disease (CLD)/ Bronchopulmonary dysplasia (BPD)	Transient tachypnea of newborn Meconium aspiration syndrome Respiratory distress syndrome Persistent pulmonary hypertension of newborn Pneumonia Pneumothorax Aspiration pneumonia Pleural effusion including chylothorax Pulmonary hemorrhage Surfactant protein deficiency syndromes Alveolar capillary dysplasia	Congenital diaphragmatic hernia Tracheoesophageal fistula Pulmonary sequestration Congenital lobar emphysema Choanal atresia Pulmonary agenesis Pulmonary lymphangiectasis Congenital cystic adenomatoid malformation Congenital pulmonary airway malformations Asphyxiating thoracic dystrophy	CVS: Heart failure due to congenital heart disease CNS: Perinatal asphyxia, hypoxic ischemic encephalopathy and neuromuscular disorders Metabolic: Inborn errors of metabolism including organic acidemia Hematologic: Anemia, polycythemia Infections: Sepsis, pneumonia

PATHOGENESIS AND PATHOPHYSIOLOGY

The pathophysiology of respiratory failure will vary in newborn depending on the underlying cause. Developmental disorders of the lung, effects due to transition from fetal to neonatal mode of ventilation, or complications during peripartum period significantly influence the pathogenesis of respiratory failure. Since lung development continues till at least 2 years of life, developmentally related causes due to extrauterine exposures to inflammation medicated injury as in chronic lung disease (or Bronchopulmonary dysplasia) can also contribute to neonatal respiratory failure. In the case of RDS, it is due to a deficiency of surfactant, which then leads to alveolar atelectasis resulting in decreased compliance and increased work of breathing. In MAS, it is a combination of airway obstruction, surfactant dysfunction, and chemical pneumonitis, all of which contribute to an increase in airway resistance and altered compliance; consequently, resulting in respiratory distress in the newborn. In TTNB, it is due to retained fluid in the lung, a phenomenon related to alteration in the normal transition at birth. Altered pulmonary mechanics, either as a result of increased airways resistance, decreased lung compliance or both, contributes to the clinical manifestations of respiratory distress in the newborn and the consequent respiratory failure.

CLINICAL FEATURES

Recognition of Respiratory Distress

Respiratory distress in newborn is recognized by the presence of one or more of following signs:

- *Tachypnea*: It is an increase in respiratory rate above 60/minute, It can be a compensatory mechanism for hypoxemia, or acidosis (metabolic and respiratory). It therefore is a nonspecific sign for respiratory failure.
- *Grunting*: This is an audible sound due to forced expiration against a partially closed glottis and signifies decreased lung compliance. It may be viewed as a compensatory mechanism to improved compliance by increasing end expiratory pressure. It is a definite sign of a lung pathology.
- *Chest retraction*: Subcostal, intercostal, supraclavicular, and sternal indrawing indicate increased work of breathing due to altered pulmonary mechanics.
- *Nasal flaring*: It may be seen as a compensatory mechanism to decrease airway resistance by increasing the diameter of the upper airway.
- *Central cyanosis*: This is a sign of severe hypoxemia.

Severity of Respiratory Distress

It is of paramount importance to identify the severity of respiratory distress. There are several clinical scoring tools that can be used to assess the severity of respiratory distress in newborns. The Silverman Anderson Score (SAS) is ideal for preterm infants **(Table 2)**.[9] The Downes and Vidyasagar score can be used in all newborn infants (**Table 3**).[10]

Identification of etiology: Useful information on history that would point to the possible underlying etiology is outlined in **Table 4**.

Clinical examination: The newborn infant may also be lethargic, with poor feeding and hypothermic.

Table 3: Downes and Vidyasagar score for term newborn

	RR	*Retractions*	*Cyanosis*	*Grunt*	*Air entry*
Score 0	< 60	None	None	None	Equal
Score 1	60–80	Mild to moderate	Room air	On stethoscope	Decreased
Score 2	>80	Severe	On FiO_2 > 40%	Audible	Absent

Note*: Interpret Downes and Vidyasagar scores with the status of sensorium. An improving score with alert newborn suggests improvement. An improving score with worsening sensorium suggests deterioration. Onetime assessment is not enough. Look at the trends every hour to grade the respiratory status.*

Table 2: Silverman Anderson score for preterm newborn

	Upper chest retraction	*Lower chest retraction*	*Xiphoid retraction*	*Nasal flaring*	*Expiratory grunt*
Grade 0	Synchronized	None	None	None	None
Grade 1	Lags on inspiration	Just visible	Just visible	Minimal	On stethoscope
Grade 2	See saw	Marked	Marked	Marked	Audible

Note*: Interpret Silverman and Anderson score with the status of sensorium. An improving score with alert newborn suggests improvement. An improving score with worsening sensorium suggests deterioration. Onetime assessment is not enough. Look at the trends every hour to grade the respiratory status.*

Table 4: Information to be sought in clinical history

Ask for	*Suggestive of*
Age at onset	• Onset within 6 hours of birth suggests birth process related cause • Late onset (> 3d) may suggest congenital heart disease • Abrupt onset suggests an air leak
Duration of illness	• Respiratory distress of short duration may suggest a transient problem such as TTNB • Duration of more than 2 weeks suggests a chronic problem
Progress of illness	• It may help determine whether the disease state is the same, worsening or improving
Worsening on bag and mask resuscitation	Congenital diaphragmatic hernia (CDH), air leak
Prolonged labor, difficult labor, assisted delivery, fetal distress, meconium stained liquor	Asphyxial lung disease, MAS
Positive pressure ventilation in delivery room	Air leak
Elective cesarean section	TTNB
Maternal fever, foul liquor, prolonged labor, multiple per vaginal exams, PROM > 12 hours, PPROM, assisted delivery	Congenital pneumonia, sepsis
No antenatal steroids to mother in preterm baby, infant of diabetic mother (IDM), Rh isoimmunization, perinatal asphyxia	RDS
Polyhydramnios	CDH, tracheoesophageal fistula (TEF)
Oligohydramnios	Pulmonary hypoplasia
Maternal hypertension, pre-eclampsia	Asphyxia, MAS
Placenta previa or abruption	Shock
Family history of unexplained neonatal deaths, stillbirths	RDS, IDM, congenital heart disease (CHD), inborn error of metabolism (IEM)
Post feed worsening	Gastroesophageal reflux disease (GERD), isolated cleft palate, TEF, IEM
Relation with crying	Crying worsens cyanosis (CHD), crying relieves cyanosis (choanal atresia)
Chronic course, oxygen dependency	BPD, CHD (TAPVC), atypical infection (CMV, fungus, *Pneumocystis carinii*, chlamydia), Wilson-Mikity syndrome, recurrent aspiration (GER, pharyngeal incoordination, H type TEF), osteopenia of prematurity

(TTNB: transient tachypnea of newborn; RDS: respiratory distress syndrome; PROM: prolonged rupture of membrane; PPROM: preterm premature rupture of membranes; MAS: meconium aspiration syndrome; CMV: cytomegalo virus; CHD: congenital heart defect; TAPVC: total anomalous pulmonary venous return)

As respiratory failure worsens, the infant tends to become more drowsy, perfusion begins to get impaired (cool extremities, prolonged capillary refill time beyond 3 secs, hypotension), becomes hypotonic. Additional clinical findings that may provide a clue to etiology include a scaphoid abdomen (CDH), heart sounds better heard on right than left (CDH, air leak, dextrocardia), inability to negotiate a feeding tube (esophageal atresia/TEF).

Box 1: Clues to congenital heart disease

- Cyanosis disproportionate to clinical status
- Differential cyanosis (Upper limb SpO_2> Lower limb SpO_2 by 10 mm Hg)
- Single second heart sound
- Murmur
- Isolated hepatomegaly
- Sudden deterioration and shock (possible ductus dependent lesion)
- Lack of response to oxygen (fail hyperoxia test)
- Cardiomegaly (radiological)

Pulse oximetry

In all neonates with respiratory distress, a pulse oximeter must be attached preferably in the right hand (pre-ductal region). Healthy newborns should normally maintain an SpO_2 value between 94% and 100% at room air.[11] In practice, the threshold at which oxygen supplementation is provided is often SpO_2 < 90%.[12] A labile saturation reading (on crying or movement) should suggest a right to left shunt as in PPHN.

Clues to cardiac etiology

Box 1 provides clues to a possible cardiac etiology to the respiratory distress. Hyperoxia test may be used

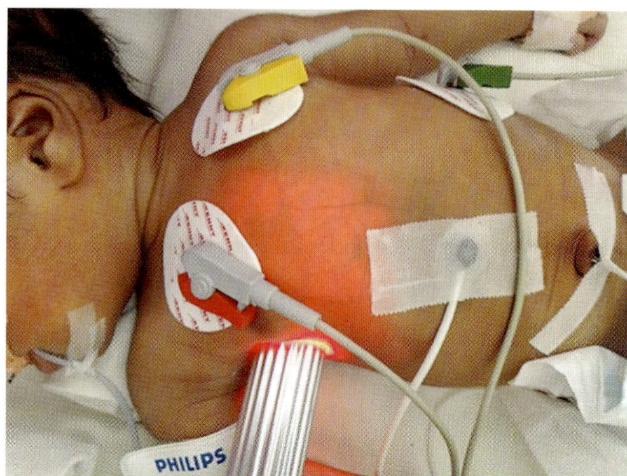

Fig. 1: Brilliant transillumination of chest indicating pneumothorax

to distinguish a respiratory from cardiac disease in a cyanosed infant. Arterial PaO_2 from a preductal arterial sample of more than 250 mm Hg after allowing the neonate to inspire 100% oxygen for 10–15 minutes virtually excludes a structural heart disease as the cause of cyanosis. Neonates who fail the hyperoxia test should undergo echocardiographic evaluation to exclude a structural cardiac defect.

Transillumination of the chest

Transillumination can be done at the bedside, which in an emergency will allow one to detect air leaks. Brilliant transillumination would indicate an air leak (**Fig. 1**)

LABORATORY INVESTIGATIONS

Investigations that could help in identifying the etiology are summarized here.

Hematological

Hemoglobin <12 g/dL should suggest anemia. A hematocrit >65% would suggests polycythemia. Sepsis screen would include total leukocyte count, absolute neutrophil count, immature-mature neutrophil ratio (I/T), acute phase reactants (C-reactive protein, procalcitonin). Neutropenia, I/T > 0.2, elevated CRP or procalcitonin are indicative of an infection if at least two of the laboratory values are abnormal. It should be done when history and clinical examination suggest pneumonia/sepsis as a possible etiology. In such cases, blood cultures should also be prior to initiation of antibiotic therapy.

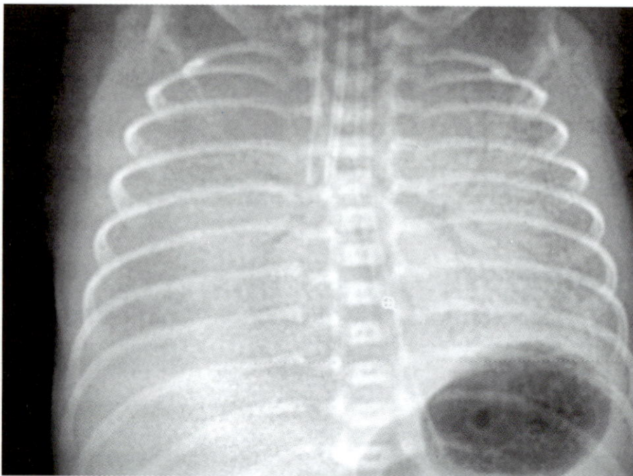

Fig. 2: Respiratory distress syndrome (RDS). Note the decreased lung volume, air bronchogram and reticulogranular pattern and complete opacification of lung fields (white out lung). ET tube is placed

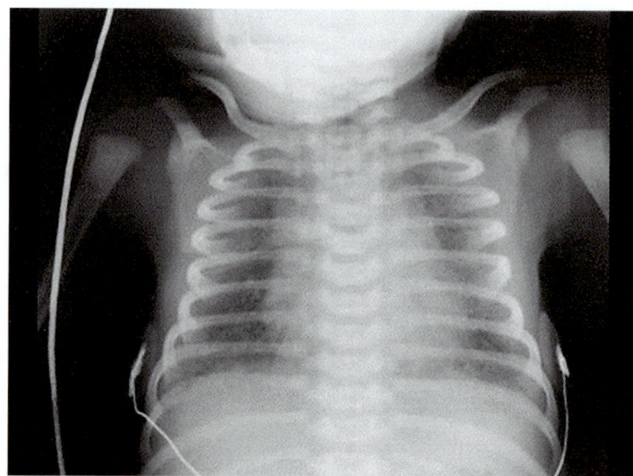

Fig. 3: Transient tachypnea of newborn (TTNB). Note the increased lung volume, fluid in the fissures. There is apparent cardiomegaly. At times, pleural effusions may be present

Imaging

X-ray chest

It is probably the most important investigation in a neonate with respiratory distress. It is indicated in all cases with respiratory distress (**Figs. 2 to 6**). **Table 5** provides a summary of radiological clues to determine etiology of respiratory distress.

USG chest

Ultrasonography has the advantage of being a bedside procedure. It can be used to detect/evaluate the following

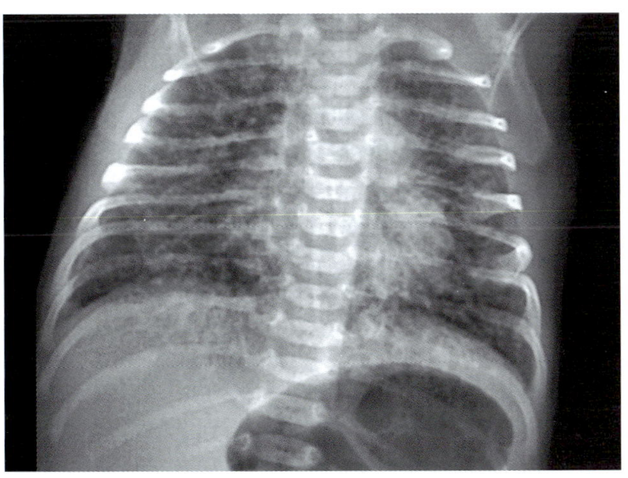

Fig. 4: Meconium aspiration syndrome (MAS). Note the diffuse, patchy/nodular infiltrates, asymmetric with hyperinflated lung fields. Presence of air leaks and cardiomegaly suggests complications

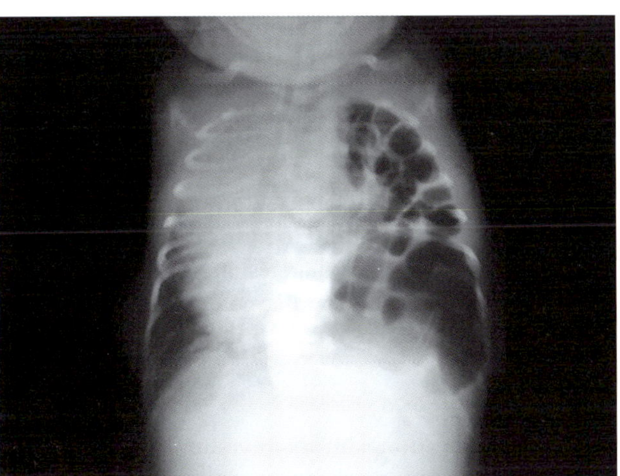

Fig. 6: Congenital diaphragmatic hernia. Note the bowel loops and the stomach bubble is present in the left hemithorax. There is shift of mediastinum

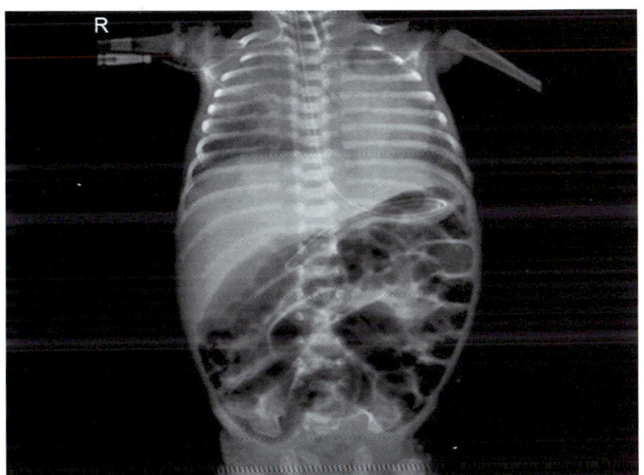

Fig. 5: Pneumonia. Note the patchy infiltrates in the right upper/ middle lobe

conditions: (i) pleural diseases, pleural effusion, (ii) distinction of solid from cystic intrathoracic masses, and (iii) evaluation of diaphragmatic excursion.

CT thorax

The utility of a CT image of the chest would be to determine (i) the anatomical sites of areas of cystic change, (ii) evaluation of mediastinal masses and their relationship to normal vascular structures, and (iii) in cases of suspected vascular ring or sling with airway obstruction.

Table 5: Radiological clues to etiology of respiratory distress in newborn

Radiological signs	*Etiology (see Figs. 2 to 6)*
Decreased lung volume	RDS, pulmonary hypoplasia
Increased lung volume	MAS, TTNB, cystic lung disease, congenital lobar emphysema
Air bronchogram	RDS, pneumonia
Diffuse parenchymal infiltrates	TTN, MAS, pneumonia decreased
Lobar consolidation	Pneumonia, congenital cystic adenomatoid lung maformation
Pleural effusion	Pneumonia, pulmonary lymphangiectasia
Reticular granular pattern	RDS, pneumonia
Hyperinflation	TTN, MAS, pulmonary lymphangiectasia
Fluid accumulations in interlobar spaces	TTN, pulmonary lymphangiectasia
"Cystic" mass	CCAM, CDH, pulmonary sequestration
Pneumothorax/ pneumomediastinum	Spontaneous, MAS, RDS, pneumonia

MRI chest

The MRI chest would be of value in the following situations – (i) pulmonary sequestration (to show the vascular supply from below the diaphragm, as well as the relationship of the sequestration to the diaphragm) and (ii) evaluation of presence and size of the pulmonary arteries when they cannot be delineated by cardiac catheterization or echocardiography.

2D echocardiography

In all neonates with suspected cardiac etiology, echocardiography should be done to confirm the presence of structural cardiac lesion. It can also provide useful information about cardiac contractility and cardiac function.

Arterial blood gas

This should be done in all neonate with significant respiratory distress or clinical suspicion of respiratory failure. It will provide information about the metabolic status (acidosis/alkalosis), oxygen levels and carbon dioxide levels. It will not only aid in diagnosis when combined with clinical and other laboratory data, but also aid in the management of respiratory failure.

MANAGEMENT

Management of respiratory distress involves both the supportive care, which is common to all newborns with respiratory distress, and the specific care which is etiology-specific. **Flowchart 1** provides an algorithm for the management of neonates with respiratory distress.

Supportive Care

Thermal care: Ensure normothermia (36.5–37.5°C) by placing infant under a radiant warmer. In infants <32 weeks evaporative losses must be minimized (by clothing or using polythene wraps).

Flowchart 1: Management approach in a case of respiratory distress in a newborn

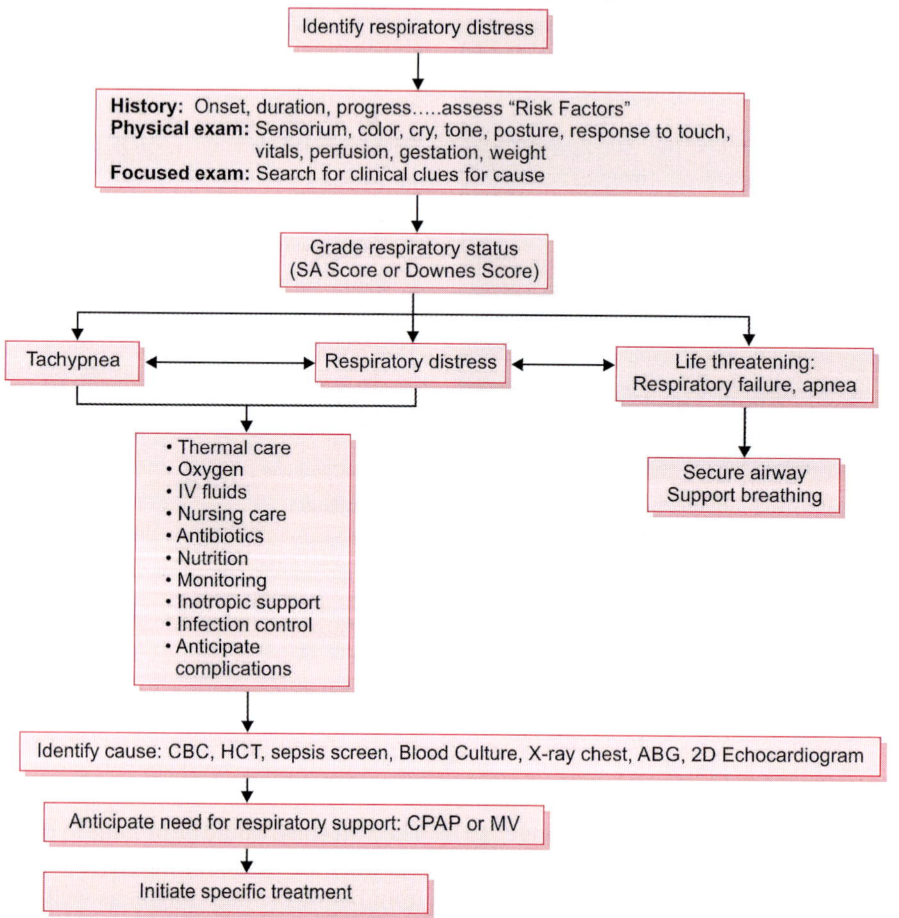

(CBC: complete blood count; HCT: hematocrit; ABG: arterial blood gas; CPAP: continous positive airway pressure; MV: mechanical ventilation)

Oxygen therapy: It may be administered by nasal prongs or oxygen hood. Oxygen must be warm and humidified. SpO_2 targets must be set to maintain between 90% and 95%.

Inotropic support: In neonates where shock is fluid-resistant consider ionotropic support. Dopamine is the drug of choice. Dobutamine is preferred if there is myocardial involvement.

Intravenous fluids: Provide fluids and electrolytes as per age, gestation to ensure adequate hydration. There is no evidence for routine restriction of fluids. Blood glucose should be monitored to prevent both hypo- and hyper-glycemia. Also monitor perfusion and urine output.

Nursing care: These babies must have minimal handling. Babies must be placed in a position of maximum comfort. Ensure airway is clear and visible secretions must be suctioned. Use pain-control measures like touch, swaddling, and sucrose—for IV insertion, pricks for blood collection, and gastric tube insertion. Efforts must be made to club nursing procedures together.

Nutrition: During the unstable phase, avoid enteral feeding. Trophic feeds should be initiated as early as feasible. Feeds should be increased in a graded manner once the newborn is stable. Consider parenteral nutrition if it is unlikely that the newborn could be fed over the next 72 hours.

Antibiotics: If sepsis/pneumonia is suspected, appropriate antibiotics should be initiated. However, there should be an exit policy based on clinical course, sepsis screen and blood culture.

Monitoring

Monitoring should be performed at regular interval and should include sensorium, vital parameters, respiratory status and perfusion. Investigations and clinical course need to be reviewed multiple times in a day to refine management plan.

Specific Therapy

Specific therapy for various etiologies is summarized in **Table 6**.

Respiratory Support

Besides supplemental oxygen, many neonates with respiratory distress would need additional respiratory support either as CPAP or mechanical ventilation.

Continuous positive airway pressure

This modality should be considered in the following circumstances:

- Preterm with onset of respiratory distress within the first 6 hours of birth;
- Presence of any two of the following: respiratory rate >60/min, chest retractions, grunting;
- Term and late preterm infants with SA score >5 or Downes score >5.

Noninvasive or invasive mechanical ventilation

The modalities of ventilation could include synchronized intermittent mandatory ventilation (with or without pressure support) or High frequency ventilation. Mechanical ventilation should be considered in the following circumstances:

- Gasping or poor respiratory efforts
- If on CPAP support with FiO_2>70% and CPAP pressure >7 cm of water
- Shock
- Recurrent apnea on CPAP.

The initial settings for neonate needing mechanical ventilation (non-high frequency) is provided in **Table 7**. **Table 8** summarizes the management of a preterm neonate with respiratory distress. **Boxes 2 and 3** provide practical illustrations of the management of a preterm and term neonate with respiratory distress.

Table 6: Specific treatments for etiologies of respiratory distress

Condition	*Treatment*
Pneumonia	Antibiotics, CPAP, NIMV, MV
RDS	Surfactant, CPAP, MV
Air leak	Intercostal drain
Polycythemia	Partial exchange transfusion
Anemia	Packed RBCs transfusion
CCF	Diuretics and digoxin
Ductus dependent cardiac lesion	Prostaglandin
TEF	Emergency surgery
CDH, CLE, CCAM, cleft palate	Elective surgery
Refractory hypoxia	HFV, iNO, ECMO

(NIMV: noninvasive mechanical ventilation; RBC: red blood cell; CCF: congestive cardiac failure; CLE: congenital lobar empphysema; HFV: high frequency ventilation; iNO: inhaled nitric oxide; ECMO: extra-corporeal membrane oxygenation)

Table 7: Suggested initial settings for common conditions

Ventilator parameter	*Clinical adequacy*	*Normal lung*	*RDS*	*MAS*
PIP	Gentle chest rise	13–15	20–25	20–25
PEEP	Absent chest indrawing	5	5–7	5
FiO_2	10% higher prior to intubation, titrated with SpO_2			
Rates	Mimics patients clinical status	30–40	40–60	40–60
Flow (L/min)	Depends on minute ventilation	8–10	8–10	8–10
I-time (sec)	Based on rates ensuring, ensure I:E 1.2	0.4	0.4	0.4

Table 8: Management of a preterm neonate with respiratory distress

Initiate: Thermal care, oxygen, IV fluids, nursing care, antibiotics, nutrition, monitoring, infection control, anticipate complications

Identify cause: CBC, HCT, sepsis screen, B culture, X-ray chest, ABG

Silverman Anderson score <3	**Silverman Anderson score 4–6**	**Silverman Anderson score ≥7**
Oxygen	Early CPAP	Exit from CPAP
	If FiO_2 >0.3, consider surfactant (INSURE)	If apnea, FiO_2>0.6, CPAP pressure ≥8, respiratory failure = Consider intubation and ventilation

(INSURE: intubate, surfactant, extubate)

Box 2: Case management of preterm baby with respiratory distress

A 30 weeks, 1.2 kg, male baby was born to a primigravida with severe hypertension by emergency LSCS delivery. Mother had received 1 dose of dexamethasone about 5 hrs prior to delivery. The Apgar scores were 3 and 7 at 1 and 5 minutes respectively. The baby was noted to have lower chest and xiphoid retraction with audible grunting. The baby's temperature was checked and noted to be 36°C. As the baby was hypothermic, the baby was placed under the radiant warmer for re-warming. The baby had an SA score of 4 with an SpO_2 of 88% in room air. The blood glucose was 47 mg/dL (indicative of hypoglycemia), therefore the baby was given a bolus of 200 mg/kg of 10% dextrose and initiated on IV dextrose infusion @ 6 mg/kg/min. In view of prematurity, and incomplete course of antenatal steroids a clinical diagnosis of RDS was made. The baby was initiated on bubble CPAP with nasal prongs, with PEEP of 5 cm H_2O, FiO_2 of 0.5 and flow rate of 5 liters/min (see Table 8). After 30 minutes the SA score was noted to be 5. PEEP was increased to 6 cm H_2O in view of persistent chest indrawing. In view of worsening respiratory status the infant was administered intratracheal surfactant (100 mg/kg) while continuing CPAP. Vital parameters, color, SA score, breath sounds and air entry was monitored hourly. X-ray chest revealed low lung volumes with air bronchogram suggestive of RDS. By 12 hours, trophic gavage feeds were initiated. At 34 hours the baby was removed from CPAP support with grading up of enteral feeding.

Box 3: Case management of term baby with respiratory distress

A 39 weeks, 3.18 kg, male baby delivered vaginally to a 28-year-old multigravida mother after an uneventful antenatal period. There was meconium stained amniotic fluid at delivery. The baby was born vigorous at birth but developed respiratory distress at 1 hour of age with a respiratory rate of 90/min and chest retractions with an SA score of 6. The baby had a temperature of 36.9°C, The SpO_2 on room air was 84%. Infant was initiated on oxygen by hood. The SaO_2 reached 92% at 60% FiO_2. The blood glucose was 60 mg/dL. The infant was initiated on IV fluids @ 60 mL/kg/day of 10% dextrose. A clinical diagnosis of meconium aspiration syndrome was made (later confirmed on chest skiagram). Arterial blood gas (ABG) from the right radial artery revealed pH of 7.25, PaO_2 57 mm Hg and PCO_2 of 56 mm Hg. In view of the respiratory acidosis on ABG, the baby was intubated and mechanically ventilated in SIMV mode. The initial ventilatory settings needed were - PIP of 25 cm H_2O, PEEP of 4 cm H_2O, RR of 60/min, and $FIO_2$of 0.6. A 2-D ECHO revealed structurally normal heart with no evidence of pulmonary hypertension. The infant was monitored regularly for vitals, oxygenation, blood gases and glucose. The baby improved and was extubated from ventilator to nasal prong oxygen 0.5 L/min on day 5 of life. Gavage feeds were introduced on day 3 of life and were graded to full feeds on day 7 of life. Infant was discharged on day 9 on breast feeds.

Referral Criteria

If the facility does not have the capacity to provide intensive care for a baby, then infants need to be referred. The criteria for referral could include one or more of the following:

- In utero transfer for high-risk fetus inability to maintain SpO_2 > 90% room air
- Worsening sensorium
- Respiratory distress with poor circulation
- SA score/Downes and Vidyasagar score > 7.

OUTCOME AND PROGNOSTIC FACTORS

Recovery from RDS is dependent on the severity of illness. This is affected by gestational age and birth weight. Historically 50% mortality from RDS was seen in infants <1000 g birth weight. RDS is rarely an isolated pathology affecting extreme preterm infants. Respiratory insufficiency, due to immaturity of the lungs, limits the viability in extremely preterm infants. Impact of CLD/BPD is thought to be life-long, with survivors having reduced lung function persisting later in life. The routine use of antenatal corticosteroids, exogenous surfactant replacement therapy, CPAP and more gentle ventilation methods have substantially improved the outcomes of premature newborns. TTNB generally has good prognosis. An alternative diagnosis should be sought in cases requiring prolonged respiratory support or oxygen supplementation.

Infant with MAS not requiring mechanical ventilation usually do better, as compared to those who need to be mechanically ventilated. Outcomes of neonates with pneumonia vary greatly and are dependent upon the organism and its virulence. Early identification and treatment of neonates at risk of infection or with symptoms of infection reduces both morbidity and mortality.

PREVENTION

The interventions that can prevent respiratory distress or an adverse outcome consequent to it include one or more of the following:

- Preventing preterm births.
- Use of antenatal steroids. It decreases RDS most consistently between 28 and 34 weeks of gestational age (RR- 0.65; 95% CI 0.47–0.75) with NNT 12. When used <27 weeks, there is no reduction in RDS. At <32 weeks, antenatal steroids and surfactant therapy act synergistically in reducing severity of RDS, decrease mortality and decreases air leak when compared to either intervention alone or no intervention.
- Delivery room CPAP and early rescue surfactant.
- Improved antenatal and intrapartum surveillance to prevent development of perinatal asphyxia and MAS.
- Early detection of life-threatening surgical conditions.
- Early and prompt referral.

KEY MESSAGES

- The newborn infants are vulnerable to a range of respiratory disorders, all presenting with signs of respiratory distress.
- The most common cause of respiratory distress in preterm newborn is respiratory distress syndrome (RDS) and in-term newborn are transient tachypnea of the newborn (TTNB) and meconium aspiration syndrome (MAS).
- Severity of respiratory distress is assessed by the Silverman Anderson score in preterms and Downes score in term neonates.
- A chest radiograph is crucial to assist in diagnosis of an underlying cause. 2D-Echo helps in timely diagnosis of suspected congenital heart disease.
- Management consists of supportive care, respiratory support (CPAP, noninvasive/invasive ventilation, and prompt referral, if needed.

REFERENCES

1. Thakre R. Approach respiratory distress. In: Thakre R, Murki S, editors. Protocols in Neonatology. New Delhi: Jaypee Brothers Medical Publishers; 2016. p. 14-23.
2. Hermansen CL, Lorah KN. Respiratory distress in the newborn. Am Fam Physician. 2007;76:987-94.
3. Edwards MO, Kotecha SJ, Kotecha S. Respiratory distress of the term newborn infant. Paediatr Respir Rev. 2013;14:29-37.
4. Warren JB, Anderson JM. Newborn respiratory disorders. Pediatr Rev. 2010;31:487-96.
5. Aly H. Respiratory disorders in the newborn: Identification and diagnosis. Pediatr Rev. 2004;25:201-8.
6. Rimensberger PC. Neonatal respiratory failure. Curr Opin Pediatr. 2002;14:315-21.
7. Gnanaratnem J, Finer NN. Neonatal acute respiratory failure. Curr Opin Pediatr. 2000;12:227-32.
8. Kumar A, Bhat BV. Epidemiology of respiratory distress of newborns. Indian J Pediatr. 1996;63:93-8.
9. Silverman WA, Anderson DH. A controlled clinical trial of effects of water mist on obstructive respiratory signs, death rate and necropsy findings among premature infants. Pediatrics. 1956;17:1-10.
10. Downes JJ, Vidyasagar D, Boggs TR Jr, *et al.* Respiratory distress syndrome of newborn infants. I. New clinical scoring system (RDS score) with acid-base and blood-gas correlations. Clin Pediatr. 1970;9:325-31.
11. Levesque BM, Pollack P, Griffin BE, *et al.* Pulse oximetry: what's normal in the newborn nursery? Pediatr Pulmonol. 2000;30:406-12.
12. Oxygen therapy for children: A manual for health workers. Geneva: World Health Organization; 2016. p. 4.

CHAPTER

71

Shock in the Newborn

Shiv Sajan Saini

INTRODUCTION

Shock is a state of acute circulatory insufficiency, leading to inadequate delivery of oxygen and nutrients to the tissues relative to their metabolic demands. Under these conditions, the tissues are unable to sustain aerobic metabolism, and they resort to anaerobic metabolism. This leads to energy deficiency, increased production of lactic acid and other inorganic acids. Progressively worsening cellular hypoxemic and acidotic conditions lead to deterioration in organ-system(s) functioning including metabolic, hematological, endocrine and cardiac functions. Continued progression of shock leads to the irreversible alteration in organ functions leading to multiorgan failure and ultimately death.

Defining Shock

In day-to-day clinical practice, shock is identified by presence of either hypotension (BP <5th centile) or a constellation of clinical signs such as cool extremities, prolonged CFT, decreased urine output and low volume pulse (*see* **Table 1**). However, many of the above signs are subjective and therefore may cause interobserver variability in identification of shock. **Table 1** provides a more objective definition of shock. Although it is designed for septic shock, these criteria can be used for defining shock of non-septic etiology.[1]

Table 1: Definition of shock according to international pediatric sepsis consensus conference[1]

Either one or more of following		
A.	Blood pressure <5th percentile for age[3] OR	
B.	Need for vasoactive drug to maintain BP in normal range (dopamine >5 µg/kg/min or dobutamine, epinephrine, or norepinephrine at any dose) OR	
C.	Presence of two or more of following	• Base excess worse than -5.0 mEq/L • Arterial lactate >2 times upper limit of normal • Urine output <0.5 mL/kg/hr in past 6–12 hours • Capillary refill time >3 secs • Core to peripheral temperature gap >3°C

In the early stages of hemodynamic compromise, the body tries to preserve the function of vital organs especially brain, heart and adrenal glands at the expense of non-vital organs like skin, gastrointestinal tract and muscles. At this stage, the skin perfusion is compromised but the blood pressure is maintained. This is also known as ***compensated shock***. However, if this stage is not aggressively managed, blood pressure falls and condition rapidly deteriorates. This is known as ***uncompensated shock***. The chances of shock reversal decrease as the baby progresses from compensated shock to uncompensated shock. Irrespective of the etiology, the recognition of shock involves dysfunction of vital organs, e.g. hypotension; dysfunction of non-vital organs, e.g. impaired skin perfusion, decreased urine output, etc.; and derangement in acid-base disturbances.

EPIDEMIOLOGY AND ETIOLOGY

Neonates develop shock mainly due to four reasons—(a) Decreased intravascular volume (Hypovolemic shock)

Table 2: Etiologies of various forms of neonatal shock

Types of shock	*Etiology of shock*	*History*	*Clinical clues*	*Investigative parameters**
Hypovolemic	Loss of body fluids (blood, water/ electrolyte)	Concealed or revealed hemorrhage, diarrhea, polyuria	Clinical signs of dehydration may be present	Serum sodium and osmolality may be raised, functional echocardiography can help in doubtful situations
Cardiogenic	Birth asphyxia; congenital heart diseases, cardiomyopathies, arrhythmias; electrolyte abnormalities: hypocalcemia; severe anemia; drugs, e.g. opioids, magnesium sulfate	Birth asphyxia; antenatal diagnosed congenital heart diseases; interrupted feeding/perspiration during feeding, history of maternal/ neonatal drug use, maternal diabetes, antenatal scans	Signs of congestive cardiac failure, murmurs, hydrops, severe pallor	Biomarkers (CK-MB), serum electrolytes, ECG abnormalities, echocardiography
Obstructive	Increased intrathoracic pressure: tension pneumothorax, increased intrathoracic ventilator pressure; ventricular outflow obstruction: ductal dependent CHDs, pulmonary embolism; pericardial tamponade	Resuscitation details, positive pressure ventilation, antenatal scans, known congenital heart diseases	Asymmetric chest rise/ auscultaory findings, feeble femoral pulses, presence of central lines	Chest X-ray, blood gas analysis, upper and lower limb BP, echocardiography
Distributive/septic	Early septic shock with decreased afterload (bacterial, viral or fungal), anaphylaxis, loss of sympathetic vascular tone secondary to spinal cord or brainstem injury, drugs, e.g. β_2 agonists	Maternal or postnatal risk factors of infection, drugs administration	Signs of systemic inflammatory response syndrome (SIRS), multiple organ involvement	Sepsis markers, culture of sterile body fluids (especially blood and CSF), organ specific investigations

*This list is representative and not-comprehensive

volume leading to decreased preload and cardiac output; (b) Decreased cardiac functions (cardiogenic shock) due to poor myocardial systolic and diastolic functions; (c) Obstruction to cardiac output (obstructive) or restrictions of cardiac chambers; (d) Distributive due to shock abnormalities of vasomotor tone as a result of infectious or non-infectious processes. The etiologies of these four forms of shock are given in **Table 2**.

PATHOGENESIS/PATHOPHYSIOLOGY

There are three main components of circulation: preload, myocardial contractility and afterload. The preload is the end diastolic volume that stretches the ventricles of the heart to its maximum dimensions. The pressure generated by end-diastolic volume in the left atrium (left atrial pressure) is estimated indirectly by the pulmonary capillary wedge pressure (PCWP). Myocardial contractility is estimated by echocardiography. Afterload depends on the systemic vascular resistance, which is clinically inferred by the blood pressure (as there is no direct way to measure SVR). Blood pressure is the product of cardiac output and the systemic vascular resistance (SVR). In the initial stages of circulatory compromise, blood pressure (BP) is maintained by either increase in SVR or cardiac output. However, with the loss of compensatory phenomena, BP falls eventually. One or more of these parameters get affected in individual pathophysiological category of shock. **Table 3** shows the change in the alteration in hemodynamic parameters among four main categories of neonatal shock.[2]

The common causes of neonatal shock include birth asphyxia, sepsis, congenital heart diseases with ductal dependency or congestive cardiac failure, transitional circulation, hypovolemia and adrenal insufficiency. The salient changes in preload, myocardial contractility and afterload in the common causes of neonatal shock is tabulated in **Table 4.**[3]

Table 3: Hemodynamic parameters in main categories of neonatal shock

		Preload		*Myocardial*		*Afterload*	
Shock type		*Central venous pressure*	*Left atrial pressure*	*Contractility*	*Cardiac output*	*Systemic vascular resistance*	*Blood pressure*
Hypovolemic		↓↓↓	↓↓↓	↔ or ↑	↓	↑	↔ or ↓
Cardiogenic	Systolic	↑↑	↑↑	↓↓↓	↓↓	↑↑	↔ or ↓
	Diastolic	↑	↑↑	↔	↔ or ↓	↑↑	↔ or ↓
Obstructive		↑↑	↑↑	↓	↓	↑	↔ or ↓
Septic	Early	↓	↓	↔ or ↑	↑↑↑	↓↓↓	↔ or ↓
	Late	↔ or ↑	↑	↓	↓↓	↓↓	↓↓

(Adapted from Nelson Textbook of Pediatrics)

Table 4: Pathophysiology in main etiologies of neonatal shock

Etiology	*Preload*	*Myocardial contractility*	*Afterload*
Asphyxia	Increases, may decrease in advanced stages due to capillary leak	Depressed due to hypoxemic/ischemic injury to myocardium	Increase in early stages, decreases at later stages
Transitional circulation in ELBW neonates	Increases	Depressed due to sudden increase in left ventricular afterload after birth	Increases in early stages
Intracardiac shunts, e.g PDA	Increases	Increased myocardial work (hyperdynamic circulation)	Decreased (systemic to pulmonary shunts)
Ductal dependent circulation (e.g. LV obstruction)	Increases in LVO and decreases in RVO obstruction	Decreases after brief increase in initial period	Increases
Septic shock	Decreases, relative hypovolemia due to increased capacitance	Depressed myocardial function, more pronounced in the later stages	Decreased vasomotor tone
Hypovolemia	Decreased	Not affected	Slightly increased to maintain BP
Adrenal insufficiency	Not affected or increased	Depressed	Decreased
Raised intrathoracic pressure	Decreased as poor venous return	Slightly decreased; affected due to poor capacity to distend	Increases in markedly increased intrathoracic pressure

CLINICAL FEATURES

At the bedside, hemodynamic status is assessed by evaluation of following signs:

- *Heart rate*: Heart rate outside the normal range (120–160 bpm) is one of the early indicators of hemodynamic disturbance. It is nonspecific and can be out of range in a number of clinical conditions. Nevertheless, a trend of heart rate abnormality can alert physician about the impending hemodynamic instability.
- *Capillary filling time (CFT)*: Normal value is <3 sec. It is studied as the time of return of pink color after the skin is pressed (preferably against sternum or forehead) for 5 seconds and released. Values of 3 sec or more are abnormal.
- *Temperature (core and peripheral temperature)*: Core temperature of <36.5°C and a core-periphery difference of 3°C or more is associated with hemodynamic instability.
- *Pulse volume*: Usually central pulses (brachial or femoral pulses) should be evaluated for pulse-volume assessment.
- *Urine output*: A urine output of <1 mL/kg/hr in preceding 6 hours could be due to poor circulation.

Blood pressure: BP is measured either noninvasively by oscillometry or invasively by intra-arterial catheters attached to invasive BP monitors. Generally, noninvasive BP tends to overestimate the BP especially in lower ranges. The reference range of BP in neonates is published by few authors. One such example is Zubrow's charts.[4] Normal levels of mean BP on day 1 are generally taken as equivalent to gestational age.

Color: The pale color of neonate suggests poor peripheral circulation.

Individually CFT and core periphery temperature difference may not correlate very well with organ perfusion.[1,5] It is well known that BP is a late marker of shock. It is product of cardiac output and systemic vascular resistance. If cardiac output is decreased, the tissue perfusion decreases. Decreased cardiac output may be masked if systemic vascular resistance is elevated. Thus, despite BP being stable during shock, the tissue perfusion may be compromised. Furthermore, the "normal" range of blood pressure is not clear for various gestational ages. Thus, we should not rely on single parameter for detection and management of shock and use collective information, i.e. heart rate, capillary refill time, color, urine output, temperature (core and peripheral temperature), and blood pressure for assessment of circulation.[6]

Complications

Neonates presenting with shock can additionally have various organ dysfunctions. The spectrum of organ dysfunction includes but not limited to the following manifestations given in **Table 5**.

Table 5: Spectrum of non-cardiac organ dysfunction in critically sick neonates

System	*Disorders*
Respiratory	Respiratory distress, failure, hypoventilation and apnea
Neurological	Lethargy, encephalopathy, seizures
Renal	Pre-renal or Renal failure
Hematologic	Thrombocytopenia, consumptive coagulopathy (disseminated intravascular coagulation), thrombosis
Gastrointestinal	Abdominal distension, stress ulcers, septic ileus, peritonitis, necrotizing enterocolitis
Endocrine	Hypoglycemia, adrenal insufficiency
Metabolic	Metabolic acidosis, dyselectrolytemia
Liver	Transaminitis, cholestasis

DIFFERENTIAL DIAGNOSES

The differential diagnosis of neonatal shock includes hypovolemic shock, cardiogenic shock, obstructive shock and distributive or septic shock (**Table 2**). History of blood loss in peripartum or in postnatal life, instrumental delivery, difficult delivery, internal bleeding diarrhea, urine output, birth asphyxia; antenatal suspicion of congenital heart diseases, drugs administration, e.g. opioids, magnesium sulfate, positive pressure ventilation, interrupted feeding/perspiration during feeding, fetal heart rate abnormality, antenatal features of hydrops, and antenatal or postnatal risk factors of infections should be evaluated. Clinical examination should involve vital signs, screening for signs of dehydration, pupils, femoral pulses, congestive failure, cardiac rhythm, severe pallor, asymmetric air entry, cardiac murmurs and signs of peripheral/central circulation, abdominal distension, skin pustules/vesicles, genital examination and neurological examination including fontanels and sutures. Additionally screening of other organ systems should be performed to identify multiorgan dysfunction.

LABORATORY INVESTIGATIONS

The investigations in a case of shock should include the following:

- *Microbiological investigations*: Following tests are required to identify the infective organism in septic shock and performed whenever sepsis is considered. A rule of thumb is to obtain blood culture before giving the first dose of antibiotics.
    - Culture of sterile body fluids (especially blood and CSF): All cases
    - Culture of site-specific infective focus (aspirates, swabs, etc.): Wherever indicated
    - Serologies/PCR if viral infections are suspected (wherever indicated).
- *Biochemical investigations*: To be obtained in all cases of shock.
    - *Blood glucose*: Hypoglycemia is frequently observed, and it must be treated aggressively as it is associated with poor long-term outcomes.
    - *Serum electrolytes* (especially serum sodium, potassium, ionized calcium): They are important as they are frequently deranged in various etiologies and are required for optimal cardiac performance.

- *Blood gas analysis* (capillary or preferably arterial) to assess metabolic acidosis and lactate levels. Standard base excess and lactate can help in diagnosis and shock management. Current ABG machines can provide other useful data like electrolytes and hematocrit.
- *Renal function tests*: Acute kidney injury is frequently observed in such neonates and is independently associated with mortality.

- *Hematological investigations*
  - *Complete hemogram*: It is required to ascertain need for optimal hematocrit and platelet count. During shock it would be desirable to maintain ≥40% hematocrit to optimize oxygen carrying capacity of the blood. Thrombocytopenia is frequently observed in septic shock and therefore must be evaluated.
  - *Coagulation studies* must be done if bleeding tendency is present. Shocked neonates may have disseminated intravascular coagulation, especially in neonates with septic shock.
  - Crossmatching for blood/component therapy should be considered.
- Depending on physical examination findings, other tests may be required to define the cause of shock. These tests include but not limited to thoracic trans-illumination, chest X-ray, neuroimaging, drug levels, etc.
- ECG for continuous monitoring and to detect rhythm and electrolyte abnormalities.
- Functional echocardiography may be used for hemodynamic assessment for the assessment of preload assessment (e.g. IVC collapsibility), myocardial contractility and cardiac output. Additionally, functional echocardiography can help to exclude certain causes of shock like hemodynamically significant PDA, duct dependent systemic circulation.[7]

MANAGEMENT

Initial Stabilization

The case fatality rate in shock is very high in neonates. Therefore, early recognition and appropriate intervention is the key for improved survival and better neurodevelopmental outcomes. Management of shock begins with maintenance of euthermia. The airway is stabilized and breathing generally requires support with either CPAP or mechanical ventilation, based on severity of respiratory distress. Elective positive pressure ventilation should be considered in advanced shock, e.g. if more than two vasoactive drugs are required. An intravenous line is required for fluid resuscitation and/or vasoactive drugs administration. If vasopressors are needed, they should preferably be given through central venous lines. Blood glucose should be maintained above 50 mg/dL in first 48 hours and above 60 mg/dL thereafter. Serum sodium and calcium should be normalized, if found low.

Goals of Therapy[2]

Successful management requires early and aggressive therapy with supportive measures and control of the underlying cause. The goals of circulatory stability include:

- Normal skin perfusion—CFT <3 sec
- BP within normal centiles
- Improved central pulses—femoral and brachial
- Improved acid base status.

Other parameters such as urine output, sensorium and organ dysfunctions may take time for normalization. The goals of supportive care for various other organ function is given in **Table 6**.[2]

Volume Resuscitation

Volume resuscitation is the first line of therapy during management of shock. Normal saline bolus of 10 mL/kg irrespective of gestational age is infused over 15–30 minutes (longer duration chosen in VLBW neonates). For term neonates, fluid volume up to 40 mL/kg and for preterm neonates 10–20 mL/kg is advised.[1-3,5,8] The fluid resuscitation in preterm neonates is cautiously given as there is risk of fluid overload, Hs-PDA and intraventricular hemorrhage with excess fluids. In neonates, absolute hypovolemia is unlikely except in conditions of blood or water losses. Therefore, if shock is secondary to asphyxia, congenital heart diseases and ELBW neonates in first 12 hours of life without any obvious reason, fluids should be cautiously used.

Pharmacologic Therapy

Pharmacotherapy of shock involves three classes of drugs—inotropes, vasopressors and lusitropes.[9] Inotropes increase myocardial contractility, vasopressors improve systemic vascular resistance and lusitropes improve myocardial relaxation, improve systemic blood flow. Appropriate vasoactive agent(s) should be chosen based on underlying

Table 6: Goals and supportive care therapies for various non-cardiac organ dysfunction in critically sick neonates

System	*Goals*	*Therapies*
Respiratory	• Prevent/treat: hypoxia and respiratory acidosis • Prevent hyperoxia, barotrauma/ volutrauma • Decrease work of breathing	• Oxygen (target SpO_2 <34 weeks 90–95% and 94–98% thereafter) • Appropriate breathing support: Noninvasive ventilation, early endotracheal intubation and mechanical ventilation, high-frequency ventilation • Permissive hypercapnia once stabilized • Extracorporeal membrane oxygenation (ECMO)
Renal	• Prevent/treat: hypovolemia, hypervolemia, hyperkalemia, metabolic acidosis, hypernatremia/hyponatremia, and hypertension	• Appropriate fluid resuscitation • Circulatory stability • Furosemide (not during active shock) • Dialysis, ultrafiltration, hemofiltration
Hematologic	• Prevent/treat: anemia, bleeding tendency or clotting tendency	• Vitamin K • Platelet concentrate • Fresh-frozen plasma • Heparinization
Gastro-intestinal	• Prevent/treat: altered aspirates • Avoid abdominal distention • Avoid mucosal atrophy	• Continuous nasogastric drainage • Saline gastric washes • H2-receptor–blockers • Trophic feeding • Early enteral feedings after stabilization
Endocrine	• Prevent/treat: Hypoglycemia, adrenal crisis	• Consider stress-dose hydrocortisone in patients previously given steroids • Hydrocortisone for catecholamine resistance
Metabolic	• Correct underlying etiology • Normalize pH	• Treatment of hypovolemia (fluids), myocardial dysfunction (vasoactive drugs) • Improvement of renal acid excretion • Low-dose (0.5–2.0 mEq/kg) sodium bicarbonate if the patient is not showing response, pH <7.0, and ventilation (PCO_2) is adequate

Table 7: Vasoactive drugs, dose and important actions

Agent	*Dose µg/kg/min*	*Action*	*Special features*
Dopamine	5–20	5–10: ↑contractility and HR (inotropy), >10: increases SVR in addition (vasopressor)	Acts mainly on β-receptors by releasing norepinephrine from presynaptic vesicles. Caution in presence of PPHN.
Dobutamine	5–20	↑ contractility thereby improve BP, ↑ HR (inotropy)	Direct actions on β-receptors, effective in myocardial dysfunction
Epinephrine	0.1–0.5	<0.3 ↑contractility and HR (inotrope), ≥0.3 predominantly vasopressor actions	Direct actions on adrenergic receptors. Adverse effect include ↑ HR, serum lactate and hyperglycemia
Milrinone	Loading: 75 µg/kg IV over 60 min, Maintenance: 0.5 to 0.75 µg/kg/min	Both inotropy and lusitropy. ↓vascular tone in both pulmonary and systemic circulation	More effective than dobutamine in presence of diastolic dysfunction. Useful adjunct to iNO in presence of PPHN. Cautious in presence of hypotension
Vasopressin	0.01 to 0.04 units/kg/hr	↑ SVR and releases cortisol in presence of ACTH	Indicated in catecholamine resistant warm shock. Caution in myocardial dysfunction. Watch for oliguria as ↓ renal blood flow is known
Noradrenaline	0.2–1.5 µg/kg/min	↑SVR (vasopressor) but also acts on β-receptors	Limited evidence of efficacy. Considered as last resort in refractory shock
Levosimendan	0.05–0.2 µg/kg/min	Lucitrope, inotropy and ↓SVR	Limited evidence of efficacy. Useful in postoperative care of congenital heart diseases

pathophysiology. As a general rule, inotropes are given in peripheral circulatory failure with normal blood pressures and vasopressors are required for hypotension. **Table 7** summarizes commonly used vasoactive drugs in neonatal shock.[2,6,9] The algorithm of management of shock is given in **Flowchart 1**.

Flowchart 1: Stepwise, time sensitive management of neonatal shock

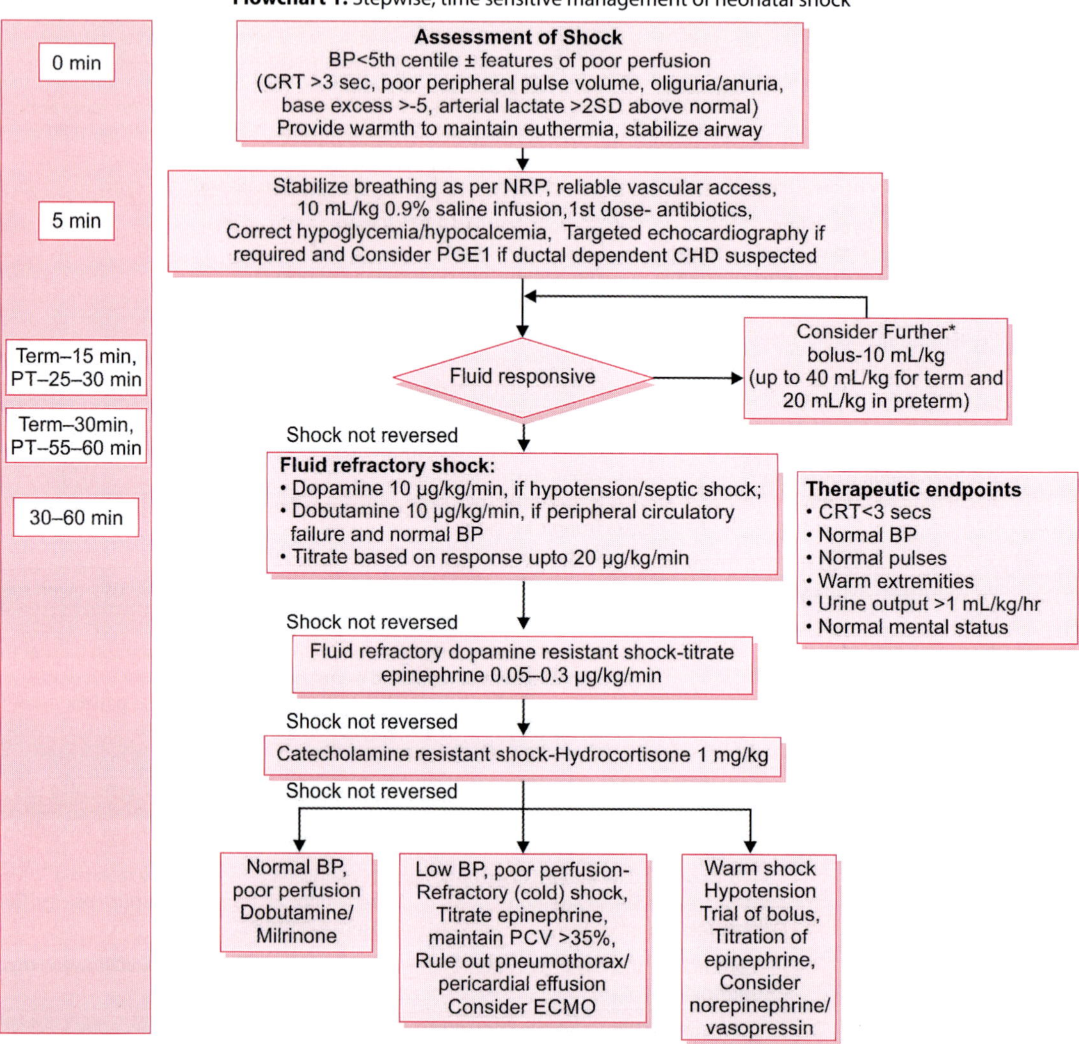

(Modified from The Handbook of Neonatology, Davis et al.)[3,13]

Steroids

Steroids are indicated in vasopressor resistant shock. They are shown to increase blood pressure and decrease vasopressor requirement in such neonates. The dose followed in neonatal studies is quite variable but 1 mg/kg/dose every 6 hourly can be given for 5 days. A loading dose of 2 mg/kg of hydrocortisone may be considered.

Supportive Management

Keeping low threshold for sepsis, broad-spectrum antibiotics should be initiated as soon as possible. First dose should be administered as early as possible within the first hour of shock. Trophic feeding can be continued unless there are altered GI aspirates/GI pathology. Once shock is stabilized, parenteral nutrition can be continued with low lipid dose of 1 g/kg/day and warrants close monitoring with triglyceride and platelets. The electrolytes including calcium and glucose levels must be maintained in their normal range. Hematocrit should be maintained above 35%. Appropriate supportive measures should be instituted as per **Table 6**. For refractory shock, veno-arterial ECMO may be considered where facilities are available.[2,3] Prostaglandin (PGE_1) should be started in duct dependent systemic/pulmonary circulation.

OUTCOMES/PROGNOSTIC FACTORS

The outcomes of neonatal shock depend on the underlying etiology. Invariably the worst outcomes are obtained in septic shock especially gram-negative septic shock. Mortality rate among neonatal septic shock in developed countries has been documented as 40% and in developing countries mortality rates are exceedingly high (~75–80%).[6,10-12] Neonates with shock are predisposed for growth failure, chronic lung disease, retinopathy and adverse neurodevelopmental outcomes. An early recognition and prompt management of shock is the key to improved outcome.

KEY MESSAGES

- A practical definition of shock is presence of either hypotension (BP <5th centile) or a constellation of clinical signs such as cool extremities, prolonged CFT, decreased urine output and low volume pulse.
- Common causes of shock in the newborn include perinatal asphyxia, sepsis and ductus dependent congenital cardiac defects.
- The mainstay of therapy include volume resuscitation, pharmacotherapy, steroids and supportive care.
- In refractory shock ductus dependent cardiac defects, air leaks must be considered and use of PGE1 should be considered early rather than late.
- Use of an algorithm can help a systematic approach to management of shock.

REFERENCES

1. Goldstein B, Giroir B, Randolph A. International Consensus Conference on Pediatric Sepsis. International pediatric sepsis consensus conference: Definitions for sepsis and organ dysfunction in pediatrics. Pediatr Crit Care Med. 2005;6(1):2-8.
2. Turner DA, Cheifetz IM. Shock. In: Kleigman RM, Stanton, BF, St Geme III, JW, Schor, NF, Behrman RE, editors. Nelson Textbook of Pediatrics, 20th edition. Philadelphia: Elsevier; 2016. p. 516-27.
3. Saini SS, Aradhya AS. Shock in neonates. In: Bhat R, Kumar P, Vidyasagar D, editors. The Handbook of Neonatology. New Delhi: Indian Journal of Pediatrics; 2018. p. 377-84.
4. Zubrow AB, Hulman S, Kushner H, *et al.* Determinants of blood pressure in infants admitted to neonatal intensive care units: A prospective multicenter study. Philadelphia Neonatal Blood Pressure Study Group. J Perinatol. 1995;15:470-9.
5. Wynn JL, Wong HR. Pathophysiology and treatment of septic shock in neonates. Clin Perinatol. 2010;37:439-79.
6. Singh Y, Katheria AC, Vora F. Advances in diagnosis and management of hemodynamic instability in neonatal shock. Frontiers in Pediatrics. 2018;6:2.
7. Mertens L, Seri I, Marek J, *et al.* Targeted neonatal echocardiography in the neonatal intensive care unit: Practice guidelines and recommendations for training. Eur J Echocardiogr. 2011;12:715-36.
8. Singh Y. Commentary: Echocardiographic evaluation of hemodynamics in neonates and children. Frontiers in Pediatrics. 2018;6:76.
9. Noori S, Seri I. Neonatal blood pressure support: The use of inotropes, lusitropes, and other vasopressor agents. Clin Perinatol. 2012;39:221-38.
10. Baske K, Saini SS, Dutta S, *et al.* Epinephrine versus dopamine in neonatal septic shock: A double-blind randomized controlled trial. Eur J Pediatr. 2018;177(9):1335-42.
11. Saini SS, Kumar P, Kumar RM. Hemodynamic changes in preterm neonates with septic shock: A prospective observational study. Pediatric Critical Care Medicine. 2014;15:443-50.
12. Skinner JR. Echocardiography on the neonatal unit: A job for the neonatologist or the cardiologist? Arch Dis Child. 1998;78:401-2.
13. Davis AL, Carcillo JA, Aneja RK, et al. American College of Critical Care Medicine. Clinical practice parameters for hemodynamic support of pediatric and neonatal septic shock. Crit Care Med. 2017;45:1061-93.

CHAPTER

72

Neonatal Convulsions

Neeraj Gupta

INTRODUCTION

Neonatal seizures (NS) often represents the first sign of neurological dysfunction[1] and constitutes one of the common neonatal neurological emergencies. Developmental immaturity of the brain predisposes newborns to high risk of seizure than any other age group. These may manifest in isolation or along with other systemic symptoms including encephalopathy. However, a large number of seizures in newborn period may get missed due to their subtle nature.[2] Moreover, few non-epileptic movements may get easily confused with seizures.

Focused history, targeted examination supplemented with basic investigations and neuroimaging helps in clinching the diagnosis in large number of patients. Prompt evaluation is a must to institute etiology-specific therapy, as not only these neonates are at high risk of early death but may also develop long-term neurological impairment including epilepsy, motor and cognitive deficits.[3] Moreover, seizures themselves can contribute to ongoing brain injury. The long-term prognosis is highly variable and is primarily dependent on the underlying etiology and its severity.

EPIDEMIOLOGY AND ETIOLOGY

The true incidence of NS is difficult to estimate due to the subclinical nature of these events and method of ascertainment used. The preterm and low birth weight newborns are much more at risk of NS as compared to their term counterparts. The estimated incidence in term infants range between 1 and 5 per 1000 neonates[4] whereas it is as high as 57.5 per 1000 in very low birth weight (VLBW) infants.[5] The overall incidence of NS in India is reported to be 1% as per National Neonatal-Perinatal Database 2003 report.[6] The median prevalence of seizures among commonly reported etiologies is 38–48% in hypoxic-ischemic encephalopathy (HIE); 3–7.5% in hypoglycemia; 2.3–9% in hypocalcemia and 5.5–10.3% in central nervous system infections.[7]

Neonatal seizures may arise due to variety of pre-, peri- or postnatal insults to the central nervous system (CNS).[8] The etiology may vary from benign to life-threatening disorder. Majority of the NS are "symptomatic" seizures occurring as consequence of identifiable underlying etiology and are rarely idiopathic in nature. The current International League Against Epilepsy classifies seizure causes as *genetic, structural, metabolic, infectious, immune and unknown.*[10] Within that classification scheme, the majority of neonatal seizures are structural or metabolic in etiology.

Identification of the underlying etiology not only helps in acute management but also plays an important role in prognostication. A good history followed by relevant examination and investigations help in picking up the underlying etiology (See section 'approach to diagnosis'). While there are many underlying etiologies of NS, however, the common ones includes hypoxic-ischemic encephalopathy (HIE), metabolic derangements (hypoglycemia, hypocalcemia, and hyponatremia), CNS infections and structural brain injuries including ischemic and hemorrhagic strokes. HIE is the most common cause accounting NS in almost 40–50% of the cases. **Table 1** depicts the common etiologies of NS along with the respective salient clinical features.

Table 1: Common etiologies of neonatal seizures

Etiology	*Time of onset*	*Seizures*	*Clinical features*	*Remark*
Hypoxic-ischemic encephalopathy (HIE)	Within the first 12–24 hours after birth in moderate to severe HIE. May occur during rewarming phase of therapeutic hypothermia	Usually focal and may be multifocal All types of seizures with subtle being the most common	Signs of HIE including altered mental status, hypotonia, depressed to absent primitive reflexes and need of invasive ventilation (in severe HIE) in the context of fetal distress and perinatal depression Evidence of hypoxic injury to other organs (cardiovascular, renal, pulmonary, etc.)	Most common cause in both term and preterm neonates Always rule out associated metabolic causes (hypoglycemia, hypocalcemia, hyponatremia) too which coexist EEG is invaluable in identifying ongoing subclinical seizures
Ischemic stroke	Between 12 and 72 hours of age	Focal clonic seizures	Mental status is usually preserved unlike in HIE Usually there is no asymmetry in the motor examination in the acute phase	Second most common cause of neonatal seizures in full-term newborns
Cerebral sinus venous thrombosis	Between 12 and 72 hours of age		Have diffuse or focal neurological deficit	
Intracranial hemorrhage (Subarachnoid hemorrhage)	Between 24 and 48 hours of age	Focal seizures	Appears clinically well between seizures	Probably more common than realized Most do not produce any symptoms
Subdural hemorrhage	Between 24 and 48 hours of age	Focal seizures	May have altered mental status with large subdural hemorrhage	
Intraventricular haemorrhage	Within first week of life especially in first 72 hours	All types but predominantly subtle and generalized tonic seizures		Primarily seen with grade III or IV intraventricular hemorrhage More common in preterm infants
Intracranial infections • TORCH infection	Within first 72 hours in severe infection (CMV infection and toxoplasmosis) After first week in HSV encephalitis	Not specific	May have other stigmata of intrauterine infections like intrauterine growth restriction, microcephaly and other skin, ophthalmic, and systemic findings	
• Meningitis	Any time in the setting of meningitis	Not specific	Altered mental status along with systemic symptoms	
Malformations of the brain	Any time in neonatal period	All types	Neuro-cutaneous markers may be seen	Includes tuberous sclerosis, focal cortical dysplasia, hemimegalencephaly, lissencephaly, subcortical band heterotopia, peri-ventricular nodular heterotopia, schizencephaly, and polymicrogyrias. Most patients with these malformations do not have seizures in the neonatal period Seizures are often very refractory to medications

Contd...

Contd...

Etiology	*Time of onset*	*Seizures*	*Clinical features*	*Remark*
Metabolic disturbances	Hypoglycemia: Usually 2nd day of life Hypocalcemia (early onset): 24–72 hours Hypomagnesemia: 24–72 hours Hypocalcemia (late onset): 1–2 weeks of life Hypernatremia: Especially during correction Hyperbilirubinemia: 48–96 hours Local anesthetic Intoxication	All types	Manifestations include lethargy or irritability, jitteriness, tachypnea, apnea, hypotonia and vomiting	
Inborn error of metabolism	Can occur at any time in neonatal period Folinic acid-responsive seizures, pyridoxine dependency: as early as few hours after birth Organic acidemias, urea cycle defects and other disorders causing accumulation of toxic products: after 36–48 hours of birth	All types	Presentation is variable including lethargy, poor feeding, vomiting, altered mental status, apnea, hiccups, hypotonia and seizures The onset of clinical manifestations depends upon underlying disorder There may be associated metabolic derangements including hyperammonemia, metabolic acidosis and hypoglycemia	Shows poor response to anti-epileptic drugs Disorders include enzyme defect in metabolic pathways of carbohydrates, proteins, fat, mitochondrial or peroxisomal disorders, GLUT-1 transporter deficiency, nonketotic hyperglycinemia, pyridoxine dependency, folinic acid-responsive seizures and sulfite oxidase deficiency
Epilepsy syndromes				
Benign familial neonatal convulsion:	Day 2 or 3 of life	Focal clonic, focal tonic or apnea	Newborns appears well in the inter-ictal period	Autosomal dominant channelopathy involving voltage-gated potassium channels Favorable prognosis
Benign infantile neonatal seizures (Benign nonfamilial neonatal convulsion/ fifth-day fits)	Day 5 of life (4–6th day of life)	Focal clonic	Newborns appears well in the inter-ictal period	Favorable prognosis
Early myoclonic epilepsy	First few weeks to few months of life	Myoclonic (also focal motor clonic and tonic)		Etiology is usually underlying metabolic disease (e.g. Glycine encephalopathy) and are rarely structural or genetic Seizures are refractory to therapy with poor prognosis
Early infantile epileptic encephalopathy (Ohtahara syndrome)	First few weeks to few months of life	Tonic spasms (also focal motor clonic)		Etiology is usually structural brain lesion and are rarely genetic or metabolic Seizures are refractory to therapy with poor prognosis
Malignant migrating partial seizures in infancy (Coppola syndrome)	First few weeks to few months of life	Focal motor seizures occur and escalate aggressively, shifting clinically and electrographically from side to side		Unknown etiology Highly refractory to anti-convulsant medications

CLINICAL FEATURES

Definition

Seizure occurs due to excessive synchronous electrical discharge of the neurons within the central nervous system. A seizure is defined clinically as a paroxysmal alteration in neurological function, i.e. motor, behavioral or autonomic function.[8] These events are often associated with electrical ictal discharges identified on electroencephalography (EEG).

Classification of Neonatal Seizures

EEG based

As per American Clinical Neurophysiology Society,[9] NS have been classified into following three categories:

1. *Electroclinical seizure*: The clinical paroxysmal event is associated with synchronous electrical ictal discharges on EEG.
2. *EEG-only/Subclinical seizure*: The electrical ictal discharges occur in absence of clinical paroxysmal event. These are also known as nonconvulsive, or occult seizures.
3. *Clinical-only seizure*: The clinical paroxysmal event is not associated with electrical ictal discharges on EEG, e.g. generalized tonic posturing and motor automatism.

Neonatal EEG seizures are described as having[8] all of the following: *sudden EEG change, repetitive waveforms that evolve in morphology, frequency, and/or location, amplitude of at least 2 μV, and duration of at least 10 seconds*. However, if there is associated clinical event along with the electrical activity on EEG, it is still labeled as electroclinical seizure despite of duration being less than 10 seconds.

Clinical

Neonatal seizures have been classified into following four categories based on their clinical recognition:[8]

1. *Subtle seizures*: These are named so because of the subtle clinical manifestations, which may be easily missed even by a skilled observer. Subtle seizures are the most common neonatal seizures and occur more frequently in preterm neonates as compared to term newborns. These are often associated with EEG changes. They may manifest as:
   a. *Ocular movements*: Tonic horizontal deviation of eyes with or without jerking of eyes or sustained eye opening with ocular fixation.
   b. *Oral-buccal-lingual movements*: Chewing movements, lip smacking or tongue thrusting.
   c. *Limb movements*: Resembling cycling, boxing, swimming or hooking movements of the limbs.
   d. *Autonomic phenomena*: Tachycardia, bradycardia or flushing of skin.
   e. *Apnea*: Apnea being a manifestation of seizure activity is more common among term neonates as compared to preterm newborns. Convulsive apnea is associated with tachycardia but not bradycardia. However, if it gets prolonged then there may be associated bradycardia.
2. *Clonic seizures*: Clonic seizures manifest as repetitive, rhythmic contractions of specific muscle groups of a focal area involving limbs, face or trunk. There is a fast contraction phase followed by a slow relaxation phase. Typically, they have slow frequency of repetition around 1–3 per second unlike jitteriness and cannot be stopped by passive restraint. These are of two types as follows:
   a. *Focal clonic seizures* involve the face, extremities or axial structures like neck or trunk on one side of the body.
   b. *Multifocal clonic seizures* exhibit asynchronous clonic activity of several body areas that occurs simultaneously or migrate in a non-Jacksonian marching pattern like clonic movement of right upper limb followed by left lower limb involvement.

   Rarely, there can be generalized clonic seizures. Both types of clonic seizures are consistently associated with EEG changes.
3. *Tonic seizures*: Tonic seizures manifest as sustained contraction (flexion or extension) of axial or appendicular group of muscles. These are of two types as follows:
   a. *Focal tonic seizures* manifest as sustained posturing of a limb or asymmetrical posturing of neck or trunk. They are commonly associated with EEG changes.
   b. *Generalized tonic seizures* manifest as either flexion of both upper limbs and extension of bilateral lower limbs (like decorticate posturing) or extension of all the four limbs (like decerebrate posturing). These are not usually associated with EEG changes unlike focal tonic seizures. Thus, these events may represent "brainstem release" phenomena.
4. *Myoclonic seizures*: Myoclonic seizures manifest as very rapid jerks affecting one or multiple muscle groups. These are different from clonic jerks in terms of rapid

speed, absence of slow return and predilection for flexor group of muscles. These are of three types as follows:

a. *Focal myoclonic seizures* involve flexor muscles of an extremity.
b. *Multifocal myoclonic seizures* involve asynchronous twitching of several parts of the body.
c. *Generalized myoclonic seizures* manifest as bilateral jerks of flexion of upper and occasionally of lower extremities and appear similar to infantile spasm witnessed in older infants.

All the three types have poor correlation with EEG changes except with generalized type of myoclonic seizures, which has a somewhat better association.

APPROACH TO DIAGNOSIS

The first step while approaching such patients is to identify and differentiate these abnormal movements from non-epileptic neonatal movements (seizure mimics). One should take quick relevant history; do focused examination followed by basic investigations to determine the underlying etiology. One must ensure temperature, airway, breathing and circulation (TABC) first if required, before proceeding for establishing diagnosis and starting treatment. The stabilization of the neonate takes precedence over any other task.

Differentiate from Non-epileptic Movement (Seizure Mimics)

Before initiating treatment for neonatal seizures, one must differentiate the non-epileptic neonatal movements from true seizures, which in itself is a tedious task, sometimes requiring EEG assessment. Jitteriness is occasionally confused with neonatal seizures. The other close seizure mimics include tremors, benign neonatal sleep myoclonus, spasms due to tetanus, fragmentary myoclonic jerks and benign paroxysmal neonatal motor phenomena (e.g. roving/dys-conjugate eye movements). Some non-ictal movements are benign entities, while others, although not seizures, are nonetheless abnormal and indicative of underlying brain injury or dysfunction. Some of these are described briefly:

- *Jitteriness*: It is characterized by movements with qualities primarily of tremulousness but occasionally of clonus. The most consistently defined causes of jitteriness are hypoxic-ischemic encephalopathy, hypocalcemia, hypoglycemia, and drug withdrawal. **Table 2** describes the salient features differentiating seizures from jitteriness.
- *Spasm due to tetanus*: The spasms appear after 48 hours of age and are triggered by any stimulus like touch, light or sound. Fists are often tightly clenched. The neonate is conscious throughout often crying with pain. One may find trismus and opisthotonus posture in severe spasm.
- *Benign sleep myoclonus*: Unlike such other forms of myoclonus, myoclonic seizures are not induced by stimuli and cannot be suppressed by pressure to the affected body part. Furthermore, newborns with myoclonic seizures almost always have abnormal neurological exams, whereas newborns with benign myoclonus are otherwise normal.

Hyperekplexia/startle disease/congenital stiff-man syndrome: This disorder is characterized by episodes of tonic stiffening that is often confused with epilepsy in the neonatal period. Clinical diagnosis of hyperekplexia is

Table 2: Differentiating seizure and jitteriness

	Seizure	*Jitteriness*
Type of movement	Clonic/myoclonic/ tonic movements with low frequency and high amplitude Predominant movement is clonic jerking	High frequency, low amplitude and oscillatory Predominant movement is tremor (i.e. the alternating movements are rhythmic and of equal rate and amplitude)
Provoked by stimulus	No (spontaneous in onset)	Yes
Aborted by passive flexion of limb	No	Yes
Associated with autonomic changes (tachycardia, fluctuation in blood pressure)	Yes	No
Ocular phenomena (eye fixation or deviation), automatism	Yes	No
Examination in between abnormal movements	Normal or abnormal	Normal
EEG	Abnormal	Normal

made by a nose-tapping test. Tapping the nose of a normal baby will elicit either a blink response or no response and habituation to the response will be present but in a baby with hyperekplexia, nose-tapping results in exaggerated startle and stiffening episodes without habituation.

It is important to differentiate seizures from these non-epileptic movements because of all-together different management and outcome. Inappropriate treatment of non-epileptic conditions may cause more harm. Occasionally, these conditions may pose diagnostic challenge. Meticulous history, close observation and EEG helps in differentiating these non-epipleptic movements from seizures. It is important to note that apnea may be the sole manifestation of seizures in term neonates. Presence of associated tachycardia may support the diagnosis in presence of underlying setting.

Determining Etiology

History

History is the first step in identifying the underlying etiology. However, it may not be possible to take a detailed history in an emergency setting especially when the neonate is seizing. The priority is to stabilize the neonate and then proceed as highlighted earlier. One may take simultaneous history if possible. **Table 3** describes

Table 3: Key points in the history in a case of suspected neonatal seizure

History	*Key point*	*Possible etiology*
Gestation	Term	HIE, metabolic disorders, developmental defects, intracranial infections and epilepsy syndromes
	Preterm	HIE, Intracranial hemorrhage, intracranial infections, hypoglycemia, hypocalcemia
Birth weight and current weight	To determine excessive postnatal weight loss which is usually due to poor/faulty feeding	Hypernatremia, cortical sinus thrombosis, meningitis, hypoglycemia
Intrauterine growth status (AGA/SGA/LGA)	SGA LGA	SGA – Hypoglycemia LGA – Hypoglycemia, hypocalcemia
Day of onset of seizure	0–3 days	HIE, ICH, intracranial infections, hypoglycemia, early onset hypocalcemia, accidental LA injection, NKH, pyridoxine dependant seizure, developmental defects, usually present within 72 hours
	>3 days	Late onset hypocalcemia, late hemorrhagic disease of newborn (beyond 1 week), infections, development defects and epilepsy syndromes
Antenatal history	H/s/o intrauterine infection (fever, rash, arthralgias, neck swelling, genital ulcer especially in first trimester)	TORCH infection especially CMV and toxoplasma
	Drug, X-ray or teratogen exposure	Brain malformation
	Vesicles around genitalia in peripartum period	HSV infection
	PIH and chronic illness (RHD, CKD, etc.)	SGA infant
	HELLP syndrome	Fatty acid oxidation defects
	Diabetes (Pre-existing)	Brain malformation, hypoglycemia, hypocalcemia
	Gestational diabetes mellitus	Hypoglycemia, hypocalcemia
	H/o intra-uterine infection/chorio-amnionitis	Meningitis
	Beta- blockers	Hypoglycemia
	Narcotic addiction	Withdrawal syndrome
	Excessive fetal movements/hiccups on ultrasound – suggesting intra-uterine seizures	IEMs like non-ketotic hyperglycinemia
	Clotting or bleeding tendencies	Neonatal stroke or hemorrhage

Contd...

Contd...

History	*Key point*	*Possible etiology*
Perinatal history	H/o fetal distress, decreased fetal movements, abnormal cardio-tocograph, passage of meconium, instrumental delivery, need for resuscitation at birth, Apgar scores, abnormal cord blood gas	Perinatal asphyxia ± IVH in preterms
	Accidental injection of local anesthetic agent in the fetal scalp	Lignocaine toxicity (due to inadvertent injection of lignocaine into infant's scalp, at the time of placement of paracervical, pudendal, or epidural block or LA for episiotomy)
Place of delivery	Home delivery	Intracranial hemorrhage (Hemorrhagic disease of newborn due to non-administration of Vitamin K at birth) Perinatal asphyxia
Postnatal history		
Feeding history	Difficulty in feeding causing excessive weight loss	Hypernatremic dehydration IEM
	Mixed feeding especially cow's milk	Late onset hypocalcemia
General well-being	Poor feeding, decreased activities, vomiting, fever	IEM Meningitis
Family history	Consanguinity, family h/o convulsions/ mental retardation, unexplained neonatal deaths	IEM Epileptic syndromes Genetic epilepsies Benign familial neonatal convulsions

the specific points in the history, which one should seek to pick up the underlying etiology of neonatal seizures. However, an important aspect is to describe the event—the pre-ictal phase (awake/sleeping), semiology of seizure including associated eye movements, autonomic phenomenon, restraint ability of the episode, any skin mottling or cyanosis and post-ictal phase (duration of unconsciousness if any) and subsequent level of alertness (normal or depressed). It is best to see the video of seizure if available and always counsel parents to video record these episodes in future.

Examination

Focused examination including vitals, general and systemic examination plays a pivotal role. It not only helps in picking up the likely etiology but also in the overall management. **Table 4** highlights key findings that should be actively looked for in cases of neonatal seizures.

MANAGEMENT

Investigations

The basic laboratory work up in a case of suspected NS includes the following:

- Blood glucose
- Serum electrolytes primarily serum sodium, ionized calcium and magnesium
- Sepsis screen parameters including complete blood count with its differential
- Cerebrospinal fluid (CSF) examination including counts, sugar and proteins
- Microbial cultures (blood, urine and CSF samples)
- Coagulogram (PT/aPTT) and platelet count in case of suspected bleeding disorder
- Serum bilirubin
- Cranial ultrasound
- Arterial blood gas (ABG), plasma ammonia and plasma lactate in suspected inborn errors of metabolism (IEM).

The clues from the history and examination helps in choosing the appropriate investigations however, blood glucose, serum electrolytes and CSF examination are required in almost all cases of NS. Most of these basic investigations can be easily done in an emergency room. CSF examination may be withheld in case of severe cardiorespiratory compromise till the infant gets stabilized and may be omitted in case of severe perinatal asphyxia with a clear sentinel event explaining perinatal asphyxia with no risk factor for early onset sepsis. However, in doubtful cases of sepsis and metabolic disorders, it should be done

Table 4: Key examination findings in case of suspected neonatal seizure

Examination	*Key findings*	*Possible etiology*
General physical examination	Vitals	To first maintain TABC
	Microcephaly	TORCH infection
	Macrocephaly	Hydrocephalus
	Pallor	Intracranial bleed
	Icterus with sole staining	Acute bilirubin encephalopathy
	Cataract	TORCH infection Metabolic (storage) disease
	Malformation or dysmorphism	Chromosomal abnormalities like trisomy
	Neuro-cutaneous marker	Ash leaf macule in tuberous sclerosis Port wine stain of the forehead/eyelid – in Sturge-Weber syndrome
	Petechiae or ecchymosis	TORCH infection, intracranial bleed
	Blueberry muffin skin lesion	Congenital rubella syndrome (or other TORCH infection)
	Vesicular lesion	HSV infection
	Abnormal body or urine odor	IEM
	Hiccups	IEM like non-ketotic hyperglycinemia
	Tremulousness, sweating	Withdrawal symptoms
	Sclerema	Sepsis
Abdominal examination	Hepatosplenomegaly	IEM, TORCH infection
Central nervous system examination	Bulging anterior fontanel	Intracranial bleed, meningitis
	Level of alertness (alert/drowsy/unconscious)	Decreased alertness in sepsis or encephalopathy due to any cause like HIE and IEM
	Fundus	Chorioretinitis in TORCH infection Hypoplastic optic nerve in cerebral dysgenesis
	Spontaneous movements and tone	Asymmetry suggesting structural lesion of brain or neonatal stroke

to rule out intrauterine infection and metabolic conditions like glycine encephalopathy/glucose transporter defects predisposing to perinatal asphyxia.

Additional investigations are required in setting of refractory or unexplained seizures or in presence of specific clues. These investigations include the following:

- Herpes simplex virus (HSV) PCR in case of suspicion of HSV encephalitis
- Work up for TORCH infections
- CT head, MRI brain including MRA, MRV in cases of suspected intracranial hemorrhage and sinus venous thrombosis and echocardiography in setting of ischemic stroke
- MR spectroscopy in suspected inborn error of metabolism (IEM)
- EEG – conventional or amplitude integrated EEG
- Lactate/pyruvate ratio in blood and CSF, tandem mass spectrometry (TMS), blood and urine ketones, urine for reducing substance and urine organic acids in suspected IEM
- Thrombophilia studies
- Genetic studies
- Urine drug test in cases of intoxication or withdrawal.

It is important to realize that neuroimaging except bedside neurosonogram needs transportation, which poses a risk of destabilization. Therefore, this investigation should be deferred until the neonate is stabilized and treatment has been initiated.

Neuroimaging

There is a limited role of neuroimaging in an emergency room, with following exceptions.

- *Neurosonogram*: A bedside neurosonogram may help in picking up gross intracranial parenchymal bleed including intraventricular hemorrhage, hydrocephalus, cerebral edema or gross structural malformations of the brain.
- *Computed tomography (CT) head*: It can pick up even small intracranial bleed including axial bleeds like subdural and sub-arachnoid hemorrhage, infarcts, cerebral sinus venous thrombosis and calcification apart from hydrocephalus, cerebral edema and few structural brain malformations. However, it leads to significant radiation exposure. The advantage of CT head over magnetic resonance imaging (MRI) brain is that only few seconds are required to get it done unlike MRI where it takes at least 20–30 minutes. However, getting CT or MRI carries an inherent risk of destabilization. Therefore, these investigations are done in selected patients.
- *Magnetic resonance imaging (MRI) brain*: Though it is a time consuming investigation, it offers advantages over CT head in terms of picking up posterior fossa lesion, minor brain structural malformations especially neuronal migration disorder and better delineation of gray and white matter for identifying any pathology including IEMs and disorders of myelination. Moreover, there is no radiation exposure. MRI brain is usually not possible in emergency setting and done later on while investigating the underlying etiology of seizure in cases where the baseline work-up is non-contributory.

Electroencephalography (EEG)

The EEG is an important diagnostic and prognostic tool in neonatal seizures; however, it is not possible to get it done in an emergency setting. Video EEG is the gold standard modality; however, its availability is very limited. World Health Organization (WHO) guidelines on neonatal seizures recommend confirmation of all clinical seizures by EEG if the facility is available.[7]

The EEG helps in differentiating seizures from nonepileptic movements and picks up subclinical seizures. Moreover, it helps in identifying seizures in neonates who are paralyzed but at high risk of seizures and helps in assessing response to therapy. Moreover, background abnormalities in EEG provides important prognostic information about long-term neurodevelopmental outcome. Because of these reasons, there is an increasing emphasis on continuous EEG monitoring to aid in the management of neonatal seizures. Continuous EEG is possible only once the neonate is shifted to neonatal intensive care unit (NICU) or in EEG rooms after stabilization.

Amplitude-integrated EEG (aEEG)/cerebral function monitoring (CFM)

The aEEG uses the conventional EEG data obtained through single or dual-channel, compress it and generate the final tracing showing several hours of EEG data on a single screen. It is an easily accessible technique available to neonatologist to monitor cortical electrical activity at bedside in NICU. One can easily interpret without specialized training. It shows both electrical seizures and background abnormalities like conventional EEG however, with slightly low sensitivity and specificity. It should be recorded for 24 hours in high risk neonates and continued for 24 hours after the last seizure.

Treatment

It is important to treat seizures due to two reasons. First, seizures per se may cause acute deterioration in the ventilator function and circulation thus causing hemodynamic compromise. Second, the available evidence suggests that the repeated seizures may cause secondary brain injury leading to less favorable long-term neurodevelopmental outcome. Therefore, seizures needs to be treated aggressively. WHO guidelines[7] on neonatal seizures recommend treatment of all clinically apparent seizures (lasting more than 3 minutes) and electrographic seizures. The systematic approach for treating NS is as follows:

First step: Initial medical management

1. The first and the foremost requirement in an emergency room is to ensure the stability of the neonate. Place the neonate in thermoneutral environment; ensure patent airway, effective breathing and adequate circulation (TABC). Start oxygen if required, secure intravenous (IV) access and draw blood samples for checking blood sugar and other first line investigations including hemogram and electrolytes **(Flowchart 1)**.
2. This is followed by quick relevant history and focused clinical examination as discussed in previous sections to identify the underlying etiology. The treatment and the evaluation goes hand in hand in the initial phase of management. **Flowchart 1** describes the overall treatment algorithm in case of neonatal seizure.

Flowchart 1: Algorithm for acute management of neonatal seizure

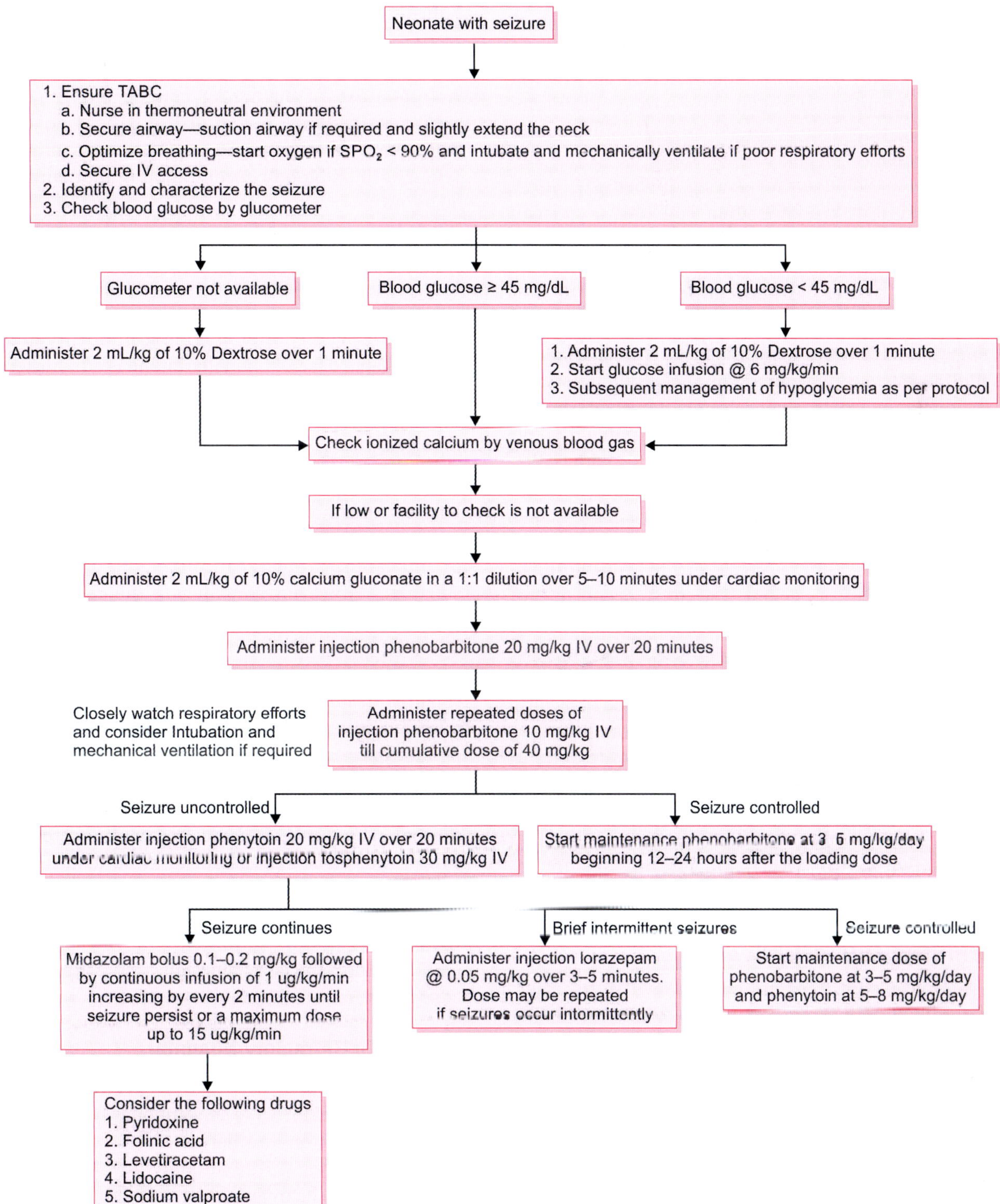

Second step: Correct hypoglycemia (if present)

1. After ensuring TABC, correct hypoglycemia (blood sugar <45 mg/dL by glucometer) if present, by a bolus of 2 mL/kg of 10% dextrose followed by maintenance glucose infusion of 6–8 mg/kg/min to maintain blood sugar between 70 and 100 mg/dL. Subsequent management of hypoglycemia should be as per the protocol. If facility for measuring the bedside blood glucose is not available then consider empirical treatment with glucose bolus and see its response.

Third step: Correct hypocalcemia (if present)

1. In case the seizure continues despite normal blood sugar levels to begin with or after its correction, then ionized calcium (iCa) should be checked in blood gas estimation machine. Hypocalcemia if present, should be corrected by infusing calcium gluconate (10%) at the dose of 2 mL/kg (200 mg/kg; 1:1 diluted with D5W/D10W/DW) slowly over 5–10 minutes under strict cardiac monitoring (withhold infusion if heart rate <100/min and wait for it to recover) followed by maintenance calcium. In case seizures persist due to hypocalcemia, give second dose of calcium. If seizure reoccurs due to hypocalcemia, consider administration of 0.2 mL/kg of 50% magnesium sulfate intramuscularly (IM). One can repeat the same dose every 12 hours until normal level of magnesium is achieved. In absence of facility for measuring ionized calcium, calcium infusion may be considered if seizures persist despite normal glucose level in a neonate. It is important to first evaluate and treat hypoglycemia and hypocalcemia in that order if present, rather than directly administering anti-epileptic drug (AED) for aborting seizure in neonates.

Fourth step: Anti-epileptic drugs

If a neonate continues to have convulsions after ensuring TABC and taking care of correctable metabolic disturbances like hypoglycemia and hypocalcemia, then AED should be considered.

First line drug

1. Phenobarbitone is the first AED administered for treating neonatal seizures and the same has been reinforced in WHO guidelines.[7] The loading dose of 20 mg/kg is necessary to achieve a blood level of approximately 20 µg/mL, which achieves a significant anticonvulsant effect in the newborn. Additional dose of 10 mg/kg of phenobarbitone can be administered if the initial dose is ineffective in controlling seizures. A total dose of 40 mg/kg can be administered until seizures have seized or the patient develops dose limiting adverse effects (Maximum targeted phenobarbital blood concentration is approximately 40 µg/mL).
2. It can be given by both intravenous (preferred) and intramuscular route. To achieve the same blood level, the intramuscular dose must be approximately 10–15% greater than the intravenous dose.
3. If seizures cease after phenobarbitone loading, maintenance dose of phenobarbitone is administered at the dose of 3–5 mg/kg/day, the first maintenance being given 12 hours after loading in case of a term neonate.

Second line drug

1. Based on the available evidence, the WHO guidelines on neonatal seizures recommend either midazolam or lidocaine as the second-line AED in neonatal seizures.[7] However, considering the restraints in providing respiratory support in most neonatal units in India, phenytoin or fosphenytoin is used as the second line agent in neonates who continue to have seizures despite the administering of the maximal tolerated dose of phenobarbital. The use of phenytoin or lidocaine requires cardiac monitoring facilities.
2. Phenytoin precipitates in dextrose containing intravenous fluids and hence should be diluted in normal saline only. It should be administered at a slower rate of <1 mg/kg/min to avoid disturbances of cardiac rhythm. *Fosphenytoin*, a phosphate ester prodrug of phenytoin, has advantages over phenytoin with higher water solubility, safe intramuscular administration and faster allowable rate of intravenous administration.

Drugs used in Refractory Neonatal Seizures (Table 5)

If the seizures are refractory to conventional AEDs then the following drugs may be considered.

- *Benzodiazepines*: Approximately 20% or more of newborns with electrographic seizures do not respond to the sequential administration of phenobarbital

Table 5: Anti-epileptic drugs–dosage, efficacy and adverse reactions

Drug	*Dose*	*Adverse effects*	*Special remarks*
Phenobarbitone	• Loading dose: 20 mg/kg over 20 mins • Maintenance: 3–5 mg/kg/day OD	Impairs neurodevelopment, promotes neuronal apoptosis, a/w drug interactions by induction of CYP450	The therapeutic level in the neonatal period is 20–40 mg/L
Phenytoin	• Loading dose: 20 mg/kg over 20 mins • Maintenance: 5–8 mg/kg/day OD in <7days neonates • >7 days infant: up to 8 mg/kg/dose q 8–12 hourly	Extravasation causes tissue inflammation and necrosis due to high pH and osmolality. Promotes neuronal apoptosis and drug-drug interactions	Precipitates with dextrose solution
Lidocaine	• Loading: 2 mg/kg i/v over 10 mins, f/b • Maintenance: 6 mg/kg per hour for 6 hours, then 4 mg/kg per hour for 12 hours, then 2 mg/kg per hour for 12 hours	Arrhythmias and significant bradycardia	Because of the cumulative risk of toxicity, lidocaine must be stopped within 36 hours The dose must be reduced in premature infants or if the newborn is undergoing therapeutic hypothermia, as clearance decreases by 24% during hypothermia
Benzodiazepines • Lorazepam • Midazolam	• Lorazepam: 0.05–0.1 mg/kg over 3–5 mins • Midazolam: 0.15–0.2 mg/kg over 5 mins, f/b continuous infusion @1–15 μg/kg/min	Associated with severe respiratory depresssion, so not advised in non-critical care setting	
Levetiracetam	• Loading: 40 mg/kg • Maintenance: 30–60 mg/kg/day in 2 divided doses	Sedation and irritability No serious side effects are noted	It does not induce cell death in the developing brain which might offer a theoretical benefit over older established anticonvulsants
Topiramate	3 mg/kg/day (oral)	Acute myopia, secondary angle-closure glaucoma, hyperthermia, decreased sweating and metabolic acidosis have been reported with topiramate	Also used as an adjunct for neuroprotection against HIE
Valproate	Loading: 20 mg/kg Maintenance: 10 mg/kg every 12 hourly	Elevated ammonia levels, hepatotoxicity	Watch for hyperammonemia during the first week of administration and suspend treatment if the serum ammonia level exceeds 350 μmol/L
Paraldehyde	IM: 0.1–0.2 mL/kg/dose PR: 0.3 mL/kg/dose mixed with coconut oil in 3:1 by rectal route	Pulmonary hemorrhage, pulmonary edema, hypotension, liver injury	Additional doses may be given after 30 mins and q 4–6 hrly
Vigabatrin	15–20 mg/kg/dose twice daily, hiked up to 75 mg/kg/dose q 12 hourly	Hyperkinesia, weight gain, insomnia, visual field defects	Vigabatrin is the drug of choice for infantile spasms associated with tuberous sclerosis

and phenytoin. Lorazepam and midazolam are the frequently used benzodiazepines in neonatal seizures. Lorazepam enters the brain rapidly and is effective in treatment of neonatal clinical seizures. The onset of action is seen within 2 to 3 minutes and the duration extends up to 24 hours. Midazolam is the short-acting benzodiazepines, useful in refractory neonatal seizures with the advantage of less respiratory depression and sedation than lorazepam and diazepam. However, due to its potential risk on neurological maturation of newborns, it should not be used as the first line to abort seizures.[11]

- *Levetiracetam*: Levetiracetam is a relatively new AED which is proposed to act through synaptic vesicle protein 2A (SV2A), by preventing calcium influx through N-type calcium channels which in turn reduces exocytosis and reduces the release of glutamate from intracellular vesicles. It has a very favorable pharmacokinetic and safety profile in neonates.[12] Levetiracetam has been a preferred second line AED in certain neonatal units, considering its safe administration and proposed neuroprotective role by preventing neurotransmitter release.
- *Lidocaine*: Lidocaine can be used as a second or third-line agent for refractory neonatal seizures.[7] The medication has good CNS penetration and acts as a depressant. Full term newborns had a better response rate than did preterm newborns. Lidocaine can cause arrhythmias and bradycardia. It should be avoided in newborns who have congenital heart issues, unstable serum potassium or have received other pro-arrhythmic drugs like phenytoin.
- *Topiramate*: Topiramate reduces the frequency of action potential firing by altering GABA neurotransmission, blocking voltage-gated sodium channels and by weakly blocking AMPA glutamate receptors. It was shown to have potent anticonvulsant effects and neuro-protective properties for neuronal or pre-myelinating oligodendrocyte injury. Intravenous preparations are not available, thereby limiting its use in acute seizure control.
- *Valproate*: Valproate can occasionally be used in refractory neonatal seizures. It should be used with caution in hepatocellular failure, suspicion of neurometabolic disorder and mitochondrial cytopathy.
- *Bumetanide*: Bumetanide is a potential adjunct to AED treatments for neonatal seizures, inhibiting the chloride co-transporter responsible for the elevated neuronal chloride levels and restores the inhibitory response of GABA receptor activation.[8] However, due to its poor CNS penetration and possible risk of ototoxicity, the use is restricted.
- *Vigabatrin*: Vigabatrin acts by inhibition of GABA transaminases. It is useful as a monotherapy in infantile spasms and as an adjunct therapy in refractory partial epilepsy. Visual field defects is the most commonly encountered side effect. It can aggravate absence and myoclonic seizures.
- *Thiopental*: The dose is 10 mg/kg, administered intravenously over 2 minutes, and response occurs promptly. However, it has serious adverse effects in form of severe hypotension, requiring vasopressors.
- *Carbamazepine*: The use of carbamazepine in HIE showed an excellent clinical response. Therapeutic levels were achieved within 2 to 4 hours after a loading dose of 10 mg/kg administered by nasogastric tube. However, variability in blood levels suggests that more data are needed to determine the value of this agent.

In neonates where there is no apparent cause of refractory seizures, possibility of IEM should be considered and a trial of following drugs should be given.

- *Pyridoxine*: A therapeutic trial with 100 mg of pyridoxine is given intravenously and a simultaneous response is assessed electrographically or clinically. If the response is present, one should get the urine test done for alpha-AASA or plasma pipecolic acid levels followed by mutation analysis to confirm the diagnosis of pyridoxine-dependent seizures. In case the response is equivocal, trial of repeated doses of 100-mg of pyridoxine infusions may be given to maximum of 500 mg. Some infants do not respond to pyridoxine and may require pyridoxal-5-phosphate (PLP), the active form of vitamin B_6. A dose of 50 to 100 mg/kg of PLP divided six times per day is administered for at least 3 to 5 days. PLP is only available in enteral forms and has side effects similar to pyridoxine. The positive response in form of clinical or electrical subsidence of seizures points towards pyridoxal-phosphate responsive seizures, which should be confirmed by mutation analysis.
- *Folinic acid*: If there is no response to pyridoxine or PLP, then a trial of folinic acid (leucovorin) should be considered, with a dose of 3 to 5 mg/kg per day administered orally for at least 3 to 5 days. Positive response (electrical or clinical) suggests folinic acid responsive seizures.
- *Biotin*: Biotinidase deficiency presents little later than neonatal period however, a trial of 10 mg of oral biotin may be considered in suspected cases.
- *Ketogenic diet*: The ketogenic diet is the optimal treatment for newborns with a *glucose* transporter defect with onset of seizures in the neonatal period.

Etiology-specific therapy

It is equally important to treat the underlying cause of seizures apart from giving AED. Therefore, apart from the overall management as highlighted in **Flowchart 1**, etiology-specific therapy needs to be strongly considered in each case based on the suspected underlying cause. The initial management of hypoglycemia and hypocalcemia has already been highlighted in the **Flowchart 1**. Thereafter, these should be managed as per their protocol. CNS infections should be treated with the prompt antimicrobial administration. Therapeutic hypothermia is the standard of care for moderate to severe HIE and should be given as per standard protocol.

End-point of acute therapy

Considering the adverse effect of repeated seizures on long-term brain development, the ideal goal of acute therapy is to eliminate the electrographic seizures. Moreover, administration of AEDs in neonates may cause electroclinical dissociation leading to vanishing of clinical seizures with persistence of electrical activity. Therefore, ideal management includes EEG confirmation of the treatment response, which is seldom available in the developing countries. The current practice mostly consists of AED therapy until clinical seizures are controlled. It is important to understand that in some cases the ideal goal of complete elimination of electrographic seizure is not possible due to the potentially dangerous adverse reactions of AED in form of disturbances in the cardiac and ventilator function. So underlying etiology must be taken into account while treating seizures. Complete electrographic control is appropriate in a neonate with HIE whereas the goal may be to reduce clinical seizures as much as possible in a neonate with brain malformation thus retaining acceptable alertness in long-term.

Duration of therapy

The optimal duration of AED in neonatal seizures revolves around the likelihood of seizure recurrence/epilepsy and impairment in long-term neurological outcome after discontinuation of these drugs. On the contrary, both animal and preliminary human data has raised possibility of deleterious effect of AEDs in particular of phenobarbitone on the developing brain by causing apoptotic neurodegeneration. This effect is much more pronounced with the combination of various AEDs including phenytoin, valproate and clonazepam.

Traditionally, underlying etiology of the neonatal seizures (transient metabolic disturbances vs. HIE/cerebral dysgenesis/IEM), neurological examination at discharge/follow-up (normal vs. abnormal) and EEG (normal vs. abnormal) are the three important factors, which have been considered while deciding the timing of withdrawal and stoppage of AEDs. However, sedation and potential neurotoxic effect of AEDs on the developing brain as highlighted above has now led clinicians to err on the side of stopping these drugs early. Lack of well-defined criteria due to the lack of robust evidence regarding the ideal timing for considering stoppage of AEDs has resulted in wide variation in the practices among the clinicians.

The WHO guidelines on "when" AEDs should be discontinued clearly states that *"In neonates with normal neurological examination and/or normal electroencephalography, consider stopping antiepileptic drugs if seizure-free for >72 hours; the drug(s) should be reinstituted in case of recurrence of seizures (weak recommendation)".*[7]

Once the decision has been taken to stop the drug, then "how" should the medication be discontinued is the next question. As per WHO guidelines, in neonates in whom the seizure control has been achieved with a single antiepileptic drug, then the drug can be discontinued abruptly without any tapering of the dose. However, in neonates requiring more than one antiepileptic drugs for seizure control, the drugs may be stopped one by one, with phenobarbital being the last drug to be withdrawn.[7]

PROGNOSIS

There is increased risk of mortality as well as poor long-term neurodevelopmental outcome among neonates with seizures. The current incidence of mortality is around 7–16% in term neonates in contrast to preterm neonates where it as high as 22–58%.[3] Moreover, there is a high risk of mortality among survivors during childhood especially in those with cerebral palsy and global developmental delay.

Neurological impairment in form of motor deficits, cerebral palsy, intellectual disability, global developmental delay, cognitive deficits and postneonatal epilepsy develops in as high as 20–50% of the survivors.[13] Postneonatal epilepsy including West syndrome develops in 10–30% of the survivors and majority have the onset within first year of life. High seizure burden, refractory seizures, abnormal neurological examination, abnormal neuroimaging and persistently abnormal interictal EEG background activity are the important risk factors for development of postneonatal epilepsy. Infants developing postneonatal epilepsy are also at high risk of cognitive and motor deficits.

The two most important factors determining long-term neurodevelopmental outcome is the underlying etiology of neonatal seizures and the EEG findings (background abnormalities and seizure burden). Moderate to severe HIE, IEMs, cerebral malformation and meningitis carries high risk of disability as compared to seizures due to subarachnoid hemorrhage, transient electrolyte/metabolic disturbances or idiopathic seizures. Moderate background EEG abnormalities like voltage asymmetries, "immaturity", and severe background abnormalities like burst-suppression pattern and marked voltage suppression results in neurological sequelae in almost 50% and 90% of the infants respectively. Persistence of abnormal findings in repeated EEGs also predicts poor long-term outcome. In general, neonates with frequent seizures or status epilepticus have poor outcome.[3] Gestational age also influence the outcome with increasing risk of both morbidities and mortality with decreasing gestational age.

PREVENTION

Improving basic perinatal practices like antenatal steroids in eligible population, institutional deliveries with timely resuscitation if required thus avoiding of perinatal asphyxia, early initiation of breastfeeding, screening and prompt treatment of hypoglycemia and jaundice and prevention of infection may help in preventing neonatal seizures to a large extent in low- and middle-income countries like ours.

KEY MESSAGES

- Neonatal seizures are one of the most common neonatal neurological emergencies and should be treated promptly.
- The incidence increases with decreasing gestational age.
- These are of three types: electroclinical, EEG only/subclinical seizures and clinical only.
- Clinically, neonatal seizures are of various types with different manifestations; one should learn to distinguish between them.
- The most common cause of neonatal seizures is hypoxic-ischemic encephalopathy.
- Focused history, targeted examination supplemented with basic investigations helps in clinching the diagnosis in large number of patients.
- One should always rule out hypoglycemia and hypocalcemia before administering phenobarbitone, which is still the first anti-epileptic drug to be used.
- Continuous video-electroencephalogram is the gold standard in detecting and monitoring neonatal seizures.
- One should consider trial of pyridoxine and/or folinic acid in case of refractory seizure.
- Underlying etiology and the EEG findings are the two most important prognostic factors determining long-term neurodevelopmental outcome.

REFERENCES

1. Glass HC. Neonatal seizures: Advances in mechanisms and management. Clin Perinatol. 2014;41:177-90.
2. Panayiotopoulos CP. Neonatal Seizures and neonatal syndromes. In: Panayiotopoulos CP, editor. The Epilepsies: Seizures, Syndromes and Management. Oxfordshire (UK): Bladon Medical Publishing; 2005.
3. Uria-Avellanal C, Marlow N, Rennie JM. Outcome following neonatal seizures. Semin Fetal Neonatal Med. 2013;18:224-32.
4. Vasudevan C, Levene M. Epidemiology and aetiology of neonatal seizures. Semin Fetal Neonatal Med. 2013;18:185-91.
5. Wusthoff CJ. Seizures in infants born preterm: Defining the scale of the problem. J Pediatr. 2017;187:7-8.
6. NNPD Nodal Center at Department of Pediatrics, WHO Collaborating Centre Newborn Training and Research, All India Institute of Medical Sciences, India. 2005. Report of National Neonatal-Perinatal Database (NNPD) 2002-2003. Available from: *https://www.newbornwhocc.org/pdf/nnpd_report_2002-03.PDF*. Accessed August 30, 2019.
7. WHO. 2011. Guidelines on neonatal seizures. Available from: *https://apps.who.int/iris/bitstream/handle/10665/77756/9789241548304_eng.pdf;jsessionid=9D603BD5B451D831726B4E8203C12E50?sequence=1*. Accessed August 30, 2019.
8. Abend NS, Jensen FE, Inder TE, *et al.* Neonatal seizures. In: Volpe JJ, editor. Volpe's Neurology of the Newborn, 6th edition. Philadelphia: Saunders Elsevier; 2018. p. 342-402.
9. Tsuchida TN, Wusthoff CJ, Shellhaas RA, *et al.* American clinical neurophysiology society standardized EEG terminology and categorization for the description of continuous EEG monitoring in neonates: Report of the American Clinical Neurophysiology Society Critical Care Monitoring Committee. J Clin Neurophysiol. 2013;30:161-73.
10. Scheffer IE, Berkovic S, Capovilla G, *et al.* ILAE classification of the epilepsies: Position paper of the ILAE Commission for Classification And Terminology. Epilepsia. 2017;58(4):512-21.
11. Khanna A, Walcott BP, Kahle KT. Limitations of current GABA agonists in neonatal seizures: Toward GABA modulation via the targeting of neuronal Cl^- transport. Front Neurol. 2013;4:78.
12. Merhar SL, Schibler KR, Sherwin CM, *et al.* Pharmacokinetics of levetiracetam in neonates with seizures. J Pediatr. 2011;159:152-4.e3.
13. Brunquell PJ, Glennon CM, DiMario FJ Jr, *et al.* Prediction of outcome based on clinical seizure type in newborn infants. J Pediatr. 2002;140:707-12.

CHAPTER 73

Neonatal Hypoglycemia

Jogender Kumar, Sourabh Dutta

INTRODUCTION

Hypoglycemia in newborns is one of the most commonly encountered metabolic problems. It is commonly associated with other neonatal illnesses. The incidence of hypoglycemia varies with gestation, intrauterine growth status, sickness level, feeding patterns, the definition used for defining hypoglycemia and the timing of screening.[1,2] A large cohort study of 4000 neonates, found that 3.4% babies had blood glucose < 40 mg/dL and 12.1% had blood sugar < 47 mg/dL.[2] The major risk factors for hypoglycemia are infant of diabetic mother (IDM), large for gestational age (LGA), small for gestational age (SGA) infants, and late preterm. The estimated incidence of hypoglycemia in SGA infants can vary from 20% to 70%.[3]

PATHOGENESIS

The brain utilizes glucose as its primary fuel. Hence, the supply of glucose to the fetal and neonatal brain is a critically important activity. During fetal life, the brain receives a constant and adequate supply of glucose. Glucose crosses the placenta by facilitated diffusion. Fetal glucose levels are approximately two-thirds of maternal levels. This happy state of affairs continues till the umbilical cord is clamped, after which the newborn blood glucose levels plummet to a nadir at 1 to 2 hours of life. The levels then increase and stabilize at mean levels of 65 to 71 mg/dL by 3 to 4 hours of life. It takes time for the newborn baby to establish effective feeding. The period between the cessation of glucose supply from the maternal circulation and the resumption of effective supply by enteral nutrition is akin to a period of fasting. The neonatal metabolic pathways quickly adapt to this period of fasting in order to preserve fuel supply to the brain. There are 5 key metabolic pathways (**Flowchart 1**) and 5 key hormones that are involved in glucose homeostasis. The five hormones that regulate glucose homeostasis are insulin, glucagon, adrenaline, cortisol and growth hormone (**Table 1**).

Flowchart 1: Metabolic adaptation to fasting

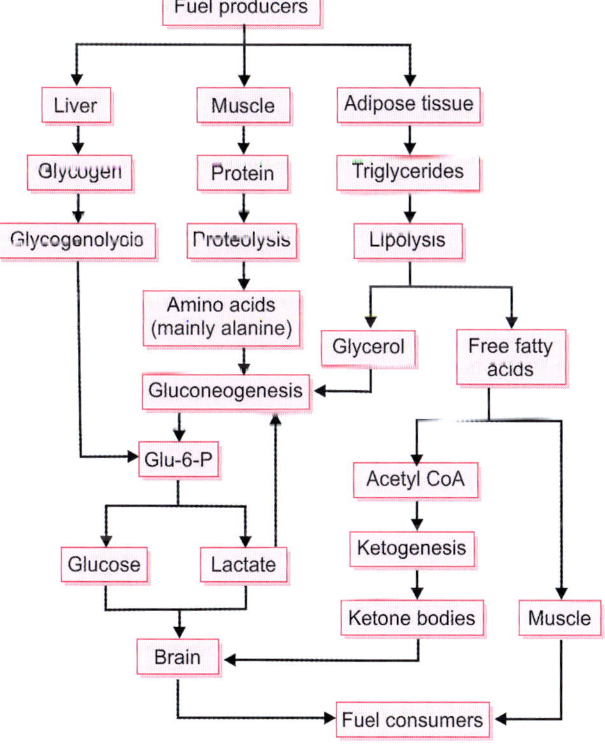

Table 1: Action of various hormones involved in glucose metabolism

Hormone	*Glycogenolysis*	*Gluconeogenesis*	*Proteolysis*	*Lipolysis*	*Ketogenesis*
Insulin	–	–	–	–	–
Glucagon	+	+	0	0	0
Adrenaline	+	+	0	+	+
Cortisol	0	+	+	0	0
Growth hormone	0	0	0	+	0
+: Stimulates; –: Inhibits; 0: No effect					

The effect of the later four counters the effects of insulin; hence, they are called counter-regulatory hormones.

ETIOLOGY

The causes of neonatal hypoglycemia could be classified either on the basis of pathogenesis or clinical presentation. The classification based on the pathogenesis shall be discussed first as this follows directly from the concept of the metabolic pathways and the regulatory hormones (**Table 2**).

Small for gestational age (SGA) babies, preterm infants and sick infants with sepsis, hypothermia or shock can have multiple reasons for hypoglycemia. The causes can also be classified in a more clinically relevant system, according to whether the baby has transient, prolonged or persistent hypoglycemia. This system is enumerated here with a brief explanation, wherever applicable.

Transient Neonatal Hypoglycemia

It lasts up to 72 hours of life.

Maternal causes

- *Maternal diabetes mellitus or gestational diabetes*: The persistently raised maternal blood glucose levels lead to fetal hyperglycemia, which in turn stimulates the islet cells and leads to hyperinsulinism. After birth, the maternal source of glucose is suddenly cut off, but the hyperinsulinism persists. This period of mismatch between insulin production and glucose availability leads to hypoglycemia.
- *Tocolytic therapy* (Terbutaline, Isoxsuprine, Salbutamol).
- *Oral hypoglycemic agents.*
- *Intrapartum glucose infusion* leads to higher insulin and lower glucagon in the neonate.
- *Beta-blocker therapy* (Labetalol, Propanolol, etc.) leads to blunting of the catecholamine response in neonate and predisposes to hypoglycemia.

Neonatal causes

- *Hyperinsulinism*: Erythroblastosis fetalis, malpositioned umbilical catheters, abrupt cessation of a high glucose infusion, post-exchange-transfusion.
- *Decreased stores*: Prematurity, intrauterine growth retardation, inadequate calorie intake in late preterm's, babies born to primigravida mother, elective cesarean section and who finds it difficult to feed.
- *Increased consumption and/or decreased production*: Sepsis/Shock (The increased metabolic demands result in greater glucose consumption without commensurate glucose production), asphyxia (increased consumption and inefficient glycolysis results in hypoglycemia), Hypothermia (glucose is rapidly consumed to generate heat), polycythemia (glucose is consumed rapidly by the increased RBC mass).

Prolonged Neonatal Hypoglycemia

Prolonged neonatal hypoglycemia is usually secondary to dysregulated insulin production lasting for 72 hours to a few weeks. It is seen in SGA, preterm and asphyxiated neonates.

Persistent/Refractory Neonatal Hypoglycemia

Hypoglycemia is said to be persistent if the need for glucose infusion persists for weeks and is considered refractory if the infant remains hypoglycemic despite receiving glucose infusion rate >12 mg/kg/min. It needs evaluation for endocrine and metabolic disturbances (**Table 3**).

Congenital hyperinsulinism

It is the most common cause of persistent hypoglycemia. Its major causes involve defects in *ABCC8* and *KCNJ11* genes, which encode sulfonylurea1receptors (SUR1) and killer cell inhibitory receptors (KIR6.2) of the pancreatic

Table 2: Classification of hypoglycemia based on pathogenesis

System affected	*Condition*	*Mechanism*	*Lactate*	*Ketones*
Glycogenolysis	SGA	Decreased stores	+/–	+
	Preterm	Decreased stores	+/–	+
	Most GSDs	Enzyme defect	–	+
Gluconeogenesis	Preterm	Immature enzyme	+	+
	Galactosemia	Inhibition by galactose	++	+
	Fructose intolerance	Inhibition by fructose	++	+
	GSD type 1	G-6 Phosphatase defect	++	+
	Glycolytic pathway defects	Enzyme defects	++	+
Proteolysis	SGA	Decreased stores	+/–	+
	Preterm	Decreased stores	+/–	+
	Amino acidopathies	Enzyme defects	+	+
Lipolysis	SGA	Decreased stores	+	+/–
	Preterm	Decreased stores, immature	+	+/–
	Beta-blockers	Inhibits adrenaline action	+	–
Ketogenesis	Non-ketotic hypoglycemia	Immature enzyme	+	–
	Fatty acid oxidation defects	Enzyme defects	+	–
Hormonal regulation	Infant of diabetic mother	Hyperinsulinism	–	–
	PHHI	Hyperinsulinism	–	–
	Beckwith-Wiedemann syndrome	Hyperinsulinism	–	–
	Islet cell tumors	Hyperinsulinism	–	–
	Malpositioned umbilical artery catheters	Hyperinsulinism	–	–
	Post-exchange transfusion	Hyperinsulinism	–	–
	Adrenal insufficiency	Cortisol deficiency	+	+
	Panhypopituitarism	GH, cortisol deficiency	+	+
Glucose consumption	Hypothermia	Increased consumption	++	+
	Sepsis	Increased consumption	++	+
	Polycythemia	Increased consumption	++	+
	Shock	Increased consumption	++	+

(GH: growth hormone; GSD: glycogen storage disease; PHHI: persistent hyperinsulinemic hypoglycemia of infancy; SGA: small for gestational age. Clinically, the causes are classified as transient, prolonged or persistent)

β-cell ATP-sensitive K1 channel, respectively. It should be suspected in the presence of severe and persistent hypoglycemia, symptomatic hypoglycemia, and requirement of high glucose infusion rate (>10 mg/kg/minute) and/or absence of ketonemia or acidosis. The **diagnostic criteria** (in critical blood sample with plasma glucose <45 mg/dL) are: (i) Hyperinsulinemia (plasma insulin >2 μU/mL) and/or (ii) Plasma free fatty acids <1.5 mmol/L (iii) Plasma beta-hydroxybutyrate <2 mmol/L (iv) Glycemic response to injection glucagon ≥ 30 mg/dL (pathognomic).[4,5]

HYPOGLYCEMIA AND THE BRAIN

The newborn brain adapts to hypoglycemia by increasing cerebral blood flow and by using alternate metabolic substrates, particularly ketone bodies and lactate. The healthy term newborn has an enormous capacity to increase ketone body production in the face of hypoglycemia and is able to reach blood levels of ketone bodies in hours, which adults would take days to achieve. Breastfed infants have lower blood glucose, but higher concentrations of ketone bodies than formula-fed infants.[6] Ketone body concentration appears to be

Table 3: Etiological work-up for evaluation of persistent/refractory hypoglycemia

Etiology	*Investigations to be sent*
▪ **Hormone excess (hyperinsulinemic state)**	**First line investigations**
• Beckwith-Wiedemann syndrome	Insulin
• Hereditary defects of pancreatic islet cells (Congenital hyperinsulinism)	Cortisol
• Insulin-producing tumors	Thyroid profile
▪ **Impaired conversion of glucose**	Urine for ketone and reducing substances.
• *Fatty acid oxidation defect*	**Second line investigations**
– Carnitine palmitoyl transferase deficiency type I/II	Growth hormone levels
– Acyl CoA dehydrogenase deficiency	ACTH
– HMG CoA lyase deficiency	17-OH-P
– Beta-ketothiolase deficiency	Blood ammonia
• *Amino acid metabolism defects*	Blood lactate levels
– Maple syrup urine disease	Galactose 1 phosphate uridyl transferase levels
– Propionic acidemia	Urine aminoacidogram
– Methylmalonic acidemia	TMS
– Tyrosinemia	Free fatty acid levels
– Glutaric acidemia type II	
– Ethylmalonic adipic acidemia	
– Glutaric acidemia	
▪ **Decreased production of glucose**	
• Defects in carbohydrate metabolism	
– Glycogen storage disease	
– Galactosemia	
– Hereditary fructose intolerance	
– Glycogen synthase deficiency	
– Fructose-1,6-diphosphatase deficiency	
• *Endocrine deficiency*	
– Adrenal insufficiency	
– Hypothalamic deficiency	
– Congenital hypopituitarism	
– Glucagon deficiency	
– Epinephrine deficiency	
• *Ketotic hypoglycemia*	

directly proportionate to the degree of postnatal weight loss.

The MRI data from term neonates with symptomatic hypoglycemia shows that white matter abnormalities occurred in 94% cases, being severe in 43% and a predominantly posterior pattern in only 29% cases.[7] Cortical abnormalities occur in 51%, white matter hemorrhage in 30% and basal ganglia lesions in 30%. For a long time, researchers have been trying to pinpoint the level of blood glucose below which neural injury starts occurring in the human neonate and determining whether this injury is reversible or leads to long-term sequel. Since the brain is the major consumer of glucose, the majority of symptoms of hypoglycemia are related to neuronal dysfunction.

CLINICAL FEATURES

Hypoglycemia may or may not manifest with clinical symptoms. In symptomatic cases the adrenergic signs and symptoms (**Table 4**) appear earlier and at a higher glucose value, compared to neuroglycopenic.[8]

The definition of hypoglycemia on the basis of clinical signs excludes a large group of infants who have no clinical manifestations despite very low blood glucose levels. The significance of this "asymptomatic hypoglycemia" group has been a matter of debate for a long time. Studies have shown that asymptomatic hypoglycemia is associated with neurodevelopmental sequelae. The increased risk of adverse neurodevelopmental sequelae following symptomatic hypoglycemia is fairly well established, but the evidence for a direct causal link between glucose

Table.4: Clinical signs associated with hypoglycemia	
Neurogenic/ Adrenergic (Due to activation of sympathetic system)	*Neuroglycopenic (Due to CNS deprivation of glucose)*
Sweating	Lethargy
Pallor	Stupor
Hypothermia	Apnea
Irritability	Hypotonia
Jitteriness	Seizure
Tremors	Coma
Tachycardia	Death (if uncorrected)
Cyanotic spells	

Table 5: Definitions of hypoglycemia

Statistical Definition: It assumes that any value <2 standard deviations from the mean is abnormal. This is the most inappropriate way to define hypoglycemia as it completely ignores the clinical condition of the baby.

Metabolic Definition: It refers to the blood glucose level below which the counter-regulatory response becomes activated. Thus, this definition cannot boast of a definite numerical blood glucose level as yet. The ability of premature newborn to mount a counter-regulatory response or generate alternative fuels is less than term babies.[10] Thus, the "safe" value, if any, ought to be higher in preterms than terms.

Neurophysiological Definition: A threshold blood glucose level below which the neurophysiology will get disturbed. An old study that evaluated infants with spontaneous and insulin-induced hypoglycemia concluded that brainstem auditory evoked potentials were deranged below 47 mg/dL. However, it could not be replicated in further studies.

Neurodevelopmental Definition: In symptomatic hypoglycemia any value of less than 45 mg/dL is significant. A recent meta-analysis of 11 studies comprising 4041 infants concluded that hypoglycemia has a definite adverse impact on neurodevelopmental outcome.[9] Children having hypoglycemia in the first week of life are at increased risk of visual-motor impairment (RR 3.46 (1.13–10.57) and executive dysfunction (RR 2.50 (1.20–5.22) in early childhood (2–5 years). In mid childhood (6–11 years) they are at increased risk of neurodevelopmental impairment (RR- 3.62 (1.05–12.42), low language/literacy (RR- 2.04 (1.20–3.47) and low numeracy (RR- 2.04 (1.21–3.44). Although the overall quality of evidence was low to very low, the existing evidence suggests that neonatal hypoglycemia have important long-term adverse effects on neurodevelopment and reinforces the need of early identification of at-risk infants and meticulous management for the prevention of hypoglycemia. The neonatal hypoglycemia increases the risk of impaired executive function and visual motor function in a dose-dependent fashion, even if not detected clinically, and there is no exact "magic number" which can be considered as a safe threshold at all ages. A value < 45 mg/dL is likely to be more important after 48 hours than it is in the first 48 hours of life.

Operational Definition: The concentration of blood glucose at which "intervention should be considered". The operational threshold is different from therapeutic goals, do not define normal or abnormal but provide a margin of safety. For practical purposes and uniformity of definition, a blood glucose value of <40 mg/dL (plasma glucose < 45 mg/dL) should prompt intervention for hypoglycemia in all newborns.

levels and outcome is weak.[9] The ability to successfully adapt may explain the lack of symptoms in some babies and also explain why asymptomatic hypoglycemia does not show a consistent relationship with neurological outcome.

Definition of Hypoglycemia

There is lot of controversy on the optimal definition of neonatal hypoglycemia. There are multiple ways to define hypoglycemia **(Table 5)** in neonates. The operational definition is most widely used for the management of neonatal hypoglycemia. **Table 6** gives the threshold for intervention at various time points.

Screening for Hypoglycemia

Screening refers to the scheduled measurement of blood glucose in asymptomatic neonates. Healthy term neonates without risk factors should not be screened. This is because they can utilize substrates other than glucose; no safe cut-off has ever been defined in this group, and reagent strips tend to over-diagnose hypoglycemia in this group leading to overtreatment.[11] There is no evidence that transient asymptomatic hypoglycemia (<36 mg/dL) is detrimental in this group. The at-risk infants (**Table 7**) and the frequency of screening in them are given in **Table 8**. The bulk of these cases comprise one of the

Table 6: Comparison of AAP and PES guidelines for neonatal hypoglycemia

	Clinical condition	Threshold blood glucose values (mg/dL)			
		0–4 hrs	4–24 hrs	24–48 hrs	>48 hrs
AAP	Symptomatic	Treat if < 40			
	Asymptomatic	25	35	45	60
PES		50			60

(AAP: American Academy of Pediatrics; PES: Pediatric Endocrine Society)

Table 7: Indications for routine blood sugar monitoring

Neonatal conditions	*Maternal conditions*
• Prematurity (< 34 weeks) • Low birth weight (< 2000 g) infants • Small or large for gestational age • Sick neonate (Hypothermia, Asphyxia, Sepsis) • Polycythemia • Congenital heart diseases (TGA) • Total parenteral nutrition • Hyperinsulinism • Rh isoimmunization • Blood exchange transfusion • Suspected inborn errors of metabolism • Suspected endocrine disorders	• Insulin-dependent/Gestational diabetic mothers • Morbid obese mothers • Maternal drug ingestion, e.g. Beta blockers, oral hypoglycemics, sympathomimetic • Mothers received large amounts of dextrose in the intrapartum period

Table 8: Frequency of monitoring of blood sugar

Condition	*Frequency of monitoring*
Hyperinsulinemic states	0, 1, 2, 3, 6 and 6 hourly for 48 h of life
Birth weight (< 2000 g), SGA and Preterm (<34 weeks)	1, 2, 3, 6 and 6 hourly for 72 h of life
Babies on IVF and TPN, sick neonates	6 hourly
Primigravida mother delivered by LSCS	6 hourly for first 24 h of life

following three situations: Preterm infants, SGA infants, and infants of diabetic mothers.

MEASURING BLOOD OR PLASMA GLUCOSE

The common laboratory methods for measuring glucose are the *glucose oxidase* method and the *hexokinase* method. In the former method, hydrogen peroxide concentrations are measured following the oxidation of glucose, whereas in the latter NADPH levels are following the reduction of glucose-6-phosphate.

Capillary blood glucose is unreliable if peripheral circulation is poor or if the heel has been squeezed. Contamination with alcohol used for preparing the skin can raise glucose values. Hematocrit affects measured glucose levels. The plasma glucose concentration on an average is 18% higher than whole blood glucose and the difference keeps widening with rising hematocrit. Hemolysis and hyperbilirubinemia also interfere with glucose estimation resulting in falsely low values.

Reagent Paper Strips

These are widely used for bedside glucose estimation. It must be remembered that these strips were developed for diabetics and were originally not meant to be used for the blood glucose ranges encountered in neonatal hypoglycemia. Attempts have been made to improve the level of precision by shifting from the older colorimetric method to a reflectance metering system (e.g. Reflolux).

Reagent strips often over-diagnose hypoglycemia and that too in an unpredictable and erratic manner. Of the various reagent strips available in the world market, the most reliable appear to be Glucometer Elite XL and the Ames Glucometer Elite.[12] There are very few head-to-head comparisons between reagent strips. Hence, it has been recommended that, although emergent treatment can be started on the basis of a reagent strip report, the final diagnosis must be based on a laboratory method.

Laboratory Diagnosis

This is the most accurate method. In the laboratory, glucose can be measured by either the glucose oxidase (calorimetric) method or by the glucose electrode method (as used in blood gas analyzer). Blood samples should be analyzed quickly to avoid erroneously low glucose levels. The blood sample must be stored in fluoride/citrate vial and processed within the shortest possible turnover time. Delayed processing may lead to lowering of blood glucose as high as 14–18 mg/dL/h.

Continuous Glucose Monitors (Subcutaneous/Transdermal)

Subcutaneous CGM devices measure the glucose concentration of the interstitial fluid with the help of biosensors introduced in subcutaneous space. Transdermal sensors are still in the development process. They rely on diffusion of glucose into the transdermal fluid leading to a conformational change in the specialized glucose binding proteins which is reflected as glucose concentration.[13] While the use of CGM in neonates seems to be attractive in improving neonatal glycemic control and reducing the numbers of sampling and blood loss, there is currently little direct evidence of the benefits and risks of this technology in neonates.[13,14] One small randomized trial found that CGM reduced the median duration of hypoglycemic episodes by 50% and the number of blood samples by 25% in very low birth weight infants.[15] However larger rigorous trials are needed before introducing into routine clinical care.

TREATMENT

Concurrent with the treatment of hypoglycemia should be a prompt consideration of the cause. Term breastfed babies never develop symptomatic hypoglycemia as a result of simple underfeeding. An underlying illness must be looked for, such as sepsis.

Moderate, *asymptomatic hypoglycemia* (20–35 mg/dL) should be first treated by giving frequent and measured supplementary feeds. This should preferably be in the form of expressed human milk by cup and spoon.

Dextrose Gel

It has been explored in asymptomatic hypoglycemia. It is simple and inexpensive and can be applied directly to the buccal mucosa for rapid correction of hypoglycemia. Studies have shown that the use of dextrose gel along with continuation of milk feeding leads to decrease in number of hypoglycemic episodes, decrease in recurrence rate of hypoglycemia, decrease in the need for admission to the neonatal intensive care unit to treat hypoglycemia leading to reduced incidence of mother-infant separation for treatment and increased exclusive breastfeeding rates at discharge.[16–18] However, there were some concerns regarding the adverse neurodevelopmental outcome due to higher dextrose concentration.

Intravenous Therapy

It should be instituted if the "moderate; asymptomatic hypoglycemia" fails to improve on milk feeds, or if the blood glucose is less than 25 mg/dL or if it is symptomatic (**Flowchart 2**). The role of a routine "minibolus" of 2 mL/kg 10% dextrose prior to starting the dextrose infusion is still controversial. Even with the "minibolus", there are fears that since the rate of administration exceeds the rate of cellular uptake it may cause rebound hypoglycemia and the rapid administration may be detrimental to the brain of a preterm baby. However, there is agreement that of the three indications for intravenous therapy, it is the symptomatic hypoglycemia group that merits the "minibolus" the most. In any case, the minibolus must be followed by a glucose infusion providing 6 to 8 mg/kg/min. There is complete unanimity that there is no place for treatment with intermittent "miniboluses" alone.

The *objective of intravenous therapy* in the vast majority of cases is to maintain a blood glucose level >45 mg/dL. It must be noted that the glucose level which is the objective of therapy is higher than the indications for starting therapy (i.e. single value < 20 mg/dL or persistently <35 mg/dL). For symptomatic infant with documented profound, recurrent or persistent hyperinsulinemic hypoglycemia the objective

Flowchart 2: Operational algorithm for management of neonatal hypoglycemia

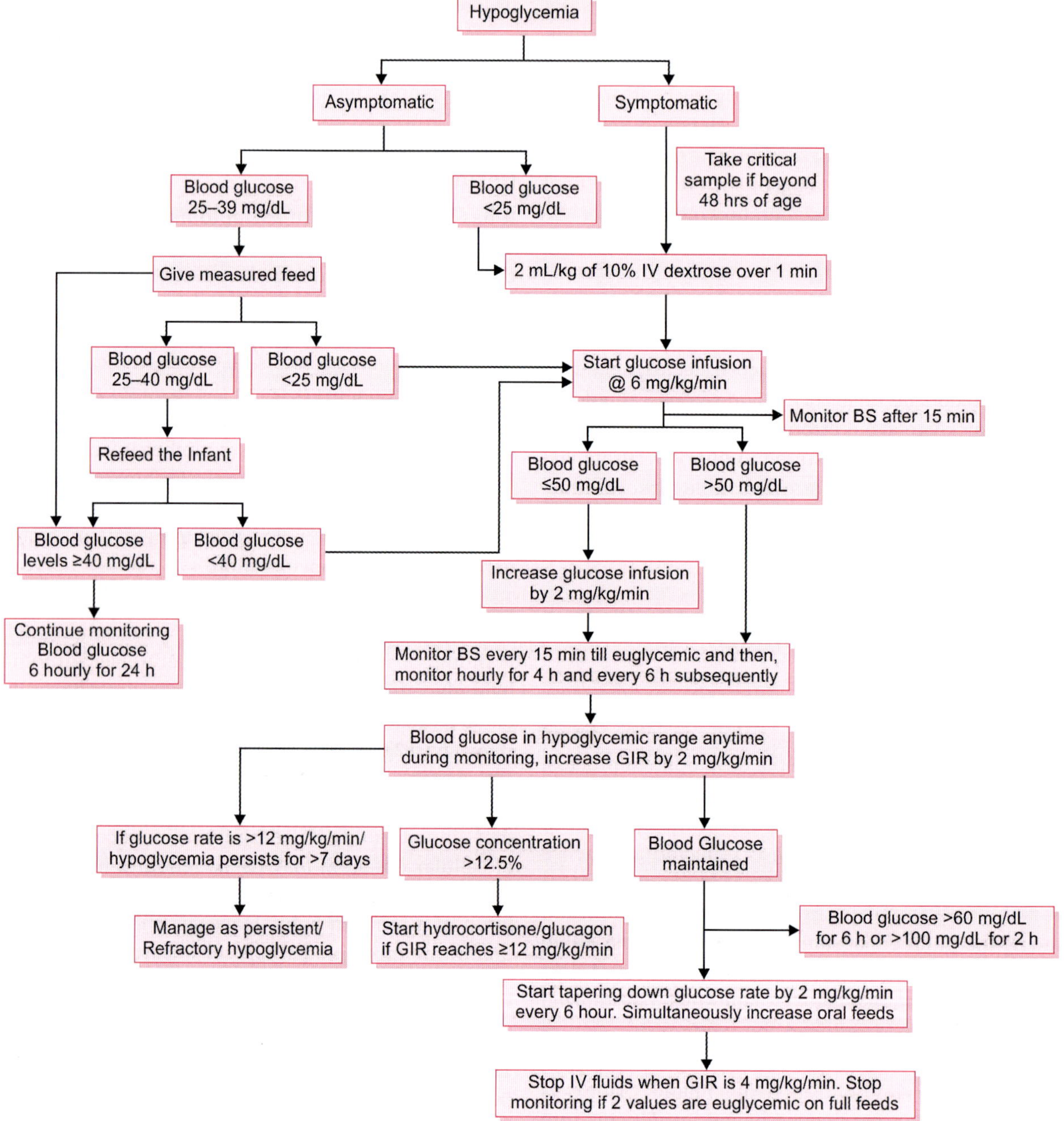

of therapy is to maintain blood glucose about 60 mg/dL. After starting glucose infusion, blood glucose should be monitored as shown in **Flowchart 2** and glucose infusion rate should be adjusted accordingly. A central venous line is required if glucose concentration exceeds 12.5% as higher concentration may lead to thrombophlebitis. It is a good idea to continue breast milk feeds, especially if the anticipated fluid therapy will be brief and the combined volumes does not become unphysiological.[19] This is because breast milk has beneficial effects on hormonal regulation and release of ketones and free fatty acids. Once glucose levels have stabilized, tapering of infusion rate with a concomitant increase in feed volume should be done.

PERSISTENT/ REFRACTORY HYPOGLYCEMIA

Besides increasing GIR for persistent hypoglycemia, certain drugs should be used depending upon etiology/ available workup. The place of glucagon in the treatment of hypoglycemia is controversial. A dose of 200 µg/kg intravenous bolus can increase glycogenolysis, gluconeogenesis and ketogenesis for several hours.[20] Glucagon seems to act even in situations where glycogen stores are expected to be depleted, such as preterm and small for gestational age infants. The side effects of glucagon include vomiting, diarrhea, and hypokalemia.[20]

Similarly, the exact indication of hydrocortisone in the treatment of hypoglycemia is ambiguous. Usually, 5 mg/kg of hydrocortisone is administered 12 hourly if glucose infusion rates exceed 12 mg/kg/min. After normoglycemia is attained for 48 hours, first the intravenous fluids should be tapered and the baby should be kept on hydrocortisone for another 48 hours off intravenous fluids. Diazoxide, octreotide, nifedipine, and somatostatin are required in conditions of persistent hyperinsulinism.[21]

PREVENTION OF HYPOGLYCEMIA

Prevention consists of avoiding certain peripartum risk factors, instituting feeding or intravenous fluids in those who cannot be fed. Maternal glucose infusion during labor should be restricted. Hypothermia should be prevented at birth, the baby must be effectively resuscitated at birth and skin-to-skin must be encouraged. The most effective way of preventing hypoglycemia is ensuring milk feeding (preferable breast milk) as soon as possible after delivery. Any form of pre-lacteal feeds should be avoided.

Healthy preterm infants between 32 and 36 weeks gestation: They should be allowed to feed as soon as possible after birth and at 2-3 hourly intervals. If the baby is awake but requirements are not met by direct breastfeeding the alternative is to offer expressed human milk by cup and spoon feeds.

Healthy preterm babies between 28 and 32 weeks of gestation: They can be started on expressed human milk by gavage feeding from day 1. Infants less than 28 weeks gestation have immature bowel motility and needs dextrose infusion.

Small for gestational age infants: They must be started on enteral feeds as soon as possible. SGA babies have higher endogenous glucose production rate, therefore require higher volume and timely feeds.

Infants of diabetic mothers: They should be breastfed immediately after birth and frequently (at 1–2 hour intervals) thereafter. If pre-feed blood glucose at 3 hours is normal, it is unlikely that baby will need supplementary feeds.

There are not enough well-designed studies to endorse the practice of adding powdered sugar or glucose to milk to prevent hypoglycemia. However, there is some evidence that supplementing the milk feed with fat (medium chain triglycerides) can prevent hypoglycemia.

Intravenous fluids have to be started in the presence of cardio-respiratory distress, gastrointestinal malformations, ileus and gestational age <28 weeks. Glucose infusion should be started at the rate of 6 mg/kg/min in all neonates irrespective of gestation and underlying etiology. There is no role of a "minibolus" of glucose for preventing hypoglycemia.

LONG-TERM OUTCOME AND FOLLOW-UP

Long term outcome of hypoglycemia is determined by factors like the degree and duration of hypoglycemia, cerebral utilization of glucose, and associated comorbidities. These infants are at risk of seizures, hypotonia, microcephaly, visual/hearing impairment, and delayed neurodevelopment. These infants should be assessed at one month corrected age for vision/hearing evaluation. Thereafter periodically they should be followed up for growth, neurodevelopment, vision, and hearing loss. Recent studies have shown that they should be followed till adulthood for executive functions and visuomotor integration skills, MRI at 4–6 weeks provide a good estimate of hypoglycemic injury and therefore should be considered in follow-up of such infants subject to affordability.

KEY MESSAGES

- Symptomatic hypoglycemia has been associated with an increased risk of the adverse neurological outcome. The relationship of asymptomatic hypoglycemia with the neurological outcome is still controversial.
- Early and frequent milk feeds are the best way to prevent hypoglycemia. Breast milk is superior to formula milk.
- Persistent and refractory hypoglycemia should be evaluated for underlying etiology. The drugs like glucagon, hydrocortisone and diazoxide are useful in such cases.
- Laboratory enzymatic methods are the gold standard for the measurement of hypoglycemia. Reagent strips may be used for starting treatment, but are too unreliable to be used for diagnosing neonatal hypoglycemia.
- Prevention of hypoglycemia is the best strategy to mitigate the consequences

REFERENCES

1. Hosagasi NH, Aydin M, Zenciroglu A, *et al.* Incidence of hypoglycemia in newborns at risk and an audit of the 2011 American Academy of Pediatrics guideline for hypoglycemia. Pediatr Neonatol. 2018;59:368-74.
2. Bromiker R, Perry A, Kasirer Y, *et al.* Early neonatal hypoglycemia: Incidence of and risk factors. A cohort study using universal point of care screening. J Matern Fetal Neonatal Med. 2019;32:786-92.
3. Sharma A, Davis A, Shekhawat PS. Hypoglycemia in the preterm neonate: Etiopathogenesis, diagnosis, management and long-term outcomes. Transl Pediatr. 2017;6:335-48.
4. Arnoux JB, Verkarre V, Saint-Martin C, *et al.* Congenital hyperinsulinism: Current trends in diagnosis and therapy. Orphanet J Rare Dis. 2011;6:63.
5. De León DD, Stanley CA. Determination of insulin for the diagnosis of hyperinsulinemic hypoglycemia. Best Pract Res Clin Endocrinol Metab. 2013;27:763-9.
6. Bilgen H, Kültürsay N, Türkyılmaz C. Turkish Neonatal Society guideline on nutrition of the healthy term newborn. Turk Pediatri Ars. 2018;53(Suppl 1):S128-37.
7. Burns CM, Rutherford MA, Boardman JP, *et al.* Patterns of cerebral injury and neurodevelopmental outcomes after symptomatic neonatal hypoglycemia. Pediatrics. 2008;122: 65-74.
8. Thompson-Branch A, Havranek T. Neonatal hypoglycemia. Pediatr Rev. 2017;38:147-57.
9. Shah R, Harding J, Brown J, *et al.* Neonatal glycaemia and neurodevelopmental outcomes: a systematic review and meta-analysis. Neonatology. 2019;116-26.
10. Avenarius HA, Versteege CWM, Engelshove HA. Cerebral damage due to neonatal hypoglycemia. JBR-BTR. 2003;86: 136-7.
11. Committee on Fetus and Newborn. Postnatal Glucose Homeostasis in Late-Preterm and Term Infants. Pediatrics. 2011;127:575-9.
12. Michel A, Küster H, Krebs A, *et al.* Evaluation of the glucometer elite XL device for screening for neonatal hypoglycaemia. Eur J Pediatr. 2005;164:660-4.
13. McKinlay CJD, Chase JG, Dickson J, *et al.* Continuous glucose monitoring in neonates: A review. Matern Health Neonatol Perinatol. 2017;3:18.
14. Galderisi A, Facchinetti A, Steil GM, *et al.* Continuous glucose monitoring in very preterm infants: A randomized controlled trial. Pediatrics. 2017;140:e20171162.
15. Uettwiller F, Chemin A, Bonnemaison E, *et al.* Real-time continuous glucose monitoring reduces the duration of hypoglycemia episodes: A randomized trial in very low birth weight neonates. PloS One. 2015;10:e0116255.
16. Rawat M, Chandrasekharan P, Turkovich S, *et al.* Oral dextrose gel reduces the need for intravenous dextrose therapy in neonatal hypoglycemia. Biomed Hub. 2016;1(3). pii: 448511.
17. Newnam KM, Bunch M. Glucose gel as a treatment strategy for transient neonatal hypoglycemia. Adv Neonatal Care. 2017;17:470-7.
18. Weston PJ, Harris DL, Battin M, *et al.* Oral dextrose gel for the treatment of hypoglycaemia in newborn infants. Cochrane Database Syst Rev. 2016;(5):CD011027.
19. American Academy of Pediatrics section on breastfeeding. Breastfeeding and the use of human milk. Pediatrics. 2012; 129:e827-e41.
20. Welters A, Lerch C, Kummer S, *et al.* Long-term medical treatment in congenital hyperinsulinism: A descriptive analysis in a large cohort of patients from different clinical centers. Orphanet J Rare Dis. 2015;10:150.
21. Kumar J, Singh A. A brief review of hyperinsulinism in small for gestational age infants. J Med Sci Clin Res. 2017;05:15379-83.

CHAPTER

74

Emergencies in Inborn Errors of Metabolism

Sunita Bijarnia-Mahay

INTRODUCTION

Inborn errors of metabolism are genetically determined metabolic disorders which are usually diagnosed (IEM) using specific biochemical tests. The IEMs occur due to deficiency of an enzyme or co-factor or transporter resulting in biochemical derangements and symptoms related to it. As many of the biochemical processes are dynamic and fluctuating, based on the requirement of the body, hence there is often an episodic phenomenon of presentation of IEMs.

The biochemical processes serve multiple purposes in the body-energy production, essential maintenance of our internal milieu, or getting rid of toxic metabolites that are formed as a result of the intermediary metabolism. Some defects have a slow and long term effect (e.g. storage disorders), others have an immediate effect (e.g. hypoglycemia - lack of energy, hyperammonemia causing acute toxicity to the brain leading to cellular edema and damage). It is these "acutely presenting IEMs" that are episodic and usually present as emergencies.

IEMs can present at any age, depending upon the severity of the genetic defect and the biochemical process involved. The moment of birth marks an important switch in the body's biochemistry, as the baby has to deal with abnormal metabolites on its own, without the protective cape of the placenta. Thus, a large majority of the acutely presenting IEMs would manifest in the neonatal period.

EPIDEMIOLOGY AND ETIOLOGY

There are over 1000 IEMs known, occurring due to genetic alterations in nuclear as well as mitochondrial genome.[1] The incidence of all IEMs is about 1 in 1000.[2] Individually, they occur with variable frequencies in different populations in the world. Newborn screening has facilitated in ascertaining the prevalence of some of the IEMs across the world.[3-5] In the absence of a universal newborn screening program in India we are uncertain of the exact disease burden. Date collected from symptomatic children give us some clue to the IEM disease burden.[6-9] **Table 1** provides the relative

Table 1: Frequency of IEMs in India

	Sir Ganga Ram Hospital (9) (n = 1556)	*National Institute of Mental Health & Neurosciences (6) (n = 23000)*
Total samples tested	1556	23,000
Total positives identified	122 (7.8%)	752 (3.2%)
Amino acid disorders	**38 (31.1%)**	**329 (43.8%)**
MSUD	9	73
Phenylketonuria	6	101
Urea cycle disorders (mainly citrullinemia type 1)	16	34
Tyrosinemia type 1	1	41
Others	4	80
Total organic acidemias	**60 (49.1%)**	332 (44.5%)
Methylmalonic acidemia	24	48
Glutaric aciduria type 1 (GA 1)	8	108
Propionic acidemia	8	96
Others	16	Nil
FAOD/Gluconeogenetic pathway	19 (15.5%)	85 (11.3%)
Primary lactic acidemia (Others)	5 (4%)	Nil

frequencies of IEMs from two large data sets from amongst symptomatic children in India.[6,9]

The inheritance of inborn errors of metabolism is largely autosomal recessive, while some are X-linked. With improved genetic diagnostics, more than 300 IEMs have been in the past 7–8 years.[10,11] Most of the IEMs have presented predominantly with neurologic manifestations. Treatment is available for less than a hundred of these disorders, but the numbers are improving.[12]

PATHOPHYSIOLOGY

The pathophysiologic basis of each individual IEM is unique, depending upon the biochemical process that is disrupted. According to one classification, they are either small molecule or large molecule type of IEM, depending upon the mass of the toxic/accumulating or offensive substrate in the body.[13] Saudubray has proposed a pathophysiological classification according to which there are two categories of IEM.[11] The first includes IEMs affecting either only one system (such as the endocrine system, or immune system) or only 1 organ or anatomic system (such as the liver, intestine, renal tubules, erythrocytes, or connective tissue) where a single functional system or organ system is involved (e.g. renal tubular acidosis, coagulation system). The disorders are relatively easy to predict as symptoms are uniform (e.g. Crigler-Najjar Syndrome presenting with unconjugated hyperbilirubinemia). The second category is the one where the basic biochemical defect either affects 1 metabolic pathway *common* to a large number of cells or organs (e.g. storage disorders) or is restricted to one organ (e.g. liver) but has larger secondary consequences (e.g. hyperammonemia). These are more complex and require expertise as well as multiple metabolic investigations to make a diagnosis. Within this second category, there are 3 groups:

1. Disorders of the intermediary system affecting the small molecule - usually acute and intermittent toxicity-related symptoms
2. Disorders involving primary energy deficiency - acute or chronic or intermittent symptoms related to lack of energy
3. Disorders involving complex molecules caused by storage or other mechanism leading to progressive and chronic symptoms.

This classification is an over simplification, as it does not cover many other IEMs, especially those that are now being detected by direct genetic testing via exome sequencing.[11] Only the those conditions that present as an emergency are discussed in this chapter.

CLINICAL FEATURES

Clinical features tend to be common and non-specific especially in a neonate who has a limited repertoire of presentation, mainly lethargy, poor feeding, respiratory distress, jaundice or seizures. Understanding of a few basic principles outlined below will enable better appreciation of the clinical manifestations:

- The symptom-free period could vary from hours to months to years. The exception to this rule are the chronically presenting complex molecule disorders.
- The clinical signs of intoxication may be acute (vomiting, coma, liver failure, thrombosis, etc.) or chronic (failure to thrive, developmental delay, ectopia lentis, cirrhosis, ichthyosis, cardiomyopathy, etc.), or even progressive (neurodegeneration).
- The acute "metabolic" attacks are usually provoked or triggered by fasting, catabolism, fever, intercurrent illness, or food intake.
- The diagnosis of IEMs, requires a high index of suspicion which could be flagged by a previous or a family history of a similar occurrence, or presence of consanguinity.
- IEMs should be suspected in parallel with (or along with) other more common conditions like infection, intoxication etc., so as not to lose the crucial time window where emergency treatment could save the baby's life.

The various patterns of clinical presentations are outlined in the following section.

Acute Neurological Presentations

These include encephalopathy, seizures, abnormal movements or abnormalities of body tone. A baby/child's condition deteriorates after a period of lethargy and poor feeding with or without other symptoms. Some of the accompanying features include the following:

Metabolic acidosis: Encephalopathy with/without seizures is frequently seen in organic acidemias, lactic acidemias, gluconeogenetic (Fructose-1-6-bisphosphatase deficiency - FBPD, glycogenolytic defects (Glycogen storage disorder type 1) or certain endocrine disorders.

Seizures: Seizures may be predominant in disorders that respond to vitamins like pyridoxine, folinic acid or biotin, or due to non-ketotic hyperglycinemia (NKH), sulfite oxidase/molybdenum co-factor (SO/MoCF) deficiency or peroxisomal disorders. Seizures may not be due to a primary IEM and could be due to other genetic disorders such as channelopathies, etc.

Hypotonia: Among the metabolic causes, NKH, peroxisomal and SO/MoCF may in fact present initially with hypotonia only. Other conditions are mitochondrial respiratory chain disorders, trifunctional enzyme deficiencies, congenital disorders of glycosylation (CDG) and disorders of cholesterol biosynthesis. Other than IEMs, there are several genetic conditions such as spinal muscular atrophy and other neuromuscular disorders that can present as a floppy infant or baby.

Hypoglycemia: Presence of hypoglycemia may indicate a gluconeogenetic, glycogenolytic or a fatty acid oxidation defect. Hyperinsulinemia is an important cause of difficult-to-treat hypoglycemia.

Hyperammonemia: This is a specific pointer towards urea cycle disorder or an organic acidemia.

Hepatic Involvement

Liver is the most commonly involved organ in IEMs, after the brain. The various hepatic presentations include:

Hepatomegaly with hypoglycemia: The most common disorders presenting with these features are glycogenosis types I and III, fructose -1-6 bisphosphatase deficiency (FBPD), hereditary fructose intolerance (HFI)(history of exposure to fructose, such as table sugar or honey), or fatty acid oxidation disorders (FAOD). All except FAODs are usually also associated with high lactate and ketones. Low ketones with hypoglycemia suggest FAOD or hyperinsulinism.

Hepatomegaly with jaundice: The liver dysfunction in this category may vary from minor transaminitis to fulminant hepatic failure. This group includes disorders such as HFI, galactosemia, tyrosinemia type 1, mitochondrial respiratory chain disorders or mitochondrial DNA (mt DNA) depletion syndromes or other mitochondriopathies. Crigler-Najjar syndrome & G-6-PD deficiency may be categorized here because of unconjugated hyperbilirubinemia, however, there is no associated liver dysfunction. Neonatal hemochromatosis also presents with hepatic failure, but this is not an IEM, but an alloimmune disorder.

Hepatomegaly with cholestatic jaundice with or without failure to thrive and/or diarrhea: This group includes various disorders like inborn errors of bile acid metabolism including peroxisomal disorders, Niemann-Pick disease type C, urea cycle disorders such as citrullinemia type 1 and 2, argininosuccinate deficiency (hyperammonemia present in all), CDG type 1 and 2, and other disorders of cholesterol metabolism. A proven case of alpha-1-antitrypsin deficiency has not been reported from the Indian population so far.

Hepatomegaly and splenomegaly with or without hydrops or coarse facies: Disorders of lysosomal storage such as GM1 gangliosidosis, galactosialidosis, sialidosis type II, I-cell disease or mucolipidosis type 2, Niemann-Pick type A/C, mucopolysaccharidosis especially type 7, Gaucher disease, and disorders of glycosylation are the common disorders likely to present in neonatal period. Erythropoietic porphyria also usually presents in the neonatal period with hepatosplenomegaly with hemolytic anaemia.

Cardiac Involvement

Cardiac involvement may present as a rhythm disturbance, shock-like symptoms, cardiomegaly or cardiomyopathy leading to cardiac failure. Glycogen storage disease type 2 (Pompe disease), fatty acid oxidation defects – medium-chain acyl-CoA dehydrogenase (MCAD), very long chain acyl CoA dehydrogenase deficiency (VLCAD), Carnitine palmitoyl transferase I and II (CPT I and II), carnitine acyl-carnitine translocase CAT deficiency, tyrosinemia type 1, CDG type Ia, Barth syndrome and mitochondrial respiratory chain disorders may present with cardiac symptoms. There would usually be other associated findings to suggest the etiology such as hypoglycemia in glycogenosis and FAOD, raised lactate with or without cataracts in mitochondrial disorders, hepatic and renal dysfunctions in tyrosinemia type 1, CDG, and mitochondrial disorders and an extreme hypotonia with suggestive ECG, raised creatine phospho kinases (CPK) in Pompe disease.

Renal Involvement

Renal involvement is usually in the form of renal tubular acidosis (RTA) or polyuria. For example, Bartter syndrome presents with failure to thrive with metabolic acidosis or alkalosis. RTA is frequently proximal in disorders such as galactosemia, tyrosinemia type 1, HFI, cystinosis, and mitochondrial respiratory chain disorders. Occasionally, a cystic renal disease may be due to peroxisomal disorders.

Cataract

Cataracts detectable in the newborn period can be seen in Galactosemia (Galactose-1-phosphate uridyl transferase [GALT], galactokinase [GALK] or uridine diphosphate galactose-4-epimerase deficiency), Lowe syndrome, Cockayne syndrome, peroxisomal biogenesis disorders (Zellweger variants, rhizomelic chondrodysplasia punctata), phosphoglycerate dehydrogenase deficiency, sorbitol dehydrogenase deficiency, and mitochondrial disorders like Senger's syndrome.

Gastrointestinal

These include chronic diarrhea, vomiting and dehydration or failure to thrive. Syndromes such as congenital chloride diarrhea, glucose-galactose malabsorption, lactase and sucrose isomaltase deficiency, acrodermatitis enteropathica, MNGIE (mitochondrial neurogastrointestinal encephalopathy) syndrome, CDG type 1b, HFI, Wolman syndrome and others present with such symptoms. Cystic fibrosis and other malabsorption syndromes may also present as chronic diarrhea and failure to thrive.

Hematologic

Anemia is a frequent feature of many IEMs. Hemolytic anemia may be a presentation of deficiency of glycolytic and pentose phosphate shuttle, erythrocyte membrane disorders, porphyrias or disorders of lipid metabolism. Macrocytic anemia along with other symptoms may suggest either maternal or inherited disorders of Vitamin B12 and folate metabolism, with exception of severe methyl tetra hydrofolate reductase (MTHFR) deficiency. Leucopenia/neutropenia and thrombocytopenia are also frequently observed in organic acidemias.

Abnormal Urine/Body Odor

Urinary odor is best appreciated on drying urine soaked filter paper, or from a container opened after allowing it to remain closed with urine in it for at least a few minutes. Some disorders present with distinctive smell: maple syrup or burnt sugar in MSUD, boiled cabbage in hypermethioninemia, tomcat urine smell in multiple carboxylase deficiencies and sweaty feet odor in glutaric aciduria type 1 & isovaleric aciduria. A unique fishy body odor is recognizable in trimethylaminuria, especially in breast fed babies after their mothers ate egg or fish.

Fetal or Neonatal Hydrops

Non-immune hydrops is often a presentation in IEMs of the storage type, most commonly Mucopolysaccharidosis type 7 (or 1/2/3), Gaucher disease, Niemann-Pick disease and GM1 gangliosidosis. A host of other metabolic disorders can present as hydrops, which is impossible to enumerate here.

APPROACH TO DIAGNOSIS

The most important step to diagnosing a metabolic disorder is to consider the possibility since there are no specific symptoms or signs as pointers to the diagnosis. **Table 2** lists some of the basic and advanced metabolic investigations that need to be done. **Flowcharts 1 to 4** provide algorithms which could aid in the diagnosis.[13,14]

Sample Collection, Storage and Transport

Urine: Collect 10–15 mL of urine, preferably the first-morning specimen. Tests should include:

- Routine biochemical tests, protein, glucose, reducing substances, pH.
- Chemical tests like di-nitro phenyl hydrazine DNPH, ferric chloride test, sulfite dipstick test etc.
- Amino acid chromatography and quantitative estimation.
- Organic acids (collect on filter paper)

Blood

- For ammonia estimation, a free-flowing fresh sample (preferably arterial) should be drawn in a vial and transported directly to the lab on ice as soon as possible. This is critical, as ammonia tends to rise falsely if the sample is not processed immediately. For lactate and pyruvate, a fluoride vial is used and the same precautions as for ammonia are to be taken. The sample for ammonia is required in EDTA vial.
- Collect in EDTA if plasma is required for testing or for DNA storage.
- For galactosemia and tyrosinemia testing, heparinized blood is required.
- For enzyme assays on blood leukocytes, a blood sample should be collected in heparinized vial.
- For tandem mass spectrometry (TMS) or MS/MS, take fresh blood on filter paper, or 1 mL of blood in heparin or EDTA vial and put on filter paper.

Table 2: Investigations for the diagnosis of inborn errors of metabolism

A. Initial investigations	**Blood:** • Complete blood count: Hemoglobin, white blood count, differential, platelets • Arterial blood gas • Plasma electrolytes [anion gap (Na + K) – (HCO_3 + Cl) = normal <20 nmol/L] • Glucose • Calcium, magnesium • Blood urea nitrogen, creatinine • Liver function tests (Prothrombin time, liver enzymes, albumin, etc.) • Ammonia • Lactate *Additional tests, indication based*: • CPK (Creatine kinase), uric acid • Lipid profile • Prolactin **Urine:** • Color, odor, specific gravity, pH • Proteins • Sugar, reducing substances (Benedicts and uristix) • Ketones, ketoacids (DNPH) • Sulfites • Microscopy
B. Specialized investigations	**Blood:** • Amino acid analysis, quantitative (by high performance liquid chromatography [HPLC], ultra high performance liquid chromatography [UPLC] or liquid chromatography-mass spectrometry/mass spectrometry [LC-MS/MS] - may be needed in CSF in specific situations like in NKH*) • Galactosemia screening test (galactose metabolite or GALT Beutler spot) • Carnitine, total and free (Tandem Mass Spectrometry or TMS also known as MS/MS, on dried blood spots or DBS) • Acylcarnitine profile (TMS or MS/MS) • Plasma very long chain fatty acid analysis (VLCFA) • Serum transferrin isoforms (using any technique such as Iso electric focusing (IEF), and capillary zone electrophoresis (CZE), or HPLC) • Plasma for storage at -20°C: 2–5 mL **Urine:** • Organic acids (GC-MS) • Succinyl acetone (can be done on DBS) • Urine thin layer chromatography for aminoacid profile/quantitative amino acid levels • Urine for storage at -20°C: 10–20 mL **Imaging:** MRI brain with or without MR spectroscopy Echocardiography Ultrasound abdomen, especially for liver, spleen, kidneys, etc.
C. Highly specialized investigations	• **Biochemical enzyme assays:** For lysosomal storage diseases, galactosemia, biotinidase deficiency, glycogenosis and others depending upon need and availability (blood, skin fibroblasts and sometimes liver biopsy*) • **Neurotransmitter analysis:** For diagnosis of neurotransmitter and pterin disorders (sample required is CSF in specific conditions*) **Molecular tests** (blood/skin/other tissue derived DNA): • Single gene sequencing, copy number part/whole gene • Next generation sequencing – for group of genes/panel/exome sequencing

*Sampling conditions specific, and described in the text

CSF examination: CSF examination is recommended to be done as a paired sample, with simultaneously drawn plasma sample. The CSF and plasma should be done for glucose, lactate and amino acid quantitation. An additional sample for CSF neurotransmitters, if indicated, is to be immediately frozen in -80°C, and sent to a laboratory in dry ice.

Flowchart 1: Initial approach to a sick neonate/infant[10]

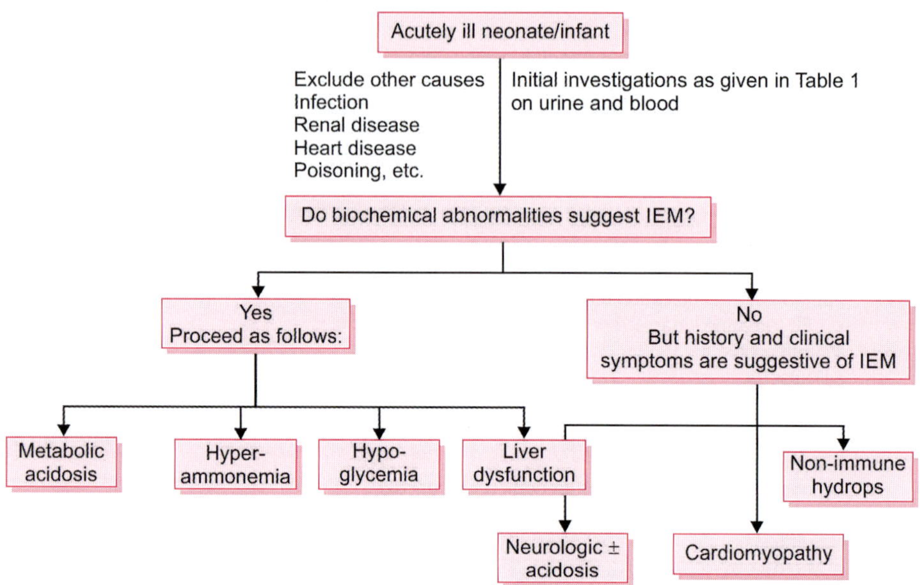

Flowchart 2: Algorithmic for metabolic acidosis

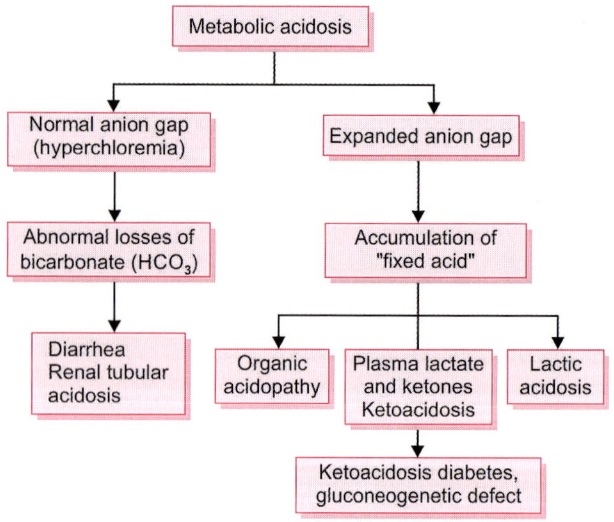

Source: Modified from JTR Clarke.[13]

Tissue Biopsy for Enzymology

Enzymology requires a fresh frozen sample to be sent to a lab in frozen condition, with dry ice used for transportation– this is usually needed for liver, skin and muscle biopsies often sent for mitochondrial respiratory chain enzymology. Liver biopsy in dry ice is also required for certain enzyme assays such as HFI, FBP and glycogenosis. Sometimes, for skin fibroblast, one requires culturing followed by transporting the skin fibroblasts in transport medium in ambient temperature.

Transport of urine and blood samples on Whatman® no. 903 filter paper and DNA can be done in room air, while plasma samples and blood for enzyme assays need to be cooled during transportation, especially in summer.

Storage of Samples for Postmortem Investigations

Every suspect case of IEM who is very sick should have following samples collected and stored for making a precise diagnosis and prevent recurrence of the disorder in future pregnancy by carrying out the prenatal diagnosis in the family's subsequent pregnancies. **Table 3** indicates the critical samples to be collected in the event of neonatal death.[15]

MANAGEMENT

Initial Emergency Management

As for any sick neonate, the first basic principle of general management in any baby is the initial stabilization. Most babies may require ventilatory and/or circulatory support as well as correction of acid-base balance, dyselectrolytemia and other measures immediately.

Flowchart 3: Algorithm for diagnosis of hyperammonemia

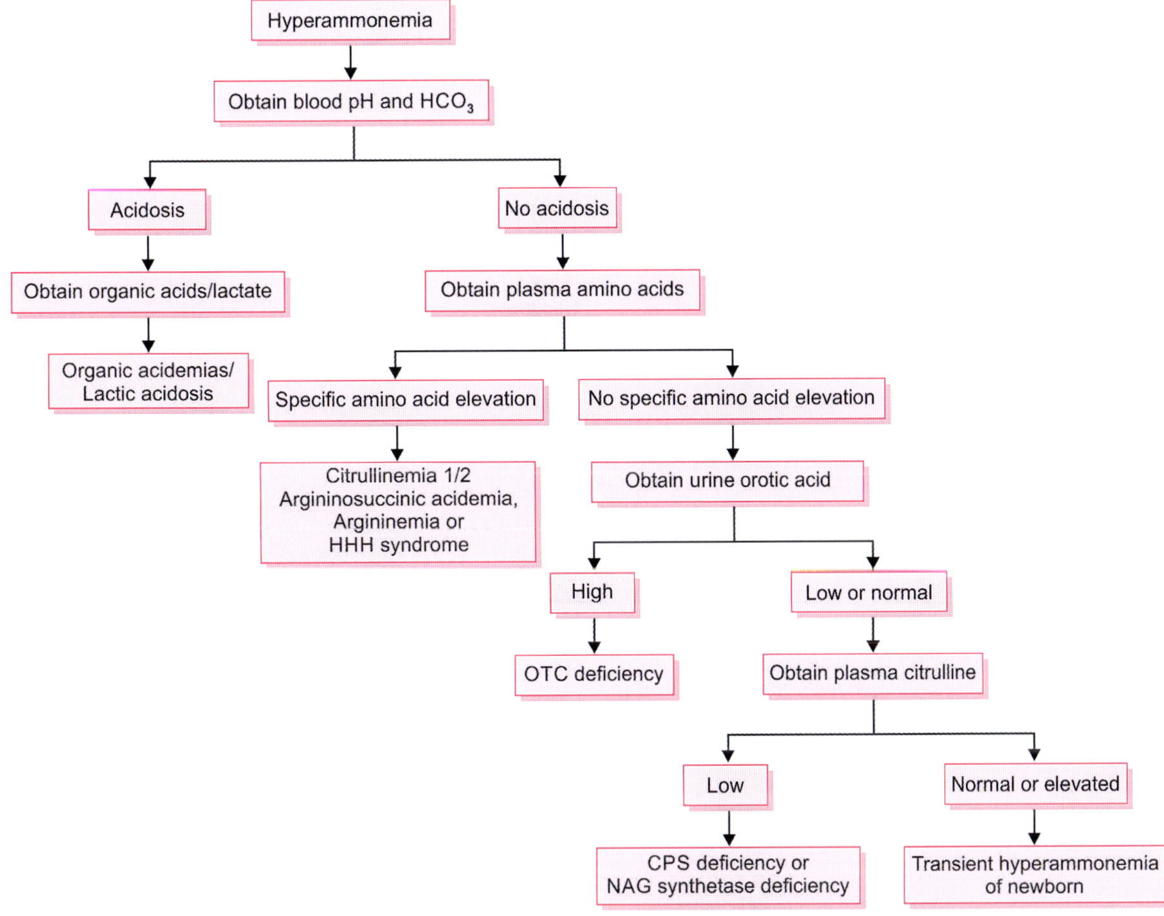

(OTC: ornithine transcarbamylase; CPS: carbamoyl phosphate synthetase)
Source: Modified from Nelson's Textbook of Pediatrics[14]

Table 3: Samples for postmortem investigations

Sample (storage conditions)	*Test to be performed*
Urine (–20°C)	Amino acids, organic acids, tubulopathy markers
Blood (–20°C)	DNA (EDTA vial), amino acids (Heparin vial), uric acid, etc.
Dried blood spots (room temperature)	Acylcarnitine profile, DNA
CSF sample (–80°C)	Neurotransmitters, amino acids
Skin biopsy (fibroblasts, culture medium at room temperature)	Enzyme analysis, DNA

Babies who present with actual sepsis are even sicker as the catabolic state is enhanced and requires more urgent intervention and treatment simultaneously.

Nonspecific Interventions

After initial stabilization, collect appropriate samples: blood, urine and other body fluids wherever necessary.

- *Stop protein intake/external source of toxin*: Oral milk may be stopped temporarily (24–48 hours only) to prevent further accumulation of toxic metabolites generated by oral proteins. In case of galactosemia – breastfeeding to be stopped altogether, substituted with another appropriate milk which is completely lactose/galactose free.
- *Reverse the process of catabolism in body*: High dose energy substitutes in form of 10–12.5% dextrose infusions @150 mL/kg/day (to provide ~10–12.5 mg/kg/min glucose, ~60–75 kcal/kg/24 hours) to be given IV or exceptionally via NG tube; add insulin IV to

Flowchart 4: Algorithmic approach for diagnosis of hypoglycemia

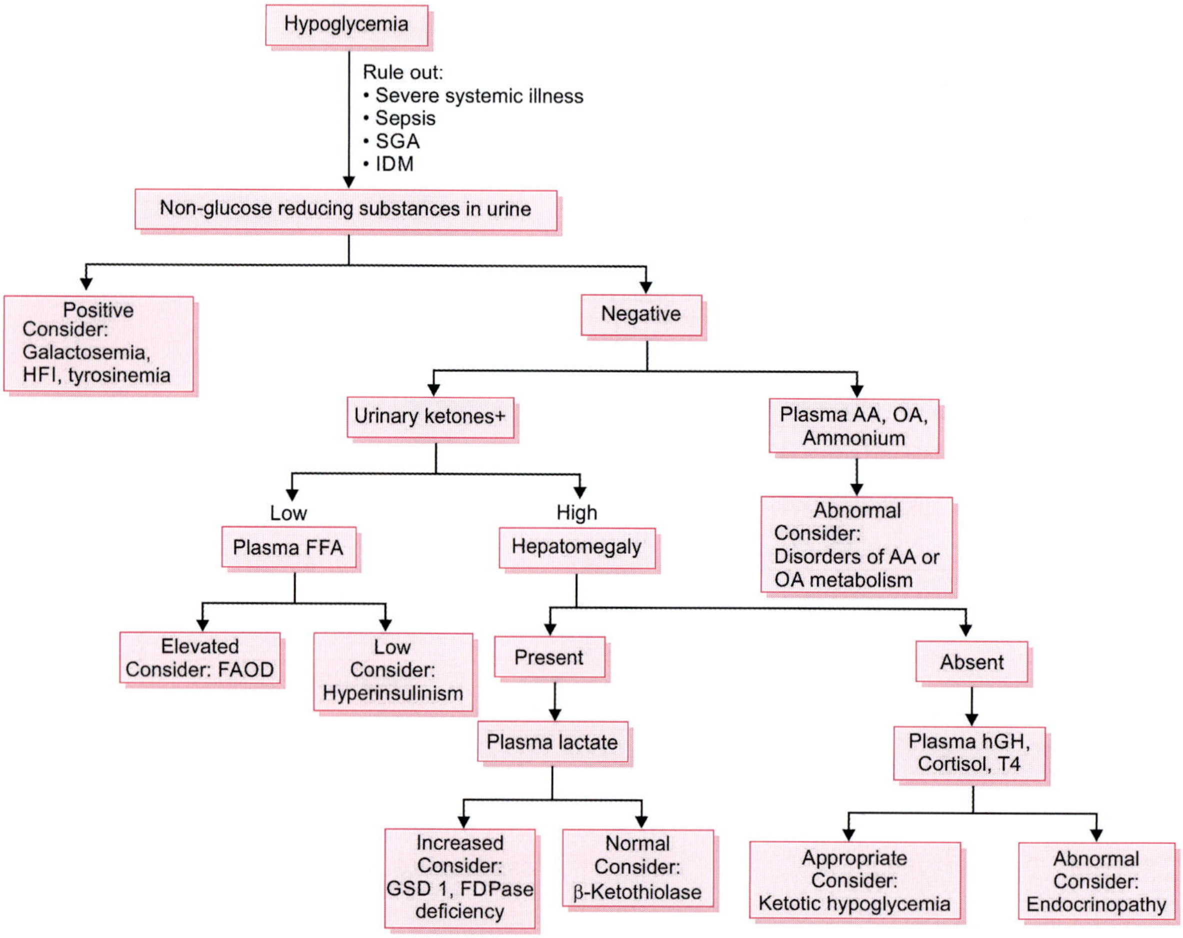

Hypoglycemia
↓ Rule out:
- Severe systemic illness
- Sepsis
- SGA
- IDM

Non-glucose reducing substances in urine
- Positive: Consider: Galactosemia, HFI, tyrosinemia
- Negative
  - Urinary ketones+
    - Low → Plasma FFA
      - Elevated: Consider: FAOD
      - Low: Consider: Hyperinsulinism
    - High → Hepatomegaly
      - Present → Plasma lactate
        - Increased: Consider: GSD 1, FDPase deficiency
        - Normal: Consider: β-Ketothiolase
      - Absent → Plasma hGH, Cortisol, T4
        - Appropriate: Consider: Ketotic hypoglycemia
        - Abnormal: Consider: Endocrinopathy
  - Plasma AA, OA, Ammonium → Abnormal: Consider: Disorders of AA or OA metabolism

(FFA: free fatty acids; SGA; small-for-gestational age; IDM; infants of diabetic mothers; HFI: hereditary fructose intolerance; AA: amino acid; HA: hyaluronic acid; OA: organic acids)
Source: Modified from Clarke JTR[13]

neutralize hyperglycemia if needed (check lactate). Add parenteral lipid infusion @ 1-3 g/kg/24 hours (not if fatty acid oxidation disorders are suspected).

- *Ensure adequate fluid and electrolyte intake*: aim for sodium concentration of 140 mmol/L to reduce the risk of cerebral edema.
- Carry out detoxification measures depending upon the disease and toxicity (*see* below)
- Give appropriate antibiotics if there is any suspicion of an infectious cause.
- Consider specific drug treatments according to presentation (vitamins, carnitine, carbamyl glutamate, etc.)
- All infants suspected of IEMs should be transferred to a tertiary care center where genetic/metabolic studies can be performed and consultants are available.

Nutrition

A basic principle for treatment in a suspected IEM baby is to provide enough calories so as to break the catabolic cycle in the body and revert back to the anabolic state. This is best achieved by the provision of the highest possible "safe calories". The source of these calories will depend upon the suspected group of IEM. For urea cycle disorders and organic acidemias where babies have acute sickness due to protein catabolism, the initial nutrition provided is through a 'non-protein' source, mainly carbohydrate (10–15% IV glucose, with insulin neutralizing drip if needed, through central line) and sometimes with fat infusion (IV intralipid infusions @ 2–4 g/kg/24 hours) through parenteral route if oral or enteral is not possible. Special protein-free formula feeds are now available which can be started orally or by NG feeds as soon as the baby is in a condition to accept. In babies where clinical suspicion is of a fat oxidation disorder, it is prudent to withhold fat in feeds or parenteral nutrition, while providing enough calories through carbohydrates and proteins.

Detoxification Procedures

Extra-corporeal detoxification methods are the most effective techniques. The various methods used are:

- Continuous venovenous hemodiafiltration (CVVH) - best technique, most efficient in clearing the body of a toxic metabolite.
- Hemodialysis (HD).
- Peritoneal dialysis (PD)–ease of performance, more widely used, less efficient than CVVH or HD.
- Exchange transfusion (ET)– not preferred as it increases the protein and ammonia load on the body.

Emergency Management in Specific Scenarios

Hyperammonemia

Ammonia >180 μmol/L in all neonates requires intervention. Extracorporeal methods to be employed at levels >500 without delay. Acute management includes:

- Stopping protein intake
- Starting intravenous (IV) 10% glucose
- Initiation of first-line medications as
  - *Ammonia scavengers*: Sodium Benzoate (@250 –500 mg/kg/24 hours in 6 to the hourly interval, oral or via NG tube, mixed in 5–10% dextrose). Sodium benzoate is freely available at established pharmacies as well as local grocery stores (used as preserving). Other medications in Sodium Phenylbutyrate (@250–500 mg/kg/day (Not available in India) CVVH if ammonia >500 μmol/L– CVVH available only at few tertiary care centers, peritoneal dialysis is a more practical and feasible alternative, available at most tertiary care centers.
  - *L-Arginine* @ 250–350 mg/kg/24 hours, oral divided in 6–8 hourly dose. Can be mixed with Sodium benzoate and given together.
  - *Oral carbamyl glutamate* is specifically used for reducing ammonia in suspected organic acidemias and N-acetyl glutamate synthase (NAGS) deficiency (dose 100–300 mg/kg/day in divided doses).

Metabolic acidosis

Normal blood pH - 7.37–7.43; HCO_3-21–28 mmol/L; anion gap 7-16 mmol/L. Metabolic Acidosis with increased anion gap (suspected organic acidemia-accumulation of organic anions and/or lactate):

- Check for associated ketones, glucose and ammonia.
- Given initial volume replacement, if metabolic acidosis persists, start sodium bicarbonate infusion. If severe metabolic acidosis (pH<7.2, HCO_3^-<10), extracorporeal methods of toxin removal are recommended.
- *L-Carnitine therapy*: IV or oral carnitine therapy should be initiated as early as possible, after taking necessary blood samples like for MS/MS. Dose: oral or NG 100–200 mg/kg/day, IV 50–100 mg/kg/24-hours in 4 divided doses. Contraindicated in long-chain fatty acid oxidation disorders.
- *Vitamin therapy*:
  - Inj. Hydroxocobalamin 1 mg/IM or IV per 24 hours (for suspected MMA/cobalamin disorders).
  - Tab. Thiamine 100 mg/day oral or IV for suspected MSUD/mitochondrial disorders.
  - Tab Riboflavin 100 mg/day oral or IV for suspected Glutaric aciduria type 1 or 2/other.
  - Tab Biotin 5–10 mg twice daily oral for suspected multiple carboxylase deficiency.
- *Additional drugs:*
  - Syr. Metronidazole 10 mg/kg/day oral or iv for gut bacterial clearance (in propionic acidemia).
  - Glycine amino acid–in suspected Isovaleric acidemia and methyl crotonyl-CoA deficiency.

Neonatal seizures

Refractory seizures, in high-risk situations such as previous neonatal deaths or consanguinity could need emergency management of seizures.

- Treat with anticonvulsants, but avoid sodium valproate.
- Therapeutic trials of following drugs may be attempted.
  - Tab Biotin 5–10 mg twice to three times a day, orally or via NG tube.
  - Tab Pyridoxine 15–30 mg/kg/day divided into 6–8 hourly intervals orally. IV dose for same is

Box 1: Case scenario with a healthy baby born to a couple with previous neonatal deaths suspected to have IEM

This is a common scenario in tertiary care NICUs as the awareness increases, yet with no accurate diagnosis in the deceased babies. The neonate should be managed on lines of an acute IEM unless proved otherwise since most often the risk of disease is as high as 25–50%. The baby would need a careful observation in NICU, with monitoring of general parameters, and metabolic parameters (glucose, electrolytes, lactate, ammonia, blood gas, ketones) and a gradual introduction of feeds (mother's milk is the best choice), followed by metabolic screening using TMS and GC-MS 12–24 hours after introduction of feeds. Any symptom should be taken seriously and acted upon pre-emptively and treatment continued until the diagnosis of IEM is either proven or ruled out. Close collaboration with a metabolic specialist is strongly recommended, whether onsite or telephonically.

100 mg IV infusion, repeat after 6–8 hours if no response. Oral use of pyridoxal-5-phosphate is also recommended in pyridoxine unresponsive babies at a dose of 30–50 mg/kg/day at 6 hourly intervals. Pyridoxal-5-phosphate is now available in India through online portals or few specific pharmacies.

- Tab Folinic acid 7.5 mg in two divided doses (or 2.5 mg IV infusion once in 24 hours).
- Inj. Hydroxocobalamin 1 mg/mL– 1 mL intramuscular or iv every 24 hours, especially for inherited cobalamin disorders.

Box 1 provides an outline of managing a neonate in the neonatal care unit.

NEWBORN SCREENING

India does not have a universal newborn screening program, for metabolic disorders.[7,16,17] However, newborn screening is being carried out in many private institutions and a few government hospitals. Most centers test for congenital hypothyroidism, congenital adrenal hyperplasia and for G-6-PD deficiency, and some include TMS for metabolic disorders.

What to do is a Newborn has a Positive NBS Result?

This result does not always mean that the baby will be affected by that disease. As NBS is a "screening test", hence the most important aspect is to confirm the diagnosis before moving on with management. NBS for metabolic disorders can be done for more than 50 disorders in the expanded program with the use of Tandem Mass Spectroscopy (TMS). The NBS results always need to be confirmed using various methods before "labeling" a baby with a diagnosis. The confirmation of organic acidurias (MMA, Propionic acidemia, glutaric aciduria type 1 or GA1 etc.) is done by urine GC-MS, amino aciduria by plasma quantitative amino acids by HPLC or UPLC, urea cycle disorders by HPLC/UPLC amino acids and urine GC-MS based orotate levels and FAOD by enzyme assay on skin fibroblasts or DNA based gene studies. All the disorders can be confirmed using gene studies.

Follow-up

If the baby is already symptomatic by the time the results arrive, then the acute management is essentially the same as for any "symptomatic" baby. If the baby is asymptomatic but proven with a metabolic disorder or IEM, then immediate treatment for that specific disorder needs to be started, preferably with a metabolic specialist.

OUTCOME AND PROGNOSTIC FACTORS

The outcome following acute management in the emergency is variable and dependent on the time taken to recognize a particular disorder, as well as initiation of emergency management regimen subsequent to initial suspicion. The earlier it is done, the better is the prognosis–as the disorder tends to progress relentlessly unless measures are taken to halt the process by intervention as detailed above. The emergency situation also arises in infants or children who have already been diagnosed, either via previous symptoms or by newborn screening. Thus, it is important for the treating pediatrician/metabolic specialist to provide an "emergency letter" to the family and instruct them to show it to the doctors on arrival in an emergency unit. This would not only save time but also provide the emergency physician with a quick line of management as would be mentioned in the letter.

PREVENTION

As all IEMs are inherited, with recessive inheritance (X- or autosomal) being the most common mode, thus there is a risk of recurrence in the families –25% in autosomal and up to 50% in X-linked disorders. After a definitive diagnosis in the affected patient, a cascade testing within the families is advisable to look for more affected or carrier individuals. As parents of an affected child are carrier by default, hence a prenatal diagnosis is advised in all subsequent pregnancies in the couple. PND is done via either enzymology (wherever feasible) or molecular genetic analysis at a minimum of 11 weeks of pregnancy or later, up to 20 weeks of pregnancy.

KEY MESSAGES

- Inborn errors of metabolism (IEMs) present in common and non-specific presentations mostly summarized as "sepsis-like".
- There is usually a symptom-free period varying from hours to days or even more for all the acutely presenting IEMs.
- The acute "metabolic" attacks are usually provoked or triggered by fasting, catabolism, fever, sepsis, and sometimes even food intake.
- Most of these disorders can be diagnosed usually simple and basic metabolic investigations such as glucose, electrolytes, lactate, ammonia, acid-base (blood gas), and ketones.
- Treatment is possible, at least partially for most of these disorders as they require emergency removal of the toxin by special diets, extracorporeal procedures, vitamins or cleansing drugs (carnitine, sodium benzoate, penicillamine, etc.) or supplementation of a crucial product, such as glucose or biotin, the deficiency of which is the major cause of symptoms.

REFERENCES

1. Scriver C, Beaudet A, Sly W, Valle D, editors. The Metabolic and Molecular Bases of Inherited Disease, 8th edition. New York: McGraw-Hill; 2001. p. 6338.
2. Applegarth DA, Toone JR, Lowry RB. Incidence of inborn errors of metabolism in British Columbia, 1969-1996. Pediatrics. 2000;105:e10.
3. Sanderson S, Green A, Preece MA, *et al.* The incidence of inherited metabolic disorders in the West Midlands, UK. Arch Dis Child. 2006;91:896-9.
4. Wilcken B, Wiley V, Hammond J, *et al.* Screening newborns for inborn errors of metabolism by tandem mass spectrometry. N Engl J Med. 2003;348:2304-12.
5. Lehotay DC, Hall P, Lepage J, *et al.* LC-MS/MS progress in newborn screening. Clin Biochem. 2011;44:21-31.
6. Christopher R, Natarajan A. Screening for inborn errors of metabolism by tandem mass spectrometry: an eight year experience. Techagappe. 2016;2:21-3.
7. Kapoor S, Thelma BK. Status of newborn screening and inborn errors of metabolism in India. Indian J Pediatr. 2018;85: 1110-17.
8. Bijarnia-Mahay S, Puri RD, Verma IC. Screening for inborn errors of metabolism. In: Sachdeva A, Dutta AK, editors. Advances in Pediatrics, 2nd edition. New Delhi: Jaypee Brothers Medical Publisher; 2012; p. 265-72.
9. Bijarnia-Mahay S, Verma IC. Inborn errors of metabolism. In: The Handbook of Neonatology, 1st edition. New Delhi: Indian Journal of Pediatrics Publication; 2018. p. 144-59.
10. Saudubray JM, Baumgartner M, Walter J, editors. Inborn Metabolic Diseases Diagnosis and Treatment, vol. 1, 6th edition. Heidelberg (Germany): Springer; 2016. p. 658.
11. Saudubray JM. Inborn errors of metabolism overview pathophysiology, manifestations, evaluation, and management. Pediatr Clin N Am. 2018;65:179-208.
12. van Karnebeek CDM, Stockler S. Treatable inborn errors of metabolism causing intellectual disability: A systematic literature review. Mol Genet Metab. 2012;105:368-81.
13. Clarke JTR. Acute metabolic illness in the newborn. In: Clarke JTR, editor. A Clinical Guide to Inherited Metabolic Diseases. 2nd edition. Cambridge: Cambridge University Press; 2002. p. 176-204.
14. Rezvani I, Yudkoff M. Defects in metabolism of amino acids-urea cycle and hyperammonemia. In: Kliegman RM, Stanton BF, Schor NF, St Geme III JW, editors. Nelson's Textbook of Pediatrics, 20th edition. Philadelphia: Saunders; 2016. p. 671.
15. Marín-Valencia I, Vilaseca MA, Thió M, *et al.* Assessment of the perimortem protocol in neonates for the diagnosis of inborn errors of metabolism. Eur J Paediatr Neurol. 2010;14:125-30.
16. Verma IC, Bijarnia S. Inborn errors of metabolism in the neonatal period - is it time to change our practice? Indian J Pediatr. 2012;79:528-9.
17. Verma IC, Bijarnia Mahay S, Jhingan G, *et al.* Newborn screening: Need of the hour in India. Indian J Pediatr. 2014; 82:61-70.

CHAPTER

75

Neonatal Jaundice

Srinivas Murki, Deepak Sharma

Jaundice is visible manifestation of yellowness of the skin and sclera due to elevated serum bilirubin levels. It is seen in neonates when serum bilirubin level exceeds 5–7 mg/dL. The prevalence of neonatal jaundice is 50–60% in term and nearly 80% in preterm infants.[1] In most infants, unconjugated hyperbilirubinemia reflects a normal transitional phenomenon however epidemiological evidence suggests that severe neonatal jaundice (SNJ) results in substantial morbidity and mortality. SNJ has been recognized to cause deafness, learning difficulties, cerebral palsy, auditory neuropathy and cognitive impairment. A recent report noted that at least 0.48 million term/near term neonates are affected by SNJ each year worldwide with around 0.11 million dying of the same.[2] Nearly 65% to 75% of very low birth weight (VLBW) infants require treatment for neonatal jaundice. The most common cause of readmission after discharge from birth hospitalization is neonatal jaundice.[3]

Though neonatal jaundice is a global clinical problem, the incidence is highest in Asian and south east Asian regions.[4] High prevalence of late preterm births, exclusive breastfeeding rates, G6PD deficiency and poor prevention of Rh isoimmunization are the reasons for high incidence of jaundice in these regions. Genetic and environmental factors also contribute to the high incidence of jaundice in South East Asian population.[4]

Delayed referral, improper phototherapy and high prevalence of co-morbid conditions such as asphyxia, intrauterine growth restriction and sepsis contribute to the increased incidence of bilirubin encephalopathy in developing countries.

ETIOLOGY

Most of the newborn babies have elevation in serum bilirubin level during first week of life because of their physiological immaturity to handle increased production of bilirubin. When this rise in bilirubin does not warrant treatment than it is called physiological jaundice. Appreciable jaundice starts appearing at around 24 to 72 hours of life. Serum bilirubin level in term infants rises to peak value of around 12 to 15 mg/dL by 72 hours of life and then gradually decreases. In preterm neonates, the peak level of TSB reaches by day 3 to 7 of life and can rise to peak value of more than 15 mg/dL. It may take a prolonged period up to weeks both in term and preterm neonates before TSB values decline to the normal adult level. The term physiological hyperbilirubinemia should be used cautiously in preterm neonates because such values can be dangerous in these babies. When the jaundice of the newborn does not conform to the timeline of physiological jaundice or jaundice is severe enough to warrant therapy, it is designated as pathological jaundice.

Etiology of neonatal hyperbilirubinemia is depicted in **Table 1**.

PATHOGENESIS AND PATHOPHYSIOLOGY

Bilirubin is produced in the reticuloendothelial system, transported in the blood by albumin, conjugated in the liver to mono or diglucuronide, enters the gastrointestinal tract as conjugate bilirubin and then excreted in the stool. In the absence of gut bacteria, beta-glucuronidase (intestinal enzyme) converts conjugate bilirubin back to

Table 1: Causes of pathological jaundice

Increased bilirubin load	*Decreased bilirubin clearance*	*Increased enterohepatic circulation*
Feto-maternal blood group incompatibility • Rh incompatibility • ABO incompatibility • Minor blood group incompatibility **RBC membrane defects** • Hereditary spherocytosis • Elliptocytosis • Stomatocytosis • Pyknocytosis **RBC enzyme abnormalities** • Glucose-6-phoshate dehydrogenase deficiency • Pyruvate kinase deficiency **Polycythemia** *Extravasated blood* • Cephalhematoma • Subgaleal hemorrhage *Hemoglobinopathies* • Alpha thalassemia	Mutations in genes encoding "UGT1A1" • Crigler-Najjar syndrome type I&II • Gilbert syndrome **Hormonal defects** • Hypothyroidism • Hypopituitarism **Metabolic defects** • Galactosemia	• Breast milk jaundice • Not breastfeeding jaundice • Intestinal atresia • Meconium ileus • Hirschsprung disease

the unconjugated form and is reabsorbed into the blood (enterohepatic circulation) (**Fig. 1**).

Bilirubin production: Bilirubin is an end product of heme catabolism. Degradation of heme is the primary source of bilirubin. Lysis of red blood cells releases heme which in the presence of heme-oxygenase is converted to biliverdin. This rate limiting step results in release of iron and carbon monoxide (CO) in equimolar amounts. Biliverdin is converted to bilirubin in the presence of biliverdin reductase. The degradation of 1gram of heme forms 34 mg of bilirubin.

Bilirubin transport: Unconjugated bilirubin released into circulation is rapidly bound to albumin as it is insoluble in water at the body pH of 7.4. Each gram of albumin binds to 8 mg of unconjugated bilirubin. Unconjugated bilirubin not bound to albumin is the free bilirubin. It is the free (unbound) bilirubin that crosses the blood-brain barrier and causes neurological dysfunction or damage.

Conjugation of bilirubin: Excretion of bilirubin into the bile requires it to be converted to a water-soluble compound. Bilirubin dissociates from albumin before entering the liver. Bilirubin enters the liver cell by carrier mediated diffusion. Inside liver cells, bilirubin binds with α-ligandin (intracellular cytoplasmic protein) which helps transferring bilirubin to endoplasmic reticulum where conjugation of bilirubin takes place. Conjugation of bilirubin with two molecules of glucuronic acid in the presence of UDPG-glucuronyl transferase facilitates this process.

Enterohepatic circulation: α-glucuronidase hydrolyzes conjugated bilirubin to unconjugated bilirubin in intestinal lumen. This unconjugated form is readily absorbed from the intestine. Intestinal bacteria convert conjugate bilirubin to urobilinoids which are not the substrates for α-glucuronidase thus preventing enterohepatic circulation.

Risk Factors for Hyperbilirubinemia

- *Excessive bilirubin production*
  - Increased red blood cell volume
  - RBC survival in newborn infants is less compared to adults (90 days versus 120 days).
  - Ineffective erythropoiesis also significantly contributes to increased bilirubin production.
- *Decreased bilirubin uptake by liver*
  - Decreased membrane transport.
  - Decreased Ligandin levels
  - *Defective conjugation* because of decreased uridine diphosphoglucuronide transferase (UDPGT) activity. At birth the activity of UDPG-glucuronyl transferase is 5% of adult activity but increases significantly after 24 hours to handle the bilirubin load. In North Indian population, polymorphism in the promoter sequence of UDP-glucuronyl

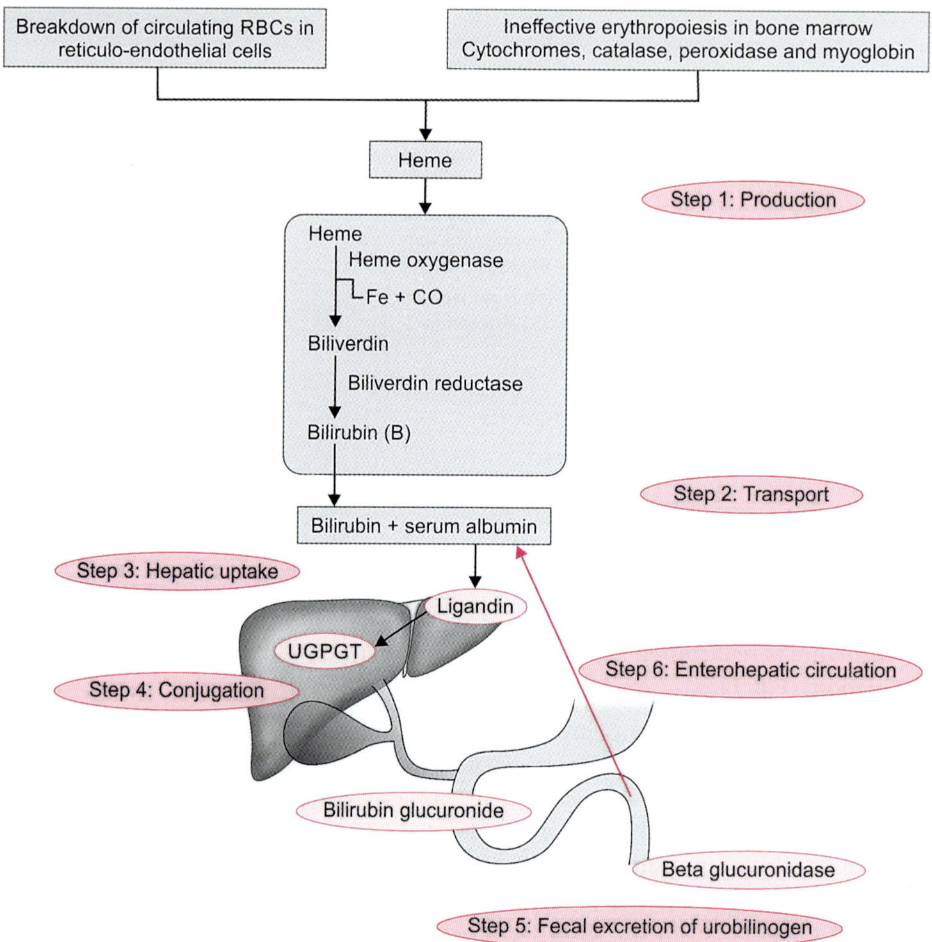

Fig. 1: Metabolism of bilirubin

transferase is associated with increased risk of hyperbilirubinemia.[5]

- *Increased enterohepatic circulation*
  - High levels of beta-glucuronidase in neonatal intestine.
  - Conjugation of bilirubin to monoglucuronide rather than diglucuronide.
  - Less number of bacteria in neonatal intestine.
  - Poor gut motility with decreased evacuation of meconium laden with bilirubin.

CLINICAL FEATURES

Clinical evaluation: When a jaundiced neonate presents to the health care provider, one must attempt to answer the following questions:

- Is the jaundice physiological or pathological?
- Is it possible to predict that jaundice will rise to a level needing treatment?
- If pathological jaundice is suspected what are the possible causes?
- Does the infant have clinical signs of bilirubin encephalopathy?
- Which infants require further investigations and what investigations are needed?
- When and how to treat jaundiced neonates?

Pathological Jaundice

The following guidelines will aid in differentiating physiologic from pathologic jaundice:

- Any value of TSB more than 5 mg/dL within first 24 hours, more than 10 mg/dL on day 2 of life or anytime any value greater than 12–13 mg/dL is regarded as pathological jaundice.[6]
- Jaundice visible within first 24 hours of birth, on day 2 appreciable jaundice on limbs, anytime yellowish staining of palms and soles, increase in TSB concentration by more than 0.2 mg/dL/hour or 5 mg/dL/day, features of acute bilirubin encephalopathy are the features indicating pathological jaundice thus warranting further evaluation and management.
- Conjugated bilirubin >20% of total serum bilirubin or more than 2 mg/dL at any age is not physiological.
- Jaundice lasting for more than 2 weeks in term and more than 3 weeks in preterm neonates should also be considered as pathological jaundice necessitating adequate management and evaluation.

Clinical judgment is widely used and utilizes the principle that jaundice first appears on the face and then progresses cephalocaudal from trunk to limbs as the intensity increases. Staining of palms and soles can be seen when bilirubin levels exceed 15 mg/dL. Transcutaneous bilirubin estimation offers an objective method of assessing the degree of hyperbilirubinemia. It may be used as a screening tool in the initial assessment of jaundice and for expected bilirubin values < 14 mg/dL.[7]

Prediction of severe jaundice. In healthy term and late preterm infants (gestation of 34–36 weeks), hour specific serum bilirubin nomogram predicts the development of subsequent severe jaundice in the first week after birth (**Fig. 2**). If the TSB value at any age is falling in the high-risk zone (>95th centile) or in the intermediate risk zone (40th to 95th centile) the chance of subsequent hyperbilirubinemia is significant. If the hour specific TSB is in the low risk zone (<40th centile), there is no measurable risk of subsequent severe jaundice.[8] In term healthy neonates if serum bilirubin at 24 ± 8 hours is <6 mg/dL the risk of subsequent hyperbilirubinemia is almost negligible.[9]

A detailed history, examination (**Table 2**), and the age at onset of jaundice (**Table 3**) along with investigations can provide us the likely etiology for jaundice.

Prolonged Jaundice

Clinical jaundice persisting for >2 weeks in term neonates and for >3 weeks in preterm neonates is termed as prolonged jaundice. Most common etiology in these

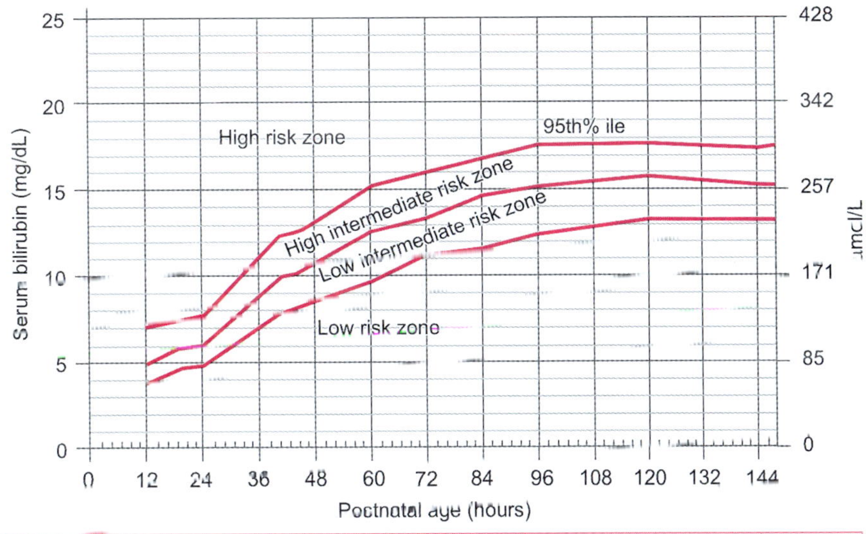

Designated risk status	Evaluation	Follow-up
High	For hemolysis and risk factors	In 6–12 hours, Intervention strategy
High-intermediate	For risk factors	May repeat TSB in 24 hours
Low intermediate	For risk factors	May repeat TSB in 48 hours
Low	Assess well being	May not need repeat testing

Fig. 2: Prediction of severe hyperbilirubinemia and hour specific TSB

Table 2: History and clinical examination and relevance in neonatal jaundice	
History	
• Previous sibling with neonatal jaundice, family history of anemia, splenectomy	• Blood group incompatibility (Rh, ABO), G6PD Deficiency, Hereditary spherocytosis, • Crigler-Najjar yndrome
• Maternal fever and rash during pregnancy	• Intrauterine infections
• Labor and delivery events • Maternal drugs	• Asphyxia, trauma, oxytocin, delayed cord clamping • Sulfonamides, nitrofurantoin and antimalarials may cause hemolysis in G6PD deficient infa
• Liver disease in the family	• Galactosemia, Alpha 1 antitrypsin deficiency
• Prolonged parenteral nutrition	• Cholestatic jaundice
Examination	
• Small for date	• IU infections, polycythemia
• Microcephaly	• IU infections
• Pallor	• Hemolysis, extravasation of blood
• Petechia	• IU infection, Rh immunization, sepsis
• Hepatosplenomegaly	• IU infections, hemolytic jaundice, liver disease
• Chorioretinitis	• IU infections
• Urine diaper staining and acholic stools	• Cholestatic jaundice

Table 3: Etiology based on the age at onset of jaundice		
Less than 24 hrs of birth	*24–72 hrs of age*	*After 72 hrs of age*
• Rh isoimmunization • ABO and minor blood group incompatibility • Intrauterine infections (TORCH), malaria, bacterial • G6PD deficiency	• Physiological • Sepsis • Polycythemia • Extravasations • Increased enterohepatic—Circulation • Hypertrophic pyloric stenosis, intestinal obstruction	• Sepsis • Neonatal hepatitis • Extrahepatic biliary atresia • Breast milk jaundice • Metabolic (galactosemia, tyrosinemia, fructosemia, alpha 1 antitrypsin deficiency, organic acidemias, cystic fibrosis)

babies is breast milk jaundice but one needs to rule out more sinister causes such as hypothyroidism and biliary atresia. Staining of diapers and pale stools suggest cholestasis. Relevant investigations are necessary to rule out hypothyroidism, urinary tract infection, galactosemia, sepsis, malaria, ongoing hemolysis, Crigler-Najjar syndrome, pyloric stenosis and neonatal cholestasis syndromes.

COMPLICATIONS

Bilirubin Encephalopathy

The important step in bilirubin induced neuronal injury is the entry of bilirubin into brain and subsequent exposure of bilirubin to neurons (**Fig. 3**). Hypoalbuminemia, impaired binding of albumin to bilirubin, increased concentration of H^+ ions, i.e. metabolic acidosis, increased permeability of blood brain barrier (BBB) due to injury and increase in susceptibility of neurons to bilirubin toxicity contribute to bilirubin induced neuronal damage. Unbound bilirubin in presence of hydrogen ions forms bilirubin acid. Bilirubin acid ultimately leads to neuronal injury. Experimental studies suggest a direct relationship between level of free bilirubin and occurrence of neuronal injury.[10] More the duration of severe neonatal jaundice, more are the chances of neuronal damage. The major neurological features of acute bilirubin encephalopathy (ABE) are due to involvement of neurons of reticular formation, basal ganglia (predominantly globus pallidus nucleus and subthalamic nuclei) and brainstem nuclei.

Bilirubin Induced Neurological Dysfunction

The clinical presentation of ABE is usually considered in 3 phases of increasing severity which gradually evolve over

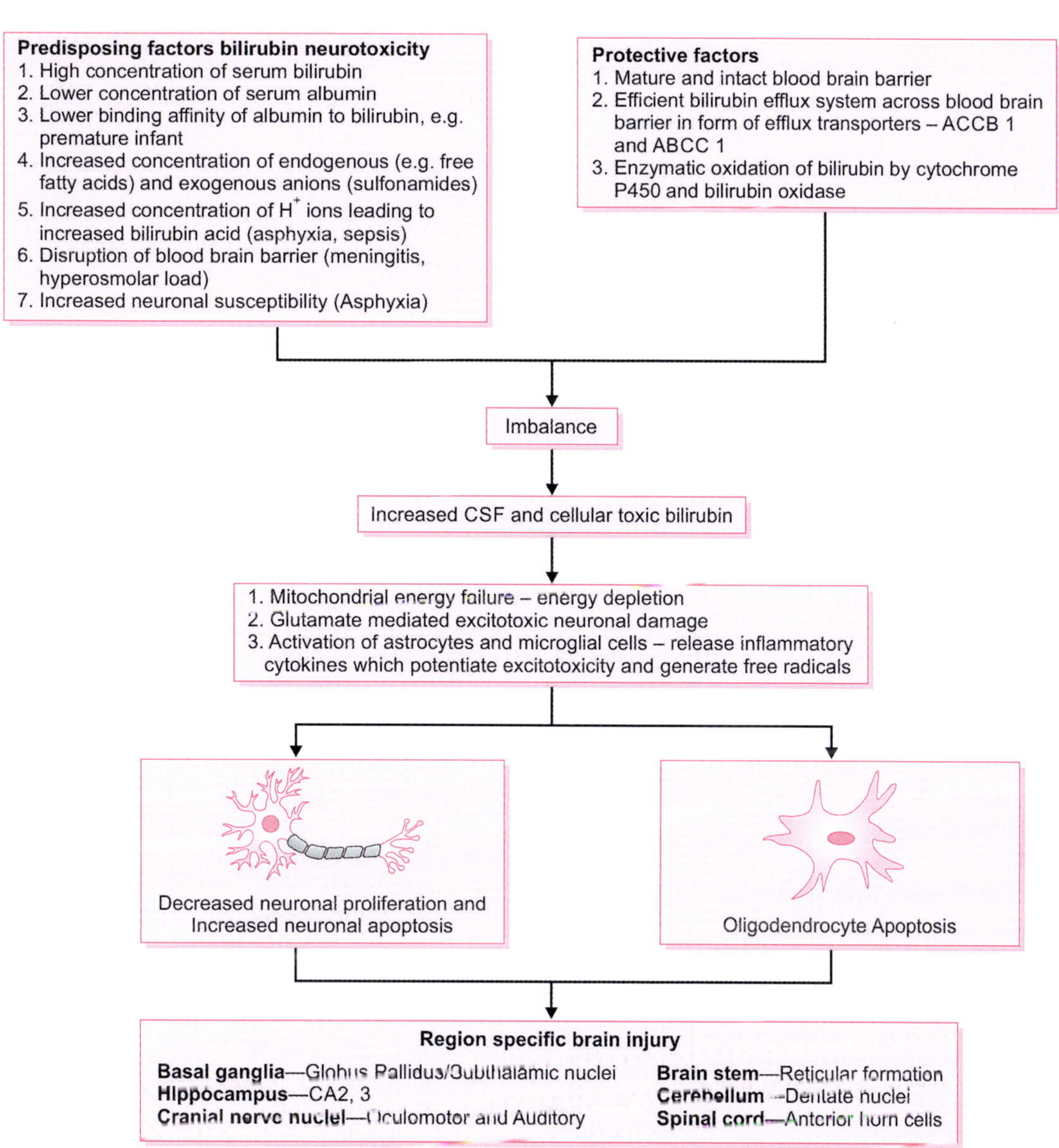

Fig. 3: Pathogenesis of bilirubin Induced neurological damage

several days BIND scoring is used to describe the intensity of the clinical features associated with acute bilirubin encephalopathy and quantifies the severity of the clinical manifestations and their association with developmental outcome. Original BIND score was based on mental status, tone abnormalities and cry pattern which was later modified by addition of gaze abnormalities. Modified BIND score is shown in **Table 4**.

Important for clinicians is to recognize bilirubin encephalopathy early before the neonate progresses to irreversible stage. Early detection of BE may be possible by use of brainstem evoked response audiometry (BERA). BERA in acute bilirubin encephalopathy may present with abnormalities of threshold for all waves, latency for wave I, and increased interwave I - III and I -V intervals. BERA appears to be a sensitive method of detecting

Table 4: Modified BIND (bilirubin-induced neurological dysfunction) score

Clinical sign		*Score*	*Severity*
Mental status	Normal-awake alert	0	None
	Sleepy but arousable or decreased feeding	1	Mild
	Lethargy or poor suck and/or irritable/jittery	2	Moderate
	Unable to feed or apnea or seizures or coma	3	Severe
Tone pattern	Normal flexed tone	0	None
	Persistent mild hypotonia	1	Mild
	Moderate hypotonia or hypertonia, beginning of arching of neck or trunk	2	Moderate
	Severe tone abnormality, persistent retrocollis or opisthotonos	3	Severe
Cry pattern	Normal	0	None
	High pitched	1	Mild
	Shrill	2	Moderate
	Weak or absent cry or inconsolable cry	3	Severe
Oculomotor or eye movements	Normal	0	None, mild
Sunsetting or paralysis of upward gaze		3	Severe

Proposed interpretation: total score 1 to 3 indicates mild ABE, 4 to 6 indicates moderate ABE and score more than 7 indicates severe ABE

bilirubin induced neuronal dysfunction and probable imminent neuronal damage. MRI of the brain may show acute abnormalities as hyperintense signals in the globus pallidus and subthalamic nucleus.

Chronic Post-kernicteric Bilirubin Encephalopathy

Clinical features characteristic of chronic post-kernicteric bilirubin encephalopathy may not become apparent before the age of 6 to 12 months. The characteristic features of fully developed chronic bilirubin encephalopathy are extra-pyramidal movement disorders, gaze abnormalities, auditory dysfunction and dental dysplasia. Usually Intellectual functions are preserved.

MEASUREMENT OF SERUM BILIRUBIN

- *Transcutaneous bilirubinometer (TcB)* ***(Fig. 3)***
  - Transcutaneous bilirubin estimation is a useful alternative to serum bilirubin measurement. Its routine use can decrease the need for blood sampling.
  - TcB can be used in infants with gestation ≥35 weeks after 24 hours of birth. It becomes unreliable if baby is already receiving phototherapy, is more than 2 weeks old, gestation is <35 weeks, within 24 hours of birth and when serum bilirubin is >13 mg/dL.
  - Whenever TcB value is >12 to 14 mg/dL, confirmatory serum bilirubin assessment should be done.
- *Serum bilirubin measurement*
  - *Indications for (total serum bilirubin) TSB assessment*
    - Visible icterus during first 24 hours of life
    - After 24 hours of life if clinical jaundice is likely to be > 12–14 mg/dL.
    - In conditions where TcB is not reliable or TcB is not available.
    - When not sure of clinical assessment
    - TcB> 13 mg/dL
    - During ongoing phototherapy for monitoring purpose and to check for rebound after stopping phototherapy (hemolytic jaundice).
  - *Methods for measurement of serum bilirubin*
    - Biochemical: for measurement of serum bilirubin level, high performance liquid chromatography remains the gold standard test. However, Van den Bergh reaction is routinely used for laboratory estimation of TSB and it has marked inter laboratory variability.[11]
    - Serum bilirubin measurement by micro method is based on spectrophotometery and is useful in neonates as bilirubin is predominantly unconjugated in newborns.

INVESTIGATIONS

Investigations are required for assessing the severity of jaundice, to differentiate conjugated from unconjugated jaundice, to identify the etiology and to predict the risk of bilirubin encephalopathy.

- As a routine, in all neonates with severe jaundice a total serum bilirubin with direct and indirect fractions, packed cell volume, reticulocyte count, direct coombs test (DCT), peripheral smear, serum albumin and G6PD screening are advised.
- When sepsis is clinically suspected, a sepsis screen along with blood and urine culture is recommended.
- In Rh isoimmunized mothers, cord blood should be screened for total serum bilirubin, hematocrit, blood grouping and DCT.
- For jaundice lasting for greater than 2 weeks in term neonate and more than 3 weeks in a preterm, a thyroid profile, liver function tests, urine culture, and galactosemia screen are the needed investigations.

PCV <40%, reticulocyte count >5% after day 3, peripheral smear showing marked aniso-poikilocytosis, heterochromia and nucleated RBC's suggest hemolysis as the cause of jaundice. Plenty of micro spherocytes on the peripheral smear is suggestive of ABO incompatibility. A positive indirect comb's test in the mother or positive DCT in the baby is indicative of immune hemolysis.

TREATMENT

Management of neonates for hyperbilirubinemia using phototherapy or exchange transfusion is generally based on the American academy of pediatrics (AAP) guidelines.[12] There are two age specific bilirubin nomograms provided by AAP, one for phototherapy and the other for exchange transfusion (**Figs. 4 and 5**).

The nomograms provided by AAP have 3 different action lines for 3 different risk categories of neonates and these include:

- Neonates at low risk (≥ 38 weeks gestation without risk factors)

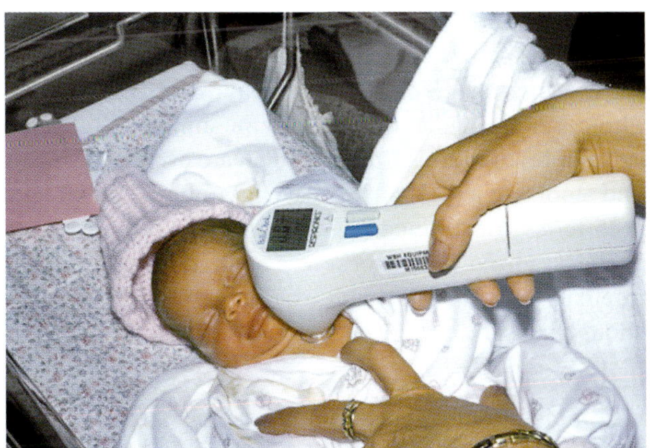

Fig. 4: Transcutaneous bilirubinometer

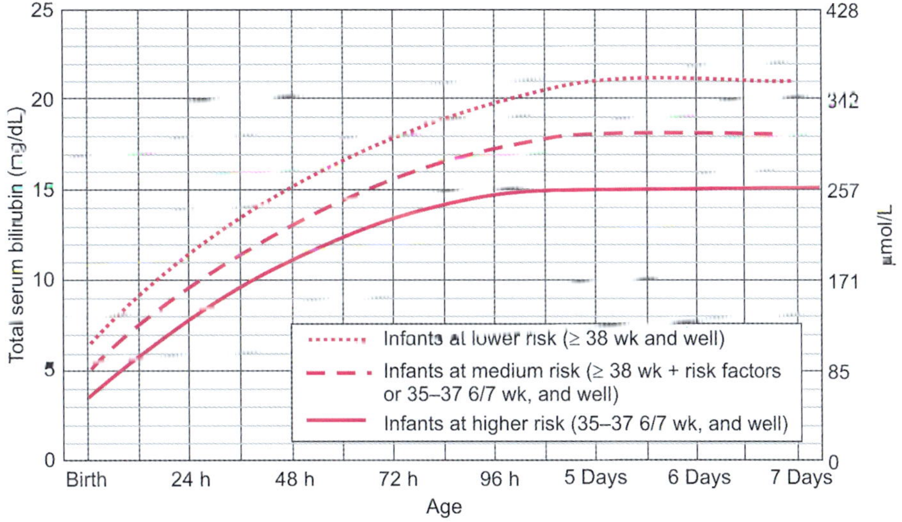

Fig. 5: Guidelines for phototherapy in hospitalized infants ≥ 35 weeks of gestation

- Neonates at intermediate risk (≥38 weeks gestation with presence of risk factors or with gestation 35 to 37 weeks 6 days without any risk factor)
- Neonates at high risk (neonates with gestation 35 to 37 weeks 6 days with presence of 1 risk factor).

Risk factors taken into consideration before assigning risk category include presence of isoimmune hemolytic disease, sepsis, acidosis, hypoalbuminemia, G6PD deficiency, asphyxia, hypothermia and temperature instability. For the purpose of management, total serum bilirubin concentration should be considered and direct fraction should not be subtracted.

Phototherapy

Phototherapy (PTx) at present is the mainstay therapy for managing neonates with hyperbilirubinemia. Phototherapy acts by converting unconjugated bilirubin (insoluble) to soluble isomers which are excreted in urine and stools. At a particular wavelength of blue green light (425 to 475 nm), unconjugated bilirubin isomerizes to harmless forms. In case of severe neonatal jaundice high-intensity phototherapy with irradiance >30 $\mu W/cm^2/nm$ should be used.

Care during phototherapy:

- Ambient room temperature should be optimum (25 to 28°C).
- Maximum body surface area should be exposed by removing all clothes except diapers. Cover the eyes with patches during phototherapy.
- Keep the distance between baby and light as close as possible to improve irradiance but to allow visualization and monitoring (or as per manufacturer recommendation).

Maximizing phototherapy efficacy: There should be periodic assessment of irradiance of phototherapy lights.

- Expose maximal surface area of the baby and ensure frequent change of posture.
- Ensure correct spectrum of the light exposed (425 to 475 mm)
- Ensure good hydration and nutrition of the baby.

Monitoring and stopping of phototherapy

- Temperature of the neonate should be monitored at least every 4 hours while under PTx.
- Measure bilirubin level every 12 to 24 hours or more frequently if needed.
- Stop PTx if two consecutive TSB values at least 12 hours apart are below age specific cut offs at that point of time.
- After stopping PTx do remember to check for rebound increase in TSB level within 24 hours especially for infants with immune hemolysis or severe jaundice.

Side effects

- Impaired maternal infant bonding (most important and common)
- Increased insensible water losses
- Watery diarrhea and increased fecal water losses
- Skin rashes
- Hypocalcemia
- Bronze baby syndrome (in the presence of raised direct fraction).

Lately there has been some concern that blue green wavelengths of PTx may cause DNA damage, thereby increasing the risk of cancers in later life [California Late Impact of Phototherapy (CLIP) study and Late Impact of Getting Hyperbilirubinemia or Phototherapy (LIGHT) study]. Keeping possible long-term adverse effects in consideration, it seems prudent that intensive phototherapy be reserved for neonates with severe hyperbilirubinemia.

Exchange Transfusion

Exchange transfusion (ET) is typically reserved for symptomatic infants, those with severe jaundice, and those at risk for severe jaundice who fail to respond adequately to intensive PTx. The procedure of exchanging newborns blood involves removing of blood having high bilirubin levels, antibody coated RBCs, partially lysed RBCs and simultaneous replacement with blood having fresh albumin with binding sites for albumin.

Indications for exchange transfusion

- Isoimmune hemolytic disease with hydrops, cord Hb <11 g/dL and cord TSB > 5 mg/dL, increasing TSB at a rate > 1 mg/dL/hour despite PTx, rate of rise of TSB >0.5 mg/dL/hour despite PTX if hemoglobin is between 11 and 13 g/dL
- Any baby having features of acute bilirubin encephalopathy
- TSB level in exchange range on the age specific nomograms (AAP charts, **Fig. 6**).

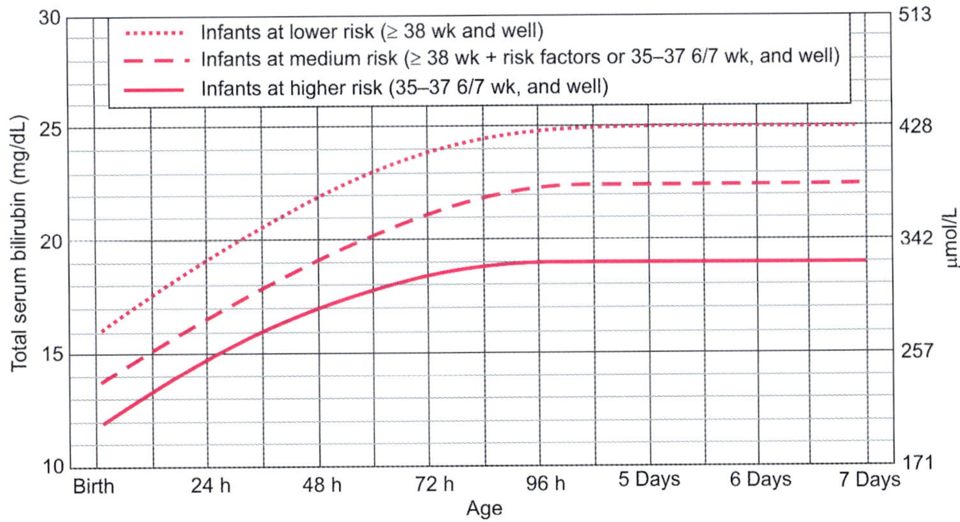

- The dashed lines for the first 24 hours indicate uncertainty due to a wide range of clinical circumstances and a range of response to phototherapy
- Immediate exchange transfusion is recommended if infant shows signs of acute bilirubin encephalopathy (hypertonia, arching, retrocollis, opisthotonos, fever, high pitched cry) or if TSB is ≥ 5 mg/dL (85 µmol/L) above these lines
- Risk factors isoimmune hemolytic disease, G6PD deficiency, asphyxia, significant lethargy, temperature instability, sepsis, acidosis
- Measure serum albumin and calculate B/A ration (See legend)
- Use totoal bilirubin, do not subtract direct reacting or conjugated bilirubin
- If infant is well and 35–37 6/7 wk (median risk) can individualize TSB levels for exchange based on actual gestational age

Fig. 6: Guidelines for exchange transfusion in hospitalized infants ≥ 35 weeks of gestation

Blood for exchange transfusion

Amount of blood required for exchange transfusion depends on the circulating blood volume in the neonate.

- *For double volume exchange transfusion (DVET)*
  - Twice the circulating blood volume is required (e.g. for 3 kg term neonate, circulating blood volume = 240 mL, volume for DVET = 2 × 240 = 480 mL)
  - Mostly used to remove bilirubin and antibodies
  - DVET replaces around 85% of circulating blood volume.
- *Single volume exchange transfusion (SVET)*
  - Blood needed = circulating blood volume
  - SVET replaces around 60% of circulating blood
  - SVET is preferred when etiology is not hemolytic
  - In case of hydrops or CCF with low PCV (<35%) at birth, SVET should be preferred to quickly restore oxygen carrying capacity of blood as it is unlikely that baby will tolerate DVET in such situations.

Blood product

Blood to be used for ET should satisfy the following criteria:

- Should have a hematocrit of 0.5 to 0.6.
- Matched with both mother and baby's blood group.
- Depleted of leukocytes.
- Should be irradiated and used within 24 hours of irradiation.
- Preferably the blood should be collected within last 5 days.

Best method is to use irradiated and leukocyte depleted packed red cells crossed matched with mother and baby's blood group suspended in AB positive plasma in 70:30 ratio. Selecting the type of blood needed for exchange transfusion is depicted in **Table 5**.

Exchange transfusion procedure

Exchange transfusion should be performed slowly over 45 to 60 minutes and more slowly in preterm infants to avoid

Table 5: Blood type to be used for exchange transfusion

Condition	*Blood type to be used*
Rh incompatibility	• Rh negative O type or baby's blood group suspended in AB positive plasma, cross matched with baby's and mother's blood
ABO allo-immunization	• O type blood group, Rh compatible and suspended in AB positive plasma • Should be cross matched with baby's blood and mother's blood
Other conditions (G6PD deficiency, non-hemolytic, other isoimmune hemolytic jaundice	• Baby's group and Rh type • Cross matched with baby's and mother's blood

major fluctuations in blood pressure. **In and out method** is the commonest method but is being used less often now. Equal amount of baby's blood is taken out and donor blood is infused via umbilical venous catheter. **Continuous flow method** is being increasingly used. Peripheral venous and arterial lines are inserted. Donor blood is infused at a constant rate through vein and baby's blood is constantly removed through artery. It is essential to match the rate of removal to rate of infusion. Complications with this method are less as compared to in out method.

Monitoring during exchange transfusion

- A constant monitoring of volume of blood withdrawn and injected during each cycle should be documented.
- General condition and vitals (heart rate, respiratory rate, blood pressure, oxygen saturation) of the neonate should be monitored every 10 to 15 minutes and should be documented on a predesigned proforma.
- Serum glucose level of the baby should be monitored before procedure, at least once during the procedure and post procedure as indicated.
- In case condition of the baby deteriorates during the procedure, stop the procedure and call for assistance.
- Strict asepsis should be maintained during the procedure.
- Routine antibiotic use during or after procedure is not indicated.
- When using whole blood, settling of RBCs in the blood bag is prevented by frequently turning blood bag upside down.

A checklist would help to prevent errors and optimizing the outcomes of this complex procedure **(Table 6)**.

Table 6: Exchange procedure checklist

Procedure checklist
• Umbilical cannulation done
• Umbilical catheter in-situ
• Proper aseptic precautions taken during cannulation
• Back flow checked
• Need of peripheral artery
• Phototherapy continued during procedure
• Blood bag no. and blood group cross-checked
• Three way connected to umbilical catheter
• Blood bag sufficiently warm
• Transfusion set and IV set properly connected
• Cycle started with pull out
• Same volume pushed in
• Bag missing done intermittently
• Hemodynamics monitored
• Desired number of cycles done
• Blood volume was sufficient for cycles
• IVIG dose administered
• Last aliquot sent for PCV, TSB and calcium
• Procedure notes written

Post-procedure care of the infant

- Vital signs to be monitored regularly post procedure.
- Measure blood glucose level immediately after completion of procedure and later as indicated till blood sugars are stable.
- Post-exchange serum bilirubin should be measured once after one hour of procedure and subsequently as indicated.
- Phototherapy should be continued until serum bilirubin levels are within acceptable zone.
- Catheter sites should be observed frequently for signs of bleeding.
- Post-procedure baby should be kept nil oral for a minimum of four hours.
- Immediately post-procedure, electrolytes should be measured to identify dyselectrolytemia.

Complications: During or following exchange transfusion most commonly seen adverse events include hypo or hyperthermia, hypo or hyperglycemia, hypocalcemia, hyperkalemia, acidemia, arrhythmias, bradycardia, coagulopathy, feed intolerance (necrotizing enterocolitis), septicemia, air emboli, thrombosis, hemorrhage, hemodynamic (hypo or hypertension) and intraventricular hemorrhage (preterm).

Adjuvant Therapies

Intravenous immunoglobulin

High dose IVIg in a single dose or dual dose of 500 mg/kg or 1 g/kg early in the course of jaundice is useful in decreasing the need for exchange transfusion and in preventing significant hyperbilirubinemia in babies with isoimmune hemolytic disease of newborn (HDN). A recent meta-analysis has shown that usefulness of IVIg remains uncertain in cases of Rh isoimmune HDN since studies with low risk of bias indicated no benefit and studies with high risk of bias suggested benefit.[13] Late anemia may be a problem in infants treated with IVIg. Since IVIg is a pooled blood product, there is a risk of transmission of blood born infections. In addition, IVIg can cause immune reactions and can lead to aseptic meningitis.

Intravenous fluids

In some centers it is a routine practice to give intravenous or oral fluid supplementation (50–100 mL/kg) for neonates with severe neonatal jaundice approaching exchange range or associated with dehydration. However, in healthy term newborn babies with unconjugated hyperbilirubinemia, the routine use of IV fluid supplementation has not shown any effect on important clinical outcomes such as ABE, kernicterus, cerebral palsy or hearing impairment.[14] IV fluid supplementation may result in rapid decline of TSB during initial hours of treatment but overall duration of intensive PTx or need for exchange transfusion is not changed.[15]

Metalloporphyrins

Metalloporphyrins (Tin, zinc, chromium) are analogs of heme which inhibit heme oxygenase (HO), the rate limiting enzyme in heme metabolism. By inhibiting HO they can reduce bilirubin production thereby decrease the risk of bilirubin induced neurotoxicity. Although promising, but due to insufficient evidence on their usefulness and unknown long term safety profile, currently metalloporphyrins are not recommended for routine use.[16]

Phenobarbitone

Phenobarbital in a dose of 5 to 8 mg/kg/day acts by inducing microsomal enzymes, increasing conjugation of bilirubin and by increasing excretion of bile. However, it takes 3 to 5 days to induce the liver enzymes. Hence, it is not a useful drug for treatment of acute jaundice but can be effective as a prophylactic agent in very low birth weight infants and chronic cases like hyperbilirubinemia due to Crigler-Najjar syndrome Type II and direct hyperbilirubinemia associated with hyperalimentation.[17] In case of erythroblastic fetus, if given to mother during antenatal period, phenobarbitone can reduce bilirubin levels. If given antenatally to the mother, phenobarbitone is also effective in lowering bilirubin levels in erythroblastic infants. It is neither effective for prevention of severe jaundice in G6PD deficient neonates nor for augmenting the efficacy of phototherapy.[18]

Probiotics

Probiotics role in the management of NNJ is in the new area of research for clinicians. A recent meta-analysis on role of probiotic supplementation in pathological neonatal jaundice has shown that the use of probiotics (Bifidobacterium, *S. boulardii, Bacillus subtilis* for 3 to 7 days) reduced the duration of phototherapy and hospitalization in neonates with jaundice.[19]

Albumin infusion

Infusion of albumin 0.5 to 1g/kg, 1 to 4 hours prior to exchange transfusion may potentially increase the removal of bilirubin by the exchange, by chelating out bilirubin from the tissues. This may decrease the duration of phototherapy and need for subsequent exchange transfusions. However, the current evidence is not strong enough for routine recommendation of albumin infusion.[20]

Other medications that of doubtful utility and currently are not recommended for treatment of jaundice include agars, activated charcoal, cholestyramine polyvinyl pyrrolidine, Clofibrate and D-Penicillamine.

PREVENTION

Prevention of severe jaundice and bilirubin encephalopathy are the continuum of management of neonatal jaundice. The prevention of severe neonatal jaundice would include:

- Rh Isoimmunization
  - Screening of mothers for Rh isoimmunization.
  - Timely use of anti-Rh immune globulin in women with Rh negative pregnancy.
  - Fetal blood transfusion in infants affected with Iso-immune jaundice.

Flowchart 1: Approach for surveillance and early detection of neonatal jaundice

Step 1: Does the baby has serious jaundice*?#

- Yes → Start phototherapy → Measure TSB level and determine if baby requires phototherapy or exchange transfusion
- No → Step 2: Does the infant have significant jaundice to require TSB measurement?#
  - Yes → Measure TSB level and determine if baby requires phototherapy or exchange transfusion
  - No → Continued observation every 12 to 24 hrs for initial 3 to 5 days

Measure TSB level and determine if baby requires phototherapy or exchange transfusion → Determine the cause of jaundice and provide supportive and follow up cares

***Serious jaundice:**
- Presence of visible jaundice in first 24 hours
- Yellow palms and soles anytime
- Signs of acute bilirubin encephalopathy or kernicterus.
- TcB value more than 95th centile as per age specific nomogram

#Measure serum bilirubin if:
- Jaundice in first 24 hours
- Beyond 24 hours: if on visual assessment or by transcutaneous bilirubinometry, TSB is likely to be more than 12 to 14 mg/dL or approaching phototherapy range or beyond
- If you are unsure about visual assessment

- Surveillance and early detection of any jaundice (**Flowchart 1**):
  - Pre-discharge identifying infants at risk of severe jaundice
  - Screening neonates with transcutaneous or total serum bilirubin
  - Evaluation of serum bilirubin level in the context of hour-specific nomograms (**Fig. 2**).

KEY MESSAGES

- Visible jaundice within 24 hr of birth, extending up to palms/soles, or persisting beyond 2 weeks of life signify non-physiologic jaundice and must be investigated and treated urgently.
- To identify appropriate treatment – phototherapy or exchange transfusion, appropriate reference charts (such as the hour specific bilirubin charts) must be used.
- Delay in diagnosis or initiating appropriate treatment, can result in bilirubin encephalopathy with long term risk of disability.
- Severe jaundice and its sequelae can be prevented by screening for infants at risk for severe jaundice prior to discharge and keeping them under surveillance for development of significant jaundice.

REFERENCES

1. Kumar RK. Neonatal jaundice: An update for family physicians. Aust Fam Physician. 1999;28:679-82.
2. Bhutani VK, Zipursky A, Blencowe H, *et al.* Neonatal hyperbilirubinemia and Rhesus disease of the newborn: incidence and impairment estimates for 2010 at regional and global levels. Pediatr Res. 2013;74 Suppl 1:86-100.
3. Maisels MJ, Gifford K. Normal serum bilirubin levels in newborns and effect of breast-feeding. Pediatrics. 1986;78:837-43.
4. Ho NK. Neonatal jaundice in Asia. Baillieres Clin Haematol. 1992;5:131-42.
5. Agarwal SK, Kumar P, Rathi R, *et al.* UGT1A1 gene polymorphins in North Indian neonates presenting with unconjugated hyperbilirubinemia. Pediatr Res. 2009;65:675-80.
6. Madan A, Mac Mohan JR, Stevenson DK. Neonatal hyperbilirubinemia. In: Taeush HW, Ballard RA, Gleason CA, editors. Avery's Diseases of the Newborn, 8th edition. Philadelphia: WB Saunders; 2005. p. 1226-56.
7. Ip S, Chung M, O'Brien R, *et al.* An evidence based review of important issues concerning neonatal hyperbilirubinemia. Pediatrics. 2004;114:e130-53.
8. Bhutani VK, Johnson L, Sivieri EM. Predictive ability of a predischarge hour specific serum bilirubin for subsequent

significant hyperbilirubinemia in healthy term and near term newborns. Pediatrics. 1999;103:6-14.

9. Agarwal R, Kaushal M, Aggarwal R, *et al.* Early neonatal hyperbilirubinemia using first day serum bilirubin level. Indian Pediatr. 2002;39:724-30.
10. Ip S, Chung M, Kulig J, *et al.* An evidence-based review of important issues concerning neonatal hyperbilirubinemia. Pediatrics. 2004;114:e130-e153.
11. Van Imhoff DE, Dijk PH, Weykamp CW, *et al*; BARTrial Study Group. Measurements of neonatal bilirubin and albumin concentrations: A need for improvement and quality control. Eur J Pediatr. 2011;170:977-82.
12. American Academy of Pediatrics Subcommittee on Hyperbilirubinemia. Management of hyperbilirubinemia in the newborn infant 35 or more weeks of gestation. Pediatrics. 2004; 114:297-316.
13. Alcock GS, Liley H. Immunoglobulin infusion for isoimmune haemolytic jaundice in neonates. Cochrane Database Syst Rev. 2002;CD003313.
14. Kamar AA, Choo YM, Kong JY, *et al.* Fluid supplementation for neonatal unconjugated hyperbilirubinaemia. Cochrane Database Syst Rev. 2017;(2):CD011891.
15. Goyal P, Mehta A, Kaur J, *et al.* Fluid supplementation in management of neonatal hyperbilirubinemia: A randomized controlled trial. J Matern Fetal Neonatal Med. 2018;31: 2678-84.
16. Suresh GK, Martin CL, Soll RF. Metalloporphyrins for treatment of unconjugated hyperbilirubinemia in neonates. Cochrane Database Syst Rev. 2003;(2):CD004207.
17. Kumar R, Narang A, Kumar P, *et al.* Phenobarbitone prophylaxis for neonatal jaundice in babies with birth weight 1000-1499 grams. Indian Pediatr. 2002;39:945-51.
18. Murki S, Dutta S, Narang A, *et al.* A randomized, triple-blind, placebo-controlled trial of prophylactic oral phenobarbital to reduce the need for phototherapy in G6PD-deficient neonates. J Perinatol. 2005;25:325-30.
19. Chen Z, Zhang L, Zeng L, *et al.* Probiotics supplementation therapy for pathological neonatal jaundice: A systematic review and meta-analysis. Front Pharmacol. 2017; 8:432.
20. Dash N, Kumar P, Sundaram V, *et al.* Pre exchange albumin administration in neonates with hyperbilirubinemia: A randomized controlled trial. Indian Pediatr. 2015;52: 763-7.

CHAPTER

76

Approach to a Bleeding Neonate

Arun Kumar

INTRODUCTION

Pediatricians throughout the world are faced from time to time with potentially life-threatening bleeding in infants. A systematic approach with appropriate laboratory support should lead to a successful outcome in the majority of infants.

This chapter will provide readers with an overview of this topic from a clinician's viewpoint. The focus would be on the neonate presumed to have abnormal hemostasis. It will not delve into details of site specific bleeding such as intracranial or pulmonary hemorrhage. Thrombosis in the newborn is also beyond its scope. While the broad principles of treatment are discussed, these would ultimately be governed by local policies and resources.

EPIDEMIOLOGY

There is paucity of information on the prevalence of bleeding episodes in neonates. Venkatesh *et al.*[1] reported figures from the first prospective study on prevalence in a multi-centric study in the UK, Australia and USA. Bleeding occurred in 25% of infants and was most common in preterm infants. Major or severe bleeds were seen in 11% infants, 1% had moderate and 13% had minor bleeds. Of the 11 babies within the major bleeding group, two infants developed rectal hemorrhage, two had pulmonary hemorrhages and seven had intracranial hemorrhage. In the severe group of five infants, three had pulmonary hemorrhage and two had sub-aponeurotic bleeds with intracranial hemorrhages. Among infants with minor bleeding episodes, bleeding from the nasogastric tube was the most common source. Intracranial hemorrhage was also a commonly observed form of bleeding and 17% infants developing this in some form.

In developing countries, severe sepsis and hypoxic injury are common, and are often accompanied by bleeding from associated disseminated intravascular coagulation and liver dysfunction. Also, prophylactic vitamin K may not be used consistently and hemorrhagic disease of the newborn remains an important problem. Institutional data from India support these observations.[2,3] The prevalence of conditions associated with thrombocytopenia does not vary significantly across the globe. Coagulation disorders are relatively uncommon but more prevalent in communities with high levels of consanguinity.

PHYSIOLOGY OF NEONATAL COAGULATION

Any discussion on bleeding requires an understanding of the concept of developmental hemostasis in neonates, which reflects the fact that the hemostasis system is incompletely developed at birth and matures throughout infancy until adulthood.

Published literature including a paper by Kenet G[4] indicate that the concentration of vitamin-K dependent coagulation factors (II, VII, IX, X) and contact factors (XI, XII, pre-kallikrein and high molecular weight kininogen) is low in neonates and gradually increases with age and gestation. The activated partial thromboplastin time (APTT) is prolonged in neonates due to decreased plasma concentrations of the contact factors. Prothrombin time (PT) is also prolonged reflecting decreased plasma levels of vitamin-K dependent factors. The level of factors V, VIII and XIII are normal. Plasma concentrations of fibrinogen may be raised but thrombin C time (TCT) is prolonged, due to the presence of "fetal" fibrinogen, which has different properties to normal fibrinogen. Platelet counts are similar to adult ranges. Bleeding time is shorter in healthy neonates probably because of high hematocrit and increased concentrations and enhanced function of Von-Willebrand factor (vWF) and higher levels of vWF large multimers. The capacity of newborns to generate thrombin, dependent upon plasma concentrations of pro-coagulants, is reduced. Thus, the theoretically increased risk of bleeding from decreased coagulation factors is balanced by the protective effects of physiologic deficiencies of the inhibitors of coagulation, as well as by the decreased capacity of the fibrinolytic system in infants. This implies that an abnormal result on tests of coagulation may not necessarily require treatment and needs interpretation in the clinical context.

ETIOLOGY

Most bleeding in neonates is secondary to other disease processes. In a minority, the problem arises from congenital defects in hemostasis. A broad classification of causes is given in **Table 1**.

Table 1: Causes of bleeding in neonates

Cause	*Examples*
Thrombocytopenia, or disorders of platelet function	Alloimmune and isoimmune thrombocytopenia, sepsis, congenital infection, perinatal asphyxia, Glanzmann's thrombasthenia
Vitamin K deficiency	Breastfed infants not receiving prophylactic vitamin K, maternal medication
Disseminated intravascular coagulation	Sepsis, perinatal asphyxia, hypotension, acidosis, hypothermia, single twin demise
Liver cell failure	Herpes simplex infection, septicemia, primary liver disease, metabolic errors
Coagulopathies	Hemophilia A and B, von Willebrand disease Type 3 and some Type 2, congenital deficiencies of fibrinogen, prothrombin, Factor V, VII, XI, XIII
Iatrogenic	Total body hypothermia, ECMO, bleeding from arterial and central lines
Perinatal	Vasa previa, feto-maternal hemorrhage, cord avulsion
Congenital anomalies	Vascular malformations

A brief discussion of some of the important causes follows.

Hemorrhagic Disease of the Newborn (Vitamin K Deficiency Bleeding - VKDB)

This is a bleeding disorder resulting from a deficiency of vitamin K dependent coagulation factors II, VII, IX and X. vitamin K is essential for γ-carboxylation of these proteins, which converts them to their active form. Newborn babies are relatively vitamin K deficient for a variety of reasons including low vitamin K stores at birth, poor placental transfer of vitamin K, low levels of vitamin K in breast milk, and sterility of the gut. The daily requirement of vitamin K is 1 µg/kg/day. VKDB is exceedingly rare in formula-fed infants for whom intakes are typically 50 µg/day compared to 1 µg/day in breast-fed infants. Typical clinical manifestations include bruising, cephalohematomas, gastrointestinal and umbilical hemorrhage, as well as oozing from mucous membranes, circumcisions and venipuncture sites. Intracranial bleeding remains the main cause of mortality and long-term morbidity.

Three forms are recognized:

1. Early onset, at less than 24 hours after birth, is caused by vitamin K deficiency in utero, and is usually as a result of maternal medications that interfere with vitamin K, such as anticonvulsants (phenobarbitone, phenytoin), anti-tuberculous therapy and oral anticoagulants. This risk can be minimized by giving such mothers vitamin K during the last four weeks of pregnancy.
2. The classic onset, 2–6 days after birth, occurs almost exclusively in breastfed infants who have not received vitamin K supplementation.
3. Late onset, which occurs between 8 days and 6 months of life. In addition to breastfeeding, risk factors include diarrhea, hepatitis, cystic fibrosis, celiac disease, and alpha-1-antitrypsin deficiency. Late onset VKDB tends to be more severe than early or classic onset and has a high incidence of intracranial hemorrhage.

A coagulation screen will typically show prolongation of the prothrombin time (PT). Factor VIII, Factor V, platelet count and fibrinogen levels are within normal limits.

Treatment is with 1 mg of vitamin K given intravenously given 8 hourly if required.[5] Decreased hemorrhage and return of vitamin K dependent factor levels to normal usually occurs within 2–3 hours. If significant hemorrhage has occurred, an infusion of 10-15 mL/kg of fresh frozen plasma is also indicated to rapidly correct the coagulation defects.

Prophylaxis is the key to prevention of this disorder. The recommended policy is to offer intramuscular vitamin K to all infants at birth. The dose is 1 mg for term infants and 400 μg/kg (maximum 1 mg) in preterm infants. Where parents decline intramuscular vitamin K, oral vitamin K can be offered. Two doses of 2 mg each are required, given at birth and one week with a further dose at one month of age for breastfed infants.[5] Konakion MM Paediatric® which is solubilized using natural components can be given IM, IV with dilution or orally.[5]

Thrombocytopenia

The normal platelet count in neonates is the same as in adults - 150 to 400 × 10^9/L. Infants with significant thrombocytopenia will develop petechiae but in addition could bleed from any site including into the cranium. In term infants, thrombocytopenia is extremely uncommon and the most common clinically important cause in term infants is alloimmune thrombocytopenia. In preterm neonates, early-onset thrombocytopenia (<72 h) is usually secondary to antenatal causes, has a characteristic pattern and resolves without complications or the need for treatment. By contrast, late-onset thrombocytopenia in preterm neonates (>72 h) is nearly always due to post-natally acquired bacterial infection and/or necrotizing enterocolitis, which rapidly leads to severe thrombocytopenia.[6] Other causes such as those associated with congenital malformations and genetic conditions are relatively rare, as are thrombasthenias. 15–20% of neonatal thrombocytopenias occur secondary to transplacental passage of maternal platelet allo- and autoantibodies.

Treatment of thrombocytopenias is dependent on the underlying mechanism and conditions. There are no evidence-based guidelines for platelet transfusion but consensus-based guidelines exist.[7] These recommend transfusions when counts fall below 20–30 × 10^9/L in the absence of bleeding, below 50 × 10^9/L in case of bleeding, current coagulopathy, planned surgery or exchange transfusion, and below 100 × 10^9/L for major bleeding and major surgery.

Alloimmune Thrombocytopenia

In this condition, fetal and neonatal thrombocytopenia results from transplacental passage of maternal platelet specific antibodies. Severe thrombocytopenia occurs in the fetus or in the early neonatal period with a 10% risk of intracranial hemorrhage. In Caucasian populations, 80% result from antibodies to HPA -1a and most of the rest to HPA -5b platelet antigens.

Therapy during pregnancy comprises close monitoring, fetal platelet transfusions, maternal intravenous immunoglobulin and corticosteroid administration.

Following delivery, if the platelet count is less than 30 × 10^9/L, or if there is evidence of bleeding, the infant will need transfusing with HPA compatible platelets (usually HPA -1a and HPA 5b negative ABO and RhD compatible) until the platelet counts stabilize. If this is not available, washed maternal platelets can be considered. HPA incompatible platelets or intravenous immunoglobulin can be used if HPA compatible platelets are not available. The aim is to keep platelet counts above 30 × 10^9/L for the first 72–96 hours without active bleeding and above 50 × 10^9/L if there is evidence of active bleeding.[6]

Neonatal Autoimmune Thrombocytopenia

Maternal autoantibodies in women with idiopathic thrombocytopenic purpura and SLE can similarly cross thrombocytopenia but it is quite infrequent, occurring in only 10% of cases. Major morbidity is rare. Platelet transfusions of any antigen type are usually ineffective. In those with thrombocytopenia, a platelet count should be repeated after 2–3 days as platelet counts are often at their lowest at this time before rising spontaneously by day 7 in most cases. If platelet count is below 30 × 10^9/L in the first week of life and <20 × 10^9/L thereafter, treatment with IVIG 400 mg/kg per day given over 2–4 hours for 5 days or 1 g/kg per day for 2 days may be useful.[6]

Disseminated Intravascular Coagulation (DIC)

This is commonly encountered with severe sepsis, hypoxia, hypotension, acidosis or hypothermia. There is activation of the coagulation cascade with consumption of platelets and coagulation factors, and secondary activation of fibrinolysis. The clinical presentation typically is bleeding from multiple sites including heel pricks and sites of insertion of intravenous lines. Laboratory tests will reveal a low platelet count, prolonged prothrombin and partial thromboplastin times, and decreased fibrinogen levels, with schizocytes in a peripheral blood smear. D-dimers are elevated but not diagnostic as these can be elevated in healthy neonates, particularly preterms, with no evidence of coagulopathy.

Treatment comprises elimination of the trigger factor, with replacement of factors using cryoprecipitate or fresh frozen plasma and platelet concentrate as required. Packed cells may be indicated if the infant is anemic. One recommended approach is to maintain the platelet count > 50 × 10^9/L (100 × 10^9/L if ventilated, with recent surgical sites or actively bleeding), PT ≤ 3 seconds above the upper limit of normal and the fibrinogen > 100 mg/dL.[8] Although inhibiting the activation of the coagulation system with prophylactic dosing of heparin (5–10 U/kg/hour) has been considered, trials of anticoagulation in neonates have not been conclusive and the risk of bleeding may be increased.[8] There is little experience with using antithrombin III in neonates. Management of DIC is complex and blood products need to be used judiciously in consultation with hematologists. A review of DIC in the pediatric population has been published recently.[9]

Liver Cell Failure

This is seen in neonates secondary to infection, including bacterial sepsis, neonatal herpes simplex infection, other viral infections, primary liver disease or hypoxic injury, or inborn errors of metabolism. Neonatal herpes simplex (HSV) infection is an emerging important cause and this diagnosis should always be considered in any unwell infant presenting with a prolonged prothrombin time, jaundice and raised liver enzymes who may also be encephalopathic. Treatment consists of addressing the cause and correction of the coagulopathy, if there is bleeding, with vitamin K, fresh frozen plasma or cryoprecipitate. If a diagnosis of HSV is considered, intravenous acicyovir 20 mg/kg/dose 8 hourly should be commenced immediately pending the results of HSV PCR on blood and CSF samples.

Coagulation Disorders

These are relatively uncommon but can cause significant hemorrhage. Hemophilia A and B are the most frequently encountered conditions. Other disorders such as afibrinogenemia and deficiencies of other factors are rare but need to be considered in the differential diagnosis. von Willebrand disease(vWD) presents unusually in the neonatal period because of their higher vWF factor levels. Only Type 3 or some infants with Type 2 vWD present with bleeding in neonates, due to their higher severity.[10,11]

Hemophilia

Hemophilia A and B are X-linked disorders characterized by deficiency of coagulation factors VIII and IX respectively. Hemophilia A occurs in 1 in 5,000 live male births, and is about six times as common as Hemophilia B. As awareness has increased and prenatal diagnosis has become available, diagnosis during the neonatal period has increased significantly.

Kenet G *et al.*[12] have reported figures from the US Hemophilia Centre Network via the Universal Data Collection (UDC) surveillance project. Of the 864 male infants aged 0–2 years with hemophilia, 633 (73%) were diagnosed within one month of birth; reasons for diagnosis were carrier mother (47.2%), family history (23.2%) and bleeding events (28.8%). The sites of neonatal bleeding included circumcision site (15.49%), intracranial bleeding (17.69%), heel pricks (14.8%) and venipuncture sites (3.61%). The condition should always be suspected if major sub-galeal bleeding is encountered.

Where a family history is available, strategies available for management in pregnancy include pre-implantation diagnosis, and offering fetal sexing to couples who wish to consider this option, either by chorionic villus sampling or ultrasound. There is also the option for third trimester amniocentesis, as this may allow the diagnosis of an unaffected pregnancy.[13] There is controversy regarding the merits of normal delivery versus an elective cesarean section. UK guidelines recommend that this should be informed by both obstetric and hemostatic factors, including maternal morbidity with cesarean section for hemophilia B carriers.[13] Data from the UDC cohort suggests that when infants were grouped by presence or absence of family history, intracranial hemorrhage occurred more in vaginal births than cesarean births.[12] Invasive monitoring with scalp electrodes and fetal scalp blood sampling should be avoided as should application of obstetric forceps and Ventouse extraction. On delivery, a sample of cord blood collected carefully without contamination from maternal blood, or a peripheral venous blood sample should be processed as soon as possible for coagulation screen and coagulation factor assay.

The diagnosis of severe and moderate hemophilia can also be confirmed in the neonatal period. However, confirmation of mildly affected cases could be problematic due to overlap with the normal range necessitating repeat testing at around 6 months of age.

These infants should not have any arterial stabs, and heel pricks should be kept at a minimum. Intramuscular injections should be avoided and Vitamin K can be given orally. Circumcision if requested should be performed only with adequate preparation. Details of management appear later in this chapter.

Those with suspected intracranial bleeding on ultrasound scan will usually need an MRI scan to establish the diagnosis.

Following confirmation of diagnosis, short-term prophylactic replacement therapy should be given in neonates at increased risk of bleeding, e.g. following traumatic delivery, instrumental delivery, or a prolonged second stage of labor,[13] and considered following preterm delivery.[14] Children and neonates with severe hemophilia who have had a spontaneous central nervous system bleed should continue long-term prophylaxis.

Other coagulation disorders

Congenital deficiencies of fibrinogen, prothrombin, Factor V, VII , XI and XIII are very rare but can be encountered in communities with high prevalence of consanguinity. These can present with cord bleeding (especially fibrinogen and Factor XIII deficiency) or intracranial hemorrhage. Treatment is with the appropriate concentrate where available including fibrinogen, recombinant Factor VIIa, and Factor XIII. Cryoprecipitate or FFP are alternatives. For Factor II and X deficiencies, there are no specific concentrates available and prothrombin complex concentrates are the treatment of choice. Factor V deficiency can be isolated or co-exist with Factor VIII deficiency. Treatment is with FFP and Factor VIII concentrates if applicable. Alternatives to these products are cryoprecipitate or FFP. Alpha 2 antiplasmin deficiency is treated with Tranexamic acid or EACA but there is no neonatal data available for its use. Further information is available in References 8,15 and 16. As with hemophilia, expert guidance should always be sought from the local hematology team.

Iatrogenic

Disastrous bleeding can occur in neonates from dislodged arterial and umbilical lines. Therapeutic hypothermia potentially can affect coagulation and platelet function in infants who are already at high risk for these disturbances from the hypoxic etiology of their encephalopathy. Close attention should be paid to platelet count, coagulation measures (PT, aPTT, fibrinogen), and clinical signs of bleeding when neonates undergo hypothermic cooling protocols. If derangements in the coagulation measures are found and bleeding is present, they should be replaced with FFP or cryoprecipitate as indicated.[11]

Recombinant tissue plasminogen activator used for thrombolysis in neonates has an associated risk of mild to severe bleeding. There is a significant risk of hemorrhagic complications after ECMO and cardiopulmonary bypass in neonates undergoing corrective heart surgery. These are secondary to anticoagulation, activation of the coagulation and fibrinolytic systems with consumption of coagulation factors, together with dilutional thrombocytopenia. Management includes careful monitoring of heparinization, replacement therapy with hemostatic factors and platelets, and use of drugs such epsilon-aminocaproic acid and recombinant Factor VIIa.[17] A detailed discussion on this complex subject is beyond the scope of this chapter.

Hemorrhage in the Perinatal Period

Massive fetal bleeding may result following placenta previa, placental abruption or incision of the placenta at cesarean section. Accidental hemorrhage can occur following slippage of a cord clamp. Rupture of the umbilical cord and hematomas into the cord can occasionally lead to severe neonatal anemia with a high perinatal mortality rate. Feto-maternal hemorrhage can occur spontaneously and may be increased by invasive procedures such as fetal blood sampling and cesarean section. Another potential problem is vasa previa. This can be associated with catastrophic fetal bleeding at the time of delivery.

Infants with massive perinatal bleeding can be in shock at the time of delivery and require extensive resuscitation including transfusion of packed cells. Most maternity units stock O negative packed cell units in the labor ward, which can be used without cross-matching in such emergencies. Unlike in adults, neonatologists are accustomed to waiting for results of coagulation screening before transfusing fresh frozen plasma, a practice that is being called into question.[18] Please also refer to the section on Major Hemorrhage Protocols later in this chapter.

There is evidence that with successful identification of vasa previa antenatally with planned cesarean section, outcome for the infants can be excellent.[19]

CLINICAL FEATURES

In the history, particular attention must be paid to birth details, risk factors for sepsis, use of instruments to augment labor, maternal drugs or illnesses during pregnancy, history of genital herpes, family history of coagulation disorders, and any previously affected siblings. A history of consanguinity would increase the risk of autosomal recessive conditions. Where there is prior information available indicating the possibility of a bleeding disorder in the neonate, meticulous planning of the care in labor and postnatal periods is essential.

In addition to bleeding, the affected neonate may have other features indicating the etiology including the following:

- *Petechiae* are suggestive of low platelets
- *Ecchymosis*, may indicate a coagulopathy
- *Bleeding from umbilicus, circumcision site, large sub-galeal bleeding*, could all indicate a possible coagulopathy
- *Oral mucous membrane bleeding, or an ooze* rather than active bleeding from any site, is suggestive of thrombocytopenia
- *Intracranial hemorrhage* is usually associated with prematurity, traumatic delivery, arteriovenous malformations, and secondary to coagulopathies or thrombocytopenia
- *Jaundice* indicates a possible underlying liver dysfunction
- Signs of sepsis, including poor capillary refill and sclerema, full anterior fontanelle
- Blistering lesions over presenting part, site of insertion of scalp electrodes or elsewhere, and seizures are seen in herpes simplex infection
- Hepatosplenomegaly is seen in congenital infections
- A relatively well infant with bleeding could have immune thrombocytopenia, vitamin K deficiency, an inherited coagulation factor deficiency, or bleeding from anatomic lesions such as a hemangioma. A sick infant with bleeding may have disseminated intravascular coagulation (DIC), sepsis or liver failure.

DIFFERENTIAL DIAGNOSIS

Some entities can masquerade as neonatal bleeding. Pinkish-orange urate crystals deposited from urine into the nappies of normal babies could be misinterpreted as bleeding. Sometimes, the newborn will swallow large quantities of maternal blood especially in the setting of antepartum hemorrhage and then either vomit dark brown maternal blood or pass large quantities of tarry stools. These infants would be clinically very well and laboratory tests would all come back as normal. An Apt test could help differentiate fetal from maternal blood but it is not reliable and persistent bleeding would merit investigation.

INVESTIGATIONS

If there is clinically significant bleeding, the following tests will need to be performed as soon as possible:

- Full blood count, including hemoglobin/hematocrit (for diagnosis of anemia). If laboratory samples cannot be processed swiftly, a laboratory centrifuge if available would help with quick estimation of packed cell volume. Modern blood gas analyzers can measure hemoglobin and provide an initial guide while awaiting laboratory results.
- Peripheral blood smear.
- *Coagulation screening*: Prothrombin time, partial thromboplastin time, fibrinogen, thrombin clotting time. Measurement of individual coagulation factors is usually dependent on outcome of this initial screening. Ideally, the sample for coagulation should be taken from a free flowing vein and it is important to ensure that the right volume of blood is collected to maintain the correct ratio with the anticoagulant in the sample bottle. Sometimes, the sample may be taken from an arterial line particularly in the NICU setting. This is acceptable as long as sufficient blood has been drawn into a syringe beforehand to minimize heparin contamination, and the laboratory is informed about this, as they may be able to perform a Reptilase Time to help interpretation in the event of heparin contamination. Sampling from heel pricks is best avoided for clotting studies.
- Blood for group and cross matching.
- *Investigations relevant to suspected etiology*: Blood culture, herpes simplex PCR.
- If a lumbar puncture is contemplated due to concerns with sepsis, this should NOT be performed until a coagulopathy has been excluded or corrected, and platelet count is above 100×10^9/L.
- A bedside ultrasound scan of the head helps to check for intracranial hemorrhage. This test is not reliable and if there is strong clinical suspicion, further neuroimaging will be required.

Interpretation of Coagulation Tests

The normal values for full blood count and coagulation screen are different in newborn babies and also vary with age and gestation. **Table 2** gives accepted values for these parameters from widely quoted sources in the literature for term infants and those between 30-36 weeks gestation.[20,21] **Table 3** is a general guide to interpreting the results.

Published normal reference ranges for infants at lower gestations have been sparse but most neonatologists are aware that these are wider for these infants.

Christensen *et al.*[22] published values for coagulation tests from cord samples of 175 infants including those less than 28 weeks gestation, and between 28 and 34 weeks. For those below 28 weeks, the 5-95th percentile for PT was 14.9-20.9 secs, APTT 27-64 secs; and for gestation between 28 and 34 weeks, the range for PT was 13.9-20.4 secs, APTT 30-57 secs. Based on their data and that from previous studies, they have recommended a cutoff of >21 and 64 secs for PT and APTT respectively for gestations below 28 weeks, and 21 and 57 secs for those between 28 and 34 weeks. They mention the need to substantiate their data through screening of large numbers of infants.

Neary *et al.*[23] published values from 116 infants in Ireland for coagulation parameters between 23.7 and 29.9 weeks gestation. Median (5th-95th percentile) day 1 PT, APTT and fibrinogen were 17.5 (12.7-26.6) s, 78.7 (48.7-134.3) s and 1.4 (0.72-3.8) g/L, respectively. Preterm PT and APTT were prolonged compared with results obtained using cord blood from term infants ($n = 15$, $p < 0.001$); however, no difference in plasma fibrinogen between the two groups was observed. Serial analysis in infants who did not receive plasma revealed reduction of median (10th-90th percentile) PT

Table 2: Normal values for hemostasis screening tests in the newborn*

	30–36 weeks gestation	*30–36 weeks gestation*	*Term infant*	*Term infant*
TEST	*Day 1*	*Day 30*	*Day 1*	*Day 30*
Prothrombin time (sec)	Mean: 13.0 Range: 10.6–16.2	Mean: 11.8 Range: 10.0–13.6	13.0 ± 1.43	11.8 ± 1.25
Activated partial thromboplastin time (sec)	Mean: 53.6 Range: 27.5–79.4	Mean: 44.7 Range: 26.9–62.5	42.9 ± 5.8	40.4 ± 7.42
Thrombin clotting time (sec)	Mean: 24.8 Range: 19.2–30.4	Mean: 24.4 Range: 18.8–29.9	23.5 ± 2.38	24.3 ± 2.44
Fibrinogen (g/L)	Mean: 2.43 Range: 1.50–3.73	Mean: 2.54 Range: 1.50–4.14	2.83 ± 0.58	2.70 ± 0.54
Platelet count (x 10^9/L)	Range: 150–400	Range: 150–400	Range: 150–400	Range: 150–400

*Data from Andrew M *et al.*[20,21] All infants received vitamin K at birth

Table 3: Results of hemostasis screening tests in bleeding disorders

PT	*aPTT*	*TT*	*Fibrinogen*	*Platelets*	*Diagnosis*
↑	↑	↑	↓	↓	Disseminated intravascular coagulation
↑	N/↑	N	N	N	Vitamin K deficiency bleeding
N	↑	N	N	N	Hemophilia A, B, C
↑	N	N	N	N	Factor VII deficiency
N	N	N	N	↓	Thrombocytopenia
↑	↑	N	N	N	Factor V, X deficiency
↑	↑	↑	N/↓	N/↓	Liver disease
N	N	N	N	N	Factor XIII deficiency* Qualitative platelet disorder, alpha 2 antiplasmin deficiency
↑	↑	↑	Absent	N	Afibrinogenemia
N/↑	↑	↑	N	N	Heparin contamination**

*Diagnosis requires clot solubility test. **Reptilase Time is prolonged in DIC but not with heparin contamination
(PT: prothrombin time; aPTT: activated partial thromboplastin time; TT: thrombin time; FDP: fibrinogen degradation products; N: normal)

from 17.1 (13.2–20.5) s on day 1 (n = 84) to 13.7 (11.6–16.2) s on day 3 (n = 46) and 12 (11.2–16.2) s in week 2 of life (n = 23), and reduction of median (10th–90th percentile) APTT from 74.7 (53.8–97.9) s on day 1 (n = 85) to 49.3 (35.3–68.3) s on day 3 (n = 46) and 47.4 (31.9–68) s in week 2 (n = 23).

Mixing studies such as 50:50 test with normal plasma is helpful to differentiate abnormal clotting from situations such as presence of a coagulation factor inhibitor or a phospholipid antibody such as lupus anticoagulant, where such mixing will not significantly correct the abnormal coagulation result.

If no abnormality is found in these tests and the infant is bleeding, rarer causes may need to be considered such as FXIII deficiency, α2-antiplasmin deficiency or a platelet function disorder. Be wary of over-interpreting borderline abnormal results and always discuss with an expert hematologist first.

MANAGEMENT

There is evidence and increasing consensus that in well preterm infants, abnormal clotting values are not predictive of IVH, pulmonary hemorrhage or GI bleeding in the first week of life,[24] and that routinely checking clotting values increases the use of FFP and clotting products with no evidence of benefit.[25,26]

Sometimes, bleeding is mild and the laboratory parameters are stable. A typical example is small amounts of hemorrhagic gastric aspirates from the nasogastric tube after perinatal stress, which can be managed expectantly or with a short course of H2 receptor antagonists.

If bleeding is significant, time is of the essence for clinical intervention and is essential to maintain active liaison with the laboratory and hematology services.

While a member of the team collects information from the parents to help establish the diagnosis, other members should concentrate on examining the infant, to ensure that there is no life-threatening situation that requires immediate assistance. In the context of bleeding, checking for hemodynamic stability is of paramount importance.

Rapid intravenous access must be obtained, using an umbilical venous catheter if peripheral cannulation proves difficult. If the infant is actively bleeding and in shock, an intra-osseous needle could be used to obtain vascular access. After the relevant blood samples are collected, an initial bolus of 0.9 % saline 10 mL/kg body weight may be needed if there are concerns about a slow capillary refill time. If the infant is pale and shocked at birth and born in a setting of possible severe bleeding, such as placenta previa, immediate transfusion of O negative blood, 10-20 mL/kg as a slow intravenous push may be given without cross matching from emergency "flying squad" blood units kept in many delivery suites for obstetric hemorrhage. You would need to follow local blood banking policies in this regard.

In a less urgent situation, start treatment for possible associated illnesses such as sepsis while awaiting results of blood tests and administer further treatment based on the results.

Initiate supportive treatment as indicated by the infant's condition.

Once results of initial tests become available, appropriate therapy for the bleeding diathesis can be given. These could include:

1. *Vitamin K_1*, 1 mg intravenously for vitamin K deficiency. Intramuscular injections should be avoided in any bleeding diathesis.
2. *Packed cell transfusion*, 10–20 mL/kg body weight given at the rate of 5 mL/kg/hour for significant hemorrhage. If profuse, proportionately larger volumes may be required more quickly.
   Red cells for IUT or neonatal transfusion must be ABO and D compatible with both maternal and neonatal groups, and must be IAT crossmatch-compatible with clinically significant red cell antibodies present in maternal or neonatal plasma. In general, group O D-negative red cells are used for most neonatal top-up and exchange transfusions. If hospitals use group-specific red cells, most commonly for elective large volume transfusions, they must be ABO and D compatible with both maternal and neonatal groups.[27] In addition to routine screening for Hepatitis B, syphilis and HIV, blood for neonatal transfusions should be obtained from cytomegalovirus negative donors and should also be leucodepleted. Blood from related donors especially parents should be avoided as it could pose potential immunological risks and a greater likelihood of graft versus host disease.[28] Irradiated blood is indicated when the infants have received intrauterine transfusions or are known to be immunocompromised.
3. *Fresh frozen plasma* obtained from screened donors, is used where rapid correction of coagulation defects is desired as in bleeding associated with vitamin K deficiency, DIC and in coagulation deficiencies where factor concentrate is not available. One infusion of 12-15 mL/kg infused at the rate of 10-20 mL/kg/hour with careful monitoring for acute transfusion reactions or circulatory overload.[7]

4. *Platelet concentrates* are indicated in clinically significant thrombocytopenia which is discussed in a separate section. A platelet concentrate obtained from one donor is suspended in 50–75 mL of plasma. The dose is 10–20 mL/kg, which would be expected to increase the platelet count by 100×10^9/L. In sick neonates, however, such increases in platelet numbers are seldom seen due to rapid consumption or sequestration. It should be given as soon as possible usually at a rate of 10-20 mL/kg/hour.[7]
5. *Factor VIII or IX concentrates* are indicated in hemophilia. Acute management of the bleeding infant requires recombinant Factor VIII or IX as applicable to be administered as soon as possible. There is little information on the pharmacokinetics of replacement therapy in neonates and treatment is based on guidelines for older children. For Hemophilia A, the usual dose for recombinant Factor VIII for severe bleeding is 40–50 units per kg body weight rounded to the nearest vial size given every 8 hours.[29] For Hemophila B, the dose of recombinant Factor IX is 80-100 IU/kg (round total to nearest vial size), and repeated at least every 24 hrs until bleeding has resolved.[29] Guidelines published by the World Federation of Hemophilia[30] constitute another excellent resource and also includes advice on duration of therapy where there are resource constraints.
   If recombinant factor concentrate is not available, highly purified virally inactivated plasma derived Factor VIII or IX products can be administered. Cryoprecipitate should only be used if factor concentrates are not available. If the diagnosis is not known, fresh frozen plasma, 15–25 mL/kg can be administered.[13] The administration of desmopressin (DDAVP) may result in dilutional hyponatremia with consequent seizures, and should not be used for the treatment of neonates with mild hemophilia A.[13]
6. *Cryoprecipitate*: Cryoprecipitate is used as a more concentrated source of fibrinogen than FFP and is primarily indicated when the fibrinogen level is <0.8–1.0 g/L in the presence of bleeding from acquired or congenital hypofibrinogenemia. The dose is 5–10 mL/kg of body weight.[7]
7. *Exchange transfusion* can be performed in disseminated intravascular coagulation especially if associated with sepsis.
8. *Recombinant activated Factor VII* is a novel therapeutic alternative for bleeding associated with coagulation factor deficiencies.[8] Use in neonates is based solely on case reports, case series, and prospective uncontrolled studies. In most cases, treatment was effective in controlling hemorrhage. Doses of 40 to 300 μg/kg were used, but further investigation of neonatal rFVIIa pharmacokinetics is required to determine an optimal dose. The safety of rFVIIa in neonates remains a concern as thrombotic complications have been observed. In the majority of these reports, rFVIIa was used as a desperate final measure, after standard measures had failed to control life-threatening hemorrhage.

The laboratory tests may need to be repeated 8–12 hourly until stable. If bleeding is severe in areas such as the gut, or in the brain, urgent consultation with a pediatric surgeon or neurosurgeon would be needed to plan management. Bleeding in the setting of severe liver failure may need the input of a pediatric hepatology team.

Bleeding from the lung (pulmonary hemorrhage) requires intubation and ventilation, or manipulation of ventilator settings to control pulmonary edema in addition to treatment of coagulopathy. A dose of surfactant may help to improve pulmonary function.

The use of all blood products requires to be balanced with potential risks. If large amounts of blood are transfused, this by itself can carry the risk of further hemostatic and metabolic complications which require to be anticipated and managed.[31]

Major Hemorrhage Protocols

Major hemorrhage protocols, which automatically alert blood banks to trigger the release of pre-determined packs of packed cells, fresh frozen plasma and platelets, are used in adult practice particularly in the context of catastrophic hemorrhage as in trauma. Apart from the coagulopathy associated in trauma from tissue injury and hypoperfusion, massive transfusion itself carries the risk of coagulopathy from dilutional effects, hypothermia, acidosis and hypocalcemia, hence transfusion of balanced proportions of packed cells, fresh frozen plasma and platelets in a 1:1:1 ratio is now common practice. Some institutions have developed pediatric protocols based on extrapolation from adult data. The definition of major hemorrhage has to be related to circulating blood volume in children, with one suggested definition being a situation where 1–1.5 blood volumes may need to be infused either acutely or within a 24-hour period.[32] Consideration for such an approach may be required in some neonatal situations such as feto-maternal hemorrhage, vascular malformations, twin-to-twin transfusion,sub-galeal bleeding secondary to Ventouse

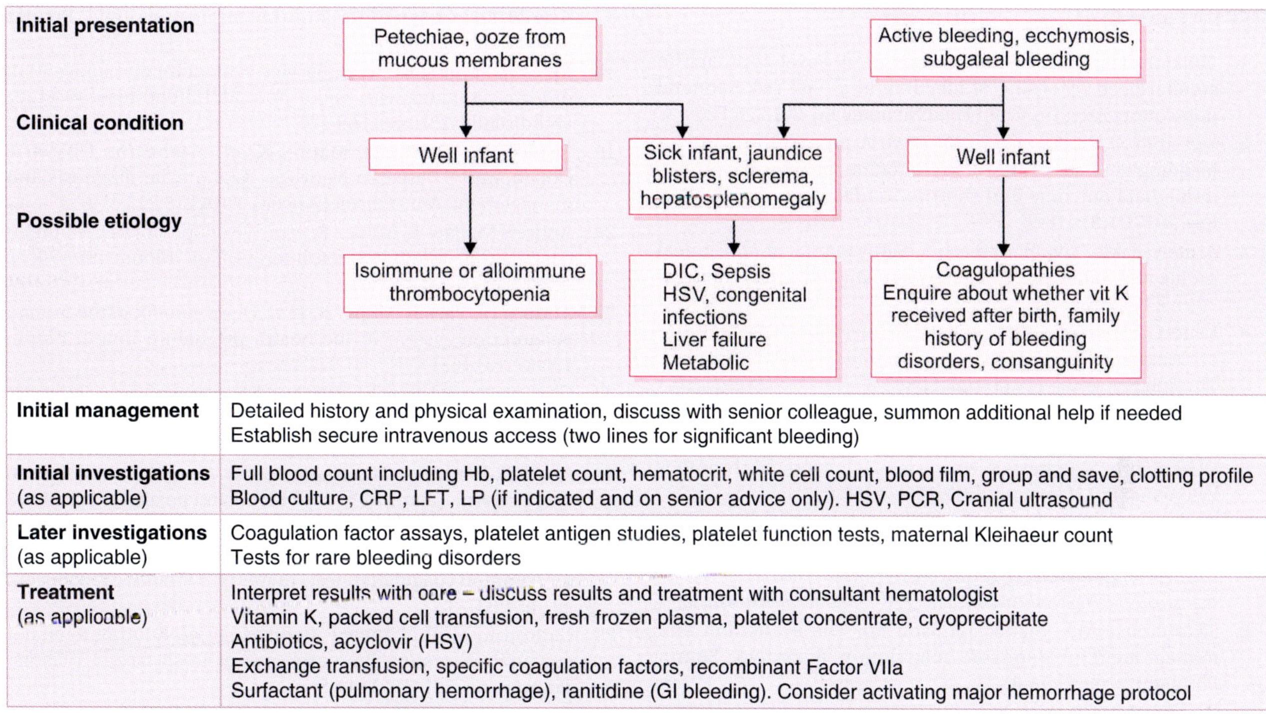

Fig. 1: General principles for managing a bleeding neonate

delivery, bleeding from dislodged arterial catheter, etc.[31] Cryoprecipitate may also be required, and recombinant Factor VIIa has been used in some situations. The reader can refer to the relevant references for more information.[31-34]

Figure 1 provides a structured plan for managing the bleeding infant. Please always maintain a broad approach and consider all possibilities. Thrombocytopenia and coagulopathy, for example, are not exclusive and often co-exist in sepsis, DIC, etc.

OUTCOME AND COMPLICATIONS

Most episodes of bleeding can be managed effectively. Intracranial hemorrhage carries a guarded prognosis with risk of long-term neurological handicap. Neonatal herpes simplex infection with liver failure also carries a poor prognosis. Those with congenital coagulopathies require a lifetime of follow-up and treatment.

PREVENTION

Universal administration of vitamin K in newborn infants would be a cost effective strategy for prevention of severe bleeding. Wherever possible, careful planning prior to delivery of high risk infants would invariably improve the outcome.

Genetic counseling should be arranged for couples of infants affected with inheritable coagulation disorders. Pre-implantation genetic diagnosis is available for hemophilia and prenatal diagnosis is possible for several congenital coagulopathies allowing parents the option for termination or proceeding towards early intervention and therapy.

KEY MESSAGES

- Neonatal bleeding is usually secondary to other medical conditions, but could be due to a primary problem with hemostasis.
- Laboratory ranges for neonatal coagulation parameters differ from other age groups.
- Liaison with hematology is vital to ensure correct interpretation of test results, and appropriate management, especially the use of blood products.
- Wherever possible, an antenatal plan for management of the high-risk infant would ensure smooth delivery of care.
- The evolution of major hemorrhage protocols may improve care when dealing with catastrophic bleeding.

REFERENCES

1. Venkatesh V, Curley A, Khan R, *et al.* A novel approach to standardised recording of bleeding in a high risk neonatal population. Arch Dis Child Fetal Neonatal Ed. 2013;98:F260-3.
2. Swarnim S, Rai BK, Divya M, *et al.* A prospective study of bleeding neonates: Clinical presentation, aetiological profile, immediate outcome and short term follow up. Curr Pediatr Res. 2017;21(3):416-9.
3. Arutsivasakthi siva S, Ramesh S, Saravanan S, *et al.* Clinical profile and follow up of bleeding neonate. Int J Curr Med Sci. 2015;5(10):51-5.
4. Kenet G. Bleeding in the neonate. 2nd International Symposium on Women's Health Issues in Thrombosis and Hemostasis. Thromb Res. 2007; 119 (Suppl. 1):S82-4.
5. Available from: *https://bnfc.nice.org.uk/drug/phytomenadione.html*
6. Chakravorty S, Roberts I. How I manage neonatal thrombocytopenia. Br J Haematol. 2012;156(2):155-62.
7. Norfolk N. Handbook of Transfusion Medicine United Kingdom Blood Services, 5th edition,2013. Wed edition. *https://www.transfusionguidelines.org/transfusion-handbook/10-effective-transfusion-in- paediatric-practice/10-2-neonatal-transfusion*
8. Saxonhouse MA, Manco-Johnson MJ. The evaluation and management of neonatal coagulation disorders. Semin Perinatol. 2009;33:52-65.
9. Rajagopal R, Thachil J, Monagle P. Disseminated intravascular coagulation in paediatrics. Arch Dis Child. 2016;0:1-7. doi:10.1136/archdischild-2016-311053
10. Donnér M, Holmberg L, Nilsson IM. Type IIB von Willebrand's disease with probable autosomal recessive inheritance and presenting as thrombocytopenia in infancy. Br J Haematol. 1987;66(3):349-54.
11. Jaffray J, Young G, Ko RH. The bleeding newborn: A review of presentation, diagnosis, and management. Semin Fetal Neonatal Med. 2016;(21):44-9.
12. Kenet G, Chan AKC, Soucie JM, et al. Bleeding disorders in neonates. Hemophilia. 2010;16(Suppl 5):168-74.
13. Chalmers E, Williams M, Brennan J, *et al.* Guideline on the management of hemophilia in the fetus and Neonate. Brit J Haematol. 2011;154:208-15.
14. Richards M, Williams M, Chalmers E, *et al.* A United Kingdom Hemophilia Centre Doctors' Organization guideline approved by the British Committee for Standards in Haematology: Guideline on the use of prophylactic factor VIII concentrate in children and adults with severe hemophilia A. Brit J Haematol. 2010;149:498-507.
15. Mumford AD, Ackroyd S, Alikhan R, *et al.* Guideline for the diagnosis and management of the rare coagulation disorders. A United Kingdom Haemophilia Centre Doctors' Organization guideline on behalf of the British Committee for Standards in Haematology. Br J Haematol. 2014;167:304-26.
16. Hanmod SS, Jesudas R, Kulkarni R, *et al.* Neonatal hemostatic disorders: Issues and challenges. Semin Thromb Hemost. 2016;42:741-51.
17. Arnold PD. Coagulation and the surgical neonate. Pediatr Anesth. 2014;24: 89-97.
18. Jones R, Sayge J, Evans D. Service evaluation of management of term neonates with major perinatal blood loss. 10.1136/archdischild-2015-308599.120
19. Swank ML, Garite TJ, Maurel K, *et al.* and the Obstetric Collaborative Research Network. Vasa previa: diagnosis and management. Am J Obstet Gynecol. 2016;215:223.e1-6.
20. Andrew M, Paes B, Milner R, *et al.* Development of the human coagulation system in the full term infant. Blood. 1987;70(1):165-72.
21. Andrew M, Paes B, Milner R, *et al.* Development of the human coagulation system in the health premature infant. Blood. 1988;72(5):1651-7.
22. Christensen RD, Baer VL, Lambert DK, *et al.* Reference intervals for common coagulation tests of preterm infants. Transfusion. 2014;54:627-32.
23. Neary E, McCallion N, Kevane B, *et al.* Coagulation indices in very preterm infants from cord blood and postnatal samples. J Thromb Haemost. 2015;13:2021-30.
24. Christensen RD, Baer VL, Lambert DK, *et al.* Reference intervals for common coagulation tests of preterm infants. Transfusion. 2014;54:627-32.
25. Catford K, Muthukumar P, Reddy C, *et al.* Routine neonatal coagulation testing increases use of fresh frozen plasma. Transfusion. 2014;54:1444-5.
26. Stanworth SJ, Grant-Casey J, Lowe D, *et al.* The use of fresh frozen plasma in England: High levels of inappropriate use in adults and children. Transfusion. 2011;51:62-70.
27. New HV, Berryman J, Bolton-Maggs PHB, *et al.* on behalf of the British Committee for Standards in Haematology. Guidelines on transfusion for fetuses, neonates and older Children. Br J Haematol. 2016;175(5):784-828.
28. Guidelines on gamma irradiation of blood components for the prevention of transfusion associated graft versus host disease. BCSH Blood Transfusion Task Force. Transfusion Med. 1996;6:261-71.
29. Available from: *http://www.clinicalguidelines.scot.nhs.uk/ggc-paediatric-guidelines/ggc-guidelines/emergency-medicine/haemophilia-protocol/*
30. World Federation of Hemophilia. Guidelines for the management of Hemophilia, 2nd edition. Blackwell Publishing, 2012. Available from: *http://www1.wfh.org/publications/files/pdf-1472.pdf*
31. Diab YA, Wong ECC, Luban NLC. Massive transfusion in children and neonates. Brit J Haematol. 2013;161:15-26.
32. Available from: *https://www.transfusionguidelines.org/document-library/documents/tracy-shackleton-paediatric-massive-haemorrhage-188-kb-18-slides*
33. Blain S, Paterson N, 1.Paediatric massive transfusion. BJA Education. 2016;16(8):269-75. https://doi.org/10.1093/bjaed/mkv051
34. Available from: *https://www.transfusionguidelines.org/transfusion-handbook/10-effective-transfusion-in-paediatric-practice/10-4-major-haemorrhage-in-infants-and-children*

CHAPTER

77

Neonatal Cardiac Emergencies

Kuntal Roy Chowdhuri, Parvathi U Iyer

INTRODUCTION

Most cardiac emergencies in children present during the neonatal period or in infancy. A recent Japanese report comparing neonatal cardiac surgical outcomes across the world reported a hospital mortality of less than 10%.[1] In India too, many centers have comparable results—surgical survival in d-transposition of great arteries with intact ventricular septum (dTGA.IVS), total anomalous pulmonary venous connection (TAPVC) being more than 90%.[2–4] However, these outcomes are feasible only with early diagnosis, appropriate stabilization and timely referral of sick cardiac newborns. Managing "cardiac emergencies" in the newborn infant can be a challenging experience particularly for the novice junior doctor in the emergency room.

EPIDEMIOLOGY AND ETIOLOGY

Cardiac malformations are probably the most common of all congenital anomalies and are responsible for most deaths due to congenital defects. The current prevalence of congenital heart disease (CHD) is 4–8/1000 live births, so approximately 150,000 to 200,000 infants with congenital heart disease (CHD) are born each year In our country.[5] Of these, about a third (~70,000) would need some sort of cardiac intervention in the first year of life in order to reach their first birthday.[5] What is less well known is that about 10–20% of newborns with cardiac defects (~30,000 neonates annually) have potentially lethal cardiac abnormalities which lead to circulatory collapse and death in the newborn period if not appropriately managed.[6] dTGA.IVS is the commonest congenital heart defect presenting with cyanosis in the newborn period comprising about 25–30% of all critical neonatal heart defects. Tetralogy of Fallot is the commonest of the congenital cyanotic heart defects and constitutes nearly 10% of all congenital cardiac defects. Duct dependent systemic circulation comprises nearly 50% of all critical neonatal cardiac defects. Coarctation of aorta and HLHS together form 90% of those presenting with neonatal shock.[6] Saxena estimates that only a very small proportion of these sick cardiac newborns get any form of care in our country.[5]

PATHOPHYSIOLOGY

The neonatal myocardium is relatively noncompliant, with a restrictive physiology, being poorly responsive to increased preload and highly intolerant of increased afterload. Neonates rely on chronotropy to maintain cardiac output and intense vasoconstriction to sustain blood pressures, maintaining blood pressures till the very end. Thus, a baby who has tachycardia and intense vasoconstriction is a sick newborn. Newborns also respond rapidly to stress with profound changes in pH, serum lactate, acid base status and glucose levels, becoming desperately sick very quickly. Newborns with critical CHD are extremely fragile and vulnerable, rapidly developing uncompensated low cardiac output state (LCOS) and multiple organ dysfunction.[7,8]

Transitional Circulation (Figs. 1A and B)

It is useful to look at neonatal heart disease as (1) *urgent or critical heart disease,* i.e. those who need urgent or

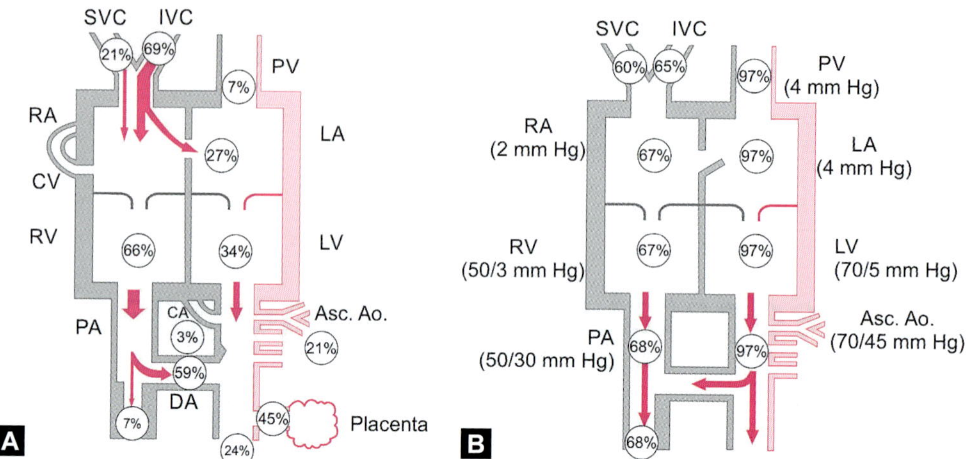

Figs. 1A and B: (A) Fetal circulation—showing relevance of ductus arteriosus, patent foramen ovale (PFO). A predominant ductal systemic circulation; (B) Transitional circulation—changes at birth, ductal and PFO closure

Source (B): Transitional circulation (Modified from Rudolph AM: Congenital Diseases of the Heart. Chicago, Year Book Medical Publishers, Inc, 1974)

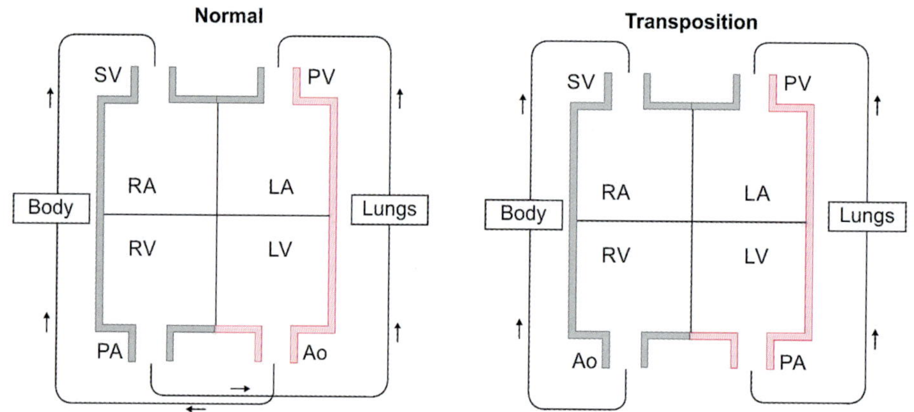

Fig. 2: Transposition of great arteries with intact ventricular septum (dTGA.IVS)—two parallel non-mixing circulations

immediate intervention, or (2) *nonurgent heart disease*, i.e. those who can wait.

Most neonates with structural heart disease have urgent or critical heart disease and present in a dramatic fashion at the time of ductal closure and hence are also considered to have "duct dependent heart disease".[6–8] Ductal constriction followed by ductal closure occurs in the first few days after birth. At the same time, the foramen ovale also undergoes functional closure followed by anatomic closure. So, very little blood then shunts across the ductus or the foramen ovale during the early post natal period. These changes in fetal circulation or transitional circulation, as it is called, causes profound hemodynamic instability in neonates who depend on adequate ductal flow or flow across the foramen ovale for a stable circulation.

Duct Dependent CHD

These newborns rely on a patent ductus arteriosus to ensure: (i) adequate inter circulatory mixing in parallel non-mixing circulations, e.g. d-transposition of great arteries (dTGA.IVS) **(Fig. 2)**; (ii) adequate pulmonary blood flow in right sided obstructive lesions (RVOTO) i.e. duct dependent pulmonary circulation—pulmonary atresia **(Fig. 3)** or tricuspid atresia **(Fig. 4)**; (iii) adequate systemic perfusion as in left sided obstructive lesions (LVOTO) or aortic arch obstructive **(Fig. 5)** or hypoplastic lesions, i.e. duct dependent systemic circulation.

All these conditions worsen rapidly with ductal closure and present in a dramatic fashion to the emergency if undiagnosed before ductal closure. Pediatricians and other caregivers need to be familiar with these circulatory

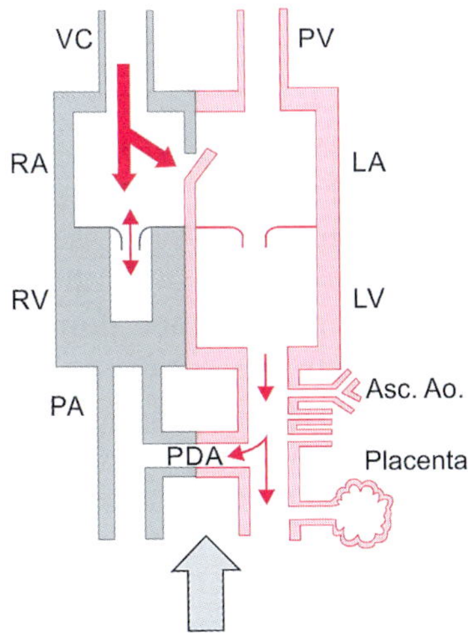

Fig. 3: Pulmonary atresia with intact ventricular septum

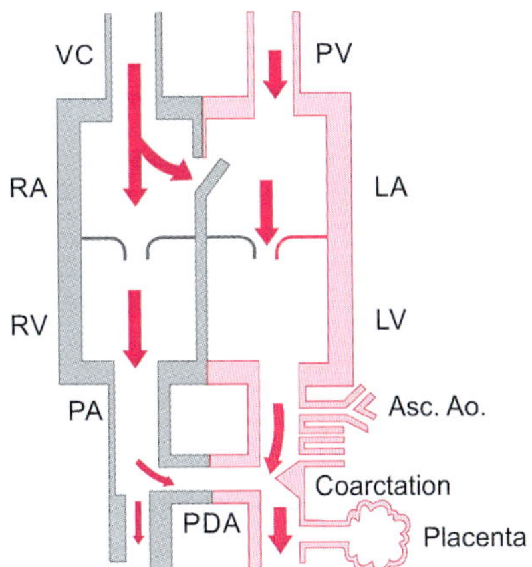

Fig. 5: Aortic coarctation

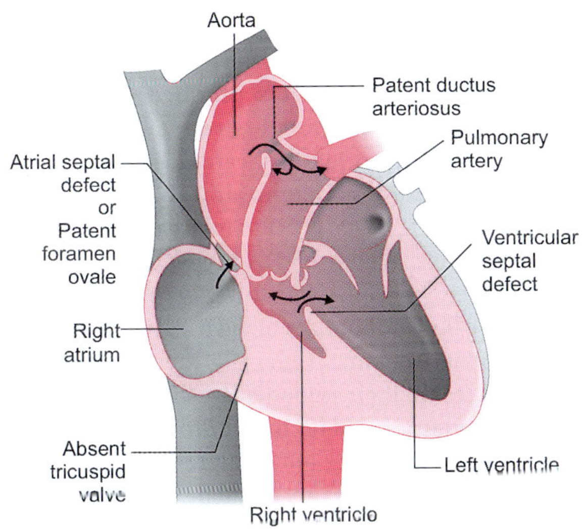

Fig. 4: Tricuspid atresia

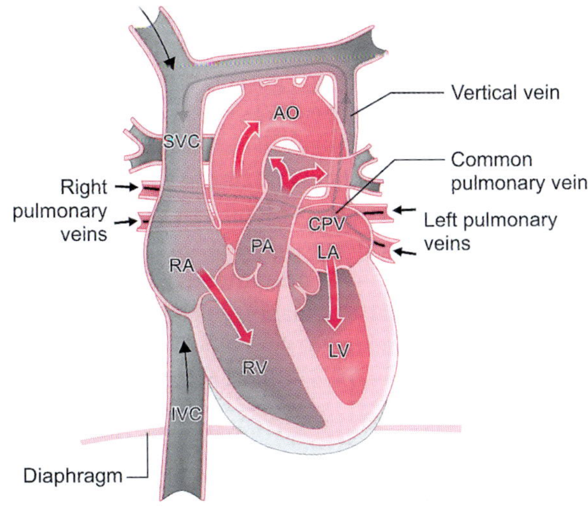

Fig. 6: Supracardiac total anomalous pulmonary venous connection (pulmonary veins connecting via vertical vein to superior vena cava)

changes and consequent hemodynamic effects in order to provide immediate stabilization and speedy referral to a cardiac center.

Non-duct-dependent Critical CHD

Important "Non-duct-dependent" neonatal cardiac emergencies include: (i) obstructed total anomalous pulmonary venous connection (TAPVC) **(Fig. 6)**, and (ii) destabilizing cardiac arrhythmias. Both these conditions are potentially lethal, but the majority of these infants can be readily salvaged with meticulous management.

CLINICAL PRESENTATION[6-12]

It is useful to have a diagnostic approach based on clinical presentation. Neonates with *urgent heart disease present to the emergency with major problems like cyanosis, shock or cardiovascular collapse, heart failure with respiratory distress, mixed presentation, e.g. cyanosis with respiratory distress and arrhythmias.* These categories are not always comprehensive and symptoms may often overlap. All of these symptoms indicate "critical heart disease" and need immediate stabilization followed by an appropriate

Table 1: Congenital heart disease presenting with cyanosis

- **Transposition of great arteries (dTGA)—commonest**
- Right sided obstruction (RVOTO)
  - Pulmonary atresia intact ventricular septum
  - Tricuspid atresia with pulmonary atresia
  - Tetralogy of Fallot
  - Pulmonary atresia with ventricular septal defect
  - Ebstein's anomaly with functional pulmonary atresia
- Total anomalous pulmonary venous connection (TAPVC)
- Truncus arteriosus
- Complex single ventricle

intervention for survival. On the other hand, newborns without urgent heart disease usually have been found to have a murmur on routine examination.

- *Cyanosis at presentation*: Deepening or progressive cyanosis is the commonest manifestation of "Critical or Urgent heart disease" in the newborn infant. Cyanosis is usually noticed by the parents after discharge from the postnatal ward, i.e. at 2–3 days of life. Newborns who present with *progressive cyanosis* have either (a) impaired intercirculatory mixing or (b) cardiac defects with reduced pulmonary blood flow **(Table 1)**.
  - *Impaired intercirculatory mixing* occurs in d-transposition of great arteries (dTGA.IVS) where the pulmonary circulation and systemic circulation are in parallel rather than in series as in the normal body. About 50% of all infants with dTGA present in the first few hours of life with cyanosis and mild tachypnea, and 90% are symptomatic by the first 24–48 hours of life. These babies deteriorate rapidly and develop worsening hypoxemia with profound metabolic and lactic acidosis if the parallel circulations are allowed to continue indefinitely without ensuring adequate mixing.

    Clinically, in the early stages, the baby is relatively comfortable, i.e. has "peaceful cyanosis", the second heart sound is split and a murmur may or not be audible. Some babies with dTGA have a very tiny ductus at birth, or the ductus may have closed in utero either spontaneously or due to maternal intake of medications, e.g. indomethacin. Thus, a newborn with dTGA.IVS and a tiny or closing ductus and a very small PFO or no PFO at birth tends to deteriorate very rapidly after birth due to inadequate mixing between the two parallel circulations. This subset of babies with dTGA. IVS present very early—within a few hours of birth with marked cyanosis, which increases very dramatically and rapidly over a very short period of time.
  - *Right sided obstruction or right ventricular outflow tract obstruction (RVOTO)*: The second group of babies who present with cyanosis are those with right sided obstructions. Cardiac defects with reduced pulmonary blood flow or right sided obstruction include critical pulmonary valvar stenosis with right to left shunting, pulmonary valvar atresia with intact ventricular septum or functional pulmonary atresia, e.g. Ebstein's anomaly, tricuspid atresia with pulmonary atresia and a small ventricular septal defect and severe tetralogy of Fallot or pulmonary atresia with ventricular septal defect.

    Of these, the commonest is critical pulmonary stenosis, which is often a part of tetralogy of Fallot. Sometimes, the pulmonary stenosis is so severe that the pulmonary artery is virtually atretic. These cardiac defects produce cyanosis and hypoxemia with progressive metabolic acidosis due to right-to-left intracardiac shunting. These lesions are dependent almost entirely on the ductus arteriosus (DA) to maintain blood flow to the lungs. When the DA finally closes, the baby suddenly become visibly and noticeably cyanotic since their pulmonary blood flow is almost entirely duct dependent.[6–8] Clinically, they are not in heart failure and their second heart sound is single.

  Pulse oximetry is useful in confirming cyanosis, the saturation often being not greater than 80–85%, often in the fifties to sixties in neonates who present late in their natural history of CHD. If there is evidence of heart failure, i.e. puffiness and hepatomegaly, it is more likely to be a dTGA.IVS than due to reduced pulmonary blood flow.

  Cardiovascular collapse or Shock ***(Table 2)***: Some newborns present with circulatory collapse or clinical features of shock with varying degrees of lactic acidosis due to severely impaired systemic circulation. These infants usually present in the first 2 weeks of life and have structural heart defects associated with critical LVOTO or left ventricular outflow tract obstruction, i.e. severe coarctation of the aorta, aortic arch interruption, aortic valvar stenosis or hypoplastic left heart syndromes (HLHS).[6–8,10]

Table 2: Congenital heart disease causing circulatory collapse
• Severe coarctation of aorta
• Interrupted aortic arch
• Hypoplastic left heart syndrome (HLHS)
• Critical aortic valvar stenosis

These babies have duct-dependent systemic circulation and manifest features of greatly reduced peripheral circulation or shock as the ductus begins to close during the first few days of postnatal life. Once the ductus closes, the systemic blood flow is greatly diminished. Thus, initially, when the ductus is open and systemic perfusion adequate the baby appears relatively well with normally felt central pulses, and so are discharged from the maternity ward or neonatal unit. As the ductus begins to constrict, these babies become dull, lethargic and feed poorly. On examination, they look unwell, are often tachypneic, tachycardic and have a mottled ashen gray color with cool, clammy peripheries and delayed capillary refill.[7,8,10] The femoral pulses are feeble or impalpable and often all central pulses are poorly felt.

Early clinical signs of coarctation or aortic arch interruption include brachio-femoral pulse discrepancy; differential upper and lower limb blood pres-sures may also be useful. If the coarctation is severe and has been undetected for a prolonged period, the left ventricle becomes steadily dysfunctional. Severe left ventricular dysfunction with poor ejection fractions of 10–15% at presentation are not unusual in our country. *Hypoplastic left heart syndrome (HLHS)* is the commonest cause of death due to heart disease in the first week of life. These babies present with circulatory collapse soon after ductal closure and are often desperately ill. Many of these babies have subtle signs on careful examination, e.g. tachycardia, tachypnea, cyanosis and occasionally steadily weakening peripheral pulses before ductal closure.[7,8,10]

Similarly, neonates with *critical aortic stenosis* have severely compromised systemic circulation after ductal closure and present in much the same manner as babies with hypoplastic left ventricle. In addition clinically, the second heart sound is single, there is often a well audible ejection systolic murmur and a third heart sound.

- *Respiratory distress and heart failure*: Some babies present predominantly with tachypnea and respiratory distress.[7,8,10] The *causes of heart failure in the newborn are listed in **Table 3***. Important causes include large patent ductus arteriosus (PDA), myocarditis, sepsis, anomalous origin of coronary artery from pulmonary artery (ALCAPA) and various arrhythmias. An important and commonly missed cause of tachypnea and respiratory distress is coarctation of aorta or arch interruption (with or without an associated ventricular septal defect) before obvious decompensation occurs. These babies typically present at 5–7 days of age and can be easily diagnosed by the discerning physician due to relatively impalpable or poorly felt femoral pulses. Unfortunately, routine examine of the femorals is not often done, and the differential pulses are missed. Babies with large left to right shunts develop heart failure once pulmonary over circulation occurs, i.e. when the pulmonary vascular resistance begins to fall. Thus, typically most large left to right shunts (ventricular septal defects, i.e. VSDs, VSDs with large PDA, large aortopulmonary windows) usually present after 6 weeks of age when the pulmonary vascular resistance falls to permit pulmonary overflow. In some infants, the pulmonary vascular resistance falls soon after birth, particularly in preterm infants and those with trisomy 21. These infants present much earlier—by the 3rd to 4th week of postnatal life. Many babies with large VSDs who develop early onset heart failure invariably have shunting at multiple levels or have associated severe coarctation or arch interruption. These infants usually develop florid heart failure with severe respiratory distress and become dangerously unwell quickly. Thus, they need to be very cautiously evaluated and swiftly stabilized. Causes of *congenital heart disease (CHD) causing heart failure in the newborn period or early infancy is shown in **Table 4***. This group of infants tire easily during feeding, nurse more frequently, are tachypneic at rest, have a diastolic

Table 3: Causes of neonatal heart failure
• Large patent ductus arteriosus
• Birth asphyxia
• Hypoglycemia, hypocalcemia
• Severe anemia
• Sepsis
• Arrhythmias
• Myocarditis/Cardiomyopathy
• Congenital heart disease
• Arteriovenous malformations

Table 4: Congenital heart disease causing heart failure

- **Large L-R Shunt (Pulmonary over circulation) without cyanosis**
  - Large patent ductus arteriosus
  - Large ventricular septal defect
  - Large ventricular septal defect + coarctation
  - Left to right shunt at multiple levels
  - Complete atrioventricular canal
  - Aortopulmonary window
  - Arteriovenous malformations
- **Left sided obstruction**
  - Coarctation of aorta
  - Critical aortic valvar stenosis
- **Diminished left ventricular function**
  - Myocarditis
  - Dilated cardiomyopathy
  - Anomalous origin of left coronary artery from pulmonary artery—often missed
- **Pulmonary over circulation with cyanosis**
  - d-Transposition with ventricular septal defect and or coarctation
  - Double outlet right ventricle + ventricular septal defect
  - Truncus arteriosus
  - Complex single ventricle
  - Ebstein's anomaly

apical flow rumble and frequently a gallop rhythm due to left ventricular failure. Babies with more florid failure have clinical signs of poor peripheral perfusion like decreased toe temperature and poor capillary refill. In addition, babies with a VSD have a heaving precordium, a harsh pan systolic murmur while those with an AVSD have similar clinical findings but in addition the second sound has a fixed split. Babies with an ASD have a soft systolic ejection murmur, and again a fixed split of the second sound with or without a diastolic rumble depending on the degree of shunting. Babies with a systemic AV malformation can present with very severe heart failure and shock like state, and may be symptomatic even in the first few hours of life if the systemic run off is very large. Careful examination in these babies usually reveals a cerebral bruit, or a bruit over the liver and sometimes bounding pulses.

- *Mixed presentation*: There is a small group of newborns who present with mild to moderate cyanosis and rapidly increasing respiratory distress due to heart failure. Neonates who have respiratory distress along with cyanosis are likely to have dTGA.IVS, hypoplastic left heart syndrome (HLHS), obstructed TAPVC or Ebstein's anomaly. Conditions which present with tachypnea and cyanosis after the first few weeks of life include dTGA.VSD, dTGA.VSD with coarctation or arch interruption, truncus arteriosus, double outlet right ventricle, ventricular septal defect (DORV.VSD) or complex single ventricle.
  Some of these babies have total anomalous pulmonary venous connection (TAPVC), i.e. all the pulmonary veins are draining into the right side of the heart, the SVC, the right atrium or the IVC. If the pulmonary venous drainage is obstructed, these babies can deteriorate very rapidly unless the pulmonary veins are urgently re-routed surgically. There are very few specific diagnostic signs clinically except for a fixed split of the second heart sound. The diagnosis is readily confirmed on 2D echocardiography. TGA.VSD and DORV.VSD are important causes of mixed presentation, i.e. cyanosis with tachypnea. The tachypnea is due to heart failure secondary to increased pulmonary flow.
  Another cause of mild cyanosis and cardiac failure is *truncus arteriosus*. These infants have tachypnea and a prominent systolic murmur with a systolic ejection click. The pulses are usually bounding due to a run off into the pulmonary artery. These babies are usually symptomatic by 3 to 4 weeks of age or later, i.e. whenever the pulmonary vascular resistance falls and pulmonary overcirculation occurs.
  A very unusual cause of structural heart defect in the newborn is *Ebstein's anomaly* of the tricuspid valve. These babies presents with cyanosis, florid right heart failure, a systolic murmur due to tricuspid valve regurgitation, loud third and fourth sounds, massive cardiomegaly on chest X-ray and right ventricular hypertrophy on EKG. These findings along with massive cardiomegaly on X-ray confirms the diagnosis. Sometimes, they have functional pulmonary atresia due to elevated pulmonary vascular resistance.
- *Arrhythmias*: Some babies present predominantly with an arrhythmia, i.e. *tachyarrhythmia* (heart rate persistently >200/min) or a *bradyarrhythmia* (heart rate <70/*min*). Both conditions if unrecognized and allowed to persist can rapidly lead to heart failure, secondary low output state and cardiogenic shock. Birth asphyxia, hypothermia, sepsis, hypothyroidism are some conditions associated with rhythm disturbances. Ventricular dysfunction and electrolyte imbalance may cause various ventricular arrhythmias. Most often, there is no underlying structural heart disease. Thus, it is important to get an electrocardiogram (ECG) done in all sick newborns presenting to the emergency.

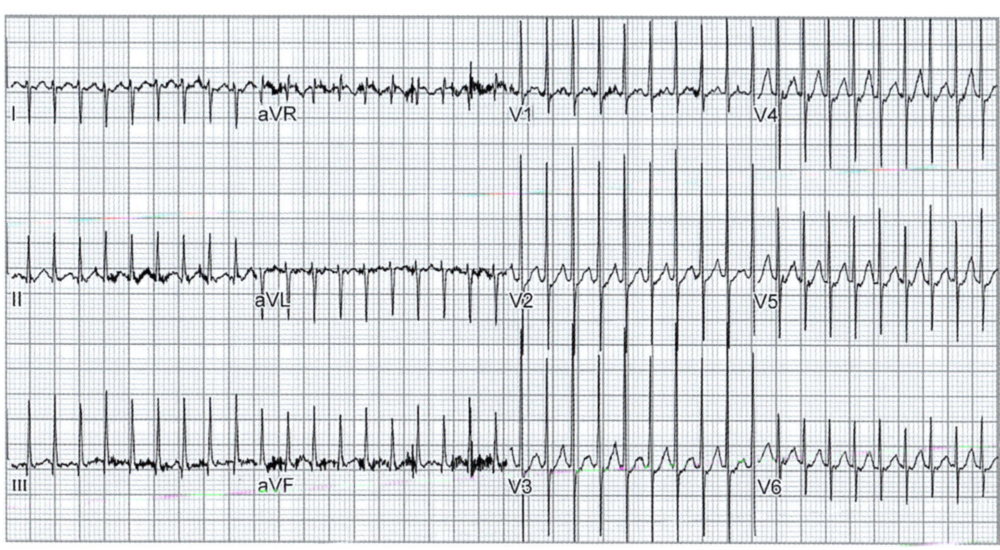

Fig. 7: ECG of a neonate with supraventricular tachycardia (HR > 250/min)

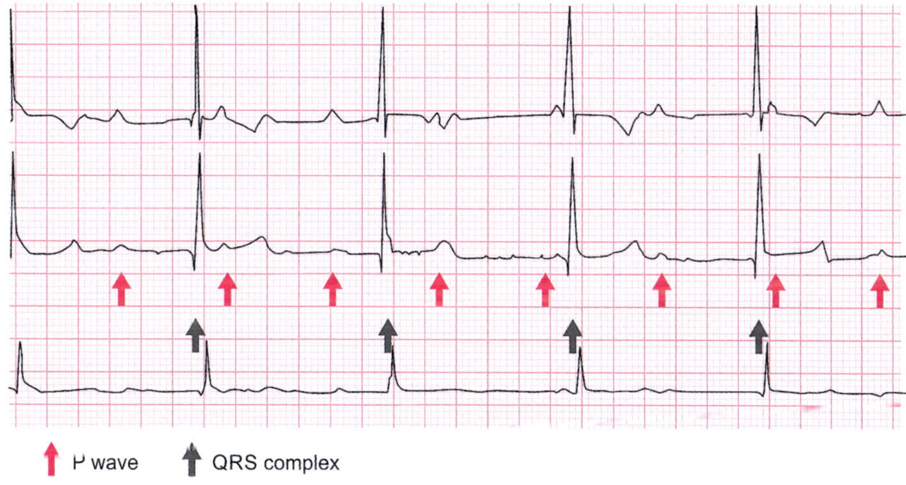

Fig. 8: ECG of a neonate with congenital complete heart block. Note that the HR < 60/min
Upper arrows P wave; Lower arrows QRS complex

Likewise, if an arrhythmia is suspected an ECHO should be done to assess both ventricular function and to exclude structural heart disease.

Tachyarrhythmias: These are more common than bradyarrhythmias. Newborns who have tachyarrhythmia constitute a serious medical emergency since no baby can sustain heart rates of over 200/min for a long period of time. The commonest type is supraventricular tachycardia (SVT) or narrow ventricular complex tachycardia **(Fig. 7)**. This is suspected when heart rates are more than 200/min, usually over 250/minute, with a narrow QRS complex and no beat to beat variability.

Bradyarrhythmias: These are due to congenital heart block occurring either de novo or due to maternal lupus **(Fig. 8)**.

DIFFERENTIAL DIAGNOSIS

Cyanosis

In a cyanotic infant, it is often difficult to decide whether the cyanosis is due to an underlying respiratory disorder

Flowchart 1: Approach to a cyanotic newborn

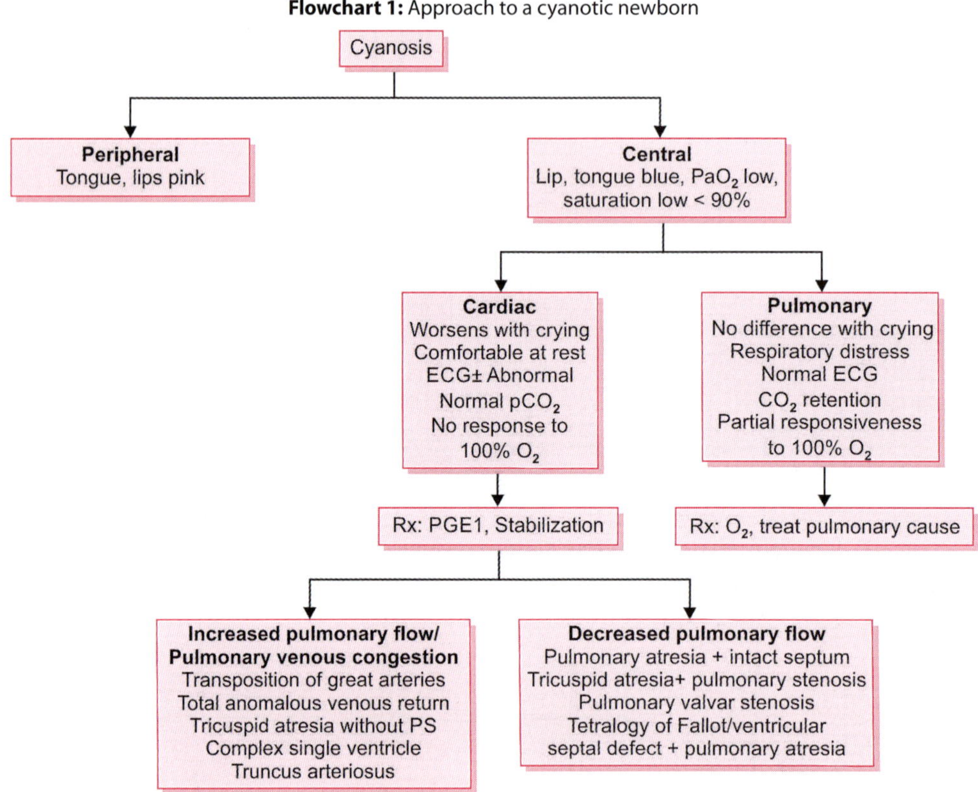

or due to a cardiac defect. The classical and traditional *hyperoxia test* is often still useful. If the PaO_2 is <150 mm, after being in 100% oxygen, the infant is likely to have a cardiac defect causing right to left shunting. Persistent pulmonary hypertension (PPHN) is an important differential and often mimics cyanotic heart disease. These babies often have a setting for PPHN-like aspiration syndromes, or maternal diabetes. Babies with PPHN are often sicker and have greater respiratory distress. Some babies with severe PPHN may not show a good response to hyperoxia, and occasionally PPHN and dTGA may coexist. Thus, definitive diagnosis may be extremely difficult in an individual baby. **Flowchart 1** provides a useful diagnostic algorithm for a cyanotic neonate.

Respiratory Distress

A chest X-ray often confirms or excludes major lung disease, e.g. pneumonia, bronchiolitis, aspiration which can cause respiratory distress in the newborn.

INVESTIGATIONS

2D and Color Doppler Echocardiography (ECHO)

It is the most informative diagnostic tool today in congenital heart disease and should be done in all cases to confirm the diagnosis.

Chest X-ray

dTGA.IVS: The chest skiagram reveals cardiomegaly with increased pulmonary artery markings with a narrow mediastinum—an "egg on string" appearance. Often, the X-ray may not be typical or diagnostic, but the lungs fields are either normal or have increased vascularity **(Fig. 9)**.

Pulmonary stenosis or atresia: The chest skiagram reveals a normal sized or small cardiac shadow with oligemic lung fields **(Fig. 10)**.

TAPVC: It often shows a normal heart size and pulmonary venous congestion, i.e. a mottled look or diffuse haziness **(Fig.11)**; the typical snowman appearance hardly ever seen.

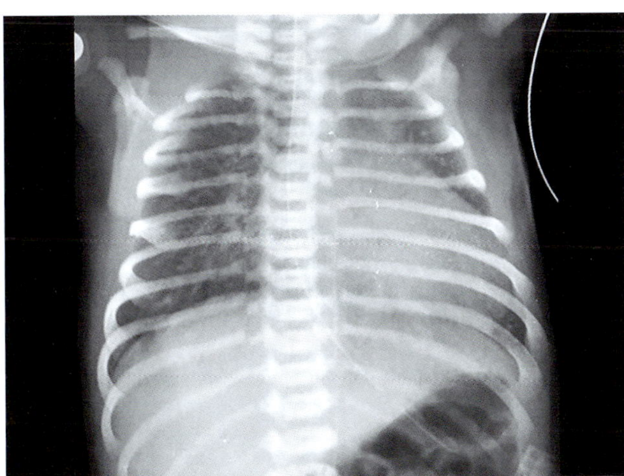

Fig. 9: X-ray chest of a neonate with dTGA.IVS

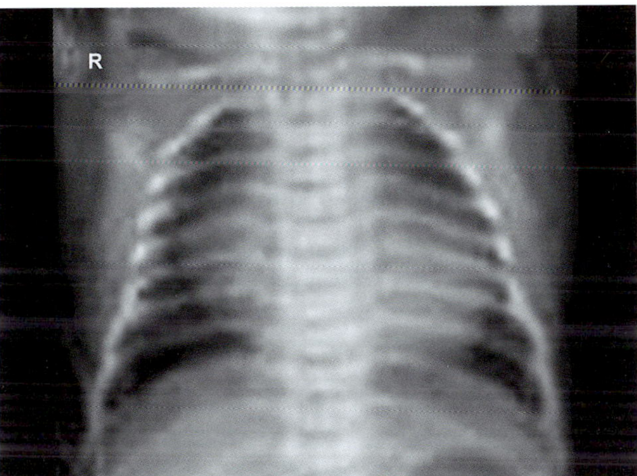

Fig. 10: X-ray chest of a neonate with pulmonary atresia

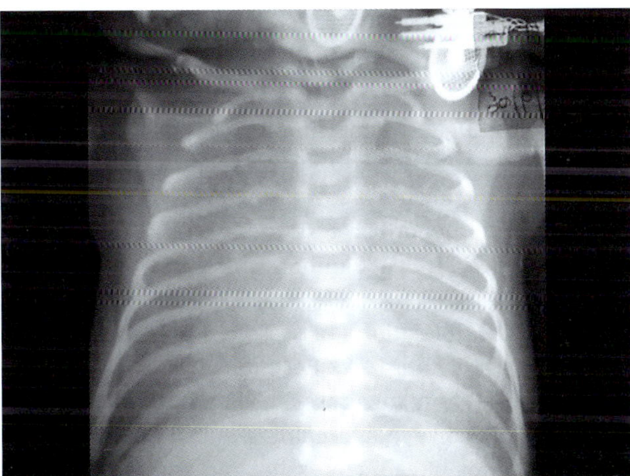

Fig. 11: Chest X-ray of a neonate with obstructed TAPVC

These features on chest X-ray should prompt an urgent echocardiographic study to confirm the diagnosis.

LVOTO: In coarctation and aortic stenosis, it is unremarkable with a normal heart size, cardiomegaly only being present when the infant presents with heart failure. Babies with HLHS invariably have features of cardiomegaly with pulmonary congestion.

Left to right shunts: The chest skiagram in all instances shows cardiomegaly, plethora and sometimes patchy atelectasis.

Electrocardiogram (ECG)

It is typically useful in certain instances—in tricuspid atresia, the ECG shows left axis deviation. Likewise in HLHS the ECG shows diminished left ventricular forces and in significant LVOTO the ECG shows left ventricular hypertrophy. Typical, pathologic Q waves are seen in the lateral leads in ALCAPA, though a normal ECG does not exclude ALCAPA.

CT Angiogram

It may be useful to delineate pulmonary venous anatomy in TAPVC or branch pulmonary arteries, or the coronary artery in ALCAPA. CT angiograms is also useful to confirm AV malformations, their exact location and other vascular details.

Cardiac MRI is useful to confirm myocarditis and to quantify ventricular dilatation.

MANAGEMENT

The initial management of a newborn with critical heart disease greatly affects the outcome of surgery or catheter intervention. A baby who reaches a specialized unit in a stable condition has much better chances of intact survival than a baby who arrives in a moribund, preterminal state.[6-12] Delayed diagnosis of neonatal heart disease and presentation in a sick state with circulatory collapse, severe metabolic acidosis or organ dysfunction has been shown to be associated with both higher postoperative morbidity and mortality.[13] Emergency management and initial stabilization of the sick cardiac neonate is depicted in **Flowcharts 2 and 3**.

Prompt referral and safe transport to a tertiary center is necessary. In many instances road transport may be

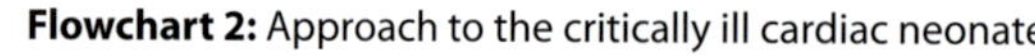

Flowchart 2: Approach to the critically ill cardiac neonate

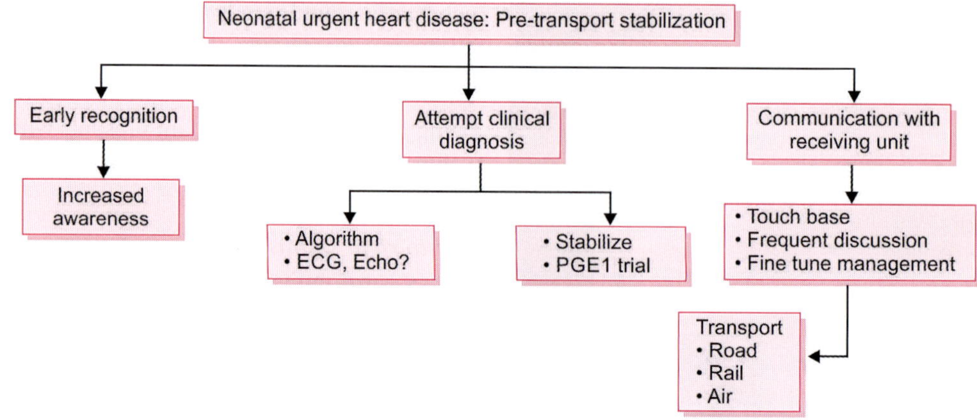

Flowchart 3: Stabilization of the critically ill cardiac newborn

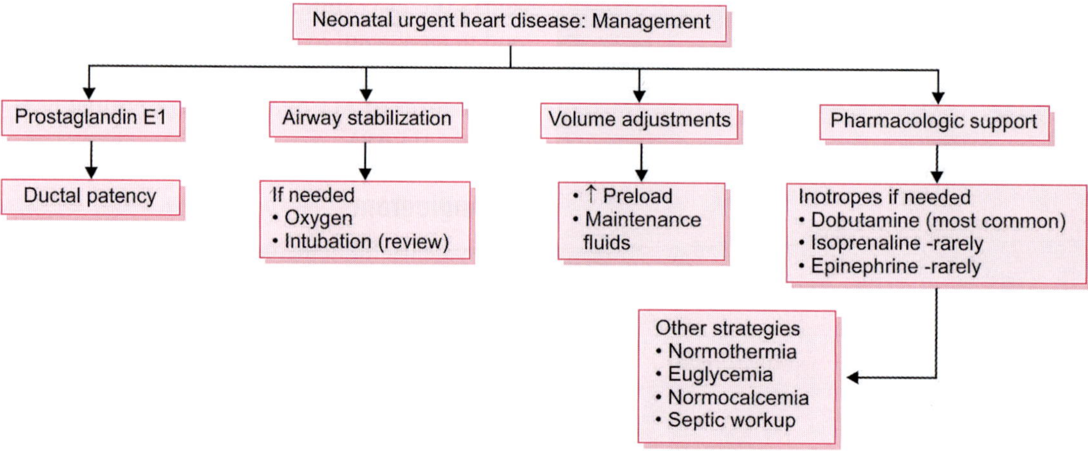

feasible, but increasingly transfer by rail or air has been successfully accomplished in our country. The safety of transfer would depend on the nature of the cardiac defect, the clinical status of the neonate and the distance to be traveled. Ideally transfer is best organized as in most centers across the world, in close consultation with the receiving cardiac team, so that optimal stabilization, within the resources of the referring doctor or team, is done prior to transfer.[6-12]

Essential principles of management include *measures to rapidly improve cardiac output and tissue perfusion.*

- *Restoration of ductal circulation*: Stabilization involves in most instances timely restoration of ductal circulation to maintain systemic or pulmonary blood flow or to enhance intercirculatory mixing. If the newborn is not too unwell, very often this is all that is needed to stabilize the baby.[6-12]

Prostaglandin E1 (PGE1) should be initiated to establish ductal patency in doses of 0.025–0.1 µg/min. PGE1 is commenced on clinical suspicion in a neonate in shock during the first week of life, is visibly cyanotic or fails the hyperoxia test. A neonate should ideally be watched for 30–60 minutes prior to transport after commencing PGE1. Side effects described are apnea (12%), vasodilatation (10%), fever (14%), bradycardia (7%), and seizures (4%). Recent reviews of PGE 1 have shown that very low doses 0.003 µg/kg to 0.02 µg/kg may be effective in maintaining ductal patency. These lower doses have been associated with significantly reduced rates of apnea.[14,15] PGE1 has occasionally been found to be effective weeks after ductal closure.[16] Sometimes it might be worth trying PGE1 even in the *older infants in shock or with cyanosis.* Occasionally clinical deterioration is seen following commencement of PGE1. This may occur in the absence of a ductus, an unresponsive ductus or in the presence of obstruction at the PFO or pulmonary veins. Structural heart defects associated with clinical deterioration with PGE1 include obstructed total anomalous pulmonary veins, d-transposition of great arteries and intact ventricular septum with restrictive patent foramen ovale, hypoplastic left heart syndrome or mitral atresia with restrictive patent foramen ovale. *In the event of deterioration, PGE1 should be immediately ceased and the baby re-evaluated by ECHO if possible.*

If the baby appears to stabilize, it is useful to use this window and swiftly organize a transfer to the receiving cardiac unit. Ongoing communication with the receiving unit cardiologist, intensivist or surgeon is the key to a stable and smooth transfer.

- *Advanced life support*: Basics of advanced life support really implies good airway management. It is tempting to give supplemental oxygen to a cyanotic newborn. However, oxygen has little benefit in a cyanotic neonate baby unless the baby has severe pulmonary hypertension, e.g. TAPVC.[7,8] Oxygen therapy may cause pulmonary overcirculation and pulmonary edema due to the pulmonary vasodilator effect of oxygen leading to severely reduced peripheral circulation in HLHS and complex single ventricle situations, where the goal of stabilization is to maintain a Qp:Qs of close to 1. *Supplemental oxygen should be given only after consultation with a pediatric cardiologist, since it may confer no benefit but actually harm the baby.*

  Intubation may be needed if the baby is apneic after PGE1, deeply cyanosed or has significant respiratory distress. The potential complications of elective intubation prior to transport has been recently reviewed.[17] The benefits of elective intubation needs to be carefully balanced against the possible risks of accidental tube dislodgement, overventilation and air leaks that may occur during transport.[17,18]
- *Maintain euvolemia*: Normal or reduced maintenance fluids is needed in these neonates to maintain euvolemia. Additional volume augmentation may be required in some babies due to the non-compliant neonatal myocardium or PGE1 induced vasodilatory hypotension. Volume repletion may be with normal saline, dextrose saline or albumin.
- *Inotropic support*: Inotropes may often be needed to improve myocardial contractility and improve tissue perfusion once intravascular volume status is replete especially when babies present late. Delayed diagnosis is often associated with right ventricular, left ventricular or biventricular dysfunction. *Dobutamine is the usual preferred inotrope.* Very occasionally, epinephrine or isoprenaline is used when the heart rate is slow.
- *Correction of metabolic derangements*: The negative inotropic effect of hypoglycemia, acidosis and hypocalcemia are often underestimated, and if uncorrected these metabolic derangements may lead to progressive and irreversible deterioration. In fact profound and sustained hypocalcemia has been shown to cause severe, potentially lethal systolic and diastolic ventricular dysfunction. The ventricular dysfunction may be easily reversed with timely correction of hypocalcemia. Likewise, hypothermia and hyperthermia need to be corrected due to their adverse effects on the myocardium.[7,8]

  All these measures usually help in improving perfusion and secondary tissue and metabolic acidosis. *Sodium bicarbonate correction is usually not required – in fact sodium bicarbonate administration has been associated with poor outcomes. In the event of refractory acidosis half correction may be cautiously administered.*
- *Management of sepsis and other comorbidities*: Many desperately sick neonates have coexisting gram negative, gram positive or fungal sepsis. It is appropriate to initiate broad spectrum antimicrobial and or antifungal therapy after drawing blood cultures, so that the window of timely management of sepsis is not missed.[7,8] Later, if cultures are negative, the receiving unit can cease antimicrobial therapy. Additional malformations, e.g. esophageal atresia, various syndromes and chromosomal abnormalities, e.g. trisomy 21 need to be looked for, so that other system abnormalities can be appropriately addressed. Families, then can be suitably counseled to have realistic expectations.

  Older neonates with heart failure should be managed with heart failure medications, i.e. diuretics, spironolactone and occasionally digoxin. Acute deterioration may need myocardial support with an inotrope and intravenous diuretics. If the baby tires while feeding, the infant may need assisted feeding by a feeding tube. The reader is referred to a chapter on heart failure management to understand current concepts of heart failure management.[19]

Treatment of Arrhythmia

Tachyarrhythmia

- *Clinically stable*: Standard vagal maneuvers may be tried, at all times ensuring that the airway is not compromised.[11] Various emergency options include crushed ice in a plastic bag placed on the forehead (eyes need to be protected), insertion of an anal thermometer or anal probe or a nasogastric tube. *Eyeball pressure and carotid massage in newborns are no longer recommended as they can acutely compromise cerebral circulation.* If there is no response within 10–20 seconds, then adenosine (dose 100 µg/kg rapid push) may be tried. Adenosine should be given through a large central vein or through the antecubital vein for optimal effect. If not effective, adenosine dose may be increased in increments of 50 µg/kg up to a maximum of 500 µg/kg. Since adenosine acts by blocking the atrioventricular node, occasionally the baby may develop ventricular tachycardia needing resuscitation. Sometimes if there is no response, esmolol or amiodarone may be tried. Doses are given in **Table 5.**
- *Sick or unstable* or unresponsive to above measures, restore sinus rhythm by synchronized cardioversion. Once sinus rhythm is restored, it is important to remember that in many instances, the tachyarrhythmia will recur. So, the baby needs to be seen by a pediatric cardiologist who is familiar with arrhythmias since the infant is likely to need some long-term medications (beta blocker, e.g. propranolol or metoprolol or amiodarone or sometimes both).

Table 5: Approach to neonatal supraventricular tachycardia

- **Hemodynamically stable**
  - Vagal maneuvers (ice in plastic bag, anal thermometer)
  - Adenosine 100 µg/kg rapid IV push; may be increased to 500 µg/kg in 50 µg increments until response
  - Esmolol at bolus dose of 200 to 500 µg/kg over 10 minutes, followed by 50–100 µg/kg/min
  - Amiodarone (bolus infusion of 25 µg/kg/min infused over 60 to 90 minutes followed by continuous infusion of 5 to 15 µg/kg/min)
  - Synchronized DC Cardioversion at 0.5 to 4 Joules/kg
- **Hemodynamically unstable**
  - Immediate synchronized DC Cardioversion at 0.5 to 4 Joules/kg
  - Transesophageal pacing if available

Bradyarrhythmia

These infants need to be swiftly transferred to a cardiac unit where a permanent pacemaker can be placed if required. Current indications for pacemaker in a neonate include (1) ventricular dysfunction, (2) heart failure, (3) heart rate < 55–60/min. Pacemakers are placed surgically in the epicardial area and most surgical units today perform these procedures with relatively few complications.

Common Pitfalls in Management

Some common pitfalls in diagnosis and management[12] need to be emphasized. Many frequently employed treatment strategies in the emergency room like oxygen, bronchodilators, liberal fluid therapy, diuretics may actually cause the infant to worsen. Neonates with heart failure frequently have wheezing and may be administered bronchodilator therapy, which leads to deterioration with increasing tachycardia, heart failure and metabolic acidosis. Babies with critical RVOTO may have hyperinflated lung fields and again may inadvertently be given bronchdilators with serious consequences.

Many cyanotic babies are administered oxygen at high flow rates leading to ductal closure in duct dependent critical heart disease. Oxygen therapy is a pulmonary vasodilator, increasing pulmonary blood flow in conditions with pulmonary overcirculation causing pulmonary edema with systemic steal, impaired systemic perfusion and clinical deterioration. Many babies look sick with apparent dehydration and are given inappropriate large fluid boluses precipitating heart failure and pulmonary edema. Some hypovolemic infants are given injudicious furosemide worsening intravascular hypovolemia.

PROGNOSIS

It is important that the pediatrician and the neonatologist is familiar with current advances in neonatal cardiac care, so that he or she can guide, counsel and support families of babies with various cardiac defects.

dTGA.IVS: The arterial switch operation is the surgery of choice for this condition. This surgery is considered to be the most physiologic solution—anatomic normalcy

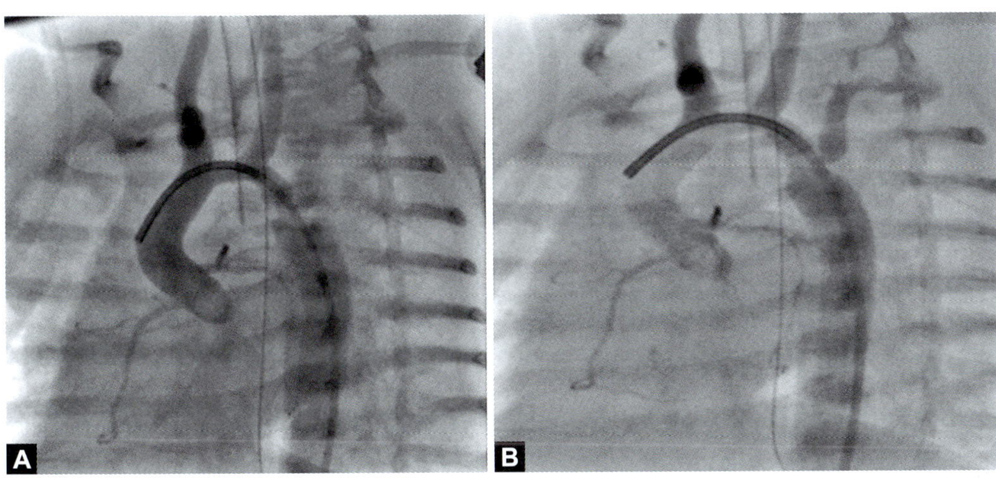

Figs. 12A and B: Cardiac catheterization images of treatment of coarctation of aorta by ballooning: (A) Preballooning; (B) Post-ballooning

is restored, i.e. the aorta is re-connected to the left ventricle (LV) and main pulmonary artery to the right ventricle (RV). The outcome depends on early surgical intervention. The morphologic left ventricle begins to regress rapidly after birth and currently it is unclear when the regression becomes irreversible. If the left ventricle regresses significantly, it is unable to support the systemic circulation and these babies develop severe refractory low cardiac output states after an arterial switch. *So, the arterial switch operation should be done in the first month of life and preferably in the first two weeks of life.* If an arterial switch is performed at the ideal age in an infant with stable hemodynamics, current mortality rates are between 0% and 5%.[1] Long-term outcomes are also excellent with good quality of life and reasonable mainstream integration of the survivors.[20,21]

dTGA with ventricular septal defect has relatively prepared left ventricles due to the associated ventricular septal defect, so surgery (arterial switch with ventricular septal defect closure) can be safely performed in the first few months of age—ideally before 3 months of age. The surgical mortality is less than 5%.

Right sided obstruction (RVOTO) can be divided into two broad groups—biventricular physiology and single ventricle or SV or univentricular physiology. Babies with severe RVOTO whatever the underlying anatomy, need an urgent alternate source of pulmonary blood flow in the form of a surgically placed communication between the systemic and pulmonary circulation-most often a modification of the Blalock-Taussig shunt.[22] In the event of isolated pulmonary valve stenosis, a balloon valvotomy (catheter intervention) is often enough and is usually lifesaving. Those with ventricular septal defect and pulmonary atresia need a shunt followed by a right ventricle to pulmonary artery conduit, i.e. an artificial connection or tube between the right ventricle and branch pulmonary arteries. Thus, these children need multiple life-long surgeries—since the conduit needs to be replaced as the child grows. Both these conditions, i.e. tetralogy and pulmonary atresia, VSD have two functioning ventricles and are categorized as biventricular physiology.

Pulmonary atresia intact ventricular septum, tricuspid atresia with diminutive right ventricle have SV or univentricular physiology since they are born with a small or hypoplastic right ventricle and have only one functioning ventricle, i.e. the left ventricle. These infants need multiple palliative staged surgeries—the final surgery being the Fontan operation.[22,23] These babies even after palliation have effectively only a single pumping ventricle (the left ventricle) and so are called single ventricle physiology. Published literature reports steadily improving long-term outcomes but 10 years and 20 years survival rates remain only at about 75% and 60%.[23-25] Thus, parents and families need to be very clear whether they are willing to pursue a treatment option which involves a steady attrition.

Critical coarctation and arch interruption are again one of the commoner critical cardiac defects presenting in the neonatal period.[6] Definitive surgery is imminently possible with excellent early outcomes.[6,26] Infants with a hypoplastic aortic arch tend to develop re-coarctation and may need re-surgery or catheter ballooning **(Fig. 12)**. Nowadays, aortic valvar stenosis is relieved by catheter ballooning of the aortic valve in the catheterization laboratory with high initial success rates. Many need repeated procedures, since the valve tends to restenose and finally about half will need aortic valve replacement in later life.[6]

The last two decades have witnessed great improvements in management of HLHS. HLHS again falls into the group of single ventricle physiology, the functional ventricle being the right ventricle. Management involves multiple staged surgeries, hybrid procedures, with high interstage attrition rates and finally culminating in the Fontan operation. Long-term survival continues to be low.[6,10,25] Babies with **obstructed total anomalous pulmonary venous connection** do not benefit from any form of stabilization. They need urgent surgical rerouting of the pulmonary veins to the left atrium. Initially, a high mortality procedure (nearly 20% surgical mortality) due to late diagnosis, severe postoperative pulmonary hypertension and low cardiac output, current survival has improved to 90–95% with improvements in surgical technique, cardiac intensive care and mechanical support.[27,28] Our early survival is currently greater than 95%. It is not feasible to discuss outcomes of every cardiac condition and the reader is referred to published literature on current surgical and catheter outcomes.[1,6,10]

Problems associated with late diagnosis: Late diagnosis of critical neonatal heart disease has significant adverse prognostic implications. Brown *et al.* showed that delayed diagnosis of neonatal heart disease was associated with increased preoperative cardiovascular compromise and organ dysfunction both of which adversely affected surgical outcomes.[13] Delayed neonatal diagnosis was associated with increased postoperative mortality, increased duration of ventilation and postoperative length of stay.[13]

Delayed diagnosis may cause multiorgan dysfunction (kidney, bowel, liver, heart and the brain may all be affected) if the cardiovascular compromise is significant. These infants may develop acute kidney injury, necrotizing enterocolitis, transaminitis, varying degrees of myocardial dysfunction and or brain injury.

PREVENTION AND EARLY DETECTION

Antenatal or fetal diagnosis of CHD has evolved greatly over the last many years. There is increasing evidence that prenatal diagnosis of complex CHD is associated with improved postoperative morbidity and mortality. In the absence of universal prenatal diagnosis, our goal should be early neonatal diagnosis of critical congenital heart disease. A prospective Swedish study[29] showed that a predischarge comprehensive neonatal screening (a thorough physical examination including femoral pulses + pulse oximetry screening) diagnosed more than 80% of duct dependent heart disease and 100% of duct dependent pulmonary circulation. Screening pulse oximetry has now become the standard of care in many countries in Europe, South East Asia and the USA after endorsement by the Department of Health and Human Services in 2011 for early detection of neonatal critical heart disease.[30]

KEY MESSAGES

- The burden of neonatal heart disease is huge in our country. 150,000–200,000 infants are born with cardiac defects every year in India.
- Commonest neonatal heart disease are dTGA and coarctation of the aorta. These two lesions have excellent early surgical survival and good long-term outcomes.
- Critical neonatal heart disease usually has duct dependent systemic circulation, duct dependent pulmonary blood flow or impaired circulatory mixing.
- A sick cardiac neonate typically presents with cyanosis, respiratory distress, heart failure, cardiovascular collapse or arrhythmias.
- Early stabilization involves restoration of ductal circulation with PGE1 along with other measures of advanced life support.
- Comprehensive neonatal screening (examination of femorals and pulse oximetry screening) reduces the incidence of missed diagnosis.
- Delayed diagnosis is associated with organ dysfunction, brain injury and adverse surgical outcomes.
- Outcome of neonatal heart disease is steadily improving. So, serious efforts should be made to detect them either prenatally or soon after birth.

REFERENCES

1. Hasegawa T, Masuda M, Okumura M, *et al.* Trends and outcomes in neonatal cardiac surgery for congenital heart disease in Japan from 1996 to 2010. Eur J Cardiothorac Surg. 2017;51:301-7.
2. Kumar G, Iyer PU. Management of perioperative low cardiac output state without extracorporeal life support: What is feasible? Ann Pediatr Cardiol. 2010;3(2):147-58.
3. Kumar G, Iyer PU. Neonatal cardiac emergencies. In: Choudhury P, Bagga A, Chugh K, Ramji S, Gupta P, editors. Principles of Pediatric and Neonatal Emergencies, 3rd edition. New Delhi: Jaypee Brothers Medical publishers (P) Ltd; 2011. p. 579-90.

4. Jenkins KJ, Castaneda AR, Cherian KM, *et al.* Reducing mortality and infections after congenital heart surgery in the developing world. Pediatrics. 2014;134(5):1422-30.
5. Saxena A. How to deliver the best: A call for action for congenital heart disease treatments in India. Future Cardiol. 2014;10:359-66.
6. Mellander M. Diagnosis and management of life-threatening cardiac malformations in the newborn. Semin Fetal Neonatal Med. 2013;18:302-10.
7. Wessel DL, Fraisse A. Preoperative care of the pediatric cardiac surgical patient. In: Nichols DG, Rogers MC, Ackerman AD, editors. Rogers's Textbook of Pediatric Intensive Care, 4th edition. Philadelphia: Lippincott Williams and Wilkins; 2008. p. 1149-58.
8. Wernovsky G, Chang AC, Wessel DL, et al. Cardiac intensive care. In: Allen HD, Shaddy RE, Feltes TF, Driscoll DJ, editors. Moss and Adams' Heart Disease in Infants, Children, and Adolescents, Including the Fetus and Young Adult, 7th edition. Philadelphia: Lippincott Williams and Wilkins; 2008. p. 448-80.
9. Stevenson DK, Benitz WE. A Practical approach to diagnosis and immediate care of the cyanotic neonate. Stabilization and preparation for transfer to level III nursery. Clin Pediatr. 1987;26:325-31.
10. Andropoulos DB, Shekerdemian LS, Checchia PA, et al. Cardiovascular intensive care. In: Allen HD, Shaddy RE, Penny DJ, Feltes TF, Cetta F, editors. Moss and Adams' Heart Disease in Infants, Children, and Adolescents, Including the Fetus and Young Adult, 9th edition. Philadelphia: Wolters Kluwer; 2016. p. 665-713.
11. Yates MC, Rao PS. Pediatric cardiac emergencies. Emergency Med. 2013;3(6):1-7.
12. Sarnaik S, Cashen K, Sarnaik AP. Emergency presentation of heart disease. In: Sarnaik AP, Ross RD, Lipshultz SE, Walters III HL, editors. Cardiac Emergencies in Children: A Practical Approach to Diagnosis and Management, 1st edition. Switzerland: Springer International Publishing AG; 2018. p. 1-16.
13. Brown KL, Ridout DA, Hoskote A, *et al.* Delayed diagnosis of congenital heart disease worsens preoperative condition and outcome of surgery in neonates. Heart. 2006;92:1298-302.
14. Alprostadil (Prostaglandin E1). Royal Hospital for Women. Newborn Care Guidelines; 2016.
15. Huang FK, Lin CC, Huang TC, *et al.* Reappraisal of the prostaglandin E1 dose for early newborns with patent ductus arteriosus-dependant pulmonary circulation. Pediatr Neonatol. 2013;54:102-6.
16. Freed MD, Heyman MA, Lewis AB, *et al.* Prostaglandin E1 in ductus arteriosus-dependent congenital heart disease. Circulation. 1981;64:899-905.
17. Meckler GD, Lowe C. To intubate or not to intubate? Transporting infants on prostaglandin E1. Pediatrics. 2009;123: e25-30.
18. Browning Carmo KA, Barr P, West M, *et al.* Transporting newborn infants with suspected duct dependent congenital heart disease on low-dose prostaglandin E1 without routine mechanical ventilation. Arch Dis Child Fetal Neonatal Ed. 2007;92:F117-9.
19. Iyer PU, Dutta N, Roy Chowdhuri K. Congestive heart failure. In: Gupta P, Menon PSN, Ramji S, Lodha R, editors. PG Textbook of Pediatrics, 2nd edition, New Delhi: Jaypee Brothers Medical Publishers (P) Ltd; 2018. p. 2125-35.
20. Raju V, Burkhart HM, Durham LA 3rd, *et al.* Reoperation after arterial switch: A 27-year experience. Ann Thorac Surg. 2013; 95:2105-13.
21. Tobler D, Williams WG, Jegatheeswaran A, *et al.* Cardiac outcomes in young adult survivors of the arterial switch operation for transposition of great arteries. J Am Coll Cardiol. 2010;56:58-64.
22. Alwi M, Geetha K, Bilkis AA, *et al.* Pulmonary atresia with intact ventricular septum percutaneous radiofrequency-assisted valvotomy and balloon dilation versus surgical valvotomy and Blalock Taussig shunt. J Am Coll Cardiol. 2000;35(2):468-76.
23. Yoshimura N, Yamaguchi M. Surgical strategy for pulmonary atresia with intact ventricular septum: Initial management and definitive surgery. Gen Thorac Cardiovasc Surg. 2009;57: 338-46.
24. Pundi KN, Johnson JN, Dearani JA, *et al.* 40-year follow-up after the Fontan operation: Long-term outcomes of 1,052 patients. J Am Coll Cardiol. 2015;66:1700-10.
25. Iyengar AJ, Winlaw DS, Galati JC, *et al.* The extracardiac conduit Fontan procedure in Australia and New Zealand: Hypoplastic left heart syndrome predicts worse early and late outcomes. Euro J Cardiothorac Surg. 2014;46(3):465-73.
26. Fesseha AK, Eidem BW, Dibardino DJ, *et al.* Neonates with aortic coarctation and cardiogenic shock: Presentation and outcomes. Ann Thorac Surg. 2005;79:1650-5.
27. St Louis JD, Harvey BA, Menk JS, *et al.* Repair of "simple" total anomalous pulmonary venous connection: A review from the Pediatric Cardiac Care Consortium. Ann Thorac Surg. 2012;94(1):133-8.
28. Kelle AM, Backer CL, Gossett JG, *et al.* Total anomalous pulmonary venous connection. Result of surgical repair of 100 patients at a single institution. J Thorac Cardiovasc Surg. 2010; 139:1387-94.
29. De-Wahl Granelli A, Wennergren M, Sandberg K, *et al.* Impact of pulse oximetry screening on the detection of duct-dependent congenital heart disease: A Swedish prospective screening study in 39,821 newborns. BMJ. 2009;338:a3037.
30. Mahle WT, Martin GR, Beekman RH 3rd, *et al.* Endorsement of Health and Human Services recommendation for pulse oximetry screening for critical congenital heart disease. Pediatrics. 2012;129(1):190-2.

CHAPTER

78

Acute Kidney Injury in Newborn

Mukta Mantan, Shipra Agrawal

Acute kidney injury (AKI) previously known as acute renal failure (ARF) is an important emergency where prompt and appropriate management is lifesaving whereas injudicious treatment may result in life-threatening complications. AKI usually occurs in patients with previously normal renal function but may occasionally be superimposed on pre-existing renal disease (acute-on-chronic renal failure). The incidence of AKI in neonatal units varies from 20% to 50%. Neonatal AKI is associated with poor outcomes; also these babies are predisposed to develop chronic kidney disease in future.

NEONATAL RENAL PHYSIOLOGY

Neonates are born with immature kidneys, the number of glomeruli at birth ranges from 0.3 million to 1.8 million. Nephrogenesis begins by 7–8 weeks and fetal kidneys begin to produce urine by 12 weeks of gestation. The maximum numbers of glomeruli are achieved by 36 weeks of gestation and after that only the size of the glomeruli increases.[1] During fetal life, renal blood flow is less and renal vascular resistance is high owing to low mean arterial pressure (MAP). GFR is maintained by efferent arteriolar constriction mediated by angiotensin II and this is reflected by high plasma renin activity in newborns. Endothelin is another potent vasoconstrictor, which is expressed more in the neonates, and high levels are seen in immediate postnatal period. There is high level of atrial natriuretic peptide, which help in reducing the expanded extravascular volume. Apart from these, there are high circulating levels of vasodilatory prostaglandins. Inhibition of angiotensin due to use of ACE inhibitors or ARBs in mother during antenatal life or use of prostaglandin inhibitors in early neonatal period can predispose to neonatal AKI.

The glomerular filtration rate (GFR) at birth is about 20 mL/min/m^2 in term neonates and there is a rapid increase in GFR in first 2 weeks of life. The preterm infants have a slower rate of rise in GFR. GFR reaches the adult value by 2 years of age. Also the tubular development is immature in the first few months and this predisposes to decreased reabsorption of sodium and water resulting in higher fractional excretions and greater urinary volumes. Maximum urinary concentrating ability is achieved by 6–12 months of age. The total body water in neonate is around 80% and the average urine output varies from 1 to 3 mL/kg/h.

EPIDEMIOLOGY AND ETIOLOGY

The reported incidence of neonatal AKI from different neonatal intensive care units varies from 20% to 50%.[2] Higher incidence has been reported from post-cardiac surgery neonatal units (up to 60%). A recent multicentric, multinational observational cohort study reported an incidence of 30% for neonatal AKI from 24 participating NICUs. The same study reported a higher (48%) incidence among babies below 29 weeks of gestation. Most AKI reported in these studies developed within the first 7 days of nursery stay.[3]

Better chances of survival of sick and low birth weight babies have resulted in increasing recognition of neonatal AKI in NICUs. Perinatal exposures and events leading to neonatal AKI are predominantly maternal exposure to drugs like nonsteroidal anti-inflammatory agents, angiotensin convertase enzyme inhibitors (ACEI) and birth asphyxia. Other causes include hypovolemia, septicemia, respiratory distress syndrome and intravascular volume depletion following surgery. Birth asphyxia and sepsis are the chief causes of neonatal AKI especially in developing countries. Mathur *et al.* from India described 200 term neonates with sepsis of whom 52 developed AKI. Those who developed AKI had a lower birth weight and were more likely to have meningitis, disseminated intravascular coagulation, and septic shock.[4] Bilateral renal artery thrombosis may occur after umbilical artery catheterization. Nephrotoxicity due to commonly used medications like aminoglycosides, vancomycin, amphotericin-B, indomethacin, captopril and furosemide also contributes to the occurrence of neonatal AKI. Urinary tract abnormalities, like posterior urethral valves, bilateral pelviureteric junction obstruction, multicystic dysplastic kidneys, and neurogenic bladder may also present as AKI though they would be classified as CKD later.

CLINICAL FEARURES

Classification of AKI

Acute kidney injury is defined as an increase in serum creatinine by ≥0.3 mg/dL within 48 hours; or an increase in serum creatinine to ≥ 1.5 times baseline, which is known or presumed to have occurred within last 7 days; or a urine volume < 0.5 mL/kg/h for 6 hours. AKI is further classified into 3 stages based on rise of serum creatinine or change in urine volume **(Table 1)**. It is recommended to use Kidney Disease: Improving Global Outcomes (KDIGO) classification for an early diagnosis of AKI so that measures are taken to prevent the progression of the condition.[2]

Suspecting AKI in the Neonate

AKI should be suspected if any of the following are present:

- Plasma creatinine > 1.5 mg/dL for at least 24–48 hrs.
- Rise in serum creatinine by 0.3 mg/dL over baseline.
- Serum creatinine fails to fall below the maternal levels by 5–7 days (in preterm babies may take longer).
- Oliguria defined as UO <1 mL/kg/hr after first day of life.

Criteria based on urine output may not be very reliable in first 3 days as newborns have a low GFR and the urine output is less during this period. Roughly about 17% neonates have their first void in the delivery room, 90% void by 24 hours and 99% by 48 hours. AKI can also present with normal renal output in one third of the cases. This can happen especially in asphyxiated neonates. Hence, it is essential to monitor plasma creatinine apart from urine output.

History and Examination

Specific history should be sought regarding the use of medications such as ACE inhibitors, ARBs and beta blockers by the mother in the antenatal period. The use of these medications is associated with neonatal AKI. Details of antenatal ultrasound done especially in 2nd or third trimester showing evidence of oligohydramnios and/or hydronephrosis or distended bladder in the fetus could indicate the presence of an underlying obstructive structural defect. Increased bladder wall thickness also indicates the presence of posterior urethral valves. Evidence of intrauterine anoxia in the form of requirement

Table 1: Classification of acute kidney injury (KDIGO Classification)

AKI severity	*Serum creatinine criteria*	*Urine output criteria**
Stage I	1.5–1.9 times baseline OR ≥0.3 mg/dL increase	< 0.5 mL/kg/hr for 6–12 hrs
Stage II	Increase ≥2–2.9 times baseline	<0.5 mL/kg/hr for ≥12 hrs
Stage III	3.0 times baseline OR Increase in serum creatinine to ≥4.0 mg/dL OR Initiation of renal replacement therapy OR, In patients <18 years, decrease in eGFR to < 35 mL/min per 1.73 m^2	<0.3 mL/kg/hr for 24 hrs or anuria for 12 hrs

*urine output criteria may not be very reliable in first 3 days after birth

Table 2: Pointers in history for acute kidney injury

History	*Remarks*
Antenatal history • History of medications use in mother, e.g. ACE inhibitors, ARBs, NSAIDs • Antenatal USG showing hydronephrosis, renal anomaly, oligohydramnios • Maternal fever, prolonged leaking, foul smelling, vaginal discharge	Increase risk of AKI in neonate Structural anomaly Risk factors for early onset sepsis
Gestational age, birth weight Birth asphyxia, Apgar score Respiratory distress syndrome	Increased risk of AKI in preterm and LBW Increased risk of renal injury
Blood loss, diarrhea, hyperthermia	Decreased extracellular fluid volume
Fever, lethargy, irritability	Sepsis induced AKI
Poor urinary stream, dribbling	Posterior urethral valve
Medications use, e.g. aminoglycosides, NSAIDs	Drug induced AKI

of resuscitation after birth with an Apgar score of ≤ 6 at 5 minutes or signs and symptoms of chorioamnionitis in the mother place the baby at a higher risk of AKI. Family history of fetal or neonatal deaths or renal failure may indicate a familial etiology such as congenital cystic diseases of the kidney, congenital nephrotic syndrome and tubulopathies. The pointers in history and conditions predisposing to neonatal AKI are given in **Table 2**.

Findings such as single umbilical artery, lumbar meningomyelocele, bladder exstrophy, cloacal abnormalities, palpable urinary bladder and genitourinary abnormalities should be looked for. Such babies may have underlying structural renal anomalies as a cause of AKI and are also predisposed to urinary tract infections. Blood pressure should also be recorded to identify any hypertension (neonatal cuff with an oscillometric device). Urine output of all babies at risk should be monitored carefully for early identification of AKI.

INVESTIGATIONS

Hematological, Biochemical and Urinalysis

Blood investigations required to identify AKI and its complications are complete blood counts, blood urea and serum creatinine levels. Serum sodium, potassium, calcium, phosphate should also be done. A venous blood gas should be done to detect metabolic acidosis.

Table 3: Indices to differentiate pre-renal from established renal acute kidney injury

	Pre-renal	*Renal*
Urinary sodium (mEq/L)	<20	>40
Urinary osmolality (mOsm/kg)	>500	<300
Blood urea-creatinine ratio	>20: 1	<20: 1
Urine-plasma osmolality ratio	>1.5	<1.0
Fractional excretion of sodium*	<l	>3

$$\text{*FeNa (\%)} = \frac{\text{Urine sodium} \times \text{serum creatinine}}{\text{Serum sodium} \times \text{urine creatinine}} \times 100$$

In addition, tests like C-reactive protein (CRP), procalcitonin and micro-ESR are useful in detecting sepsis in neonates; appropriate blood, urine and CSF cultures should be sent in infants suspected of sepsis. Investigations like urine osmolality, fractional excretion of sodium may be useful in differentiating pre-renal from renal AKI. The indices that help in differentiating pre-renal from renal AKI are given in **Table 3**.

Urinalysis is often bland in neonates with AKI and a culture may come positive if there is an underlying urinary tract infection.

Imaging

Radiological investigations like a chest X-ray may detect cardiomegaly/effusions due to fluid overload. An ultrasound of the abdomen helps in identifying structural anomalies of the kidneys like hydronephrosis, posterior urethral valves, single kidney, etc. Antenatal ultrasounds of the mother especially in the third trimester showing unilateral or bilateral hydronephrosis suggest congenital structural renal anomalies. Postnatal ultrasound is done to confirm hydronephrosis followed by a micturating cystourethrogram in such babies to identify lower tract anomalies.

Radionuclear scans like DTPA (diethylene triamine pentaacetic acid), MAG-3 (mercapto acetyl triglycine) and DMSA (dimercaptosuccinic acid) should not be done in the first 10–12 weeks of life as the low GFR does not allow good radiotracer uptake resulting in poor films.

Role of Biomarkers

Currently the diagnosis of AKI is based on identifying either decreased urine output or an elevation in serum creatinine values. However, serum creatinine rises in blood only after 48–72 hours of renal injury. There is an emerging need of new biomarkers that can detect AKI early so that its progression can be stopped.

Recent research has focused on identifying early and more specific indicators of AKI, e.g. plasma neutrophil gelatinase-associated lipocalin (NGAL) and cystatin C and urinary NGAL, interleukin 18 (IL-18), and kidney injury molecule 1 (KIM)-1 which get markedly upregulated in proximal tubules after ischemic injury.[5] A rise of NGAL up to 10 fold has been seen within 6 hours of cardiac surgery in those patients that later developed AKI. Elevated NGAL levels have been seen in neonates with birth asphyxia. Elevated NGAL levels correlate well with AKI and appear to be a sensitive marker of asphyxia related AKI. However, elevated levels of NGAL are also seen in neonates with sepsis and interpretation of the levels may be difficult in complex situations when multiple etiologies are contributory to AKI. Kits are commercially available for detection of blood and urinary NGAL and serum cystatin C. However, they are expensive and not routinely used in clinical practice. A recent study found cystatin C to be a superior marker for early detection of AKI in preterm neonates with respiratory distress syndrome.[6]

MANAGEMENT

The management of neonatal AKI includes managing complications and planning renal replacement therapy when required. Fluid and electrolyte imbalances are common since kidneys are the principal organ handling them. Over hydration, pulmonary edema and congestive heart failure may result from excessive fluid retention due to a fall in glomerular filtration rate and inappropriate fluid administration. On the other hand, hypotension should also be adequately treated; hypotension is common in critically ill neonates with sepsis and septic shock.

Fluid Management

Fluids must be restricted to insensible water loss plus the urinary volume. The insensible water loss in a term neonate is around 25 mL/kg/day. In preterm neonates, this can vary between 40 and 100 mL/kg/day depending upon the gestation, postnatal age, use of radiant warmers, phototherapy, etc. Phototherapy alone may increase the insensible losses by 10–20 mL/kg.

The insensible losses should be replaced with 5 or 10% dextrose solution. The urinary losses can be replaced with 0.2N saline. Potassium should not be added to these fluids till normal levels are documented in the blood samples. Besides if there is metabolic acidosis that needs correction (serum bicarbonate levels <8 mEq/L), sodium bicarbonate solution can be added to 5 or 10% dextrose solution. Urine output should be carefully monitored by taking diaper weights. Bladder catheterization should be avoided for monitoring the urine output. Baby should be weighed each day to identify any excess fluid overload.

Electrolyte Imbalance

Hyponatremia

Hyponatremia in AKI is primarily dilutional and responds well to fluid restriction. However, if there are accompanying seizures the baby should be administered 3% saline (should be given over 2 hours). The rate of rise of serum sodium should not be more than 10–12 mEq/L every 24 hours. Rapid correction of hyponatremia predisposes to intracellular dehydration especially of brain cells and can precipitate CNS symptoms and intracerebral hemorrhage.

Hypernatremia

Hypernatremia associated with AKI would require early initiation of peritoneal dialysis as extra free water administration in this situation can be detrimental.

Hyperkalemia

The emergency management of hyperkalemia causing ECG changes is administration of intravenous calcium gluconate (10%) 0.5–1 mL/kg over 5–10 minutes. This counteracts the effects of K on cardiac cells. Subsequently nebulization should be started with salbutamol (β2 agonist) in doses of 0.15–0.2 mg/kg. Salbutamol redistributes the K in the blood by promoting its entry into cells. The doses can be repeated at frequent intervals (2 hourly). Less urgent measures include administration of 7.5% sodium bicarbonate in doses of 1–2 mL/kg over 15 minutes or starting dextrose (10%) 0.5–1 g/kg and insulin 0.1–0.2 U/kg neutralizing drip. However, sodium bicarbonate should be administered very carefully in neonates as it has a high osmolality (1800 mOs/L) and its infusion is associated with occurrence of intracerebral hemorrhage especially in preterm infants. Calcium or sodium resoniums (kayexalate) can be given in doses of 1 g/kg every 12 hours, orally mixed with breast milk. They exchange potassium with sodium or calcium in the gut. Action of these resins takes a longer time to start (4–6 hours).

Table 4: Management of complications

Complication	*Treatment*	*Remarks*
Fluid overload	Fluid restriction. Insensible losses (400 mL/m^2/d); add urine output and other losses; 5–10% dextrose for insensible losses; N/5 saline for urine output	Monitor other losses and replace as appropriate; consider dialysis
Pulmonary edema	Oxygen; furosemide 2–4 mg/kg IV	Monitor using CVP/umbilical pressures; consider peritoneal dialysis
Hypertension	Symptomatic: Sodium nitroprusside 0.5–10 μg/kg/minute infusion; furosemide 2–4 mg/kg IV; nifedipine 0.3–0.5 mg/kg oral/sublingual Asymptomatic: amlodipine, prazosin or atenolol	In emergency, reduce blood pressure by one-third of the desired reduction during first 6–8 hr, 1/3 over next 12–24 hr and the final 1/3 slowly over 2–3 days
Metabolic acidosis	Sodium bicarbonate (IV or oral) if bicarbonate levels <8 mEq/L or pH<7.2	Watch for fluid overload, hypernatremia, hypocalcemia; consider dialysis
Hyperkalemia	**Emergency** Calcium gluconate (10%) 0.5–1 mL/kg over 5–10 minutes IV Salbutamol 0.5 mg nebulized (repeated 2 hourly; maximum 12 doses) **Less urgent** Sodium bicarbonate (7.5%) 1–2 mL/kg over 15 minutes Dextrose (10%) 0.5–1 g/kg and insulin 0.1–0.2 U/kg Calcium or sodium resonium (kayexalate) 1 g/kg mixed in 25% sorbitol solution (for rectal administration)	Stabilizes cell membranes; prevents arrhythmias Shifts potassium into cells Shifts potassium into cells Requires monitoring of blood glucose Given orally or rectally, can be repeated every 6 hours
Hyponatremia	Fluid restriction; if sensorial alteration or seizures 3% saline 6–12 mL/kg over 30–90 minutes	Hyponatremia is usually dilutional; 12 ml/kg of 3% saline raises sodium by 10 mEq/L
Severe anemia	Packed red cells 3–5 mL/kg; consider exchange transfusion	Monitor blood pressure, fluid overload
Hyperphosphatemia	Phosphate binders (calcium carbonate or acetate; aluminum phosphate)	Avoid high protein infant formulas

The management of complications of AKI is given in **Table 4**.

Nutrition Management

Optimal calorie and protein intake is essential for the management as hypercatabolism occurs in AKI. The nutrition may be provided via enteral or parenteral route depending upon the clinical status of the baby. The recommended calorie intake of 100-120 Kcal/kg/day and protein intake of 1-2 g/kg/day should be provided. For those on parenteral nutrition, the calorie requirement is around 90-100 Kcal/kg/day due to lack of diet induced thermogenesis. A glucose infusion rate of 4-6 mg/kg/min should be given to maintain euglycemia. In case of fluid restriction, higher glucose concentrations can be provided by placing a central venous catheter/umbilical catheter (maximum dextrose concentration of 15%). For the neonates on enteral nutrition, expressed breast milk is ideal. However, if enteral feeding is not feasible total parenteral nutrition can be provided.

Role of Drugs

Diuretics

Diuretics mainly furosemide has been extensively used in AKI. Rationale behind its use was to increase urine output and since it inhibits Na-K ATPase, it will limit oxygen consumption in already damaged tubules. However, recent studies have shown that use of diuretics only helps in fluid overload and may ease fluid administration. The use of diuretics has not shown an improvement in mortality or reduction in the use of RRT for neonatal AKI. A furosemide challenge with 1–1.5 mg/kg can be given to oliguric neonates after a fluid bolus and those not responding to this should not receive further doses. Lack of response to furosemide challenge is associated with higher chances of progression to severe AKI and need for renal replacement therapy.[7]

Mannitol

Mannitol is ineffective in management of AKI primarily due to its hyperosmolarity and may cause volume overload and precipitate congestive heart failure. The current KDIGO guidelines do not support the use of mannitol for the management of AKI.

Vasopressors

The AKI is frequently accompanied by septic shock in critically ill children. It should be managed by judicious use of fluids and vasopressors. Low doses of dopamine 1–5 µg/kg/min have been found to cause selective renal vasodilatation and found to increase urine output. However, recent studies have shown that it has no beneficiary role in clinical outcome and its use in AKI is no longer recommended. Fenoldopam is newer drug which has lesser toxicity, some pediatric reports and adult studies have shown beneficial effect of this drug in AKI, however currently no recommendation has been made regarding the use of this drug in management of AKI.[8,9]

Theophylline

The AKI occurs in almost 40% of neonates suffering from perinatal asphyxia.[10] One of the mechanisms for this AKI is adenosine mediated vasoconstriction. Theophylline being adenosine receptor antagonist is shown to have renoprotective action. When given in first hour of life, the rise in serum creatinine is lower and creatinine clearance and GFR is better. Two RCTs (n = 40; n = 70) showed benefit of low dose (5 and 8 mg/kg) theophylline in post asphyxiated neonates in preventing AKI.[11,12] A recent study from India in term neonates with birth asphyxia showed similar results.[13] Another RCT in preterm neonates with respiratory distress syndrome showed beneficial role of theophylline in prevention of AKI.[14] Based on the results of these studies the KDIGO guidelines suggest the use of single dose of theophylline in severe birth asphyxia preferably within first hour after birth to prevent neonatal AKI. While the renal outcome improves with the use of the drug, it does not have any implication for better neurological outcome.

Management of Underlying Etiology

Hypotension

Hypotension should be managed appropriately to prevent progression of AKI. In case of hypovolemia, volume replacement is required and should be done carefully as rapid fluid boluses may precipitate intraventricular hemorrhage. Inotropes should be used in cases of fluid resistant shock, dopamine is usually the first choice followed by dobutamine. Noradrenaline and adrenaline should be used in conditions associated with systemic vasodilation, e.g. sepsis, necrotizing enterocolitis. Hydrocortisone should be given in cases of inotrope refractory shock or in situations of adrenocortical insufficiency.

Sepsis

Appropriate management of sepsis using appropriate antibiotics is essential for the management of sepsis induced AKI. Avoid using nephrotoxic medication as far as possible. If they need to be administered, the doses should be reduced depending upon the calculated GFR values.

Others

Stopping nephrotoxic medications or modifying their doses in case of AKI due to drugs can prevent the progression of the condition. Premature and low birth weight infants are at a higher risk of developing AKI. Special points to be considered while managing these neonates with AKI are high insensible water loss, presence of comorbidities like respiratory distress syndrome, patent ductus arteriosus, necrotizing enterocolitis, hyperbilirubinemia, which contribute to AKI. Early attention to these conditions helps in preventing the progression of AKI.

RENAL REPLACEMENT THERAPY

The AKI requiring dialysis can be managed with a variety of modalities, including peritoneal dialysis, intermittent hemodialysis and continuous hemofiltration or hemodiafiltration. The choice of dialysis modality to be used in managing a specific patient is influenced by several factors, including the age of patient, the goals of dialysis, the unique advantages and disadvantages of each modality and institutional resources.

Peritoneal Dialysis

It is the most common modality employed in neonates as it does not require invasive vascular access or systemic anti-coagulation and has less risk of hemodynamic instability. It is a modality of choice in resource constraint setting due to easy availability and being less expensive. The indications for initiating renal replacement therapy include:

- Severe or persistent hyperkalemia (>7 mEq/L), Or
- Fluid overload (pulmonary edema, severe hypertension), Or
- Uremic encephalopathy, Or
- Persistent severe metabolic acidosis (TCO_2 <10-12 mEq/L), Or
- Hyponatremia (120 mEq/L or symptomatic) Or
- Hypernatremia.

The access for peritoneal dialysis is achieved mostly using a stiff trocar catheter. The smallest neonatal size should be used. In small sized babies, large bore intravenous catheters (16, 14 gauze) can be used. A recent report from China has described the use of 14 Fr central venous catheter as the PD access with successful outcome.[15] The peritoneal dialysis through the stiff catheter should not be continued beyond 48 hours. The risk of peritonitis rises exponentially after this period. Soft peel off catheters are available for neonates but are expensive. Tenckhoff soft catheters can also be surgically placed for neonates and the subcutaneous tunneling reduces the risk of peritonitis. The decision to start dialysis should be based on an overall assessment of the patient keeping in view the likely course of AKI. The dialysate for neonate is the available dextrose (1.7%) and lactate based PD fluid. However, in presence of liver dysfunction and certain inborn errors of metabolism lactate may not be converted to bicarbonate in the body. In such situations, a bicarbonate based fluid should be used. The fill volumes are generally 20-30 mL/kg and the dwell time varies from 20 to 30 minutes. One mL of KCL should be added to 1 liter of PD fluid once the serum potassium is normal or low. Electrolytes, blood sugar and calcium should be monitored after every 6-8 cycles. Serum creatinine can be monitored every 12-24 hours. The practical details of peritoneal dialysis are given in **Box 1**.

PROGNOSIS

The mortality due to AKI varies from 25% to 75 % in oligoanuric AKI/sepsis.[16,17] Nonoliguric AKI has a better prognosis in neonatal period. The risk factors for mortality are presence of intrinsic renal disease, use of ventilation, need for RRT and prolonged anuria. The long-term abnormalities in GFR and tubular functions can persist in up to 25% of the neonates and may progress to chronic kidney disease. All neonates with AKI should be followed up for at least for 1 year for the detection of chronic kidney disease. The KFT and urine protein analysis should be done every 3 months to look for the resolution of AKI. If they have an established CKD, then they would require more prolonged follow-ups.

Box 1: Steps of peritoneal dialysis in newborn

- A rigid peritoneal dialysis (PD) neonatal catheter can be used for access to peritoneal cavity. Besides neonatal PD catheter other catheters like 16F IV cannula, suction catheters, neonatal chest drains can also be used
- The common site for insertion is usually midline below the umbilicus, or right/left lower quadrant of the abdomen. All aseptic precautions should be used before catheter insertion. Once inserted, the head of the catheter should face up and it should be connected to a three way stop valve. The infant should have a urinary catheter to evacuate the bladder prior to insertion of PD cannula
- Once the catheter is inserted, the PD fluid should be introduced into the abdomen through an IV set attached to PD fluid bottle through one port of three way stop valve. Another end of the valve should drain an IV set into an empty bottle to collect the effluent dialysate fluid
- The initial exchange volume should be 10 mL/kg and when this volume is tolerated it can be increased up to 30–40 mL/kg subsequently
- Each PD cycle can be of 45–60 minutes with 20–30 minutes of dwell time and 10–15 minutes each for inflow and outflow. The PD is done for a maximum of 48 cycles as complications especially peritonitis are very common after this duration
- Heparin is added to the PD fluid especially after the first 10 cycles for preventing blockage by fibrin strands. 250–500 IU heparin are added to 1 liter of PD fluid. A lower dose may be used if bleeding is anticipated. Potassium 1.5 to 2 mL is added to 1 liter of PD fluid after about 10 cycles
- Monitoring during PD - blood glucose every 4–6 hrs, sodium and potassium after every 12 hours, serum creatinine every 12 hours and weight of the baby every 12 hours. Also strict monitoring of IV fluids, urine output and the inflow and outflow volume of the dialysate fluid.

KEY MESSAGES

- Incidence of neonatal AKI varies from 20% to 50% in NICUs.
- Common causes of AKI are sepsis, birth asphyxia, CAKUT and hypovolemia.
- Avoid use of nephrotoxic medications in high risk neonates (aminoglycosides, vancomycin, amphotericin B, etc.).
- Most patients with neonatal AKI improve on conservative management.
- Peritoneal dialysis is the most common modality for renal replacement therapy in neonates.
- Nonoliguric AKI has a better prognosis.
- Long-term abnormalities in GFR and tubular functions can persist in up to 25% of the neonates.

REFERENCES

1. Nada A, Bonachea EM, Askenazi D. Acute kidney injury in the fetus and neonate. Semin Fetal Neonatal Med. 2017;22:90-7.
2. Kidney Disease: Improving Global Outcomes (KDIGO) Acute Kidney Injury Work Group. KDIGO Clinical Practice Guideline for Acute Kidney Injury. Kidney international Suppl. 2012:1-138.
3. Jetton JG, Boohaker L, Sethi SK, *et al.* Incidence and outcomes of neonatal acute kidney injury (AWAKEN): A multicenter, multinational, observational cohort study. Lancet Child Adolesc Health 2017;1:184-94.
4. Mathur NB, Agarwal HS, Maria A. Acute renal failure in neonatal sepsis. Indian J Pediatr. 2006;73:499-502.
5. Nguyen MT, Devarajan P. Biomarkers for the early detection of acute kidney injury. Pediatr Nephrol. 2008;23:2151-7.
6. El-Gammacy TM, Shinkar DM , Mohamed NR, *et al.* Serum cystatin C as an early predictor of acute kidney injury in preterm neonates with respiratory distress syndrome. Scand J Clin Lab Invest. 2018;78:352-7.
7. Chawla LS, Davison DL, Mitchell EB, *et al.* Development and standardization of a furosemide stress test to predict the severity of acute kidney injury. Crit Care. 2013;17:R207
8. Brienza N, Malcangi V, Dalfino L, *et al.* A comparison between fenoldopam and low-dose dopamine in early renal dysfunction of critically ill patients. Crit Care Med. 2006;34:707-14.
9. Moffett BS, Mott AR, Nelson DP, *et al.* Renal effects of fenoldopam in critically ill pediatric patients: A retrospective review. Pediatr Crit Care Med. 2008;9:403-6.
10. Kaur S, Jain S, Saha A, *et al.* Evaluation of glomerular and tubular renal function in neonates with birth asphyxia. Ann Trop Paediatr. 2011;31:129-34.
11. Bakr AF. Prophylactic theophylline to prevent renal dysfunction in newborns exposed to perinatal asphyxia–a study in a developing country. Pediatr Nephrol 2005;20:1249-52.
12. Bhat MA, Shah ZA, Makhdoomi MS, *et al.* Theophylline for renal function in term neonates with perinatal asphyxia: A randomized, placebo-controlled trial. J Pediatr 2006;149: 180-4.
13. Raina A, Pandita A, Harish R, *et al.* Treating perinatal asphyxia with theophylline at birth helps to reduce the severity of renal dysfunction in term neonates. Acta Paediatr. 2016;105: e448-51.
14. Cattarelli D, Spandrio M, Gasparoni A, *et al.* A randomised, double blind, placebo controlled trial of the effect of theophylline in prevention of vasomotor nephropathy in very preterm neonates with respiratory distress syndrome. Arch Dis Child Fetal Neonatal Ed. 2006;91:F80-4.
15. Ao X Zhong Y, Yu X, Marshall MR, *et al.* Acute peritoneal dialysis system for neonates with acute kidney injury requiring renal replacement therapy: A case series. Perit Dial Int 2018;38(s2):s45-s52.
16. Agras PI, Tarcan A, Baskin E, *et al.* Acute renal failure in the neonatal period. Ren Fail. 2004;26:305-9.
17. Durga D, Rudrappa S Clinical profile and outcome of acute kidney injury in neonatal sepsis in a tertiary care centre. Int J Contemp Pediatr. 2017;4:635-44.

CHAPTER

79

Disturbances of Temperature in Newborns

Ruchi Rai

INTRODUCTION

Newborn babies, particularly those who are low birth weight, preterm or sick, are at relatively high risk of developing thermoregulatory disturbances. Neonates have difficulty in maintaining their body temperature due to an immature thermoregulatory system. The consequences of disturbed thermoregulation, if not promptly identified and treated, are increased morbidity and mortality. The normal temperature of a newborn ranges from 36.5°C to 37.5°C. **Table 1** provides a classification for temperature disturbances in neonates.[1] Hypothermia is relatively more common than hyperthermia in neonates. Hypothermia has far reaching consequences in newborns. Each 1°C drop in axillary temperature from 36.5°C increases the mortality by 28%.[2] This is one of the most important prognostic factors for the outcome of sick newborns admitted in a hospital.

EPIDEMIOLOGY AND ETIOLOGY

Hypothermia

Hypothermia in newborns is an important problem observed globally. Studies from India[3-6] have reported a prevalence of 32–85% among newborns admitted to neonatal intensive care unit (NICU). The case fatality rates due to hypothermia have been reported to vary from 8.8% to 15.4% in different studies and all showed a significantly higher mortality in hypothermic babies.[7-9] It is difficult to ascertain the direct causality of hypothermia to mortality, but it is certainly an important contributor. The major causes of neonatal mortality, which include perinatal asphyxia, sepsis, and preterm related complications, have been observed to have hypothermia as a significant associated complication.[10]

The reasons for predisposition of newborns to hypothermia are outlined in **Box 1**. For every 100 g decrease in

Table 1: Classification of temperature disturbances in neonates

<32°C (<89.6°F)	Severe hypothermia
32°–35.9°C (89.6°F–96.6°F)	Moderate hypothermia
36.0°–36.4°C (96.8°C–97.5°C)	Cold stress/Mild hypothermia
36.5°–37.5°C (97.7°F–99.5°F)	Normal temperature
>37.5°C (>99.5°F)	Hyperthermia

Box 1: Physiological handicaps for hypothermia in newborn

1. They have a higher body surface area per unit body weight when compared to older children or adults which increases *radiant* heat loss
2. The skin of preterm neonates is very thin, immature and permeable which facilitates trans-epidermal water loss and thus the *evaporative* heat loss. The decreased subcutaneous fat contributes to less insulation
3. Neonates produce heat essentially by a non-shivering thermogenesis mechanism. Brown fat is the primary source of heat production. The decreased amount of brown fat in preterm and low birth weight babies increases their risk for hypothermia
4. The body tone in preterm and sick newborns is decreased resulting in an extended posture. This results in exposure of more body surface area for heat loss
5. At birth the baby is born wet and naked, resulting in increased risk of evaporative loss. In addition the gradient between the baby's temperature (37°C) and the ambient delivery room temperature (25–26°C) contributes to heat loss from the baby if not adequately wrapped/dried.

birth weight, the risk of hypothermia increases by 31.3% in babies weighing < 2000 g, by 13.5% in babies weighing 2000–2500 g and by 7.4% in babies > 2500 g.[7]

Fever/Hyperthermia

The incidence of hyperthermia is higher in tropical countries especially in the summer months. The neonate tends to get hyperthermic in high environmental temperature due to immature thermoregulation. The baby may develop hyperthermia due to reasons other than high ambient temperature, which are discussed later.

The aim should be to maintain the newborn in a ***thermoneutral environment***, which is the range of environmental temperature in which the baby maintains a normal body temperature with minimum basal metabolic rate and oxygen consumption. The thermoneutral range varies inversely with the baby's gestational age and postnatal age—the thermoneutral range of temperature being higher as the gestational age decreases, and higher during the earlier postnatal days of life.

CLINICAL FEATURES

Temperature disturbances can be identified by either measuring the actual body temperature or feeling the coolness/warmth of the body by touching the baby's skin.

Temperature Measurement

Routinely temperature in a newborn is measured in the axilla, but it can be done on the skin or in the rectum.

Axillary temperature: The digital thermometer is kept deep into the axillary roof (axilla should be dry) and the arm of the baby held close to its body to prevent the thermometer getting displaced (**Fig. 1**). The temperature is read when the thermometer gives a beep/alarm.

Skin temperature: This is measured by placing a thermistor probe on the skin of the baby over the right upper quadrant of the abdomen (**Fig. 2**).

Rectal temperature: This is measured by a special, low reading thermometer with a rounded bulb to prevent trauma (the routine thermometer should not be used) (**Fig. 3**). The bulb of the thermometer is greased and gently inserted into the rectum directed towards the sacrum for half to one inch and temperature is read after 3 min. The baby should never be left unattended with a rectal thermometer in place. It carries a risk of rectal perforation.

Rectal temperature is not the usual method of measuring neonatal temperature. It is usually restricted to sick neonates or during therapeutic cooling in babies with hypoxic ischemic encephalopathy.

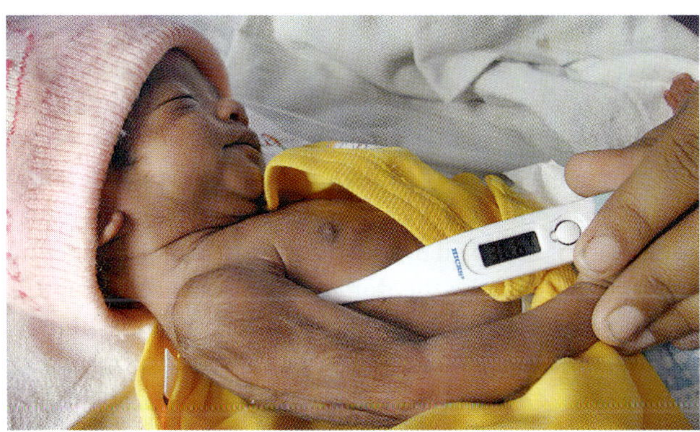

Fig. 1: Correct method for measuring axillary temperature

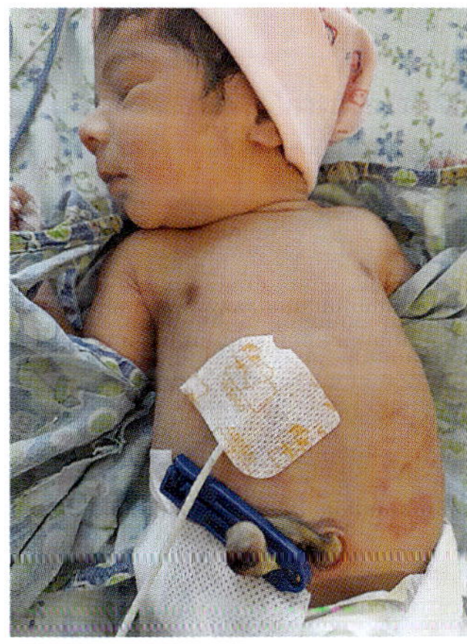

Fig. 2: Thermistor probe attached to the abdomen of the baby

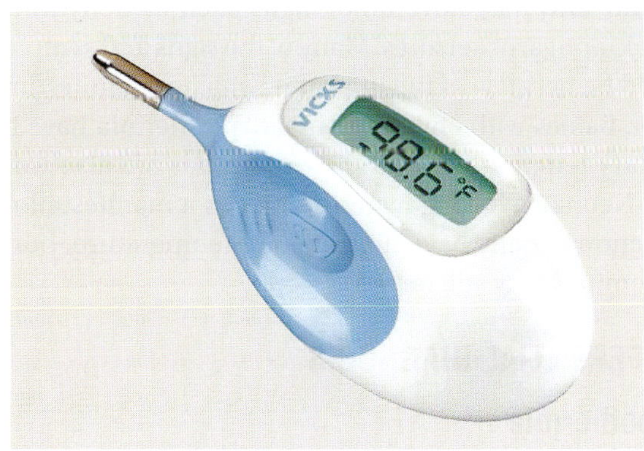

Fig. 3: Digital rectal thermometer

Table 2: Assessment of temperature by touch

Peripheries	*Trunk*	*Temperature*
Warm	Warm	Normal
Cold	Warm	Cold stress/mild hypothermia
Cold	Cold	Moderate/severe Hypothermia
Warm	Warm	Fever

Assessment by touch: Assessment of warmth/coolness can also be done by the touch method. This is very important for educating mothers for temperature maintenance at home and early identification of hypothermia. The temperature of the baby is assessed by touching the peripheries and the trunk of the baby by the dorsum of the hand. Using this technique, the baby's thermal status can be classified as outlined in **Table 2**.

Hypothermia

A hypothermic baby will be cold to touch and may be lethargic, have a poor suck and even be comatose. The baby may appear to be pale, bradycardic, have apnea, peripheral and/or central cyanosis and be hypotensive or in shock. Hypoglycemia is an important associated biochemical abnormality.[11]

Fever/Hyperthermia

The temperature of the baby is >37.5°C. Although hypothermia is more commonly encountered in neonates, but hyperthermia is also not infrequent. Baby may appear well, active, alert and warm to touch. The baby may present with flushed appearance, irritability and excessive crying; the baby may also have tachycardia and tachypnea. If the temperature is very high (>40.5°C), the baby may be red, hot with dry skin; may be unresponsive, breathing rapidly and may have other signs such as dehydration, shock, apnea, or seizures. Many of the signs and symptoms could be because of the infection, which is manifesting as fever. Babies with environmental hyperthermia have high axillary temperature and the extremities are also warm/hot. Neonates having hyperthermia as a manifestation of infection usually have high axillary temperature, but the extremities may still be cold.

DIFFERENTIAL DIAGNOSIS

Hypothermia

Hypothermia may be due to a variety of conditions:

- *Low ambient temperature.*
- *Sepsis*: Hypothermia may be an early sign of sepsis. A hypothermic baby who does not improve after adequate measures have been taken should be managed as sepsis.
- Other neonatal illnesses such as birth asphyxia, hypoglycemia, respiratory distress syndrome, necrotizing enterocolitis, etc. may have hypothermia associated with them.

Hyperthermia

Dehydration fever

The baby during the first 3–4 days of life may develop fever especially during the hot summer months. This is more commonly seen in exclusively breastfed babies. As the breastfeeding has not been properly established by this time and the mother is still producing only thick colostrum so the fluid intake of the baby is less. Decreased fluid intake along with high environmental temperatures are the incriminating factors. The fever subsides in 2–3 days when the lactation is well established and the fluid intake of the baby improves. These babies are otherwise well and active.

Overclothing

Hyperthermia may sometimes be due to overzealous efforts to prevent hypothermia. The baby is clothed more than is required and the room where the baby is kept may also be hot and uncomfortable.

Central cause

The newborn may develop fever due to abnormal thermoregulation due to central nervous system involvement such as birth asphyxia.

Sepsis

Sepsis in neonates especially in their first week presents with hypothermia rather than hyperthermia. But sometimes fever may be a manifestation of infection.

Iatrogenic

Hyperthermia is many times seen in neonates admitted to NICU. This may be due to malfunctioning of radiant warmer, probe displacement, phototherapy, placing a baby close to a heat convector when radiant warmers/incubators are not available.

COMPLICATIONS

Hypothermia

Metabolic acidosis: When the baby gets hypothermic, the body increases the basal metabolic rate (BMR), there is peripheral vasoconstriction and tissue ischemia, ultimately leading to metabolic acidosis.

Respiratory acidosis and hypoxia: Decreased respiratory effort and recurrent apnea can result in respiratory acidosis and hypoxia.

Jaundice: The liver also suffers ischemia and the hepatic functions are compromised leading to hyperbilirubinemia.

Hypoglycemia: The combination of increased BMR resulting in increased glucose consumption and decreased feeding contributes to hypoglycemia.

Others: Pulmonary hemorrhage and disseminated intravascular coagulopathy.

Hyperthermia

Dehydration, metabolic acidosis, hypernatremia, and intracranial hemorrhage.[12]

INVESTIGATIONS

- Blood sugar should be done immediately on receiving the baby to rule out hypoglycemia
- Arterial blood gas analysis to evaluate for metabolic and respiratory acidosis
- Serum electrolytes especially for hypernatremia
- Serum bilirubin
- Kidney function tests should be done especially if the baby is suspected to be in acute renal failure
- If sepsis is suspected, sepsis screen, CRP and blood culture should be sent before starting antibiotics. A lumbar puncture should be done if meningitis is suspected especially in babies with hyperthermia
- Cranial ultrasound should be done to rule out an intracranial bleed, especially in infants with neurologic features.

MANAGEMENT

Hypothermia

When a baby is detected to be hypothermic, the first step is to ensure that any wet clothing is removed and rewarming is initiated. Blood sugar should be checked to identify hypoglycemia, which if present, needs to be managed.

Rewarming

Cold stress (36.0°–36.4°C): The room where the baby is kept should be warm. Factors leading to hypothermia should be identified (like wet clothes, open window) and rectified. The simplest means of rewarming the neonate is by initiating skin to skin contact as in Kangaroo mother care (KMC). The clothes of the baby are removed but the baby should be wearing cap, socks and mittens even when being given KMC (**Fig. 4**). Baby's temperature should be monitored every 30 minutes till normal and thereafter 2–3 hourly. After the baby's temperature becomes normal, it can be dressed in appropriate clothing and wrapped warmly **(Fig. 5)**. The mother should be encouraged to frequently breastfeed the baby. These measures are usually sufficient for management of cold stress in term, good weight babies who are otherwise healthy. If the baby is preterm/low birth weight or sick, then one needs to be more alert and the baby may need admission and provision of external heat as described for moderate and severe hypothermia.

Moderate hypothermia (32°–35.9°C): Such babies need external source of heat, such as from a radiant warmer or an incubator. The baby should not be clothed as this may interfere with rewarming, but should be wearing cap, socks and mittens. The set temperature in the warmer/incubator should be 36.5°C. The probe should be firmly attached to the right upper quadrant of the baby. During rewarming, the baby's heart rate (HR), respiratory rate (RR), capillary refill time (CRT) and oxygen saturation (SpO_2) should be constantly monitored, besides the temperature. The baby should be initiated on enteral feeding as early as

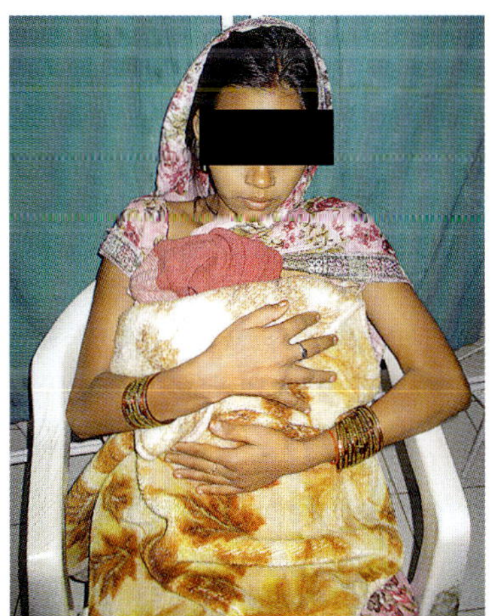

Fig. 4: Mother doing KMC

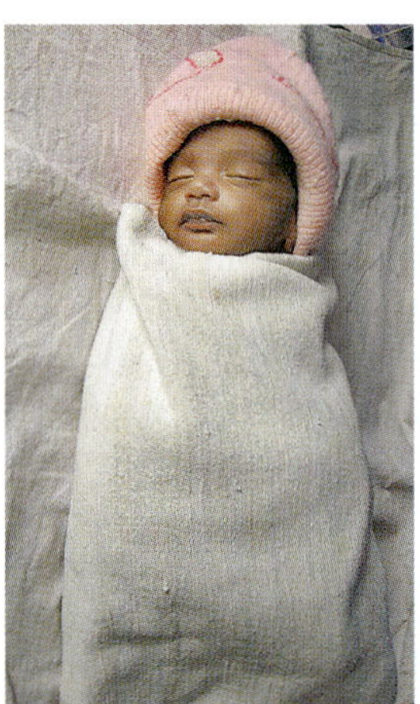

Fig.5: Well covered baby

possible; if not fit for enteral feeding and/or hypoglycemic, intravenous glucose/electrolytes solution should be started. If warmer/incubator is not available, then skin to skin care should be initiated till the baby can be referred to a facility which can provide appropriate care.

Severe hypothermia (<32°C): Babies with severe hypothermia need to be managed with extreme care. The baby should be rewarmed using servo-controlled heat source like a radiant warmer or an incubator. The baby should be given supplemental oxygen and oxygen saturation monitored continuously. Baby should be started on intravenous fluids and Vitamin K_1 should be administered. Room temperature should be maintained between 25° and 28°C. Vitals like the HR, RR, CRT, SpO_2 should be monitored and hypoglycemia should be ruled out. The temperature of the warmer should be set at 36.5°C and the skin probe firmly attached. Axillary temperature should be measured every 15–30 minutes till normal and then every 2 hours. Rate of rewarming in a hypothermic baby is controversial. Rapid rewarming (rise of temperature of >0.5°C/hr) till the baby's temperature is 34°C followed by slow rewarming (rise of temperature of <0.5°C/hr) is recommended by some.[13] There was no significant difference between rapid and slow warming in major neonatal outcomes of extremely low birth weight babies admitted in NICU in one such published study.[14]

Treat infections and complications

Infection is often associated with hypothermia. All babies must be screened for infection and in case of severely hypothermic babies, appropriate antibiotics should be started after appropriate laboratory samples have been taken. *Complications* such as hypoglycemia, hypotension, hypoxia, apnea, bleeding should also be managed appropriately, if present.

Hyperthermia/Fever

The extra clothing of the baby should be removed and the baby shifted to a room with temperature 25–28°C. If the axillary temperature is >39°C (102.2°F), tepid sponging should be done (temperature of water should be around 35°C) till the temperature comes below 39°C.

If the baby is already under a radiant warmer, then one must check whether the warmer is functioning properly or not. If the warmer is malfunctioning, it may give heater output in spite of the displayed temperature being more than normal. The probe should also be checked and fixed securely to the skin, if loose or dislodged. If a heater/blower was giving direct heat to the baby it should be immediately removed.

Dehydration: The baby's hydration should be checked. If the baby is well hydrated and active, breastfeeding should be continued and provided more frequently. If the baby is dehydrated, then appropriate intravenous rehydration should be initiated. In case the baby is suspected to be having dehydration fever and was exclusively breastfed, these babies are likely to have hypernatremic dehydration. In such cases, rehydration must be carried out more slowly over 24–36 hrs as hypernatremic dehydration based on laboratory serum electrolyte reports.

If blood sugar is <40 mg/dL, then appropriate steps should be initiated to correct hypoglycemia. If ***sepsis*** is suspected, appropriate antibiotics should be started and relevant investigations sent. ***Complications*** such as acidosis, hypotension, bleeding, jaundice, etc. should be managed appropriately.

Flowchart 1 summarizes management of temperature disturbances in the newborn.

PREVENTION OF HYPOTHERMIA

A warm chain should be maintained throughout in the delivery room, neonatal intensive care unit or the postnatal ward and even at home. WHO recommends a warm chain to be followed while handling a newborn. Steps for maintaining a warm chain for prevention of hypothermia in newborns are:

Flowchart 1: Management of thermal disturbances in newborns

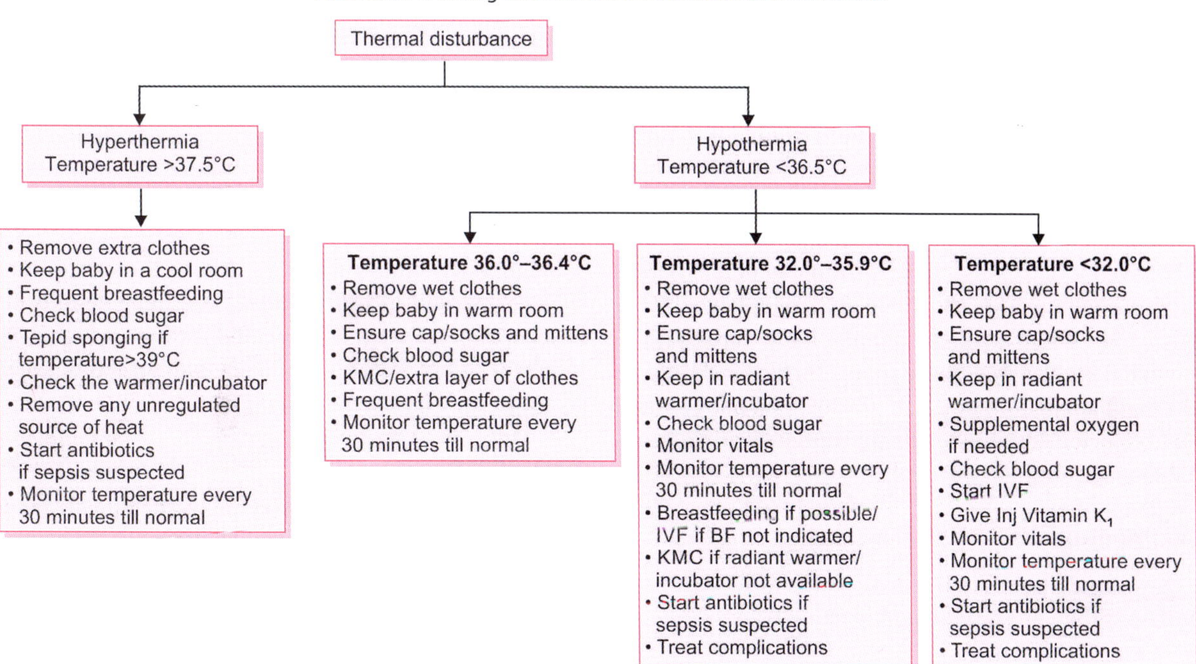

(IVF: intravenous fluids; BF: breastfeeds; KMC: kangaroo mother care).

Warm Delivery Room

The delivery room should be kept warm. The temperature of the room should be kept at 26–28°C even it feels warm to the mother and the health personnel. The temperature of the neonatal intensive care unit should be maintained at 28 ± 2°C. The temperature of the baby area inside the delivery room should be maintained before the baby is born. Ideally a radiant warmer should be available in every delivery area, which should be switched on when a delivery is anticipated, so the ambient temperature under the warmer is maintained by the time baby is delivered. The warmer should be set on the air mode/manual mode. Babies with lesser gestational age and birth weight need higher ambient temperature to maintain their temperature. When the baby is delivered and brought under the warmer the mode can be changed from air mode to baby/skin mode and the temperature set at 36.5°C.

Preterm babies <28 weeks should be immediately wrapped in food grade plastic bag even before drying, to reduce evaporative heat loss and placed under a radiant warmer. Cochrane analysis showed that use of plastic wraps or bags compared to routine care led to higher temperature on admission to NICU with less hypothermia in extremely low birth weight (ELBW) babies.[15]

Warm Resuscitation

In the entire process of resuscitation, temperature needs to be maintained. The towels used for drying and wrapping, oxygen if needed, the baby tray, pan of the weighing machine and all other equipment needed should be warm.

Immediate Drying

The baby should be immediately dried after birth using a sterile, warm and dry towel. This towel, which becomes wet should be removed immediately after drying and the baby should be wrapped in another warm and dry towel.

Skin to Skin Contact

In a term, healthy baby who does not need resuscitation, skin to skin contact should be started immediately after birth. The baby should be kept on the mother's abdomen even before the cord is cut in case of a vaginal delivery or over the chest of the mother in case of cesarean section.

KMC should be done in the NICU or the postnatal wards also to prevent hypothermia.[16]

Postpone Bathing

The baby should not be given bath soon after birth. The vernix which keeps the baby warm, should not be removed. Bathing can be postponed till the baby is a week old in low birth babies and good weight, healthy babies can be given a bath on second or third day of life. Babies with birth weight < 2 kg, should be given a bath when they weigh > 2 kg. While giving bath to the baby, care must be taken that it is given in a closed room. The water should be warm and bath should be given quickly. The baby should be quickly dried and dressed in appropriate warm clothes and the head should be covered.

Breastfeeding

The baby should be started on breastfeeds within one hour of birth and then given frequent breastfeeds.

Rooming In

The mother and the baby should be kept together in the same room and on the same bed in close contact. The room should be warm and free from air draughts.

Cover the Baby Well

The baby should be covered well and made to wear appropriate clothes according to the season and temperature. Special emphasis should be laid on covering the head, hands and feet.

Warm Transport

Utmost care must be taken for temperature maintenance while transporting newborn babies, whether from delivery room to NICU, hospital to home or from one hospital to another hospital. Special electrical blankets or phase change material wraps, which keep the baby warm on the way can be used. The baby should be well covered and transported in a closed vehicle. Skin to skin contact is a useful method of maintaining temperature during transport. The baby if being admitted to the NICU, should be transported from the delivery room in a transport incubator. The transport incubator should be prewarmed and the warmer in the NICU should also be prewarmed before the baby is transferred.

PREVENTION OF HYPERTHERMIA

The clothing of the newborn should be appropriate for the environmental temperature. In summer months, the baby should wear light clothes and multiple layering of clothes should be avoided. The room temperature should be cool and comfortable, which can be done using a fan, cooler or an air conditioner. The mother should breastfeed the baby frequently.

The baby should never be left in direct sunlight or in a car parked in hot weather. The baby should never receive direct, unregulated heat as through a room heater, a blower or hot water bottle. This may sometimes lead to hyperthermia and heat injury (**Fig. 6**).

Awareness

It is essential to build awareness among healthcare workers and the family members of the baby regarding prevention, identification and management of hypothermia. The mother and the family should be counseled at discharge regarding the steps for prevention of hypothermia. Education of mothers regarding package of neonatal care practices at the community level, which included hypothermia prevention practices like early breastfeeding, skin to skin care, delayed bathing, immediate drying and wrapping and other infection prevention practices resulted in decrease in neonatal mortality by 54%.[17] The risk factors for hypothermia in neonates at admission to NICU were found to be prematurity, age ≤ 24 h, no skin to skin care after delivery, delayed initiation of breastfeeds and resuscitation at birth.

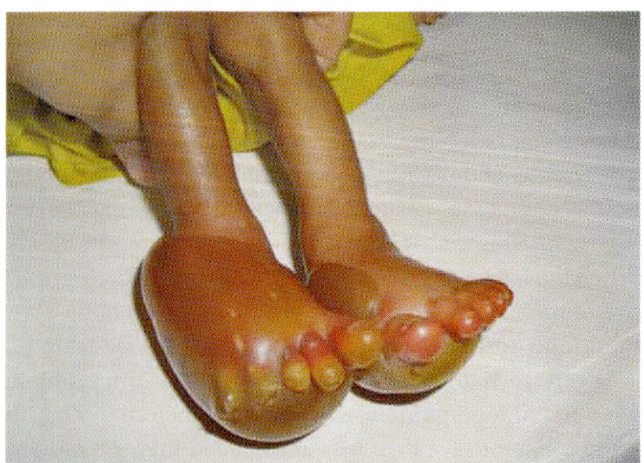

Fig. 6: Heat injury when a baby was kept very close to burning fire to treat hypothermia

KEY MESSAGES

- Hypothermia is common in newborns, especially in preterm, low birth weight and sick babies, resulting in increased morbidity and mortality.
- Mild hypothermia/cold stress can be managed at home by KMC/covering the baby well and raising the room temperature.
- Moderate to severe hypothermia needs extra heat by a radiant warmer or incubator.
- Warm chain should be maintained while handling all neonates for prevention of hypothermia. Temperature maintenance is crucial while transportation of all newborns.
- It is essential to bring about awareness regarding prevention, identification and management of hypothermia amongst the healthcare workers and the family members.

REFERENCES

1. World Health Organization. Maternal Health and Safe Motherhood Programme & Meeting of Technical Working Group on Thermal Control of the Newborn 1993. Thermal control of the newborn: A practical guide. Geneva: World Health Organization. Available at URL: *http://www.who.int/iris/handle/10665/60042,* Accessed on February 7, 2019.
2. Laptook AR, Salhab W, Bhaskar B. Neonatal Research Network. Admission temperature of low birth weight infants: Predictors and associated morbidities. Pediatrics. 2007;119:643-9.
3. Datta V, Saili A, Goel S, *et al.* Reducing hypothermia in newborns admitted to a neonatal care unit in a large academic hospital in New Delhi, India. BMJ Open Qual. 2017;6:e000183.
4. Bang AT, Reddy HM, Baitule SB, *et al.* The incidence of morbidities in a cohort of neonates in rural Gadchiroli, India: seasonal and temporal variation and a hypothesis about prevention. J Perinatol. 2005;25:S18-28.
5. Darmstadt GL, Kumar V, Yadav R, *et al.* Introduction of community-based skin-to-skin care in rural Uttar Pradesh, India. J Perinatol. 2006;26:597-604.
6. National neonatal perinatal database, Report 2002-2003. Available at: *https://www.newbornwhocc.org/pdf/nnpd_report_2002-03.PDF.*
7. Mullany LC, Katz J, Khatry SK, *et al.* Hypothermia during the neonatal period and associated risk of mortality in southern Nepal. Arch Ped Adolesc Med. 2010;164:650-6.
8. Mullany LC. Neonatal hypothermia in low-resource settings. Semin Perinatol. 2010;34:426-33.
9. Mathur NB, Krishnamurthy S, Mishra TK. Evaluation of WHO classification of hypothermia in sick extramural neonates as predictor of fatality. J Trop Pediatr. 2005;51:341-5.
10. Lunze K, Bloom DE, Jamison DT, *et al.* The global burden of neonatal hypothermia: systematic review of a major challenge for newborn survival. BMC Med. 2013. doi.org/10.1186/1741-7015-11-24.
11. Chatson KE. Temperature control. In: Eichenwald EC, Hansen AR, Martin CR, Stark AR, editors. Cloherty and Stark's Manual of Neonatal Care, 8th edition. Philadelphia; Wolters Kluwer; 2017. p. 185-191.
12. Zhao CL, Mao HJ, Xia F, *et al.* Fourteen cases of neonatal ultrahyperpyrexia syndrome induced by improper care. Adv Ther. 2007;24:101-5.
13. Agarwal A, Deorari A, Paul V, Sankar MJ, Sachdeva A, editors. Thermal care. Common Issues in Care of Normal and High-risk Newborns. AIIMS protocols in Neonatology, 2nd edition, Vol 1. Delhi; Noble Vision; 2019.p. 15-35.
14. Rech Morassutti F, Cavallin F, Zaramella P, *et al.* Association of rewarming rate on neonatal outcomes in extremely low birth weight infants with hypothermia. Pediatr. 2015;167:557-61.
15. McCall EM, Alderdice F, Halliday HL, *et al.* Interventions to prevent hypothermia at birth in preterm and/or low birth weight infants. Cochrane Database Syst Rev. 2018;12:2:CD004210.
16. Suman RP, Udani R, Nanavati R. Kangaroo mother care for low birth weight infants: a randomized controlled trial. Indian Pediatr. 2008;45:17-23.
17. Kumar V, Mohanty S, Kumar A, *et al.* Study Group. Effect of community-based behavior change management on neonatal mortality in Shivgarh, Uttar Pradesh, India: A cluster-randomized controlled trial. Lancet. 2008;372:1151-62.

CHAPTER

80

Neonatal Surgical Emergencies

Satish Kumar Aggarwal, Aparajita Mitra

INTRODUCTION

Many of the conditions that present in the neonatal age group are heralded by certain findings on antenatal imaging. In such cases, the team of physicians including the obstetrician, neonatologist and the pediatric surgeon are prepared with a set of protocols according to the information gathered before the birth of the baby. But more often than not, and especially in a country like ours, we are faced with unanticipated medical or surgical emergencies. In such cases, the diagnostic work up has to be started simultaneously with initial resuscitative measures. The pediatrician/neonatologist is the pivot around which the perioperative care of these babies revolves. This chapter aims to give an overview of common surgical emergencies in the newborn under the following headings—intestinal obstruction, abdominal wall defects, respiratory distress and obstructive uropathy.

EPIDEMIOLOGY AND ETIOLOGY

Intestinal obstruction: The causes of neonatal intestinal obstruction are listed in **Table 1**. *Duodenal atresia* is the commonest cause of duodenal obstruction and occurs in 1 per 5000 live births. About 25% of affected children have associated Down syndrome, and in 80% cases, the obstruction is distal to the ampulla of Vater. *Meconium ileus* is seen in 15% cases of cystic fibrosis. Pancreatic deficiency and cystic fibrosis are known to be associated in about 80% cases. In *anorectal malformations*, associated malformations are seen in 50–60% cases—60% are genitourinary, 25% vertebral, 20% cardiac, 10% gastrointestinal, and 15% have VACTERL/CHARGE association. *Necrotizing enterocolitis* is predominantly a disease seen in preterm infants and is 10 times more common in babies who have been fed.[1]

Abdominal wall defects: *Exomphalos* has an incidence of about 1:13,000 births and may be associated with cardiac defects, chromosomal (Trisomy 18) anomalies, or Beckwith Wiedemann syndrome in 40% cases. *Gastroschisis* has an incidence between 1:6000–1:10000 live births. It has definite associations with low maternal age, maternal smoking and use of aspirin.[2]

Respiratory distress: **Table 2** lists the common surgical causes of respiratory distress in the newborn. *Congenital diaphragmatic hernia* (CDH) occurs in about 1 in 2000 live births. Males and females are equally affected, and it is largely sporadic and non-syndromic. The incidence of *esophageal atresia and tracheoesophageal fistula* (EA/TEF) is 1 in 5000 live births. *Congenital lobar emphysema* (CLE) is relatively uncommon but an important cause of respiratory distress. It is characterized by overdistension of a lung lobe by air trapping, causing compression of the normal lobes and herniation of the affected lobe to the opposite hemithorax. *Pneumothorax* is invariably acquired and the common predisposing conditions are hyaline membrane disease, meconium aspiration syndrome, TEF, CDH, and babies on mechanical ventilation.[3]

Posterior urethral valves (PUV): This is the most common obstructive uropathy of the lower urinary tract in a male neonate with an incidence between 1:5000–1:8000.[4] About 30% of all patients of PUV present in the neonatal period. Of them, 50% will have antenatal ultrasound diagnosis suggested by bilateral upper tract dilatation, distended bladder, distended posterior urethra (key-hole sign).

Functional Gastrointestinal Disorders (FGID)

Children present frequently to the emergency department with severe recurrent abdominal pain along with associated features like distension, nausea, vomiting, irregular bowel movements.[19] On many occasions, these recurrent episodes are not associated with detectable organic pathology. These are classified as functional abdominal pain syndrome or functional abdominal pain disorder (FAPD) according to Rome IV criteria.[20,21] It has been proposed to label these as gut-brain disorders to avoid the stigma of being "functional".[22] Functional abdominal pain disorders include entities like functional dyspepsia, irritable bowel syndrome, abdominal migraine[23] and functional abdominal pain-not otherwise specified (FAP-NOS). These entities can be diagnosed on the basis of clinical features only without requirements of additional investigations.

Management of FGID includes developing a proper communication between the physician and patients or parents. Non-pharmacological approaches including dietary modifications, probiotic supplementation and bio-psychosocial interventions; placebos; and pharmacological interventions like antispasmodics, antidepressants, antireflux drugs and antihistaminics.[20]

KEY MESSAGES

- The key consideration in acute abdominal pain is the differentiation between surgical and non-surgical causes.
- Analgesia should be used and will not mask potentially serious causes of pain.
- Repeated examination is useful to look for the persistence or evolution of signs and evaluate response to treatment.
- True bilious vomiting is dark green and warrants urgent surgical input.
- Clinician should identify the red-flag signs and seek early surgical referral. Nonspecific abdominal pain is very common but is a diagnosis of exclusion once red flags are considered.

REFERENCES

1. Kim JH, Kang HK, Han KH, *et al.* Systemic classification for a new diagnostic approach to acute abdominal pain in children. Pediatr Gastroenterol Hepatol Nutr. 2014;17:223-1.
2. Kim JS. Acute abdominal pain in children. Pediatr Gastroenterol Hepatol. 2015;219-24.
3. Yen K, Karpas A, Pinkerton HJ, *et al.* Interexaminer reliability in physical examination of pediatric patients with abdominal pain. Arch Adolesc Pediatr Med. 2005;159:373-6.
4. Reust CE, Williams A. Acute abdominal pain in children. Am Fam Physician. 2016; 93:830-6.
5. Leung AK, Sigalet DL Acute abdominal pain in children. Am Fam Physician. 2003;67:2321-6.
6. Hijaz NM, Friesen CA. Managing acute abdominal pain in children: Current perspectives. Pediatric Health Med Ther. 2017;8:83-91.
7. Panebianco NL, Jahnes K, Mills AM. Imaging and laboratory testing in acute abdominal pain. Emerg Med Clin N Am. 2011; 29;175-93.
8. Yilmaz G, Pekindil G, Akpinar S, *et al.* The radiologic evaluation of pediatric acute abdomen; Results of tertiary referral center. J Belg Soc Radiol. 2015;99:34-42.
9. Hryhorczuk AL, Mannix RC, Taylor GA. Pediatric abdominal pain: Use of imaging in the emergency department of United States from 1999- 2007. Radiology. 2012;63:778-85.
10. Hampson FA, Shaw AS. Assessment of the acute abdomen: Role of the plain abdominal radiograph. Rep Med Imaging. 2010;3:93-105.
11. Scammell S, Lansdale N, Sprigg A, *et al.* Ultrasound aids decision-making in children with abdominal pain. Ann R Coll Surg Engl. 2011;93:405-9.
12. Draghici I, Draghici L, Popescu M, *et al.* Laparoscopic exploration in pediatric surgical emergencies. J Med Life. 2010;3:90-5.
13. Fein JA, Zempsky WT, Crevaro JP. Committee on Pediatric Emergency Medicine, Section on Anesthesiology and Pain Medicine. Relief of pain and anxiety in emergency medical systems. Pediatrics. 2012;130:e1391-e1405.
14. Poonai N, Cowie A, Davidson C, *et al.* Reported provision of analgesia to patients with acute abdominal pain in Canadian paediatric emergency departments. CJEM. 2016;18:323-30.
15. Sabal S, Poswal L, Gediya S, *et al.* Mesenteric lymphadenopathy in children with recurrent abdominal pain. Int J Contemp Pediatr. 2017:4:1525-8.
16. Suzuki M, Sai JK, Shimizu T. Acute pancreatitis in children and adolescents. World J Gastrointest Pathophysiol. 2014;5: 416-26.
17. Kumar B, Upadhyaya VD, Rahul SK, *et al.* Acute presentation of Koch's abdomen in children: Our experience. Afr J Pediatr Surg. 2017;14:43-8.
18. Mohta A, Bagga D, Malhotra CJ, *et al.* Intestinal obstruction due to round worms. Pediatr Surg Int. 1993;8:226-8.
19. Devanarayana NM, Rajindrajith S, de Silva HJ. Recurrent abdominal pain in children. Indian Pediatr. 2009;46:389-99.
20. Brusaferro A, Farinelli E, Zenzeri L, *et al.* The management of pediatric functional abdominal pain disorders: Latest evidence. Pediatr Drugs. 2018;20:235-47.
21. Tringali A, Thomson M, Dumonceau JM, *et al.* Pediatric gastrointestinal endoscopy: European Society of Gastrointestinal Endoscopy (ESGE) and European Society for Paediatric Gastroenterology Hepatology and Nutrition (ESPGHAN) Guideline Executive summary. Endoscopy. 2017;49:83-91.
22. Drossman DA, Hasler WL. Rome IV-functional GI disorders: Gut-brain disorders. Gastroenterology. 2016;150:1257-61.
23. Mani J, Madani S. Pediatric abdominal migraine: Current perspectives on a lesser known identity. Pediatric Health Med Therap. 2018:9:47-58.

CHAPTER

83

Urological Emergencies

Ajay N Gangopadhyay, Vaibhav Pandey

INTRODUCTION

Pediatricians and pediatric surgeons encounter children with urological emergencies quite often.[1] The urological emergencies can have a vast spectrum of presentation and may mimic common abdominal conditions. A detailed history and clinical examination are extremely important in order to avoid misdiagnosis and complications.[2] A rapid assessment and management of these conditions is imperative to limit the morbidity and mortality. Common urological emergencies in children are listed in **Table 1**.

APPROACH TO A CASE WITH SUSPECTED UROLOGICAL EMERGENCY

Symptoms

Abdominal pain: Colicky abdominal pain in flanks radiating to groin is one of cardinal symptoms of urological emergency. It is associated with vomiting which is non-bilious (due to pyloric spasm) and fever. This presentation is difficult to assess in smaller children as child will only cry and may not be able to complain of pain at all.

Fever: Fever is a sign of underlying systemic inflammatory response syndrome (SIRS) or sepsis. In case of upper or lower urinary tract infection the fever is usually of high grade and can be associated with chills and rigor. Neonates can become lethargic with fever and there is also a high risk of febrile seizure, which can hide underlying urological problem.

Dysuria: Dysuria is described as painful micturition. The dysuria in smaller children is usually difficult to assess. The child usually cries while micturating or can hold penis in males or vulva in females. In older children it can typically radiate to tip of penis and can be associated

Table 1: Urological emergencies in children

Neonatal	
Congenital • Congenital urinary ascites • Obstructive uropathy • Exstrophy-epispadias complex • Disorders of sex development	**Acquired** • Testicular torsion • Incarcerated inguinal hernia
Pediatric	
Non-traumatic • *Infectious*: Lower UTI, upper UTI, Fournier's gangrene • *Vascular emergencies*: Acute scrotum, renal artery embolism and renal vein thrombosis, urinary tract hemorrhage, priapism • *Acute urinary tract obstruction*: Urolithiasis, non-urolithiasis causes	**Traumatic** • Renal trauma • Ureteral trauma • Bladder trauma • Urethral trauma • Trauma to external genitalia

with strangury. Strangury is frequent severe urge of urination with passage of only small amount of urine.

Dribbling: Dribbling is passage of urine in the form of drops. It can be present throughout (bladder outlet obstruction) or can occur at the end of micturition (vesicoureteric reflux). Dribbling is often associated with dysuria.

Hematuria: The nature, amount and associated symptoms are very important to understand the cause of hematuria. A profuse hematuria in a child which is painless and throughout the stream points toward a mass or malignant pathology in bladder. A hematuria with dysuria is common in lower UTI. An episode of hematuria followed by severe abdominal pain and acute retention of urine may suggest a moving stone in urinary tract which has stuck in urethra. The presence of blood at the meatus with urinary retention in a child is suggestive of underlying urethral injury.

Clinical Suspicion

A thorough understanding of the chief complaint, history of the present illness, and past medical history is vital. The physical examination will identify abnormalities and narrow the differential diagnosis; however, because other acute processes, such as appendicitis, may mimic genitourinary disease, the clinician must be alert for evidence of disease in other organ systems.

- A neonate presenting in emergency department with parents complaining of excessive irritability or lethargy with fever in presence of previous history of dribbling should raise suspicion of underlying **urinary tract infection** and or urosepsis. In case of a male neonates, the most common diagnosis is **posterior urethral valves**. Congenital vesicouretric reflux with UTI and or pyelonephritis can also present with similar symptoms.
- A neonate with history of progressive constipation and features of bladder outlet obstruction, i.e. straining, dribbling, recurrent UTI must be examined for spinal anomalies and a **neurogenic bladder**. Per rectal examination in such cases can clinch diagnosis with presence of mass arising from bladder and bulging into anterior rectal wall resulting in **bladder outlet obstruction**.
- A child with a history of colicky abdominal pain (may be radiating) followed by fever, vomiting one should have high index of suspicion for **urolithiasis**.
- A child with recurrent abdominal or flank pain, vomiting followed by purge of urine in ED should raise suspicion of underlying **uretropelvic junction obstruction**. Vomiting in such cases is more common with left side lesion compressing the duodenum.
- Any painful swelling in groin with features of abdominal distension and vomiting can be a case of incarcerated, obstructed or even a **strangulated hernia**. Similar swelling with redness and tenderness can be a case of **undescended testis with torsion**. Painful swelling of prepuce or pain and discharge from tight prepuce can lead to diagnosis of phimosis, balanitis or paraphimosis.

OBSTRUCTIVE UROPATHY

Obstruction to urinary tract at any level causing deterioration in renal function is defined as obstructive uropathy. Almost one in 100–500 pregnancies have fetus with obstructive uropathy. Around 30% of these children will need intervention postnatally.

Pathogenesis

The fetal kidneys start functioning around 10–12 weeks post-conceptionally. Any obstruction in the urinary tract leads to increase pressure. A number of growth factors like prostaglandins, renin-angiotensin, fibroblast growth factors, increased reactive oxygen species and various other pathways are activated. The interplay of these factors gradually leads fibrosis of renal tubular cell and also renal tubular apoptosis.[3]

Clinical Presentation

With the advent of prenatal ultrasound, lot of cases are now being detected antenatally. The most common clinical features postnatally are abdominal distension, dribbling of urine, fever and in few cases with acute urinary retention. On examination there may be palpable bladder, renal lump and ascites. The pattern of dilatation reflects on the site of obstruction: *Infravesical*: bilateral hydroureteronephrosis; *Vesicoureteric junction*: hydroureteronephrosis; and *Pelviureteric junction*: hydronephrosis.

Management

Ultrasound can identify level of obstruction, and hydronephrosis while voiding cysto-urethrogram is helpful for diagnosis of vesicoureteric reflux, diverticulum. Renal scan is indicated to document degree of renal dysfunction.

Management depends on the etiology. The most common diagnoses are bladder outlet obstruction (BOO) and pelviureteric junction obstruction. The common causes of BOO are posterior urethral valve, ureterocele, anterior urethral valve, congenital urethral stenosis, dysfunctional voiding, vesicoureteric junction obstruction, and pelviureteric junction obstruction. Intrauterine intervention is used in cases with infravesical obstruction with deterioration of renal function. Criteria for antenatal intervention are as follows: (a) dilatation before 24 weeks gestation; (b) moderate/severe hydroureteronephrosis (Pelvis AP diameter >10 mm); (c) thick walled bladder with oligohydramnios; (d) echo bright renal cortex with microcystic changes; and (e) fetal urine Na >100 meq. Vesico-amniotic shunt is the most commonly performed intervention.

Postnatally, the most important priority is to relive the obstruction and decrease the pressure. Patients is started on prophylactic antibiotic based on the culture and sensitivity, potassium free fluid and nutrition is maintained. Once urea and creatinine are normalized, the patient is further worked up with VCUG (**Fig. 1**) and renal scan. The definitive management depends on the type of obstruction.[4] Management of posterior urethral value is shown in **Flowchart 1**.

NEONATAL URINARY ASCITES

Urinary ascites is a rare cause of congenital ascites. It accounts for one-third of cases of isolated ascites in neonatal period. Male to female ratio is 7:1. Lower urinary tract obstruction accounts for 70% of cases.[5] Other important obstructive causes are ureteroceles, ureteral stenosis, neurogenic bladder, and urethral stenosis or atresia.

Pathogenesis/Pathophysiology

In obstructive uropathy, the upper tracts are subjected to high pressures in the intrauterine life. The posterior fornix is the weakest part of the urinary system. Thus, the site of perforation is most commonly located in the renal

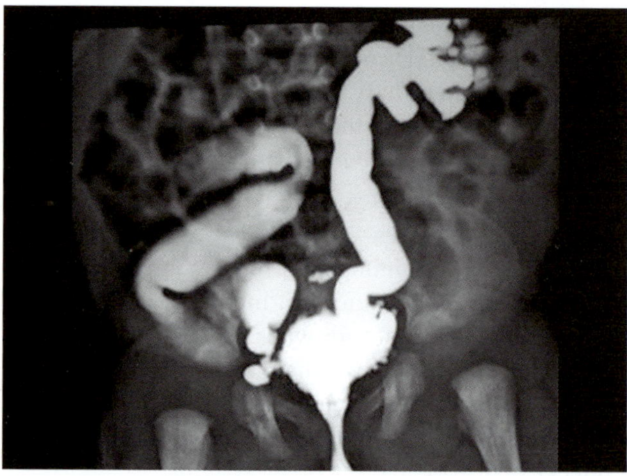

Fig. 1: VCUG demonstrating dilated and elongated posterior urethra, suggestive of posterior urethral valves, hypertrophied small bladder with bilateral grade V VUR

Flowchart 1: Management of posterior urethral valves and /or upper urinary tract dilatation with renal dysfunction

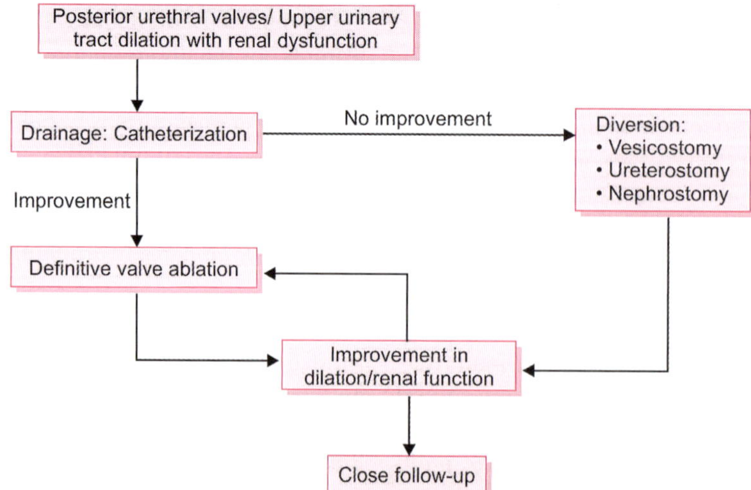

pelvis, although bladder perforation is also common. The rupture of posterior fornix is one of the pop-off protective mechanism.[6]

Clinical Features

The child presents with gross ascites at birth. They usually have respiratory distress due to splinting of diaphragm. There is usually bilateral palpable lump of hydronephrotic kidney and a third lump, distended hypertrophied bladder. There can be features of Potter syndrome (maternal oligohydramnios, renal, pulmonary, and chest wall hypoplasia) or Prune-belly syndrome. Complications such as respiratory distress and acidosis (absorption of urine from the peritoneal cavity) may be present. Hyponatremia, hyperkalemia, and an elevated serum blood urea nitrogen (BUN) level and creatinine level are also common.

Approach to Diagnosis and Management (Flowcharts 2A and B)

Prognosis

There is a risk of compromised long-term renal function due to the chronic obstruction. However, spontaneous decompression of the obstruction that results in urinary ascites is considered to protect renal function.

GENITOURINARY TRAUMA

One-fourth of traumatic injuries occur in children between age 1 and 14 years.[7]

Epidemiology

Genitourinary injury rates are relatively low and account for approximately 10% of traumatic injuries. Blunt abdominal trauma is responsible for 90% of pediatric genitourinary tract injuries, with the kidney being injured in 10% to 20% of all blunt trauma cases. Iatrogenic trauma is most common cause of ureteral injuries. Injury of the posterior urethra occurs in 10–20% of all cases of pelvic

Flowchart 2A: Approach to diagnosis of neonatal ascites

Neonatal ascites

History/Examination
- Male child
- Dribbling of urine
- Three lumps
- Ascitic tap: Raised urea, creatinine, F/S/O urinary ascites

Workup
Serum: Raised urea creatinine
Ultrasonography: Bilateral hydroureteronephrosis, with hypertrophied bladder
Voiding cystourethrography (VCUG): Posterior ureteral valves with vesicoureteral reflux [Flowchart 1]

Renal scan:
Diethylenetriamine pentaacetic acid (DTPA) or mercaptoacetyltriglycine (MAG 3): may provide information about the degree of renal parenchymal damage caused by long-standing obstruction and may show the point of extravasation

Flowchart 2B: Approach to treatment of neonatal urinary ascites

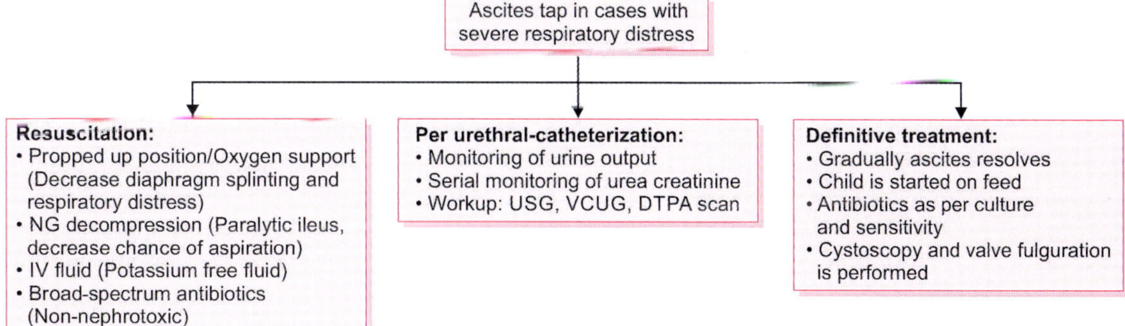

fractures with associated bladder injury occurs in 18% of patients with urethral disruptions.[8]

Pathogenesis/Pathophysiology

Children are considered at increased risk for genitourinary tract trauma. The kidneys are larger relative to the size of the child's body and are positioned lower in the abdomen, making them more exposed and vulnerable to injury. They are also less protected because of decreased perirenal fat, weaker abdominal wall musculature, and a poorly ossified thoracic rib cage. Some cases with congenital malformations with obstructed and dilated pelvis are prone for trauma.[9]

Investigations

Urine should be examined for hematuria. Focused assessment with sonography for trauma (FAST) is indicated in hemodynamically unstable patient to rapidly exclude the presence of intra-abdominal hemorrhage. Computed tomography with intravenous contrast is highly sensitive and specific for detection of parenchymal contusions/lacerations, perinephric/retroperitoneal hematoma, in delayed images 5 to 20 minutes after the contrast injection. Also, may identify urine extravasation associated with injury to the collecting system. *Retrograde urethrography* showing presence of filling defects or extravasation of the contrast agent indicates urethral disruption. Cystogram should follow the retrograde urethrogram (normal), 10% to 15% of patients will have a concomitant bladder injury.

Management

The patient should be managed as a case of polytrauma **(Flowchart 3)**.[10]

Renal injury: The patient is managed according to the hemodynamic stability **(Flowchart 4)**.

Ureteral trauma: If general condition is poor, percutaneous drainage should be performed. Later a surgical exploration and reconstruction should be done.[8]

Bladder/urethral trauma: In case of intraperitoneal rupture, surgical exploration and repair should be done. In extraperitoneal trauma if catheterization is possible most cases will heal, or in non-responder repair has to be done.[11] In urethral trauma in emergency no attempt should be made to catheterize. Maximum one attempt can be given gently by most senior and experienced surgeon. A diversion is performed and later urethra is assessed for extent of damage and length of stricture. Accordingly, definitive repair is performed.

Perineal trauma: In a female child, all cases should be suspected as sexual abuse. A proper medical examination should be done and all such cases should be reported. There is controversy regarding single staged or staged repair. All cases of Grade IV perineal tear require a staged repair or a protective colostomy. In other cases, a single staged repair or staged repair can be done as per experience of surgery, general condition of child and contamination of wound and delay in presentation.[12]

ACUTE SCROTUM

Acute scrotum is defined as acute onset pain, swelling and tenderness in the scrotum. The differential diagnosis of acute scrotum includes a few conditions which mimic each other in terms of Presenting symptoms and clinical findings.[13]

Etiology/Epidemiology

Torsion of the appendix testis is the most common diagnosis (40% to 60%), followed by spermatic cord torsion (20% to 30% excluding neonates), epididymitis (5% to 15%), and other or no pathology (10%).

Clinical Presentation

Torsion present in neonates or in adolescents as sudden onset of pain in the testis, lower abdomen, or groin, associated with nausea and vomiting. There may be history of recurrent pain or a more gradual less severe pain. The testis may be horizontally lying with severe tenderness, redness, edema a with mild hydrocele.[14]

Pathophysiology

Extratunical or extravaginal torsion is less common and is confined to the perinatal period. During descent of the gubernaculum and testis into the scrotum, there is a loose areolar plane around these moving structures, which allows the entire tunica vaginalis and spermatic cord to twist. In the normal testis, the short mesorchium attaches to the full length of the epididymis and allows testicular movement within the tunica vaginalis but prevents complete torsion. Intratunical or intravaginal torsion is more common and is predisposed to by an abnormally

Flowchart 3: Approach to management of genitourinary trauma, as a part of polytrauma management

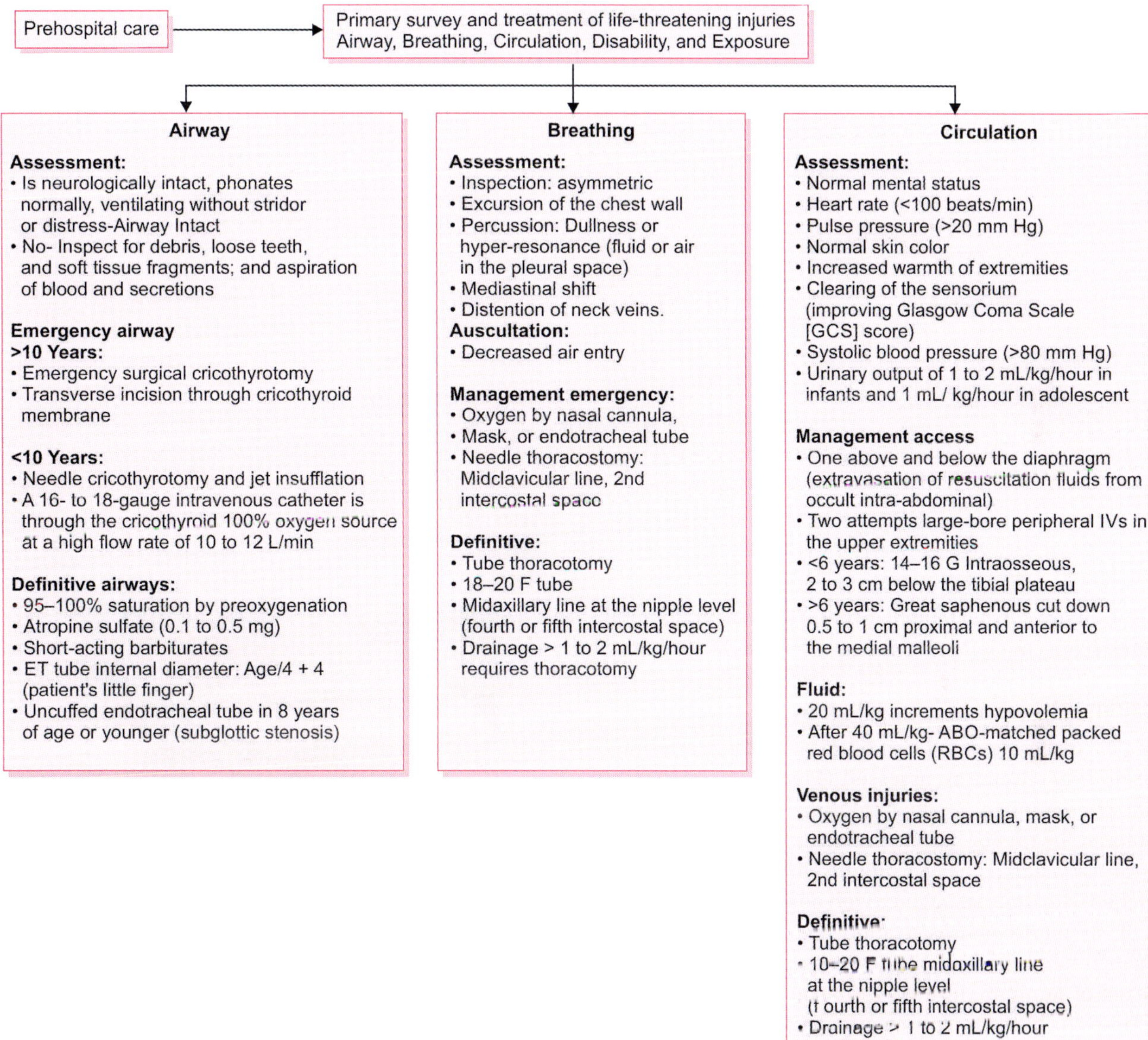

high investment of the spermatic cord by the tunica vaginalis (bell-clapper anomaly). The ischemia may occur in 4–8 hours but it can vary, a complete turn produced no ischemia in up to 12 hours.

Differential Diagnosis

- Extravaginal torsion
- Intravaginal torsion of testis
- Testicular appendage torsion
- Epididymo-orchitis
- Idiopathic scrotal edema
- Fat necrosis of scrotum

Approach to Diagnosis

Color Doppler ultrasound is the investigation of choice. It helps to demonstrate vascularity to the testis. In high index of suspicion, immediate surgical exploration should not be delayed for radiographic investigations. Treatment of a

Flowchart 4: Management of renal trauma

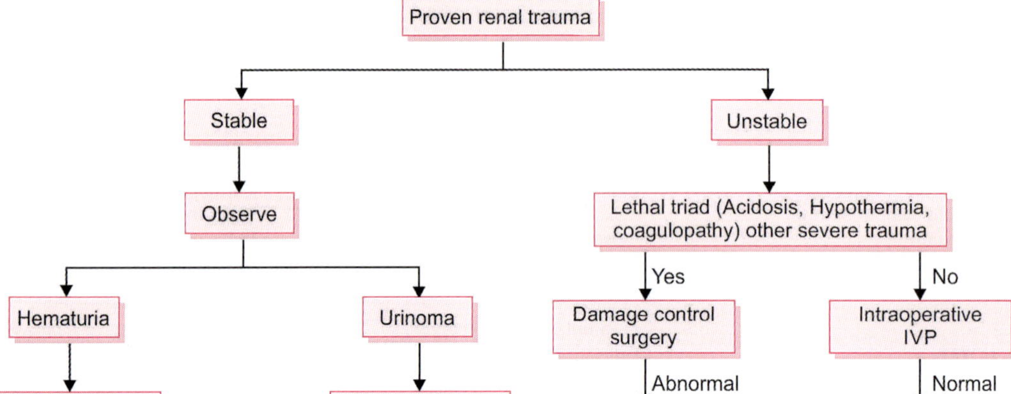

true testicular torsion requires prompt surgical exploration, before significant ischemic damage occurs at 4 to 8 hours.

Treatment

Surgical exploration of the scrotum should be performed. Vascularity should be assessed (**Fig. 2**). A warm pack should be applied. Meanwhile the opposite scrotum is explored for torsion. If it is present a window is created in tunica vaginalis by excising its part and its margin is stitched with tunica albuginea with nonabsorbable sutures

If vascularity returns, fixation should be done. In case of gangrene, (a) in children <10-year testis should be left as the risk of autoimmunization related to ischemia is low (no blood-testis barrier before spermatogenesis commences); (b) In older children orchiectomy should be done.[15]

Fig. 2: Gangrenous right testis following torsion presenting after 12 hours of pain

PEDIATRIC UROLITHIASIS

Introduction

Pediatric urolithiasis is prevalent in some geographical regions popularly known as the stone belt. Many factors are responsible for this endemic nature, namely nutritional deficiencies in vitamin A, magnesium, phosphates and vitamin B_6, low-protein and high-carbohydrate diet, dehydration, and urinary tract infection. The pattern of urinary tract involvement is quite distinct. In developed countries, it is mostly the upper urinary tract where calculi are found while reverse is noted in children from developing countries where poverty prevails.[16]

Epidemiology and Etiology

Approximately 7% of all stones occur in children younger than 16 years. Traditionally, urolithiasis was characterized by bladder calculi in children of developing countries;

the incidence of upper tract calculi, occurring mainly in industrialized areas, was much lower in children than in adults. The common etiological factors are metabolic anomalies, UTI, anatomic abnormalities, and surgical alterations in the urinary tract.[17]

Clinical Presentation

Upper tract calculi present in a characteristic fashion in the form of renal colic with severe, intermittent, refractory pain, often accompanied by nausea and vomiting. Pain may be nonspecific. It can also present as urinary tract obstruction (urethral stone). Children with vesical calculus present with dysuria, hematuria and pain.[18]

Approach to Diagnosis

Family history is present in 37% cases. History should also be sought for evidence of hyperparathyroidism, renal tubular acidosis, inflammatory bowel disease, seizure disorders treated with a ketogenic diet. Urinalysis and urine culture should be done at baseline. Serum electrolytes, blood urea nitrogen, creatinine, calcium, uric acid, phosphorus, and magnesium levels are obtained. A 24-hour urinalysis for stone risk assessment should be obtained after treatment of the presenting stone. Radiological investigations include plain abdominal radiography, ultrasonography, non-contrast CT and intravenous urography.

Management

The management in emergency is management of infection with broad-spectrum antibiotics, analgesics and maintenance of hydration. The medical therapy depends on type of stone. The most common composition of upper tract calculi is calcium oxalate. The stones are radiopaque and do not respond to dissolution therapy. Uric acid calculi are radiolucent and can be dissolved and prevented by alkalinization of the urine (pH > 6.5) using sodium bicarbonate or potassium citrate as they form at a low urinary pH. Calcium oxalate monohydrate stones may be resistant to ESWL, whereas calcium oxalate dihydrate calculi, which are more common, generally respond well. The management further depends on clinical scenario, stone size and location of stone (**Flowchart 5**).[19]

Prognosis

Children are at higher risk of recurrence as the cumulative time after 1st presentation is more. Therefore, a thorough metabolic evaluation is strongly encouraged in children after their first presentation with urolithiasis. The cornerstones for preventing stone recurrence as the child enters adulthood are the ability to render the patient stone free, elucidate and treat metabolic abnormalities, control urinary infection, and correct anatomic anomalies.

Flowchart 5: Management of urolithiasis

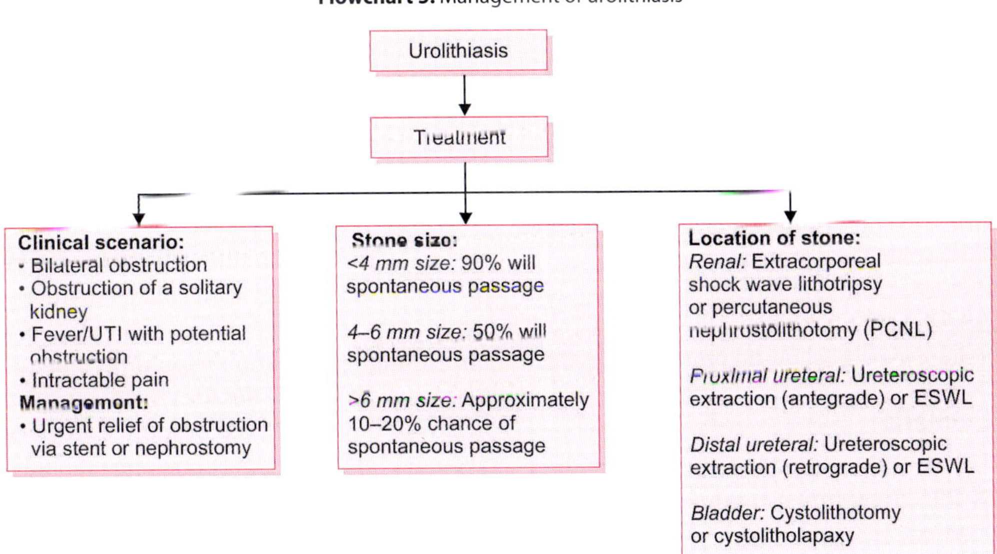

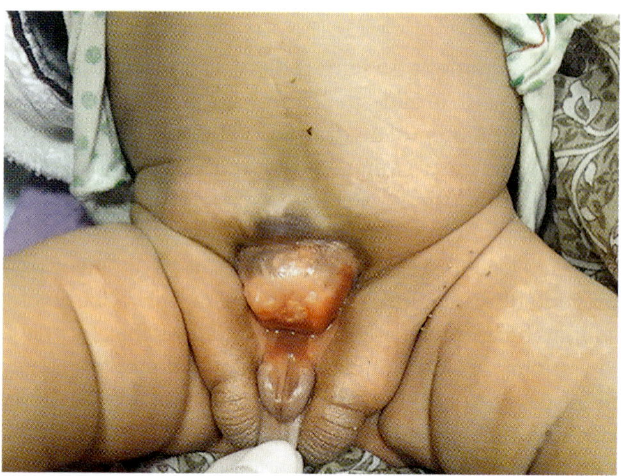

Fig. 3: Child with complete exstrophy-epispadias complex

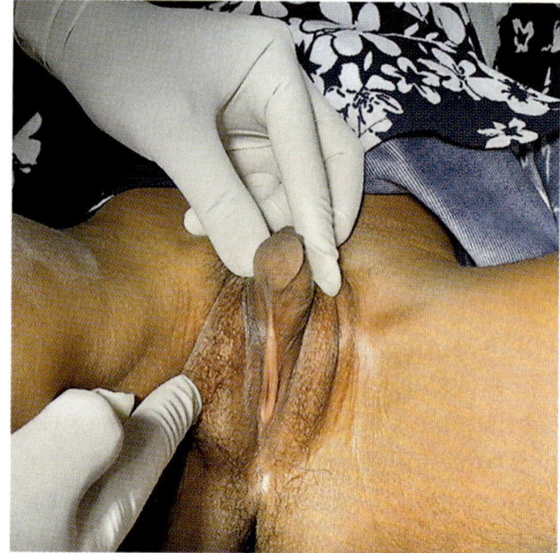

Fig. 4: Child with congenital adrenal hyperplasia with clitoral hypertrophy, empty scrotum

CONGENITAL ANOMALIES IN THE NEONATE

Few urological conditions present at birth in emergencies like bladder exstrophy, epispadias complex, patent urachus with umbilical discharge, and ambiguous genitalia. These conditions may not be surgical emergencies but may cause great concern in parents. These children need admission and proper planning and counseling by parents.

Exstrophy-Epispadias Complex

The condition presents as spectrum of disorder from simple epispadias to complete exstrophy bladder in which the posterior bladder wall is visible through a midline defect in the abdominal wall and a pubic diastasis is appreciated (**Fig. 3**). The child is allowed feeds and a workup is done to rule out associated anomalies. The treatment can require staged and multiple procedures. Team of Pediatric surgeons, orthopedician, neonatologist should plan the treatment and parents should be involved. If early surgery is not planned, parents are taught about the care of exposed bladder with moist dressing and pads and child is discharged with follow up protocol.[20]

Ambiguous Genitalia

Infants with ambiguous genitalia require immediate evaluation for life threatening anomalies which can cause severe dyselectrolytemia (**Fig. 4**). The child needs admission followed by vital monitoring to rule out hypotension and other associated congenital anomalies. The child is evaluated for serum electrolytes, urea, creatinine, 17-OH progesterone, testosterone, luteinizing hormone, and follicle stimulation hormone levels. An ultrasound abdomen is performed to see for upper urinary tract anomalies and also to see for intra-abdominal testes and to assess Mullerian structures. A karyotype is extremely useful in diagnosis. Once the karyotype is determined, serum analysis will assist in narrowing the differential diagnosis. Because congenital adrenal hyperplasia (CAH) may result in salt wasting, which can be life-threatening infants with suspicion of CAH. Other conditions need staged treatment and follow up. The treatment should be discussed with parents and team of treating doctors including pediatric surgeon, neonatologist, endocrinologist, geneticist, and psychologist.[21]

Antenatal Hydronephrosis

Neonates with prenatally detected hydronephrosis can present in emergency with worried parents. The evaluation should begin within the first few days of life. Postnatal ultrasound examination should be repeated within the first week of life. In neonates with suspected posterior urethral valves, oligohydramnios or severe bilateral hydronephrosis, an ultrasonography should be performed within 24–48 h of birth. In other cases, USG should be done preferably within 37 days or before discharge as early USG underestimates the degree of pelvic dilatation due to dehydration. In cases with normal USG examination in first week life, USG should be repeated at 46 weeks[22] as a single ultrasound in the first week of life might not detect all abnormalities.

KEY MESSAGES

- Suspect urological emergency in presence of cardinal symptoms of abdominal pain, dysuria, hematuria, fever, dribbling and acute urinary retention.
- Infravesical obstruction presents with bilateral hydroureteronephrosis; vesico-ureteric junction obstruction presents as unilateral hydroureteronephrosis; and uretero-pelvic junction obstruction presentation as isolated hydronephrosis.
- In neonates, decompression of urinary tract should be achieved as early as possible, either by per urethral catheterization or diversion.
- Genitourinary trauma is more common in children compared to adults due to unique anatomical factors and associated congenital anomalies.
- A high index of suspicion and low threshold for surgical exploration should be kept in all cases of acute scrotum in order to avoid gangrene of testes in cases with torsion.

REFERENCES

1. Lambert SM. Pediatric urological emergencies. Pediatr Clin North Am. 2012;59:965-76.
2. Bettex M. Urological emergencies in infants. J Pediatr Surg. 2004;4:730.
3. Caione P1, Nappo SG. Posterior urethral valves: Long-term outcome. Pediatr Surg Int. 2011;27:1027-35.
4. Sharma S, Joshi M, Gupta DK, *et al.* Consensus on the management of posterior urethral valves from antenatal period to puberty. J Indian Assoc Pediatr Surg. 2019;24:4-14
5. Cass AS, Khan AU, Smith S, *et al.* Neonatal perirenal urinary extravasation with posterior urethral valves. Urology. 1981;18:258-61.
6. Chilakala SK, Boulden TF, Pourcyrous M. Ruptured remnant of urachal diverticulum: An unusual cause of congenital urinary ascites. J Perinatol. 2012;32:978-80.
7. Kohler JE, Chokshi NK. Management of abdominal solid organ injury after blunt trauma. Pediatr Ann. 2016;45:e241-6.
8. Au J, Janzen N. Pediatric genitourinary trauma. In: Wesson DE, Naik-Mathuria B, editors. Pediatric Trauma: Pathophysiology, Diagnosis, and Treatment, 2nd edition. CRC Press; 2017.
9. Buckley JC, Mc Aninch JW. Pediatric renal injuries: management guidelines from a 25-year experience. J Urol. 2004;172:687-90.
10. Lynch TH, Martínez-Piñeiro L, Plas E, *et al.* European Association of Urology. EAU guidelines on urological trauma. Eur Urol. 2005;47:1-15.
11. Pichler R, Fritsch H, Skradski V, *et al.* Diagnosis and management of pediatric urethral injuries. Urol Int. 2012;89:136-42.
12. Merritt DF. Genital trauma in children and adolescents. Clin Obstet Gynecol. 2008;51:237-48.
13. Youssef FR, Shipstone D. The acute scrotum. Surg. (United Kingdom). 2014;32:310-3.
14. Yin S, Trainor JL. Diagnosis and management of testicular torsion, torsion of the appendix testis, and epididymitis. Clin Pediatr Emerg Med. 2009;10:38-44.
15. Taskinen S, Taskinen M, Rintala R. Testicular torsion: Orchiectomy or orchiopexy? J Pediatr Urol. 2008;4:210-3.
16. Edvardsson V. Urolithiasis in children. Pediatr Nephrol, 7th edition. 2015.
17. Trinchieri A. Epidemiology of urolithiasis: An update. Clin Cases Miner Bone Metab. 2008;5:101-6.
18. Persaud AC, Stevenson MD, McMahon DR, *et al.* Pediatric urolithiasis: Clinical predictors in the emergency department. Pediatrics. 2009;124:888-94.
19. Türk C, Knoll T, Petrik A, *et al.* Guidelines on urolithiasis. Eur Assoc Urol. 2014;1-98.
20. Tokhiian AD. Treatment of ectopia vesicae. Urol Mosc. 1955;2:79-82.
21. Lambert SM, Vilain EJN, Kolon TF. A practical approach to ambiguous genitalia in the newborn period. Urol. Clin. North Am. 2010;37:195-205.
22. Nguyen HT, Herndon CD, Cooper C, *et al.* The Society for Fetal Urology consensus statement on the evaluation and management of antenatal hydronephrosis. J Pediatr Urol. 2010; 6:212-31.

CHAPTER

84

Approach to Injured Child

Prerna Batra, Neha Thakur

INTRODUCTION

Trauma has been emerging as a concern in pediatric population in recent years. As per an estimate by WHO in the year 2015, injury specific mortality rate among under-five age group was 73 per 1,00,000 population.[1] Though, the problem is known to be widespread globally, epidemiology shows a variation in pattern between developed and developing countries.

Penetrating injuries are more commonly reported from North America and Africa, as against blunt trauma from motor vehicle collisions (MVCs) from the United Kingdom. Mortality due to trauma is high in Low- and Middle-Income Countries (LMICs) with South-East Asia having the second highest mortality due to unintentional injuries in the world.

Injury specific mortality contributes to 4% of under-five mortality in India. A national survey from different Indian states report a mortality rate of 302 per 100,000 live births due to unintentional injuries.[2] Increased unsupervised movement of children after one year of age becomes a reason for a higher incidence of trauma. Increased unplanned urbanization and clustering of population in smaller geographical areas leads to an increased risk of accidental injuries.

Among children, pedestrians, automobile occupants and bicycle riders are predominant sufferers. Other types of injuries that are frequently encountered in pediatric age group include submersion injuries, fall from height and burns. For a child, with multiple emergency visits for injuries with an inconsistent history should raise the suspicion of child abuse. In these children besides medical care the treating physician must also ensure social security.

TRIAGE AND TRAUMA TEAM ACTIVATION

In ideal circumstances, injured children should be managed in a hospital having pediatric trauma team comprising of pediatrician with expertise in pediatric trauma, pediatric surgeon and nurses and staff trained to take care of children with trauma. There is paucity of highly specialized trauma centers in our country. The teams managing trauma cases should be trained and made aware of some basic principles of trauma management.[3,4]

- Age appropriate resuscitation equipment should be used. A length-based resuscitation tape such as Broselow tape should be made available in all the emergencies for quick assessment of appropriate equipment size and drug dosages. **Box 1** gives the commonly used formulas used in emergency room for calculation of weight and for choosing the right size of tubes.

Box 1: Formulas for calculating age appropriate equipment size

- Weight = Age x 2 +8 kg
- Cuffed endotracheal tube size (mm) = (Age in years/4) + 3.5
- Uncuffed endotracheal tube size (mm) = (Age in years/4) + 4
- ET tube length (in cm) at the teeth = ET tube size x 3
- ET tube depth = 6 + wt in kg
- Pediatric chest tube size = ET tube size x 4
- Pediatric NG tube or Foley size = ET tube size x 2

- Providers should have expertise in placing intraosseous lines. Intraosseous line should be inserted after two failed attempts of intravenous line.
- Providers should have knowledge of pediatric fluids and doses.
- Facilities for early pediatric surgery referral should be available.
- Appropriate counselling should be done as per the need as pediatric trauma is a condition of major stress for the family.

After initial stabilization, children should be referred early to hospitals with facilities for managing pediatric trauma patients.

PRINCIPLES OF MANAGEMENT

Unique Characteristics of Pediatric Trauma

While catering to pediatric population we must be aware of their unique anatomical and physiological differences as compared to adult population which will guide both our resuscitation and response to resuscitation. These anatomical and physiological changes and their implications are given in **Table 1**.

APPROACH TO INJURED CHILD

Primary Survey

An injured child should be assessed, and managed in a systematic approach based on rapid primary survey with simultaneous resuscitation of vital functions, followed by a more detailed secondary survey, and the initiation of definitive care.[3] The primary survey comprises of the ABCDE approach based on Advanced Trauma Life Support (ATLS) principles of trauma care.

- Airway maintenance with restriction of cervical spine motion
- Breathing and ventilation
- Circulation with hemorrhage control
- Disability (assessment of neurologic status)
- Exposure/Environmental control.

Identification of life and limb threatening injuries and their treatment is given the priority in primary survey. The management follows degree of life threat and the abnormality posing the greatest threat to life is addressed first.

Table 1: Unique anatomical and physiological characteristics in children

Primary survey	*Pitfalls*	*Prevention/Management*
Airway	• Larynx and vocal cords are more cephalad and anterior in the neck • Short length of trachea can result in intubation of right mainstem bronchus	• Proper positioning for airway maintenance by orotracheal intubation under direct vision and restriction of cervical movement
Breathing	• Hypoxia is the most common cause of pediatric cardiac arrest • Respiratory acidosis due to prolonged hypoxia is the most common acid-base abnormality encountered during resuscitation of injured children • Chest wall is thin in children • Mediastinal structures are mobile hence children are more susceptible to tension pneumothorax	• Pediatric bag-mask is recommended for children under 30 kg otherwise iatrogenic barotrauma can occur due to lower tidal volume • Respiratory acidosis to be corrected by proper ventilation • Tunneling to be done while inserting chest tube in children • Decompression by inserting needle in second intercostal space
Circulation	• Increased physiological reserve is seen in children with subtle changes in vital parameters and rapid deterioration • Difficult venous access	• Identification of tachycardia and mottled skin as early markers of hypovolemia before fall in blood pressure • Age appropriate vitals to be used along with early fluid resuscitation • Weight based fluid resuscitation along with early use of blood products • Early use of intraosseous route
Disability/ Neurological	• Larger head size with relatively smaller subarachnoid space • Children are particularly prone to secondary brain injury	• CT cranium indicated along with early neurosurgical reference to rule out surgical intervention • Maintenance of cerebral blood flow by preventing hypotension is essential
Exposure	• High ratio of body surface area to body mass in children hence increased chances of hypothermia due to heat loss	• Pre-warmed fluids, warm room and blankets to be used to decrease the heat loss

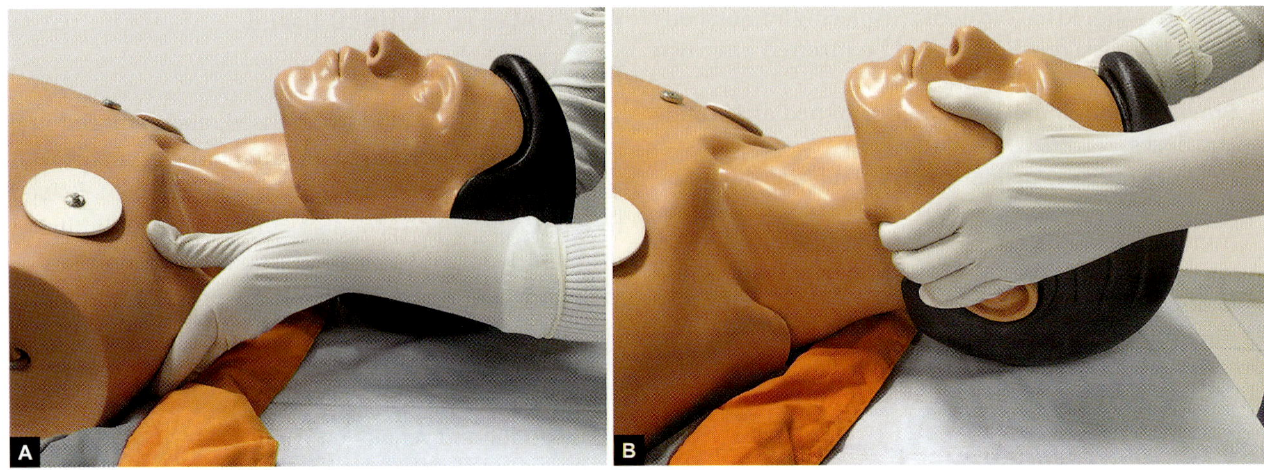

Figs. 1A and B: (A) Manual cervical inline stabilization; (B) Jaw thrust maneuver

Airway maintenance with cervical spine immobilization

One has to *LOOK* at the patient's sensorium, *LISTEN* for abnormal breath sounds and *FEEL* for position of trachea for airway assessment in an injured child. Inability to secure airway in a trauma patient can lead to lack of oxygenation and ventilation and instant death. Thus, securing airway is of utmost importance in an injured child. Oral airway (Goodle airway) should be inserted in unconscious children to prevent aspiration.

If a child is able to communicate, it virtually rules out major airway injuries. In unconscious children, GCS <8 with absent gag reflex, signs of ventilatory failure, significant hypovolemia or need for operative intervention become indication for a definitive airway. Cervical spine immobilization should be done by bimanual in-line spinal immobilization and jaw-thrust maneuver or cervical collar ***(Figs. 1A and B)***. Head tilt-chin lift carries the risk of unstabilization of cervical spine, hence is not preferred, unless cervical spine has been cleared. A one-inch padding can be placed below the infant or toddler's torso to maintain neutral alignment of cervical spine. Sniffing position should be avoided.

A potentially difficult airway can be predicted using mnemonic LEMON ***(Box 2)***. Orotracheal intubation should be performed with appropriate sized ET tube. Earlier, uncuffed tubes were preferred over cuffed ones in infants and young children, due to risk of tracheal necrosis, however with improved quality of cuffed tubes, even these can be safely used. A rough estimate of the size of ET tube can be made by using tube that approximates to the size of child's nares or little finger. One size smaller and one size bigger tube should be kept handy. ET depth should be approximately three times the internal diameter of the tube.

Box 2: LEMON assessment for difficult airway

L—Look externally for features of difficult intubation
E—Evaluate by 3-3-2 rule, to assess for the alignment of pharyngeal, laryngeal and oral anatomy
M—Mallampati classification for visual assessment of hypopharynx
O—Obstruction, e.g. conditions like epiglottitis, peritonsillar abscess and trauma
N—Neck mobility to anticipate difficulty during intubation

Drug assisted intubation (DAI), also known as rapid sequence intubation (RSI) should be done using atropine (0.01 mg/kg to 0.03 mg/kg), etomidate (0.1 mg/kg in hypovolemic children and 0.3 mg/kg in euvolemic children) and vecuronium (0.1 mg/kg), rocuronium (0.6 mg/kg) or succinylcholine (1–2 mg/kg). Patients should be preoxygenated before attempting intubation. Right placement of ET tube should be ascertained either clinically by auscultation or by colorometric capnography device or ETCO2 measurement.[4,5]

Nasotracheal intubation can be performed in spontaneously breathing patients to support ventilation. However, frontal sinus, basilar skull and cribriform plate fractures are relative contraindications. Laryngeal mask

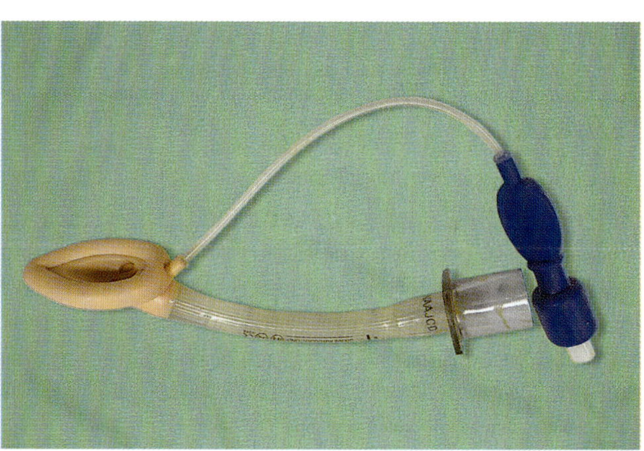

Fig. 2: Laryngeal mask airway

airway (LMA) ***(Fig. 2)***, intubating laryngeal mask airway or needle cricothyroidotomy can be used in difficult to intubate children as rescue measure, though every effort should be made to secure a definitive airway as early as possible.

Breathing and ventilation

Patent airways do not imply adequate ventilation. For adequate gas exchange and oxygenation adequate function of the lungs, chest wall, and diaphragm is required. Hence an assessment of ventilation is done keeping in mind the steps of *LOOK* for symmetrical chest rise, *LISTEN* for movement of air by auscultation and pulse oximetry. Injured children should be supplemented with oxygen using reservoir face mask. Nasal catheter, nasal canula or non-rebreather mask can also be used.

In case of ineffective ventilation, bag and mask or bag and tube ventilation should be initiated ensuring adequate seal, appropriate sized mask and ambu bag.

An injured child may have pneumothorax or hemothorax as a complication of injury or may even develop tension pneumothorax, which may hamper adequate breathing. Needle decompression should be performed in suspected tension pneumothorax in 2nd intercostal space in mid clavicular line. Chest tube should be placed in case of pneumothorax or hemothorax in 5th intercostal space, anterior to mid axillary line.

Circulation with hemorrhage control

One need to assess level of consciousness, skin colour and pulse for assessment of circulation. Shock in injured children is presumed to be due to hemorrhage unless proven otherwise. Failure to recognize hemorrhagic shock or inadequate treatment of shock is the most common cause of death in trauma. Definitive bleeding control along with appropriate replacement of intravascular volume is the key to successful management of hemorrhagic shock. Aggressive and continuous volume resuscitation without bleeding control would lead to more damage. One should try to look actively for the source of external or internal bleeding. Focused Assessment with Sonography in Trauma (FAST), chest X-ray and pelvic X-ray may be used to identify any internal source of bleeding.[6] Intravenous line should be secured with large bore cannulae and fluid resuscitation should be initiated. In case of difficulty in establishing intravenous line, intraosseous line should be secured without delay. A bolus of 20 mL/kg of warm isotonic saline should be given. Three such boluses can be given to replenish 25% of blood loss. Packed red blood cells as 10 mL/ kg can be considered while third crystalloid bolus is being considered. One can go for type specific or O negative blood. Severely injured children are also at risk of coagulopathy hence early use of blood products is recommended.

Disability (assessment of neurologic status)

A rapid neurologic evaluation establishes the patient's level of consciousness and pupillary size and reaction; identifies the presence of lateralizing signs; and determines spinal cord injury level, if present. AVPU is a simple scale to assess and monitor sensorium of a child. It determines the response of child to stimulus. A more objective Glassgow coma scale can be used, though it is more elaborate. AVPU stands for A-Alert; V-Responsive to verbal stimulus; P-Responsive to painful stimulus; and U-Unresponsive.

Exposure/Environmental control

It is important to expose the patient completely and look for any bleeding or penetrating wounds at the sites like back and chest. Hypothermia can be present on patient's arrival or can develop in the hospital while examining. It is a potentially lethal complication in injured patients as it will escalate the coagulopathy associated with trauma. This can be prevented by using prewarmed fluid for resuscitation, examining the patient in warm room and quickly covering the patient with blankets after examination and resuscitation.

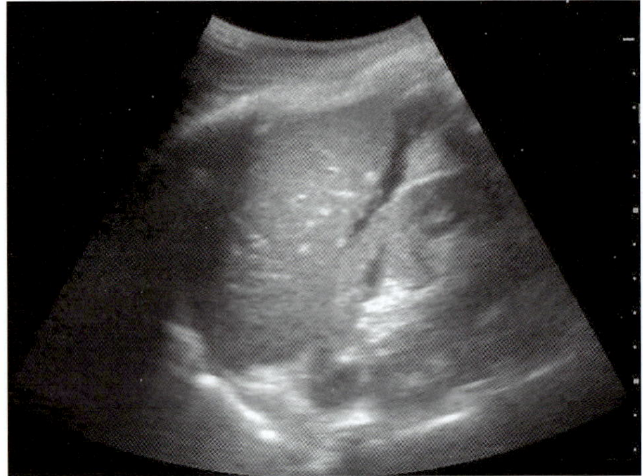

Fig. 3: Positive FAST (Fluid in hepato-renal fossa)

Adjuncts to Primary Survey

Physiologic parameters such as ventilatory rate, blood pressure, pulse pressure, body temperature, gastric aspirate and urinary output are to be recorded and monitored continuously. Values for these parameters should be obtained as soon as is practical during or after completing the primary survey and re-evaluated periodically. Electrocardiographic (ECG) recording, arterial blood gas (ABG) parameters, pulse oximetry, X-ray chest and pelvis, should be done in injured children in the ER itself. FAST is a useful adjunct to primary survey for bedside detection of intra-abdominal bleed and positive FAST indicates need for operative intervention[5,6] **(Fig. 3)**.

Secondary Survey

After completing primary survey and simultaneous stabilization, a detailed head-to-toe evaluation of the patient is done. It includes history taking with physical examination and reassessment of vitals.[4]

History

A quick *AMPLE history* has to be taken. Such a history is usually obtained by the person accompanying and may not be available all the time. AMPLE stands for

- A—Allergies
- M—Medications
- P—Past illnesses/Pregnancy
- L—Last meal
- E—Event/Environment related to injury

Examination

Head and spine: Children have larger head compared to their body with decreased subarachnoid space hence are more prone to head injuries. Their spine is more flexible with vertebral bodies wedged anteriorly and hence tend to slide forward with flexion. Children's relatively large head compared with their neck result in greater angular momentum and hence more chances of injury near occiput and upper cervical spine.

Thorax: Children have pliable and compliant chest wall which allows kinetic energy to be transmitted to the underlying pulmonary parenchyma, causing pulmonary contusion but rib fractures and mediastinal injuries are not common; if present, they indicate a severe impacting force. Children are more prone to pneumothorax due to mobility of mediastinal structures.

Abdomen: Lap belt when applied appropriately itself can prevent a number of abdominal visceral injuries. Enteric disruption due to lap belt injuries, blunt pancreatic injuries, small bowel perforations are often undiagnosed because of the vague symptoms. Hence high index of suspicion for these injuries should be kept particularly in blunt upper abdominal trauma. Bladder rupture is again more common in children as compared to adults, because of the shallow depth of the child's pelvis.

Musculoskeletal system: Children are more prone to "greenstick" fractures due to immature, pliable nature of bones. Supracondylar fractures at the elbow or knee have high chances of associated vascular injury as well as injury to the growth plate. Unlike adults, blood loss accompanying major bone fractures is less. Hence if there is hemodynamic compromise associated with isolated long bone fracture, other causes of blood loss should be promptly evaluated.

INVESTIGATIONS

Further specialized investigations can be done after secondary survey to pinpoint specific injuries. Complete cervical and thoracolumbar spine X-rays, CT scan brain and spine may be done as per indication, once the child is hemodynamically stabilized.

Table 2: Radiological anatomical normal variants in children

	Normal finding	*X-ray*
Cranium	Skeletal growth centers can mimic fractures	Apical odontoid epiphyses appear as separation on odontoid X-ray (between 5 and 11 years)
Spine	Pseudosubluxation (<7 yrs)	Anterior displacement of C2 on C3. Up to 3 mm of movement may be seen when these joints are studied by flexion and extension maneuvers Pseudosubluxation disappears by placing shoulder role
FAST	Incapable of identifying isolated intraparenchymal injuries, which account for up to one-third of solid organ injuries in children	

Box 3: PECARN criteria for CT scan in blunt head trauma

Clinical criteria	*Recommendation for CT head*
Children < 2 years	
GCS≤14 or altered mental status or palpable skull fracture	CT
GCS>14, no altered mental status, no palpable skull fracture Occipital, parietal or temporal scalp hematoma, or loss of consciousness ≥5 seconds, or severe mechanism of injury or not acting normally	Observation Vs CT depending on physician experience, multiple vs isolated findings, worsening symptoms or signs during observation, age<3 months, parental preference
Children > 2 years	
GCS≤14 or altered mental status or signs of basilar skull fracture	CT
GCS>14, no altered mental status, no signs of basilar skull fracture History of loss of consciousness or vomiting or severe headache or severe mechanism of injury	Observation Vs CT depending on physician experience, multiple vs isolated findings, worsening symptoms or signs during observation, age<3 months, parental preference

Anatomical differences between pediatric and adults reflect in radiological investigations too. **Table 2** gives some of the findings that should be given due consideration while interpreting the results of these investigations.

Role of CT Head in Childhood Trauma

Children have long term after-effects of trauma both physically and mentally. Radiation hazard is one of them which has been proved to be associated with malignancies later in life. Hence ALARA (as low as reasonably achievable) CT scans are to be considered in management of pediatric trauma. CT scans should only be advised when medically necessary, and results are likely to change management. We should preferably scan only the area of interest with the lowest radiation dose possible. Pediatric emergency care applied research network (PECARN) have given prediction rules for getting a CT scan done in case of blunt head trauma to identify clinically important traumatic brain injuries (ciTBI). These rules were validated after analyzing 42,412 children, less than 18 years of age, who presented to emergency within 24 hours of head injury and had GCS of 14–15 (**Box 3**).[7,8]

- Children also suffer a unique entity called spinal cord injury without radiographic abnormalities SCIWORA). Hence, a normal spinal radiograph does not rule out spinal cord injury.
- If we get multiple fractures in a child or fractures in different stages of healing or we get injuries which remains unexplained as per the developmental milestones e.g. fracture femur in infants, then child abuse must be suspected.

PATIENT DISPOSITION

Majority of children would respond well to treatment and would have no hemodynamic abnormalities, nevertheless there would be some children particularly those with multisystemic injuries who would require early referral to tertiary care center. Every effort should be made for safe transport of the injured child to a specialized trauma facility.

INJURY PREVENTION

The greatest pitfall in pediatric injury is the failure to prevent the injury itself. Children most commonly suffer from motor vehicle accidents either as occupant or pedestrian. Majority of injuries can be prevented by simple measures like wearing helmets while riding bicycles or wearing seat belts in car. Prevention of childhood injuries helps in avoiding social and familial disruption besides decreasing financial burden to the family and nation.[5]

CLINICAL CASE SCENARIO

A 7-year-old male child was stuck by a car while he was crossing road. At the scene patient was moaning and asking for mother. He had marked respiratory distress. Vitals at the scene of accident were Respiratory rate 30/min, Heart Rate 160/min, BP 80/40 mm Hg, and SpO_2 80%. He was transported by CATS ambulance to tertiary care hospital having facility of pediatric trauma management on face mask with rebreathing mask. He was immobilized on long spinal board with cervical collar applied. Child was assessed on reaching to hospital by emergency physician. The assessment was as follows:

	Assessment findings	*Intervention*
Airway	Moaning, able to speak	Patent
Breathing	RR 30/min, SpO_2 82%	Intubated and bag and mask ventilation started
Circulation	HR 158/min, BP 80/42 mm Hg	Two large bore canulae taken, NS bolus 20 mL/kg
Disability	Responding to painful stimulus, pupils bilaterally normal size, normally reacting	No intervention required
Exposure	No external bleed	No intervention required

Case Progression

On reassessment, airway was maintained, SpO_2 was 84%, BP 86/50 mm Hg. A detailed chest examination showed decreased breath sounds on right side of chest. Possibility of tension pneumothorax was kept. Needle decompression was done on right side in ER itself. Saturation improved to 92%. BP was 90/60 mm Hg. Another bolus of normal saline was given by 20 mL/kg. Chest X-ray and FAST was done. Chest X-ray showed right sided pneumothorax with possibility of right sided pulmonary contusion. No rib fractures were seen. FAST was negative. Using pediatric resuscitation tape, correct size chest tube was placed on right side. Reassessment of the patient showed patent airway, SpO_2 98%, PR 84/min, BP 100/60 mm Hg.

KEY MESSAGES

- Trauma is a common cause of mortality and morbidity both in developed and developing nations.
- Pediatric trauma cases should be managed in tertiary care centers capable of managing the same.
- Trauma team managing pediatric trauma must be aware of the unique anatomical and physiological characteristics of children.
- Initial assessment and management of severely injured children should follow the ABCDE approach.
- Avoid hypothermia while managing pediatric trauma patients.
- Children have both short term and long term complications of trauma particularly radiation hazard. PECARN criteria is advocated to reduce unnecessary CT Cranium.
- Early involvement of pediatric surgeon is essential.

REFERENCES

1. WHO. World Health Statistics 2015. Available from: *http://apps.who.int/iris/bitstream/handle/10665/170250/9789240694439_eng.pdf?sequence=1*. Accessed July 26, 2019.
2. Kundal VK, Debnath PR, Sen A. Epidemiology of pediatric trauma and its pattern in urban India: A tertiary care hospital-based experience. J Indian Assoc Pediatr Surg. 2017;22:33-7.
3. American College of Surgeons. Advanced Trauma Life Support (ATLS) Student Course Manual. 10th edition. Chicago: American College of Surgeons; 2018.
4. Lavoie M, Nance ML. Approach to the injured child. In: Shaw KN, Bachur RG, editors. Fleisher and Ludwig's Textbook of Pediatric Emergency Medicine, 7th edition. China: Lippincott Williams & Wilkin; 2016. p. 9-19.
5. Mikrogianakis A, Grant V. The kids are alright: Pediatric trauma pearls. Emerg Med Clin North Am. 2018;36:237-57.
6. Sola JE, Cheung MC, Yang R, *et al.* Pediatric FAST and elevated liver transaminases: An effective screening tool in blunt abdominal trauma. J Surg Res. 2009;157:103-7.
7. Kuppermann N, Holmes JF, Dayan PS, *et al.* Pediatric Emergency Care Applied Research Network (PECARN). Identification of children at very low risk of clinically-important brain injuries after head trauma: A prospective cohort study. Lancet. 2009;374:1160-70.
8. Connelly CR, Yonge JD, Eastes LE, *et al.* Performance improvement and patient safety program-guided quality improvement initiatives can significantly reduce computed tomography imaging in pediatric trauma patients. J Trauma Acute Care Surg. 2016;81:278-84.

CHAPTER

85

Traumatic Brain Injuries

Shweta Kedia, Deepak K Gupta, Ashish Suri

INTRODUCTION

Trauma remains the leading cause of death in the pediatric population age >1 year. The emotional and economic burden of a child with head trauma is immense. Nothing can be described as worse tragedy than a child losing life because of trauma. A thorough understanding of the modes of injury, injury characteristics and the management principles is needed to improvise the functional outcome. We intend to discuss the same in the forthcoming pages. We will also highlight the recent advances in the management of severe traumatic brain injuries (TBI).

EPIDEMIOLOGY

Incidence of pediatric TBI range from 47 to 280/1,00,000 children, affecting more than 3 million kids world over.[1] Almost 20% of the emergency visits by children were because of TBI in India, although a declining trend has been observed recently.[2] Dewan *et al.* studied 1,65,000 pediatric head injury patients globally and observed that they have a bimodal age presentation (0–2 years and 15–18 years).[3] After age >3 years, boys suffered more injury. Mild trauma was commonest (80%) and surgery required in only 10% of injured. However, outcome for severe TBI is 50% in the best of centers.[4] The annual death rate is 5 per 1,00,000 in kids younger than 4 years. A study at AIIMS, Delhi on 29 brain injured infants observed 10% as in-hospital mortality.[5] Younger kids succumb to injury more easily.[6]

Mode of injury: Children between 0 and 4 years presented with fall most commonly. Assault accounted for most life lost under age 4 among > 40% of TBI related deaths in USA.[7] However, only 0.4 % of visits to hospital reported assault as the mode of injury. Above age 4, motor vehicular accidents were common. Pedestrians are commonly affected in Asian countries, while vehicular occupants in USA.[8]

Low and middle income countries have almost 3.5 times the incidence of pediatric injuries.[9] Likewise, urban area and summer months had more trauma patients. Use of mobile phones while driving is a new reason for TBI.[10]

BIOMECHANICS

Two common mechanisms of injury, impact and impulsive loading are involved in TBI. Compliant skull of a child is incapable of bearing the bending loads. Any forceful impact brings in large plastic and elastic deformation in the skull resulting in varied skull fractures. A propagating wave is set distant from the point of impact producing counter coup injury. Impulsive loading is seen when a fast moving vehicle is brought to a sudden halt. Here load gets transmitted through the seat to the upper torso and neck and then to the head. Thus, the injury is witnessed in cervical spine and craniovertebral junction.

Shaken baby syndrome usually involves both the impulsive loading and the forceful impact at the cranial point. Repeated shaking results in tearing of the bridging vessels. Neck muscles are weak in infants resulting in differential motion between the brain and skull and neck producing significant cerebral as well as cervical neck trauma.

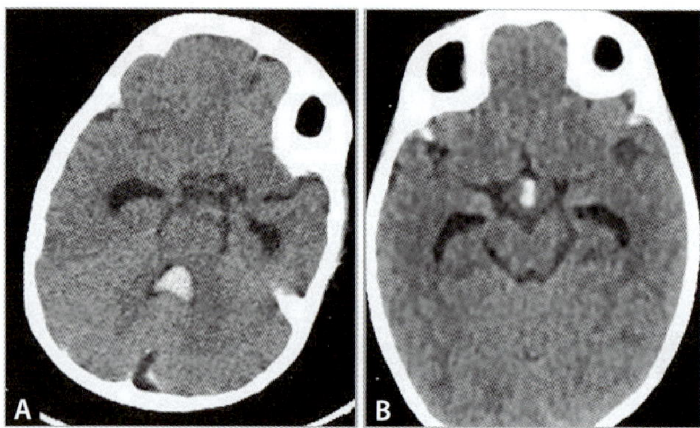

Figs. 1A and B: Child, 8 months old, with fall from stairs (2 steps), managed conservatively. NCCT head suggestive of fourth ventricular bleed

Trivial fall from bed in a child can be disastrous. Proportionately large head with respect to the rest of the body, little myelin in a neonatal brain makes the growing brain more vulnerable.[11,12] Also, immature paranasal sinuses and the protruding forehead makes the frontal bone and the parenchyma more susceptible to injury in a growing child. In a study in 1994 by Berney *et al.* concluded that younger the child, lesser the energy required to produce injuries.[13] In their study, youngest group (0–3 years) suffered most with skull fractures, subdural hematomas and had seizures. According to Jonathan Hughes *et al.*, fall from height with head center of gravity > 0.6 m, infants, point of impact at temporoparietal and occipital bone were significantly associated with underlying trauma[14] **(Fig. 1)**.

CEREBROVASCULAR PATHOPHYSIOLOGY

Understanding of cerebral blood flow (CBF), cerebral autoregulation (CA) and carbon dioxide (CO_2) reactivity post TBI is very essential for managing these patients.

Both cerebral hyperemia and hypoperfusion is detrimental in cases of severe TBI.[15] The most important factor that regulates cerebral perfusion is flow metabolism coupling. Decrease in CBF may be present in TBI, but the deleterious effect may be countered with decreasing metabolic rate, as is done with sedatives and paralytic agents.[16] Also, CO_2 is considered to be the most potent vasodilator. Small change in intra-arterial CO_2 may normalize the CBF within 1–2 mins.

Cerebral autoregulation keeps the CPP independent of CBF. However, this range of autoregulation is around 60 mm of Hg +/– 9 mm of Hg in a child.[17] Impaired CA invites the vasodilator cascade. Systemic hypotension decreases CPP, inducing vasodilatation and increasing cerebral blood volume. This results in raised ICP inducing further vasodilatation. All this is a dynamic process. CA may differ in both the hemispheres in an individual based on the focal pathology.[18] In a hyperemic brain increase in MAP may result in new hemorrhages.[19]

INJURY CHARACTERISTICS

Different age groups of the patients are susceptible to differing types of cranial injury. Cephalohematoma and caput succedaneum, for example, are seen in neonates. Caput succedaneum involves moulding of the neonatal head and often crosses the suture lines whereas cephalohematoma involves sub-periosteal bleeding and is limited by the suture lines. In low birth weight babies and those with hypoxic injuries, intraventricular bleed is seen quite often.

Injury may be focal or diffuse and usually exist in combination.

The commonest injuries picked up on CT imaging of pediatric TBI are skull fractures with or without subdural and epidural hematomas. Subarachnoid hemorrhage (SAH) is present in 50% of the patients with severe TBI. Cerebral contusions and intracerebral hematoma occur in almost one third of the patients with severe TBI.

Skull Fracture

Linear fracture is the commonest (90%), involving parietal followed by occipital, frontal and temporal bones.[20] Concurrent underlying intracranial epidural and subdural bleeds are present in 15–30% of cases.[21] May present as sutural diastasis as well (**Fig. 2**). To distinguish these fracture lines from normal suture lines typical CT findings of complex serrated edges of sutures, with signs of ossification center along suture line and classic anatomic location should be looked for. CT reconstruction with 2D and 3D images are useful in establishing the diagnosis. Most are managed with conservative approach.

Compound depressed fracture accounts for 42–66% of all fractures and uncommon in children less than 1 year because of elasticity of skull bone (**Fig. 3**). Associated dural injuries with underlying intracranial lesions are seen in almost 11% of depressed fractures. Fracture line over the sinus is managed conservatively, close watch

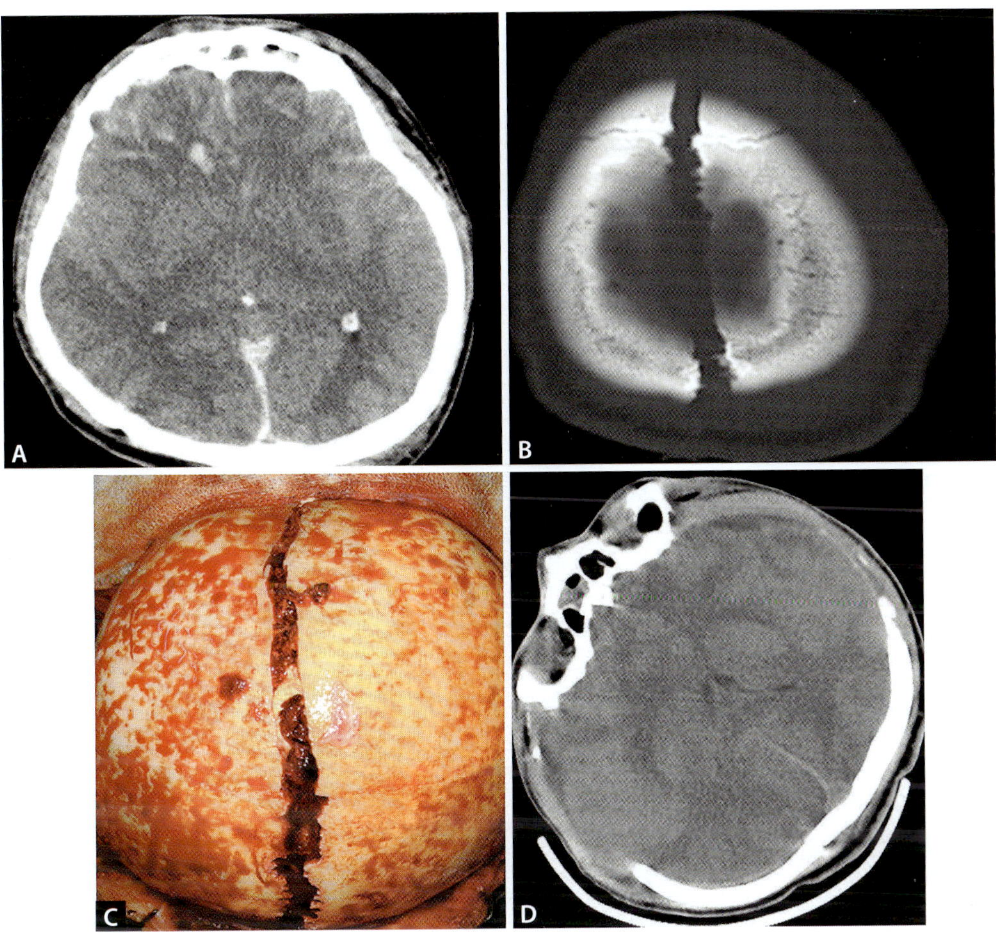

Figs. 2A to D: Classic example of bifrontal contusions with sutural diastasis. Patient was taken up for surgery in M2, discharged in M4 status. (A and B) CT imaging; (C) Intraoperative finding; (D) Postoperative after bilateral frontotemporal decompression

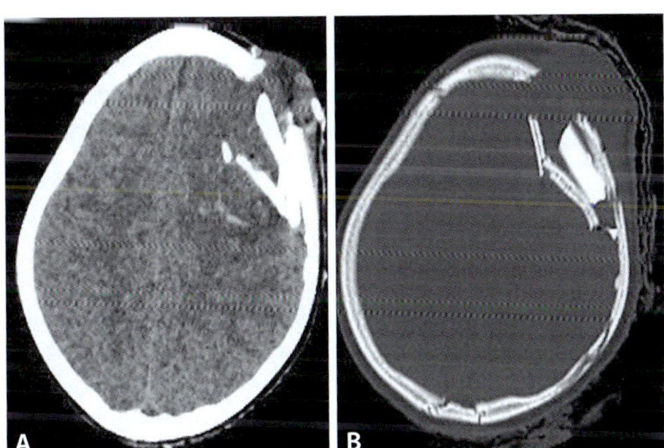

Figs. 3A and B: Clinical picture of a compound depressed fracture. (A) Brain window; (B) Bone window

kept for venous edema and enlarging epidural bleed.[22] Prophylactic anticonvulsants are given as these are commonly associated with post-traumatic seizures.

Surgery is recommended in cases with CSF leak, foreign body, contaminated wound and if there is an associated underlying large hematoma. Cosmesis may be another indication.

Basal skull fracture is not very common in pediatric age group, however, may present either with cranial and vascular injuries or at a later stage with meningitis.

Growing skull fracture (***Fig. 4***): It is seen in children usually age<3 years, with enlarging fracture line. The important pre-requisite is underlying dural tear with or without arachnoid tear. These children present with pulsatile

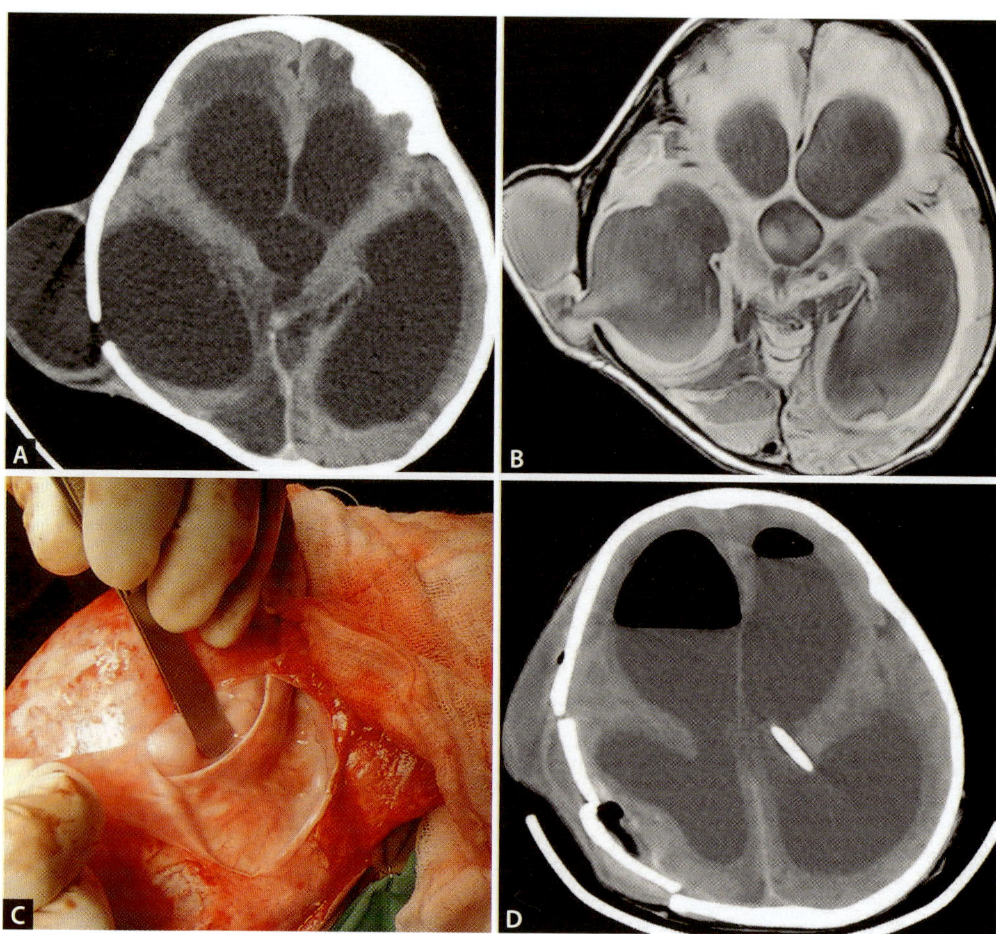

Figs. 4A to D: Two years old child with growing skull fracture. Operated for the same 4 months after primary injury. (A and B) Preoperative CT and MR (to define the dural margin); (C) Intraoperative imaging, note the retracted dura; (D) Postoperative CT scan

swelling or seizures. A retrospective review of 44 patients with growing skull fracture at AIIMS, Delhi identified important negative prognostic factors like age >8 years, female gender, defects larger than 7 cm and crossing midline, severe TBI at the time of presentation and delayed repair > 8 months.[23] Meticulous dural repair to avoid CSF leak is must.

Epidural Hematoma (EDH)

The dura is strongly adherent to the inner table of skull, making epidural hematomas not a very common injury in young children. In neonates, the middle meningeal artery is such placed, that it is unlikely to get damaged.[24] However, it may arise from the dural venous sinus injuries or tear of the emissary veins. Venous epidural may be deceptive and cross the suture line. Posterior fossa EDH because of the occipital bone fracture overlying transverse and sigmoid sinus warrants early surgery (**Fig. 5**). As per Brain Trauma Foundation (BTF) guidelines, all patients with EDH volume >30 cc, irrespective of GCS are to be surgically evacuated. Patients may be in the lucid interval phase and early surgery in indicated cases is recommended.[25]

Subdural Hematoma (SDH)

Acute SDH are usually associated with underlying vascular and parenchymal injury. Bridging veins in a wide subdural space are vulnerable.[26] Concurrent brain contusions are also commonly observed. Bilateral presentation, along the tent, calvarium and falx are typical CT findings in an unconscious child due to head trauma. SDH with thickness of more than 10 mm or a midline shift more than 5 mm are surgical candidates[27] (**Fig. 6**).

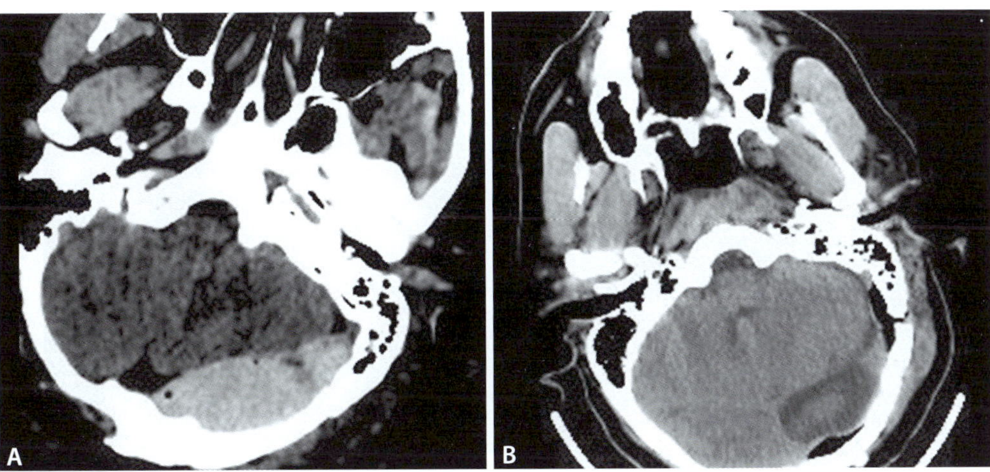

Figs. 5A and B: Posterior fossa EDH in a 17-year-old child; (A) Preoperative; (B) Postoperative

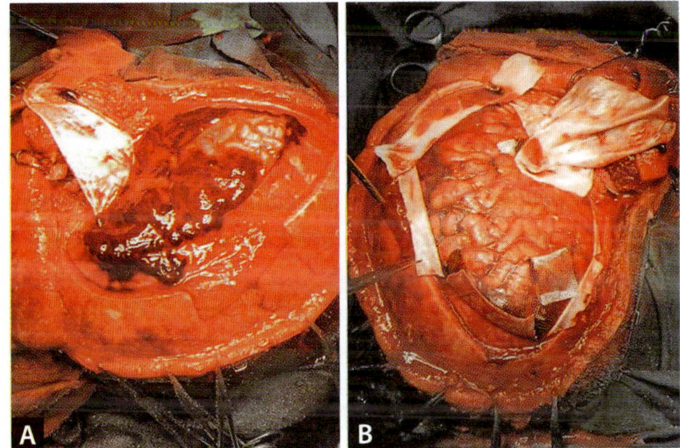

Figs. 6A and B: Subdural hematoma undergoing decompressive craniectomy. Because the brain was full and congested, bone flap was kept in abdomen

Abusive Head Trauma (AHT)

Almost 14–40 infants per 1,00,000 are suffering from AHT and is a global issue.[28] The patients may have injuries to brain and/or the spinal cord. AHT forms a very close differential to other head injury and needs a high level of suspicion for diagnosis, especially in children less than 2 years. The commonest CT picture is that of acute SDH. Acute disruption of arachnoid layer may result in hemato-hygromas. However, it may also present with SAH, ICH, and/or contusions.[29] The associated systemic presentation will help clinch the diagnosis, with the presence of apnea having a positive predictive value of 93%. Fractured ribs and multilaminar retinal hemorrhages involving both eyes, are other findings which are very common in patients with AHT (**Fig. 7**).[30]

Traumatic Subarachnoid Hemorrhages (tSAH)

Injury to the subarachnoid vessels due to varied trauma results in SAH. It may cause secondary injury by inducing inflammation and vasospasm. Patients with sTBI having SAH usually have more in-hospital complications and poor functional performance.[31] However, isolated tSAH with mild head injury have a relatively better outcome. These patients may have pituitary dysfunction and present with chronic diabetes insipidus (cDI).

Intraventricular Hemorrhage (IVH)

The prevalence for IVH for pediatric TBI is around 1.2%. These are generally associated with severe trauma and have poor outcome. The mortality/severe disability rate observed in a large prospective trial on pediatric TBI with non-isolated IVH was nearly 50%.[32] Patients with isolated IVH had a relatively better outcome, just like isolated SAH. These patients may develop post-traumatic HCP in follow-up.

Cerebral Contusions and Intracranial Hemorrhages (ICH)

Presenting as coup and counter coup injuries, frontal and temporal gray matter are usually involved.[33] These are generally associated with significant brain swelling. These lesions are known to cause focal hypoxic and

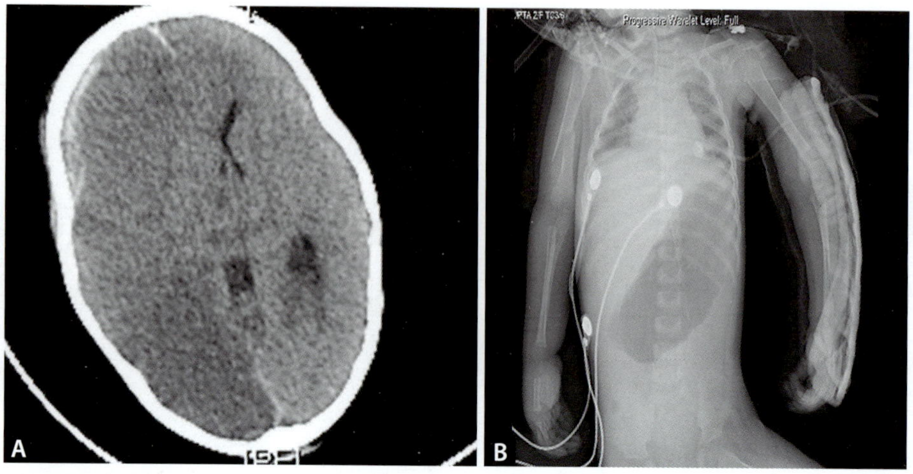

Figs. 7A and B: Battered baby with polytrauma died within 2 months of injury. (A) CT s/o ASDH and Left PCA infarct; (B) X-ray reveals bilateral upper humerus fracture, with radius, ulna fracture on left

circulatory injury, resulting in cerebral ischemia. Patients with contusions of 20 cc in volume with a midline shift of more than 5 mm or obliterated cisterns should be offered surgery. Any patient with contusion greater than 50 cc should also undergo contusectomy, irrespective of midline shift.[27] Posterior fossa contusions need early surgery as there is a high chance of brainstem compression and fourth ventricular obstruction (**Fig. 8**).

The ICH needs to differentiated for etiology, especially important to rule out aertriovenous malformations. Again, these commonly occur in frontal and temporal lobes, however may involve basal ganglia and cerebellum. May present in a delayed fashion as well, should be looked for in TBI patient with persistent or worsening neurology.[34]

Post-traumatic Hydrocephalus (PTH)

Occurs in 1% of patients with TBI, may vary from 0.7% to 45% in incidence. Nearly 30% of these require shunt diversions.[35] Other 10–15% of these patients may require external ventricular drainage (**Fig. 9**). Younger age group, SDH, SAH, septicemia, open wound and postoperative infarct are independent associated factors.[36] Although not related to increased mortality, but PTH definitely influences the length of hospital stay and costs.

Diffuse Axonal Injury (DAI)

This term diffuse is now considered a misnomer and recommended terminology is traumatic axonal injury (TAI). Almost 40% of patients presenting with severe TBI are known to have TAI.[37] It is usually a result of high impact energy causing rapid rotational and decelerating forces resulting in stretching and tearing of neurons and hemorrhage. TAI may extend to involve cranio-vertebral junction as well. Neuropathologically, there is a damage to the axonal skeleton along with secondary injury to mitochondria resulting in impaired oxidative metabolism. These lesions commonly occur in the deep white matter, ranging from 5 to 15 mm in length. The other commonly affected areas are corpus callosum, corona radiata, the rostral midbrain, and cerebellum. These lesions may be associated with punctate hemorrhages due to contiguous injuries to the adventitial vessels. Diffusion tensor imaging may help identify and quantify the white mater changes in these patients. MR Gradient echo imaging are helpful in identifying the hemorrhagic lesions (**Fig. 10**). TAI has generally been associated with poor outcome, hemorrhagic lesions and their number count doing worse in particular.[38] The classification proposed by Adam based on Ommaya Gennarelli hypothesis suggests that deeper the lesion, worse the outcome.[39] As per the classification, mild DAI involved microscopic changes in subcortical white matter, corpus callosum, brainstem, and cerebellum. Any grossly evident focal lesions in corpus callosum classified for moderate and additional lesion in the dorso-lateral rostrum of brainstem shifted it into a severe category. The mortality associated with DAI in TBI is around 40–60%.

Diffuse Cerebral Swelling (DCS)

Diffuse cerebral swelling is more often a result of poor cerebral autoregulatory mechanism resulting in cerebral

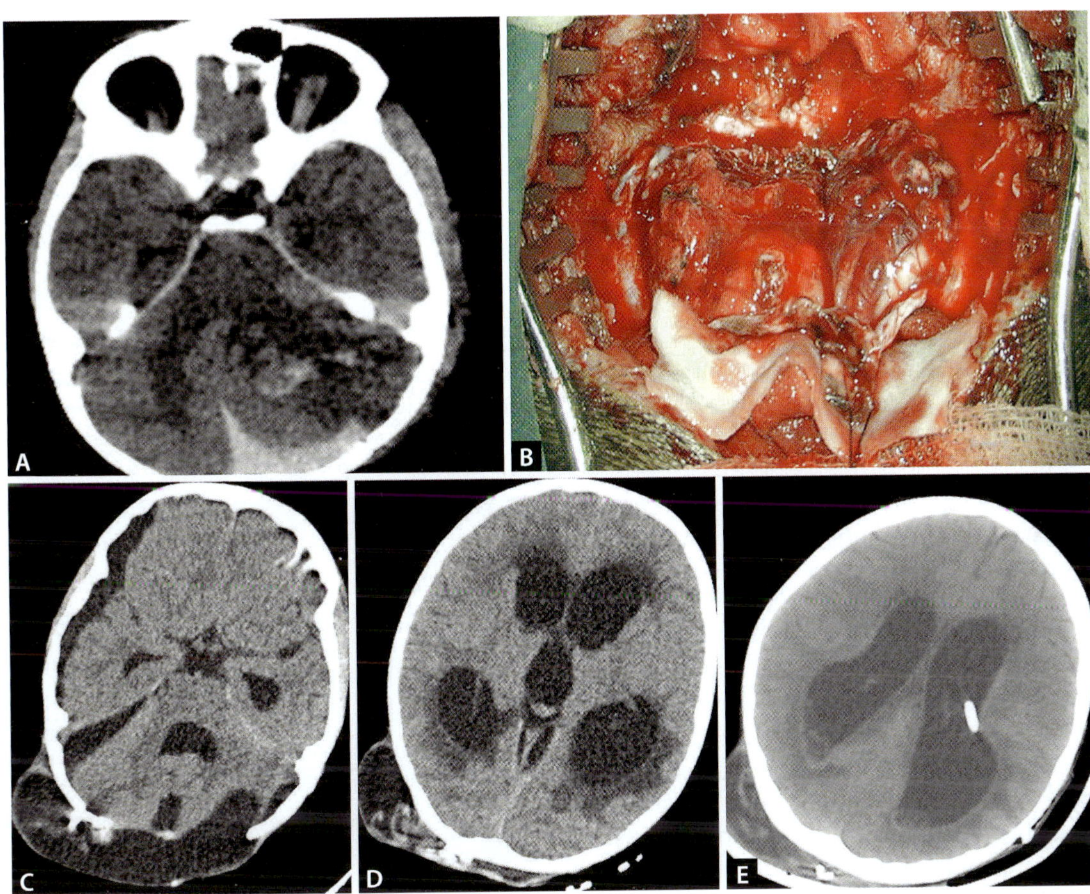

Figs. 8A to E: Posterior fossa contusion in a child, 8 years old underwent decompressive surgery, developed pseudomeningocele with hydrocephalus, LP showed meningitis and is now being managed with external ventricular drainage (EVD). (A) Preoperative CT; (B) Intraoperative imaging; (C and D) Postoperative pseudomeningocele with hydrocephalus; (E) The EVD in situ

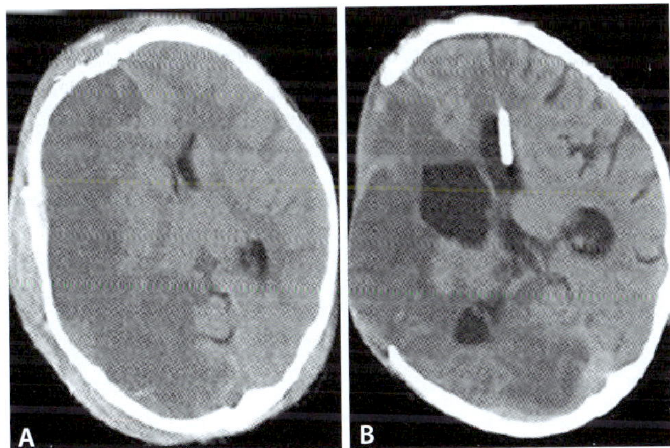

Figs. 9A and B: Clinical case of traumatic infarct with thin subdural, underwent decompressive and presented 3 months later with PTH frontal shunt. (A) Preoperative; (B) Post-decompressive hydrocephalus

hyperemia. Also, the excitatory neurotransmitters inducing inflammatory response leading to increased vascular permeability may be involved in pathogenesis. Lang et al. in 1994, suggested that children present more often with DCS because of relatively smaller amount of cerebrospinal fluid in brain.[40] CT findings where there is a poor definition of gray-white junction, obliterated cisterns with almost non-visualization of third ventricles carry a poor prognosis (**Fig. 11**). Presence of a homogeneous scan with whatsoever no normal brain architecture at the level of thalamus and ambient cistern is said to represent malignant brain swelling and patients are usually not salvageable.[41]

NEUROIMAGING

Pediatric group of patients are unable to follow instructions or cooperate in neurological assessment and hence more

Figs. 10A and B: (A) NCCT head showing lesions of TAI; (B) More hemorrhagic lesions evident on gradient echo imaging

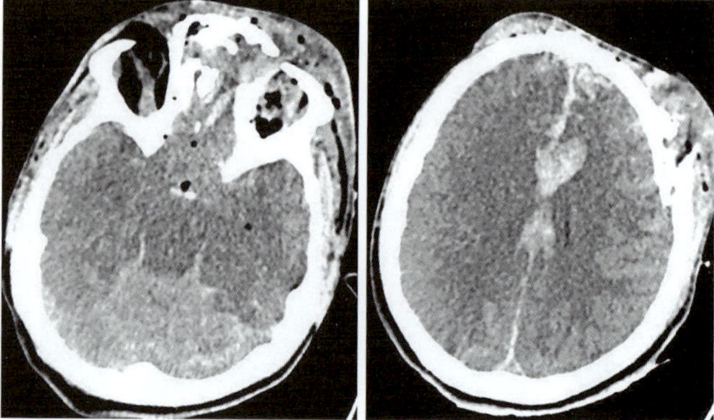

Fig. 11: A 17-year-old boy presenting in M1 status to ED, with diffuse brain edema

dependent on imaging. TBI is a dynamic process. Delayed lesions appearing in TBI occurs in almost 1% to 50% of patients, needing repeat imaging. Several clinical tools are available to guide the clinician with regards to who should be scanned, like PECARN (Pediatric Emergency Care Applied Research Network).[42] PECARN study defined clinically important TBI as those requiring hospitalization for 2 or more days, those requiring intubation for more than a day and those head injuries associated with death and the others may skip repeat imaging.[43] CT scan in a pediatric age increases the mortality risk by almost 10 times when compared to that of an adult and carries risk of cancer of 1 in 1500 in a 1 year old child.[44]

Non-contrast CT remains the screening tool for head injury. It helps in assessing the osseous and soft tissue injuries along with emergent surgical causes of raised ICP. Postoperative complications may also be well assessed on the NCCT head. Marshall's CT classification, based on cisterns, midline shift and intracranial mass, is generally used to evaluate the outcome in pediatric head injury.[45] They observed that diffuse injury type 1 was associated with 10% mortality while diffuse injury type 4 had 50% mortality rate.

The MRI avoids unnecessary ionizing radiation to the kids. The ease of accessibility in an emergency often limits the use of MR in trauma. However, currently rapid MR imaging protocol has been assessed for TBI and could be performed in less than 6 minutes.[46] Imaging protocol of even less than 3 minutes was used in a recent study, where MRI findings were found to be not inferior to that of CT. DTI and acute spin label (ASL) in MR help localize the site of lesion and also predict the cognitive outcome in children.[47] DTI has been considered as an index of

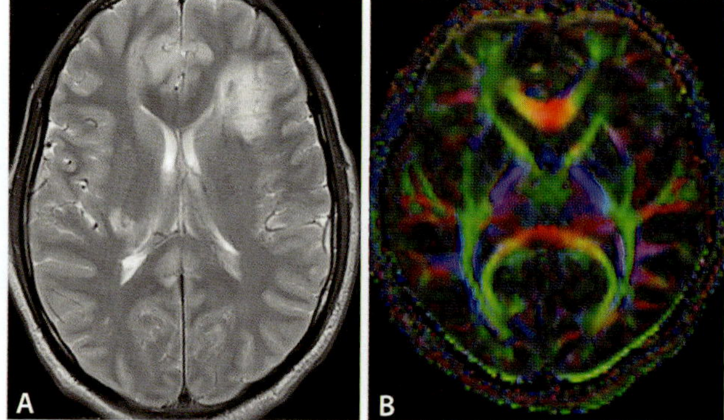

Figs. 12A and B: DTI show reduction in fractional anisotrophy (FA) at site of traumatic axonal injury, corresponds to loss of microstructural fiber integration. (A) T2 weighted; (B) DTI sequence

microstructural integrity (**Fig. 12**). f-MRI shows different areas of activation in patients with mild to moderate TBI. ASL helps in assessing the cerebral perfusion in patients with TBI. Presence of microbleeds in SWI have been shown to influence the neuro-psychological and short-term memory disturbances.

Nuclear imaging are also at times carried out to assess the metabolic (PET) and neuronal integrity (SPECT).[48]

Missed Pathologies in TBI

There have been cases where the primary pathology has been missed while managing the sTBI. Most commonly missed diagnosis is the delayed contusions and ischemia that happens 2–3 days post injury. No improvement in GCS over 48 hours warrants a repeat imaging to rule out new lesions. There are few patients presenting with trauma secondary to underlying illness. The elaborate history for

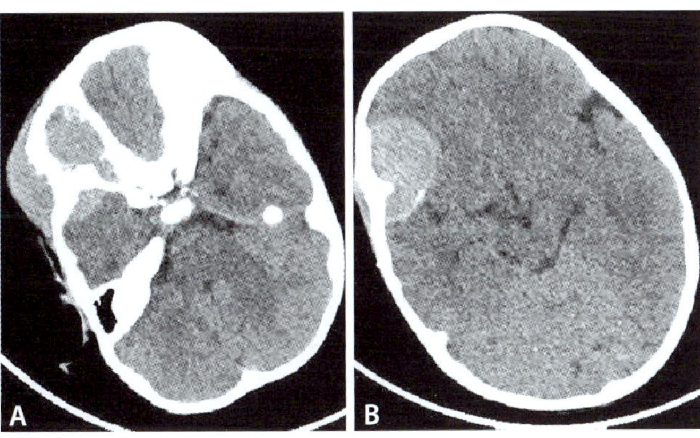

Figs. 13A and B: Six years old child with right black eye and fall from bed, CT revealed right frontal lesion, presumed to extradural hematoma in the context of trauma. A detailed exam revealed however abdominal mass, later on found to be a case of craniocerebral metastasis

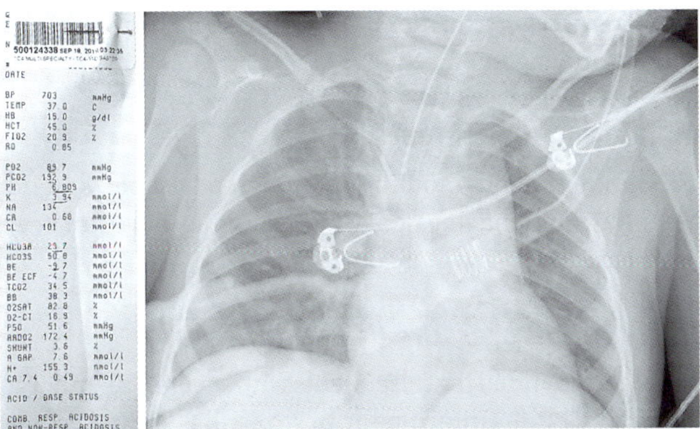

Fig. 14: Patient presented with low GCS, intubated, but could not be adequately ventilated. X-ray chest reveals tube pretty much inside in the right bronchus, readjusted the tube, but child by this time had already suffered the hypoxic injury

reason of fall must be sought. Also, cases of craniocerebral metastasis with seizures may present to trauma center with only history of trauma (**Fig. 13**).

MANAGEMENT

Classifying Head Injury

As per Centers for Disease Control and Prevention, the head injury may be classified based on the Pediatric GCS Score: Mild (GCS score 13 to 15); Moderate (GCS score 9 to 12); Severe (GCS score <9).[49]

Concussion Injury

It is a very common sports related injury and the characteristic feature is its reversibility. To call it a concussion injury, other causes like alcohol and drug abuse, vestibular or cervical dysfunction should be ruled out. Clinically these patients have dizziness, photophobia, phonophobia and vomiting with ante or retrograde amnesia. There are certain red flag symptoms like deteriorating headache, neck pain, worsening consciousness, seizure, weakness or double vision that should alert the clinician.[50] It is usually a clinical diagnosis and there are several sports concussion assessment tools available for standardized evaluation. Cognitive function evaluation is an important component as it lags behind while the other symptoms recover. Imaging is advised only when there are clinical indicators.

A gradual return in a phased manner to learn and play policy is recommended for all schools. If there is any worsening noted while attempting to return to school in the phased system, child is taken back onto the earlier stage. Involvement of a concussion specialist is recommended if symptoms persist for more than a month.

Severe TBI

Management of sTBI begins with primary and secondary survey, just like any trauma patient as described in Advanced Trauma Life Support Manual. Primary survey aims towards securing airway, establishing the need for ventilation and targeting normal systolic blood pressure. Neurologic examination comes only once the above ABCs are taken care of (**Fig. 14**).

Neurologic Evaluation

Pediatric Glasgow coma scale is used for children under 5 years because of their limited verbal and motor skills. For adolescent age group, responsiveness with the alert, verbal, pain, unresponsive (AVPU) system and Glasgow Coma Scale (GCS) is used. Pupillary response and any focal deficit is looked for. Unequal pupillary response warrants urgent imaging. Bilateral fixed dilated pupils are associated with poor prognosis. Primary survey is followed by secondary survey with head to toe examination along with a detailed neurologic evaluation.

SPECIFIC MANAGEMENT CONCERNS

Following management principles are based on various guidelines formulated by the recent brain trauma foundation regarding monitoring, thresholds, medical and surgical management.[27,51-53]

Monitoring and Thresholds

The multimodality monitoring though advisable, still not essential for managing pediatric TBI as they have not been found to influence overall outcome.

Intracranial pressure (ICP) monitoring

It is recommended that all patients with severe TBI undergo ICP and CPP monitoring for best results. ICP threshold values and duration, both are important. A sustained ICP of greater than 20 mm Hg for more than 5 minutes duration is clearly abnormal. Moderate intracranial hypertension is defined as ICP between 20 and 40 mm Hg and ICP > 40 mm Hg suggests severe TBI. Intraparenchymal monitoring is usually practized, although intraventricular monitoring is considered the gold standard. Intraventricular ICP catheters help in draining CSF as well whenever required. More than the numbers, it is the waveform analysis which shows the trend towards rising ICP. Generally a threshold of 15 mm of Hg is kept for pediatric patients in our ICU (**Fig. 15**).

Cerebral perfusion pressure (CPP)

Monitoring of CPP is essential to avoid unwanted increase in cerebral edema. It is recommended that CPP should be individualized. Brain trauma foundation guidelines however recommend CPP of 40 to 50 mm of Hg and should never go below 40 in children.

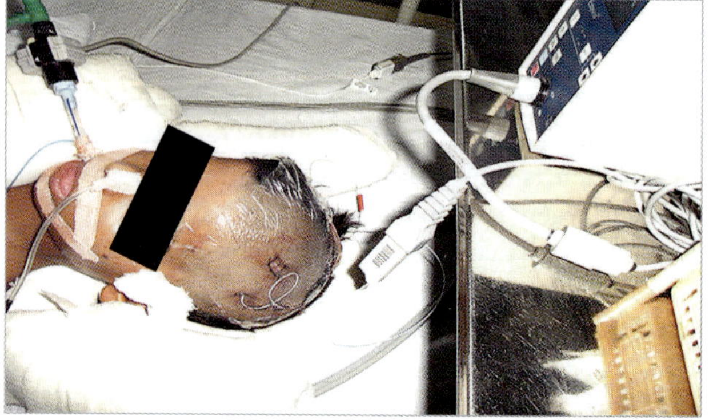

Fig. 15: Intraparenchymal placement of ICP sensors and measurement in the neurotrauma ICU. Kept for a period of 5 days or less if there is an improvement in the patient's sensorium

Continuous brain tissue oxygen ($PbtO_2$) monitoring is not a part of standard recommendations but if being used the target of > 10 mm of Hg is suggested. However, it should be noted that any invasive monitoring is to be avoided in patients with coagulopathy.

TREATMENT

Baseline care includes ABC management.

Sedatives and Analgesics

It forms a part of the general care for a pediatric patient, especially when there is a need to secure the airway and ventilate, control the ICP and need for invasive procedure. Continuous prolonged propofol infusion is to be avoided. Routine neuromuscular blocking agents can be used to reduce metabolic needs and facilitate ventilation. Bolus use of midazolam and fentanyl may result in cerebral hypoperfusion and should be used judiciously and in titrated doses.

Hyperosmolar Therapy

A lot of controversy exists between uses of mannitol versus hypertonic saline. Both are being used, while the recent reports are favoring hypertonic saline for pediatric age group. The standard treatment protocol for mannitol is interrupted dosing three times a day using 20% formulation at a dose of 0.25–1.0 g/kg. Target is to maintain plasma osmolality at ≤ 310 mOsm/L. Hypertonic saline has however shown to have fastest and sustained improvement in ICP. Target serum sodium is kept around 160 mmol/kg. Values above this make the patients more susceptible to deep vein thrombosis and very high levels increases chances of thrombocytopenia and anemia. A bolus dose of 3% hypertonic saline at 2 and 5 mL/kg over 10–20 mins is recommended. Effective doses as a continuous infusion of 3% saline range between 0.1 and 1.0 mL/kg of body weight per hour, administered on a sliding scale. Minimum dose needed to maintain ICP <20 mm Hg should be used. Serum osmolarity should be maintained below 320 mOsm/L (Level 2 evidence). Bolus of 23.4% saline may be used for refractory ICP at a dose of 0.5 mL/kg with the maximum of 30 mL.

CSF Drainage

Found to be an effective way of reducing ICP, now form an integral part of management of moderate to severe TBI,

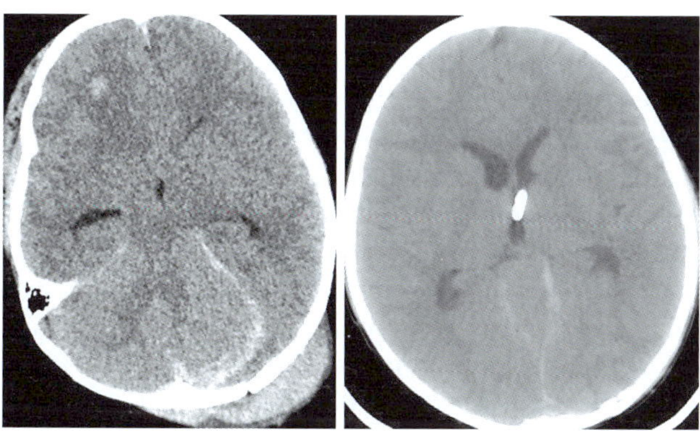

Fig. 16: Case of a patient being managed by CSF drainage. Surgery could be deferred and patient discharged in good status day 6 of injury

getting precedence over decompressive. However, there is a definite increase in the risk of cerebral hemorrhage and infection (Level III) (**Fig. 16**).

Hyperventilation

Hyperventilation can be used as a temporizing measure inducing vasoconstriction and thereby lowering ICP. However, within first 48 hours, there is a significant drop in the CBF, and therefore, caution against use of hyperventilation during this period. Mild hypocarbia with $PaCO_2$, 30–35 mm of Hg is suggested for lowering ICP in refractory cases. This also necessitates a close watch on arterial blood gases and end tidal carbon dioxide monitoring.

Barbiturates

Barbiturate coma has been recommended as the second tier measure for refractory intracranial pressure. Pentobarbital in particular is useful for children with severe trauma. However, it may be difficult to use barbiturates in the presence of hypotension. Continuous watch has to be kept on hypotension and myocardial depression.

Temperature Control

Trials have failed to satisfactorily recommend hypothermia as a treatment option for refractory intracranial hypertension. There is no questioning about deleterious effect of hyperthermia. It leads to increased metabolic needs, lipid peroxidation, inflammation and induces more seizures. As per the guidelines, in children with moderate to severe head injury, moderate hypothermia 32°C to 33°C for up to 48 hours followed by slow rewarming (0.5 to 1°C over 12–24 hours) may be used. Use of phenytoin during rewarming from hypothermia may induce toxicity and warrants dose readjustments.

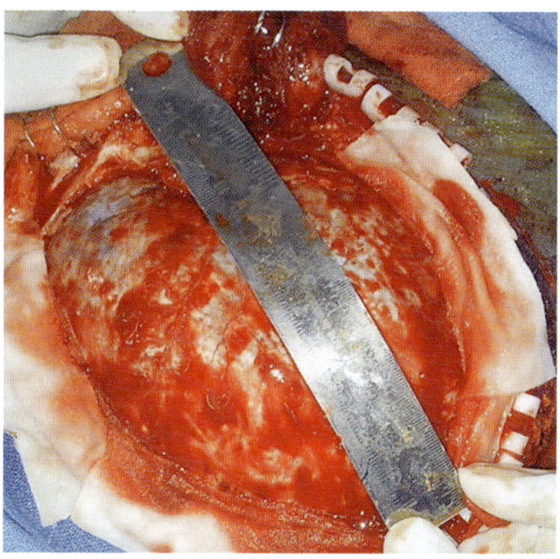

Fig. 17: Importance of adequate decompression needs to be underlined. The condition of brain determines the need to replace the bone flap back

Decompressive Craniectomy (DC)

Indications for decompressive are based on presenting GCS post resuscitation, ICP values if being monitored, CT findings suggestive of large midline shift along with herniation. Gupta *et al.* studied 71 children in an apex trauma center who underwent decompressive craniotomy and concluded that decompressive offers a survival advantage to more than 50% of patients.[54,55]

Timing of decompressive is another important factor. Longer the brain is exposed to raise ICP > 20 mm of Hg or the CPP < 50 mm of Hg, more deleterious is the outcome. Once the medical therapy on a tiered basis is exhausted, decompressive should be offered as early as possible.

Decompression can be primary when the mass lesion like EDH, contusions is evacuated or it may be secondary to treat refractory ICP. To replace the bone flap back or remove is solely decided on table based on the status of the brain intraoperatively (**Fig. 17**). It has its own list of complications, the most bothering of which is the hydrocephalus and infection (**Fig. 18**). There may also be wound dehiscence and cerebral ischemia.

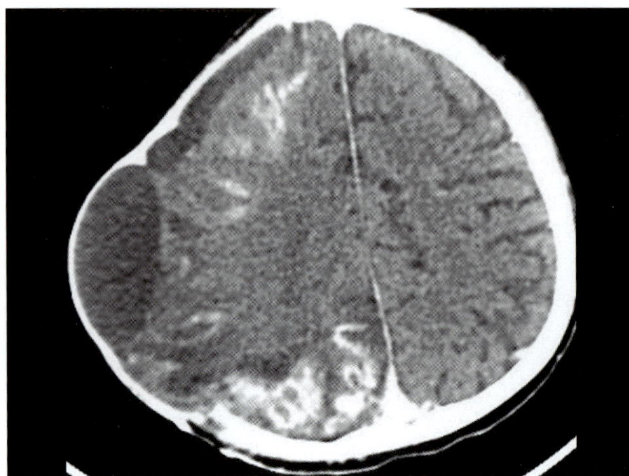

Fig. 18: Case of cerebritis in a 2-year-old child post decompressive; CECT Head

Corticosteroids

These are not recommended in any head injury patients. It is known to increase susceptibility to infectious disease.

Nutritional Management

It is recommended to start the full replacement by day 7 post injury. Calorie requirement should be 130–160% replacement to cover up for the nitrogen loss. Enteral route should be used unless contraindicated. Immune modulating diet has not shown to influence outcome.

Anticonvulsants

This group of patients is more prone to develop early seizures, particularly infants have a very low threshold. Various risk factors are identified in the literature like age less than 2, hypotension, severe TBI where prophylactic drugs are given. EEG, imaging studies are recommended for planning discontinuation of these drugs.[56]

ROLE OF BIOMARKERS IN TBI

More than 90 biomarkers identified in blood for assessing severity, prognosticating pediatric TBI. None are FDA approved for clinical use in adults or children. Ideal marker will indicate the site of involvement and the levels will be proportionate to the severity of injury. Biomarkers can be subclassified as astroglial, neuronal and axonal injury markers.[57] S100β, marker for astrocyte injury and is abnormally elevated in concussions and neurocognitive dysfunction. Need for CT is reduced by 30% when using S100β as diagnostic tool. However, it lacks specificity. Glial fibrillary acidic protein (GFAP) is another astroglial marker for moderate to severe TBI and also in mild TBI. It may help in predicting outcome at 6 months.

Neuronal marker, Neuron specific enolase (NSE) correlates well with outcome in children less than 4 years of age. In cases of sTBI with TAI, levels of NSE at 3rd post injury day suggests poor outcome.

UCH-L1 is an early marker of injury despite negative CT scans. It is detectable within an hour of injury in the CSF and remains elevated for at least 1 week post injury.

Alpha-II spectrin breakdown products, as axonal injury markers had elevated levels in moderate to severe TBI but not so much in mild TBI.

Total Tau proteins have also been shown to correlate with severe TBI. Cleaved tau proteins enter CSF after TBI and their levels are indicative of severity and outcome.

Neurofilaments (NF) are the component of neuronal skeleton and the levels of heavy subunit of neurofilaments in CSF on Day 2–4 post injury was suggestive of poor outcome. It has also been observed that the levels of NF are significantly high in children with DAI.

OUTCOME

The TBI has been listed as a major killer in the pediatric age group > 1 years old and 30% of this mortality is preventable.[58] The mortality rate for severe TBI is almost close to 55–60% at one year. Yet, almost 15% of these patients do have a good outcome at 10 years follow-up.[59] There are varied predictive factors responsible for determining the outcome in pediatric head injury. For the ease of analysis, we would like to group them as demographic, clinical and radiological factors.

Studies have shown that children with the same severity of injury fare well when compared to adults with TBI.[60] Age is one of the most important factor with children < 5 years with severe TBI having poor prognosis. In a study done at AIIMS in TBI, it was observed that while the mortality rate for age <1 year as 57%, for those above 5 years it was 12%.[61]

The nature of primary injury and presenting GCS has a significant role in outcome. Shock and coagulopathy contributes together to a poor outcome.[62] Associated injuries and secondary brain injury in the form of hypoxia, hypotension and seizures are important determinants of outcome. It has been shown that in children where there was a delay in addressing hypotension 3.4 times higher odds of death was present and almost 3.7 times more morbidities.[63] Mortality rate is reported as 61% in hypotensive alone and 85% in hypoxic and hypotensive children while only 22% in normotensive and normotoxic.

Level III evidence is there to support the target CPP of 40 mm of Hg. There are studies to show an association between raised ICP and outcome but failed to show survival advantage.[64,65] The refractory nature rather than the level of ICP was associated with worse outcome.[66] As per PEGASUS study, intervention within 30 minutes of the event (hypotension) is definitely associated with better outcome and discharge status.[67] Although the patients who were offered decompressive had a better outcome than those being managed by medical line of treatment, the difference was not statistically significant.

Neuroimaging based criteria has been used by some to predict the outcome.[68] Availability of bedside CT helps avert unwanted secondary hypoxic and hypotensive episodes that may happen in transit. Hypoxia lasting for less than 10 minutes, SAH and bilateral unreactive pupils had worse GOS-E Peds.[69]

It has been rightly observed that a dedicated pediatric neurocritical care program is definitely going to help improvise the outcome.[70] There was a definite reduction in mortality and increase discharge rates from the pediatric ICU once there was a strict adherence to the protocol-based management.[71,72]

An observational cohort study, Approaches and Decisions for Acute Pediatric TBI (ADAPT) is underway from 0 different countries, investigating ICP management strategies, ways adopted to avoid secondary insults to brain, and metabolic parameters.[73,74] The multidisciplinary rehabilitation protocol is a must for favorable long-term outcome.

CONCLUSION

Traumatic brain injury during childhood has a lot of emotional, socio-economic impact in the society. The victim grows into an adult with behavioral issues, if survived the trauma. Since last 20 years or more management of severe TBI has been revolving around the same medical and surgical entities, with little improvement on outcome. Mortality of children with severe TBI is still 50% and above. Thus, the best way to control the mortality is prevention and a good early resuscitation provided at the site of accident and emergency department. Lots of research is happening toward the inclusion of multimodality monitoring, newer MRI imaging modalities and serum biomarkers for identifying high-risk TBI. A lot more is still to be done.

KEY MESSAGES

- Pediatric TBI patients may present with normal vital signs even in presence of shock. They are known to have sudden deterioration. Watch for tachycardia.
- Post-resuscitation, in a severe head injury, all monitoring devices should be in place, which includes, ICP monitoring, LICOX and EVD. In a resource constrained area, EVD is still advisable. Continuous EEG monitoring for all paralyzed patients.
- Children with severe TBI to be kept sedated and if needed paralyzed for the first 48 hours. $PaCO_2$ of 32 mm of Hg is preferred. Volume control mode of ventilation is generally used.
- Target CPP kept with the help of fluid and if need be vasopressors. Choice of fluid normal saline.
- ICP spikes treated in a step-wise manner. EVD placed 10 cm above the midbrain level and CSF drained to lower ICP. Hyperosmolar therapy and CSF diversion is an effective way of lowering ICP. Serum osmolarity >320 and serum sodium more than 160 mmo/L can be deleterious.
- Decompressive craniotomy as an option in refractory hypertension and once the medical management fails. Hypothermia may be used as a rescue therapy in refractory hypertension.
- CT scans form the screening tool of investigation. Radiation exposure to any pediatric patient should be kept as low as possible.
- Advances in neuroimaging technique, with special sequences like DWI, DTI, SWI helps in picking up hemorrhagic lesions and DAI and prognosticate the patient.
- Biomarkers in TBI has been shown to be predictive of severity and outcome, yet none is FDA approved and are still experimental.
- Prognosis of outcome following TBI is influenced by multiple factors including injury severity, age, physiological factors, biomarkers, electroencephalogram and neuroimaging.

REFERENCES

1. Centers for Disease Control and Prevention. Rates of TBI-related emergency department visits by age group—United States, 2001–2010. CDC; 2016.
2. Kumar R, Mahapatra AK. The changing "epidemiology" of pediatric head injury and its impact on the daily clinical practice. Childs Nerv Syst. 2009;25(7):813-23.
3. Dewan MC, Mummareddy N, Wellons JC 3rd, *et al.* Epidemiology of global pediatric traumatic brain injury: qualitative review. World Neurosurg. 2016;91:497-509.e1.
4. Reid SR, Roesler JS, Gaichas AM, *et al.* The epidemiology of pediatric traumatic brain injury in Minnesota. Arch Pediatr Adolesc Med. 2001;155:784-9.

5. Vaghani G, Singh PK, Gupta DK, *et al.* Outcome of patients with traumatic head injury in infants: An institutional experience at level 1 trauma center. J Pediatr Neurosci. 2013;8(2):104-7.
6. Koepsell TD, Rivara FP, Vavilala MS, *et al.* Incidence and descriptive epidemiologic features of traumatic brain injury in King County, Washington. Pediatrics. 2011;128:946-54.
7. Schrieff LE, Thomas KG, Dollman AK, *et al.* Demographic profile of severe traumatic brain injury admissions to Red Cross War Memorial Children's Hospital, 2006 - 2011. S Afr Med J. 2013;103:616-20.
8. Agrawal A, Agrawal CS, Kumar A, *et al.* Epidemiology and management of paediatric head injury in eastern Nepal. Afr J Paediatr Surg. 2008;5:15-8.
9. De Silva MJ, Roberts I, Perel P, *et al.* Patient outcome after traumatic brain injury in high-, middle- and low-income countries: Analysis of data on 8927 patients in 46 countries. Int J Epidemiol. 2009;38(2):452-8.
10. Kumar R, Mahapatra AK. Head injury in children. In: Mahapatra AK, Raj Kamal, editors. Textbook of Head Injury, 3rd edition. New Delhi: Modern Publishers; 2005. p. 253-70.
11. Margulies SS, Thibault KL. Infant skull and suture properties: Measurements and implications for mechanisms of pediatric brain injury. J Biomech Eng. 2000;122(4):364-71.
12. Goldsmith W, Plunkett J. A biomechanical analysis of the causes of traumatic brain injury in infants and children. Am J Forensic Med Pathol. 2004;25:89-100.
13. Berney J, Froidevaux AC, Favier J. Pediatric head trauma: Influence of age and sex. II. Biomechanical and anatomo-clinical correlations. Childs Nerv Syst. 1994;10:517-23.
14. Hughes J, Maguire S, Jones M, *et al.* Biomechanical characteristics of head injuries from falls in children younger than 48 months. Arch Dis Child. 2016;101:310-5.
15. Adelson PD, Clyde B, Kochanek PM, *et al.* Cerebrovascular response in infants and young children following severe traumatic brain injury: A preliminary report. Pediatr Neurosurg. 1997;26:200-7.
16. Harper AM, Glass HI. Effect of alterations in the arterial carbon dioxide tension on the blood flow through the cerebral cortex at normal and low arterial pressures. J Neurol Neurosurg Psychiatry. 1965;28:449-552.
17. Vavilala MS, Lee LA, Lam AM. The lower limit of cerebral autoregulation in children during sevoflurane anesthesia. J Neurosurg Anesthesiol. 2003;15:307-12.
18. Vavilala MS, Tontisirin N, Udomphorn Y, *et al.* Hemispheric differences in cerebral autoregulation in children with moderate and severe traumatic brain injury. Neurocrit Care. 2008;9:45-54.
19. Aldrich EF, Eisenberg HM, Saydjari C, *et al.* Diffuse brain swelling in severely head-injured children. A report from the NIH Traumatic Coma Data Bank. J Neurosurg. 1992;76:450-4.
20. Bonfield CM, Naran S, Adetayo OA, *et al.* Pediatric skull fractures: The need for surgical intervention, characteristics, complications, and outcomes. J Neurosurg Pediatr. 2014;14(2): 205-11.
21. Orman G, Wagner MW, Seeburg D, *et al.* Pediatric skull fracture diagnosis: Should 3D CT reconstructions be added as routine imaging? J Neurosurg Pediatr. 2015;16:426-31.
22. Tamimi A, Abu-Elrub M, Shudifat A, *et al.* Superior sagittal sinus thrombosis associated with raised intracranial pressure in closed head injury with depressed skull fracture. Pediatr Neurosurg. 2005;41:237-40.
23. Prasad GL, Gupta DK, Mahapatra AK, *et al.* Surgical results of growing skull fractures in children: A single centre study of 43 cases. Childs Nerv Syst. 2015;31:269-77.
24. Leggate JR, Lopez-Ramos N, Genitori L, *et al.* Extradural hematoma in infants. Br J Neurosurg. 1989;3:533-9.
25. Carney N, Totten A, O'Reilly C, *et al.* Guidelines for the Management of Severe Traumatic Brain Injury, Fourth Edition. Neurosurgery. 2017;80(1):6-15.
26. Loh JK, Lin CL, Kwan AL, *et al.* Acute subdural hematoma in infancy. Surg Neurol. 2002;58:218-24.
27. Bullock MR, Chesnut R, Ghajar J, *et al.* Surgical management of acute subdural hematomas. Neurosurgery. 2006;58(3 Suppl):S16-24.
28. Barlow KM, Minns RA. Annual incidence of shaken impact syndrome in children. Lancet. 2000;356:1571-2.
29. Wright JN. CNS injuries in abusive head trauma. AJR Am J Roentgenol. 2017;208(5):991-1001.
30. Maguire S, Pickerd N, Farewell D, *et al.* Which clinical features distinguish inflicted from non-inflicted brain injury? A systematic review. Arch Dis Child. 2009;94:860-7.
31. Hochstadter E, Stewart TC, Alharfi IM, *et al.* Subarachnoid hemorrhage prevalence and its association with short-term outcome in pediatric severe traumatic brain injury. Neurocrit Care. 2014;21:505-13.
32. Lichenstein R, Glass TF, Quayle KS, *et al.* Presentations and outcomes of children with intraventricular hemorrhages after blunt head trauma. Arch Pediatr Adolesc Med. 2012;166:725-31.
33. Graham DI. Pediatric head injury. Brain. 2001;124:1261-2.
34. Stein SC, Spettell CM. Delayed and progressive brain injury in children and adolescents with head trauma. Pediatr Neurosurg. 1995;23:299-304.
35. Rumalla K, Letchuman V, Smith KA, *et al.* Hydrocephalus in pediatric traumatic brain injury: National incidence, risk factors, and outcomes in 124,444 hospitalized patients. Pediatr Neurol. 2018;80:70-6.
36. Chen H, Yuan F, Chen SW, *et al.* Predicting posttraumatic hydrocephalus: Derivation and validation of a risk scoring system based on clinical characteristics. Metab Brain Dis. 2017;32(5):1427-35.
37. Mittl RL, Grossman RI, Hiehle JF, *et al.* Prevalence of MR evidence of diffuse axonal injury in patients with mild head injury and normal head CT findings. AJNR Am J Neuroradiol. 1994;15:1583-9.
38. Abu Hamdeh S, Marklund N, Lannsjö M, *et al.* Extended anatomical grading in diffuse axonal injury using MRI: Hemorrhagic lesions in the substantia nigra and mesencephalic tegmentum indicate poor long-term outcome. J Neurotrauma. 2017;34(2):341-52.
39. Ommaya AK, Gennarelli TA. Cerebral concussion and traumatic unconsciousness. Correlation of experimental and clinical observations of blunt head injuries. Brain. 1974;97:633-54.
40. Lang DA, Teasdale GM, Macpherson P, *et al.* Diffuse brain swelling after head injury: More often malignant in adults than children? J Neurosurg. 1994;80(4):675-80.
41. Bruce DA, Alavi A, Bilaniuk L, *et al.* Diffuse cerebral swelling following head injuries in children: The syndrome of "malignant brain edema". J Neurosurg. 1981;54(2):170-8.
42. Burstein B, Upton J, Terra HF, *et al.* Utilization of computed tomography for pediatric head trauma from 2007–2014 in the

United States: Before and after PECARN clinical decision rules. Pediatr Child Health. 2018;23:e8.
43. Schonfeld D, Bressan S, Da Dalt L, *et al.* Pediatric emergency care applied research network. Head injury: clinical prediction rules are reliable in practice. Arch Dis Child. 2014;99(5):427-31.
44. Brenner D, Elliston C, Hall E, *et al.* Estimated risks of radiation-induced fatal cancer from pediatric CT. AJR Am J Roentgenol. 2001;176:289-96.
45. Marshall LF, Marshall SB, Klauber MR, *et al.* A new classification of head injury based on computerized tomography. J Neurosurg. 1991;75:S14-20.
46. Mehta H, Acharya J, Mohan AL, *et al.* Minimizing radiation exposure in evaluation of pediatric head trauma: Use of rapid MR imaging. AJNR Am J Neuroradiol. 2016;37(1):11-8.
47. Ferrazzano PA, Rosario BL, Wisniewski SR, *et al.* Use of magnetic resonance imaging in severe pediatric traumatic brain injury: Assessment of current practice. J Neurosurg Pediatr. 2019;23(4):471-9.
48. Goshen E, Zwas ST, Shahar E, *et al.* The role of 99Tcm-HMPAO brain SPET in paediatric traumatic brain injury. Nucl Med Commun. 1996;17(5):418-22.
49. Centers for Disease Control and Prevention. Traumatic brain injury and concussion: Severe TBI. Available from: *https://www.cdc.gov/traumaticbraininjury/severe.html.* Accessed August 31, 2019.
50. Weissman B, Joseph M, Gronseth G, *et al.* CDC's guideline on pediatric mild traumatic brain injury: Recommendations for neurologists. Neurol Clin Pract. 2019;9(3):241-9.
51. Bell MJ, Kochanek PM. Pediatric traumatic brain injury in 2012: The year with new guidelines and common data elements. Crit Care Clin. 2013;29(2):223-38.
52. Kochanek PM, Carney N, Adelson PD, *et al.* Guidelines for the acute medical management of severe traumatic brain injury in infants, children, and adolescents—second edition. Pediatr Crit Care Med. 2012;113 Suppl:S1-82.
53. Kochanek PM, Tasker RC, Carney N, *et al.* Guidelines for the management of pediatric severe traumatic brain injury, third edition: Update of the brain trauma foundation guidelines, executive summary. Neurosurgery. 2019;84(6):1169-78.
54. Sinha S, Raheja A, Garg M, *et al.* Decompressive craniectomy in traumatic brain injury: A single-center, multivariate analysis of 1,236 patients at a tertiary care hospital in India. Neurol India. 2015;63(2):175-83.
55. Prasad GL, Gupta DK, Mahapatra AK, *et al.* Surgical results of decompressive craniectomy in very young children: A level one trauma centre experience from India. Brain Inj. 2015;29(13-14):1717-24.
56. Kurz JE, Poloyac SM, Abend NS, *et al.* Variation in anticonvulsant selection and electroencephalographic monitoring following severe traumatic brain injury in children-understanding resource availability in sites participating in a comparative effectiveness study. Pediatr Crit Care Med. 2016;17(7):649-57.
57. Berger RP, Beers SR, Richichi R, *et al.* Serum biomarker concentrations and outcome after pediatric traumatic brain injury. J Neurotrauma. 2007;24:1793-801.
58. Zurek J, Bartlova L, Fedora M. Hyperphosphorylated neurofilament NF-H as a predictor of mortality after brain injury in children. Brain Inj. 2012;25:221-6.
59. Sharples PM, Storey A, Aynsley-Green A, *et al.* Avoidable factors contributing to death of children with head injury. BMJ. 1990;300:87-91.
60. Pigula FA, Wald SL, Shackford SR, *et al.* The effect of hypotension and hypoxia on children with severe head injuries. J Pediatr Surg. 1993;28:310-4.
61. Garg K, Sharma R, Gupta D, *et al.* Outcome predictors in pediatric head trauma: a study of clinicoradiological factors. J Pediatr Neurosci. 2017;12(2):149-53.
62. Patregnani JT, Borgman MA, Maegele M, *et al.* Coagulopathy and shock on admission is associated with mortality for children with traumatic injuries at combat support hospitals. Pediatr Crit Care Med. 2012;13:273-7.
63. Zebrack M, Dandoy C, Hansen K, *et al.* Early resuscitation of children with moderate-to-severe traumatic brain injury. Pediatrics. 2009;124:56-64.
64. Chesnut RM, Temkin N, Carney N, *et al.* A trial of intracranial pressure monitoring in traumatic brain injury. N Engl J Med. 2012;367:2471-81.
65. Young AM, Donnelly J, Czosnyka M, *et al.* Continuous multimodality monitoring in children after traumatic brain injury: Preliminary experience. PLoS One. 2016;11:e0148817.
66. Bennett TD, DeWitt PE, Greene TH, *et al.* Functional outcome after intracranial pressure monitoring for children with severe traumatic brain injury. JAMA Pediatr. 2017;171(10):965-71.
67. Jagannathan J, Okonkwo DO, Yeoh HK, *et al.* Long-term outcomes and prognostic factors in pediatric patients with severe traumatic brain injury and elevated intracranial pressure. J Neurosurg Pediatr. 2008;2:240-9.
68. Kannan N, Wang J, Mink RB, *et al.* Timely hemodynamic resuscitation and outcomes in severe pediatric traumatic brain injury: Preliminary findings. Pediatr Emerg Care. 2016;34:325-9.
69. Agrawal D, Saini R, Singh PK, *et al.* Beside computed tomography in traumatic brain injury: Experience of 10,000 consecutive cases in neurosurgery at a level 1 trauma center in India. Neurol India. 2016;64:62-5.
70. Rosario BL, Horvat CM, Wisniewski SR, *et al.* Presenting characteristics associated with outcome in children with severe traumatic brain injury: A secondary analysis from a randomized, controlled trial of therapeutic hypothermia. Pediatr Crit Care Med. 2018;19(10):957-64.
71. Pineda JA, Leonard JR, Mazotas IG, *et al.* Effect of implementation of a pediatric neurocritical care programme on outcomes after severe traumatic brain injury: A retrospective cohort study. Lancet Neurol. 2013;12:45-52.
72. Maas AI, Menon DK, Adelson PD, *et al.* Traumatic brain injury: Integrated approaches to improve prevention, clinical care, and research. Lancet Neurol. 2017;16(12):987-1048.
73. Lloyd J, Wilson ML, Tenovuo O, *et al.* Outcomes from mild and moderate traumatic brain injuries among children and adolescents: A systematic review of studies from 2008–2013. Brain Inj. 2015;29(5):539-49.
74. Bell MJ, Adelson PD, Wisniewski SR, *et al.* Challenges and opportunities for pediatric severe TBI-review of the evidence and exploring a way forward. Childs Nerv Syst. 2017;33(10):1663-7.

CHAPTER

86

Orthopedic Emergencies

Bhushan Sagade, Mandar Agashe

The four most common and dreaded emergent orthopedic conditions in children, *viz*: acute septic arthritis, acute osteomyelitis, supracondylar fracture of the humerus and acute compartment syndrome are discussed in this chapter.

ACUTE SEPTIC ARTHRITIS

Acute septic arthritis refers to the invasion of the joint space by various pathogenic organisms (mostly pyogenic) and the associated inflammatory response of the body. Left untreated, it has the potential to cause very significant local morbidity and in some instances, mortality.[1-3]

Epidemiology

Acute septic arthritis is most commonly a hematogenous infection. It is commonly seen in joints where the metaphysis is intra-articular, like the hip and the shoulder joint. The U-pin bends of the metaphyseal blood vessels result in a sluggish flow which in turn causes the bones to become more and more susceptible to infection.[1,2]

The incidence of acute septic arthritis is around 4–5 per 100,000 children per year in developed countries though an exact incidence in India is very difficult to determine due to paucity of data. Many a time, bone and joint infections are misdiagnosed as soft tissue abscesses and treated as such. Boys are twice more commonly affected than girls. There is a distinct bimodal distribution—the first peak being the neonatal period and infancy while the second peak is between 4 and 8 years of age. The commonly affected joints in the body are hip, shoulder, knee, and ankle followed by small joints.

Etiology

The commonest organism causing septic arthritis in children in the community is *Staphylococcus aureus*, of which, methicillin sensitive *Staphylococcus aureus* (MSSA) is still the commonest and accounts for 70–80% of all such infections. However, the incidence of methicillin resistant *Staphylococcus aureus* (MRSA) in the community has been increasing over the last few years. The other common organisms are *Streptococcus pyogenes* in neonates and *Haemophilus influenzae* in older children as well as gram negative organisms like *Pseudomonas aeruginosa*. Children who are immunosuppressed are susceptible to organisms of low virulence like *Candida* species, *Kingella kingae* and aspergillosis. Sickle cell anemia patients are prone to infections with capsulated organisms due to splenic derangement—most commonly due to *Salmonella typhi* as well as *Pneumococcus.*[1,2]

Pathogenesis

Septic arthritis is most commonly due to hematogenous origin; rarely, it can arise from direct inocultation (e.g. intra-articular penetration of needle during femoral puncture) or secondary spread from an adjacent metaphyseal osteomyelitic focus in the bone. When the bacteria gain access to the joint cavity in septic arthritis, they rapidly cause synovitis within a few hours and cause formation of fibrinous exudates and areas of synovial necrosis. Endotoxins and enzymes such as proteases, peptidases and collagenases. Collagen destruction follows. Increase in the intra-capsular pressures and thrombosis causes articular destruction resulting in decreased joint space and other sequelae.[4,5]

In infants, the metaphyseal vessels extend till the joint and hence any infection in the joint has the potential to cause involvement of the metaphyseal bone with subsequent osteomyelitis, involvement of the growth plate and high chance of growth arrest. This typically occurs in the hip and the shoulder since the metaphysis of these two joints is intra-articular.

Clinical Features

The clinical features of septic arthritis vary depending on the age of the child and the immune status of the child.

Neonates and infants

The child typically presents with features of "pseudo paralysis, i.e. paralysis with pain (painful paralysis) or inability to use or move that limb due to pain. This is usually accompanied by signs of systemic toxicity like fever, tachycardia and irritability. There may be local signs like warmth, redness, etc. though typically in superficial joints like the knee and the elbow. In NICU graduates, the clinical features of systemic toxicity are masked, and the child may even be afebrile. Remember the adage that "*any painful paralysis of the limb in an NICU graduate is septic arthritis unless proved otherwise.*"

Older children and toddlers

Septic hip typically presents with the classical finding of inability to bear weight on that limb along with other features like fever, irritability and tachycardia. The Kocher criteria are very helpful in confirming the diagnosis.[6] If all 4 of the Kocher criteria (**Box 1**) are present, then there is a 99.4% chance that we are dealing with a septic hip rather than transient synovitis of the hip. Over the years, the Kocher criteria were modified with the addition of C-reactive protein (CRP) as well as addition of radiological features.

Box 1: Kocher criteria

A point is given for each of the four following criteria
- Fever (>99.5°F)
- Inability to bear weight
- Total white blood count (WBC) > 12,000/mm^3
- Erythrocyte sedimentation rate (ESR) >40/hr

Differential Diagnosis

The commonest differential diagnosis of acute septic arthritis of the hip is transient synovitis which is basically a reactive effusion in the hip most likely as a reaction to viral illnesses like upper respiratory illnesses, viral diarrhea, etc. The course of transient synovitis is usually a very benign self-limiting one and can be treated with just anti-inflammatory medicines and rest.[6] The other differential diagnoses include scurvy, trauma, acute osteomyelitis and very rarely malignancies like Ewing sarcoma, which can present acutely.

Approach to Diagnosis

Radiographs

Radiographs are of limited value in acute septic arthritis. The feature of increase in joint space due to infective effusion is very difficult to exactly make out, especially with unossified epiphysis in very young age. The other features include osteopenia (in early metaphyseal infections) as well as joint dislocations (in late cases). In most cases, radiographs are utilized to rule out other causes of pseudoparalysis like fractures and scurvy.

Ultrasound

Ultrasound (USG) examination in very useful to detect joint effusion as well as subperiosteal edema. USG guided joint aspiration is a very important diagnostic modality. USG cannot detect intra-medullary changes and is not useful in deeper zones like the pelvis for pelvic osteomyelitis. It is also very difficult to perform the ultrasound in small neonates and an acutely tender joint since the probe pressure will be exceedingly painful for the child.[3-4]

Magnetic resonance imaging (MRI)

The MRI has emerged as the diagnostic modality of choice for the diagnosis of bone and joint infections in children. It can distinguish between joint effusion of transient synovitis versus acute septic arthritis and also is able to differentiate inflammatory arthritis from acute septic arthritis. It can help to plan the surgery as well as the extra-articular collections, if any (**Fig. 1A**). The only limitation of MRI in children is the need for general anesthesia in young kids.[3]

Laboratory investigations

A routine hemogram, ESR, CRP are helpful to diagnose and monitor the course of treatment. Serial changes in

CRP are more informative. Blood culture must be routinely performed and sometimes it can identify the pathogen. Organism identification is extremely important for both, confirmation of the diagnosis and guiding antimicrobial selection. Needle aspiration is likely to grow an organism in almost 50–60% of cases whereas blood cultures yield positive results in one third to little more than half of specimens.

Management

Septic arthritis is a "surgical condition in a medical disease". Management includes surgical drainage and debridement and prolonged antibiotics to treat the sepsis.

Orthopedic management

Prompt surgical drainage and thorough wash of the joint is necessary (**Fig. 1B**). Open surgical drainage of the joints is essential to prevent necrosis (e.g. head of the femur or humerus). In some superficial joints like knee or elbow, a joint aspiration and lavage is usually equally effective though deeper joints like the hip and shoulder require a formal arthrotomy and drainage.

Drainage of pus offers the following advantages: decompression of the joint with drainage of pus leading to increased vascularity and healing, direct instillation of antibiotics in the local site (which were otherwise unable to reach due to tight compartment like pressure) and rapid healing of joint due to clearance of tissue-destroying fluid and also due to decrease in the tamponade effect on the delicate circulation around the growth plate.

Pus or fluid obtained during surgery must be sent for Gram staining and appropriate culture, which can help in selection of proper antibiotics. Involvement of pediatric orthopedic surgeon at the onset of treatment itself is important such children need long-term follow-up.

Medical management

Antimicrobial therapy should commence immediately after drainage of pus and should be guided by Gram staining of the aspirated pus. Up to 50% of joint aspirates are sterile in septic arthritis, possibly because joint fluid is bacteriostatic or because the organisms are limited to the synovium. Broad-spectrum antibiotics like first generation cephalosporins, ampicillin-cloxacillin or amoxicillin-clavulanic acid in community-acquired infections, and vancomycin in hospital acquired infections, can be started till culture/sensitivity results are obtained and then appropriate antibiotics can be started according to sensitivity report.

Till a few years back, intravenous antibiotics were continued for prolonged period—up to 3 to 6 weeks. However, recent randomized controlled trials have proved that short course therapy of intravenous antibiotics is equally effective as compared to longer course of intravenous antibiotics. Hence, as per new protocol, intravenous antibiotics are given for around

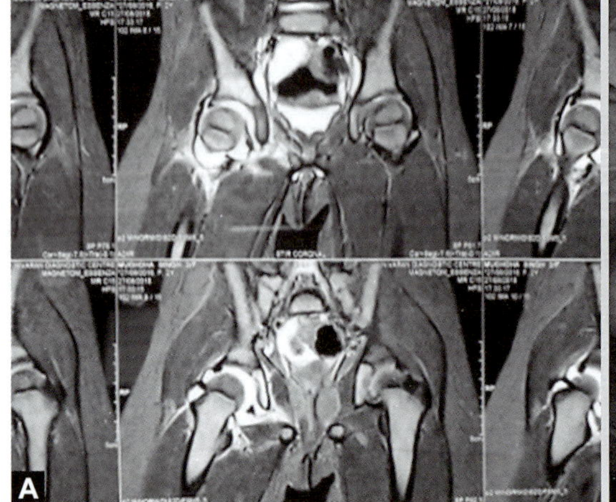

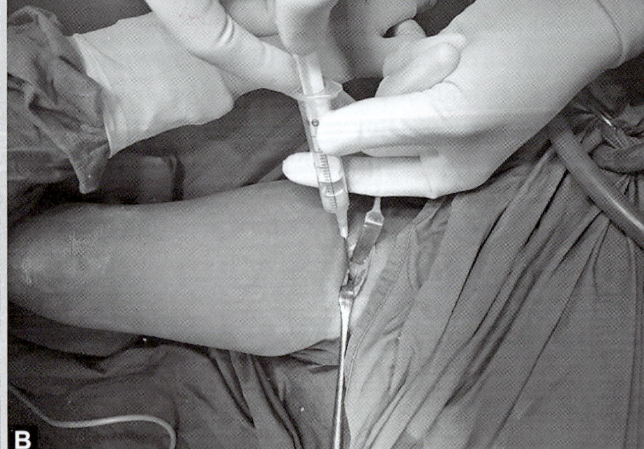

Figs. 1A and B: (A) MRI of a 5-year-old child with pain in the right hip which shows severe fluid collection in the right hip joint suggestive of septic arthritis of right hip; (B) Intraoperative photograph of the arthrotomy of the hip of the same child with aspiration of purulent fluid from the hip joint

4–5 days after which repeat complete blood count (CBC), ESR and CRP are done. Once the CRP has normalized and the ESR shows a down trending, the child may be shifted to oral antibiotics. Oral antibiotic therapy is continued for a total of 6 weeks. The exceptions to this short course of antibiotics are immunosuppression due to any cause, a very virulent organism like MRSA or *Pseudomonas*, or in patients in whom culture sensitivity shows poor sensitivity for oral antibiotics.

Close monitoring of the clinical, blood and radiological parameters is required to ensure that the treatment is effective and the outcome satisfactory. Antibiotics can usually be stopped by 6 weeks if the child has improved. Radiographs must be taken 6 monthly to see for any sequalae.

ACUTE OSTEOMYELITIS

Introduction and Epidemiology

Osteomyelitis (*Osteon*- bone, *myelo*- marrow and *itis*- inflammation) refers to the infection and inflammation of the bone and bone marrow which can lead to the reduction in the blood supply of the bone. Osteomyelitis (OM) in childhood has bimodal distribution—the first peak is during neonatal period and infancy and the second peak is between 4 and 8 years of age. Boys and girls are almost equally affected though with a slight male preponderance. The long bones of the lower limbs are most commonly involved in osteomyelitis, especially the distal end of the femur, followed by proximal tibia, proximal humerus, proximal femur and distal tibia in that order. The pelvic bones and the axial skeletal are less commonly involved.[7-9]

Pathophysiology

Depending upon the source of origin, OM is of three types:

- Acute hematogenous OM;
- OM secondary to contiguous spread of infection after trauma, puncture wounds or surgery; and
- OM due to vascular insufficiency.

Acute hematogenous OM occurs due to bacteremia with resultant seeding of the metaphyseal blood vessels due to sluggishness of blood flow in the U-pin bends of the blood vessels. *Staphylococcus aureus* is the most common organism to cause AOM.[7] In most cases, the preceding bacteremia which is the cause of the osteomyelitis is cryptic. The main nidus of infection starts in the valveless sinusoidal loops of the venules at the junction of the epiphysis and metaphysis due to the slow and non-laminar blood flow through this very unique vascular bed. It can also be after a very nonspecific antecedent trauma that causes a metaphyseal hematoma. Once this gets infected, a metaphyseal abscess is formed in the subperiosteal space of the metaphysis. The pus then tracks down through the path of least resistance, which is either along the shaft in the sub-periosteal space or bursting through the periosteum to reach the soft tissue and musculature. Once the periosteum is sheared off, then vascularity of the sub-cortical bone of the metaphysis is significantly hampered and the entire bone in that zone can get devascularized. This itself is a potential cause for the long-term complications of acute OM which include chronic OM with sequestrum formation, discharging sinus, disseminated medullary infection, Garre's or Brodie's abscess or pathological fractures.

Microbiology

The commonest organism causing OM is *Staphylococcus aureus* in all age groups. The incidence has increased over the last few years since the incidence of other hemo-invasive organisms like *H. Influenzae B* and *Streptococcus pneumoniae* has decreased over the last few decades due to successful vaccination campaigns. Like septic arthritis, MSSA is still the commonest organism in the community acquired setting while the MRSA is commonest in the hospital acquired setting. However, MRSA has become quite common in the community acquired setting over the last few years.[9] The other common organisms are *Streptococcus pyogenes, Kingella kingae, Klebsiella pneumoniae*, and *Pseudomonas aeruginosa*. *Pseudomonas aeruginosa* is commonest in penetrating trauma of the small bones of the feet, of the tarsals and metatarsals. *Salmonella typhi* causes a unique diaphyseal infection in kids who have impaired vascularity especially in kids with sickle cell anemia.

Clinical Features

Acute osteomyelitis (AOM) presents in two distinct ways: the first is an acutely ill, febrile child who has all the systemic and constitutional symptoms of septicemia with local signs of skeletal infection like local rise in temperature, warmth and redness. The other common scenario is a child who is otherwise not unwell, has low grade fever and shows a gradual progression of skeletal illness. This usually occurs along with progressive loss of function or range of motion. Overall, the hallmark of AOM of both types is localized pain with restricted movement with or without fever.[10,11] Neonatal OM is usually associated with concomitant septic arthritis due to the vascularity of the growth plate especially in joints like the hip and the shoulder. Thus, neonatal OM may present with symptoms and signs of joint involvement and increased intra-articular volume like localized tenderness at the joint, position of comfort which maximizes joint volume (for the hip, flexion, abduction and external rotation), reduced range of the motion of the joint to a much greater degree than that seen in isolated AOM, and pseudoparalysis. Neonatal OM especially in the setting of neonatal sepsis is very likely to be associated with multifocal involvement.[7]

One of the common causes of OM in our sub-continent is tuberculosis. This usually presents in a chronic manner with low grade fever, local swelling, minimal systemic features, low grade constitutional symptoms like loss of appetite and loss of weight.

Diagnosis

The diagnosis of AOM is based on clinical, hematological and radiological features. In the acute setting, a high WBC count along with elevated neutrophils, elevated ESR and a high CRP is diagnostic of AOM. Procalcitonin is an important marker of acute infection especially in presence of systemic infection, but its cost and non-availability in most centers makes it difficult to use it in widespread manner. Subtle signs of AOM disease like rarefaction at the metaphysis, periosteal elevation, etc., may be seen on radiographs. The X-ray findings start becoming obvious at around 1–2 weeks after the onset of symptoms. The typical "rat-bite" in the metaphysis is a late sign (**Fig. 2A**) and its absence does not rule out AOM. Radiographs are also useful in ruling out other causes of acute pseudoparalysis like scurvy and Ewing sarcoma.[10] USG may be helpful in some cases where the abscess has formed or when it is associated with septic arthritis. MRI has emerged as the investigation of choice in the diagnosis of acute OM in children and also helps in diagnosing any associated extra-osseous collection if present (**Figs. 2B and C**). Aseptic aspiration of the collection with a wide bore needle under USG or CT guidance is an important investigation in AOM. The aspirate should be immediately sent for culture and sensitivity and definitive antibiotics need to be started based on the culture sensitivity report.

***Differential diagnosis*:** The two main differential diagnoses of AOM are scurvy and Ewing sarcoma. X-ray, MRI and if necessary, a small incision biopsy may be performed to conclusively diagnose the condition.[9]

Treatment

Surgical management

Surgical management of AOM involves either aspiration of the fluid in early cases or formal drainage and debridement of the osteomyelitic focus.[7-11] Formal drainage and debridement of the osteomyelitic focus involves evacuation of the sub-periosteal collection by incising the periosteum widely as well as making multiple drill holes or a corticotomy to relieve the intramedullary pressure and creating an opening for free drainage of intramedullary fluid in the soft tissue (**Fig. 2D**). Intraoperative imaging should be used to know the exact extent of debridement. The wound is usually closed under a wide bore negative suction drain so as to provide prolonged drainage. The limb is protected with a plaster slab or a cast whenever possible or feasible for at least 4 weeks.

Medical management

Broad-spectrum empirical antibiotics are administered till culture reports are obtained and then definitive antibiotics are administered till normalization of CRP. A first or second generation cephalosporin like cefazolin or cefuroxime is the drug of choice for the initial management in community acquired OM. In addition, an extended spectrum antibiotic like cefepime or piperacillin-tazobactam can be started when Enterobacteriae or *Pseudomonas* are suspected. The parenteral antibiotics need to be continued for a period of at least 5–7 days depending on the type of organism isolated. In case of MSSA, the shift to oral antibiotics can happen at around 5–7 days at the time of normalization of CRP. In other organisms, especially in MRSA, IV antibiotics need to be given at least for 2–3 weeks depending on the clinical response, CRP levels as well as the antibiogram. It is to be remembered that due to diminished penetration into bone, orally administered beta-lactamase antibiotics need to be administered at higher-than-traditional doses to achieve adequate inhibitory concentrations at the site of infection.[10]

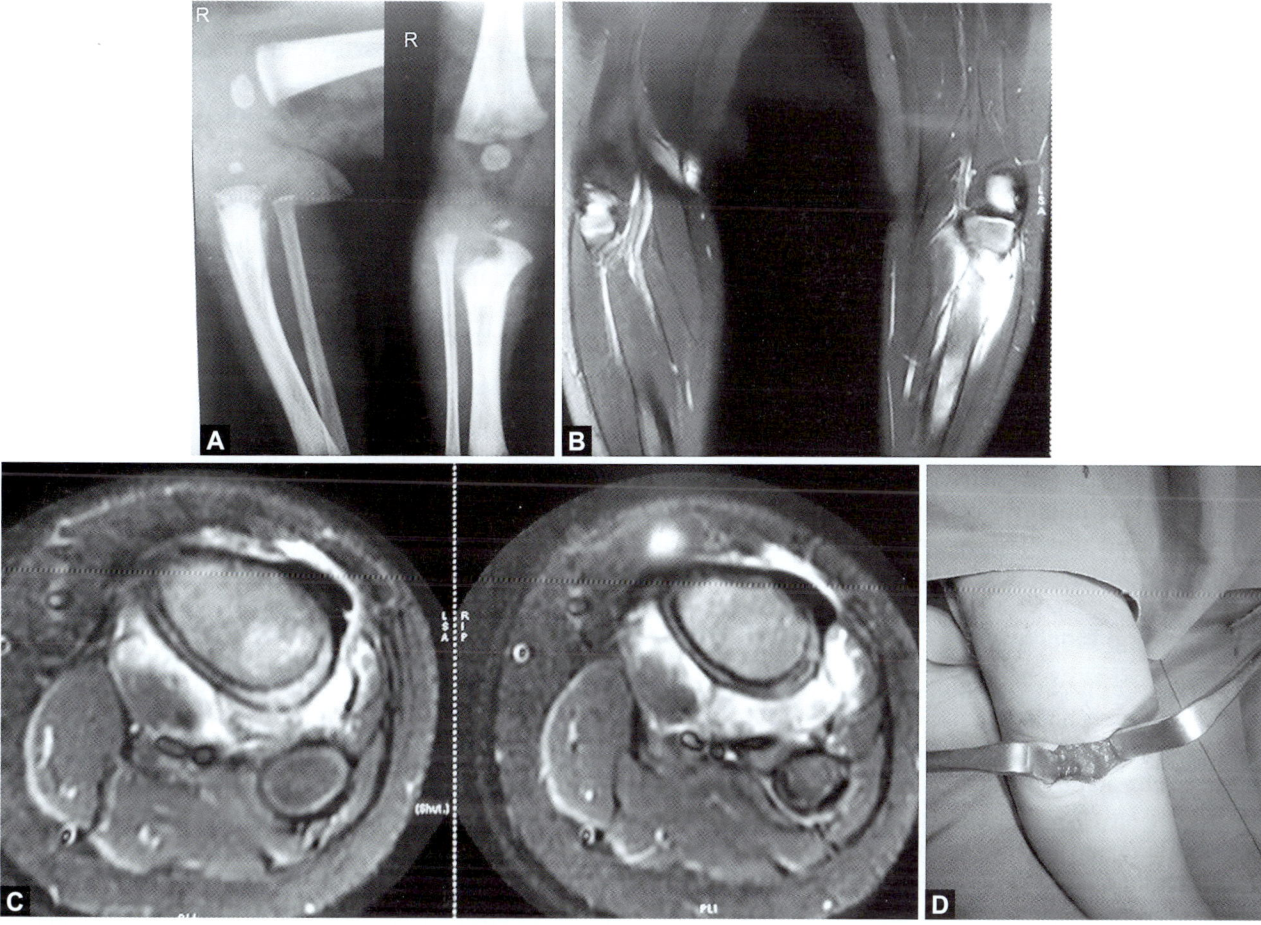

Figs. 2A to D: (A) Plain radiograph of a two-month-old child with osteomyelitis of the upper tibia showing a severe involvement of the upper tibial metaphysis and the typical "rat-bite" appearance of the metaphysis; (B and C) MRI of the same child with upper tibial osteomyelitis showing severe involvement of the metaphysis and a large sub-periosteal abscess formation; (D) Intraoperative photograph of the same child showing upper tibial metaphyseal lesion being debrided

Complications

The complications of AOM are described as under:

- *Systemic sepsis* especially in AOM due to MRSA and *Klebsiella*.
- *Chronic OM*: The segment of bone underneath the subperiosteal abscess gets avascular and becomes a dead segment known as *a sequestrum*, which continues to lie free in a pool of pyogenic tissue. The pus finds a way of coming to the exterior of the bone through an opening known as the *cloaca* and to the exterior of the skin through the opening known as the *sinus*. So long as the sequestrum is present in the medullary cavity, the external sinus is not likely to heal. Hence, its treatment involves a radical debridement and removal of the sequestrum known as sequestrectomy.
- *Pathological fracture*: This is a dreaded complication of acute as well as chronic OM. This happens due to the weakening of the bone due to the pyogenic process as well as due to inadvertent large size corticotomy performed which causes a point of weakness for the bone. This is very difficult to treat and requires eradication of infection as well as stabilization of the fracture. This process may be lengthy and may require multiple surgeries.
- *Garre's abscess*: This happens when the intramedullary abscess gets walled off and causes a thick walled collection of granulation tissue. This is typically seen in the upper tibia and is a source of chronic pain and may cause intermittent draining sinuses.

SUPRACONDYLAR FRACTURE OF HUMERUS

Introduction

Supracondylar fractures of humerus are one of the most common injuries around the elbow seen in children. They account for 7-9% of all the fractures in children and about 86% of all fractures around the elbow.[12] This fracture occurs most commonly between 3 and 10 years of age. The fracture is more common on the left or the non-dominant side. Initially, it was thought that there is a male predominance for these fractures but recent studies denote an equal incidence between males and females.[13] Associated neurovascular complications range from 5% to 19% and open fractures constitute less than 1% of all fractures.[12] Current consensus suggests that displaced supracondylar humerus fractures are best managed surgically and they are the most common pediatric fractures requiring emergent surgical intervention.[14]

Anatomy and Mechanism of Injury

The distal humerus is made up of two columns: the lateral column is made up of the trochlea and the lateral supracondylar ridge, and the medial column is made up of the trochlea and the medial supracondylar ridge. The medial and lateral columns are connected by a thin wafer of bone between the olecranon fossa posteriorly and the coronoid fossa anteriorly. By far, the most common mechanism of injury leading to supracondylar humerus fractures in fall on outstretched hand with a resultant hyperextension of the elbow causing an extension type of supracondylar humerus fracture (98%). The other way in which the fracture occurs is a direct blow to the flexed elbow which causes anterior displacement of the distal fragment leading to a flexion type supracondylar humerus fracture seen in 2-5% of cases.[15] With the extension type injuries, the distal fragment can be displaced either posteromedially (75%) or posterolaterally (25%). The posterolaterally displaced fractures are more commonly associated with neurovascular injuries.[15]

Classification

The fractures are first classified and extension type or flexion type and depending upon the degree of displacement. The supracondylar humerus fractures have been classified by Gartland into 3 types which have undergone subsequent modification into 4 types.[13]

- *Type* I: Undisplaced or minimally displaced fractures
- *Type* II: Fractures with angulation with one cortex intact
- *Type* III: Completely displaced fractures (**Fig. 3A**)
- *Type* IV: Fractures which are highly unstable and distal fragment displaces into flexion and extension both.

The type III and IV fractures are pediatric orthopedic emergencies and need urgent reduction and fixation in most cases (**Table 1**).

Diagnosis

Children usually present to the emergency room with history of fall and a tense, swollen elbow with decreased movements of the elbow. Clinical examination will reveal a swollen painful elbow and tenderness over the humeral condyles and supracondylar ridges. 'S'-shaped deformity of the elbow is sometimes evident in severely displaced fractures and an anterior puckering may also be seen if the proximal fragment has impaled the brachialis and the anterior fascia of the elbow. In such cases, an ecchymosis is also seen around the anterior aspect of the elbow (**Fig. 3B**).[14]

It is imperative to perform a thorough neurological and vascular examination to look for associated neurovascular injuries. Sensory examination of the autonomous zones of the median, radial and ulnar nerves should be done. Motor examination including active wrist finger and thumb extension (radial nerve) flexion of the thumb and index distal interphalangeal joint of index finger (median nerve) and examination of interossei (ulnar nerve) should be done. Vascular examination includes examination of the radial pulse, capillary refill, warmth and color of the hand,[16] depending on the vascularity the hand can be warm and red with a radial pulse, warm and red with absent radial pulse, or cool and blue with absent radial pulse.[15]

Carefully documented pre-manipulation exam findings and post-manipulation neurovascular deficits can alter decision making. Compartment syndrome though a rare complication of supracondylar humerus fractures is a true surgical emergency and needs a careful vigil to prevent devastating complications. The attending surgeon should keep a high index of suspicion in mind whenever a supracondylar humerus fracture is associated with swelling and ecchymosis, anterior skin puckering, absent pulse, pain on passive stretching or increasing pain/pain out of

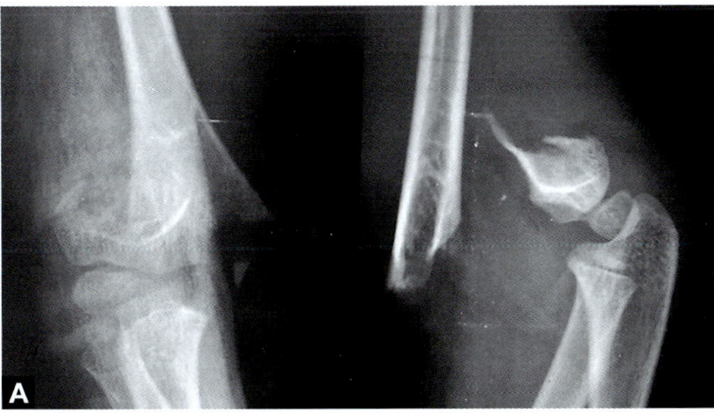

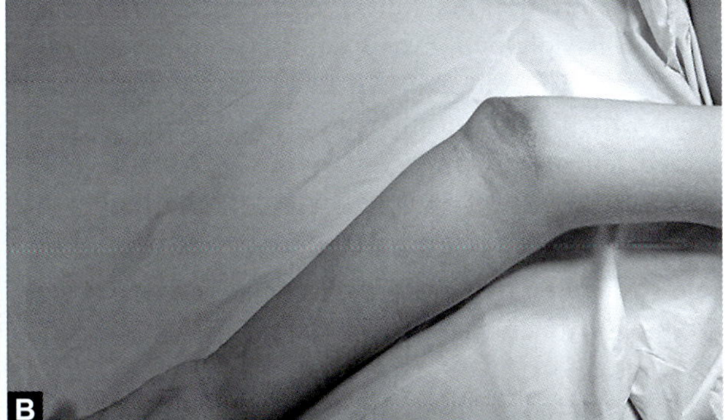

Figs. 3A and B: (A) Plain radiograph of the elbow of a 5-year-old child showing gross displacement of the fracture fragments of the supracondylar humerus fracture (Gartland type III); (B) Clinical photograph of the same child with severe ecchymosis around the elbow and the pucker sign seen

Table 1: Modified Gartland classification of supracondylar fractures of the humerus

Fracture type	*Characteristics*	*Comments*
I	Minimal displacement	Fat pad elevation on radiographs
II	Posterior hinge	Anterior humeral line anterior to capitellum
III	Displaced	No cortical contact
IV	Displaced in extension and flexion	Flexion and extension instability demonstrated radiographically
Medial comminution	Collapse of medial column	Loss of Baumann angle

proportion to the injury, apprehension or increasing need of analgesics. Lastly, the entire upper extremity should be thoroughly examined for any associated injuries.

Radiographic evaluation

Supracondylar humerus fractures are best diagnosed on standard anteroposterior and lateral X-rays of the elbow. They are assessed for evidence of fracture, degree of displacement; rotation and translation, degree of comminution of the fracture and evidence of intra-articular extension.

When no fracture line is visible the presence of the posterior fat pad sign on a lateral radiograph is suggestive of an occult fracture.[2] Anterior humeral line should intersect, the middle third of the capitellum. In cases of fractures the line passes through the anterior third or in front of the capitellum. On the AP radiograph of the elbow, the Baumann's angle formed by the line along the long axis of the humerus and the physeal line of the lateral condyle is useful to assess a coronal plane deformity.[12]

Management

Treatment consists of splinting the fracture in a long arm posterior slab with the elbow in 20–40° of flexion. It is advisable to avoid excess flexion or tight bandaging to prevent the development of vascular compromise. The distal circulation should always be checked before and after application of the splint. The child and the parents should be advised limb elevation with the fingers above the elbow and the elbow above the heart for the first 48 hours after injury.[15]

Type I fractures

These fractures are inherently stable due to intact periosteum and can usually be successfully managed conservatively. The child is given a long arm posterior splint for 5–10 days till the initial swelling subsides following which a check X-ray is taken to confirm that there is no further displacement of the fracture. Once a confirmation is made the child is given a long arm cast for 3–4 weeks. The cast can be removed after 3–4 weeks and range of motion exercises are begun gradually.[13]

Type II fractures

In these fractures, the intact posterior periosteal sleeve acts as a hinge and aids in reduction of the fracture.[14] After reduction is achieved the general consensus is to fix the fractures with K wires inserted percutaneously followed by immobilization in a long arm posterior slab in 30–60° of elbow flexion for 3–4 weeks. At the 3–4 weeks follow-up radiographs are repeated, and the wires are removed in the office without any anesthesia, immobilization is discontinued, and range of motion exercises are encouraged.[15]

Type III/type IV fractures

These fractures are inherently unstable as the periosteum around the fracture is torn and there is no cortical contact between the two fracture fragments. These fractures are associated with significant soft tissue injury or neurovascular injuries. Treatment options include open or closed reduction and fixation with K-wires.

Maneuver of closed reduction includes the assistant holding the proximal fragment to apply counter traction while the surgeon applies axial traction to the distal fragment with the elbow extended. Once length is gained the varus/valgus alignment is corrected **(Figs. 3C and D)**.

Complications

Early complications include neurovascular injury and compartment syndrome as discussed before. Delayed complications include malunion, elbow stiffness and myositis ossificans.[4] Malunion leading to cubitus varus is one of the most common complications of supracondylar humerus fractures that are not treated appropriately. Cubitus varus is a painless deformity not affecting elbow range of motion. However, O'Driscoll, *et al.*[17] identified 22 adult patients who presented with pain as well as signs and symptoms of elbow instability 20 to 30 years after sustaining supracondylar fractures in childhood. Cubitus varus requires a corrective osteotomy and fixation.

ACUTE COMPARTMENT SYNDROME

Introduction

Compartment syndrome (CS) is a limb- and sometime life-threatening condition observed when perfusion pressure falls below tissue pressure in a closed anatomical space leading to increased interstitial pressure and microvascular compromise.[18-28] Compartment syndrome is particularly important in children as the cardinal signs of compartment syndrome may be masked in children leading to difficulty and delay in diagnosis and further morbidity.

Etiology

The commonest cause of CS in children is trauma, of which the elbow is the commonest region. Displaced supracondylar humerus fracture is the most common cause, followed by forearm fractures, fracture of tibia and femoral shaft fracture.[18] Certain others like massage and tight bandaging or plasters can precipitate CS.[22] The other common causes of CS in children are soft tissue injuries without fractures, intra-compartmental bleeding due to extravasation (**Fig. 4A**), or due to snake or spider bite, and intra-compartmental bleeding in hematological disorders.[26] Another important cause of CS is muscle crushing due to fall of heavy weight, typically seen in earthquake victims.[21]

Pathogenesis

The pathophysiology of CS follows ischemic injury. When fluid is introduced into the osseo-fascial compartments which have a relatively fixed volume or when the volume

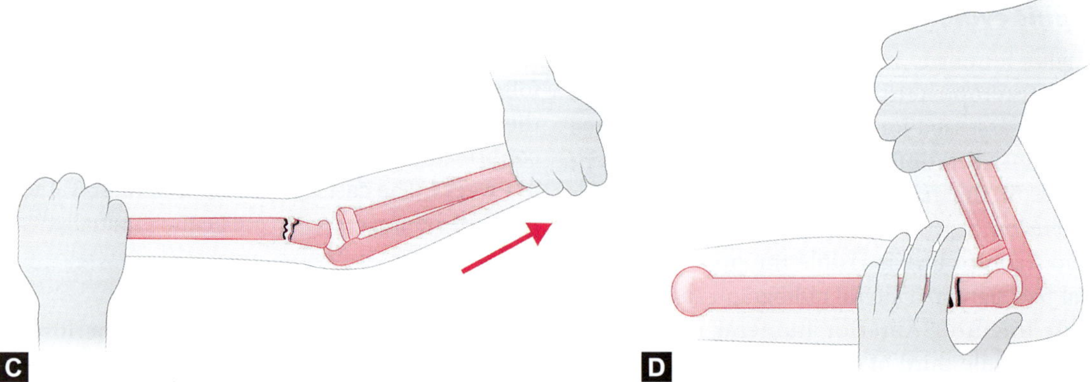

Figs. 3C and D: Schematic diagram of reduction maneuver in fracture supracondylar humerus. Initially longitudinal traction is given with the elbow extended (C) and then once length is achieved, the elbow is flexed and then definitive fixation done with k wires (D)

decreases, pressure rises above the normal average of 10 mm Hg. This in turn decreases tissue perfusion until no oxygen is available for cellular metabolism. As the intracompartmental pressure rises, venous pressure rises and exceeds the capillary perfusion pressure (CPP) causing the capillaries to collapse (**Fig. 4A**). Generally, at intracompartmental pressures exceeding 30 mm Hg, blood flow through the capillaries stops and oxygen delivery is impaired. Hypoxic injury causes cells to release vasoactive substances (histamine and serotonin) which increase endothelial permeability, which further increases tissue pressure and advances injury. Nerve conduction slows, tissue pH falls due to anaerobic metabolism, surrounding tissue suffers further damage and muscle tissue suffers necrosis, releasing myoglobin. CS occurring in earthquake victims is different than the classical CS. In this, muscle crush occurs first, which leads to early myoglobinuria causing systemic problems including renal failure.

Clinical Features

The classical clinical features of compartment syndrome in older children, adolescents and adults are described as the 6P's (Pain, pressure, paresthesia, paralysis/paresis, pallor and pulselessness).[18-20]

Pain: The pain is described to be out of proportion to the injury and is most commonly due to the ischemia of the nerves due to rise in pressure. It is exaggerated by the passive stretch of the involved muscles of the compartment. The classical sign of "passive stretch" needs to be looked for in all the patients suspected to have CS. It, however, may also be negative in obtunded children, very young children, and in late cases of CS when the neuronal damage has already set in.

Pressure: This is a very early finding and is a clinical sign **(Figs. 4B and C),** which is always to be looked for. Pressure measurements can be of two types: Clinical and

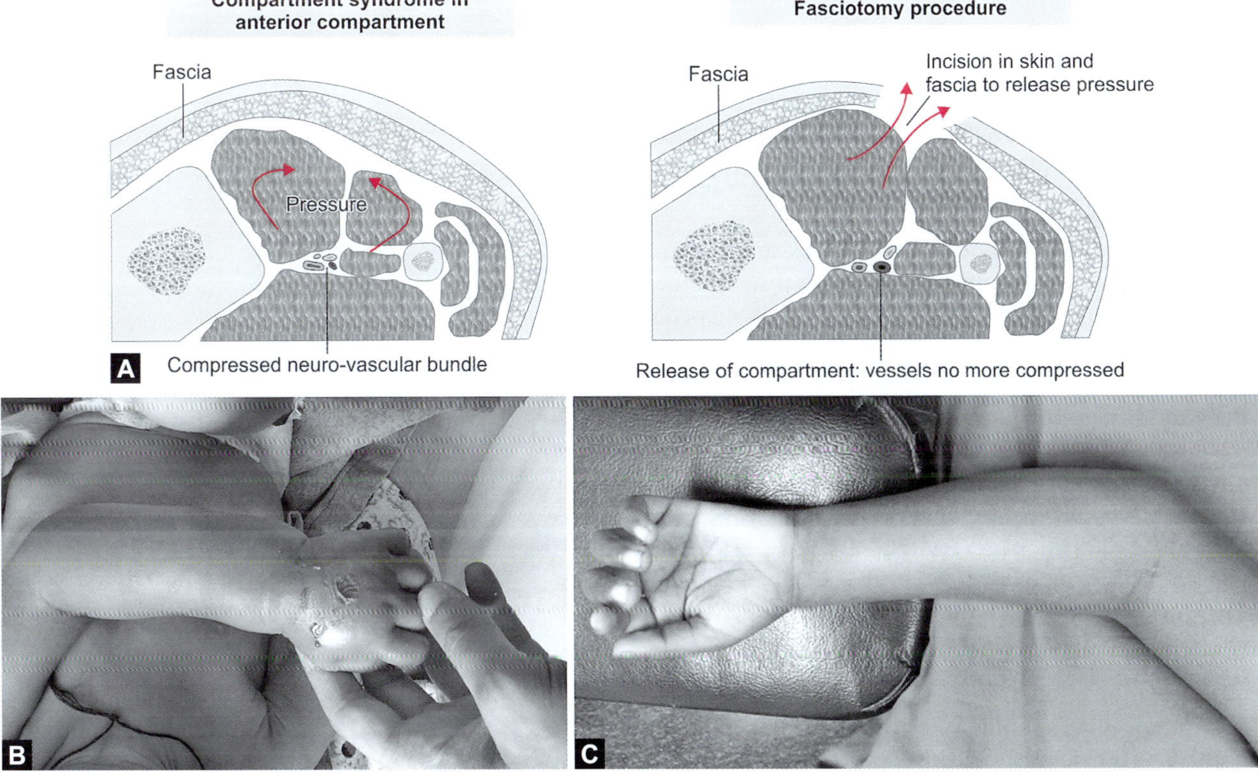

Figs. 4A to C: (A) Schematic representation of a tense closed compartment showing compression of the neurovascular structures at the onset of compartment syndrome and then the relief of the pressure after compartment release with a fasciotomy; (B) Clinical photograph of a 6-week-old child with compartment syndrome of the forearm following IV extravasation. Note the ecchymosis at the site of IV line insertion; (C) Clinical photograph of a 6-year-old child with compartment syndrome of the forearm. Note the tense swelling with shiny skin

manometric. Clinical measurement or assessment of compartment pressure and turgidity by palpation is one of the most important tests for diagnosing CS. The objective method of evaluation of compartment pressure is by using pressure measuring devices is rarely used.[22]

Paresthesia: Paresthesia is a sign or the cry of the "dying" nerves. Neuralgic pain is one of the most specific sign of rising compartmental pressures, though in young children it may not be easily interpreted.

Paralysis/Paresis: This is a late sign and in fact denotes that irreversible muscle and nerve damage has already occurred. It is sometimes difficult to interpret due to pain.

Pallor/Pulselessness: This also is a very late sign and shows that ischemic damage is quite widespread and many a time shows irreversibility.

In very young kids however, these 6 P's are very difficult to interpret and they are replaced by 3A's as under:

***A**nxiety and **A**pprehension*: These two are very sensitive features of compartment syndrome in children and are to be looked for. In a child who has a plaster, or in the post-operative period, if the child is anxious or apprehensive, then immediate intervention needs to be done, and compartment pressure reduced at least initially by removal or slitting of the plaster and definitive intervention if required may be performed later.

*Increased **A**nalgesic requirements*: This is especially true in postoperative patients, where fixation of fractures has been performed. Kids with fractures like displaced supracondylar humeral fractures usually are comfortable once the fracture is fixed and a plaster is given. If however, the child is requiring significant amount of analgesics in the postoperative period, which is not proportionate to the amount of operative trauma, then this serves as a warning sign of increased compartmental pressures and needs early intervention.

Treatment

Pre-hospital care: CS can develop very rapidly after an arterial or a major bony injury. Only essential life-saving procedures should be performed in the field and immediate transport should be done to the hospital.

Emergency department care: Irreversible nerve damage can begin within 6 hours of intracompartmental hypertension. Removal of constricting casts and bandages is of paramount importance. Almost 90% of the intra-compartmental pressures can be relieved by just removing the constricting casts and padding.[22]

Medical management

Medical management forms a minor part of the overall treatment of CS, and consists of correction of hypovolemia. Hyperbaric oxygen therapy (HBO) especially in crush syndrome is beneficial to reduce the ischemic injury.[21]

Surgical management

Surgical management forms the mainstay of treatment of CS and consists of fasciotomy, necrectomy, and management of associated skeletal injuries. Early complications/ include infection, myoglobinuria and renal failure, and irreversible neurological deficit. Volkmann's ischemic contracture due to muscle contracture is a late complication.

KEY MESSAGES

- Acute septic arthritis should be suspected in children with decreased and painful movements of limbs, and those having gait disturbance with history of fever.
- Kocher criteria of fever (>38°C), inability to bear weight, WBC >12,000/ mm^3 and ESR > 40 mm/hr are useful to diagnose acute septic arthritis. MRI is the investigation of choice.
- Empirical broad-spectrum antibiotics need to be started after drainage of the fluid and sending the fluid for microbiological analysis in treatment of acute septic arthritis. Duration of antibiotic therapy is at least 6 weeks and should be accompanied with clinical and laboratory response including falling CRP levels.
- Acute osteomyelitis may present with localized limb pain with restricted movements with or without fever. X-ray and MRI may help in diagnosis.
- It is important to assess the neurovascular status of the limb in every child with a supracondylar humerus fracture. Displaced supracondylar humerus fractures are best managed operatively.
- The classical clinical features of compartment syndrome in older children and adolescents are described as the 6P's: pain, pressure, paresthesia, paralysis/paresis, pallor and pulselessness. In very young kids however, these 6 P's are very difficult to interpret and they are replaced by 3A's: **a**nxiety and **a**pprehension and increased **a**nalgesic requirements. Surgical management is the mainstay of treatment.

REFERENCES

1. Narang A, Mukhopadhyay K, Kumar P, *et al.* Bone and joint infection in neonates. Indian J Pediatr. 1998;65:461-4.

2. Curtiss PH Jr, Klein L. Destruction of articular cartilage in septic arthritis. II. In vivo studies. J Bone Joint Surg 1965;47A:1595-604.
3. Rutz E, Brunner R. Septic arthritis of the hip - current concepts. Hip Int. 2009;19 Suppl 6:S9-12.
4. Sultan J, Hughes PJ. Septic arthritis or transient synovitis of the hip in children: The value of clinical prediction algorithms. J Bone Joint Surg Br. 2010;92:1289-93.
5. Pääkkönen M, Kallio MJ, Kallio PE, *et al.* Sensitivity of erythrocyte sedimentation rate and C-reactive protein in childhood bone and joint infections. Clin Orthop Relat Res. 2010;468:861-6.
6. Kocher MS, Zurakowski D, Kasser JR. Differentiating between septic arthritis and transient synovitis of the hip in children: An evidence based clinical prediction algorithm. J Bone Joint Surg Am 1999;81:1662-70.
7. Fox L, Sprunt K. Neonatal osteomyelitis. Pediatrics 1978;62: 535-42.
8. Syriopoulou VP, Smith AL. Osteomyelitis and septic arthritis. In: Feigin RD, Cherry JD, editors. Textbook of Pediatric Infectious Diseases, 2nd edition. Philadelphia: WB Saunders;1987. p. 759-79.
9. Conrad DA. Acute hematogenous osteomyelitis. Pediatr Rev. 2010;31:464-70.
10. Lew DP, Waldvogel FA. Osteomyelitis. Lancet. 2004;364:369-70.
11. LaMont RL, Anderson PA, Dejani AS. Acute hematogenous osteomyelitis in children. J Pediatr Orthop. 1987;7:579-83.
12. Antonioli D, Lampasi M, Stilli S, *et al.* Pediatric elbow fractures and rehabilitation. In: Porcellini G, Rotini R, Kantar S, Di Giacomo S, editors. The Elbow. Springer, Cham. 2010.
13. Abzug JM, Herman MJ. Management of supracondylar humerus fractures in children: Current concepts. J Am Acad Orthop Surg. 2012;20(2):69-77.
14. Rockwood CA Jr, Wilkins KE, King RE. Fractures in Children, Vol. 3, 3rd edition. Philadelphia: JB Lippincott, 1991. p. 526-617.
15. Herring J, Tachdjian M. Tachdjian's Pediatric Orthopedics. Philadelphia: Elsevier/Saunders. 2014.
16. Baratz M, Micucci C, Sangimino M. Pediatric supracondylar humerus fractures. Hand Clin. 2006;22:69-75.
17. O'Driscoll SW, Spinner RJ, McKee MD, *et al.* Tardy posterolateral rotator instability of the elbow due to cubitus varus. J Bone Joint Surg Am. 2001;83:1358-69.
18. Hwang RW, De Witte P, Ring D. Compartment syndrome associated with distal radius fracture and ipsilateral elbow injury. J Bone Joint Surg. 2009;91:642-45.
19. Cascio BM, Wilckens JH, Ain MC, *et al.* Documentation of acute compartment syndrome at an academic health-care center. J Bone Joint Surg Am. 2005;87:346-50.
20. Namboothri S. Compartment syndrome and systemic hypertension. J Bone Joint Surg Br. 2005;87:1420-22.
21. Reis ND, Better OS. Mechanical muscle-crush injury and acute muscle-crush compartment syndrome: With special reference to earthquake casualties. J Bone Joint Surg Br. 2005;87: 450-3.
22. Halanski M, Noonan KJ. Cast and splint immobilization: Complications. J Am Acad Orthop Surg. 2008;16:30-40.
23. Mubarak SJ, Pedowitz RA, Hargens AR. Compartment syndromes. Curr Orthop. 1989;3:36-40.
24. Klenerman L. The evolution of the compartment syndrome since 1948 as recorded in the JBJS (B). J Bone Joint Surg Br. 2007;89:1280-2.
25. Fraipont MJ, Adamson GJ. Chronic exertional compartment syndrome. J Am Acad Orthop Surg. 2003;11:268-76.
26. Bacal D, Lampman RM, Hogikyan JV, *et al.* Compartment syndrome of the arm and disseminated intravascular coagulation. Am J Orthop (Belle Mead NJ). 2001;30:422-3.
27. Kleshinski J, Bittar S, Wahlquist M, *et al.* Review of compartment syndrome due to Group A Streptococcal infection. Am J Med Sci. 2008;336:265-69.
28. Ramos C, Whyte CM, Harris BH. Nontraumatic compartment syndrome of the extremities in children. J Pediatr Surg. 2006; 41:e5-e7.

CHAPTER

87

Ocular Emergencies

Payal Gupta

While many ocular diseases have an apparent clinical presentation in the child prompting the parents to seek an ophthalmology consultation, often a pediatrician is the first healthcare professional to address these concerns. In such a scenario, it is pertinent for the pediatric specialist to keep himself well versed with the obvious as well as the not-so-obvious signs of an emergent ophthalmic disease.

NEONATAL OCULAR EMERGENCIES

Birth Trauma

Trauma to the eye can occur during aided delivery, especially with the use of forceps during delivery. Birth trauma to the eye and its adnexa include eyelid tears, injury to the facial nerve, corneal abrasions and edema, hyphema and retinal hemorrhages.[1] Eyelid tears need surgical repair. Corneal abrasions or edema would require detailed anterior chamber examination under sedation. All cases of assisted deliveries with suspected ocular trauma should be referred to an ophthalmologist at the earliest.

Acute Conjunctivitis (Ophthalmia Neonatorum/ Neonatal Conjunctivitis)

Any mucoid, mucopurulent or purulent discharge from one or both eyes in first month of life is considered neonatal conjunctivitis. Corneal ulceration and perforation resulting due to complicated or untreated cases of ophthalmia neonatorum is a totally preventable cause of childhood blindness that can be appropriately managed by timely diagnosis and intervention.

Etiology

It could be bacterial (gonococcal, chlamydial, staphylococcal, streptococcal), viral (herpes simplex virus) or chemical (rarely).

Clinical features

Associated redness, chemosis, blepharitis and keratitis may be present depending on the severity and etiology of infection.

- Gonococcal conjunctivitis usually presents within first 48 hours of life with severe bilateral affection. There is usually an intense conjunctival redness and edema with thick, yellow, sticky, purulent eye discharge causing matting of eyelashes (**Fig. 1**). Retractors may be needed to separate tense-swollen lids for ocular examination. There is a high risk of corneal perforation and thus immediate referral to an ophthalmologist is recommended in suspected cases.

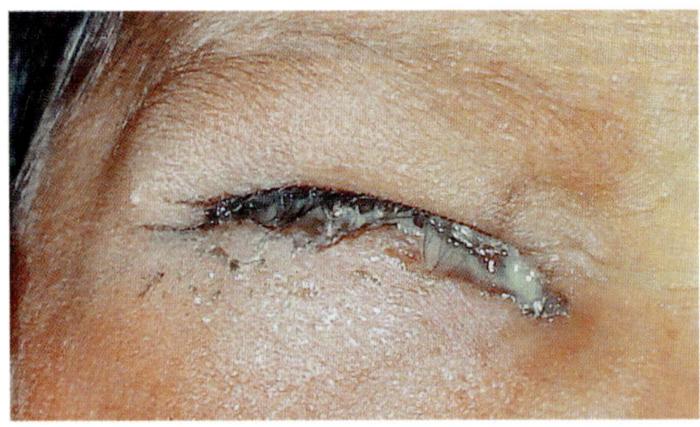

Fig. 1: Ophthalmia neonatorum

- Chlamydial conjunctivitis typically presents after 1 week of birth. There is overlap of symptoms with gonococcal conjunctivitis, but lid involvement is comparatively less.
- Viral ophthalmia neonatorum following herpes simplex virus (HSV) infection, presents 5–7 days after birth with watery discharge and associated blepharitis.
- Chemical conjunctivitis following perinatal ophthalmic prophylaxis, seen rarely, has an early presentation (within first 48 hours) with inflamed lids and conjunctiva with watery discharge.

Management

Mild conjunctivitis can be managed by treating the underlying infection with broad-spectrum topical drops like tobramycin and fusidic acid are effective. These can be used in 6 hourly dosing. Moderate to severe conjunctivitis requires conjunctival swab for staining and culture sensitivity for specific treatment, but empirical treatment (frequent eyewash with normal saline and broad-spectrum topical antibiotics) should begin at once while awaiting an ophthalmology consult. Neonates with suspected or confirmed gonococcal conjunctivitis should be hospitalized and treated with frequent irrigation of the conjunctiva and intravenous or intramuscular administration of ceftriaxone (25–50 mg/kg, to a maximum dose of 125 mg single dose), along with topical therapy (0.3% gentamicin every 15–30 minutes initially and bacitracin eye ointment 2–4 hourly). They should also be investigated for systemic gonorrheal infection like urethritis, arthritis, endocarditis, meningitis and septicemia. Chlamydial conjunctivitis requires topical as well as systemic therapy; erythromycin (50 mg/kg in 4 divided doses for 2–3 weeks) or azithromycin (10 mg/kg for 3 days) are recommended. Treatment of neonatal conjunctivitis due to HSV involves both topical and systemic parenteral acyclovir (3% acyclovir ointment 5 times a day for a week then 3 times a day till resolution along with high dose IV acyclovir is recommended for systemic involvement). Chemical ophthalmia neonatorum usually resolves spontaneously in 24–36 hours or may require erythromycin eye ointment with lubrication.

Congenital Nasolacrimal Duct Obstruction (CNLDO)

There is incomplete canalization of nasolacrimal passage, most commonly valve of Hasner, resulting in blockage of tear outflow pathway. Parents of a child with CNLDO would complain of watering from one or both the eyes (epiphora) of the baby since birth. Due to stagnation of tear fluid in lacrimal sac, there may be superadded infection leading to acute or chronic dacryocystitis (inflammation and infection of lacrimal sac) with mucoid/mucopurulent discharge and matting of lashes.

Clinical features

On examination, **r**egurgitation **o**n **p**ressure over **la**crimal **s**ac area (ROPLAS test) is positive.

Management

In less than 6 months of age, a proper hydrostatic sac massage by mother/caretaker several times a day can open up the passageway in more than 90% of children.[2] For superadded infection (mild to moderate), topical application of tobramycin eyedrops given in 6–8 hourly doses can suffice. Presence of acute or chronic dacryocystitis, dacryocele/mucocele and unresolving NLD obstruction requires urgent referral to pediatric ophthalmologist. Beyond 6 months of age, spontaneous resolution with sac massage is rare. Surgical probing is generally required, which if delayed is ineffective due to fibrosis and ossification. Continued infection in the lacrimal sac can lead to preseptal cellulitis, which is a much more serious condition requiring hospitalization. Untreated acute dacryocystitis can develop into lacrimal abscess, which may spontaneously burst out resulting in a permanent fistula over skin in lacrimal sac region.

CONDITIONS AT RISK OF AMBLYOPIA OR BLINDNESS

Congenital presentation in an infant requiring emergent attention are discussed here.[3]

Congenital Cataract

Any white reflex (leukocoria) in a newborn's eye, unilateral or bilateral, needs an immediate/emergent referral to a pediatric ophthalmologist. Etiology of congenital cataract is listed in **Box 1**.

Clinical features

Clinical features or history suggestive of any of these etiological conditions listed in **Box 1** requires screening for a congenital cataract. Clinical presentation depends on density and laterality of the lenticular opacity. Early onset, bilateral dense cataracts usually present with leukocoria (**Fig. 2**) and nystagmus or nystagmoid movements. Parents may comment that the child does not open her eyes, does not recognize mother and does not fixate or reach out for toys. Unilateral dense cataracts have a higher tendency of going into sensory deprivation amblyopia and often present with strabismus. Untreated or inadequately managed congenital cataracts can cause partial or complete blindness.

Management

Visually significant cataract needs to be operated as early as possible. Cataract extraction with intraocular lens implantation with postoperative amblyopia therapy is the treatment of choice. Early intervention and visual rehabilitation by an ophthalmologist, gives the child a chance at normal life.

Congenital Glaucoma

Childhood glaucoma can be inherited or sporadic. They may present at birth (congenital), within 3 years of life (infantile), or later (juvenile). If undiagnosed, or untreated, it can lead to irreversible optic nerve damage and permanent vision loss. Congenital glaucoma is usually associated with congenital cataract; associated syndromes (**Box 2**) are common.

Clinical features

Congenital glaucoma (**Fig. 3**) commonly presents as excessive tearing, photophobia (child typically keeps his face buried in parents' shoulder or chest) with blepharospasm, corneal enlargement (buphthalmos),

Box 1: Common causes of congenital cataract

- Idiopathic: 50% cases
- Chromosomal abnormalities
  - Trisomy 21
  - Turner syndrome
  - Cri du chat syndrome
- Congenital infections
  - Rubella
  - Toxoplasmosis
  - CMV
  - Varicella
  - Zika virus
- Inborn errors of metabolism
  - Galactosemia
  - Lowe disease
  - Fabry disease
  - Mannosidosis
  - Hypoparathyroidism
- Maternal malnutrtion
- Antenatal drug history
- Antenatal radiation exposure

Box 2: Common syndromic associations of glaucoma

- Trisomy 13-16 (Patau syndrome)
- Trisomy 18 (Edwards syndrome)
- Trisomy 21 (Down syndrome)
- Turner (XO/XX)
- Stickler syndrome (hereditary progressive arthro-ophthalmopathy)
- Zellweger (cerebrohepatorenal syndrome)
- Hallermann-Streiff syndrome (dyscephalic mandibulo-oculofacial syndrome)
- Oculodentodigital dysplasia
- Prader-Willi syndrome
- Cockayne syndrome
- Sturge-Weber syndrome: cerebral calcifications, seizures, developmental delay
- Neurofibromatosis 1
- Oculodermal melanocytosis
- Marfan syndrome
- Weill–Marchesani syndrome
- Lowe/oculocerebrorenal syndrome
- Homocystinuria
- Juvenile xanthogranuloma
- Congenital rubella syndrome
- Fetal alcohol syndrome

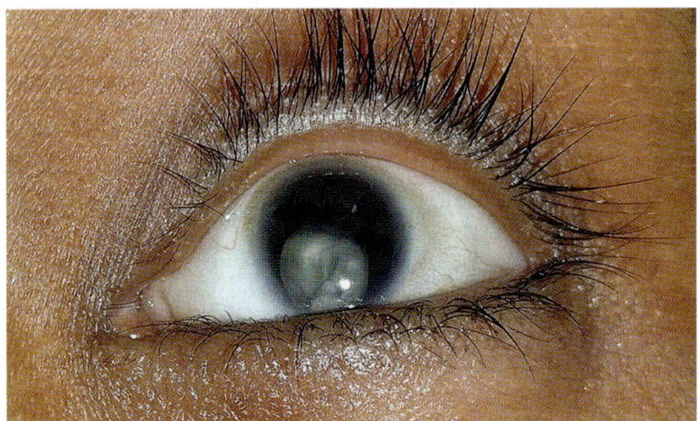

Fig. 2: White reflex (developmental cataract) with iris coloboma

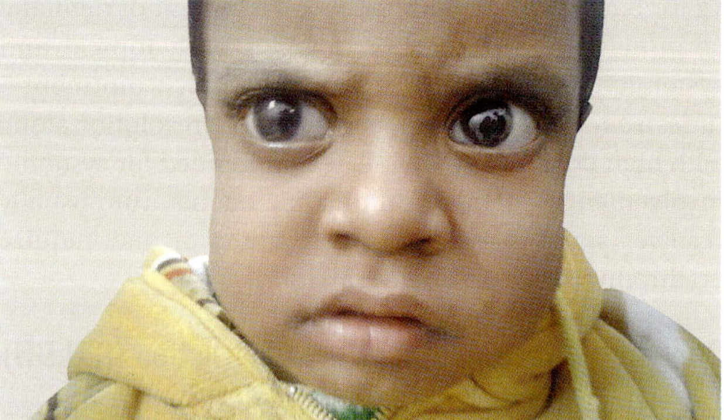

Fig. 3: Buphthalmos (late presenting congenital glaucoma)

corneal clouding or edema (bluish haze of cornea on torchlight examination), and conjunctival congestion. On fundoscopic examination, there is optic nerve damage. All these babies require a detailed examination under anesthesia for recording intraocular pressure, measurement of corneal diameter, retinoscopy for any associated refractive error and ophthalmoscopy for optic disc assessment.

Management

Treatment is mostly surgical, aided by long-term topical antiglaucoma therapy.

Congenital Corneal Opacity

Intrauterine infections, birth trauma, syndromic associations and metabolic disorders like mucopolysaccharidosis, Hurler's syndrome, glycogen storage disease, and lipidosis can cause congenital opacification of the cornea. Opacity involving visual axis results in sensory deprivation, which in early age causes arrest of visual development potential. Presentation can vary from mild cosmetic blemish to obvious amblyopic features of squint, nystagmus and vision loss. Definitive treatment is keratoplasty, with these children requiring long-term monitoring and ophthalmic care for graft survival. Long standing, unattended cases are not amenable to even keratoplasty and usually result in permanent partial or complete blindness (Amblyopia).

Persistent Hyperplastic Vitreous (PHPV)

Failure of tertiary vitreous to differentiate results in persistent fetal vasculature or persistent hyperplastic vitreous. Clinical presentation is with leukocoria and is often mistaken as congenital cataract. PHPV is usually unilateral with high risk of amblyopia, though bilateral cases have also been reported. Any child presenting with a unilateral cataract, specially a posterior capsular plaque type, and associated with microcornea or microphthalmos, should be referred to rule out PHPV.[4] Approach and principles of management are on the lines of cataract.

Retinopathy of Prematurity (ROP)

Detailed discussion of ROP is outside the scope of this textbook. However, it is essential for a pediatrician to know when and which newborn to refer for screening of ROP. Depending on the stage and zone of involvement, presentation may vary from asymptomatic to leukocoria, squint and nystagmus.

Box 3: Common risk factors for retinopathy of prematurity

- Hypoxic episodes
- Supplemental oxygen
- Sepsis
- Respiratory distress
- Hypercarbia
- Multiple blood transfusions
- Multiple births (twins/triplets)
- Intraventricular hemorrhage

Screening for ROP

In India, all preterm neonates who are born at <34 weeks' gestation and/or weighing less than 1750 grams at birth; and babies born at 34–36 weeks gestation or weighing 1750–2000 grams at birth but having risk factors for ROP (**Box 3**), need to be screened for ROP. The ideal recommended timing for first screening is within 4 weeks of age in infants born ≥ 28 weeks of gestational age and, within 2–3 weeks of age in infants born less than 28 weeks or < 1200 grams birth weight.[5] Screening is done by a dilated fundus examination using an indirect ophthalmoscope. All such cases should be followed up long-term, depending on staging of ROP, for continued screening till retina is fully vascularized.

Treatment

Laser, cryotherapy, intravitreal antivascular endothelial growth factors (anti-VGEF), or surgery is indicated depending on stage of ROP, if changes are detected. Untreated and undetected cases of ROP can rapidly progress to advanced stages resulting in retinal detachment with or without macular involvement. There can be secondary glaucoma, amblyopia, or worse, phthisis bulbi (soft, shrunken, blind eye).

OCULAR EMERGENCIES IN OLDER CHILDREN

Lacrimal System Infections (Acute Dacryocystitis, Dacryocele)

The child presents with acute onset painful swelling over the lacrimal sac area with all signs of local inflammation. Mild conjunctival congestion and mucoid to mucopurulent discharge are variable findings. There may be associated systemic features like fever and lethargy. Any attempt to perform ROPLAS test is usually thwarted due to severe tenderness, but if performed it is positive. If a pus point develops over skin, it indicates lacrimal abscess or dacryocele, which may rupture forming a fistula, if not treated in time. Immediate broad-spectrum systemic antibacterial drugs should be started after sending discharge for culture and sensitivity. Topical therapy with the same should also begin at once. In case of abscess formation, it needs to undergo incision and drainage to relieve the tension and prevent fistula formation. Acute and chronic dacryocystitis usually heal by scarring where syringing and probing are futile. The treatment of choice is then dacryocystorhinostomy.[6]

Acute Keratitis (Corneal Ulcer)

Corneal blindness is a preventable and treatable cause of childhood blindness. Corneal ulcers healing with opacification are amenable to various keratoplasty techniques. Same visual prognosis cannot be guaranteed with complicated, perforated ulcers. Common causative agents are listed in **Box 4**.

Clinical features

Clinical presentation depends on the causative agent. All cases have a common feature of acute painful red eye with discharge, loss of corneal transparency and decreased vision. Bacterial keratitis (**Fig. 4**) presents along with mucopurulent discharge and pus in anterior chamber (hypopyon). Viral keratitis due to herpes simplex has a dendritic pattern and watery discharge; there is marked photophobia, hyper-lacrimation, blepharospasm and reduced corneal sensations. Signs of fungal corneal ulcer are out of proportion to symptoms; ulcer has a feathery margin and discharge is mucopurulent but the symptoms of discomfort and pain to the child are comparatively less; there is usually a history of injury with vegetative matter. Keratomalacia (corneal ulcer or corneal melting due to vitamin A deficiency), is a serious emergent condition; the child keeps the eyes closed to any light source and examination requires lid retractors and sedation; there are associated systemic features of malnutrition.

Box 4: Etiology of acute keratitis

- Bacterial
  - *Staphylococcus aureus, albus*
  - *Streptococcus pneumoniae, pyogenes*
  - *Corynebacterium diphtheriae*
  - *Neisseria gonorrhoeae*
  - *Haemophilus influenzae*
  - *Nocardia* sp.
  - *Moraxella* sp.
  - *Pseudomonas* sp.
  - *Listeria* sp.
- Viral
  - Adenovirus
  - Herpes simplex virus
- Fungal
  - *Aspergillus*
  - *Fusarium*
  - *Candida*
- Protozoal
  - *Acanthamoeba*
- Nutritional
  - Vitamin A deficiency (Xerophthalmia)

Management

Corneal scraping from ulcer for Gram stain, KOH mount, and culture sensitivity should be taken prior to starting any treatment, whenever possible. Hence, an urgent ophthalmic consult must be taken prior to starting antibiotics. Fortified topical antibiotics (5% or 10% cefazolin with 1.4% tobramycin alternating at half hourly intervals and tapering according to response) and cycloplegics (atropine 1%, 2% homatropine/1% cylclopentolate) are mainstay of treatment in bacterial keratitis. Viral keratitis may require systemic Acyclovir along with topical therapy and antibacterial cover to prevent superadded infection. Fungal keratitis needs specific antifungal systemic as well as topical treatment (itraconazole and natamycin are commercially available antifungal eyedrops). Cases of corneal melt or keratomalacia should be considered as open globe injury and first line of therapy should be given on the lines of management of lacerating trauma (See later).

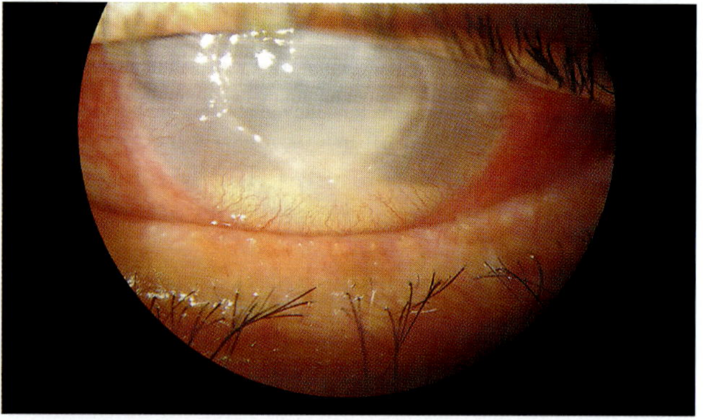

Fig. 4: Bacterial corneal ulcer with hypopyon

Box 5: Therapeutic dosing schedule of vitamin A

Age group	*Oral dose immediately*	*Oral dose next day*	*Follow-up*
0–5 months	50,000 IU	50,000 IU	Same age specific dose two weeks later
6–11 months	1,00,000 IU	1,00,000 IU	
>12 months	2,00,000 IU	2,00,000 IU	

Adapted from WHO/UNICEF/IVACG. *in case the child has diarrhea, oral vitamin A should be withheld and half the age-specific dose prescribed above should be given as an intramuscular injection.

Age appropriate doses of vitamin A (oral/intramuscular), on day 0, 1 and 14 days later (**Box 5**) should also be administered, even in early stages of vitamin A deficiency like conjunctival or corneal xerosis and Bitot spots.

Orbital/Periorbital Cellulitis

Orbital cellulitis may occur as a result of spread of infection from the paranasal sinuses (maxillary, frontal and ethmoid) into the orbital space, or spread from preseptal cellulitis. Periorbital cellulitis is caused by spread of local infection like stye, chalazion, dacryocystitis, impetigo, insect bite, and skin trauma.

Clinical features

The child complains of pain and swelling of the eyelids. On examination, there is decreased vision, local erythema of periorbital skin, swelling of eyelids limited up to superior orbital rim, proptosis, restricted ocular movements, and a chemosed and congested conjunctiva. There may also be papilledema with optic nerve involvement.

Periorbital cellulitis presents with redness, mild to moderate periorbital swelling with local rise of temperature, and tenderness. There is typically no ocular involvement and ocular movements are full and painless in all gazes.

Management

It is important to differentiate between periorbital and orbital cellulitis as the management is entirely different. Conjunctival and extraocular muscle involvement, proptosis, optic nerve involvement, periorbital edema limited up to superior orbital rim, and associated fever or sinusitis, are typically suggestive of orbital cellulitis. A CT Scan will confirm presence of paranasal sinus infection. Orbital cellulitis is an emergent condition requiring immediate hospitalization with a multidisciplinary (pediatrician, ophthalmologist, otorhinolaryngologist) approach.[6]

Parenteral antibiotics like amoxicillin with clavulanic acid, metronidazole or third generation cephalosporin, targeting common respiratory microorganisms, should immediately be started in age appropriate doses. Surgical intervention may be required.

Although preseptal cellulitis is a benign condition responding to systemic antibiotics with gram positive cover, a close watch should be kept, to monitor progression. In immunocompromised children, mucormycosis should always be suspected (**Fig. 5**). As surgical debridement is needed in such cases, urgent ophthalmological consult should be obtained.

Ocular Trauma

Ocular trauma to the eye can be classified as thermal burns (firecracker injury), chemical injury with acid or alkali (**Fig. 6**), superficial or intraocular foreign body, and mechanical trauma with blunt or sharp object. Clinical presentation depends on nature and severity of the injury. A detailed history of causative agent is usually not available in cases of very young children. Prior to an urgent ophthalmic referral, following needs to be done at first presentation with trauma.[6,7]

- In any chemical injury or superficial thermal burns, eye should be thoroughly washed with copious amount of saline, RL or tap water, whichever is available for at least 15 minutes. If there is any particulate matter or deposits in or around the eye, they should be manually removed using a cotton tipped bud or forceps.
- Superficial corneal or conjunctival foreign bodies can usually be dislodged by adequate irrigation. If not, they may be removed using cotton tipped bud or forceps under topical anesthesia. All cases, even after complete foreign body removal should be referred for ophthalmological examination for any residual material, corneal abrasions or missed penetrating trauma.
- In cases of blunt trauma, ocular movements and pupillary reflexes should be assessed for damage or entrapment of extraocular muscles. A primary radiological evaluation with an X-ray to look for any orbital wall fracture should be obtained. Racoon eyes or panda eyes are typically suggestive of basal skull fracture (**Fig. 7**). CT scan is more helpful in such cases.

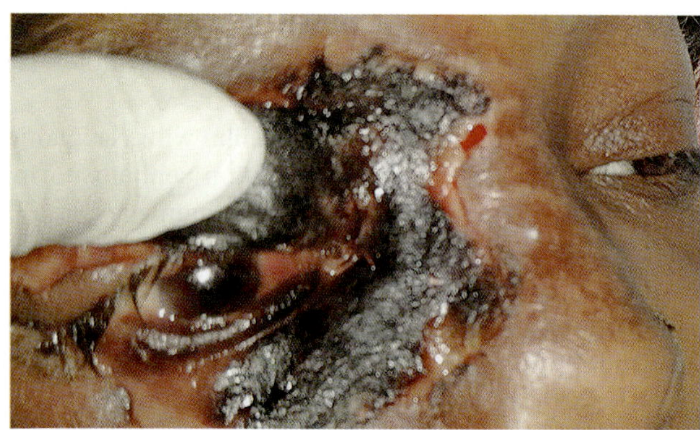

Fig. 5: Orbital cellulitis with CNS Spread in immunocompromised patient (mucormycosis)

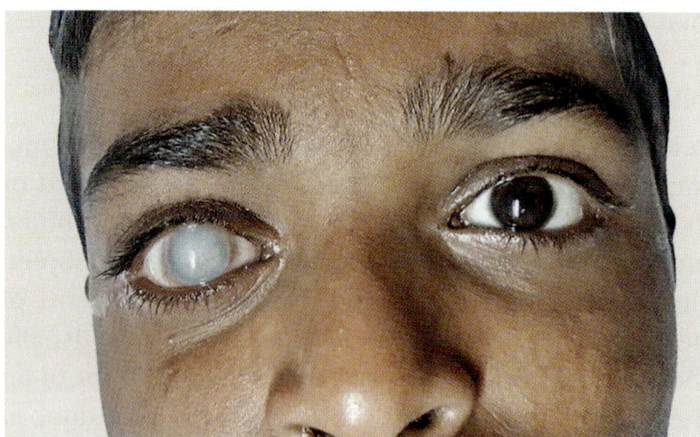

Fig. 6: Total corneal opacity following chemical injury

- In cases of lacerating trauma with open globe injury (**Fig. 8**), assess the wound carefully. If the wound is self-sealing, apply a light patch and refer the patient to an ophthalmologist. If there is tissue loss from the corneal or scleral wound, with or without extrusion of any intraocular contents, it is best to cover the eye with a rigid eye-shield available commercially. It is best to avoid contact eye patch, or any topical medication in such cases. If nothing is available, and there is bleeding from the eyelid or eyeball, a sterile pad may be applied without exerting any inadvertent pressure. Lid lacerations (**Fig. 9**), if any need to be repaired under microscope to prevent any ectropion (outward turning of lid margin) or entropion (inward turning of lid margin) which may result in ocular surface damage and tear film instability.
- Ocular imaging is required in all cases of suspected intraocular foreign body and is helpful if done prior to ophthalmic consult. Avoid ordering MRI until and unless one is sure of the non-metallic nature of foreign body.

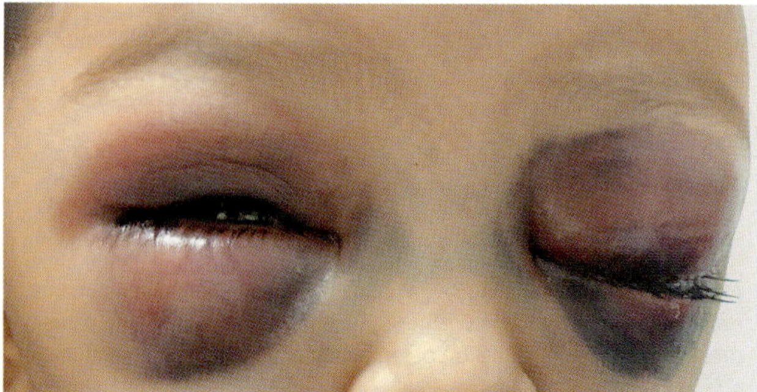

Fig. 7: Panda eyes in basal skull fracture

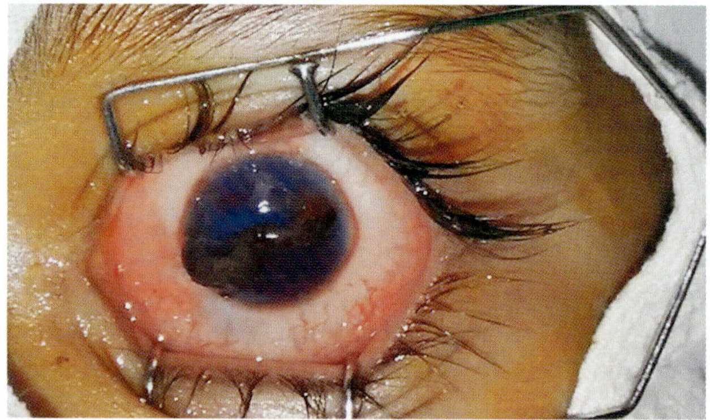

Fig. 8: Corneal perforation with iris prolapse firecracker injury

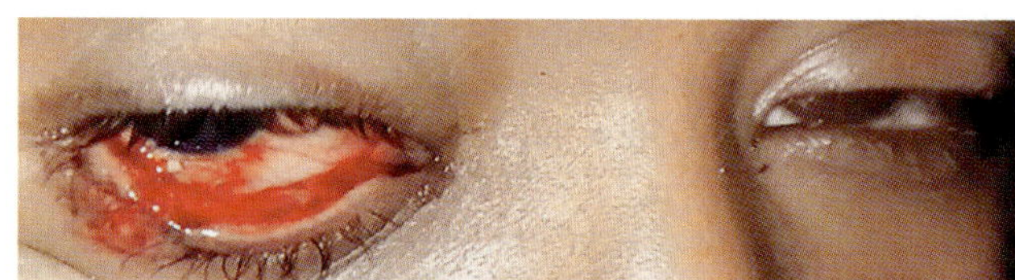

Fig. 9: Lid laceration with singeing of eyelashes after firecracker injury

Ocular Malignancies

Retinoblastoma is the most common pediatric ocular malignancy. It typically presents with leukocoria but may also present with squint, proptosis (**Fig. 10**), red-painful eye or fixed dilated pupil, with or without visual changes. Other ocular tumors like neuroblastoma, rhabdomyosarcoma, acute leukemias (especially relapsed acute lymphoblastic leukemia), and lymphomas, usually present with proptosis.[6] All cases of suspected

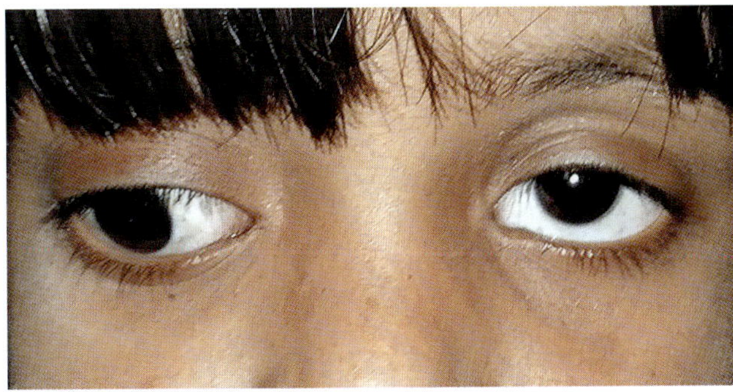

Fig. 10: Proptosis

malignancies need to be referred to ophthalmology for detailed ophthalmic examination under anesthesia. A pre-emptive neuroimaging (preferably CT scan in cases of retinoblastoma), prior to ophthalmic consult is helpful and time saving.

Ocular Misalignment

These demand urgent attention in cases of suspected third nerve palsies (child presenting with *exotropia,* outward deviation of affected eye); and suspected lateral rectus paresis or sixth nerve palsy (child presenting with *esotropia,* inward deviation and restricted lateral movements of the affected eye).

KEY MESSAGES

- Ocular diseases with media opacity (congenital cataracts, corneal opacity, PHPV, retinoblastoma) can result in dense amblyopia if left untreated. All such cases need surgical attention and should be referred at earliest possible.
- All preterm neonates with risk factors should be referred for ROP screening.
- Warning signs for an urgent ophthalmology referral include:
  - Congenital or acquired difference in the red reflex on distant direct ophthalmoscopy;
  - Leukocoria (white reflex);
  - Tearing and photophobia without associated discharge;
  - Cloudy cornea;
  - Swelling in lacrimal sac area;
  - Ocular misalignment; and
  - Proptosis.
- Ocular trauma is the most common cause of ophthalmic emergency in pediatric age group. A pediatrician should be well versed with first line of management prior to ophthalmic referral.

REFERENCES

1. Jain IS, Singh YP, Gupta SL, *et al.* Ocular hazards during birth. J Pediatr Ophthalmol Strabismus. 1980;17:14-6.
2. Qian Y, Traboulsi EI. Lacrimal sac compression, not massage. J Pediatr Ophthalmol Strabismus. 2009;46:252.
3. Clarke WN. Ophthalmic emergencies in infants and children. Paediatr Child Health. 2003;8:413-4.
4. Khokhar S, Jose CP, Sihota R, *et al.* Unilateral congenital cataract: Clinical profile and presentation. J Pediatr Ophthalmol Strabismus. 2018;55:107-12.
5. Pejaver RK, Vinekar A, Bilagi A. (2015). National Neonatology Forum's Evidence Based Clinical Practice Guidelines 2010. Retinopathy of Prematurity (NNF India, Guidelines). Available from: *https://www.ontop-in.org/ontop-pen/Week-12-13/ROP %20NNF%20Guidelines%20.pdf.*
6. Prentiss KA, Dorfman DH. Pediatric ophthalmology in the emergency department. Emerg Med Clin N Am. 2008;26:181-98.
7. Kuhn F, Pieramici DJ. Ocular Trauma: Principles and Practice. New York: Thieme; 2002.

CHAPTER

88

Ear, Nose and Throat Emergencies

Neelima Gupta, Ankit Vishwani

A study from Srinagar found emergencies related to ear to be most common followed by pharyngoesophageal and nose conditions. Foreign bodies were also found to be common emergencies. They observed that if operative intervention is required then specialist care is required especially because of need for special equipment.[1] The various common ear, nose and throat emergencies are discussed here broadly in terms of the pathophysiology, clinical features at presentation, diagnosis and management.

ACUTE OTITIS MEDIA

Acute otitis media (AOM) is inflammation of the middle ear cleft of rapid onset and infective origin, associated with a fluid collection in the middle ear. It may also be called acute suppurative otitis media. Acute otitis media is common in children. By the age of 3 years some 50–70% of all children will have had at least one episode of AOM. It is also common in toddlers attending day care centers.[2] Symptoms suggestive of AOM include fever, pain in the ear, hearing loss, excessive crying, irritability, running nose, vomiting, poor feeding and pulling at the ears. It is difficult to examine the ear drum in a crying, uncomfortable child. However, if the ear drum is visible it may be yellow, or pinkish or congested red. Other suspected diagnosis to be considered are acute mastoiditis, otitis media with effusion, otitis externa or trauma.

Streptococcus pneumoniae is the most common causative organism reported. Most children with AOM do not require antibiotics and prescribing simple analgesics and antipyretics will help. Use of antibiotics is recommended in children under 6 months of age, children under 2 years of age with recurrent episodes, children who fail to improve after 2 days of 'watchful waiting', children with severe symptoms such as high grade fever, vomiting, or any sign of a complication. Amoxicillin remains the first choice, recommended dose being 40 mg/kg/day.

FOREIGN BODIES

Foreign bodies in the ear, nose and aerodigestive tract are among the most common emergencies in children. In a study comprising of 251 infants and children, highest number of patients presented with foreign body nose, followed by foreign body ear and injuries. Nasal foreign bodies included plastic beads, pieces of chalk, rubber, color pencils, etc. Aural foreign bodies included beads, rice grains and insects. Coins were the most common esophageal foreign bodies (Sharma K *et al.*).[3] Foreign body removal from the nose and ear requires special lighting, equipment and technique of immobilizing the child. Sometimes if the child is not cooperative, it may require administering a short general anesthesia for removal of the foreign body. Foreign body of the airway may lead to respiratory distress and child may present with stridor. This part is discussed in a separate section of the book.

EPISTAXIS

Epistaxis, "bleeding from the nose", is a common problem in children although it is rarely severe enough to require hospital admission. It is more common in males than females and is most common between the ages of 3 and

8 years.[2] Bleeding from the anterior part of the nasal septum is more common in children. There is presence of Little's area on the anterior nasal septum where there is a rich arterial plexus known as the Kiesselbach's plexus just under the thin overlying nasal mucosa. Local dryness and crusting over Little's area predisposes to bleeding from the nose. Recurrent childhood epistaxis is usually attributed to digital trauma. Other causes include facial trauma, allergic, viral and bacterial rhinitis, septal deviation, neoplasms and foreign bodies. Systemic causes include bleeding disorders, hemophilia, platelet disorders, vascular abnormalities, liver disease and dengue hemorrhagic fever. Children taking antiplatelet drugs, aspirin, non-steroidal anti-inflammatory drugs and anticoagulants may also present with epistaxis.

The assessment of children with epistaxis should begin with a careful history and physical examination. The history should include the frequency, duration and side of the bleeding. Unilateral epistaxis accompanied by foul smelling nasal discharge in a young child indicates a foreign body until proven otherwise. Having excluded a nasal foreign body, unilateral epistaxis should raise suspicion of a more serious local cause in the nose such as angiofibroma in an adolescent boy. Other significant symptoms include unilateral nasal obstruction, pain and facial swelling. On examination, the most common findings are crusting and visible vessels on the anterior septum. If there is bruising, petechiae or cutaneous telangiectasia then systemic causes should be ruled out.

Most of the children respond to direct pressure over the soft cartilaginous part of the nose for 7–10 minutes along with cold cloth application on the nose for vasoconstriction. Hospital consultation is required if the bleeding is not responsive to pressure. When a child with epistaxis presents in the emergency, the first steps are to secure the child's airway, breathing and circulation.

- If the child is hemodynamically unstable, the blood loss should be assessed, intravenous line secured and blood withdrawn for grouping and coagulation profile followed by fluid replacement.
- If the child is hemodynamically stable, the nasal cavity is examined for any bleeding site. The oropharynx is examined for signs of posterior bleeding. If the bleeding does not stop despite pressure and the bleeding is diffuse, anterior nasal packing would be required and the child needs to be referred to otorhinolaryngologist.

NEONATAL NASAL OBSTRUCTION

Neonates are obligate nasal breathers for the first few months of life, therefore they can present as acute respiratory emergencies if the nose is obstructed. Other symptom may be cyclical cyanosis relieved by crying, stertor and feeding problems.[2] One of the causes of nasal obstruction in neonates is *choanal atresia*. This is a rare condition (incidence 1 in 7000 live births) in which there is complete obstruction of the posterior choanae on one or both sides. The blockage can be either bony or membranous in origin. More commonly, it is a mix of bony and membranous obstruction. It is secondary to persistence of the bucconasal membrane. If the atresia is bilateral then the neonate presents with respiratory distress and an oral airway is required. If the atresia is unilateral then presentation may be late in life.

The diagnosis may be confirmed by nasal endoscopy and radiological imaging (CT scan of the nose and paranasal sinuses), which confirms the presence of the membrane. Choanal atresia can occur in isolation, or it can be associated with other congenital anomalies in the CHARGE (coloboma, heart defects, atresia choanae, retardation of growth, genital anomalies, ear abnormalities) syndrome. Management includes supportive measures till the surgical management is done.

COMPLICATIONS OF SINUSITIS

Children may present in the emergency with any of the complications of sinusitis. With the availability of antibiotics and medical care, the incidence of complications of acute rhinosinusitis has decreased. Still a child may present with orbital, intracranial, or osseous complications of sinusitis.

Orbital complications include the various stages of inflammation of the orbit, which is in close relation to the nose and sinuses. The stages are—inflammatory edema (preseptal cellulitis), orbital cellulitis, subperiosteal abscess, orbital abscess and cavernous sinus thrombosis. The child may present with edema of the eyelid, orbital pain, fever; restricted eye movements, proptosis, headache depending upon the involvement of the orbital structures. It is most commonly due to spread of infection from the ethmoidal sinus.[2] Prompt diagnosis aided by CT scan of the orbit, nose and paranasal sinuses is important. Management is usually medical with intravenous antibiotics, analgesics and antipyretics. Neurosurgical and otorhinolaryngological consultations along with regular ophthalmic monitoring will prevent long-term sequelae.

ACUTE LARYNGEAL INFECTIONS

Epiglottitis

Infection and inflammation of the epiglottis is mainly caused by *Haemophilus influenzae* type b and commonly affects children between ages 2 and 7 years. With the advent of vaccination against Hib there is a reduction in the incidence of this infection. If the condition is not identified and treated promptly, the condition may progress and worsen rapidly and often lead to life-threatening complications.[4]

Diagnosis relies on clinical judgment and examination primarily since time is of utmost importance. The child is febrile, tachypneic and classically will be sitting upright, with the neck extended to optimize the airway, and using the arms to provide support to the shoulder girdle to maximize the efficiency of the accessory muscles of respiration. Attempts to look at the inflamed epiglottis may be dangerous since it may precipitate complete airway obstruction. Bedside evaluation in a controlled setting is advisable. Other conditions that may mimic epiglottitis are obstruction of the airway by a foreign body, acute laryngotracheobronchitis, acute hypersensitivity or allergic reactions, injury of the throat due to chemicals and tumors.

Investigative procedures that confirm the diagnosis include X-ray (lateral view) of the neck. This shows the swollen and inflamed epiglottis, called a "thumb print" sign as the inflamed epiglottis appears like a thumb. Visualization of the inflamed epiglottis via nasopharyngoscopy or laryngoscopy may be attempted by a trained person.

Treatment

Hospitalization is essential because of the danger of respiratory obstruction. Ampicillin or third generation cephalosporins are effective against *H. influenzae* and are given intravenously. Hydrocortisone or dexamethasone is given in appropriate doses. They relieve edema and may obviate need for tracheostomy. Adequate hydration, humidification and oxygen is ensured. In acute laryngeal infections, nasotracheal intubation is preferable to tracheotomy if it is possible and practical, depending on local circumstances.

Croup

Croup, or acute laryngotracheobronchitis, is an acute infectious respiratory disease of infants and children caused by infection of the larynx or the trachea alone or together. It can cause partial or severe obstruction of the airway, which results in breathing difficulties and coughing. In some children, it can be life-threatening.

Croup is most often caused by the parainfluenza virus, but may also be the result of infection with respiratory syncytial virus (RSV), adenoviruses, or the measles virus. Bacterial croup is also known to occur, as is croup due to allergic reactions, acid reflux or irritation of the airway by a foreign body. Croup usually affects children simply because their airways are narrower than in adults, making any swelling more dangerous and likely to block the air flow.[5]

The affected child is most often between 3 months and 5 years of age, with the incidence peaking at around 24 months. Croup starts usually as an ordinary cold, but worsens after a few days. It is characterized by noisy breathing and a hoarse voice, although the most salient feature is the barking cough. There may be difficulty in breathing, especially at night. Children with croup do not typically drool or appear toxic, in contrast to children presenting with epiglottitis.

Croup is diagnosed on the basis of the symptoms and the cough. Physical examination will show signs related to laryngeal inflammation and respiratory difficulty. In severe cases, a radiograph of the thoracic inlet will show characteristic narrowing of the subglottis on an anteroposterior view ("steeple" or "pencil-tip" sign).

The child should be comforted because anxiety and fear exaggerate the obstruction and increase the breathing rate. Moist air in the form of steam is used to relieve the obstruction. In some cases, antibiotics may be required. Admission is required for approximately 5% of croupy children. The mainstay of treatment for croup is corticosteroids. Nebulized epinephrine (1 mL of 1 in 1000 epinephrine diluted in 3 mL of 0.9% saline) has an established role in the acute pediatric airway in reducing mucosal edema by an alpha-agonist effect causing vasoconstriction and bronchodilation.

PERITONSILLAR ABSCESS

It is a collection of pus in the peritonsillar space, which lies between the capsule of tonsil and the superior constrictor muscle. Peritonsillar abscess usually follows acute tonsillitis though it may arise de novo without previous history of sore throats. First, one of the tonsillar crypts, usually the crypta magna, gets infected and sealed off. It forms an intratonsillar abscess, which then bursts through the tonsillar capsule to set up peritonsillitis, and then an abscess. Culture of pus from the abscess may reveal pure growth of *Streptococcus pyogenes, S. aureus* or anaerobic organisms. More often the growth is mixed, with both aerobic and anaerobic organisms.[6]

Clinical Features

Peritonsillar abscess mostly affects adults and rarely the children though acute tonsillitis is more common in children. Usually, it is unilateral. Clinical features can be general or localized.

1. *General*: They are due to septicemia and resemble any acute infection. They include fever (up to 104°F), chills and rigors, general malaise, body aches, headache and nausea.
2. *Local symptoms* include, severe pain in throat, usually unilateral; painful swallowing which is often so marked that the patient cannot even swallow his own saliva. Other symptoms include, muffled and thick speech, often called "hot potato voice" and foul breath due to sepsis in the oral cavity and poor hygiene. There is ipsilateral earache because of referred pain via CN IX which supplies both the tonsil and the ear and trismus due to spasm of pterygoid muscles which are in close proximity to the superior constrictor. The tonsil, pillars and soft palate on the involved side are congested and swollen. Uvula is swollen and pushed to the opposite side. There is bulging of the soft palate and anterior pillar above the tonsil. Mucopus may be seen covering the tonsillar region.

Treatment

Hospitalization for intravenous fluids and antibiotics. Analgesics for relief of pain and to lower the temperature. Oral hygiene should be maintained by hydrogen peroxide or saline mouth washes. If a frank abscess has formed, incision and drainage will be required by a specialist.

CERVICOFACIAL INFECTIONS

Cervicofacial infections in children usually present as a neck swelling. The majority of these infections are related to lymph nodes. Lymphadenopathy secondary to the common acute upper respiratory infections in children is usually self-limiting but may progress to cellulitis, suppuration and abscess formation. The onset of the swelling may be precipitated by an acute inflammatory episode.[2]

Cervical Abscesses

Bacterial infection within a cervical lymph node may progress to cause local cellulitis and abscess formation. The child presents with a tender neck swelling often associated with fever, difficulty and pain in swallowing and other signs. Abscesses are tender, usually reddened and exhibit the clinical sign of fluctuance, confirming their cystic nature. Imaging in the form of an ultrasound scan is helpful but not always required. Many neck abscesses require surgical drainage. A wide-bore needle aspiration may be adequate if the pus has coalesced and liquefied.

Dental Abscess

An infected molar or premolar may cause extensive swelling extending into the face and neck and should be considered in the differential of a neck abscess.

Deep Neck Space Infections

In pediatric patients, DNSIs are typically caused by the suppuration and perforation of parapharyngeal and retropharyngeal lymph nodes, which serve as a drainage pathway for adenoid and tonsillar infections in children aged 1–5 years. Deep neck space infection may lead to other severe and potentially life-threatening complications, such as mediastinitis, septic embolization, dural sinus thrombosis and intracranial abscess. If deep neck space infection is suspected, the child must be admitted for intravenous antibiotics, rehydration and careful observation. Imaging is required to confirm the suspected clinical diagnosis. In some cases, the drainage may have to be done under general anesthesia.

Ludwig's Angina

This is a rapidly progressing cellulitis of the floor of mouth, involving the submandibular neck space. It is usually secondary to concomitant dental infections. Causative organisms include *Streptococcus* species, gram-negative rods and anaerobes. Patients usually present with swelling of the neck and submandibular space as well as firm induration of the floor of mouth, resulting in elevation and protrusion of the tongue, which can lead to airway obstruction. Prompt initiation of antibiotics is usually sufficient and surgical intervention is reserved for persistent or progressive infections or when there is evidence of abscess formation.

KEY MESSAGES

- Infants and children with ear, nose, throat conditions may present in the emergency to the pediatricians.
- The treating doctor must be aware of the signs and symptoms of common emergencies in ENT.
- In many conditions, radiological investigation can further aid in making a diagnosis.
- The associated systemic symptoms should be taken care of and child should be stabilized along with referral to ENT specialist.
- Some of the conditions may potentially be life-threatening because of airway involvement so a prompt referral and management may be warranted.

REFERENCES

1. Nisar J, Khaliq BA, Hanan A, *et al.* Pediatric ear, nose and throat emergencies—prevalence and management: A hospital based study. Int J Adv Res. 2016;4(12):1983-7.
2. Watkinson JC, Clarke RW, editors. Scott-Brown's Otorhinolaryngology and Head and Neck Surgery, 8th edition. Boca Raton: CRC Press; 2018.
3. Sharma K, Bhattacharya D, Barman H, *et al.* Common ear, nose and throat problems in pediatric age group presenting to the emergency clinic—prevalence and management: A hospital based study. Indian J Clin Pract. 2014;24(8):756-60.
4. Epiglottitis. Available from: *http://www.patient.co.uk/health/Epiglottitis.htm; http://www.nhs.uk/Conditions/Epiglottitis/Pages/Diagnosis.aspx; and www.sharinginhealth.ca/conditions_and_diseases/epiglottitis.html.* Accessed September 5, 2019.
5. Croup. Available from: *www.betterhealth.vic.gov.au/health/conditionsandtreatments/croup; http://www.ncbi.nlm.nih.gov/pubmedhealth/PMH0011299/.* Accessed September 5, 2019.
6. Dhingra PL, editor. Diseases of Ear, Nose and Throat and Head and Neck Surgery, 6th edition. Chennai, India: Elsevier India; 2018.

CHAPTER

89

Oral and Dental Emergencies

VP Mathur, JK Dhillon, G Kalra

INTRODUCTION

The emergency conditions related to oral cavity in children and infants can be serious or life-threatening. Some of the common emergencies related to oral region include the following: ulcers, traumatic injuries, orofacial pain, eruption gingivitis and teething, pulp inflammations, mandibular fractures, intraoral swellings and hemorrhage. According to isolated scattered reports, the prevalence of dental trauma for children below 6 years of age is between 12% and 18% in various parts of the country.

ULCERATIONS

These may be caused by trauma, malignancy or be the result of vesiculobullous lesions.

Traumatic Ulcers

Traumatic injuries to the oral cavity can occur due to accidental biting of tongue, lips or buccal mucosa while talking, sleeping, or secondary to mastication. Thermal injuries such as due to intake of hot foods and chemical injuries can also lead to ulceration of oral mucosa.[1] Traumatic ulcers[2] present with areas of erythema surrounding a yellow-white purulent area of necrosis (**Fig. 1**). These ulcers are painful and sensitive to spicy and hot foods.

Management

Typically, traumatic ulcers resolve within three days following removal of etiologic factors such as any sharp edges of teeth, etc.[3] It takes around 10–14 days for the ulcer to heal completely[3] and during this time an anesthetic gel may be used to provide comfort to the child especially before mealtimes. Systemic workup is required to rule out nutritional deficiencies or malignancies, if a lesion persists longer.

Recurrent Aphthous Ulcers

They usually begin in childhood or adolescence, with peak onset between 10 and 19 years. The ulcers may be single or multiple and occur on nonkeratinized mucosa particularly cheek, lips, floor of mouth, ventral surface of the tongue, and soft palate. The adjacent tissues appear healthy and there are no associated systematic features. *Management* of aphthous ulcers is essentially the same as any other ulceration and includes proper oral hygiene and use of topical medications to relieve pain.

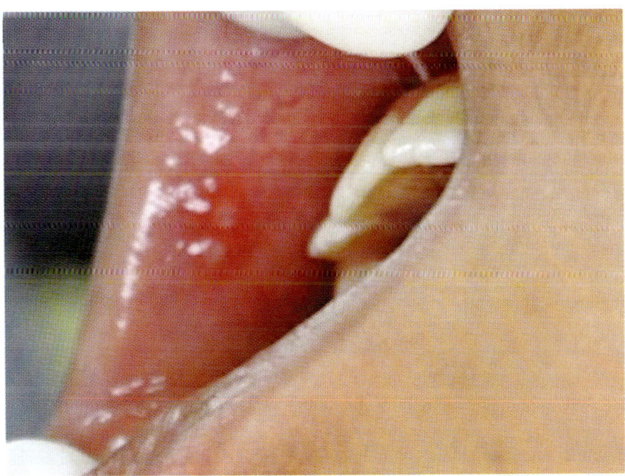

Fig. 1: Painful ulcer on the buccal mucosa near corner of mouth

Herpetic Ulcers

Acute herpetic gingivostomatitis is usually preceded by prodromal symptoms of fever, lymphadenopathy and sore throat. Within few days, vesicles appear especially on the palate, which are filled with fluid and rupture to form shallow, painful ulcers.[4] The child complaints of extreme pain resulting in difficulty in eating, drinking, or swallowing. The diagnosis is established clinically only and may be confirmed on Tzank smear.[5]

Management

The infection is self-limiting and usually lasts 10–21 days.[6] The management is directed towards symptomatic relief such as pain management, and oral intake of fluids to prevent dehydration. Acyclovir (40–80 mg/kg a day, divided in 3 or 4 doses, for 7 days) should be prescribed only if the diagnosis is made within 72 hours of onset of ulcers.[7]

TRAUMATIC INJURIES

Children get dental injuries at school, home, playground and on road. These may affect primary or permanent teeth, and are classified as follows:[8]

- *Complete avulsion*: There is complete displacement of a tooth from its socket in alveolar bone. This is quite common in young children and the patient may report with the tooth in their hand (**Fig. 2**).
- *Subluxation*: The tooth is tender to touch and exhibits increased mobility. There may be displacement of tooth from its position. There might be bleeding from the gingival crevice.
- *Intrusion*: There is apical displacement of the tooth into the alveolar bone. It is accompanied by crushing fracture of the alveolar socket. In severe injuries, the tooth may be locked into the bone. Clinical findings reveal a tooth that may appear shortened or even missing. Most of such cases have no tooth mobility or tenderness (**Fig. 3**).
- *Displacement or lateral luxation*: The tooth is displaced in a lateral, forward or backward direction. It is mostly accompanied by fracture of the supporting alveolar bone.
- *Fracture of crown*: There may be fracture of enamel alone or enamel and inner dentin (**Fig. 4**) or even exposure of the pulpal tissue (**Fig. 5**). The patient may

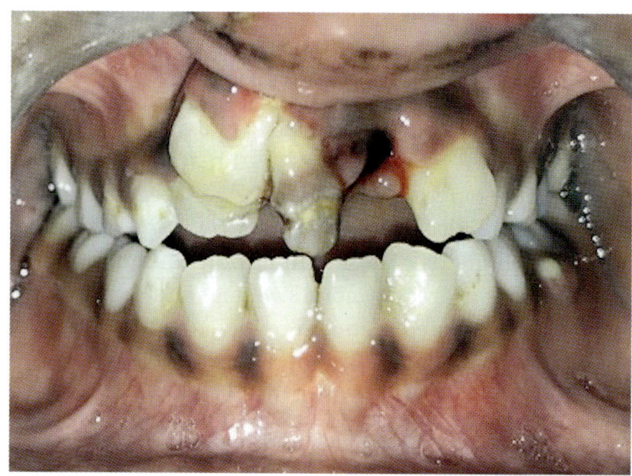

Fig. 3: Traumatic intrusion and lateral luxation of upper anterior teeth

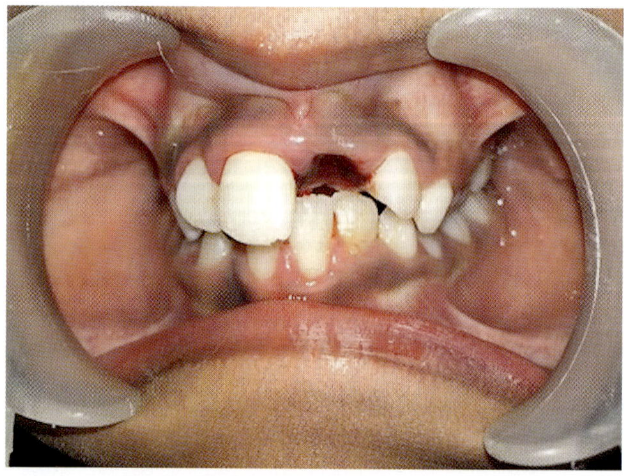

Fig. 2: Completely avulsed maxillary permanent central incisor with fresh wound

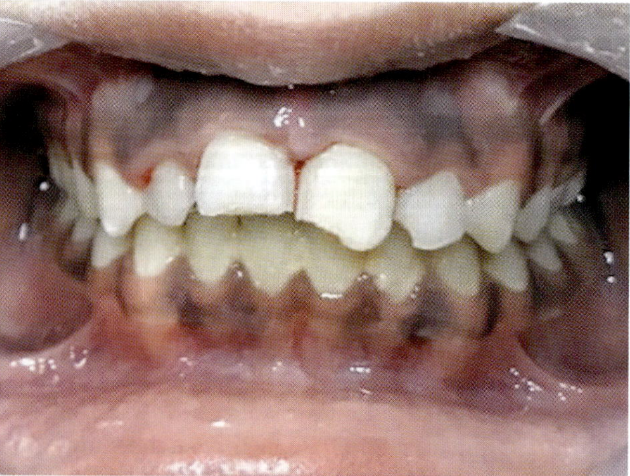

Fig. 4: Fracture of crown of upper central incisors with no pulp exposure

present with acute pain or slight bleeding from the exposed tissue, which is sensitive to thermal stimuli.

- *Fracture of root*: The diagnosis is made clinically and confirmed radiographically. The crown, i.e. the portion of tooth normally visible in the oral cavity may be mobile and/or displaced. The tooth is often tender to percussion.

Whatever is the type of trauma, obtaining a history for the time of injury is critical for management of tooth fractures, especially avulsion. After general, physical and specific examination to rule out head injury or any other major cranial/facial fractures, emergency management consists of debridement, suturing of lacerations, and pain management.

One of the most critical types of injuries is avulsion of permanent teeth. The patient reports with the tooth usually outside the mouth; this may endanger the prognosis of the tooth. The first step to be taken for preservation of the avulsed tooth is debriding it with saline by holding it using the crown. The root portion should not be touched. Following this, the clinician should try to reposition the tooth in its socket. If this is not possible, the tooth should be stored in milk, saline, coconut water or if available a physiologic media such as Viaspan. Even the patient's own saliva may be used if no other option is available. The tooth should not be kept dry and the patient should be instructed to report immediately to the dentist.[9]

All other injuries often require only pain management at the emergency visit. Definite management for dental trauma requires the expertise of a dental surgeon.

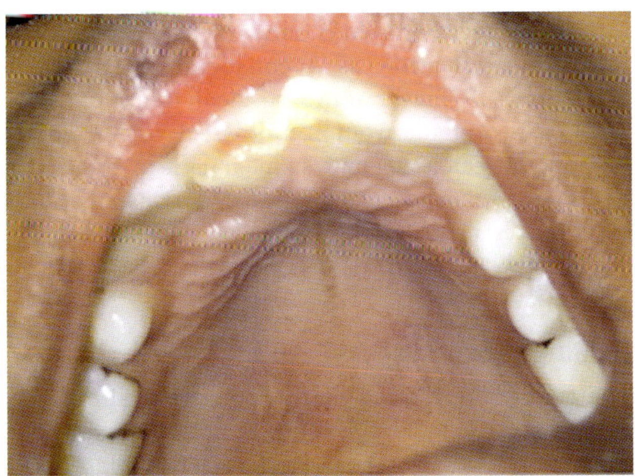

Fig. 5: Fracture of crown of upper right central incisor with pulp exposure

ACUTE NECROTIZING ULCERATIVE GINGIVITIS (ANUG)

This condition involves the gingivae of young children, mainly between 6 and 12 years. The etiology is fusiform bacteria and spirochetes. The child may report with inflamed, painful, bleeding gums; high fever, general malaise, and a bad odor. The onset is rapid and painful. Clinical diagnosis rests on identification of "punched out" ulcerations on gums with pseudomembranous necrotic slough on the marginal areas.

Management

The disease responds to intense debridement of the gingival tissues, professional plaque removal, and use of mild oxidizing solutions. If the condition is acute, antibiotics (penicillin/metronidazole) may be prescribed. Patient is instructed to follow a meticulous oral hygiene maintenance regime (rinsing with 0.5% hydrogen peroxide and 0.2% chlorhexidine twice daily after meals). NSAIDs may be given to relieve pain as and when required.[10]

ERUPTION GINGIVITIS AND TEETHING

A transient form of gingivitis may be observed in young children when their teeth erupt. This is often localized to a specific area in the mouth and associated with difficult eruption. It is mainly seen in children of ages 6 months to 3 years for primary teeth and 6–7 years when the permanent teeth erupt. The condition does not originate with eruption phenomena but is a result of an inflammatory reaction, which develops by the accumulation of food debris and bacterial plaque around/beneath the free tissue, covering the erupting tooth (**Fig. 6**). This condition can be painful and annoying. It may sometimes complicate as an abscess.

Management

Mild gingivitis requires no treatment; only maintenance of oral hygiene is enough. Adjunctive therapy including rinsing with 0.2% chlorhexidine after meals may provide a cleaner area and aid faster healing. Painful abscess may need drainage and copious irrigation with 3% hydrogen peroxide solution. Topical gels with local anesthetics may be prescribed to relieve pain. In cases of swelling and lymph node involvement, antibiotics can be prescribed.[11]

ACUTE PULPITIS

Pulp is the innermost part of tooth from where the tooth receives blood and nerve supply. In any condition like tooth decay or fracture of tooth, the pulp is exposed to

Fig. 6: Gingivitis at location of erupting tooth

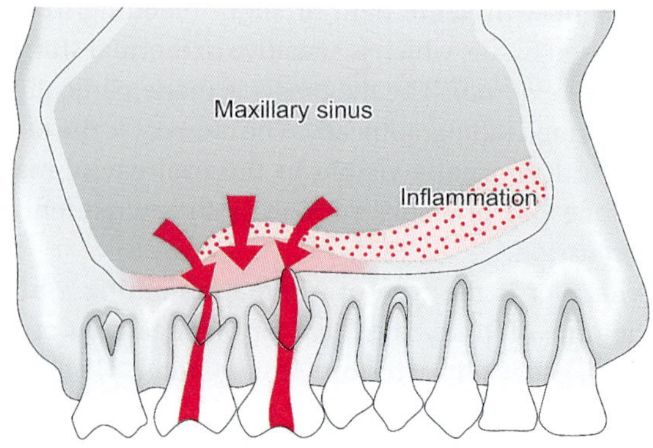

Fig. 7: Diagrammatic presentation of proximity of upper molar roots with maxillary sinus

external environment. This manifests as spontaneous, sharp, intermittent, spasmodic pain and sensitivity to cold in the affected area.

NSAIDs may relieve pain intermittently, if a dentist is not immediately available.

MAXILLARY SINUSITIS

(with Referred Pain to Upper Posterior Teeth)

Acute inflammation of maxillary sinus is one of the most common causes of referred facial pain. It may affect either or both the sides of the face. A child may complain of pain or say that "all teeth hurt" in the upper back region and the pain increases on bending. The child is often unable to point out and isolate the affected tooth/teeth adjacent to maxillary sinus (**Fig. 7**). This may occur even after several weeks of flu or upper respiratory tract infections. Patients may also exhibit typical sinusitis symptoms.

Management

Patient must be carefully examined to rule out any dental source. Digital pressure applied over the sinus wall may cause discomfort to patient and is indicative of a sinus infection. Skull PA or panoramic radiograph shows increased radiopacity in the sinus region. After confirming the history of sinus infection, thorough antibiotics and nasal decongestants for 3–5 days is recommended. In chronic condition, patient may be referred to an ENT surgeon. Symptoms generally resolve within 5–7 days if it is due to sinus infection.

MANDIBULAR FRACTURES

Mandibular fracture is involved in 33% of injuries to facial bones. The most common site is at the sub-condylar region leading to pain in opening and closing movement.[12] Along with subjective symptoms such as pain, swelling, numbness and dyspnea; restricted function of the jaw may be present with inability to chew, trismus or lockjaw. A laceration at the chin area is indicative of superiorly directive midline force suggestive of condylar damage. Accurate diagnosis is only possible with panoramic radiograph or with a CT scan.[13]

Management

In most cases, conservative treatment is preferred consisting of analgesics, soft diet and reestablishment of occlusion. This prevents possible growth disturbances during surgery. A dental surgeon can do maxilla-mandibular fixation as a conservative approach. Sometimes, it may require surgical treatment with open reduction and fixation. Untreated, undetected or improperly treated subcondyler fractures lead to ankylosis of the temporomandibular joint. Such ankylosis may have severe effects on facial growth, chewing and nutrition.

INTRAORAL SWELLINGS

Dento-alveolar Abscess

The condition presents with throbbing, localized pain along with swelling in the gums. Lymphadenopathy and fever may also be associated. Evidence of radiolucency in relation to tooth root is also evident.

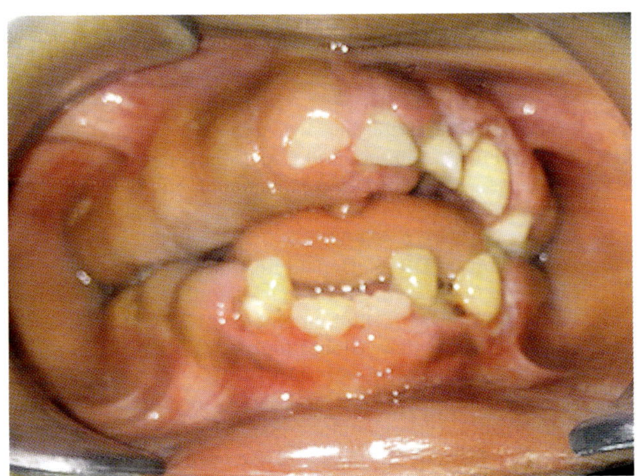

Fig. 8: Drug-induced gingival enlargement on right upper and lower gingiva

Treatment consists of use of appropriate antibiotics, analgesics, and establishment of adequate drainage either through the pulp chamber, or through incision and drainage of vestibule. Sometimes extraction may be required if the abscess has spread to a larger area.

Drug-induced Gingival Enlargements

Enlargement of gums can occur in children taking anticonvulsants (phenytoin, valproate), calcium channel blockers (nifedipine, diltiazem, verapamil), and immunosuppressive drugs. This may be accompanied with poor oral hygiene and presence of calculus and plaque. In these cases, minimal trauma like brushing may induce bleeding **(Fig. 8)**.

Discontinuation or replacement of the causative drug is the first line of treatment. Patient may be instructed to follow a meticulous oral hygiene maintenance regime. The surgical treatment of removal of hyperplastic tissue recontouring of gums is undertaken by the dental surgeons.

HEMORRHAGE

Hemorrhage from teeth or gums usually originates due to local factors. Common conditions involving intraoral bleeding may include the following:

Postextraction Bleeding from Socket/Bony Surgical Site

Post-dental extraction bleeding may include a small bleeding vessel within the bony socket or the soft tissue around the socket area. A careful history may suggest inadvertent touching of the extraction site, vigorous rinsing/gargling, or spitting immediately after the procedure leading to clot dislodgement. Children also tend to manipulate the socket with their tongue causing mechanical disruption of the clot.

Management

Site of bleeding may be identified by careful intraoral examination and the pooled saliva with blood may be suctioned appropriately. Mild bleeding may be arrested by applying pressure with cotton gauze dipped in local anesthetic solution or an anticoagulant such as 5% tranexamic acid. A pressure pack may be given for at least 20 minutes. Electrical coagulation or ligation of the bleeding site may also be done under local anesthesia. If bleeding seems to be arterial (pulsatile) in nature, then local anesthetic with a vasoconstrictor may be injected at the site followed by debridement and socket irrigation. If bleeding seems to arise from the adjacent soft tissues then a figure of eight or interpapillary sutures may be given. If bleeding fails to arrest and any underlying medical cause, is suspected, then complete hemogram with differential and platelet count is advised.

Bleeding from Gingiva

Many a time, a patient may report with bleeding gums due to periodontal infection, painful ulceration and trauma or primary herpes. Systemic factors like hemophilia, acute leukemia or coagulopathies may also result in gingival hemorrhage. Adequate history with careful examination may be done to rule out the cause.

A vasoconstrictor may be injected with local anesthetic for arresting bleeding into the affected area. Removal of granulation tissue may be done in periodontal conditions. Application of pressure with gauze may be given in cases of mild bleeding.

KEY MESSAGES

- Dental Trauma is most common emergency in children below 6 years of age with prevalence in the range of 12–18%.
- Children may suffer from pain, infections, bleeding or trauma related to oral cavity resulting in an emergency situation.
- A pediatrician should know the early signs of the such emergencies and methods to control and early referral to the specialist.

REFERENCES

1. Neville BW, Damm DD, Allen CM, *et al*, editors. Oral and Maxillofacial Pathology. St Louis, Mo, USA: Saunders; 2002.
2. Mortazavi H, Safi Y, Baharvand M, *et al*. Diagnostic features of common oral ulcerative lesions: An updated decision tree. Int J Dent. 2016;2016:7278925.
3. Wood NK, Goaz PW, editors. Differential Diagnosis of Oral and Maxillofacial Lesions. St. Louis, Mo, USA: Mosby; 1997.
4. James SH, Whitley RJ. Treatment of herpes simplex virus infections in pediatric patients: Current status and future needs. Clin Pharmacol Ther. 2010;88:720-4.
5. Taïeb A, Diris N, Boralevi F, *et al*. Herpes simplex in children: Clinical manifestations, diagnostic value of clinical signs, clinical course. Ann Dermatol Venereol. 2002;129: 603-8.
6. McCord WE. Treatment of children for primary acute herpetic gingivostomatitis with lactobacillus in aqueous suspension. Pediatr Dent. 1988;10:307-8.
7. Goldman RD. Acyclovir for herpetic gingivostomatitis in children. Can Fam Physician. 2016;62:403-4.
8. Juniper R, Parkins BJ, editors. Emergencies in Dental Practice: Diagnosis and Management, 1st edition. New Delhi: Jaypee Brothers Medical Publishers Pvt. Ltd.; 1994.
9. Andreasen JO, Andreasen FM. Avulsions. In: Andreasen JO, Andreasen FM, Andreasen L. Textbook and Color Atlas of Traumatic Injuries to the Teeth, 4th edition. Oxford: Blackwell Muksgaard; 2007. p. 444-88.
10. Dean AJ, Avery DR, McDonald RE, editors. Dentistry for the Child and Adolescent, 9th edition. Missouri: Mosby; 2011.
11. Verma D, Jhawar A, Khinda N, *et al*. Gingival diseases in childhood: A review. Global Journal of Medical Research. J Dentistry Otolaryngol. 2014;14:16-22.
12. Zhao Y, Zhang Y. Condylar fracture in children: Current knowledge and considerations. JSM Dent. 2016;4:1059.
13. Resident Manual of Trauma to the Face, Head, and Neck. Available from: *https://www.entnet.org/sites/default/files/WResidentTraumaFINALhighres.pdf*. Accessed July 26, 2019.

CHAPTER

90

Approach to a Sexually Abused Child

Chhaya Sambharya Prasad

Children who suffer from abuse in the first few years of life may undergo physical and emotional harm from which they may never fully recover. This may prevent them from reaching their full potential in the domains of cognitive, social, and emotional development. Parents may themselves force the child to keep quiet due to the societal stigma. Some parents also blame their child for the event, or its consequences.[1]

For the purpose of medical care in India, a child is defined[2] *as one who is less than 18 years of age for obtaining medical care in a health facility in India*. The UN Convention on the Rights of the Child, 1989 (Article I) also defines a child as below 18 years of age. The Juvenile Justice (Care and Protection of Children) Act, 2000 also considers a "Juvenile" or "Child" to mean a person who has not completed 18th year of age.[3]

The Protection of Children from Sexual Offences Act (POCSO Act) was formulated in 2012 to address sexual exploitation and abuse in children and adolescents. The Act defines different forms of sexual abuse, including penetrative and non-penetrative assault, sexual harassment, pornography, and also outline the punishment for the perpetrators.

WHAT IS CHILD SEXUAL ABUSE?

Sexual abuse involves forcing a child to take part in sexual activities including prostitution. The child may or may not be aware of what is happening. Sexual activities include physical contact, penetrative act (rape, buggery or oral sex) or non-penetrative acts. This includes involving children in looking at, or in the production of pornographic material. Also, involvement of children in watching sexual activities, or encouraging the children to behave in sexually inappropriate manner, constitute child sexual abuse (CSA).[4]

Other activities that amount to CSA in a child are as listed in **Box 1**.[4]

Pediatricians must be aware of the difference between the terminologies of sexual abuse and sexual assault.

- *Sexual abuse* is said to be committed by a person who is responsible for the care of the child such as a caretaker, and it has likelihood for repeated occurrences and more likely to go undetected.
- *Sexual assault* refers to the act which is committed by a stranger, a person not known to the child. Pediatricians must also remember that age determination for a child identified with sexual abuse is an important part of the examination.[5]

Box 1: Activities amounting to sexual abuse in a child

- Fondling a child's body for sexual pleasure
- Kissing a child with sexual inclinations
- Rubbing genitals against a child's body
- Sexually touching a child's body, and specifically private parts
- Includes encouraging or forcing a child to do likewise
- Making a child touch someone else's genitals, or playing sexual games
- Encouraging or forcing a child to masturbate, with the child as either a participant or observer
- Encouraging or forcing a child to perform oral sex
- Inserting objects or body parts inside the vagina, mouth, or anus of a child; includes attempts of these acts
- Looking at a child sexually or exposing one's private body parts to a child

HOW COMMON IS CHILD SEXUAL ABUSE IN INDIA?

The National Survey of Child Abuse study conducted by the Ministry of Women and Child Development in 2005 in 11 states across the country reported—21.90% children had faced severe forms of sexual abuse and 50.76% other forms of sexual abuse during their lives. 5.69% children had been sexually assaulted by persons not known to them. Children on street, children at work and children in institutional care faced highest sexual assault. 50% abusers were persons known to the child or in a position of trust and responsibility. Another study from on observational home at New Delhi among 189 boys aged 6–16 years revealed that 38% boys had suffered sexual abuse. Yet another study amongst 2211 Grade 11 students of Chennai revealed that 39% girls and 48% boys had experienced sexual abuse in some or the other form.

RECOGNIZING THE CLINICAL FEATURES OF SEXUAL ABUSE IN A CHILD[1]

Early identification of any incident of sexual abuse in a child can prevent development of severe psychosocial impairments. Early identification and early intervention can ensure a healthy physical, mental and psychosocial growth in future. Research proves that children who are subjected repeatedly to episodes of sexual abuse early in their lives, face bigger challenge in developing normal peer relationships, and face a greater risk of developing depression and or suicidal tendencies.

The information required to recognize that a child is suffering from sexual abuse can be gleaned from multiple avenues. In the healthcare setting, this will include, at the very least, the following:[6] Presenting symptoms, obtaining a detailed medical, social, behavioral, emotional and medical history, examination of child, and keeping a high index of suspicion.

Whenever a child presents with a history of physical abuse, one must keep a high index of suspicion for sexual abuse especially when the child presents with the below mentioned symptoms. Signs and symptoms for physical abuse, emotional abuse and or sexual abuse may be present in any child simultaneously, and hence a careful evaluation of history, present and past is of important.

General signs/symptoms that may suggest possibility of CSA include:[6] Loss of appetite, and or sudden changes in eating habits like compulsive eating or starving; Recurrent abdominal pain without identifiable etiology; Sudden appearance of inappropriate behaviors such as bed-wetting, thumb sucking, etc.; Internalizing/externalizing symptoms, sudden mood swings such as rage, fear, anger, or withdrawal; Self injurious behavior, suicidal tendencies, use of drugs, alcohol, and or truancy; Difficulty in falling asleep; Fear of intimacy or closeness, fear of certain people or places; Poor personal hygiene; Adult-like sexual activities with toys or other children which can be seen during play, writing, or drawings; development of new vocabulary for private body parts; showing resistance to bathing, toileting, or removing clothes even at appropriate situations; children may repeatedly say they have a secret, but may refuse to talk about it as may have been threatened by the perpetrator. Children sometimes may have a negative self-image. In addition, there are certain specific pointers towards sexual abuse to be looked out in a child,[6] and have been detailed in **Box 2**.

A pediatrician's response to a case of suspected sexual abuse in a child in outpatient setting should be based on the following cardinal principles:[7]

1. The clinic or hospital should have a *Child Centered and Child Friendly* approach—it keeps the best interest of child in mind.
2. The approach should be *Family Supportive*: Adequate medical care and response support should be provided to the family. It is important because the family child protection system is the main layer of protection system. Institutional rearing for child protection should be considered as the last option.
3. *Provision of legal safety to the doctor/Pediatrician managing the case*: Record keeping, documentation, and writing down of each and every detail identified should be impeccable to avoid professional litigation later.

Box 2: Specific pointers towards sexual abuse in a child

- Inappropriate sexual behavior
- Vaginal discharge/bleeding
- Vulvo-vaginitis
- Genital warts
- Recurrent UTI
- Recurrent abdominal pain with unidentifiable etiology
- Rectal bleeding
- Bites/bruises around genitals/anus/oral/breast/thighs
- Lacerations/tears around these areas
- Mutilation of genitals

APPROACH AND COMPREHENSIVE MEDICAL ASSESSMENT FOR A SEXUALLY ABUSE CHILD[6]

The rapidity of response to a child with suspected child sexual abuse (CSA) can be categorized as follows:

1. *Urgent response*: An urgent response may be needed if the child is brought dead or brought with a life threatening injury or with acute and grievous sexual assault. The child may require emergency medical care. The police may require collecting forensic samples immediately so that a strong case can be booked against the perpetrator. Such cases are best managed in a government hospital setting or at an One Stop Center (OSC) with a multi-disciplinary medical team available. The District Hospitals, Civil Hospitals also run the OSC Centers through the Rashtriya Bal Swasthya Karyakram (RBSK) by the Ministry of Health and Family Welfare.
2. *Admission*: To the hospital is needed if the child has serious injuries. Hospitalization is also indicated if there is an immediate threat to the child's safety at home. The siblings should also be evaluated and provided safe shelter.
3. *Reporting the case*: The Juvenile Police Unit and or the Child Welfare Committee (CWC) and Child Helpline (#1098) should be contacted for any case of child sexual abuse. The caretaker or the family may refuse to follow the treatment plan, still urgent attention must be given to these matters, and immediate reporting must be done to the Juvenile Police Unit.
4. When there is no immediate threat to the life of the child, then the interaction for an interview can be planned. The interview and examination are performed in a child friendly atmosphere with the appropriate equipment and health personnel (developmental pediatrician, social worker, psychologist, and or gynecologist if needed). A child friendly atmosphere should be responsive, caring empathetic, and sensitive to the needs of the child. The child should also feel, comfortable, relaxed, and feel at ease to confide his/her problems. Play material like dolls, and paper and colors for drawing can be provided.

   The goals of a doctor's handling the child with suspected sexual abuse are detailed in **Box 3**, and should be aligned to the best interests of the child, along with keeping oneself safe, and following all legal procedures.

Box 3: Goal of a doctor's response to CSA

Short-term goals

- To ensure safety and provide emergency care if needed.
- Provision of immediate emotional (counseling) and social support to the child and family and treating physical problems like injuries, providing immunization, STD prophylaxis and emergency contraception.
- Comprehensive medical assessment including history taking, examination and investigations and ensuring proper documentation.
  Marking on a paper with body diagram—to show areas which appear injured or damaged.
- In hospitals where service of specialists from Department of Pediatrics, Gynecologists, Orthopedics, Pediatric Surgery, Forensic Medicine, are available (for example medical colleges/institutes), the examination must be jointly conducted by them. The doctor from the forensic department, if available, must take the responsibility of all medicolegal aspects (i.e. forensic medical examination, sample/forensic evidence collection, medicolegal report preparation, etc.).

Long-term goals

Include complete physical and psychosocial well-being of the child and safety as well as ensuring reintegration into the family and social system.

History-Taking

A detailed medical and social history should be obtained from the caretaker. Keep a high index of suspicion. Ask for any history of fall, fracture or injury (including head injury), cuts and bruises, erythema, or burn marks. History of recurrent UTIs should be obtained and any abdominal, perianal pain and mouth or genital sores or discharge should be noted. Any signs of stunting should be noted and parameters of growth should be recorded. It is essential for a nurse (of the same sex as victim) to be present during the assessment. Record the assessment in a special pre-formatted proforma. A case of CSA should be managed with the same urgency as any other medical emergency.

History obtained from the primary caregiver should be recorded separately. The history told by the child should be documented verbatim. Repeated interviews should be avoided. The family should be treated with respect without making assumed accusations. The doctor must remember that he is not the investigator and that he is there to treat the child, not to investigate the case.

While obtaining history of the event, proper documentation of place, time, name of witness, noticeable behaviors as observed, developmental and immunization history should be recorded. A Pedigree chart drawn is useful. HEEADDSS assessment can be done whenever the patient is an adolescent. The HEEADDSS assessment includes asking questions about home, education, eating behavior, activities and peers, drugs, suicide, depression, sleep pattern and sexual history.

Procedure for Examination in a Suspected Child Sexual Abuse

Conduct the examination in a well-lit room.

- Consent should be obtained always from the parents as well as the adolescent for physical examination.
- A head to toe examination is essential.
- Presence of a Chaperone is essential.
- Growth parameters should be recorded.
- Sexual maturity rating (SMR).
- Physical examination of the head, face, hair, lips, perioral region, nares, chest and breasts, external genitalia, perianal area, inner thighs, pubic hair, buttocks, anal folds and any area indicated by the child's history should be carried out. If the child allows, it is best to examine the genitalia in the lithotomy or knee-elbow position.
- Examination of the vulva for any redness and or tenderness is important. Examination of the hymen can be carried out to check if there are any injured edges or bleeding, and if there is any matting of pubic hair due to presence of seminal fluid. (One must remember that in most cases the examination of genitals and anal areas will be normal).
- One should record if there is resistance to physical examination or if the child appears to go into a state of dissociative amnesia.
- A small child with suspected CSA can be examined in the mother's lap.
- One must look for an abnormal gait - if it is broad based or painful.
- Examine the clothes for any blood stains, semen, hair, etc. and the nails for tags of epithelium, blood, etc.
- Look out for oral ulcers, warts, fungating lesions.
- Age of bruises/injuries should be noted as they appear to be in their color, size, etc.

Maintain notes and records to all consultations with the patient. This should be supplemented with written notes, diagrams, and body charts. The specimens collected should be carefully preserved in refrigerator or suitable place. Take a photograph if possible. Determination of age may require multidisciplinary consultations. All opinions received from experts should also be recorded.

MANAGEMENT

The investigations that need to be done are listed in **Box 4**. Management should be child friendly and family members should be involved while planning future plan of action. Contact with the offender need to be terminated immediately.

1. Accelerated hepatitis B vaccination schedule (0, 1, 2, 12) should be considered if the child is not vaccinated.
2. Immunization protocol should be followed for a non-vaccinated child.
3. Prophylaxis for STD should be considered.
4. Emergency contraception should be considered for an adolescent girl who has attained menarche or is above the age of pubertal period.
5. Postexposure prophylaxis (PEP) is advised.
6. *PEP Regimens Guidelines*: Recommended regimen for the Antiretroviral Drugs is 3 drugs regimen. The first dose is given immediately within the first hour of exposure and not later than 72 hours. The drugs are given once daily for 28 days. A regular follow-up is essential.
7. All efforts should be made to reduce the risk of HIV in a child with sexual abuse. The first dose of medicine be administered as soon as possible. Best chance of prevention is within an hour of exposure not later than 72 hours. The drugs are to be given for 28 days. Do regular follow-up of this child.

Box 4: Investigations required in a suspected CSA

- Age assessment if a valid document not available
- Sexually transmitted disease screening, including low and high vaginal (in post pubertal girls) swabs and urethral swabs in boys and serology for HIV. Hepatitis B and Syphilis are done in cases of:
- Acute sexual assault
- Penetrative abuse
- Vaginal/ urethral discharge
- STD in abuser
- Pregnancy test is a must for an adolescent girl
- Forensic samples maintaining the chain of evidence including skin, hair, clothing, saliva, oral and genitourinary secretions to be collected in cases of acute sexual assault
- Skeletal survey (mandatory for children below 2 years) for associated injuries
- Detailed hematological studies in case of multiple bruising (including bleeding and coagulation profile)
- Neuroimaging and ultrasonography of abdomen are indicated in a case of head and abdominal injury respectively.

8. Child and the family need to be counseled appropriately.
9. The family must be made aware of existing support structure in the hospital and in the community.
10. The doctor must listen carefully to all concerns and fears associated with the disclosure. The hospital must arrange for the counselors to teach coping life skills to the child.
11. Referrals to appropriate specialties such as psychologist, psychiatrist, gynecologist, orthopedic surgeon, surgeon, social services and police should be arranged within the hospital as far as possible.

Prophylaxis for STIs and Hepatitis

Protocol for Gonorrhea (male and female adolescents)
- Ceftriaxone 250 mg intramuscular, single dose; plus azithromycin, 1 g, orally, single dose;

Protocol for Chlamydia (male and female adolescents)
- Tab azithromycin, 1 g, orally, single dose or doxycycline, 100 mg, orally, twice a day for 7 days.

Protocol for Trichomonas (female adolescents)
- Tab metronidazole, 2 g, orally, single dose or tinidazole, 2 g, orally, single dose

Reproduced from Ref. 5.

HEALTH CONSEQUENCES OF SEXUAL ASSAULT

Sexual assault may lead to several direct and indirect health consequences. These include recurrent abdominal pain, burning micturition, repeated urinary tract infection, unwanted pregnancy, and STD (sexually transmitted diseases/infections). Psychological Health Consequences are either short-term like fear and shock. Feelings of worthlessness, guilt, blame, shame, and powerlessness may occur. Long-term psychological effects include depression, chronic anxiety, post-traumatic stress disorder, nightmares, and suicidal tendencies.

Follow-up

The child needs to be re-assessed after 2 weeks. Repeat the pregnancy test if the sexual assault involved an adolescent girl. Repeat serology for HIV at 3-6 months and for syphilis at 4–6 weeks.

A single episode of non-contact sexual abuse by a stranger may just need reassurance and letting out feelings in one or two counseling sessions. It usually has a good outcome. Prolonged abuse by a close family member requires longer and multiple counseling sessions to heal completely in the form of cognitive therapies.

Regular follow-up of the child may be required to verify if the abuse has stopped; It is also essential to monitor growth, physical and mental health and early identification and early referral for therapy (counseling, cognitive behavior therapy or medication) for delayed presentation of symptoms should be suggested. This should be arranged through the legal system using child psychologists and counselors.

Guidelines for Medical and Health Professionals Under Section 27 of POCSO Act

Doctors should not demand legal document or magisterial requisition for providing first aid to children with sexual abuse. The registered medical practitioner providing medical care shall attend to the first aid needs of the child if any needed such as cuts, bruises, etc.

Recording of the statement of the child

The statement of the child shall be recorded by a woman police officer not below the rank of a Sub Inspector, at a place where the child is comfortable—residence usually. The police officer should not be in uniform, should not allow contact of the child with the accused, and identity of the child should be protected from public and media. Statement can also be recorded with the District Magistrate. The POCSO Act directs all hospitals to provide first-aid or medical treatment free of cost to the victims of a sexual assault. Emergency medical care shall be rendered in such a manner as to protect the privacy of the child, and in the presence of the parent or guardian or any other person in whom the child has trust and confidence.

Mandatory reporting

Whenever there is a medical or psychological reason to suspect that a child has been or is being sexually abused, the medical professional is required to report this to the appropriate authorities. Failure to do this would result in imprisonment of up to 6 months, with or without fine. A suggested model for CSA control and prevention consists of addressing, in-parallel, 8 distinct issues involved with the problem.[7] These are: Education and awareness, helpline, implementation of laws and policies, self-defense, identifying and punishing the perpetrator, training of personnel (healthcare providers, law-enforcement, legal personnel and counselors), medicolegal services, and support for the survivor.[7]

KEY MESSAGES

- Sexual abuse is equally common in boys as in girls.
- The treating doctor must remain the person of science and should not try to become the investigator.
- There should be provision of Legal safety to the reporting Doctor and the clinical Team treating the child.
- Record keeping, documentation, and writing down of each and every detail should be exact (POCSO Guidelines must be followed).
- Doctors must not only be aware of the Medical Protocols for managing a case of sexual assault but also the psychosocial and mental health consequences that follows.
- Every child suffering from acute or chronic abuse or from old unidentified episode of assault must be given the doubt of HIV and STD infections and must be investigated and managed accordingly.

REFERENCES

1. National Commission for Protection of Child Rights. Resource Book for Commissions for Protection of Child Rights, 1st edition. Delhi; 2016.
2. UNICEF. 2005. Convention on Rights of the Child. Available from: *http://www.unicef.org/crc/index_30229.html.* Accessed August 31, 2019.
3. Ministry of Law and Justice. The Juvenile Justice (Care and Protection of Children) Act, 2015. New Delhi; 2016. Available from: *http://cara.nic.in/PDF/JJ%20act%202015.pdf.* Accessed August 31, 2019.
4. Ministry of Women and Child Development. Model Guidelines under Section 39 of the Protection of Children from Sexual Offences Act, 2012: Guidelines for the Use of Professionals and Experts under the POCSO Act, 2012. Available from: *https://wcd.nic.in/sites/default/files/POCSO-ModelGuidelines.pdf.* Accessed August 31, 2019.
5. Study on Child Abuse: India 2007. Ministry of Women and Child Development, Government of India, New Delhi; 2007. Available from: *http://wcd.nic.in/childabuse.pdf.* Accessed August 31, 2019.
6. McIntosh N, Forfar JO, Arneil GC, editors. Forfar and Arneil's Textbook of Pediatrics, 6th edition. Edinburgh: Churchill Livingstone; 2003.
7. Aggarwal K, Dalwai S, Galagali P, *et al.* Recommendations on recognition and response to child abuse and neglect in the Indian setting. Indian Pediatr. 2010;47:493-504.

CHAPTER 91

Emergency Procedures

91.1 Vascular Access

Deepak Kumar, Garima Gupta

Vascular access is an essential element for managing sick children. Children are often not cooperative for the procedure. Moreover, in chubby babies, it is often very difficult to visualize peripheral veins. Neonates and early infants have small and fragile veins. The vascular access means access to the vessels. It can be through a peripheral vein (peripheral venous access), central vein (central vascular access), peripheral artery (arterial access) or through intraosseous compartment (intraosseous route). The access is required to deliver injectable drugs, fluids, and blood products. It can also be used to conduct hemodialysis, exchange transfusion, withdrawing blood samples, and for hemodynamic monitoring in critically ill patients.[1,2]

PERIPHERAL VASCULAR ACCESS

It is the most common route used for vascular access. Peripheral vascular access (PVA) is a simple and rapid procedure, needs less expertise, is cost effective and has fewer complications. However, it cannot be used for a longer duration of therapy. It is also difficult to visualize the veins for access in patients with obesity, severe dehydration or shock. Parenteral nutrition, infusates with pH less than 5 or more than 9 and fluids with osmolarity > 600 mOsm/L cannot be infused through the peripheral line.

There are three main types of peripheral venous access devices: (i) scalp vein needle or butterfly needle, (ii) intravenous cannula, and (iii) midline catheters. Butterfly needle usually have small gauze and short needle usually less than an inch with a small tube connected at one end (**Fig. 1A**). They are mainly used for single time withdrawl of sample or delivery of one dose of a drug. These butterfly cannulas are usually not secured in the place for the risk of infiltration. In contrast, peripheral IV cannula or "over the needle catheter" could be used for prolonged periods up to a week. They are available in various sizes and are color coded (**Fig. 1B**). For more prolonged access of 3–4 weeks, midline catheters (**Fig. 1C**) are the preferred choice. They have longer in the length in such a form that if they are inserted at antecubital fossa, their tip reaches the level below axilla. However, there is an increased risk of phlebitis with the latter.

Technique

Checklist before the procedure

- The patient has been identified with his/her name and date of birth.
- A written informed consent must be obtained from the parents or the legal guardian for the procedure.
- Parents must be offered to stay in procedure room, if they are comfortable with the same.
- The procedure should be performed with all aseptic precautions including hand wash.

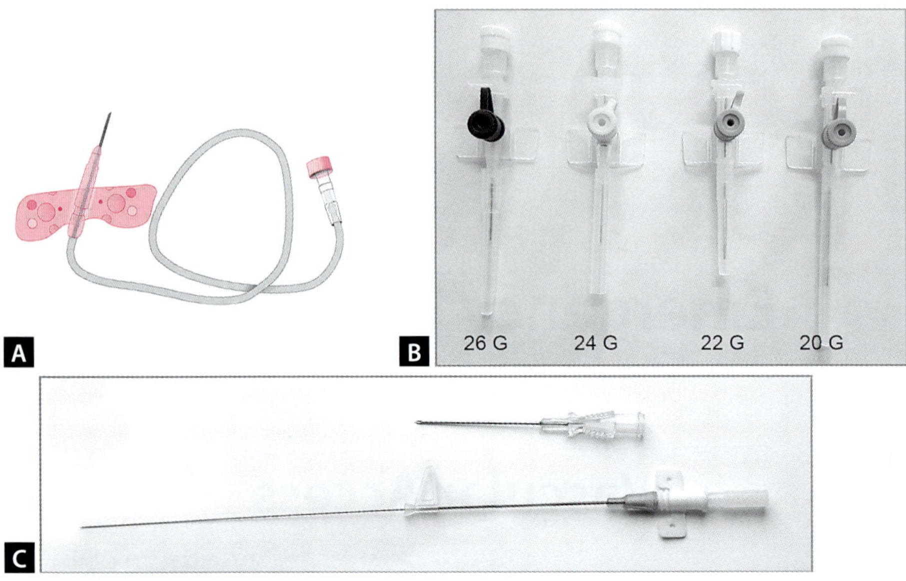

Figs. 1A to C: (A) Butterfly (scalp vein) needle; (B) Peripheral intravenous cannula; (C) Midline catheters

Table 1: Methods for pain management

Method	*Details*
Behavioral method	Soft toys Favorite cartoon character Decorated procedure roon Favortie television show Videos on mobile phone Rattle toy
Drugs	25% sucrose solution (2 mL) Topical EMLA (lidocaine + prilocaine)# Topical lidocaine cream^ Topical tetracaine cream

The use of EMLA or prilocaine is not recommended in preterms and infants receiving methemoglobin inducing drugs as metabolite of prilocaine, o-toluidine can induce methemoglobinemia

^The cream can be applied 30–45 minutes prior to the procedure.

- Ensure all the equipments required for the procedure are ready.
- Procedural sedation and pain management are essential steps before the procedure, which is often overlooked. This would ease the procedure, ensure good compliance from the patient and would allay the parental worry. It also ensures that fragile veins are not repeatedly pricked for the lack of cooperation or lack of restraint.[3] The methods used for procedural sedation are enumerated in **Table 1**.

Procedure

- *Site selection*: Distal sites are usually preferred over the proximal sites. Avoid sites that may interfere with the patient's activity like flexor areas of upper limb and dominant hand. Areas with burns, infections, cellulitis, and trauma are also to be avoided. The selected vein should be of adequate size to accommodate the cannula gauze. The commonly accessed veins include antecubital vein, median or basilic vein in the upper limbs and saphenous vein in the lower limbs (**Fig. 2**). Scalp vein should be used only in the patient below 18 months of age with no other peripheral access. Hair follicles, and epidermis over scalp usually mature beyond this age making scalp vein cannulation difficult and more painful.[4]
- *Catheter selection*: For neonates, 24G or 26G size are often used for peripheral venous access. In infants and young children, 22G to 24G size cannula is commonly used. Midline catheters are preferred if therapy is required beyond 6 days.
- *Site preparation*: If the selected site is dirty, wash it with soap and water. If the scalp is selected for cannulation, clip the hairs using scissors; do not shave the area as this may produce microabrasions, which increases the risk of infection at the site. Chlorhexidine/alcohol solution is the preferred antiseptic beyond 2 months

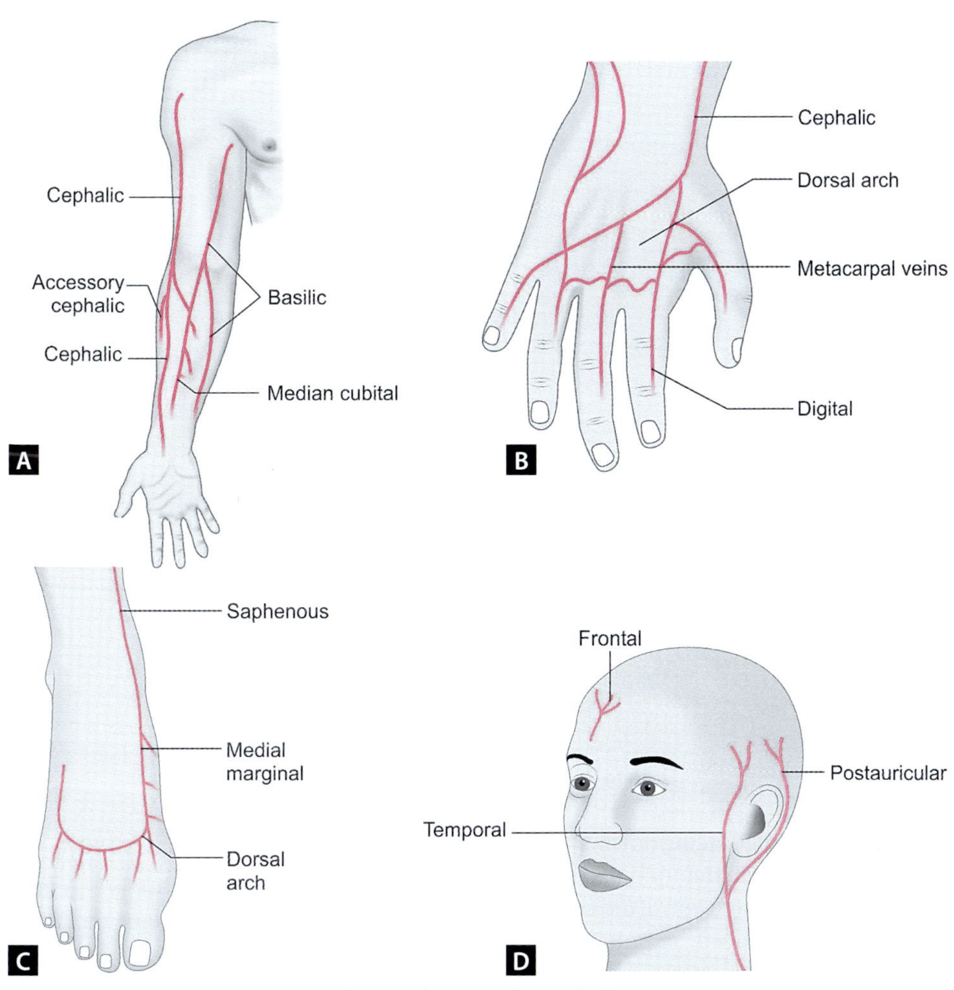

Figs. 2A to D: Commonly accessed veins for intravenous access

of age. Use of chlorhexidine below 2 months is not recommended for the risk of skin damage/burns. In babies younger than 2 months, alcohol solution can be used.[5] Apply the solution for minimum of 30 seconds at the site and allow it to dry before the procedure. There is always a risk of the solution tracking along with cannulae during insertion resulting in phlebitis if not allowed to dry. The veins can be made prominent by tapping the selected area, use of tourniquet (always check distal arterial pulsations after applying a tourniquet to the limb) and by local warming using a warm towel over the area for 7–10 minutes.[6] The veins can be visualized better using direct light illumination or infra-red-light sources (**Fig. 3**).

- *Steps in cannulation*: Fix the desired vein by applying traction on the overlying skin (**Fig. 4A**). Insert the catheter at

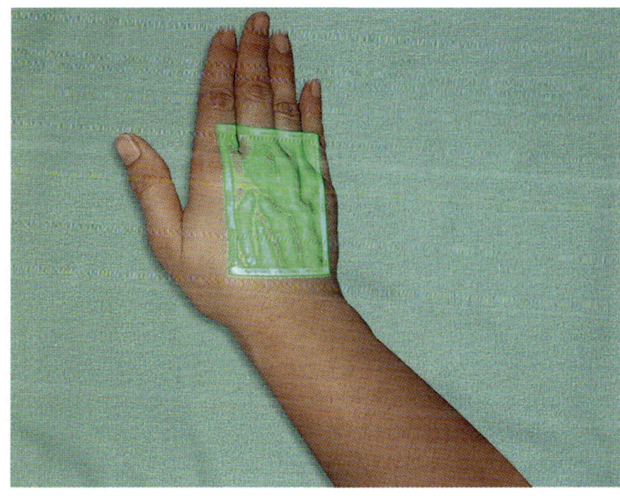

Fig. 3: Vein viewer for visualizing the vein

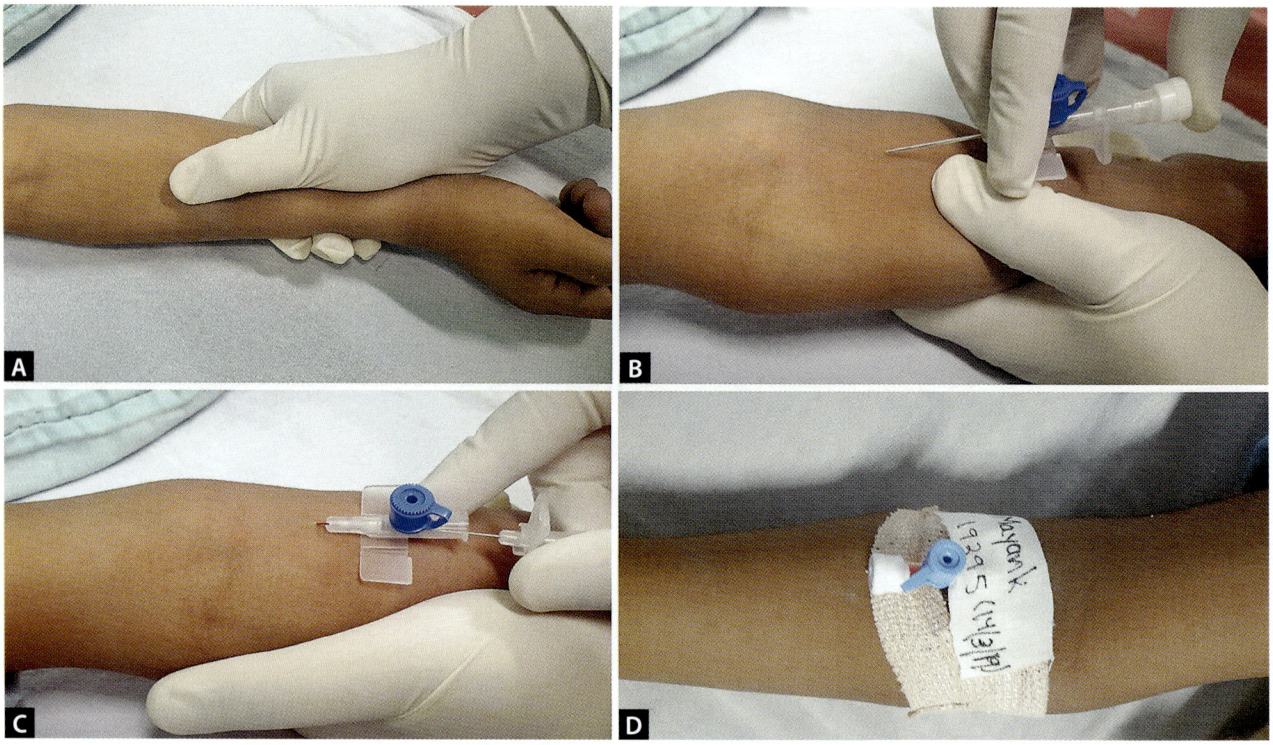

Figs. 4A to D: Steps of intravenous cannulation

an angle of 30° with beveled edge facing down to avoid counter insertion (**Fig. 4B**). Once the tip breaches the vein there will be flow of blood in the hub of the cannula. The stylet can be slowly removed, simultaneously pushing forward the cannula into the vein (**Fig. 4C**). The blood samples may be collected if required and the catheter may be fixed firmly to the skin using skin-friendly adhesive tapes or if available use Tegaderm fixators. It is essential to stabilize the joint and label the cannula with date and time of insertion (**Fig. 4D**).

CENTRAL VASCULAR ACCESS

We consider the access to lower 1/3rd of superior vena cava above the atrium to be a central venous access. It can be used for longer duration (months to years), and infusate of varied pH and higher osmolarity can be administered. These devices provide access for hemodynamic monitoring and repeated blood sampling. The procedure is better when performed by a trained expert in an intensive care setting. There are four main types of CVADs: Peripherally inserted central catheter (PICC) (**Fig. 5A**), non-tunneled CVAD (**Fig. 5B**), and subcutaneously tunneled CVAD (**Fig. 5C**) (**Table 2**).

Procedure (Seldinger Technique)

Checklist before the procedure is the same as for PVAD. All the CVAD require Seldinger technique for catheter insertion.[7] This technique uses a small gauze needle and a guidewire. Small bore needle is introduced into the vein; once free flow blood is achieved via the needle then insert the guidewire into the bore of the needle and thread it into the vein. After that take out the needle slowly over the guidewire holding the guidewire in position. Then use dilator that comes with the catheter set and inserts it over the guidewire, slowly using twisting movements insert it into the tissue till it reaches the vein. Once tract dilates, then insert catheter over guidewire and withdraw the guidewire (**Figs. 6A to C**). Sites for central cannulation, its advantages and disadvantages are outlined in **Table 3**.

STEPS IN VENOUS CANNULATION

Femoral Vein Cannulation

Step 1: Extend the leg with slight external rotation. Place a small sterile cloth under the buttocks to flatten the inguinal area. This position facilitates catheter entry easily into the vein (**Fig. 7A**).[8]

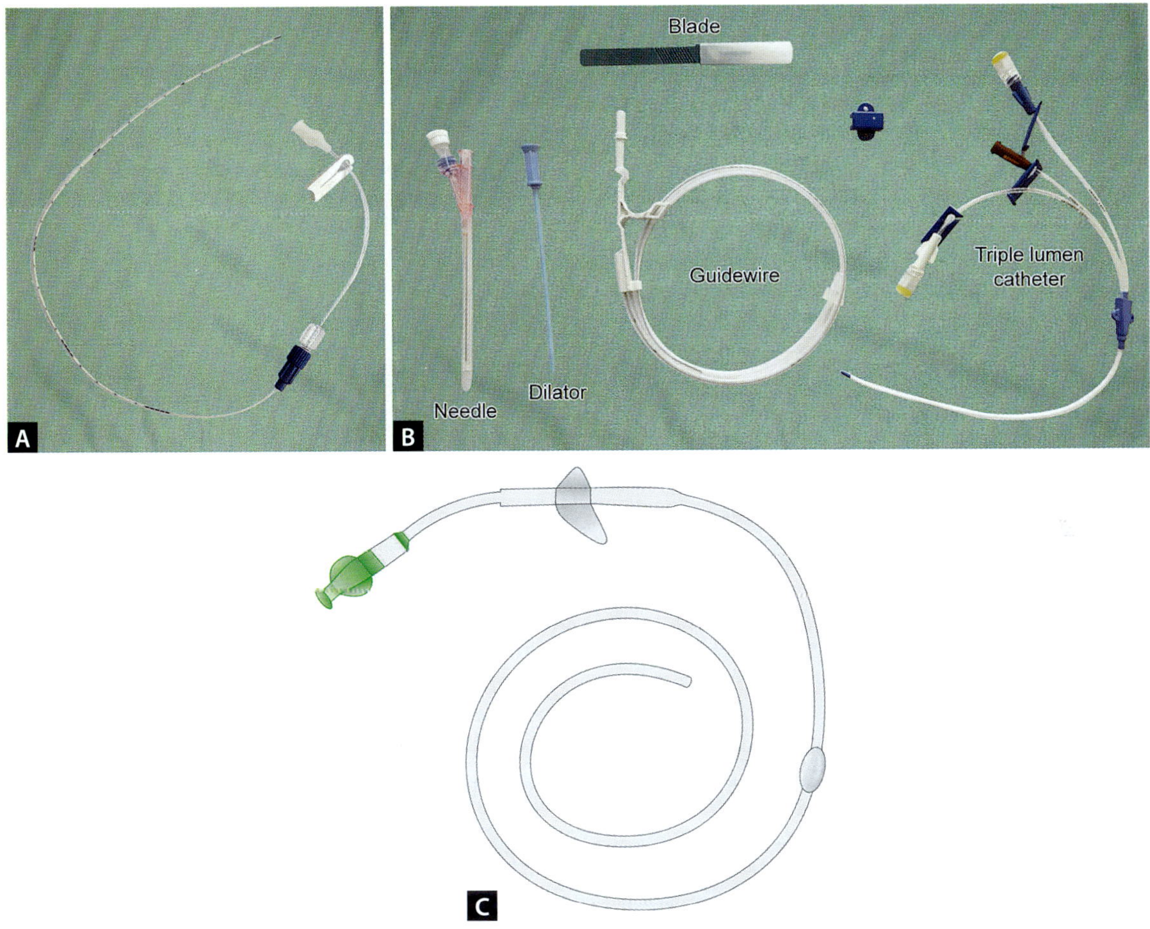

Figs. 5A to C: Central vascular access devices

Table 2: Key features of central venous access devices (CVADs)

Central venous access devices	*Key features*
Peripherally inserted central catheter	• Size can vary from 16G to 23 Gauge • Length can range from 50 to 60 cm • Most common vein is basilica vein in antecubital fossa • Other sites: Placed above antecubital fossa via cephalic, median vein or via an internal/external jugular vein • Requires frequent flushing to maintain patency
Non-tunneled CVAD	• Used for short-term (days to week) • It is inserted percutaneously via internal jugular vein or subclavian vein • Catheters with minimum lumen is preferred
Subcutaneous tunneled CVAD	• Broviac and Hickman catheter are the commonly used ones • Sizes from 17 to 22G and are of 20 to 30 inches in length • Available in single, double, triple and quadruple lumens • The catheter is surgically tunneled into subcutaneous tissue between entrance near clavicle and exit site near chest wall for stabilization • The procedure is performed in surgical operation theaters • Preferred for very long-term use (months to year) • Less risk of infection as the entry and exit are sealed

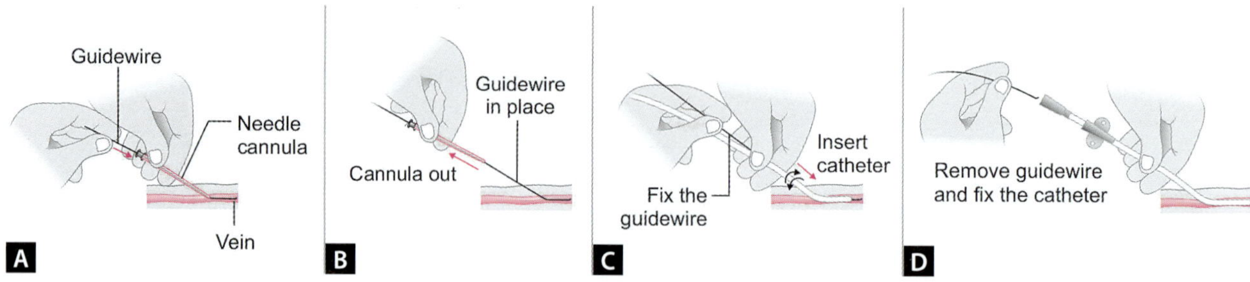

Figs. 6A to D: Seldinger technique

Table 3: Sites for central venous catheterization

Site of insertion	*Precautions*
Femoral vein	• It is easily accessible site especially with ongoing resuscitation • It is used for emergency vascular access
External jugular vein	• It has much easier access as the vein is visible • Cannulation is more difficult with repeated failures considering the acute angle for entry • Risk of airway compromise as it requires neck extension and rotation
Right internal jugular vein	• Left side avoided to prevent air leak and thoracic duct injury
Subclavian vein	• It is very difficult technically, hence avoided in children as far as possible

Step 2: Administer local anesthesia subcutaneously, and using the same needle and syringe locate the femoral vein.

Step 3: Insert the needle one fingerbreadth below the inguinal ligament. Just medial to the femoral artery, apply gentle pressure on a syringe, and insert it slowly at 45° angle.

Step 4: Once the free flow of blood is seen in the syringe hub, detach the syringe from the needle; and advance the guidewire through the needle and follow the Seldinger technique for catheter insertion.

External Jugular Vein Catheterization[9]

Step 1: Place the child in 30° head down position (Trendelenburg); turn the head opposite to the site of the puncture (**Fig. 7B**). Auscultate chest for air entry.

Step 2: Occlude the vein just above the clavicle with the middle finger of the non-dominant hand.

Step 3: Allow the vein to distend and stabilize it with the thumb.

Step 4: Cannulation techniques are the same as described in over the needle cannula or Seldinger for catheter insertion.

Internal Jugular Vein

Step 1: Place a rolled cloth beneath shoulders, hyperextend the neck (rule out cervical spine injury) (**Fig. 7C**).

Step 2: Place the child in a Trendelenburg position; auscultate chest for breath sounds.

Step 3: Identify the triangle formed by sternocleidomastoid muscle head and base of the clavicle. Insert the needle at the apex of the triangle at 30–45° angle, direct the needle towards the nipple. If the vein is not entered withdraw the needle, keep the needle subcutaneously and reattempt along the sagittal plane (less lateral). Do not proceed medially as it may puncture carotid.

Step 4: Use Seldinger technique to insert the catheter. Keep the hub of catheter obstructed with the fingertip to prevent air embolism and try to insert guidewire or cannula during expiration.

Subclavian Vein[10]

Step 1: Position the patient as described in internal Jugular vein cannulation; auscultate the chest for breath sounds.

Step 2: Identify the middle and medial 1/3rd of the clavicle. Now insert the needle under the clavicle

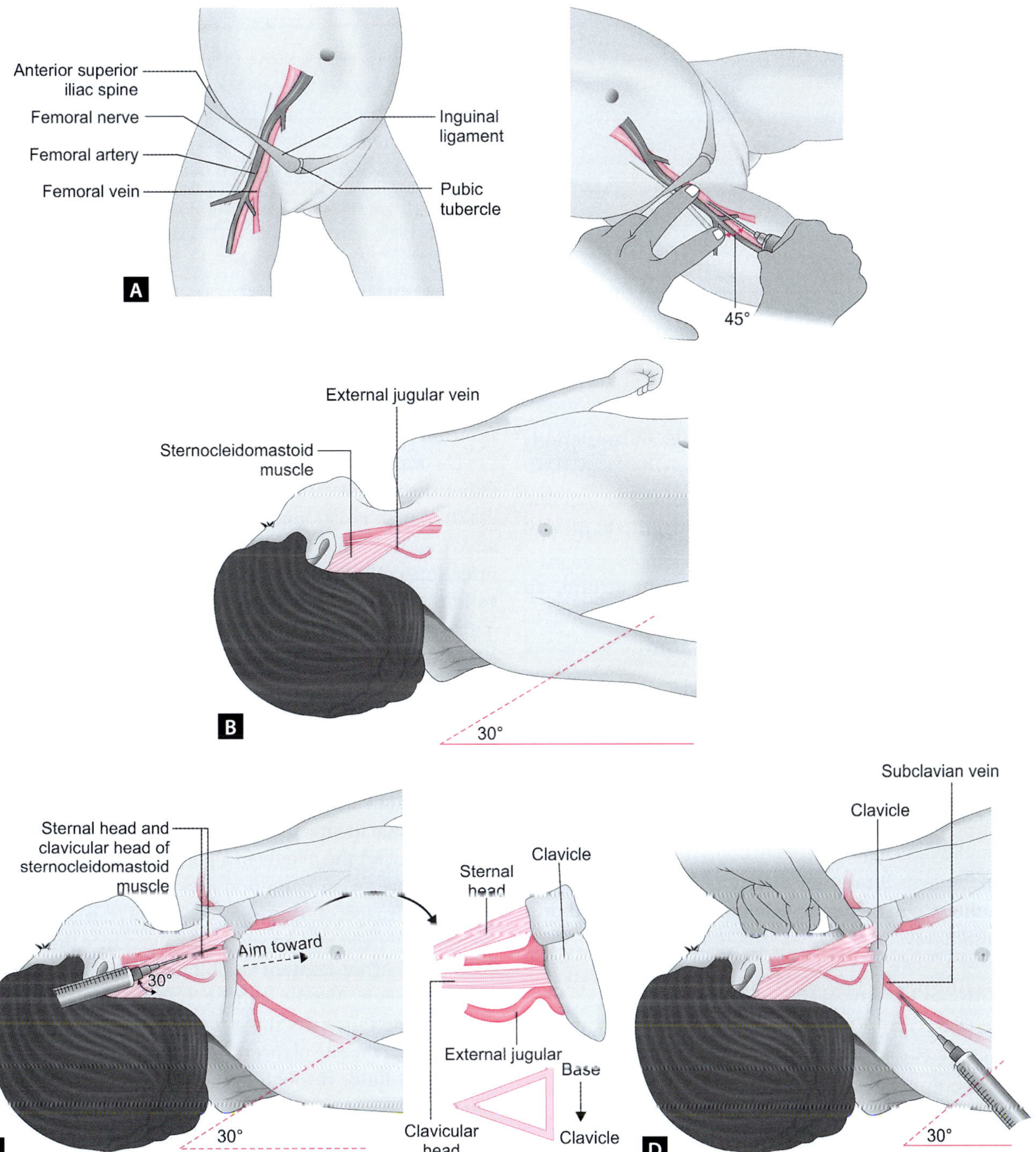

Figs. 7A to D: Cannulation of (A) Femoral vein; (B) External jugular vein; (C) Internal jugular vein; (D) Subclavian vein

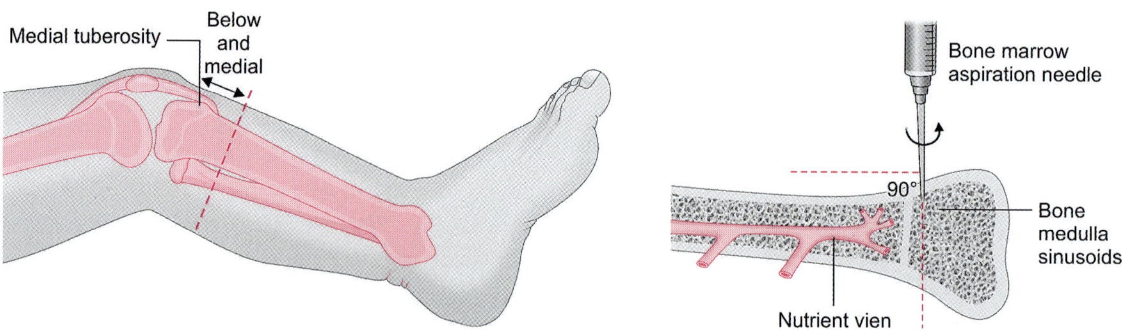

Fig. 8: Site of intraosseous access

at this junction. Slowly insert the needle by gentle negative pressure with a syringe, direct the needle toward suprasternal notch (**Fig. 7D**).

Step 3: Direct the needle medially, cephalic and posteriorly to the sternal end of the clavicle.

Step 4: Observe for free flow in the hub, remove syringe and obstruct the needle hub with a fingertip to prevent air embolism.

Step 5: Insert the guidewire into the right atrium, an entrance of guidewire into the atrium produces premature atrial contractions. If arrhythmias occur, withdraw the wire.

Step 6: Complete catheter insertion using Seldinger's technique.

If the central vein is cannulated on an urgent basis in the emergency area when procedure done under asepsis is doubtful, then it should be replaced as soon as possible and within 48 hours to prevent infection. After the procedure, obtain the chest X-ray immediately to check the position of the catheter and any complications like—pneumothorax or hemothorax.

INTRAOSSEOUS ROUTE

In an emergency, we commonly face the situation when immediate vascular access is required, and peripheral veins are not accessible as in children with shock or severe dehydration. Venous cut-down or insertion of central venous devices can be performed if resources and expertise are available immediately. Delay in initiating vascular access and therapy can be dangerous. Intra-osseous cannulation can be useful in such situations. The intra-osseous venous compartment is stiff and does not collapse under such situations. Insertion of a needle into bone marrow venous plexus provides a route for drug therapy, intravenous fluids and blood transfusion. It can be achieved very quickly; the procedure is easy and requires less expertise and resources. This route of vascular access is meant for short duration only < 24 hours.

The most common site used is proximal tibia **(Fig. 8)**. Other sites are distal tibia, distal femur and ASI spine. In children with crush injury, previous attempt at the same site, fragile bones as in osteogenesis imperfecta and infection/cellulitis at the insertion site are contraindications for intra-osseous access.

Procedure

For access to proximal tibia, the leg is placed in slight external rotation. The overlying skin is prepared. Identify tibial tuberosity located just below the knee joint, insertion site should be about 1–3 cm below and medial to tuberosity (flat area below growth plate). The stylet should be kept inside the needle while inserting to prevent tissue clogging. Insert the needle in a perpendicular direction to the tibia, use twisting motion and gentle pressure while inserting till a feel of "give away" or loss of resistance is felt. Remove the stylet and attach the syringe. Once the syringe is pulled, marrow content and blood can be seen coming in the syringe. Needle can be stabilized using gauze padding and tapes. Fix the intravenous fluid tubing over the skin near the site of insertion for stabilization. Delivery of drugs or fluids through the needle which is displaced can cause tissue necrosis or compartment syndrome, so, frequent check at the site for swelling and displacement is required.

ARTERIAL ACCESS

In a critically ill child, more specifically those who require cardiopulmonary support, continuous monitoring, and frequent blood sampling (both venous and arterial) is required for management. To prevent multiple arterial pricks and for intra-arterial blood pressure monitoring, arterial catheterization should be achieved. Another common indication for arterial access is to create a withdrawal site for exchange transfusion.

Sites for Arterial Cannulation

- *Upper limb*: Radial artery is the preferred site, it is most superficially located, distal to the limb and is easy to cannulate. Axillary artery has a low risk of ischemia due to the presence of collateral arteries but being close to aortic arch, it carries a risk of cerebral embolism secondary to flushing through the catheter.
- *Lower limb*: Dorsalis pedis, posterior tibial, and femoral artery can be used. The femoral artery carries the risk of ischemia to the distal limb. It also has a risk of contamination with urine and stools, which may cause infections.

Technique (Fig. 9)

Dorsiflex the hand at wrist joint to 45°, place a rolled cloth beneath the joint to stabilize. Palpate the radial pulse, breach the skin using the tip of the cannula, now puncture the anterior wall of the artery with a cannula. Move forward the needle until bright red blood is seen in the hub of a cannula, arterial pulsations can also be seen, now lower the needle to 10° angle, move catheter slowly anteriorly and remove the needle gently. Fix the catheter, use the heparinized saline infusion to prevent catheter block. The use of heparin 1 U/mL and papaverine (30 mg/250 mL) to the catheter infusion solution (0.9% NaCl) decreases the incidence.

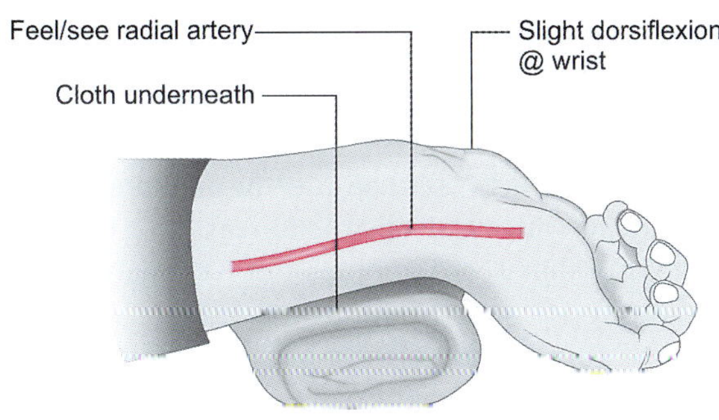

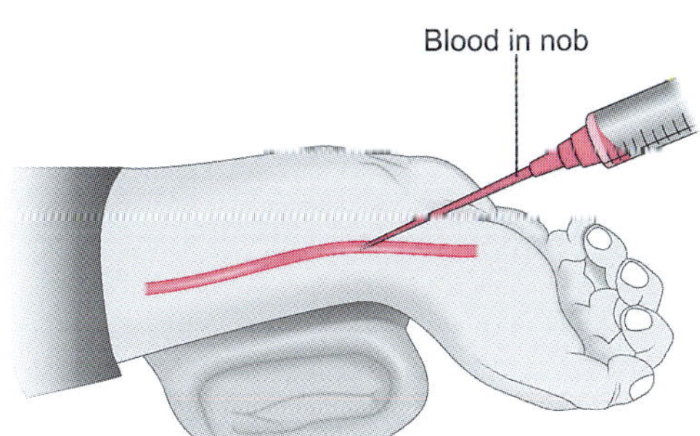

Fig. 9: Intra-arterial access

Thrombosis and vasospasm are the main reasons for arterial catheter failure. If the catheter leads to thrombosis evident by ischemia in distal tissue, then it should be removed immediately, and systemic unfractionated heparin should be started. If perfusion does not improve by 24 hours, start thrombolytic therapy with tissue plasminogen activator. If medical management fails then limb can be salvaged by balloon thrombectomy via an arteriotomy. The catheter should be removed as early as possible once the patient stabilizes and does not require monitoring.

KEY MESSAGES

- Venous access can be through peripheral vein for short-term use and central venous is desired when long-term use is required.
- Central venous catheterization requires expertise and must be performed by trained experts in intensive care setting.
- Intra-osseous access should be explored among sick babies with no venous access.
- There is restricted use of intra-arterial cannulation except in cases which require repeated arterial blood gas sampling.

REFERENCES

1. Stovroff M, Teague WG. Intravenous access in infants and children. Pediatr Clin North Am. 1998;45:1373-93.
2. Rosetti VA, Thompson BM, Aprahamian C, *et al*. Difficulty and delay in intravascular access in pediatric arrests. Ann Emerg Med. 1984;13:406.
3. O' Grady NP, Alexander M, Burns LA, *et al*. Healthcare Infection Control Practices Advisory Committee (HICPAC). Guidelines for the prevention of intravascular catheter-related infections. Am J Infect Control. 2011;39:S1-S34.
4. Frey AM, Pettit J. Infusion therapy in children. In: M Alexander, A Corrigan, L Gorski, J Hankins, R Perucca, editors. Infusion Nursing: An Evidence-Based Practice. St. Louis: Saunders/ Elsevier Publication; 2010. p. 550-70.

5. Ponnusamy V, Venkatesh V, Clarke P. Skin antisepsis in the neonate: What should we use? Curr Opin Infect Dis. 2014;27: 244-50.
6. Crowley M, Brim C, Proehl J, *et al.* Emergency nursing resource: Difficult venous access. J Emerg Nurs. 2012;38(4):335-43.
7. Seldinger SI. Catheter replacement of the needle in percutaneous arteriography: A new technique. Acta Radiol. 1953;39:368-76.
8. Kanter RK, Gorton JM, Palmieri K, *et al.* Anatomy of femoral vessels in infants and guidelines for venous catheterization. Pediatrics. 1989;83:1020-2.
9. Taylor EA, Mowbray MJ, McLellan I. Central venous access in children via the external jugular vein. Anaesthesia. 1992;47:265-6.
10. Venkataraman ST, Orr RA, Thompson AE. Percutaneous infraclavicular subclavian vein catheterization in critically ill infants and children. J Pediatr. 1988;113:480-5.

91.2 Lumbar Puncture

Sharmila B Mukherjee, Dipti Kapoor

INTRODUCTION

Lumbar puncture (LP) is a procedure in which a sample of cerebrospinal fluid (CSF) is withdrawn for diagnostic and therapeutic purposes (**Table 1**). Since the sample is collected from the spinal cord, it is also referred to as a "spinal tap," LPs have been performed to evaluate CSF in the diagnosis and management of neurologic diseases for more than a century. Despite the advent of advanced methods of neuroimaging, this procedure still retains its significant role in understanding the pathophysiology and planning further management of central nervous system (CNS) disorders.

SITE OF A LUMBAR PUNCTURE

The lower end of the spinal cord, the conus medullaris, lies at the L1–L2 vertebral interspace in most subjects and above the L3 vertebral body in all individuals without a spinal deformity (**Fig. 1**). Hence, CSF should be withdrawn from the interspaces below L3 to avoid damaging it.

CONTRAINDICATIONS

It is assumed that the clinician must have taken a detailed history and performed a thorough examination based on which a clinical diagnosis has been made, and an LP planned. Nevertheless, it is essential that a focused examination of the vital parameters and neurological status should be repeated immediately before the procedure and investigations reviewed to rule out any of the absolute or relative contraindications (**Table 2**).

Increased intracranial tension: This is an absolute contraindication for an LP, as it can alter the pressure dynamics in individuals with a CSF obstruction resulting in cerebral herniation or spinal cord compression. A cranial computed tomography (CT) or preferably magnetic resonance imaging (MRI), should always be performed before an LP (even in the absence of papilledema), if the patient has altered sensorium, clinical signs of raised intracranial tension and focal neurological signs. Radiological findings of a midline shift, cerebral edema, posterior fossa mass

Table 1: Indications for a lumbar puncture

Diagnostic	*Therapeutic*
• Clinical suspicion of meningitis or encephalitis • Subarachnoid hemorrhage • Leptomeningeal carcinomatosis • Demyelinating and inflammatory CNS disorders: GBS, ADEM, MS • Some neurodegenerative disorders	• Infusion of anesthetic, contrast or chemotherapeutic agents into the spinal canal • Treatment of benign Intracranial hypertension (Pseudotumor cerebri)

(ADEM: acute disseminated encephalomyelitis, CNS: central nervous system, GBS: Guillain-Barré syndrome, MS: multiple sclerosis)

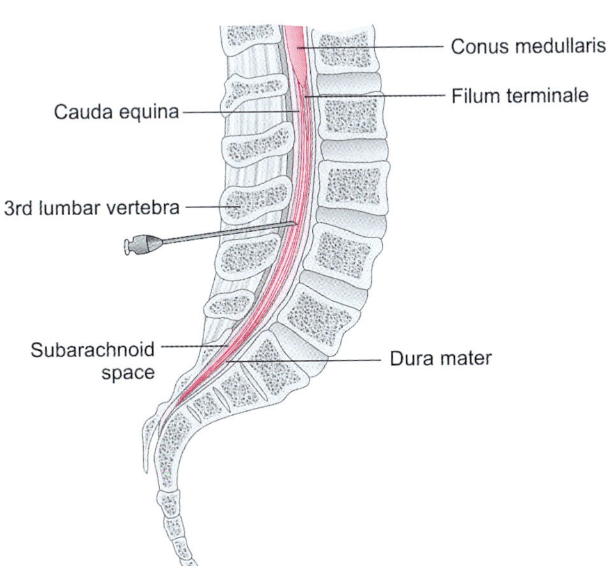

Fig. 1: Anatomy of the lower end of the spinal cord

Table 2: Contraindications for a lumbar puncture

Absolute	*Relative*
• Raised intracranial pressure	• Soft tissue infection at the site • Spinal deformity • Acute spinal injury • History of pre-existing lower back pain, lower limb neuralgias or previous lower back surgery • Thrombocytopenia • Deranged coagulation profile • Hemodynamic instability • Respiratory distress • Brain abscess

or loss of suprachiasmatic and basilar cisterns, superior cerebellar cistern or quadrigeminal plate cisterns are reasons for deferring the LP.

Local contraindications: If an LP is done at a site overlying soft tissue infection, it may lead to meningitis, epidural abscess, or osteomyelitis. Performing a conventional LP in a patient with spinal deformity is challenging. In these instances, an alternative approach may be required.

Bleeding tendencies: Patients with platelet count lower than 50,000/mm^3 and an international normalized ratio (INR) more than 1.5 are at risk of localized epidural, subdural, or subarachnoid bleeding. These abnormalities should be corrected before an LP.

Hemodynamic instability/respiratory compromise: The neck and upper back of a patient is flexed during positioning of a patient for an LP. This can cause acute worsening in a patient with existing cardio-respiratory instability.

PROCEDURE

Pre-LP procedure

This comprises of the following steps:

1. *Reviewing indications and contraindications*
2. *Obtaining informed consent/informed assent*: Parents should be involved in the decision-making process by providing them with verbal or written information regarding the purpose, benefits, risks, and possible consequences of the LP. Taking written informed consent is mandatory. Informed assent should also be obtained from children older than 7 years who are mature enough to understand the process.
3. *Sedation*: Moderate to deep sedation is often necessary for younger children or the uncooperative older child. The drugs commonly used are midazolam and fentanyl. Drugs like Ketamine should be avoided for sedation as this may result in raised intracranial pressure.
4. *Hemodynamic monitoring*: The probe of a pulse-oximeter should be attached to the patient for continuous monitoring. Pre-procedure vitals should be recorded.
5. *Preparation of the LP tray*: This (**Fig. 2**) includes three sterile cotton swabs, povidone solution, spinal needle, 25-gauge and 20-gauge needle for anesthetic infiltration (if required), 3 cc syringe, 1% lidocaine, four CSF collection vials, and sterile gloves. The recommended spinal needles are 20- or 22-gauge Quincke needles, which are beveled and fitted with a stylet. Atraumatic needles have blunt, pencil point tips and a side port for injection or collection.[1] The most common needles that are used for LP are 20 or 22-gauge needles (usually $1^1/_2$ inch in length for infants, $2^1/_2$ inch for children between 2 and 8 years, and $3^1/_2$ inches for older children. Also, keep *cardio-pulmonary resuscitation (CPR) equipment ready.*
6. *Preparation of environment and personnel*: The place where the LP is performed should be quiet and free of disturbance. Apart from the person performing the LP, there should be an assistant to hold the child in position, another to label and handle the collected CSF samples and a staff nurse for administration of medication.

LP Procedure

1. *Positioning the patient*: This is one of the factors that determine the success of an LP. It depends on the

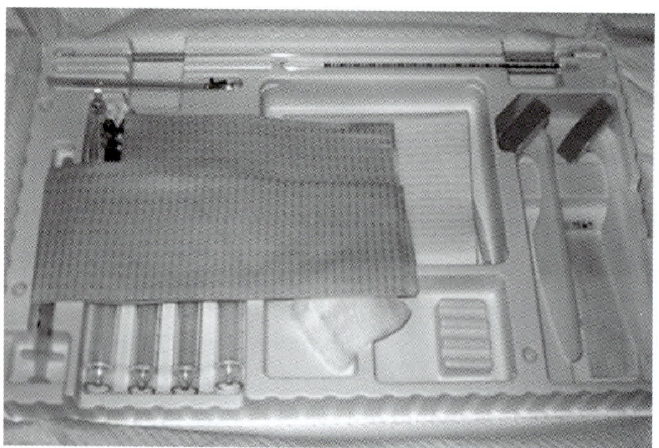

Fig. 2: Lumbar puncture tray

relaxation of the patient and the experience of the assistant. The procedure can be performed in the following positions:

a. *Lateral recumbent position*: The patient should be curled with the neck and hips flexed to maximize the size of the interspace (**Fig. 3A**). The shoulder and hips should be perpendicular to the table with the back at the edge of the bed to allow easy collection of CSF. The L3–L4 interspace is at the level of the superior iliac crests. This area should be carefully palpated and marked to ensure that it can be identified even after the patient is cleaned and draped.
b. *Sitting position (**Fig. 3B**)*: An alternative method of positioning involves placing the patient in an upright seated position with the help of an assistant or prop. This can be particularly useful in obese patients.

2. *Cleaning and draping*: The skin should be prepared using a microbicidal agent, i.e. 10% povidone-iodine. It should be given enough time to dry and then draped with a sterile towel or cloth.
3. *Local analgesia*: This may be sufficient for cooperative older children (with or without an additional anxiolytic). Theoretically, the injection of a local anesthetic (1% lidocaine) into the area should minimize pain, but the pain of injection often equals or exceeds that of the insertion of the spinal needle. Hence, use of a topical analgesic cream, such as EMLA (eutectic mixture of local anesthetics) is a better option.
4. *Positioning the needle*: The sharply beveled tip of the needle should be inserted in the midline of the desired inter-vertebral space, in the direction of the umbilicus with the bevel pointing towards the ceiling (lateral decubitus position) or to the side (sitting). As the needle is gradually advanced, the ligamentum flavum and dura mater get pierced resulting in a slight popping sensation as the subarachnoid space is entered. The stylet is removed to allow CSF to drain to the needle hub. If no fluid appears, the needle should be rotated 90° in case a nerve rootlet or strand of arachnoid is obstructing the opening. If this does not initiate CSF flow, the needle can be advanced a few millimeters more. If there is still no CSF, the stylet should be replaced and the needle slowly withdrawn and redirected in the same interspace or a higher interspace is selected for a second tap.
5. *Collection of CSF*: At least three vials of 1–2 mL of CSF are routinely collected sequentially for biochemistry, culture and cytology respectively. A fourth sample can be taken if additional studies (biochemical, microbiologic, immunologic, or metabolic) are required. The vials should be kept labeled beforehand.
6. *Removal of the needle*: If a Quincke needle has been used the stylet should be replaced before the withdrawal of the needle to avoid pulling a strand of arachnoid through the dura mater, inadvertently creating a channel for CSF leakage and increasing risk of a post-procedural headache.
7. *Management of puncture site*: This should be covered with a sterile or occlusive bandage.
8. *Documentation*: The details of the procedure and post-procedure vitals should be recorded.

Post-LP Procedure

1. *Post-procedure monitoring and care*: Time should be provided for the child to recover from the procedure in a comfortable supine position. Vitals should be monitored. The puncture site should also be monitored for blood or CSF leakage.
2. *Waste material disposal.*
3. *Transfer of samples*: The samples should be sent to the appropriate laboratory.
4. *Management of complications*:
    a. *Post-procedural headache*: This is a common complication (seen in one-third patients) that may occur within 72 hours of the LP.[2] It may worsen in an upright position and get relieved in a recumbent position. It may rarely be associated with neck stiffness, nausea, vomiting, and cranial nerve palsies. These symptoms usually resolve within a few days. The incidence and severity of

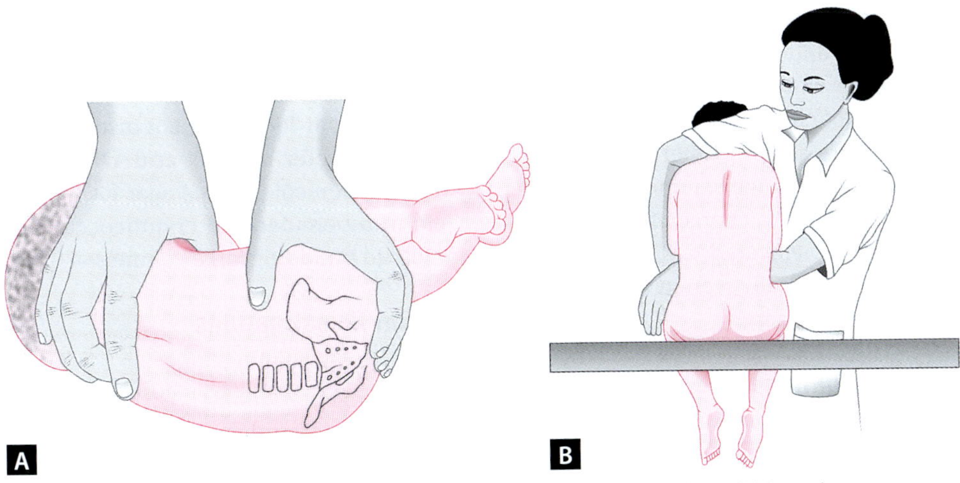

Figs. 3A and B: Positions for performing LP (A) Lateral recumbent; (B) Seated

headache can be reduced by using small-diameter or atraumatic needles. Bed rest does not prevent headache, but helps in reducing it. Although there is no evidence for the use of increased fluids to prevent headache, it is commonly practiced. Simple analgesics can be helpful.

b. *Local pain and paresthesias*: This may occur in the distribution of a lumbar nerve root resulting from contact with the needle.
c. *Infections*: Meningitis, epidural abscess, and osteomyelitis may result if asepsis is not maintained.
d. *Local bleeding*: Subarachnoid, subdural, or epidural hematomas may result from a breach of the epidural venous plexus, radicular arteries, or radicular veins. These are rare but serious complications.
e. Subarachnoid epidermal cyst.

CSF ANALYSIS

Appearance

Normal CSF is clear. Xanthochromia, a yellowish discoloration of the CSF, is seen in the presence of hyperbilirubinemia or red blood cell breakdown products. Reddish color suggests subarachnoid hemorrhage or a traumatic LP. The way of differentiating between both is by examining the color in 3 vials. In case of traumatic tap, there is a sequential clearing of CSF from first to the third vial, whereas the reddish color remains the same in all three vials in subarachnoid hemorrhage. That is why cytology is done on the 3rd vial.

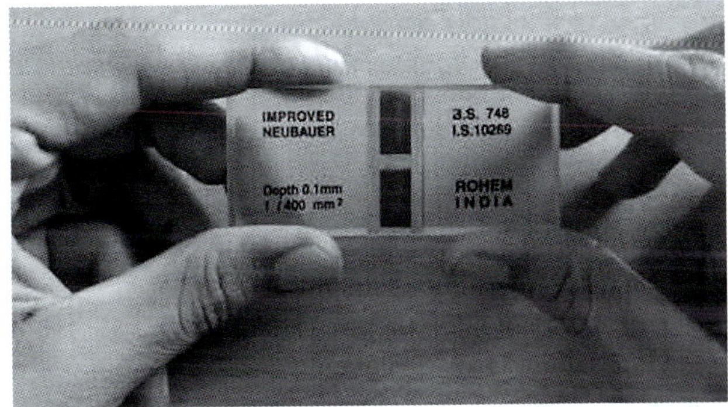

Fig. 4: Nuebauer chamber

Cytology

Counting chambers like the Neubauer chamber and the new version (**Fig. 4**) are used for quantification of red blood cells (RBC) and white blood cells (WBC) in the CSF. A few RBC can be found in normal CSF, even in the absence of a traumatic LP. The normal WBC count in CSF count varies with age (**Table 3**) with a differential of 70% lymphocytes and 30% monocytes. An elevated WBC above the upper limit may indicate inflammation or infection within the CNS, but not further differentiation of etiology. It may also be seen immediately following a status epilepticus.

Biochemistry

This includes the measurement of protein and glucose content in CSF **(Table 4)**. Blood should be collected at the same time as the LP is performed so that the CSF glucose can be compared with the blood glucose levels.

High CSF protein concentrations (>500 mg/dL) occur in patients with meningitis and subarachnoid hemorrhage. A very low CSF glucose value (hypoglycorrhachia) is characteristic of acute bacterial meningitis. Mildly to moderately low values are seen in tuberculous, fungal, protozoal, and spirochetal meningitis. It may also be seen in GLUT2 deficiency disorders. A characteristic albumin-cytologic dissociation, i.e. elevated CSF protein level without increased WBC is typically seen in Guillain-Barré syndrome (10 days after the onset).

Microbiological Examination

Intimation should be sent to the laboratory to centrifuge the CSF and stain the sediment according to the suspected microorganism, which is deduced from the age of the child and clinical scenario. These include Gram stain (bacteria), Ziehl-Nielsen stain (*Mycobacterium*), India Ink preparation (*Cryptococcus*) and Wright or Giemsa stain (Toxoplasmosis). Wet mounts are indicated in suspected protozoal and helminthic infections.

The first vial is never used for culture to avoid contamination. Culture media differ according to the suspected organism; 5% sheep blood agar and enriched chocolate agar for bacteria, Lowenstein-Jensen medium for Mycobacterium TB and Dichloran Rose-Bengal Chloramphenicol (DRBC) agar for *Cryptococcus*. Culture yield in tubercular and cryptococcal meningitis can be increased by adding large volumes of CSF to the media.

Special Investigations

These include the following:

- *Latex agglutination (LA)*: This allows rapid detection of bacterial antigens in pyogenic meningitis due to *Haemophilus influenzae* and *Streptococcus pneumonia*.
- *Polymerase chain reaction*: This is useful in suspected viral meningoencephalitis. CSF PCR has a sensitivity of 95–100% and specificity of 100% for Herpes simplex virus type 1, Epstein-Barr virus, and enterovirus.
- *Metabolic tests*: This may be useful in some specific inborn errors of metabolism. CSF lactate may be

Table 3: Normal white blood cell count, protein and glucose content of CSF

Age	*WBC count/ mm³ Mean ± SD*	*Protein*	*Glucose*
Neonate			
Preterm	5.1 ± 5.8	Up to 180 mg/dL	80% of blood glucose
Term	4.5 ± 3.6	Up to 100 mg/dL	75% of blood glucose
Infant		40–80 mg/dL	50–80 mg/dL or two-third of blood glucose level
Less than 6 weeks	3.7 ± 3.4		
6 weeks to 3 months	2.9 ± 2.9		
3–6 months	1.9 ± 2.0		
6–12 months	2.6 ± 2.5		
Child	1.9 ± 2.7	10–40 mg/dL	

Table 4: CSF abnormalities in bacterial, viral and tubercular meningitis and subarachnoid hemorrhage

Parameter	*Bacterial meningitis*	*Tubercular meningitis*	*Viral meningitis*	*Subarachnoid hemorrhage*
Opening pressure	Elevated/normal	Elevated/normal	Elevated/normal	Elevated/normal
Appearance	Clear/cloudy	Normal/cobweb	Clear	Clear/bloody
Xanthochromia	Absent	Absent	Absent	Present
RBC	< 5/HPF	< 5/HPF	< 5/HPF	> 50/mm³
WBC	Increased ~ > 100/μL, Predominantly neutrophilic	Increased ~ 50–500/μL, early neutrophilic then lymphocytic	Increased, 10–1000/μL, Predominantly lymphocytic	May be increased. Normal differential maintained
Glucose	Very low	Low	Normal/low	Normal
Protein	Elevated	Elevated	Elevated	Elevated

increased in mitochondrial but is not pathognomic. CSF organic acid may be increased in organic aciduria. CSF glycine concentration or CSF to plasma glycine ratio is elevated in nonketotic hyperglycinemia.

- *CSF gamma globulin level and oligoclonal bands*: These are elevated in acute demyelinating inflammatory conditions like acute disseminated encephalomyelitis. CSF oligoclonal bands may be present in pediatric multiple sclerosis.
- *Antibodies*: IgG anti-measles antibodies are seen in subacute sclerosing panencephalitis. IgG anti-NMDA receptor antibodies are detected in autoimmune encephalitis.
- *Biomarkers*: Several specific proteins accompany brain injury from inflammatory, traumatic, cerebrovascular, epileptic, and neurodegenerative disorders.[3] Some of these that being currently investigated, include heat shock protein (HSP70), aggregated beta-amyloid, neuron-specific enolase, S-100 beta, vascular endothelial growth factor, glial fibrillary acidic protein, brain-derived growth factor and nerve growth factor, apolipoprotein E, interleukin-6, soluble FAS receptor, and BCL2 and excitatory neurotransmitters glutamate and glycine. Their roles are still under evaluation.

KEY MESSAGES

- Lumbar puncture plays a significant role in the diagnosis of CNS disorders, despite the availability of advanced modalities of neuroimaging.
- A detailed history and examination (with special focus on vital parameters and neurological status) is essential before performing a lumbar puncture, to ensure that the clinical diagnosis is a definite indication and also to rule out any contraindication.
- The steps of pre-procedure and post-procedure management should be diligently complied with, as they are as important to follow as the lumbar puncture itself.

REFERENCES

1. Hudgins PA, Fountain AJ, Chapman PR, *et al.* Difficult lumbar puncture: Pitfalls and tips from the trenches. Am J Neuroradiol. 2017;10:1-8.
2. Hammond ER, Wang Z, Bhulani N, *et al.* Needle type and the risk of post-lumbar puncture headache in the outpatient neurology clinic. J Neurol Sci. 2011;306;21-8.
3. Shahim P, Darin N, Andreasson U, *et al.* Cerebrospinal fluid brain injury biomarkers in children: A multicenter study. Pediatr Neurol. 2013;49:31-9.

91.3 Abdominal Paracentesis

Pranav Gupta, Vyom Aggarwal

INTRODUCTION

Abdominal paracentesis refers to the procedure of obtaining or removing fluid from the abdominal cavity (ascitic fluid). Since examination of ascitic fluid can provide important clue to the etiology of myriad local and systemic illnesses, this procedure is often considered an integral part of clinical evaluation, wherever significant abdominal collection which could be "tapped" is observed.[1] While diagnostic paracentesis just aims at obtaining a small amount of fluid sample for analysis, therapeutic paracentesis involves aspiration of a significantly large amount of fluid to relieve abdominal discomfort and attendant breathing difficulty.

INDICATIONS

Diagnostic

- For determining etiology of the peritoneal fluid collection (in new onset ascites).
- For evaluation of children with ascites of known etiology presenting with symptoms suggestive of decompensation or infection such as abdominal pain, fever, gastrointestinal bleed, worsening encephalopathy, new or worsening renal or liver failure and hypotension.
- For evaluating suspected intra-abdominal malignancy.
- For evaluation of abdominal injury.
- In suspected necrotizing enterocolitis.
- In peritoneal dialysis patients with signs of infection or sepsis.

Therapeutic

- In hemodynamically stable patients with tense ascites or ascites refractory to diuretics with the aim to relieve the respiratory distress due to increased intra-abdominal pressure and/or relieving abdominal discomfort.
- For instilling drugs in the peritoneal cavity.
- Hemorrhagic pancreatitis.

Contraindications

- Absolute
  - Acute surgical abdomen
- Relative
  - Severe thrombocytopenia (platelet count < 20,000 cu mm)
  - Coagulopathy (INR > 2)
  - Distended urinary bladder
  - Distended bowel (paralytic ileus or intestinal obstruction)
  - Skin infection or cellulitis at the planned site for paracentesis
  - Severe hypoproteinemia
  - Loculated ascites due to intra-abdominal adhesions.

THE PROCESS

Prerequisites

Before undertaking the procedure, it is of utmost importance to ensure that following pre-requisites have been duly taken care of, to minimize chances of complications, errors, and potential litigations:

- *Ultrasonography*: It is ideal to do the procedure under direct sonographic guidance, if possible and feasible. Unless a dire emergency, the paracentesis should invariably be preceded by abdominal ultrasound.[2] The ultrasonographic examination helps by:
  - Confirming and quantifying the ascitic fluid
  - Suggesting the nature of fluid collection (watery, pus or blood)
  - Locating blood vessels in the trajectory of the aspirating needle
  - Determining the location and the depth of the fluid
  - Guiding the aspirating needle.
- Bladder is empty.
- Normal coagulation profile has been established.
- Informed consent has been obtained.

It is preferable, though not essential to have a pulse oximeter to monitor vitals during and after the procedure.

The instruments and supplies needed for the procedure are listed in **Box 1**.

Procedure[3]

Step 1: Positioning

Both midline and lateral approaches can be used for paracentesis. Paracentesis is usually performed with patient in supine position with heel slightly raised. Left lateral approach is also often used as the cecum is relatively fixed and lateral positioning minimizes risk of bowel injury. In case of minimal free fluid, the procedure can be performed in prone position with patient positioned on his knees and elbows allowing the ascitic fluid to gravitate to the most dependent part of the abdomen.

Step 2: Site selection

It is of paramount importance to ensure that the bladder is empty, either through voluntary micturition or by catheter drainage. The site of insertion needs careful selection. Needle can either be inserted in the midline, about 2 cm below the umbilicus or lateral to the rectus abdominis (**Fig. 1**). Lateral insertion sites are preferred to midline since collateral vessels are abundant in midline region. Areas with visible veins or surgical scars are to be avoided as scars may have tethered bowel loops increasing the chances of bowel perforation. Similarly, the areas with

Box 1: Supplies needed for ascitic tap

- Disposable paracentesis kits are readily available. In the absence of a commercially available kit, the following might serve the purpose:
  - Appropriate size sterile disposable gloves
  - Antiseptic solution (povidone iodine/chlorhexidine)
  - Isopropyl alcohol/Methylated spirit
  - Sterile swabs
  - Fenestrated drapes (cut sheets)
  - Sterile syringes of different volumes, namely, 2 mL, 5 mL, 10 mL and 50 mL
  - Hypodermic needles or intravenous cannulas: 18–26 G
  - Injection lignocaine 1%
  - Injection midazolam, ketamine (if sedation is intended)
  - Three-way cocks
  - Paracentesis catheter
  - Intravenous set
  - Specimen bottles (universal containers)
  - Waste bottle
  - Adhesive tapes
  - Tincture benzoin

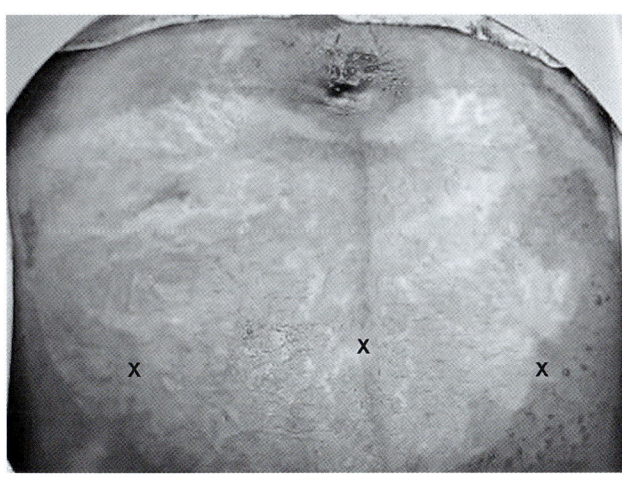

Fig. 1: Site(s) for abdominal paracentesis

visibly engorged abdominal wall vessels or abdominal wall hematomas are best avoided to minimize chances of bleeding.[4]

Preferred site is two fingerbreadths (about 3 cm) superior and two fingerbreadths medial to the anterior superior iliac spine. Ultrasound should be used to confirm the presence of fluid as well as the absence of bowel or any visceral organ at the selected site.

Step 3: Cleaning and draping

After donning sterile gloves, the selected site is cleaned with an antiseptic solution in widening circular motions beginning from the center, ensuring a large clean area, enough to fill the fenestration of the drape being used. The antiseptic solution is allowed to dry on the skin, and the site is covered with sterile fenestrated drape (cut sheet).

Step 4: Anesthesia

The selected entry site is anesthetized by injecting a small amount of lignocaine, just enough to raise a small wheal. The needle is withdrawn and after allowing some time for the effect of the local anesthetic, the needle is reinserted, perpendicular to the abdominal wall, using a "Z-track" technique. The needle is advanced in increments of 5 mm, each time followed by gentle aspiration. A small amount of lignocaine is infiltrated if no blood is aspirated, and the needle is advanced another 5 mm and the procedure repeated till the entire track is anesthetized using a total of 3–5 mL lignocaine.

Step 5: Tapping the fluid

A wide bore needle (18–20 G) attached to a 10–20 mL syringe is advanced through the anesthetized tract, into the peritoneal cavity, using "Z-track" technique. Alternatively, a paracentesis catheter may be similarly introduced if therapeutic paracentesis is intended. A small skin incision, wide enough to permit the passage of the catheter with little resistance, made using a # 11 surgical blade, may facilitate catheter insertion.

The parietal peritoneum is elastic and might tent for a few centimeters before getting pierced. Twisting the paracentesis needle a few times helps in penetrating the peritoneum. Free flow of fluid confirms that the needle has entered the peritoneal cavity. Needle or catheter is stabilized and secured to prevent its inadvertent removal.

If the free flow of fluid remains elusive despite careful maneuvering, the needle is stabilized with one hand while the aspirating syringe is detached from the needle with the other hand. It might yield a few milliliters of fluid for all critical biochemical and cytological analysis.

Bowel or omentum may at times block the tip of the needle. In such cases, a good flow obtained initially ceases almost immediately. Gently repositioning the patient to pool fluid around the needle will usually re-establish the flow.

Step 6: Diagnostic vs. therapeutic aspiration

Diagnostic aspiration: About 5 mL of fluid is enough for cytology and biochemical evaluations. About 2 mL of fluid is first collected in an EDTA vial. EDTA prevents hemorrhagic ascitic fluid from coagulation, which can alter the cell count. Rest of the specimen is transferred to a culture bottle and sterile plain vial for pyogenic culture, biochemical evaluation and special tests (if indicated). Characteristics of ascitic fluid in different conditions are shown in **Table 1**.

Therapeutic aspiration: The aspiration needle or catheter is secured with one hand, and the syringe is detached with the other. Aspiration can be done passively, with intra-abdominal pressure aiding in the removal of the ascitic fluid, by attaching the collecting bottle to the aspirating needle or cannula through a catheter. The needle or the cannula is firmly secured on the abdominal wall with adhesive tapes. Process of aspiration can be hastened by using vacuum bottles available commercially.

Table 1: Typical characteristics of ascites in different conditions (modified from Huang LL, et al)[7]

Test	*Cirrhosis*	*Congestive cardiac failure*	*Malignancy*	*Tuberculosis*	*SBP*	*Pancreatitis*
Gross appearance	Clear straw or milky	Clear to pale yellow	Milky or bloody	Milky or N	Cloudy or turbid	Milky or cloudy or turbid
TP	< 25 g/L	< 25 g/L	≥ 25 g/L	≥ 25 g/L	≥ 25 g/L	≥ 25 g/L
SAAG	≥ 1.1 g/dL	≥ 1.1 g/dL	< 1.1 g/dL	< 1.1 g/dL	< 1.1 g/dL	< 1.1 g/dL
LDH	↓	↓ or N	↑	↑ or N	↑ or N	↑ or N
Glucose	N	N	↓	↓	↓	↓
Amylase	N		↑ or N			↑
ADA	↓ or N		↓ or N	↑		
Cell counts	≥ 250/μL or N			≥ 250/uL or N	≥ 250/uL	
Smear			Malignant cells	AFB + or –		
GeneXpert				Positive for M Tb		
Bacterial culture	+ or –			+ or –	+	
Viscosity	< 1.03 cP	< 1.03 cP	≥ 1.03 cP	≥ 1.03 cP	≥ 1.03 cP	≥ 1.03 cP
Proton NMR	↑ or ↓	↑ or ↓				
VEGF	↓	N	↑	↓	↓	↓
Tumor markers	↑ or N	N	↑	↑ or N		↑ or N

(↑: increase; ↓: decrease; N: normal; +: positive; –: negative; SBP: spontaneous bacterial peritonitis; TP: total proteins; SAAG: serum ascitic albumin gradient; ADA: adenosine deaminase; VEGF: vascular endothelial growth factor)

Alternatively, fluid could be aspirated actively using a large 50 mL syringe, which is attached to the aspirating needle or the cannula through a three-way stop cock. The open end of the three-way stop cock is attached to the collection bottle through a catheter. Fluid aspirated in the syringe can be transferred to the collection bottle by diverting the flow with the three-way stop cock.

Recently, Alfapump® system has become available, which could be implanted in the subcutaneous tissue to continuously drain the ascitic fluid from the peritoneal cavity to the urinary bladder, avoiding the need for repeated punctures for therapeutic drainage.[6]

Step 7: Sealing the puncture site

The needle should be removed in one swift motion after the procedure is complete. A wisp of cotton dipped in Tincture of Iodine can be placed over the puncture site, over which a sterile dressing pad can be placed and secured with adhesive tapes.

POST-PROCEDURE INSTRUCTIONS

The patient/parents have to be instructed to monitor bleeding from the insertion site and signs of infection like pain, numbness, or discomfort in the area. They are to be trained to clean the area with warm soap and water and pat the area dry.

Watch for Complication

- The *ascitic fluid leak* occurs if "Z-track" technique is not used or if the skin incision is too broad. Such leaks are self-limiting with reduction of the volume of ascitic fluid with treatment. A stoma bag can be placed over the insertion site. This helps in quantifying the oozing fluid and prevents soiling. A large incision can be sutured to reduce the ooze.
- *Pneumoperitoneum* might occur because of the inadvertent introduction of air in the peritoneal cavity.
- *Perforation* of intra-abdominal organs (bladder, bowel, gravid uterus, and stomach) is more common in the settings of paralytic ileus or bowel adhesions. It is suspected if fecal matter or air, instead of fluid, is aspirated through the needle. When in doubt, the procedure should be abandoned, and erect X-ray of the abdomen be obtained. Presence of gas under diaphragm confirms the diagnosis of hollow viscous perforation. The risk could be minimized by the use of intracaths instead of needles for aspiration.
- *Hypotension*: Rapid removal of large amount of ascitic fluid, without adequate intravascular volume repletion can lead to profound hypotension and shock. The relief offered by therapeutic paracentesis is temporary as most fluid re-accumulates rapidly. The re-accumulated fluid is rich in albumin which might precipitate hypotension

in the already hypoproteinemic baby. Hence, it is usually advised against removing large volumes, exceeding 1.5 liters, in a single sitting. Volume support in the form of albumin or colloids minimizes such complications if larger volumes are needed to be removed.[7]

- *Electrolyte imbalance*: Large amount of fluid removal can be associated with dyselectrolytemia and attendant oliguria and renal/hepatic failure.
- Hypoproteinemia.
- Trauma to a major blood vessel(s).
- Loss of catheter or guidewire in the peritoneal cavity.
- Hematoma of the abdominal wall.
- Introduction of infection inside the peritoneal cavity (peritonitis).
- Infection of the procedure site (cellulitis).

KEY MESSAGES

- Diagnostic and/or therapeutic paracentesis is an indispensable procedure in the management of significant abdominal collection.
- This procedure is easy to perform and safe even in sick children if one is wary of very few contraindications.
- The analysis of ascitic fluid obtained by paracentesis is invaluable in managing patients with myriad of systemic illnesses.

REFERENCES

1. Bavdekar A, Thakur N. Ascites in children. Indian J Pediatr. 2016;83:1334-40.
2. Nazeer SR, Dewbre H, Miller AH. Ultrasound assisted paracentesis performed by emergency physicians vs. the traditional technique: A prospective, randomized study. Am J Emerg Med. 2005;23:363-7.
3. Thomsen TW, Shaffer RW, White B, *et al.* Videos in clinical medicine. Paracentesis. N Engl J Med. 2006;355:e21.
4. Prajapati B. Abdominal paracentesis. In: Prajapati B, editor. Essential Procedures in Paediatrics. New Delhi: Jaypee Brothers Medical Publishers; 2003. p. 232-4.
5. Huang LL, Xia HH, Zhu SL. Ascitic fluid analysis in the differential diagnosis of ascites: Focus on cirrhotic ascites. J Clin Transl Hepatol. 2014;2:58-64.
6. Bureau C, Adebayo D, Chalret de Rieu M, *et al.* Alfapump® system vs. large volume paracentesis for refractory ascites: A multicentre randomized controlled study. J Hepatol. 2017; 67:940-9.
7. Kramer RE, Sokol RJ, Yerushalmi B, *et al.* Large-volume paracentesis in the management of ascites in children. J Pediatr Gastroenterol Nutr. 2001;33:245-9.

91.4 Pericardiocentesis

Sumaira Khalil

INTRODUCTION

Pericardiocentesis is a procedure in which the fluid or blood collected in pericardial sac is aspirated. It is an emergency procedure in children who present with cardiac tamponade. The pericardial sac is a double-layered sac, which fixes the heart to the mediastinum. The two layers of the pericardium are the "Epicardium" which is a serous visceral layer and a fibrous parietal layer; enclosing the pericardial cavity.

ETIOPATHOGENESIS

Pericarditis in pediatric patients accounts for <0.2% of the emergency visits in patients presenting to a tertiary care pediatric emergency setting. Idiopathic pericardial effusions are rare in children but account for 20–40% in adults.[1] Tuberculosis is the most common cause of pericarditis seen in developing countries as opposed to viral and bacterial in developed countries.[2] Bagri *et al.* reported tuberculosis (52%) as the most common cause of pericardial effusion in children admitted in a tertiary care center followed by bacterial (23%), viral (12%) recurrent idiopathic (8%) and malignancy.[3] The pressure around the heart increases due to the accumulation of fluid in the pericardial sac. Impaired cardiac filling and decreased cardiac output occur secondary to increase in the intra-pericardial pressure. Rapid increase in the intra-pericardial

Table 1: Etiology of pericarditis

Infective	Noninfective
• *Bacterial*: Mycobacterial tuberculosis, *Staphylococcus aureus*, *Streptococcus pneumoneae*, *H. influenza*, *Streptococcus pyogenes*, Meningococcemia, *Coxiella burnetti* • *Viral*: Coxsackie B, echovirus, parvovirus B19 cytomegalovirus, human herpes virus 6 • *Parasitic*: Toxoplasmosis, *Echinococcus* sp. • *Fungal*: *Candida* sp., *Aspergillus* sp., *Histoplasma*, *Blastomyces* sp.	• Trauma • *Autoimmune*: Systemic lupus erythematosus, Sjogren's syndrome, scleroderma, rheumatoid arthritis • *Malignancy*: Primary tumors, secondary metastasis from lymphoma, lung cancer and breast cancer • Systemic vasculitides • *Drugs*: Cyclophosphamide, doxorubicin, daunorubicin, cyclosporine, thiazides, streptomycin, strptokinase • *Others*: Chronic congestive heart failure, pulmonary artery hypertension, aortic dissection, amyloidosis • Post pericardiotomy syndrome • Idiopathic

pressure secondary to acute accumulation of pericardial fluid can lead to hemodynamic compromise.

Common causes of pericarditis are listed in **Table 1**.[4]

PROCEDURE

Indications

- Cardiac tamponade secondary to pericardial effusion is the most common indication for doing pericardiocentesis in 80–90% of cases.
- Large (>20 mm) and persistent (3 months) effusions not causing hemodynamic compromise but unresponsive to medical management can be a relative indication for doing a pericardiocentesis. In small to moderate pericardial effusions (<20 mm) diagnostic pericardiocentesis is usually not indicated due to the high procedural risk and low diagnostic yield.[5]

Contraindications

- Aortic dissection and post-infarction rupture of free wall.
- Relative contraindications include uncorrected coagulopathy, anticoagulant therapy, and thrombocytopenia (platelet count <50 000/mm^3).

Technique

It is essential to monitor the vitals, central venous pressure monitoring, and baseline electrocardiogram before starting the procedure. An evaluation by echocardiography would define the size, distribution and hemodynamic effects of the pericardial effusion. In an emergency, even ultrasonography can be used to quickly localize the effusion and guide the site of aspiration.

Mayo clinic recommends deciding the approach and defining the site of entry based on echocardiographic evaluation and the place where the pericardial sac is closest to the probe with no intervening organs and maximum fluid accumulation yields most successful results. There are three main approaches used for the puncture in pericardiocentesis: apical approach, subcostal approach or parasternal approach. The parasternal approach is more preferred to the subcostal space as this is the area where the pericardial space is closest to the probe whereas in the subcostal approach, a longer path is traveled to reach the maximum fluid.

There is evidence to prove that complication rates are minimal when the procedure is conducted under echocardiographic evaluation rather than using the subxiphoid approach blindly.[6,7]

Apical approach: The site of insertion in the apical approach is within the 5th, 6th or 7th intercostals space one cm lateral to the apex. This approach has the risk of puncturing the left ventricle and has increased risk of pneumothorax.

Parasternal approach: In the parasternal approach, the needle is inserted at the level of the 5th intercostals space close to the sternal angle. The needle is advanced perpendicular to the skin but carries a high risk of puncturing the internal thoracic artery and pneumothorax. Success rates are higher when the procedure is conducted under echocardiographic visualization.

Subxiphoid approach: In the subxiphoid approach, the site of entry is between the xiphisternum and the left costal margin. Once below the cartilage, the needle is lowered at 15–30° with the abdominal wall and is directed towards the left shoulder. There is a risk of puncturing the peritoneal cavity and right atrial puncture with this approach.

Different Approaches to do Pericardiocentesis

Fluoroscopic technique

Fluoroscopic pericardiocentesis is one of the first well-standardized imaging systems used for percutaneous pericardiocentesis allowing direct visualization of the needle throughout the procedure. In this procedure, subxiphoid approach is most commonly used with the needle containing the contrast medium passes through the diaphragm and punctures the pericardial sac. Sluggish layering of the contrast medium inferiorly denotes that the needle is positioned correctly and a soft J tip guidewire is introduced; the position of which is checked at least in two angiographic views. Some disadvantages of this approach are that it requires a catheterization laboratory to perform this procedure with significant radiation exposure. Echocardiographic evaluation of the site, distribution, and maximum thickness is mandatory before the procedure.

Echocardiographic technique

There are two approaches, which are used to do pericardiocentesis guided by echocardiography. One approach is assisted by echocardiography, where the operator memorizes the pathway and advances the needle towards the pericardial space without continuous ultrasound visualization. The second approach is where the needle carrier is mounted on an ultrasound transducer, and the needle is advanced in the pericardial sac under continuous, direct visualization. The echocardiographically guided pericardiocentesis technique allows direct visualization of the pericardial effusion, site of entry, and needle trajectory effectively.

Computer tomographic (CT) guided technique

The full extent of the pericardial effusion is assessed, and the point of entry is demarcated at the entry site. The needle is then advanced to enter the pericardial effusion position of which is confirmed on a single CT scan. After entering the pericardial sac, a guidewire is introduced through the needle, and a sheath is advanced. Data published shows that this procedure has a high success rate (98.4%) and a very low rate of complications (0.3%). There is evidence to prove some advantages of CT guided pericardiocentesis over echocardiography guided. In a CT guided procedure, the exact position of the loculated effusion is very clearly demarcated, and the direction in which the needle is advanced can be clearly seen. The intrapericardial density of the effusion can be very clearly measured through CT therefore, in cases of purulent pericarditis instillation of a fibrinolytic agent can be successfully done before the procedure. CT also allows the assessment of the entire chest and other associated anomalies and can be successfully conducted in patients with poor ultrasound window. Some limitations are radiological exposure, poor logistic feasibility, time-consuming procedure, and cannot be performed during emergency situations.

Surgical approach

Surgical drainage is the gold standard for draining pericardial effusion, especially if the biopsy is also required to be taken. The subxiphoid approach involves incision under the xiphoid process, whereas in thoracotomy approach, the entry site is through the 5th intercostals space anteriorly. Thoracotomy approach prevents recurrent effusions and repeated surgeries, whereas subxiphoid approach is associated with faster extubation and less postoperative pain. In terms of long-term mortality and survival, both the procedures are known to be comparable. Some disadvantages of surgical approach are a need for general anesthesia, longer hospitalization, and risk of hypotension during impending tamponade.

COMPLICATIONS

- Cardiac arrhythmias
- Cardiac puncture, sudden death
- Pneumothorax
- Peritoneal puncture, puncture of liver or stomach, diaphragmatic injury (subxiphoid approach)
- Puncture of internal thoracic artery (parasternal approach).

KEY MESSAGES

- Emergency pericardiocentesis is a life-saving procedure in cases of cardiac tamponade.
- Echocardiographic evaluation before starting the procedure is recommended for better results and fewer complications.
- Echocardiographically guided pericardiocentesis is considered the safest and most efficacious method and lowest rate of complications as compared to the surgical approach.
- Surgical drainage is associated with higher rate of complications and longer days of hospitalization.

REFERENCES

1. Guven H, Bakiler AR, Ulger Z, *et al*. Evaluation of children with a large pericardial effusion and cardiac tamponade. Acta Cardiol. 2007;62:129-33.
2. Sagristà-Sauleda J, Mercé J, Permanyer-Miralda G, *et al*. Clinical clues to the causes of large pericardial effusions. Am J Med. 2000;109:95-101.
3. Bagri NK, Yadav DK, Aggarwal S, *et al*. Pericardial effusion in children: Experience from tertiary care center in Northern India. Indian Pediatr. 2014;51:211-3.
4. Adler Y, Charron P, Imazio M, *et al*. 2015 ESC Guidelines for the diagnosis and management of pericardial diseases: The Task Force for the Diagnosis and Management of Pericardial Diseases of the European Society of Cardiology (ESC) endorsed by: The European Association for Cardio-Thoracic Surgery (EACTS). Eur Heart J. 2015;36:2921-64.
5. Maggiolini S, Carlini CCD, Imazio M. Evolution of the pericardiocentesis technique. J Cardiovasc Med. 2018;19: 267-73.
6. Maggiolini S, Gentile G, Farina A, *et al*. Safety, efficacy and complications of pericardiocentesis by real-time echo-monitored procedure. Am J Cardiol. 2016;117:1369-74.
7. Tsang TS, Seward JB. Pericardiocentesis under echocardiographic guidance. Eur J Echocardiogr. 2001;2:68-9.

91.5 Thoracocentesis/Pleural Tap

Chandra Mohan Kumar, Nidhi Bedi

DEFINITION

Thoracocentesis is one of the common procedures in pediatric practice. It is a procedure whereby a needle or drain is inserted in the space between two pleura (parietal and visceral) to remove some fluid as a diagnostic or therapeutic measure.[1] This space contains a thin layer of fluid typically but in certain conditions like pneumonia, congestive heart failure, and malignancy, the same may be accumulated resulting in pleural effusion. Thoracentesis may also be required when this space is filled with air (termed as pneumothorax) or has a combination of two, i.e. hydropneumothorax. The procedure has been known by various names in the literature as thoracentesis, thoracocentesis, pleural aspiration and pleural tap.

INDICATIONS

- Empyema/Complicated parapneumonic effusions
- Tension pneumothorax/recurrent or persistent pneumothorax/Large pneumothorax
- Malignant pleural effusion
- Post-traumatic hemothorax/pneumohemothorax
- Diagnostic tap for infections such as tuberculosis.

CONTRAINDICATIONS/PRECAUTIONS

- Platelet count <50,000/mm^3
- Clotting abnormalities (INR >1.5 times normal)
- Patient already on anticoagulant therapy.

Equipment Required

- 1% lignocaine for local anesthesia
- Alcohol-based skin cleanser
- Sterile drapes, gown, gloves
- Needles, syringes, gauze swabs
- Scalpel, suture (0 or 1-0 silk), chest tube kit, closed system drain (including water) and tubing, dressing clamp in case of chest tube drain placement.

GENERAL PRINCIPLES

- An informed written consent should be taken unless done in emergency situation.
- Full aseptic precautions need to be followed during pleural tap.
- Sedation may be required in small children who do not cooperate.

- At least two applications of alcohol-based skin disinfectant (allowing it to dry in between applications) are suggested. While cleansing the aspiration site, the site should be wiped centrifugally from inside out.[2]
- A recent chest radiograph should be available before performing a pleural aspiration.
- Thoracic ultrasound-guided aspiration is strongly recommended for all pleural fluid aspirations. It has been observed that the failure rates and complication rates are significantly less in ultrasound-guided aspiration. Dry taps or procedure failure is associated with risk of visceral injury.[2]
- Thoracentesis with large-bore needles should be avoided as it increases the risk of post-procedure pneumothorax as well as visceral and vascular injury.
- All aspirations should be best attempted within the triangle of safety (**Fig. 1**). The triangle is bordered anteriorly by the lateral edge of the pectoralis major, laterally by the lateral edge of latissimus dorsi, inferiorly by the line of the fifth intercostal space and superiorly by the base of the axilla.[3]
- A post-procedure chest X-ray is required in case of dry tap with aspiration of air alone, difficult procedure with multiple failed attempts or if the patient becomes symptomatic immediately following the procedure.
- The procedure should be stopped when no more fluid or air can be aspirated, or if the patient develops symptoms of cough or chest discomfort. Aspiration of more than 1.5 liters of fluid may increase the risk of pulmonary edema.
- Antibiotic prophylaxis is not recommended following the procedure.

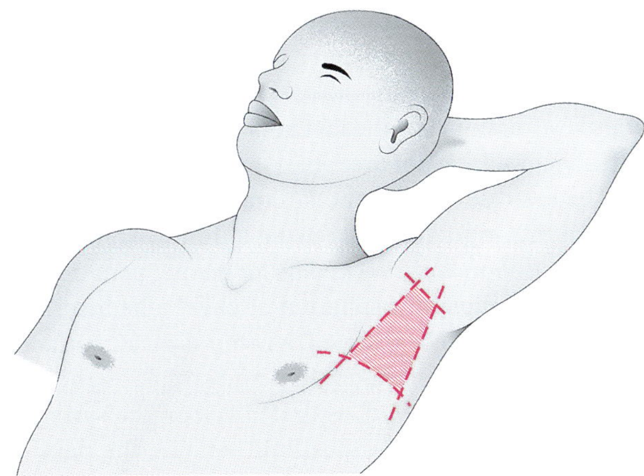

Fig. 1: Triangle of safety. Bounded anteriorly by the lateral border of pectoralis major, posteriorly by the lateral border of latissimus dorsi, inferiorly by 5th ICS and superiorly by base of the axilla

PROCEDURE

The patient should be positioned ideally in the semi-reclining position with hands behind the head or arms and head resting supported on an adjustable bedside table to make the triangle of safety most visible. If unable to sit, the patient should lie at the edge of the bed on the affected side with the ipsilateral arm over the head and the midaxillary line accessible for the insertion of the needle.[3,4]

Clean the skin twice with an alcohol-based disinfectant, starting centrifugally and moving outwards giving time for the disinfectant to dry between two applications.

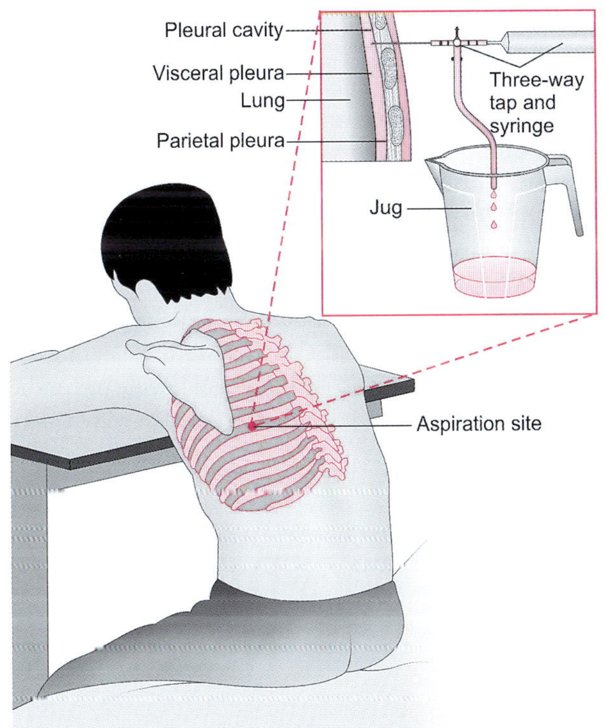

Fig. 2: Site of aspiration and technique

The site of aspiration is best identified using an ultrasound. Pleural tap is classically performed in 5th intercostal space in the mid-axillary line or 7–9th space in posterior axillary line or scapular line in affected side (**Fig. 2**). The ideal site for pleural tap in effusion is one space below the point where vocal fremitus is reduced and percussion note becomes significantly dull. Second intercostal space in the midclavicular line for tension pneumothorax is ideal especially when the facility for ultrasonography is not available.

The selected site may be infiltrated with 1% lidocaine maximum 3 mg/kg initially using a thin 25 G needle for skin penetration and 21 G needle for deeper penetration if required (therapeutic aspiration or chest tube insertion). The needle should be inserted over the superior surface of the lower rib to avoid injury to neurovascular structures. As the needle is inserted, aspirate back on the syringe to check for pleural fluid. Once fluid returns, the depth of needle should be marked with an artery forceps so as to give an approximate depth for insertion of thoracentesis needle, and after that the anesthetizing needle should be removed.

The thoracentesis needle or angiocath should then be inserted after measuring the same depth. The needle should be advanced over the superior aspect of the rib, and a constant gentle suction should be applied over the syringe as the needle is advanced. A sense of giveaway is felt once the needle enters the pleural cavity. As the pleural fluid returns, the necessary amount of fluid should be aspirated using a stopcock and tubing. For therapeutic tap, a wide bore cannula should be preferably passed over the needle after which needle is withdrawn and flow of fluid confirmed. The cannula should be attached to a three-way stopcock, tubing and closed system collecting bag. After the draining of fluid is completed needle or cannula should be gently removed and insertion site with a sterile occlusive dressing.

COMPLICATIONS

These can be minor or major:

- Pain and bruising at the site of aspiration
- Coughing
- Pneumothorax
- Pulmonary edema
- Infection at the local site
- Nerve and blood vessel damage at the local site
- Visceral lung injury
- Air embolism
- Anaphylactic or allergic reaction to anesthetic agents.

KEY MESSAGES

- All aspirations should be best attempted within the triangle of safety.
- Aspiration of pleural fluid more than 1.5 L increases the risk of pulmonary edema.
- No antibiotic prophylaxis is needed post-procedure.

REFERENCES

1. ATS Patient Education Series. American Thoracic Society 2016. Available from: <*https://www.thoracic.org/patients/patient-resources/resources/thoracentesis.pdf*. Accessed July 26>, 2019.
2. Havelock T, Teoh R, Laws D, *et al.* Pleural procedures and thoracic ultrasound: British Thoracic Society pleural disease guideline 2010. Thorax. 2010;65(Suppl 2):ii61eii76.
3. NHS Trust. Northern Devon Healthcare. Pleural Procedures Guidelines. Available from: *https://www.northdevonhealth.nhs.uk/2015/12/pleural-procedures-guidelines/*. Accessed July 26, February 2019.
4. ACI respiratory network. Consensus guidelines. Pleural drains in adults. Available from: *https://www.aci.health.nsw.gov.au/resources/respiratory/pleural-drains/pleural-drains-in-adults/introduction*. Accessed July 26, 2019.

91.6 Tube Thoracostomy and Needle Decompression

Shalu Gupta, Ankita Goel Sharma

INTRODUCTION

Tube thoracostomy is a standard procedure in which a chest tube or small catheter is placed through the chest wall into the pleural cavity primarily to drain air, fluid, and pus. It is used as an emergency procedure in cases of thoracic trauma and tension pneumothorax.

Chest tubes are silicone or polyvinyl chloride tubes that have a radiopaque strip with a gap that serves to mark the most proximal drainage hole.

INDICATIONS[1]

- Evacuation of pneumothorax-including tension, spontaneous, traumatic, iatrogenic (following central venous line placement), or bronchopleural fistula
- Empyema and complicated parapneumonic pleural effusion
- Traumatic hemo/pneumothorax
- Malignant pleural effusions—drainage, chemical pleurodesis
- Post-surgical, e.g. thoracotomy, esophagectomy, and cardiac surgery.

CONTRAINDICATIONS

Anticoagulation drugs, coagulopathy, overlying infection, or bleeding diathesis are relative contraindications for chest tube placement. In children with coagulopathy prefer needle thoracostomy.

PROCEDURE

Site and Size of Drain

The preferred position in a young or acutely ill patient is supine with arms behind the head on the affected side. The insertion site can be decided based on findings on chest X-ray, dull note on percussion and/or ultrasound chest. The best way to perform the procedure is under ultrasound guidance. The insertion should be done in "Triangle of safety," which is the area bordered by the lateral border of pectoralis major anteriorly, latissimus dorsi posteriorly and superior edge of 5th rib (**Fig. 1**). This position minimizes the risk of injury to underlying structures (e.g. internal mammary artery) and avoids damage to muscle and breast tissue. Second intercostal space in the mid-clavicular may be used for apical pneumothoraces.[1]

In infants and children, smaller chest tubes (e.g. 8–14F, including pigtail catheters) are recommended over large bore tubes, to minimize patient discomfort especially in case of pneumothorax and para-pneumonic effusions. Large bore drains (16–24Fr) may be used in empyema, hemothorax and large pneumothoraces.[1]

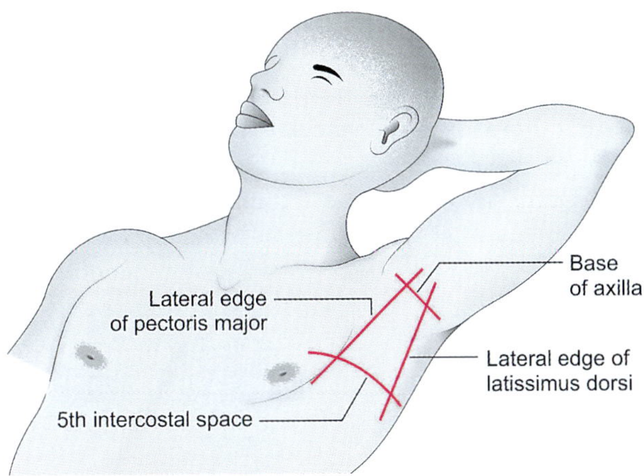

Fig. 1: Triangle of safety (Reproduced from-Emergency department guidelines for health professionals, Perth Children Hospital, Western Australia)

Technique

Two techniques are usually used to place a chest tube. The standard procedure employs blunt dissection to access the pleural space. In the Seldinger technique, pleural space is accessed with a needle and uses dilatation over a guidewire to place smaller tubes or pigtail catheters.[2]

- Attach the child to a vital sign monitor.
- Prior informed written consent should be obtained except in cases of emergency where it is not feasible.
- Prepare all the emergency drugs and check equipment.
- *Position*: Child sits comfortably in a chair leaning forward with arms and head supported on the table. In sick infants and children, supine posture is preferred.
- Identify the affected side by physical examination and chest radiograph and mark it.
- Prepare the skin around the area of insertion with chlorhexidine or povidone iodine.
- Using aseptic technique with the sterile gown, gloves, mask and body drapes, create a sterile field.
- Infiltrate the skin, subcutaneous tissue, intercostal muscles, and periosteum of the rib with a local anesthetic (1% lidocaine). Give analgesics.
- Make a skin incision parallel to the superior border of rib and at least one intercostal space below the rib. Using an artery forceps (with chest tube), bluntly dissect and create a short subcutaneous tunnel from the incision site cephalad toward the intercostal space through which the chest tube will be inserted.

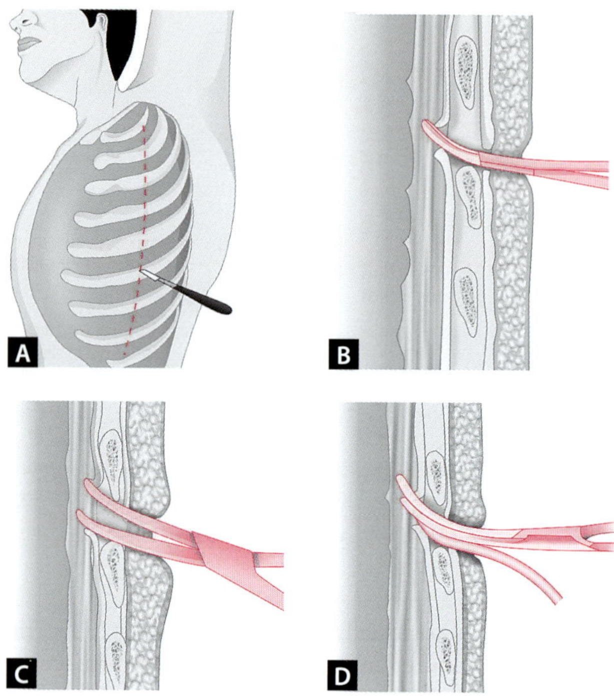

Figs. 2A to D: Steps (A to D) of insertion of inter-costal drainage tube

Clamp the distal end of the inter-costal drainage tube. Then, slide the tip over the superior rib margin, puncturing the intercostal muscles and pleura well below the neurovascular bundle of the adjacent cephalad rib. Open the forceps to spread the intercostal muscles and parietal pleura and advance the intercostal tube over it into the pleural space. A give-way feel would occur once you enter the pleural space. Advance the chest tube until the last drainage hole is fully within the thoracic cavity (**Fig. 2**).

- Connect the tube to an underwater seal placed below the patient level.
- Remove the forceps and confirm that the chest tube is in the thoracic cavity by observing column movement, or drainage from the tube.
- Place a purse string suture to anchor the chest tube. Obtain a chest radiograph to confirm tube position and assess lung expansion.
- Check daily for infection, fluid drainage volumes, and documentation for swinging and bubbling.

COMPLICATIONS

- Bleeding (local and/or perforation of major vessels)
- Pneumothorax or hemothorax
- Infection at insertion site
- Bronchopleural fistula or pleurocutaneous air leak
- Laceration or perforation of visceral organs (heart, lungs, diaphragm, spleen, liver)
- Subcutaneous emphysema
- Re-expansion pulmonary edema
- Intercostal neuralgia/neuritis.

TROUBLESHOOTING AND REMOVAL

Stoppage of fluid drainage may indicate kinking or blockage of the tube by thick exudative fluid, pus, or debris. Try stripping the tube or flushing the tube with a small amount of sterile normal saline. Ensure that the suction holes of the tube are inside the pleural space.[2]

To minimize the risk of infectious complications, the tube should be removed as soon as possible. For effusions, the chest tube should be removed once there is clinical resolution and minimal chest tube drainage (<10–15 mL per 24 hours). There is no need to do a trial of clamping the chest tube before its removal. A chest radiograph should be taken shortly after chest tube removal to check for pneumothorax. In the case of pneumothorax, the tube can be removed once the lung is expanded and no bubbling is present.

KEY MESSAGES

- Tube thoracostomy is best performed under ultrasound guidance.
- Tube should be inserted in the "triangle of safety" formed by lateral border of pectoralis major, latissimus dorsi, and upper edge of 5th rib.
- Blunt dissection or Seldinger technique are used to place a chest tube.

REFERENCES

1. Havelock T, Teoh R, Laws D, *et al.* Pleural procedures and thoracic ultrasound: British Thoracic Society pleural disease guideline 2010. Thorax. 2010;65 (Suppl 2):i61-i76.
2. Cimpello LB, Deutsch RJ, Dixon C, *et al.* Textbook of Pediatric Emergency Medicine. In: Fleisher GR, Ludwig S, editors, 6th edition. Philadelphia: Wolters Kluwer/Lippincott Williams & Wilkins Health; 2010. p. 1786.

91.7 Tracheostomy

Shalu Jain, Deepika Harit

INTRODUCTION

Tracheostomy is a potentially life-saving emergency procedure which is now increasingly performed electively in pediatric patients. It is one of the oldest described surgical procedures in medical literature. With the current improvement in medical care, ventilation strategies and improved survival of preterm newborns, the indications for tracheostomy in children have changed considerably over past 6 decades. The need for tracheostomy has shifted from diphtheria, epiglottitis, croup and polio to upper airway anomalies and for prolonged mechanical ventilation. Almost 50% of tracheostomies are performed in children less than 1 year of age.[1] Tracheostomy can be done either as an emergency procedure or as an elective procedure in a stable ICU patient requiring long-term mechanical ventilation.

ANATOMICAL CONSIDERATIONS

The anatomy of respiratory tract of a child differs from that of an adult. Children (especially infants) have a shorter and fatter neck. They have smaller air passage and the level of cricoid cartilage varies from the level of 3rd cervical vertebrae in infancy to 6th cervical vertebrae in pubertal children. Moreover, cricoid cartilage is the only identifiable landmark in children since thyroid cartilage reaches its adult size only by adolescence. Since the blood vessels are more superficial, hyperextension should be avoided during tracheostomy as it may injure the large vessels in the neck.

INDICATIONS

Tracheostomy is usually done either to relieve upper airway obstruction in patients who cannot be intubated through translaryngeal approach (e.g. supraglottic cyst/mass, glottis edema/trauma, subglottic stenosis and high tracheal stenosis) or to prevent complications of prolonged mechanical ventilation. This frequently involves extremely premature neonates, patients with chronic lung disease, congenital heart disease and neurological impairment. In contrast to adults, there is no definite recommendation in children as to when tracheostomy be performed in patients who are intubated for mechanical ventilation and therefore, the decision needs to be individualized.

TYPES OF TRACHEOSTOMY

Tracheostomy can be classified according to the site and according to the procedure.

According to the Site of Stoma

- *High tracheostomy*: At the level of 1st and 2nd tracheal rings above the isthmus of the thyroid gland.
- *Mid tracheostomy*: At the level of 3rd and 4th tracheal rings behind the isthmus.
- *Low tracheostomy*: At the level of 5th and 6th tracheal rings below the isthmus.

  Mid tracheostomy is generally the preferred site.

According to the Procedural Type

- *Open surgical technique*: In this technique after skin incision, dissection is carried out until cricoid cartilage is identified and then a vertical incision is made between 3rd and 4th tracheal ring for inserting tracheostomy tube under direct vision. This is considered an optimal technique in infants and young children.
- *Percutaneous dilational technique (PDT)*. This technique differs from open surgical technique by virtue of use of modified Seldinger technique. In PDT, after the skin incision and dissection is followed by tracheal puncture with a 22 G seeker needle. A guidewire is introduced through this needle followed by needle removal. Thereafter, stoma is created by roping in a

dilator over the guidewire. The dilator introduction technique varies according to the manufacturer. The tube is then inserted through the wire. Video bronchoscopy is recommended to aid in correct placement of tracheostomy tube. Although PDT is the recommended procedure in adults, the experience in pediatric population is very limited. This technique is recommended in older children and adolescent. Moreover, its success is highly dependent on operator experience.[2]

TRACHEOSTOMY TUBE

Tracheostomy tubes are either made up of metal (silver/stainless steel) or plastic (polyvinyl chloride/silicone) (**Figs. 1A and B**). Plastic tubes are preferred because of lesser mucosal trauma. Pediatric tubes are only available as single lumen and without any fenestrations. Both cuffed and uncuffed tubes are available in the market. Cuffed tubes are usually not used in pediatrics as they increase the risk of tracheal stenosis. However, cuffed tubes may be preferred in patients on mechanical ventilation.

Tracheostomy tubes are sized according to the diameter of the lumen of trachea, which is age-appropriate (**Table 1**). Shiley and Bivona are the commonly available tracheostomy tubes. Custom made tubes are also available in some countries.

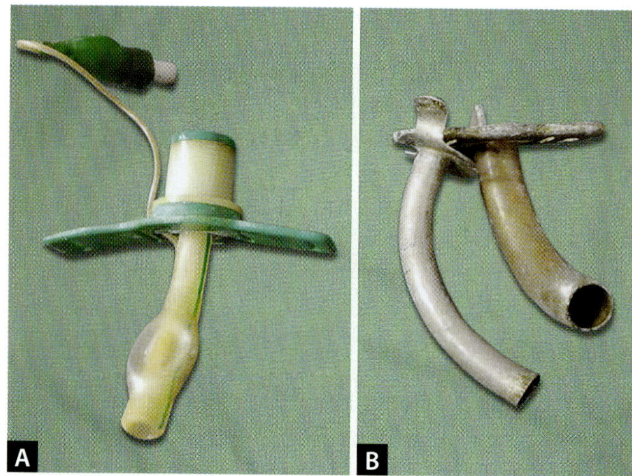

Figs. 1A and B: Tracheostomy tubes. (A) PVC cuffed tube; (B) Metal tubes

Table 1: Age-appropriate tracheostomy tube (Shiley) sizes

Age	*Tube size [internal diameter (in mm)]*
0–1 month	3.0
1–6 months	3.5
6–18 months	4.0
18 months–3 years	4.5
3–6 years	5.0
6–9 years	5.5
9–12 years	6.0

PROCEDURE

The preoperative anesthesia and analgesia is given according to the hospital protocols. No preprocedural prophylactic antibiotics are required for the procedure but antibiotics may be considered till the first change of tube. Although blood loss is minimal, in infants blood should always be ready lest accidental heavy bleeding occurs.

The child is placed supine with neck extended by placing a pillow under the shoulder and holding the head in the midline. Care should be taken while handling patients requiring cervical spine precautions. Head end of the bed is elevated to 15–20° to avoid venous engorgement in neck area. After cleaning and draping the area a 2–3 cm horizontal skin incision is made halfway between the cricoid and sternal notch. Horizontal incisions are preferred but in emergency vertical incision may be used to facilitate midline dissection. After skin incision, blunt dissection is performed longitudinally. Cricoid cartilage is identified (serves as a landmark to reach the tracheal rings) (**Fig. 2**). Strap muscles are retracted laterally to expose the pretracheal space. Most surgeons prefer using two stay sutures. For this, two 3-0 or 4-0 nylon or vicryl sutures are placed vertically on either side of tracheal area where the midline tracheostomy incision will be made. These labeled stay sutures are then taped over anterior chest wall (with labeling of left and right) until the first change of tube. Stay sutures are recommended as it helps in faster reinsertion of tube after accidental decannulation.[3]

After the identification of tracheal rings, a vertical/horizontal incision is made in the midline between 2nd and 4th tracheal rings. In infants and young children a vertical midline incision is preferred. Too high incision predisposes to subglottic stenosis. Thereafter, endotracheal tube is withdrawn proximal to the incision and an age appropriate size tracheostomy tube is inserted under direct vision and secured by suturing the flanges to the skin. A tape is tied from one end of the flange to another

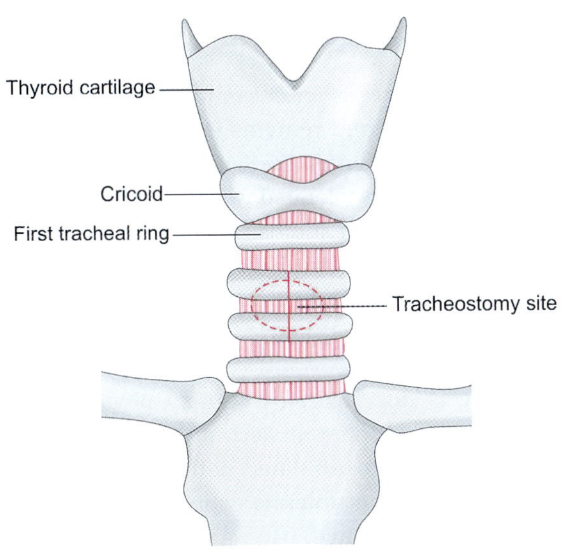

Fig. 2: Tracheostomy landmarks

by going behind the neck. Bleeding can be controlled by diathermy and direct pressure. Electrocautery should not be used when performing tracheal puncture as it may lead to airway burns. Upon successful placement of tracheostomy tube, endotracheal tube is removed. Moist gauze is placed over the tube to prevent the formation of secretions.

TRACHEOSTOMY CARE

Tube tip position should be checked by chest X-ray. The tube should be positioned in such a way that the end of the tube lies just proximal to the carina. During first 2–3 days, risk of tube displacement is highest because of immature tract formation. Any manipulation if needed in the first week must be done while keeping neck in flexed position. Frequent suctioning is required to prevent blocking of the tube with secretions. Humidified air should be used to avoid crust formation. Humidification can be easily achieved by inbuilt humidifiers in the ventilators. Other methods of achieving humidification are use of normal saline nebulization, artificial nose, trach collar and heat and moisture exchangers (HME). Tracheostomy site can also be cleaned by using hydrogen peroxide. The first change of tube can be done anytime between 3rd and 7th postoperative days (usually between 5 and 7 days).

COMPLICATIONS OF TRACHEOSTOMY

Smaller airway in children (especially <2 yrs age) predisposes them for frequent complications. A large study

Table 2: Complications of tracheostomy

Intra-procedural	*Early postoperative (<7 days)*	*Late postoperative (>7 days)*
Paratracheal insertion	Bleeding	Tracheal stenosis
Posterior tracheal wall laceration	Pneumothorax	Tracheomalacia
	Subcutaneous emphysema	Tracheo-esophageal fistula
	Airway fire	Delayed stoma closure
	Accidental decannulation	Cosmetic (unaesthetic scar)
	Stoma infection	Vocal cord paralysis
	Loss of airway	Tracheoarterial fistula
	Aspiration	Airway symptoms (hoarseness, cough, dyspnea, stridor)
		Suprastomal collapse

showed that the mortality after tracheostomy till discharge ranges from 7.7% to 8.5%.[4] Wetmore *et al.* reported 6.9% accidental decannulation in the first week.[5] Inappropriate tube length or excessive traction by ventilator circuits are commonly responsible for accidental decannulation and this can be prevented by good nursing care and surgical techniques. Decannulation before the complete maturation of the tract can be fatal because of rapid airway loss. If accidental decannulation occurs, endotracheal mechanical ventilation should be done without any delay. Only when the airway is established by endotracheal intubation, a rapid trial of tracheostomy reinsertion may be done. Other causes of mortality are tube obstruction and the complications of anesthesia. Tracheoinnominate artery fistula is also a rare but lethal complication that occurs due to erosion of the arterial wall by the tube. The complications are listed in **Table 2**.

DISCHARGE AND HOME CARE

Sending the patient home with tracheostomy is a challenge. The process of at home care starts predischarge by teaching the caregivers about tube changing and early management of complications. Daily gentle cleaning of the skin with antiseptic solution prevents infections. Tapes should be changed daily by keeping the neck in flexion to prevent accidental decannulation. Regular speech and chest physiotherapy should be continued at home.

DECANNULATION

Decannulation can be considered when the child is able to maintain airway without tracheostomy and the underlying condition due to which tracheostomy was done has improved. Decannulation protocols vary considerably. The clinical consensus statement on pediatric tracheostomy management by the American Academy of Otolaryngology and Head and Neck Surgery recommends that certain specific criteria should be met before attempting decannulation in children, provided there is resolution or improvement of the original indication for tracheostomy.[3] These criteria are:

- No ventilatory support should be required for a period of 3 months before decannulation, which could vary from 2 to 4 months.
- There should be no aspiration events, such that a tracheostomy would still be needed for suctioning to maintain pulmonary toilet.
- A flexible laryngoscopy must show a patent airway with at least one mobile vocal cord.
- Any obstructing suprastomal granulation should be removed at the time of bronchoscopy before a decannulation attempt.
- All children >2 years of age should be given a daytime tracheostomy tube capping trial. If the child tolerates capping, options before decannulation to assess for readiness may include a capped exercise test, capped sleep study or a night-time capping trial while hospitalized and being observed. In younger or smaller children, the small size of the trachea in relation to the tracheostomy tube may preclude capping, and the decannulation protocol should be tailored to the individual patient.

The ideal decannulation protocol includes following elements: tracheostomy size reduction and clinical observation; complete airway evaluation (flexible laryngoscopy and direct laryngobronchoscopy); capping trial at home during the day; capped polysomnography (PSG); admission for decannulation and post-decannulation observation for 24–48 h (along with noninvasive ventilation if required). Before attempting decannulation, a direct laryngobronchoscopy must be performed to evaluate patency of airway at all levels and trachea should be assessed for any dynamic collapse or obstruction by removing the tracheostomy tube. A favorable direct laryngoscopy is an excellent predictor of successful decannulation.[6]

Once deemed ready for decannulation, tracheostomy tube is downsized and remains in situ for 24 hours. If successful, tube is then plugged only during the daytime. If daytime capping is tolerated well, this may be followed by plugging the tube for another 24 hours. Thereafter, tube is removed while the stoma is covered with dressing. The tract usually heals on its own. Some surgeons even prefer excising of the whole tract and leaving it to heal by primary intention.

Capping is not favored by many physicians now because it does not offer an accurate physiologic representation of the decannulated child. Moreover, many small children do not tolerate capping but can still be successfully decannulated.[6]

A persistent tracheocutaneous fistula may develop after decannulation. Lower age and increased duration of tracheostomy predisposes to it. There is no consensus as to when surgery should be considered for fistula closure but most surgeons prefer after 6–12 months. During surgical repair scarred skin is excised, stoma tract is dissected and edges are approximated with sutures. For troublesome scars, a revision of tracheostomy scar may be done after 10 years of age.

KEY MESSAGES

- Endotracheal intubation is nowadays frequently done for upper airway anomalies and prolonged mechanical ventilation.
- Uncuffed plastic (PVC and silicone) tubes are preferred in children as it causes less mucosal trauma.
- Open surgical technique remains optimal in infants and young children. Role of percutaneous dilational technique is not well defined and is feasible in older children only (>10 yrs age).
- Tracheal incision should be made in midline between 3rd and 4th tracheal ring. Age appropriate tube should always be used to prevent decannulation.
- Care should be taken to prevent tube obstruction or accidental decannulation as it can be fatal. If accidental decannulation occurs in first 7 days, endotracheal mechanical ventilation should be done without any delay and thereafter only a rapid trial of tracheostomy reinsertion may be attempted.
- Suctioning and humidification are the cornerstones of good tracheostomy care.
- Complete airway assessment should be done by direct laryngoscopy before attempting decannulation.

REFERENCES

1. Berry JG, Graham DA, Graham RJ, *et al.* Predictors of clinical outcomes and hospital resource use of children after tracheotomy. Pediatrics. 2009;124:563-72.
2. Wood D, Mc Shane P, Davis P. Tracheostomy in children admitted to paediatric intensive care. Arch Dis Child. 2012;97: 866-9.
3. Strychowsky JE, Albert D, Chan K, *et al.* International Pediatric Otolaryngology Group (IPOG) consensus recommendations: Routine peri-operative pediatric tracheotomy care. Int J Pediatr Otorhinolaryngol. 2016;86:250-5.
4. Berry JG, Graham RJ, Roberson DW, *et al.* Patient characteristics associated with in-hospital mortality in children following tracheotomy. Arch Dis Child. 2010;95: 703-10.
5. Wetmore RF, Handler SD, Potsic WP. Pediatric tracheostomy. Experience during the past decade. Ann Otol Rhinol Laryngol. 1982;91:628-32.
6. Wirtz N, Tibesar RJ, Lander T, *et al.* A pediatric decannulation protocol: Outcomes of a 10-year experience. Otolaryngol Head Neck Surg. 2016;154:731-4.

91.8 Peritoneal Dialysis

Girish Chandra Bhatt, Bhupeshwari Patel

INTRODUCTION

Dialysis is a form of renal replacement therapy (RRT) which helps in removal of waste products and water in patients with acute kidney injury (AKI) or chronic kidney disease (CKD). RRT in the form of peritoneal dialysis (PD), hemodialysis (HD) or continuous renal replacement therapy (CRRT) is frequently needed for acute kidney injury in children and neonates.[1]

Peritoneal dialysis (PD) is a safe, nonvascular alternative for RRT, which is effective, inexpensive, intracorporeal renal replacement modality; with some inherent advantages over hemodialysis and no need for highly trained staff.[2] The peritoneal membrane is a natural biocompatible, internally located dialyzer that limits entry of bacteria and their products, removes uremic toxins, allows continuous, 24-hour dialysis and ultrafiltration, while avoiding the use of anticoagulants.[3] PD has been successfully used in infants and children with AKI and circulatory failure.[1]

The usual indications of the PD can be renal or non-renal as shown in **Table 1**.[1,2,4] Contraindications[5] are listed in **Box 1**.

Table 1: Indications for acute peritoneal dialysis

Renal indications	*Extra-renal indications (Rarely used)*
• RRT in the treatment of AKI in children • Hemodynamically unstable patients • Uncontrolled hyperkalemia • Uremic pericarditis or encephalopathy • Early intervention prior to significant fluid overload (Increase of more than 15% over body weight) • The presence of bleeding diathesis or hemorrhagic conditions contraindicating placement of vascular access for hemodialysis or anticoagulation • Patients with difficult vascular access placement • Removal of high molecular weight toxins (10 kD)	• Acute hemorrhagic pancreatitis: PD helps in the removal of bioactive substances presumed to be responsible for systemic inflammation • Clinically significant hypothermia or hyperthermia in patients who do not respond to conventional methods: heated or cold peritoneal solutions can be used to maintain core temperature • Liver failure • Infusion of drugs and nutrients as a supportive therapy in critically ill patients • Refractory or progressive fluid overload – Pulmonary edema – Congestive cardiac failure – Refractory hypertension • Refractory metabolic acidosis

PROCEDURE FOR PERITONEAL DIALYSIS

Preparing the Patient

- Obtain informed signed consent/assent for PD.
- Baseline vitals, weight, and serum electrolyte are recorded.
- Encourage patient to empty the bladder and bowel to reduce the risk of puncturing internal organs (catheterize in small children).
- Restraining of limbs should be considered for small uncooperative children.
- Single dose of broad-spectrum antibiotics may be used to prevent infection immediately before catheter placement.

Preparing the Equipment (Apply Strict Aseptic Technique)

- Arrangements should be made for appropriate concentration of dialysate to be used and medications.
- The dialysate should be warmed to body temperature. This will prevent patient discomfort and abdominal pain. The warmed dialysate also dilates the vessels of the peritoneum and increases the urea clearance.
- Assemble the administration set and tubing. Tubings should be primed with dialysate to reduce the amount of air entering the catheter and peritoneal cavity. This would prevent abdominal discomfort.

Box 1: Contraindications of acute PD

- Recent abdominal surgery
- Pleuroperitoneal communication
- Severe respiratory failure with diaphragmatic involvement
- Low peritoneal clearance
- Fecal or fungal peritonitis
- Abdominal wall cellulitis
- AKI in pregnancy
- Extensive adhesions from previous abdominal surgery
- Open drain in abdominal wall
- Fresh intra- abdominal vascular graft

Catheters for Acute PD

Stiff PD catheter

Polyurethane trocar catheters (Infant/Pediatric/Adult) are inserted using sharp trocar which is directed towards iliac fossa. Although, they are easy to insert, the common disadvantage of these catheters are bleeding, leakage of peritoneal fluid around the catheter insertion site, risk of peritonitis and obstruction due to small lumen and holes, if used beyond 72 hours (**Figs. 1A and B**).[6]

Soft silastic catheter (Tenckhoff/Cook)

Standard (double cuff) Tenckhoff catheter needs to be placed surgically, whereas a temporary (peel-off) catheter can be inserted bedside utilizing modified Seldinger approach. These catheters remain the gold standard for PD access.[7] Risk of injury to viscera is low and soft catheters can be used for prolonged periods (**Fig. 1**).

Femoral catheter single lumen, pigtail catheter, nasogastric tube and intercostal drainage catheter

These are improvised catheters, which are used in resource limited settings. They can be used in infants for short-term dialysis.[1]

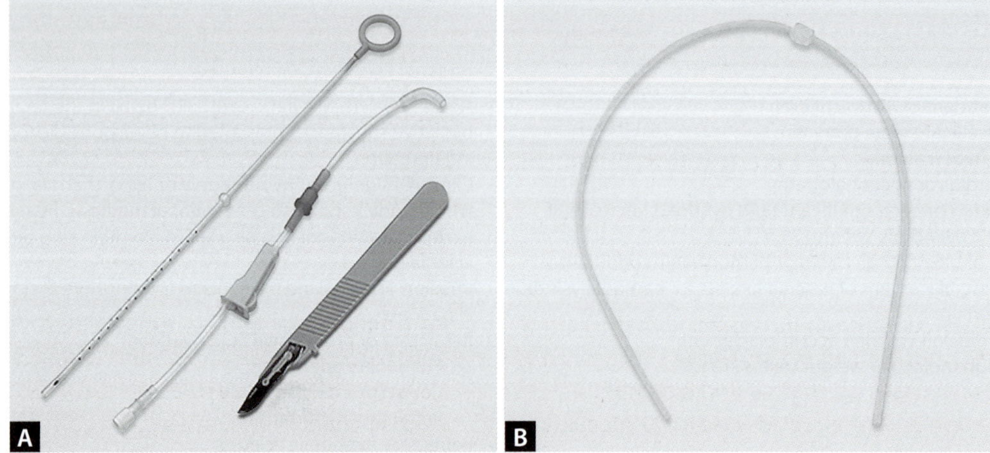

Figs. 1A and B: Different types of PD catheters: (A) Stiff PD catheter, connecting tube, blade; (B) Single cuff Tenchkoff catheter

Cycler: Cycler is a mechanized device to help in the delivery and drainage of dialysate.[7] The goal of the cycler is to provide optimal dialysis in an automated manner, during sleep thus making it a more convenient option.

Other materials required: Sterile set, surgical blade, normal saline, suture, povidone-iodine.

INSERTING THE CATHETER

In emergency situations, the physician inserts the catheter at the bedside under strict asepsis using modified Seldinger technique as shown in **Figures 2A to H**. Peritoneal dialysis catheters can be placed percutaneously, laparoscopically, or via an open surgical route.[8]

Soft PD Catheter Insertion

1. Record the vitals and catheterize the bladder.
2. In young and uncooperative children sedation is prescribed in form of first atropine 0.01 mg/kg followed by midazolam 0.1 mg/kg after 2–3 minutes followed by ketamine 1 mg/kg after 2–3 minutes. Ketamine can be repeated once or twice during the procedure.
3. Abdominal wall is cleaned using either spirit and povidone iodine or 2% chlorhexidine solution and draped with the patient supine.
4. Local anesthetic agent (1% lidocaine 2.5–5 mL) is injected into the skin and subcutaneous tissue in the midline below the umbilicus.
5. Artificial ascites (moderately tense) created by using 16–18 gauze cannula and 30 mL/kg 1.5% peritoneal fluid (this step is not needed if patient has already tense ascites).
6. Guidewire advanced through the introducing sheath of cannula.
7. Cannula removed and dilator with peel away sheath inserted over the guidewire followed by removal of dilator and guidewire leaving behind the peel away sheath.
8. Soft catheter inserted through the sheath and the sheath peeled off.
9. Subcutaneous tunnel is created with the help of artery forceps approximately 3 cm below and away from the site of insertion.
10. Catheter taken out through the tunnel with the help of artery forcep, and the cuff placed in the subcutaneous tunnel to prevent migration, leak and infection.
11. Stitch is generally not required in soft PD placement to prevent infections. Y connector (or connector with 3-way cannula) can be used for instillation and drainage of PD fluid.

Steps for Stiff PD Catheter Insertion

1. Steps 1 to 5 are same as of soft PD catheter.
2. The cannula is removed and abdominal wall punctured with surgical blade held vertically.
3. The peritoneal catheter is inserted with the stylet using a gentle boring motion. Catheter should be grasped between the finger and thumb just above the skin to control its movement and prevent excessive penetration. Entry into peritoneal cavity is indicated by a sudden decrease in resistance and a gush of dialysis fluid into the catheter.
4. As soon as the peritoneal cavity is entered, the catheter is held in vertical position and stylet is withdrawn 1–2 cm and catheter advanced at 45° angle towards the left iliac region.
5. The connecting set is attached to the catheter and dialysis fluid is run in, which should flow in a continuous stream, if the catheter is placed properly in peritoneal cavity without any kink.
6. If catheter is to be placed for more than 2 days then it is advisable to put a purse string suture around the insertion point with appropriate dressing.

PERFORMING THE EXCHANGE

An exchange involves infusion, dwell, and drainage of the dialysate.

- *Dialysate*: Peritoneal dialysis solution is available in strength of 1.5%, 2.5% and 4.25%. One may initiate PD with 2.5% dextrose solution to obtain a better ultrafiltration.[1] For hemodynamically unstable patients with moderate fluid overload, 1.5% dextrose solution should be used.
- *Infusion*: The dialysate is infused by gravity into the peritoneal cavity in about 5 to 10 minutes (also called as inflow time) to infuse 20–30 mL/kg of fluid.
- *Dwell (equilibration time)*: Time for which dialysate remains in the peritoneum, i.e. time from end of infusion to beginning of drain period. The dwell time for standard acute PD is 30 minutes to 90 minutes. A dwell time <30 minutes is not recommended. Shorter dwell time is recommended in case of peritonitis as the glucose gradient decreases more quickly due to highly permeable membrane.

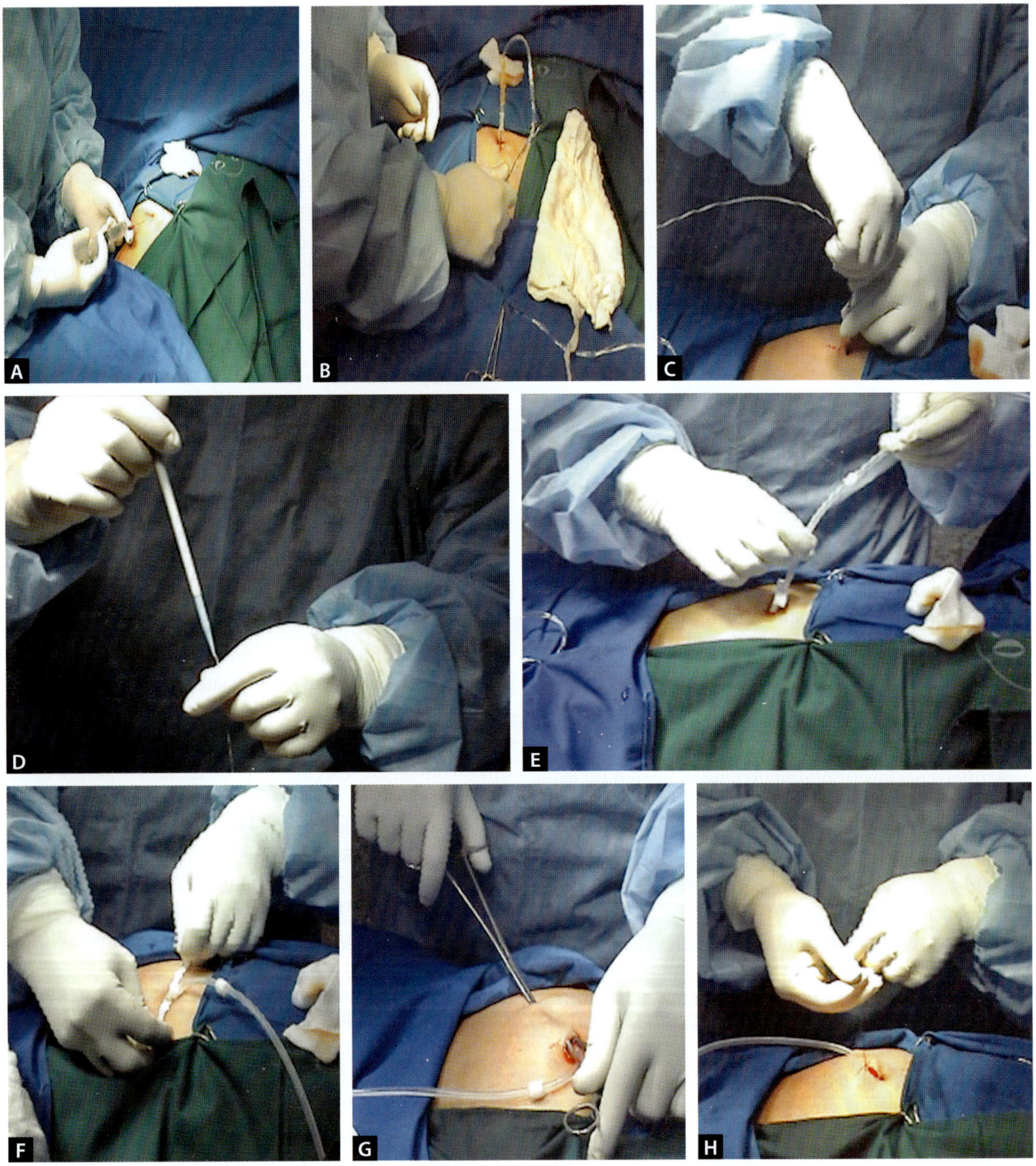

Figs. 2A to H: Sequential steps of bedside insertion of soft silastic single cuffed (Tenchkoff) peel off catheter. (A) Local anesthetic (1% lidocaine 2.5–5 mL) is injected into the skin and subcutaneous tissue in the midline below the umbilicus; (B) Artificial ascites (moderately tense) created by using 16–18 gauze cannula and 30 mL/kg 1.5% peritoneal fluid (This step is not needed if patient has already tense ascites); (C) Guidewire advanced through the introducing sheath of cannula; (D) Dilator with peel away sheath inserted over the guidewire followed by removal of dilator and guidewire, leaving behind the peel away sheath; (E) Soft catheter inserted through the sheath; (F) Sheath peeled off, leaving behind the catheter; (G) Taking out the catheter through the subcutaneous tunnel created with the help of artery forceps approximately 3 cm below and away from the site of insertion; (H) Cuff placed in the subcutaneous tunnel to prevent migration, leak and infection

- *Drainage*: The tube is unclamped and the solution is allowed to drain from the peritoneal cavity by gravity over 10 to 30 minutes. The normal drainage fluid is colorless or straw-colored and should not be cloudy. After insertion of a new catheter, the first few exchanges can be bloody owing to small capillary injury, which should become clear after few exchanges. Rapid in-out exchanges with volume 10 mL/kg until clear (about 3 exchanges) by infusing into peritoneal cavity may be considered for bloody drainage. When dialysate is clear, begin hourly exchanges. Heparin 1000 units/L in dialysate bag may also be considered in case the dialysate is hemorrhagic (250 units/L for NICU and PICU baby).[1]

Additives in Dialysis Solution

Heparin: Heparin is added 200 to 500 units/L to prevent fibrin clot. Some guidelines recommend to add heparin during initial 24 hours of PD to prevent clotting.

Insulin: High serum glucose level (>180) is independently associated with mortality in patient with acute kidney injury. Thus, the glucose measurement should be done at least 6 hourly and glucose level should be maintained between 110 mg/dL and 180 mg/dL. Intraperitoneal insulin or intravenous insulin should be used to treat hyperglycemia in PD patients.[1,5] Following units of insulin should be used for maintaining normal concentration of glucose in hyperglycemic patients:

- 4 to 5 units/L for 1.5% dextrose
- 5 to 7 units for 2.5% dextrose
- 7 to 10 units for 4.5% dextrose.

Potassium: The potassium concentration of the dialysis solution is negligible (0–2 mmol/L) at treatment initiation as many patients will have hyperkalemia along with metabolic acidosis. Potassium needs be added to dialysate when the serum potassium is below 4 mmol/L.[1]

Antibiotic Instillation in PD Fluid

Peritonitis is one of the most common complications and attributes to death in around 16% of PD patients. Antibiotic instillation in PD fluid is required in case of suspected peritonitis. The PD fluid should be sent for cytology, Gram staining and culture and peritonitis should be suspected if any two of the following is present:[9]

- Clinical features suggestive of peritonitis, i.e. abdominal pain and/or cloudy dialysis effluent;
- Dialysis effluent white blood cell count >100/µL (after a dwell time of minimum 2 hours), with > 50% polymorphonuclear (PMN) or >50% PMN even if absolute cell count is less than 100/µL.
- Positive dialysis effluent culture.

The International Society for peritoneal dialysis suggests to perform leukocyte counts daily for peritonitis surveillance in patients on acute PD. In resource limited setting, leukocyte esterase dipstick test daily should be done and in case of reading >2+, treatment should be initiated awaiting confirmatory leukocyte count and culture.

Treatment should be started when the cells are seen in cytology or a cloudy effluent is seen. Vancomycin, aminoglycosides, and cephalosporins can be administered in the same dialysis solution bag. Aminoglycoside should not be added to the same bag with penicillins because of chemical incompatibility. The antibiotic coverage should cover both gram positive and gam negative organisms. Intraperitoneal vancomycin or a first-generation cephalosporin (for gram positive) and a third-generation cephalosporin or aminoglycoside (for gram negative organism) should be used as empirical therapy.[9,10] The removal of excess water during peritoneal dialysis is achieved by using a hypertonic dialysate with high dextrose concentration. This creates an osmotic gradient across the membrane.

PD Prescription

- Dialysate composition: 1.5%, 2.5% and 4.25%
- Exchange volume: 20–30 m/kg
- Inflow time and outflow time (5–10 minutes)
- Dwell time (30–45 minutes)
- Total number of exchanges
- Dialysate additives—Heparin, potassium
- Monitoring fluid balance.

COMPLICATIONS

- Bowel perforation.
- Bleeding.
- Wound infection.
- Outflow failure results due to presence of clots or fibrin in the catheter, occlusion from omentum, or adhesions.
- Peritonitis may occur during initial period, which clinically presents as abdominal pain associated with turbid peritoneal fluid.
- Exit-site infection, tunnel infection, cuff protrusion, outflow failure and dialysate leaks, or hernias.

- *Peritonitis*: Occurs as a result of contamination with skin bacteria.

Troubleshoot for Possible Problems/ Complications during Peritoneal Dialysis

- *PD catheter leak*: If there is PD catheter leak, confirm with glucose dipstick and use low volume dialysis.
- In case of *outflow failure* due to fibrin clot of omentum, initial step should be to flush or use heparinized dialysis solution. If these measures fail, reposition of the dialysis catheter should be done.
- *Blood in the effluent*: The cause of the blood in effluent may be rupture of tiny abdominal capillaries or possible serious abdominal injury. If the fluid is blood mixed, check vitals and observe the patient. Heparin may be added to prevent blockage due to clotting. In case the fluid is having pinkish effluent as in injury to tiny capillaries, the color wil become clear in 3 to 4 exchanges.
- *Pain during dialysate* flow: This can be due to rapid infusion of dialysate, incomplete or use of hypertonic solution or omental attachment to PD catheter or peritonitis. In such cases, the dialysate flow must be decreased or reposition of PD catheter should be repositioned.

KEY MESSAGES

- Peritoneal dialysis is the modest treatment modality for acute kidney injury (AKI) in children and hemodynamically unstable patients.
- Peritoneal dialysis works by using peritoneum as a filter. There are three stages to a dialysis cycle (or exchange): Fill, dwell and drain.
- Peritonitis is one of the most important complication of PD. Abdominal pain and/or cloudy dialysis effluent are the early clinical features of peritonitis which can be timely treated with intraperitoneal antibiotics.
- PD is a safe, nonvascular, intracorporeal, effective, less expensive alternative for RRT with no need of highly trained staff.

REFERENCES

1. Cullis B, Abdelraheem M, Abrahams G, *et al.* Peritoneal dialysis for acute kidney injury. Perit Dial Int J Int Soc Perit Dial. 2014; 34:494-517.
2. Ghaffari A. Urgent-start peritoneal dialysis: A quality improvement report. Am J Kidney Dis Off J Natl Kidney Found. 2012;59:400-8.
3. Ghaffari A, Kalantar-Zadeh K, Lee J, *et al.* PD First: Peritoneal dialysis as the default transition to dialysis therapy. Semin Dial. 2013;26:706-13.
4. Daugirdas JT. Peritoneal dialysis in acute renal failure--why the bad outcome? N Engl J Med. 2002;347:933-5.
5. Ansari N. Peritoneal dialysis in renal replacement therapy for patients with acute kidney injury. Int J Nephrol. 2011;2011: 739794.
6. Henderson S, Brown E, Levy J. Safety and efficacy of percutaneous insertion of peritoneal dialysis catheters under sedation and local anaesthetic. Nephrol Dial Transplant Off Publ Eur Dial Transpl Assoc - Eur Ren Assoc. 2009;24:3499-504.
7. Wong SN, Geary DF. Comparison of temporary and permanent catheters for acute peritoneal dialysis. Arch Dis Child. 1988; 63:827-31.
8. Koch M, Kohnle M, Trapp R, *et al.* Comparable outcome of acute unplanned peritoneal dialysis and haemodialysis. Nephrol Dial Transplant Off Publ Eur Dial Transpl Assoc - Eur Ren Assoc. 2012;27:375-80.
9. Li PK-T, Szeto CC, Piraino B, *et al.* ISPD Peritonitis Recommendations: 2016 Update on Prevention and Treatment. Perit Dial Int J Int Soc Perit Dial. 2016;36:481-508.
10. Barretti P, Doles JVP, Pinotti DG, *et al.* Efficacy of antibiotic therapy for peritoneal dialysis-associated peritonitis: A proportional meta-analysis. BMC Infect Dis. 2014;14:445.

91.9 Exchange Transfusion

Dipen Vasudev Patel, Somashekhar M Nimbalkar

INTRODUCTION

Blood exchange transfusion (BET) was introduced in the late 1940s and 1950s to reduce neonatal mortality and prevent long-term neurological impairments due to kernicterus.[1,2] It involves removing aliquots of patient blood and replacing with donor blood in order to remove abnormal blood components and circulating toxins whilst maintaining adequate circulating blood volume.

It is primarily performed to remove antibodies and excess bilirubin in isoimmune disease.

Indications

The decision to perform BET is based upon the clinical judgment and a cautious extrapolation of guidelines. Indications of exchange transfusion in infants/children are summarized in **Table 1**.[3-7] Procedure should be done only after informed written consent from the parent/s or legally acceptable representatives.

Choice of Blood

Decision for choice of type of donor blood group (Both ABO and Rh) is dependent on mother's and neonate's ABO and Rh type as summarized in **Table 2**.[8] Donor blood must be cross matched against maternal plasma if infants age is less than 4 months.[9]

- For Rhesus isoimmunization, the best choice would be O (Rh) negative packed cells suspended in AB plasma. O (Rh) negative whole blood or cross-matched baby's blood group (Rh negative) may also be used. For ABO isoimmunization, O group (Rh compatible) packed cells suspended in AB plasma or O group whole blood (Rh compatible with baby) should be used.
- In other situations, child's blood group should be used.
- Use fresh whole blood or reconstituted red blood cells (RBCs of less than 5 days old) prepared in CPD (Citrate, Phosphate and Dextrose) rather than SAGM (Saline, Adenine, Glucose and Mannitol) in order to minimize osmotic shifts. In emergency, if RBCs to be prepared before the delivery, it must be O Rh negative and cross-matched against the mother's blood.
- Use saline wash if available. It reduces the risk of hyperkalemia and antigen load on the RBCs before transfusion. To prevent graft versus host disease, irradiate the donor Packed RBCs within 24 h before the transfusion.
- For sickle cell disease (SCD), preferably use leukoreduced packed RBCs of less than 15 days old

Table 2: Selection of ABO and Rh group of donor packed RBCs

Mother's blood group	*Neonate's blood group*	*Donor's blood group*
O	O / A / B / AB	O
A/ B / AB	O / A / B / AB	Neonate's Blood Group / O
Rh Negative	Rh Positive / Rh Negative	Rh Negative

For an exchange transfusion, the RBCs described above are reconstituted with AB plasma (this plasma contains no anti-A or anti-B), or with ABO-compatible plasma.

Table 1: Indications of exchange transfusion in various conditions

Condition	*Indication*
Unconjugated hyperbilirubinemia in newborns	Rh isoimmunization: Cord bilirubin: ≥ 5 mg/dL OR Cord Hb ≤ 10 g/dL For infants ≥ 35 weeks' gestation, please refer to guidelines published by American Academy of Pediatrics (2004) available online at *https://pediatrics.aappublications.org/content/114/1/297.long* For infants < 35 weeks' gestation, please refer to guidelines published by National Collaborating Centre for Women's and Children's Health (NICE Guidelines, 2010) available online at *https://www.ncbi.nlm.nih.gov/books/NBK65119/pdf/Bookshelf_NBK65119.pdf*
Severe anemia	Euvolemic partial exchange transfusion should be considered in the neonate having anemic heart failure (hematocrit <30%) Note: In hydrops, do partial exchange first and then do double volume exchange transfusion to restore oxygen carrying capacity and reduce complications
Polycythemia	a. Symptomatic child: Once other causes of illness have been considered and excluded (e.g. sepsis, pneumonia, hypoglycemia), any child with symptoms that could be due to hyperviscosity should be considered for partial exchange transfusion if the peripheral venous hematocrit is >65% b. Asymptomatic Child: The peripheral venous hematocrit between 60% and 70% can usually be managed by increasing fluid intake and repeating the hematocrit in 4 to 6 hours c. If the peripheral venous hematocrit is >70% in the absence of symptoms, partial exchange transfusion may be performed based on the treating clinician's judgment, but this is a controversial issue
Severe disturbances of body chemistry	Metabolic disorders such as aminoaciduria with associated hyperammonemia or severe electrolyte imbalance (e.g. hyperkalemia, hypermagnesemia)
Sickle cell disease	Emergency: multi-organ failure, suspected stroke, acute chest syndrome, acute severe cholestasis Routine: For regularly scheduled transfusions used in the prevention of stroke, acute chest syndrome, and recurrent painful episodes

to decrease the incidence of febrile non-hemolytic transfusion reactions. Generally, irradiation is not required, except in those undergoing hematopoietic cell transplantation.[10]

Volume of Blood to be Exchanged

Normal circulating volume at different ages and gestation:

- Premature infants—90–100 mL/kg
- Term infants—80–90 mL/kg
- Infants over 3 months of age and children—70 mL/kg.

Double volume exchange transfusion

Total volume exchanged is double the normal blood volume, i.e. 160 to 180 mL/kg in term newborns and 180 to 200 mL/kg in preterm newborns. The average volume of packed RBCs is 250 mL and that of FFP varies at different blood banks. Generally, two units of fresh whole blood or two units of packed RBCs and one unit of FFP is sufficient for term newborn. Check the volume of fresh whole blood or packed RBCs and FFP with the blood bank to order in optimum quantity.

Partial exchange transfusion in polycythemia

Volume of exchange in mL is calculated based on following formula:

[(Blood volume/kg × Weight in kg) × (Observed hematocrit – Desired hematocrit)]/Observed hematocrit

Desired hematocrit is usually considered to be 50% to 60% in polycythemia.

Example: A symptomatic 3 kg infant, hematocrit 75%, blood volume 80 mL/kg—to bring hematocrit to 50%: [(80 mL × 3 kg) × (75 – 50)]/75 = [240 × 25]/75 = 80 mL

Mixing of blood components: the reconstitution

Hematocrit of packed RBCs is approximately 60%. To ensure an optimal hematocrit (40–50%) for the donor blood, packed RBCs and fresh frozen plasma (FFP) are reconstituted in the blood bank with closed system. Certain blood banks do not provide facility of reconstitution of packed RBCs and FFP, so in this situation, it can be reconstituted at bedside in closed system in a ratio of 7:3 respectively. For example, if volume of aliquot is 10 mL, attach one more extra three-way stopcock for FFP and during BET, during each cycle, first take 7 mL of packed RBCs and then 3 mL of FFP in a syringe and infuse. Repeat the same during each cycle. Mixing is not needed if fresh whole blood is used.

Warming

During the procedure, the blood should be primed from blood warmer to body temperature (i.e. 37°C). If blood warmer is not available either a water bath or by wrapping the container in a warmed towel may be used to warm the blood.

Choice of Routes

Following options can be exercised in neonates:

- Umbilical catheter is inserted to a level that allows free flowing withdrawal of blood from the umbilical vein: Push pull method
- Catheter is inserted in both umbilical vein (for blood in) and umbilical artery (blood out): Isovolumetric exchange
- Catheter is placed in either a peripheral artery (usually radial artery) and/or a large sized peripheral vein. Usually a large peripheral or brachial vein is enough. Rarely, one may have to cannulate jugular or femoral vein if the infant is severely dehydrated and peripheral veins are collapsed.

Older children: Two large peripheral veins (one for withdrawal of blood and other for infusion) are employed.

Equipment

In addition to those for vascular access, following equipment should be available for BET.

- Gowns, sterile gloves, caps, masks, eye protectors
- Sterile surgical drapes to cover the operational area
- Two to three three-way stopcocks or one four-way stopcock
- Blood infusion tube set
- A bottle to collect withdrawn blood
- Tubings for drainage to bottle for withdrawn blood
- 5 mL, 10 mL, 20 mL syringes
- Cotton pads, gauze pieces
- Full resuscitation equipment and medications
- Monitoring equipment.

Preparation of the Infant/Child

Withhold oral feeds before the procedure and if the infant has been fed within 2 to 3 hours before the procedure, insert the gastric tube and empty the stomach. Restrain the infant if needed. Usually sedation is not needed. If ventilated, ensure the head is well stabilized.

Umbilical venous catheterization

The procedure is mentioned in detail in the section 91.10. Thorough aseptic precautions should be undertaken for the procedure. BET is usually performed through a single lumen catheter passed via the umbilical vein that has been placed in the inferior vena cava below its junction with the right atrium. If one is not able to advance the catheter in the inferior vena cava, the catheter can be withdrawn and kept at a position just far enough to obtain free flow of blood (usually no more than the distance between the xiphoid process and umbilicus). The catheter site should be covered with sterile surgical drapes and universal precautions should be taken during the procedure of catheterization.

Umbilical artery catheterization

The procedure is mentioned in detail in the section 91.10. In both the techniques, confirm the position of the tip of the catheters by X-ray.

PROCEDURE

Exchange Transfusion in Neonates for Hyperbilirubinemia

Nurse infant on an open servo-controlled warmer. During the procedure, the infant should be attached to a vital sign monitor for continuous observation of heart rate, oxygen saturations, respiratory rate, electrocardiogram and temperature. Document these parameters at completion of each cycle. Continue intensified phototherapy throughout the procedure and afterwards. Possible routes for exchange transfusion are summarized in **Table 3**. Different techniques are discussed here.

Pull-push technique

The BET is usually performed through a catheter passed via the umbilical vein. **Figure 1** shows attachments of two three-way stopcocks with umbilical vein, position of tubings for blood out and blood in and attachment of syringe for manual pull or push. First withdraw the Blood in aliquot of approximately 5 mL/kg (Aliquot size should neither be less than 2 mL nor more than 20 mL). The first withdrawn blood can be sent for pre-exchange determination of hemoglobin and hematocrit, bilirubin, electrolytes, platelet count or any other test based on clinical need (e.g. G6PD, metabolic screen, blood gas, coagulation profile). After blood out, it is replaced with equal volume from the fresh whole blood or reconstituted blood. Pull/push blood at a rate of 2 to 4 mL/kg/minute. To make it simple, a suggested rate is 30 aliquots over 2 hours, allowing 4 minutes each cycle. During the procedure document each aliquot "out" and "in".

Table 3: Possible routes for exchange transfusion

Blood out	*Blood in*
Umbilical vein	Umbilical vein
Umbilical artery	Umbilical vein
Peripheral artery	Umbilical vein
Peripheral artery	Peripheral vein
Umbilical vein	Peripheral vein
Umbilical artery	Peripheral vein

Isovolumetric exchange

This is the preferred method of exchange in nursery as it decreases the risk of wide fluctuations of blood volume and pressure. It is also called simultaneous exchange. **Figure 2** depicts the isovolumetric exchange through umbilical artery and umbilical venous catheter. If either umbilical vessel is not available, then the blood can be withdrawn via a peripheral arterial cannula and donor packed RBC + FFP should be infused through a peripheral venous cannula. Using this method, the infant's blood is

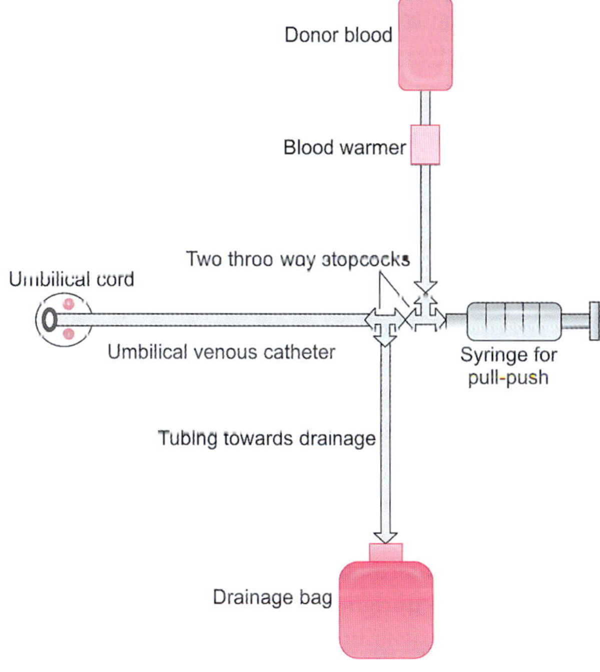

Fig. 1: Single catheter pull-push technique through umbilical venous catheter

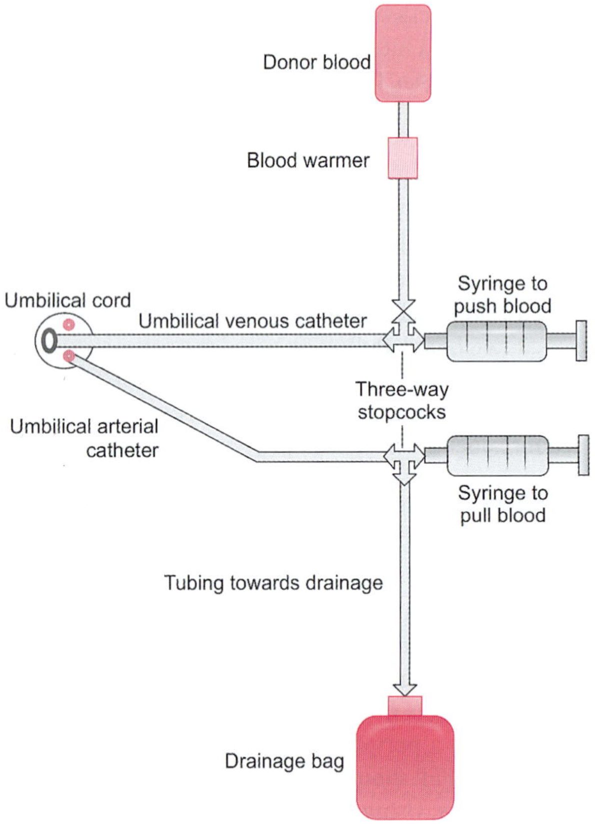

Fig. 2: Isovolumetric exchange through umbilical artery and umbilical venous catheter

slowly withdrawn from the umbilical arterial catheter (or peripheral arterial line) in aliquots of approximately 5 to 10 mL with simultaneous replacement of donor packed RBCs +FFP through the umbilical venous catheter (or peripheral venous line) using the same aliquot size at a rate of 2 to 4 mL/kg/min.

General precautions

Either of the above procedures should not be hurried and should take around 1 to 2 hours or more depending on the volume of the exchange and the physiological stability of the infant. During the procedure, the reconstituted blood or fresh whole blood should be gently shaken at every 10 minutes' interval for uniform hematocrit throughout the procedure. Avoid air bubbles in the tubing and syringe. Keep the syringe upright during pull and push to avoid inadvertent push of air in the circulation. In the middle of the procedure, send the blood out sample for electrolytes to look for hyperkalemia and hypocalcemia and check bedside blood glucose.

Use of CPD in donor blood may lead to hypocalcemia consequent to changes in calcitonin.[11,12] Incidence of symptomatic decreases in serum calcium levels is very low. Calcium infusion may lead to bradycardia, and even cardiac arrest. Thus, routine administration of calcium during BET is not justified.[13] Slow infusion from different venous line of calcium gluconate (10%) in a dose of 1–2 mL/kg may be used in presence electrocardiogram changes or in small and sick neonates, after every 50–100 mL blood exchanged under continuously electronic cardiac monitoring.[8]

Last aliquot of blood out may be used to send investigations like bilirubin, glucose, electrolytes (especially potassium and calcium), platelets, hematocrit, blood gas, coagulation profile and can also be utilized for cross match at blood bank if needed.

Serum bilirubin should be monitored at 2, 4, and 6 hours after the transfusion and then at least every 12 to 24 hours until bilirubin declines sufficiently to discontinue phototherapy. Increasing bilirubin or recurrent neurologic signs are followed to assess need for repeat exchange transfusion.

Partial Exchange Transfusion in Neonate

Partial exchange can be performed using any of the combination mentioned in **Table 3**. The procedure is almost equivalent to isovulumetric exchange transfusion except, in place of donor blood, normal saline is used for infusion in equivalent amount of the blood removed.

Manual Exchange Transfusion in Sickle Cell Disease

Reduced viscosity and HbS level are critical in potentially reversing vaso-occlusion and improving blood flow.[10,14] If the child with SCD is having Hb <5 g/dL and is critically ill, simple transfusion can be used with a goal to increase the Hb level to 10 g/dL. Since the percentage of blood volume replaced by simple transfusion in this scenario will be high, exchange transfusion generally will not be needed in such patients.

Erythrocytapheresis (automated RBC exchange) is more safe and effective method for exchange transfusion therapy in SCD; however, for technical and financial reasons, it is not widely implemented. As the manual exchange transfusion (MET) method is widely utilized with no specific need of costly equipment and that is also safe and effective, it is described below. However, for chronic transfusion, the technique to be used solely depends on the treating expert clinician's judgment, hospital protocol, local availability of resources and referral services.[15,16]

There are 3 steps in the exchange sessions: patient preparation; initial isovolemic phlebotomy (if appropriate); and whole-blood exchange, consisting of several cycles, or continuous whole-blood phlebotomy, which is associated with the infusion of diluted packed RBCs.[16] These are discussed further. Send appropriate laboratory tests, including complete blood count, reticulocytes, HbS level, serum calcium, electrolytes, liver function, and coagulation tests based on clinical need. Child should be constantly monitored during the procedure, including heart rate and rhythm, blood pressure, respiratory rate, oxygen saturation. The patient should remain in the supine position with the feet slightly raised.

Step 1: Patient preparation

Prepare two peripheral venous lines on two different limbs, one for the phlebotomy and one for the infusion of the normal saline and packed BRCs + normal saline. The venous line for phlebotomy necessitates sufficient blood flow and because of this it should be secured with large size needle, e.g. 16 or 18 F, and the one for infusion requires standard blood flow. Procedure can also be performed via double lumen central venous catheter inserted in the internal jugular vein.

Step 2: Initial isovolemic phlebotomy

If initial Hb is > 8.5 g/dL, phlebotomy is indicated to reach the Hb of 8 g/dL as per **Table 4**.[16] For patients with recent stroke, the initial phlebotomy volume should not exceed 5 mL/kg.

For example, if child's weight is 20 kg, and Hb is 10 g/dL, total amount of phlebotomy is 12 × 20 = 240 mL to be withdrawn in 60 min. Before starting the phlebotomy start infusing normal saline and after infusing 20 normal saline start phlebotomy. The amount of normal saline is same as amount of phlebotomy, i.e 240 mL in the current child. The process can also be done using 20 mL aliquots of phlebotomy and normal saline infusion. After completing this initial isovolemic phlebotomy, send last withdrawn blood for Hb estimation. If it reaches to 8 g/dL, then start exchange transfusion as below.

If child's Hb is < 8 g/dL, step 2 is not required.

Table 4: Initial phlebotomy volume for sickle cell disease

Hb level (g/dL)	*Volume of phlebotomy (mL/kg)*	*Minimal duration of bleeding (min)*
10	12	60
9.5	10	45
9	8	30
8.5	5	20

Step 3: Isovolemic blood exchange transfusion

The goal is to reduce the amount of HbS to less than 30% and to raise the hemoglobin level to approximately 10 g/dL (i.e. hematocrit of 30%). Usually total amount of volume exchanged is 35 to 45 mL/kg. This volume is both the volume of blood that will bleed during the exchange step and the volume of diluted packed RBCs (2/3 of packed RBCs and 1/3 of normal saline to reduce the hematocrit from 60% to 40%) that will be transfused to the patient during the exchange step. In place of diluted packed RBCs, fresh whole blood can also be used.

As in the scenario given above, a child with 20 kg weight needs approximately total 800 mL (20 × 40 = 800) of blood is required to be exchanged. This means 400 mL of blood to be withdrawn and 400 mL of diluted packed RBCs (i.e. 267 mL packed RBCs and 133 mL normal saline) to be infused. Please note that the dilution of packed RBCs with normal saline should be done in blood bank. If this is not possible then it can be done at bedside by adding three-way stopcock and diluting the packed RBCs before infusion using 20 mL syringe. So, first infuse 20 mL diluted packed RBCs, then phlebotomize 20 mL blood from the child and continue the cycle till the desired volume of 800 mL (400 mL phlebotomized and 400 mL infused diluted RBCs) is exchanged. Monitor the child continuously during the procedure. At the end of the procedure send Hb, electrolytes and other needed investigations based on clinical judgment from the last withdrawn aliquot.

The procedure (steps 2 and 3) takes approximately 4 hours for completion.

COMPLICATIONS

Child should be monitored periodically for following complications: hypothermia, thrombocytopenia, coagulation abnormalities, hypoglycemia, electrolyte imbalance: hyperkalemia, hypocalcemia, hypomagnesemia; and acid-base abnormalities. Less frequent complications include necrotizing enterocolitis, portal vein thrombosis, umbilical or portal vein perforation, cardiac arrhythmias especially bradycardia during procedure, apnea, infection, and all other potential complications of blood transfusion.

KEY MESSAGES

- Because of reducing need of BET, it should be performed under guidance of expert clinician.
- Select appropriate blood group of packed RBCs and FFP and decide the volume.
- Examine the infant/child to select best suitable vascular access for BET.
- Isovolumetric exchange is preferred over pull-push technique.
- Monitor continuously during and few hours after the procedure.

REFERENCES

1. Diamond LK. Erythroblastosis foetalis or haemolytic disease of the newborn. Proc R Soc Med. 1947;40:546.
2. Shamir Z, Gurevitch J. Thirty-eight cases of haemolytic disease of the newborn. Archives of Disease in Childhood. 1953;28:292.
3. American Academy of Pediatrics Subcommittee on Hyperbilirubinemia. Management of hyperbilirubinemia in the newborn infant 35 or more weeks of gestation. Pediatrics. 2004;114:297-316.
4. National Collaborating Centre for Women's and Children's Health (UK). Neonatal Jaundice. London: RCOG Press; 2010 May. PubMed PMID: 22132434.
5. Moise Jr KJ, Lopez S. Nonimmune hydrops fetalis. In: Eichenwald EC, Hansen AR, Martin CR, Stark AR, editors. Cloherty and Stark's Manual of Neonatal Care, 5th edition. New Delhi: Wolters Kluwer; 2017. p. 52-63.
6. O'Reilly D. Polycythemia. In: Eichenwald EC, Hansen AR, Martin CR, Stark AR, editors. Cloherty and Stark's Manual of Neonatal Care, 5th edition. New Delhi: Wolters Kluwer; 2017. p. 624-9.
7. US Department of Health and Human Services, National Institutes of Health, National Heart, Lung, and Blood Institute. Evidence-Based Management of Sickle Cell Disease, Expert Panel Report, 2014.
8. Murki S, Kumar P. Blood exchange transfusion for infants with severe neonatal hyperbilirubinemia. Semin Perinatol. 2011; 35:175-84.
9. New HV, Berryman J, Bolton-Maggs PH, *et al.* Guidelines on transfusion for fetuses, neonates and older children. Brit J Haematol. 2016;175:784-828.
10. DeBaun MR, Vichinsky EP. (2018). Red blood cell transfusion in sickle cell disease. Available from: *https://www.uptodate.com/contents/red-blood-cell-transfusion-in-sickle-cell-disease.* Accessed August 20, 2019.
11. Nelson N, Finnström O. Blood exchange transfusions in newborns, the effect on serum ionized calcium. Early Hum Dev. 1988;8:157-64.
12. Dincsoy MY, Tsang RC, Laskarzewski P, *et al.* Serum calcitonin response to administration of calcium in newborn infants during exchange blood transfusion. J Pediatr. 1982;100:782-6.
13. Locham KK, Kaur K, Tandon R, *et al.* Exchange blood transfusion in neonatal hyperbilirubinemia-role of calcium. Indian Pediatr. 2002;39:657-9.
14. Kwiatkowski JL. Hemoglobinopathies. In: Lanzkowsky P, Lipton JM, Fish JD, editors. Lanzkowsky's Manual of Pediatric Hematology and Oncology, 6th edition. New York: Academic Press; 2016. p. 166-96.
15. Fasano RM, Leong T, Kaushal M, *et al.* Effectiveness of red blood cell exchange, partial manual exchange, and simple transfusion concurrently with iron chelation therapy in reducing iron overload in chronically transfused sickle cell anemia patients. Transfusion. 2016;56:1707-15.
16. Koehl B, Missud F, Holvoet L, *et al.* Continuous manual exchange transfusion for patients with sickle cell disease: An efficient method to avoid iron overload. J Vis Exp. 2017;14: e55172.

91.10 Umbilical Vessel Catheterization

Shashi Kant Dhir, Praveen Kumar

INTRODUCTION

Umbilical vessels have been used as a relatively easy source of vascular access in sick neonates for sampling as well as giving intravenous infusions. The indications and contraindications for umbilical artery catheterization (UAC) and umbilical venous catheterization (UVC) are given in **Table 1**.

Table 1: Indications of umbilical vessel catheterization

	Umbilical venous catheterization	*Umbilical venous catheterization*
Indications	• Invasive blood pressure monitoring in sick neonates • Exchange transfusion • Need for frequent blood sampling – ABG analysis – Extremely preterm babies where repeated sampling is expected	• Delivery room administration of medications and intravenous fluids • Central venous pressure monitoring • Exchange transfusion • Administration of hyperosmolar fluids, total parenteral nutrition • Cardiac pacing can be done through this route
Contraindications	• Congenital malformation of the cord (e.g. omphalocele) • Localized infection (e.g. omphalitis) • Presence of necrotizing enterocolitis • Evidence of lower extremity vascular compromise	

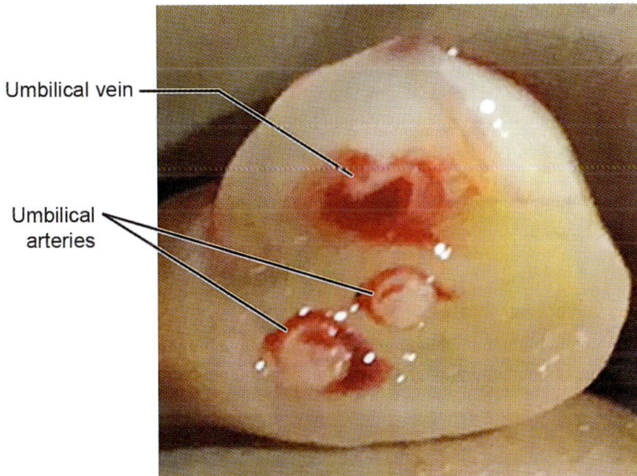

Fig. 1: Umbilical vessels

Anatomical Considerations

There are two umbilical arteries and one umbilical vein, which may be cannulated for various indications. The umbilical vein is single, thin walled, often gaping and usually is located at 12 o' clock position (**Fig. 1**). The umbilical arteries are two in number and are identified by their thick wall, closed lumen, and they usually protrude from the cut umbilical cord. The position of the umbilical arteries depends upon the site of the cutting of cord.

Preparation

Only trained and experienced persons should perform umbilical vessel cannulation and equipment required should be assembled and checked beforehand (**Table 2**). Examine the cord after the decision of UAC or UVC is taken. If the cord is shriveled or dried then saline soaked gauze should be applied 30 minutes prior to the procedure to moisten it for easy catheterization. Always calculate the length of catheter to be inserted before the procedure. Various methods of determining the required length can be used (**Table 3**). An estimate of desired length of the umbilical catheters based on the study by Dunn[1] has been given in **Table 4**.

UMBILICAL ARTERY CATHETERIZATION

Technique

The baby should be placed in a radiant heat warmer in servo control mode. Calculate precisely the length of the catheter to be inserted using **Table 3**. Ensure that all equipment is ready.

The sterile cap, mask, gown and gloves are donned as in surgical procedures. The key site and the key parts are prepared using surgical Aseptic Non Touch Technique (ANTT) using triple swab technique.[3] The umbilical tie is loosely placed across the lower part of the cord and is fastened later after putting the catheter. The cord is cut 1–2 cm above the base in a horizontal direction avoiding angulations. The base of the cord is held upright and steadied using a forceps.

The artery is identified and dilated with one or both prongs of an iris forceps. The iris forceps should be kept in the artery for minimum 60 seconds. The umbilical catheter filled with heparinized normal saline is inserted in the dilated artery. Once inside the artery, advance the catheter caudally up to the pre-decided length of the umbilical catheter. The catheter should be placed 1–2 cm beyond the calculated length and then withdrawn to the correct position. The blood should be aspirated once the desired length is reached to ensure the patency.

Table 2: Equipment required for umbilical vessel catheterization

- Sterile cap, gown, mask, gloves, drapes
- Measuring tape
- Antiseptic preparatory solution
- Sterile cotton and gauze piece
- Sponge holder forceps
- Umbilical tape
- Forceps (with and without tooth)
- Scalpel long handle with blade
- Iris forceps
- Umbilical catheters (single lumen for UAC)
  - UAC 3.5 Fr for < 1200 g and 5.0 Fr for > 1200 g
  - UVC 3.5 Fr for < 1500 g, 5.0 Fr for > 1500–3500 g and 8.0 Fr for > 3500g
- Needle or puncture device for needleless system
- Three-way stopcock
- Syringes (3, 5, 10, 50 mL)
- Normal saline for flushes
- Suture material 3-0 Mersilk
- Needle holder
- Saline heparin solution
- Infusion pump
- Transparent semi-permeable adhesive dressing
- Pressure transducer kit (for UAC)

Blood gas analysis may be done to confirm that the correct vessel is catheterized. The catheter should be secured in place using a purse string suture around the base using 3-0 Mersilk and then fixed by using Goal Post method of securing the catheter (**Fig. 2**). The catheter should then be fixed on the abdominal skin using transparent semi-occlusive dressing. The catheter is flushed with the heparinized normal saline infusion containing heparin (0.25–1.0 U per mL) and continuous infusion of same solution is started at a minimum of 0.5 mL/hour. The discoloration and blanching of the feet should be looked for during and after the procedure to assess the perfusion of the lower limbs. Attach the pressure transducer kit to the line if continuous blood pressure monitoring is required.

Table 3: Methods of determining the length of umbilical catheters*

- Shoulder umbilical length (Table 4)
  - Distance from the tip of the shoulder/lateral end of the clavicle to a point vertically below at the horizontal line drawn at level of the umbilicus
- Shukla's method[2]
  - For umbilical arterial catheter
    - Infant ≥ 1500 g (3 × BW in Kg) + 9
    - Infant <1500 g (4 × BW in Kg) + 7
  - For Umbilical arterial catheter
    - [(3 × BW in kg) + 9] ÷ 2 + 1

Note: For exchange transfusion or emergency venous access, the umbilical venous catheter is inserted to a distance where the free flow from the vessel is established.

*The length of the stump is added to the above calculation.

Catheter Tip Position

The umbilical artery catheter can be placed in two positions, i.e. either "High" or "Low". The position of catheter tip lies between the T6 and T9 vertebrae in the "High" position, i.e. between the ductus arteriosus and the origin of celiac axis, whereas in the "Low" position, the tip lies between L3 and L4 vertebrae which corresponds to the location between the inferior mesenteric artery and the bifurcation of aorta. The placement of the catheter between the T9 to L3 is avoided because aorta give rise to celiac, renal and superior mesenteric artery in this segment.

Causes of Failed UAC

- Creation of false passage
- UVC catheterization
- Inadvertent placement into ipsilateral external iliac artery/gluteal arteries or contralateral iliac artery.

In case of failed UAC, remove the catheter and place it appropriately in another umbilical artery using the same method.

Complications

The complications[4] are tabulated in **Table 4**. The most common complication noted is blanching of the lower limbs. This phenomenon is usually transient and resolves on warming of opposite limb. If the symptoms resolve, the catheter can be retained, otherwise it should be removed. Skin observation, monitoring of platelet count, blood pressure and urine examination can aid in early diagnosis of complications. Doppler ultrasonographic examination is useful for diagnosing and managing these events. The incidence of vascular complications has been shown to be less with "High" placement whereas the incidence of blanching and cyanosis is more with "Low" umbilical catheters.

Table 4: Estimated length of the umbilical vessel catheter

Shoulder umbilical length in cm*	*Low position of umbilical artery catheter (cm)*	*High position of umbilical artery catheter (cm)*	*Umbilical venous catheter (cm)*
9	4	10	4.7
9.5	4.5	10.5	5
10	5	11	5.5
10.5	5.5	11.8	5.8
11	6	12.1	6
11.5	6.5	13	6.6
12	6.8	13.3	6.8
12.5	7.2	14	7.3
13	7.5	14.5	7.5
13.5	8.0	15	8
14	8.5	15.6	8.3
14.5	9.0	16.1	8.7
15	9.5	16.7	9
15.5	9.8	17.2	9.5
16	10.0	18.0	9.8
16.5	10.6	18.3	10
17	11	19.0	10.5
17.5	11.5	19.5	10.8
18	12	20	11

*distance from the tip of the shoulder/lateral end of the clavicle to a point vertically below at the horizontal line drawn at level of the umbilicus. Adapted from Dunn PM. Localization of the umbilical catheter by post-mortem measurement. Arch Dis Child. 1966;41:69-75.2

UMBILICAL VENOUS CATHETERIZATION

Technique

The umbilical stump should be prepared in the similar way as described in the umbilical artery catheterization described above.

The vein is identified by thin wall and large gaping lumen and it is usually located at 12 'o clock position. The catheter filled with heparinized normal saline is inserted in the vein. The direction of the catheter should be in the ***cephalad*** direction. Advance the catheter up to the pre-decided length. The catheter should be placed 1–2 cm beyond the calculated length and then withdrawn to the correct position. The failure of the catheter to advance up to the desired length may indicate the lodging of the catheter in the portal vein or intrahepatic branches of the umbilical vein. The withdrawing of catheter by 2–3 cm, rotating it and then again advancing it may help in correct placement of the tip in inferior vena cava. The blood should be aspirated once the desired length is reached to ensure the patency. The fluid should be attached to the catheter. The catheter should be secured in similar method as in UAC (**Fig. 2**). Once the catheter is secured, it should not be advanced further.

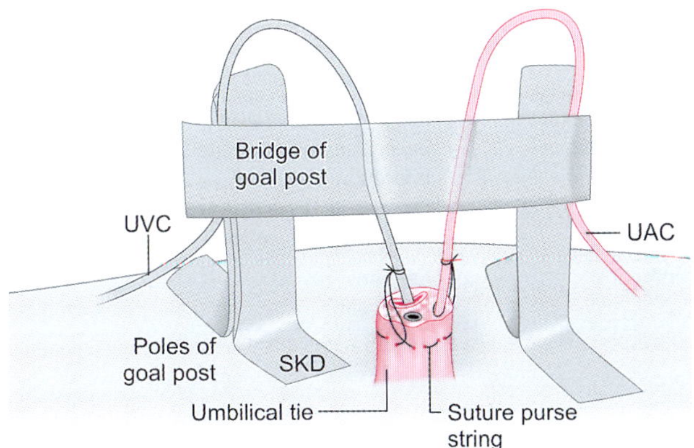

Fig. 2: The Goalpost method of securing the umbilical catheters

Catheter Tip Position

The preferred position of the umbilical venous catheter is in the inferior vena cava above the level of the diaphragm (usually 0.5 to 1 cm) and below the left atrium.[4] The radiological confirmation of the catheter tip must always be done before starting the infusions.

Complications of the UVC

The complications are tabulated in **Table 5**. The most common and serious complication noted is infection. It can be minimized by following strict asepsis and keeping the line only for the required duration. The lines are taken out if there are features of bloodstream infection. The thromboembolic complications can also occur in various organs depending upon the site of tip of the catheter. The lungs, heart and systemic organs can be involved if the tip crosses the ductus venosus, whereas hepatic and gut complications are common if the tip lies in the hepatic and the portal system.

Confirming the Position of the Catheter Tip of Umbilical Vessel Catheters

The position of the catheter should be confirmed radiologically by anteroposterior and cross table lateral

Table 5: Complications associated with umbilical vessel catheterization

	Umbilical artery catheterization	*Umbilical venous catheterization*
Thromboembolic phenomenon	• Kidney: hematuria; hypertension • Bowel: necrotizing enterocolitis or bowel infarction • Extremities: cyanosis or blanching of skin of back, buttocks, or legs	• Liver: hepatic necrosis, abscess • Bowel: necrotizing enterocolitis • Lungs: pulmonary edema, pulmonary hemorrhage
Infection	• Cellulitis • Omphalitis • Sepsis	• Cellulitis • Omphalitis • Sepsis • Endocarditis • Lung and liver abscess
Bleeding	Vessel perforation	Trauma
Other	Disseminated intravascular coagulation	Cardiac: Pericardial effusion, cardiac tamponade, cardiac perforation, pneumopericardium arrhythmias

views, or by ultrasonography. In case of doubt, radiological confirmation after injection of the contrast material should be done.

The umbilical venous catheter follows an anterior and cephalad course in the midline umbilical vein until directed posteriorly in the inferior vena cava, whereas the umbilical artery catheter is initially directed caudally and posteriorly to enter either the right or left iliac artery before coursing superiorly in the more posteriorly positioned aorta (**Figs. 3 and 4**).

If position of umbilical artery catheter tip is lower than the "High" desired position, as a rule of thumb we do not advance it upwards but in such cases, the catheter is to be pulled to "Low" position. Similarly, once secured, the umbilical venous catheter is not advanced if it is lower than the desired position because of risk of infection.

Care of the Indwelling Catheters

- Ensure proper surgical ANTT every time a central line is being handled.
- The infusions should always be running to prevent clot formation.
- Avoid introduction of air bubble in the lines.
- Avoid covering the catheter with opaque dressing as recognition of bleeding may get delayed.
- Maintain a bloodletting chart and add the flush infusates and the medication volume to the daily intake output charting.
- Ensure that the traction is not put on the catheters.

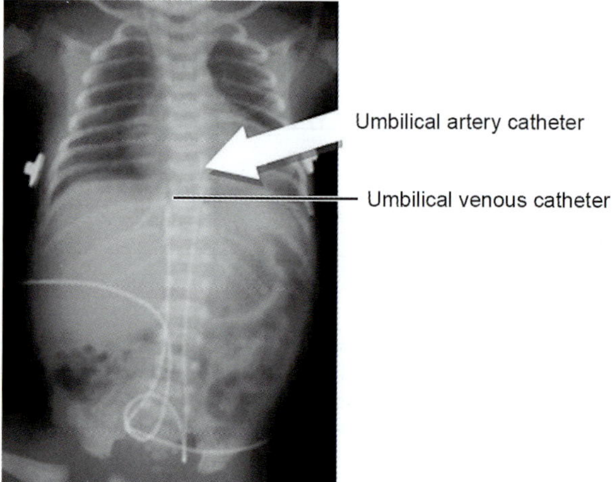

Fig. 3: Catheter tip localization in anteroposterior X-ray

For UAC

- Every time a blood sample is taken, ensure that catheter is flushed slowly (to avoid hypertension) with 0.5 to 1 mL of flush solution.
- Think of clot formation if there is difficult sampling or dampening of graph of the invasive blood pressure monitoring.

REMOVAL OF UAC AND UVC

These catheters should be removed as early as possible because of the risk of infection and colonization. The indications for the removal are as follows:

- Clinical improvement in the baby and the primary indication of putting the catheter is passive

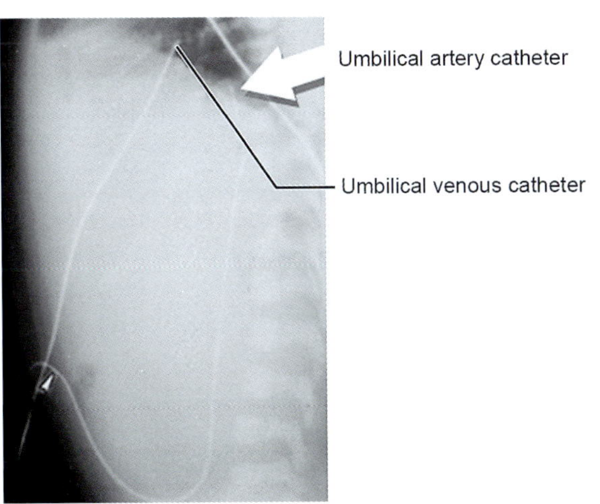

Fig. 4: Catheter tip localization in cross table X-ray

- For UAC, frequent sampling and invasive blood pressure monitoring is not required
- Occurrence of any of the complications warrants catheter removal
- CDC recommends that optimally umbilical arterial catheter should not be kept beyond 5 days and the umbilical venous catheter should not be kept beyond 14 days.[5]

Method of Removal

The umbilical tie is loosened to facilitate the pulling out of catheters. The catheter is withdrawn slowly 1 cm per 30 to 60 seconds till about 5 cm is remaining to facilitate the constriction of the proximal vessel segment. The umbilical tie is now fastened and the infusion is stopped. Holding of cord stump under pressure may be required for several minutes if the bleeding occurs from the umbilical stump. Extra care should be taken while removing the UVC as the lack of contractility may lead to more severe bleeding.

KEY MESSAGES

- Umbilical vessel catheterization is an easy source of vascular access in sick neonates but it may be associated with dangerous complications.
- Proper technique should be used to place umbilical catheters and the position of tip should be confirmed before starting infusions to avoid complications.
- Umbilical catheters should be placed as well as maintained using surgical asepsis.
- The umbilical catheters should be removed as early as possible.

REFERENCES

1. Dunn PM. Localization of the umbilical catheter by post-mortem measurement. Arch Dis Child. 1966;41:69-75.2.
2. Shukla H, Ferrara A. Rapid estimation of insertional length of umbilical catheters in newborns. Am J Dis Child. 1986; 140:786-8.
3. Rowley S, Clare S. ANTT: A standard approach to aseptic technique. Nurs Times. 2011;107:12-4.
4. Cunningham MD, Eyal FG, Gomella TL. Neonatology Management, Procedures, on-Call Problems, Diseases, and Drugs. New York, NY: McGraw-Hill Education LLC; 2013.
5. CDC. (2017). Summary of Recommendations. Guidelines for the Prevention of Intravascular Catheter-Related Infections (2011). Available from: *https://www.cdc.gov/infectioncontrol/guidelines/bsi/recommendations.html*. Accessed August 20, 2019.

Annexures

Section Editor: *Piyush Gupta*

Annexure 1

Resuscitation and Emergency Room Drugs

Arohi Gupta, Abhijeet Saha

ADENOSINE

Route of administration: IV.

Dose: Supraventricular tachycardia; Initial: 0.1 mg/kg/dose (max 6 mg/dose); Subsequent: Neonates: Increase by increments of 0.05 mg/kg to a maximum of 0.25 mg/kg/dose; Children: Increase by increments of 0.1 mg/kg/dose to a maximum of 0.3 mg/kg/dose (max 12 mg/dose). Allow 2 minutes between incremental increases. Adolescent and adults ≥ 50 kg: 6 mg rapid IV push over 1–2 seconds; if no response after 1–2 min, give 12-mg rapid IV push. If required may repeat a second 12 mg dose after 1–2 min. Maximum single dose: 12 mg.

Precautions: Administer by rapid bolus IV injection over 1–2 seconds simultaneously with a rapid saline flush of 5–10 mL with the help of 3- or 4-way stopcock. Continuous EKG and BP monitoring is required. It is contraindicated in 2nd- and 3rd-degree AV block or sick-sinus syndrome unless pacemaker placed and use with digoxin may cause enhanced depressant effects on SA and AV nodes. Half-life is <10 seconds.

Adverse effects: Headache, dyspnea, nausea, flushing, chest pain, dizziness.

Availability: Injection: 3 mg/mL.

ALPROSTADIL (PGE1)

Route of administration: IV.

Dose: Initial: neonates and infants: 0.05 to 0.1 µg/kg/minute; maintenance: 0.01 to 0.4 µg/kg/minute.

Precautions: Lowest dose which gives desired effect should be used. Apnea is a major adverse effect and may occur in neonates with congenital heart defects within first hour of infusion. It is mainly used for palliation only and continuous vital monitoring is essential.

Adverse effects: Apnea, seizures, bradycardia, hypotension, fever, diarrhea, gastric outlet obstruction. May decrease platelet aggregation.

Availability: Injection: 500 µg/mL.

AMIODARONE

Route of administration: IV.

Dose: VF/VT arrest: 5 mg/kg IV rapid push (max 300 mg/dose), arrhythmia 5 mg/kg IV over 20 to 60 minutes (max 300 mg/dose); Continuous infusion for tachyarrhythmia: 5 to 15 µg/kg/minute.

Precautions: Dilute with D5W for continuous infusion. Many drug interactions may occur due to cytochrome P450 inhibition.

Adverse effects: Cardiogenic shock, hypotension, arrhythmias, hepatotoxicity, pulmonary fibrosis, skin discoloration, interstitial pneumonitis.

Availability: Injection: 50 mg/mL.

ATROPINE

Route of administration: IV, ETT.

Dose: *Pre-intubation dose*: Neonate: 0.01–0.02 mg/kg/dose IV/IM prior to other premedication.

Child: 0.01 mg/kg/dose IV/IM; max. dose: 0.4 mg/dose; may repeat Q4–6 h as and when needed.

Cardiopulmonary resuscitation/Bradycardia: Neonate: 0.01–0.03 mg/kg/dose IV/IM Q10–15 min as needed and up to a total maximum of 0.04 mg/kg. Administer IV over 1 min. Child: 0.02 mg/kg/dose IV Q5 min × 2–3 doses on as needed basis; max. single dose: 0.5 mg in children, 1 mg in adolescents; max total dose: 1 mg children, 2 mg adolescents.

Bronchospasm: 0.025–0.05 mg/kg/dose (max. dose: 2.5 mg/dose) in 2.5 mL NS Q6–8 h via nebulizer.

Nerve agent and insecticide poisoning for muscarinic symptoms: (organophosphate or carbamate poisoning) (IV/IM/ET; dilute in 1–2 mL NS for ET administration): Child: 0.05–0.1 mg/kg Q5–10 min until bronchial or oral secretions terminate.

Ophthalmic (uveitis): *Child*: (0.5% solution; prepared by diluting equal volume of the 1% atropine ophthalmic solution with artificial tears) 1–2 drops in each eye once daily–TID.

Precautions: A minimum dose of 0.1 mg should be administered to avoid the paradoxical bradycardia that may occur with lower dosages.

Adverse effects: Fever, tachycardia, constipation, urinary retention, dizziness, hallucinations, headache, dry mouth, blurred vision.

Availability: Injection: most common concentrations are 0.4, 0.5, and 1 mg/mL.

CALCIUM CHLORIDE

Route of administration: IV.

Dose: Initial: Calcium chloride: 20 mg/kg (max 1,000 mg/dose); Subsequent: The initial dose may be repeated once, 10 minutes following initial dose. Total maximum dose 2,000 mg.

Precautions: Calcium chloride must be diluted and should be given through a central IV line whenever possible. Scalp, hand, and foot veins should not be used for administration unless in life-threatening situation. Calcium in any form should be infused slowly while monitoring the patient for bradycardia. Do not admix calcium with any solution containing sodium bicarbonate or phosphate salts (a fatal precipitation can occur). Calcium is contraindicated in digitalis toxicity. Calcium may antagonize the effects of verapamil.

Adverse effects: Hypercalcemia, cardiac arrest, venous irritation. Extravasation may cause severe necrosis and sloughing.

Availability: Injection: 1 g in 10 mL (13.5 mEq calcium/g).

CALCIUM GLUCONATE

Route of administration: IV.

Dose: Initial: Calcium gluconate: 100 mg/kg (max 3,000 mg/dose); Subsequent: The initial dose may be repeated once after 10 minutes. Total maximum dose 3,000 mg.

Precautions: Calcium gluconate should be diluted and ideally be given only through a central IV line; however, a large peripheral line may be used, if necessary. Calcium in any form should be infused slowly while monitoring the patient for bradycardia. Do not admix calcium with any solution containing sodium bicarbonate or phosphate salts (a fatal precipitation can occur). Calcium is contraindicated in digitalis toxicity. Calcium may antagonize the effects of verapamil.

Adverse effects: Hypercalcemia, cardiac arrest, venous irritation. Note: Extravasation may cause severe necrosis and sloughing.

Availability: Injection: 1 g in 10 mL (4.5 mEq of calcium/g).

DEXTROSE

Route of administration: IV.

Dose: Initial: 0.5 to 1 g/kg administered slowly (2 to 4 mL/kg of a 25% dextrose or 5 to 10 mL/kg of a10% dextrose solution). If 25% dextrose is not available, dilute 50% dextrose 1:1 with sterile water or NS for injection to yield a 25% solution. Concentrations of continuous infusions greater than 12.5% should be infused via a central line when possible. For neonates with hypoglycemia, a dose of 0.25 to 0.5 g/kg (2.5 to 5 mL/kg) of a 10% dextrose solution should be used.

Adverse effects: Hyperglycemia, hyperosmolarity.

Availability: Injection: 0.1 g/mL (10% dextrose/water), 0.25 g/mL (25% dextrose/water), 0.5 g/mL (50% dextrose/water).

DOBUTAMINE

Route of administration: IV.

Dose: 5 to 20 μg/kg/minute (titrate to desired cardiovascular effect).

Precautions: Solutions containing sodium bicarbonate should not be admixed with dobutamine as it is unstable in alkaline solutions. Central access is preferred.

Adverse effects: Tachycardia, hypertension, ventricular ectopy. Contraindicated in idiopathic hypertrophic subaortic stenosis (IHSS). Dobutamine increases cardiac output and systemic pressure in pediatric patients of every age group. In premature neonates, dobutamine is less effective than dopamine in increasing raising systemic BP without causing undue tachycardia, and has not been shown to provide any added benefit.

Availability: Injection: concentrate for IV infusion: 50 mg/mL.

DOPAMINE

Route of administration: IV.

Dose: 2 to 20 μg/kg/minute (titrate to desired renal or cardiovascular effect).

Low dose: 2–5 μg/kg/min IV; increases renal blood flow; minimal effect on heart rate and cardiac output.

Intermediate dose: 5–15 μg/kg/min IV; increases heart rate, cardiac contractility, cardiac output.

High dose: >20 μg/kg/min IV; α-adrenergic effects are prominent; decreases renal perfusion.

Precautions: Solutions containing sodium bicarbonate should not be admixed with dopamine (inactivation of dopamine may occur). May begin administration via a peripheral line, changing to central access as soon as possible.

Adverse effects: Tachycardia, vasoconstriction, hypertension, tachyarrhythmia. Newborn infants may be more sensitive to vasoconstrictive effects of dopamine. Extravasation may cause tissue necrosis; treated with phentolamine.

Availability: Injection (must be further diluted): 40 mg/mL.

EPINEPHRINE

Route of administration: IM, IV, ETT, SC.

Dose: *Cardiac uses*: Neonate: Asystole and bradycardia: 0.01–0.03 mg/kg of 1 : 10,000 solution (0.1–0.3 mL/kg) IV/ET Q3–5 min on as needed basis. Infant and child: Bradycardia, asystole, and pulseless arrest: First dose: 0.01 mg/kg of 1 : 10,000 solution (0.1 mL/kg) IO/IV; max dose: 1 mg (10 mL). Subsequent doses Q3–5 min should be the same. Must circulate drug with CPR. All ET doses: 0.1 mg/kg of 1: 1000 solution (0.1 mL/kg) ET Q3–5 min. Continuous infusion: 0.1 to 1 μg/kg/minute.

Respiratory uses: *Bronchodilator*: 1: 1000 (aqueous): Infant and child: 0.01 mL/kg/dose SC (max. single dose 0.5 mL); repeat Q15 min × 3–4 doses or Q4 h on as needed basis. Adult: 0.3–0.5 mg (0.3–0.5 mL)/dose SC Q20 min × 3 doses. Nebulization (alternative to racemic epinephrine): 0.5 mL/kg of 1: 1000 solution diluted in 3 mL NS; max. doses: ≤4 yr: 2.5 mL/dose; >4 yr: 5 mL/dose.

Hypersensitivity reactions: Child: 0.01 mg/kg/dose IM up to a max. dose of 0.5 mg/dose Q20 min–4h PRN. Hypersensitivity reactions: For bronchial asthma and certain allergic manifestations (e.g. angioedema, urticaria, serum sickness, anaphylactic shock) use epinephrine SC. Patients with anaphylaxis may benefit from IM administration.

Solution for inhalation (OTC): 2.25% (1.25% epinephrine base) (0.5 mL). <4 yr: Croup (using 2.25% solution): 0.05 mL/kg/dose up to a max. dose of 0.5 mL/dose diluted to 3 mL with NS. Given via nebulizer over 15 min.≥4 yr: 0.5 mL/dose diluted to 3 mL with NS via a nebulizer over 15 min Q3–4 h.

Precautions: Extravasations should be treated immediately with phentolamine.

Adverse effects: Hypertension, arrhythmias, tachycardia, nausea, and vomiting. Necrosis may occur at site of repeated local injection. Rare cases of serious skin and soft tissue infections, have been reported with IM or deep SC injections.

Availability: Injection: 100 μg/mL (1:10,000); 1 mg/mL (1:1,000); Autoinjector: 0.15 mg, 0.3 mg.

FENTANYL

Route of administration: IV, PO, TD, IN.

Dose: Titrate dose to effect. Neonate and younger infant: Sedation/analgesia: 1–4 μg/kg/dose IV Q2–4 h on as needed basis. Continuous IV infusion: 1–5 μg/kg/h. Older infant and child: Sedation/analgesia: 1–2 μg/kg/dose IV/IM Q30–60 min, may be repeated.

Continuous IV infusion: usual infusion ranges 1-3 µg/kg/h, titrate to needed effect.

To prepare infusion, use the following formula:

50 × Desired dose (µg/kg/h)/Desired infusion rate (mL/h) × Wt (kg) = µg Fentanyl/50 mL fluid

Breakthrough cancer pain: Buccal tabs (Fentora; ≥18 yr): Start with 100 µg by placing tablet in the buccal cavity (above a rear molar between the upper cheek and gum) and letting the tablet dissolve for 15–25 min. A second 100 µg dose, if needed, may be administered 30 min after the start of the first dose.

Lozenges (≥16 yr): Start with 200 µg by placing lozenge in the mouth between the cheek and lower gum. If needed, may repeat dose 15 min after the completion of the first dose (30 min after start of prior dose).

Transdermal: Transdermal onset of action 6–8 h with a 72-h duration of action.

Safety has not been established in children <2 yr and should be administered in children ≥2 yr who are opioid tolerant. Opioid-tolerant child receiving at least 60 mg morphine equivalents/24 h: Use 25 µg/h patch Q72 h.

Intranasal route for acute and preprocedure analgesia: ≥1 yr–adolescent: 1–2 µg/kg/dose intranasally (max. dose: 50 µg) Q1 h on as needed basis.

Precautions: Highly lipophilic and may deposit into fat tissue. IV onset of action 1–2 min with peak effects in 10 min. IV duration of action 30–60 min. Give IV dose over 3–5 min. Rapid infusion may cause respiratory depression and chest wall rigidity. Respiratory depression may persist beyond the period of analgesia. Use with caution in bradycardia and increased intracranial pressure. Adjust dose in renal failure. Buccal tabs and oral lozenges are indicated only for the management of breakthrough cancer pain in patients who are already receiving and who are tolerant to opioid therapy.

Intranasal fentanyl is equivalent to and better than morphine (PO/IV/IM) and equivalent to intravenous fentanyl for providing analgesia. Intranasal route of administration for analgesia has an onset of action at 10–30 min.

Adverse effects: Respiratory depression, chest wall rigidity, hypotension, bradycardia, hallucinations, gastritis, constipation, nausea, dry mouth.

Availability: Injection: 50 µg/mL; SR patch: 12.5, 25, 50, 75, 100 µg/h; Tabs for buccal administration: 100, 200, 400, 600, 800 µg; Lozenge on a stick: 200, 400, 600, 800, 1200, 1600 µg; Nasal solution:100 µg/spray, 300 µg/spray, 400 µg/spray (5 mL; delivers 8 sprays).

FLUMAZENIL

Route of administration: IV.

Dose: Benzodiazepine reversal: 0.01 mg/kg IV 1 dose (max 0.2 mg/dose); may repeat as needed to a max of 0.05 mg/kg or 1 mg total, whichever is less.

Precautions: Use caution if patient is dependent on benzodiazepines. May result in abrupt withdrawal precipitating hypertension, myocardial infarction, and seizures.

Adverse effects: Arrhythmias, hyper/hypotension, acute withdrawal symptoms.

Availability: Injection: 0.1 mg/mL.

HEPARIN

Route of administration: IV.

Dose: *Anticoagulation empiric dosage*: Continuous IV infusion [initial doses for goal unfractionated heparin (UFH) anti-Xa level of 0.3–0.7 units/mL].

Age	*Loading dose (IV)*	*IV infusion rate (units/kg/h)*
Neonate and infant	75 U/kg IV	28
Child ≥1–16 years	75 U/kg IV (max dose: 7700 U)	20 (max initial rate: 1650 U/h)
>16 yrs	70 U/kg IV (max dose: 7700 U)	15 (max initial rate: 1650 U/h)

Obtain APTT 4 h after the loading dose.

Heparin flush: Peripheral IV: 1–2 mL of 10 U/mL solution Q4 h; Central lines: 2–3 mL of 100 U/mL solution Q24 h; TPN (central line) and arterial line: add heparin to make a final concentration of 0.5–1 U/mL.

Precautions: Contraindicated in active major bleeding and known or suspected HIT. Use with caution if platelets < 50,000/mm^3. Avoid IM injections and other medications affecting platelet function (e.g. NSAIDs and ASA). Adjust dose with one of the following laboratory goals: Unfractionated heparin (UFH) anti-Xa level: 0.3–0.7 units/mL or aPTT level (reagent specific to reflect anti-Xa level of 0.3–0.7 units/mL): 50–80 seconds. These laboratory measurements are best measured 4–6 h after initiation or changes in infusion rate. Antidote: Protamine sulfate (1 mg/100 U heparin)

Adverse effects: Hemorrhage, heparin-induced thrombocytopenia, allergy, alopecia, thrombocytopenia.

Availability: Injection: commonly used are 1,000, 5,000, 10,000, 20,000 units/mL.

INSULIN

Route of administration: IV, SC.

Dose: *Acute management of DKA*: 0.1 units/kg SC/IV, followed by 0.1 units/kg/hour as a continuous infusion; Emergent, symptomatic hyperkalemia: Regular insulin, 0.1 U/kg IV with D25W as 2 mL/kg (0.5 g/kg) over 30 min. Repeat dose in 30 to 60 min, or begin infusion of D25W 1 to 2 mL/kg/h with regular insulin 0.1 U/kg/h. Monitor glucose hourly.

Precautions: Do not consider all clear insulin preparations to be fast acting or appropriate for IV infusion.

Adverse effects: Hypoglycemia, palpitations, tachycardia, dizziness.

Availability: Injection: 100 units/mL.

ISOPROTERENOL

Route of administration: IV.

Dose: 0.1 to 1 μg/kg/minute.

Precautions: Isoproterenol may aggravate arrhythmias associated with digitalis toxicity. In the dehydrated or hypovolemic patient, the vasodilator properties of isoproterenol may produce exaggerated hypotension. Commercially available products contain sulfites and should be used with caution in patients known to be sensitive to sulfiting agents.

Adverse effects: Tachyarrhythmia, myocardial ischemia, hypotension, hypertension, tremor, agitation.

Availability: Injection: 0.02, 0.2 mg/mL.

KETAMINE

Route of administration: IV, IM.

Dose: Rapid sequence intubation: 1 to 2 mg/kg IV or 3 to 7 mg/kg IM (1 dose).

Precautions: Avoid use in patients with suspected head trauma or seizures of unknown origin, may increase ICP.

Adverse effects: Laryngospasms, emergence reactions, tachycardia, hypertension.

Availability: Injection: 10, 50, and 100 mg/mL

LABETALOL

Dose: Child: PO: Initial: 1–3 mg/kg/24 h in two divided doses. May increase up to a maximum of 12 mg/kg/24 h up to 1200 mg/24 h; IV: Hypertensive emergency: Intermittent dose: 0.2–1 mg/kg/dose Q10 min; max. dose: 40 mg/dose; Infusion (hypertensive emergencies): 0.4–1 mg/kg/h, to a max. dose of 3 mg/kg/h; may initiate with a 0.2–1 mg/kg bolus; max. bolus: 40 mg.

Precautions: Contraindicated in pulmonary edema, cardiogenic shock, heart block, bronchial asthma. Use with caution in hepatitis. Cholestatic jaundice has been reported. Use with digitalis glycosides may increase risk for bradycardia. Onset of action: PO: 1–4 h; IV: 5–15 min.

Adverse effects: Hypotension, bradycardia, AV conduction disturbances, bronchospasm, urinary retention.

Availability: Tabs: 100, 200, 300 mg; Injection: 5 mg/mL; Oral suspension: 10, 40 mg/mL.

LIDOCAINE

Route of administration: IV, ETT.

Dose: Initial: 1 mg/kg (max 100 mg/dose) IV over 2 to 4 minutes (maximum rate 0.7 mg/kg/minute or 50 mg/minute, whichever is less) Note: If using via ETT, dose is two to four times the IV dose diluted in 3 to 5 mL of saline and followed by several positive-pressure breaths. Subsequent: Initial dose may be repeated up to two to three times at 5- to 10-minute intervals (maximum dose during a 1-hour period: 200 to 300 mg). Once the initial bolus has been given, a continuous infusion of lidocaine at 20 to 50 μg/kg/minute should be initiated. Lidocaine serum concentrations should be monitored.

Precautions: Dosage must be modified in children with CHF, shock, or liver disease.

Adverse effects: Nausea, vomiting, altered CNS status, paresthesia, seizures, cardiac toxicity (myocardial depression, arrhythmias)

Availability: Injection: various concentrations ranging from 10 to 200 mg/mL (dilute to a concentration of 10 to

20 mg/mL for IV push and 8 mg/mL for continuous infusion before use).

LORAZEPAM

Route of administration: IV, IM.

Dose: *Status epilepticus*: 0.1 mg/kg/dose (max 4 mg/dose) IV/IM q5 min 2 to 3 doses Continuous infusion: 0.05 to 0.1 mg/kg/hour.

Precautions: Contains large amounts of propylene glycol so may result in metabolic acidosis.

Adverse effects: CNS depression, respiratory depression, hypotension, bradycardia.

Availability: Injection: 2, 4 mg/mL.

METHYLPREDNISOLONE SODIUM SUCCINATE

Route of administration: IV, IM.

Dose: *Initial shock, acute SLE, multiple sclerosis, transverse mylelitis*: 30 mg/kg by IV infusion over 15 to 30 minutes, max 1,500 mg/dose; acute asthma and allergic reactions: 1 to 2 mg/kg by slow IV push over 5 to 10 minutes (usual max 80 mg/dose).

Precautions: Use of high-dose methylprednisolone in treatment of shock and spinal cord injury remains controversial.

Adverse effects: Hypotension, electrolyte abnormalities, infection.

Availability: Injection: 40, 125, 500 mg; 1 or 2 g (powder for reconstitution).

MIDAZOLAM

Route of administration: IV, IM, PO, intranasal.

Dose: *IM/IV sedation for procedures*: 0.05 to 0.1 mg/kg IM/IV just before procedure (max 2 mg/dose), may repeat every 3 minutes with a dose of 0.05 mg/kg as needed to maintain sedation (total max 0.3 mg/kg or 10 mg, whichever is less); PO sedation: 0.25 to 1 mg/kg PO 30 to 45 minutes before procedure (max dose: 15 mg); intranasal: 0.2 mg/kg using the 5 mg/mL injection administered with a needleless syringe into the nares; maintenance of sedation (i.e. post intubation): 0.05 to 0.1 mg/kg/dose IV/IM every 1 to 2 hours as needed (max 10 mg/dose); Continuous IV infusion (initial doses, titrate to effect): Infant and child: 1–2 μg/kg/min; *Refractory status epilepticus*: ≥2 month and child: Load with 0.15 mg/kg IV × 1 followed by a continuous infusion of 1 μg/kg/min; titrate dose upward Q5 min to effect (mean dose of 2.3 μg/kg/min with a range of 1–18 μg/kg/ min has been reported.

Precautions: Contraindicated in patients with narrow angle glaucoma and shock. Use with caution in renal disorder, hepatic dysfunction, and in neonates. Causes respiratory depression, hypotension, and bradycardia hence cardiovascular monitoring is recommended. Higher recommended dosage for younger patients (6 mo–5 yr) is due to the water soluble properties of midazolam and the higher percent body water for younger patients.

Adverse effects: Hypotension, bradycardia, paradoxical excitement, local pain at the injection site, laryngospasm, bronchospasm.

Availability: Injection: 1, 5 mg/mL; Oral syrup: 2 mg/mL.

NALOXONE

Route of administration: IV, IM, SC, ETT

Dose: Initial: age birth to 5 years (weight < 20 kg): 0.1 mg/kg/dose; age older than 5 years: 2 mg/dose (max initial dose: 2 mg). If giving via ETT, dose is 2 to 10 times the IV dose diluted in 3 to 5 mL of saline followed by several positive-pressure breaths. Subsequent: The initial dose may be repeated every 3 to 5 minutes up to a maximum of five doses. Graded reversal: 0.001 to 0.01 mg/kg (1 to 10 μg/kg) IV q3–5 min as needed for respiratory depression secondary to PCA/epidural or chronic opiate use.

Adverse effects: May precipitate withdrawal symptoms in narcotic-dependent patients.

Availability: Injection: 0.4, 1 mg/mL.

NICARDIPINE

Route of administration: IV.

Dose: *Hypertensive emergencies*: initial: 1 to 3 μg/kg/minute as a continuous infusion, titrate as needed to maintain BP in desired range. Max of 5 μg/kg/minute. Note: Do not use in patients at risk for increased intracranial pressure.

Adverse effects: Hypotension, reflex tachycardia, phlebitis, increased ICP.

Availability: Injection: 2.5 mg/mL.

NITROPRUSSIDE SODIUM

Route of administration: IV.

Dose: *Hypertensive emergencies*: Initial: 0.5 to 1 µg/kg/minute as a continuous infusion, titrate as needed to maintain BP in desired range. Average 3 µg/kg/minute, max of 10 µg/kg/minute. At doses higher than 4 µg/kg/minute, thiocyanate levels need to be monitored. Note: Sodium nitroprusside is only compatible with D5W and must be protected from light. Nitroprusside has an immediate onset of action. Careful hemodynamic monitoring is essential.

Adverse effects: Usually associated with excessive or rapid lowering of BP. Cyanide intoxication may occur in patients with renal dysfunction and prolonged duration of infusion. Cyanide and thiocyanate levels should be checked in patients receiving nitroprusside for more than 3 days or rates higher than 4 µg/kg/minute. Other effects may include increased ICP, disorientation, nausea, and vomiting.

Availability: Injection: 10, 25 mg/mL.

NOREPINEPHRINE

Route of administration: IV.

Dose: 0.05 to 1 µg/kg/minute as a continuous infusion. Titrate as needed to maintain BP.

Precautions: May begin administration via a peripheral line, changing to central access as soon as possible. Must be further diluted for infusion.

Adverse Effects: Hypertension, organ ischemia, decreased peripheral perfusion.

Availability: Injection: 1 mg/mL.

PHENYTOIN

Route of administration: IV, PO.

Dose: *Status epilepticus*: Loading dose (all ages): 15–20 mg/kg IV; Max. dose: 1500 mg/24 h Maintenance for seizure disorders (initiate 12 h after administration of loading dose): Start with 5 mg/kg/24 h PO/IV ÷ Q12 h; usual range 4–8 mg/kg/24 h PO/IV ÷ Q8–12 h.

Antiarrhythmic (secondary to digitalis intoxication): Load (all ages): 1.25 mg/kg IV Q5 min up to a total of 15 mg/kg; Maintenance: Child (IV/PO): 5–10 mg/kg/24 h ÷ Q8–12 h.

Precautions: Use is contraindicated in patients with heart block or sinus bradycardia. Phenytoin induces hepatic microsomal enzymes (CYP450 1A2, 2C8/9/19, and 3A3/4), leading to decreased effectiveness of fosamprenavir (used without ritonavir), quinidine, valproic acid, theophylline, and other substrates and levels may be increased by cimetidine, chloramphenicol, INH, sulfonamides, trimethoprim, etc. May also cause resistance to neuromuscular blocking action of nondepolarizing neuromuscular blocking agents. T1/2 is variable (7–42 h) and dose-dependent. Drug is highly protein-bound; free fraction of drug will be increased in patients with hypoalbuminemia. For seizure disorders, therapeutic levels: 10–20 mg/L (free and bound phenytoin) OR 1–2 mg/L (free only). Recommended serum sampling times: trough level (PO/IV) within 30 min prior to the next scheduled dose; peak or post load level (IV) 1 h after the end of IV infusion. Steady state is usually achieved after 5–10 days of continuous dosing. For routine monitoring, measure trough.

Adverse effects: Gingival hyperplasia, hirsutism, dermatitis, blood dyscrasia, ataxia, lupus-like and Stevens–Johnson syndromes, lymphadenopathy, liver damage, nystagmus, multiorgan hypersensitivity (DRESS) have been reported. An increased risk for serious skin reactions (e.g. TEN and Stevens–Johnson syndrome) may occur in few patients. IV push/infusion rate: Not to exceed 0.5 mg/kg/min in neonates, or 1 mg/kg/min in infants. Consider fosphenytoin in situations of tenuous IV access and risk for extravasation.

Availability: Chewable tabs 50 mg, Extended-release caps: 30, 100 mg, Oral suspension: 125 mg/5 mL (240 mL); Injection: 50 mg/mL (2, 5 mL).

ROCURONIUM

Route of administration: IV, IM.

Dose: RSI:0.6 to 1.2 mg/kg IV. For IM, use higher end of dosing range (up to 1.8 mg/kg/dose) if giving IM.

Precautions: Use only in the presence of personnel skilled in the management of an artificial airway.

Adverse effects: Respiratory arrest, hyper/hypotension, arrhythmias.

Availability: Injection: 10 mg/mL.

SILDENAFIL

Route of administration: IV, PO.

Dose: *Pulmonary hypertension*: Neonate: PO: 0.5–3 mg/kg/dose Q6–12 h PO. IV: Start with 0.4 mg/kg/dose IV over 3 h followed by a continuous infusion of 1.6 mg/kg/24 h (0.067 mg/kg/h) for up to 7 days. Infant and child : PO: Start at 0.25 mg/kg/dose Q6 h or 0.5 mg/kg/dose Q8 h; if needed, titrate dose up to 1–2 mg/kg/dose Q6–8 h. Child 1–17 yr: PO: ≥8–20 kg: 10 mg TID; >20–45 kg: 20 mg TID; >45 kg: 40 mg TID.

Precautions: Contraindicated with concurrent use of nitrates (e.g., nitroglycerin) and other nitric oxide donors; potentiates hypotensive effects. Use with caution in sepsis (high levels of cGMP may potentiate hypotension), with concurrent CYP450 3A4 inhibiting medications and antihypertensive medications. Hepatic insufficiency or severe renal impairment (GFR < 30 mL/min) significantly reduces sildenafil clearance.

Adverse effects: Headache, abnormal vision, flushing, rash, diarrhea, nasal congestion, hearing loss has been reported. Sildenafil is substrate for CYP450 3A4 (major) and 2C8/9 (minor) hence many drug interactions may occur.

Availability: Tabs: 25, 50, 100 mg; Oral suspension: 2.5 mg/mL,10 mg/mL, Injection: 0.8 mg/mL.

SODIUM BICARBONATE

Route of administration: IV.

Dose: Acidosis Initial: age younger than 1 month or weight less than 5 kg: 1 mEq/kg (2 mL/kg) of 0.5 mEq/mL (4.2%) solution. If only 7.5% or 8.4% solution (1 mEq/mL) is available, dilute 1:1 with D5W before administration; age older than 1 month or > 5 kg: 1 mEq/kg (1 mL/kg) of 1 mEq/mL (8.4%) solution. Subsequent: Corrective NaHCO dose (mEq) = 0.3 × body weight (kg) × base deficit (mEq/L) OR 0.5 × body weight (kg) × (24 - serum HCO_3). Note: Give one-half of this calculated estimate. Continuous infusion: Up to 1 mEq/kg/hour.

Tumor-lysis syndrome: D5W with sodium bicarbonate 75 mEq/L at 125 mL/m^2/hour to maintain urine pH 7 to 8 and SG less than or equal to 1.010. Do not use bicarbonate hydration if also using rasburicase.

Precautions: Sodium bicarbonate should be given by direct IV administration slowly (max rate for infants 10 mEq/minute) and followed by NS flush to avoid precipitation in the IV line with other drugs such as calcium. Sodium bicarbonate should not be given via the ETT because it irritates the upper respiratory tract and lung parenchyma.

Adverse effects: Hypernatremia (contains 11.9 mEq of sodium/1 g), alkalosis, hyperosmolarity.

Availability: Injection: most common concentrations are 0.5 mEq/mL (4.2%) and 1 mEq/mL (8.4%).

SUCCINYLCHOLINE

Route of administration: IV, IM.

Dose: *Intubation*: 1 to 2 mg/kg IV or 2 to 4 mg/kg deep IM (max dose: 150 mg) Use 2 mg/kg IV if younger than 2 years of age.

Precautions: Use only in the presence of personnel skilled in the management of an artificial airway. Avoid using in patients with personal or familial history of malignant hyperthermia, hyperkalemia, burns, renal failure, or myopathy associated with elevated CPK values.

Adverse effects: Hyperkalemia, muscle fasciculation, respiratory depression, malignant hyperthermia, bradycardia, hypotension, cardiac arrhythmias.

Availability: Injection: 20, 50, 100 mg/mL.

THIOPENTAL

Route of administration: IV.

Dose: RSI: 3 to 6 mg/kg IV; Reduction of ICP: 1.5 to 5 mg/kg/dose IV.

Precautions: Do not use in patients with hypotension. Extravascular injection may cause pain, swelling, ulceration, and necrosis.

Adverse effects: Pronounced hypotension, respiratory depression, apnea, delirium, nausea, vomiting.

Availability: Injection: 250 mg, 500 mg, 1 g, 2.5 g, 5 g.

VALPROIC ACID

Route of administration: IV, PO, PR.

Dose: *Status epilepticus*: Load 20 mg/kg IV over 5 minutes; epilepsy: 15 to 60 mg/kg/day in two to three divided doses. Supplemental carnitine is recommended by some experts if using high doses. Oral: Initial: 10–15 mg/kg/24 h ÷ once daily–TID. Increment: 5-10 mg/kg/24 h at weekly intervals to max. dose of 60 mg/kg/24 h. Maintenance: 30–60 mg/kg/24 h ÷ BID–TID, Rectal (use syrup diluted 1: 1 with water, given PR as a retention enema): Load: 20 mg/kg/dose, Maintenance: 10–15 mg/kg/dose Q8 h; Migraine prophylaxis: Child (limited data): 15–30 mg/kg/24 h PO ÷ BID.

Precautions: Valproic acid may interact with the following drugs: clonazepam, phenobarbital, phenytoin, salicylates, and warfarin. Serum drug concentrations should be carefully monitored in patients taking multiple drug products. Monitor liver function tests before and at frequent intervals during therapy. IV doses may need to be divided q6h to maintain adequate levels. Infusion rate is 60 minutes, unless in status epilepticus.

Adverse effects: Nausea, vomiting, hyperammonemia (with or without coma), thrombocytopenia, inhibition of platelet aggregation, hepatotoxicity, sedation.

Availability: Capsules: 250 mg, Delayed-release tablets: 125, 250, 500 mg, Injection: 100 mg/mL, Syrup: 50 mg/mL.

VASOPRESSIN

Route of administration: IV.

Dose: *VF or VT*: Adults: 40 units × 1 dose; GI hemorrhage: 0.002 to 0.005 units/kg/minute IV titrated up to a max of 0.01 unit/kg/minute; *Diabetes Insipidus*: 0.5 milliunits/kg/hour (0.005 units/kg/h) IV to a max of 10 milliunits/kg/h (0.01 units/kg/h).

Precautions: Infiltration of the IV site can result in severe necrosis.

Adverse effects: Hypertension, cardiac arrhythmias, vasoconstriction, nausea, vomiting, water intoxication.

Availability: Injection: 20 units/mL.

Rapid way to calculate:[1]

IV infusions: 6 × desired dose(μg/kg/min)/desired rate (mL/h) × weight (kg) = mg of drug/100 mL of fluid

Medication	*Dose (μg/kg/min)*	*Dilution in 100 mL in a compatible IV fluid*	*IV Infusion rate*
Alprostadil	0.05–0.1	0.3 mg/kg	1mL/h = 0.05 μg/kg/min
Amiodarone	5–15	6 mg/kg	1 mL/h = 1 μg/kg/min
Dopamine	5–20	6 mg/kg	1 mL/h = 1 μg/kg/min
Dobutamine	2–20	6 mg/kg	1 mL/h = 1 μg/kg/min
Epinephrine	0.01–0.2, up to 1 in severe circumstances	0.6 mg/kg	1 mL/h = 0.1 μg/kg/min
Lidocaine	20–50	6 mg/kg	1 mL/h = 1 μg/kg/min
Phenylephrine	0.05–2, up to 5 in severe circumstances	0.3 mg/kg	1 mL/h = 0.05 μg/kg/min
Terbutaline	0.1–4 (up to 10 has been used)	0.6 mg/kg	1 mL/h = 0.1 μg/kg/min
Vasopressin	0.5–2 milliunits/kg/min	6 milliunits/kg	1 mL/h = 1 milliunit/kg/min

Glucose infusion rate (GIR) calculation:

GIR in mg/kg/min = (dextrose% concentration × mL/kg/day)/144

OR

GIR = (D × Rate)/(6 × weight(kg)) i.e. (dextrose % conc × mL/h on the pump)/(6 × wt(kg))

REFERENCE

1. Larsen GY, Parker HB, Cash J, *et al.* Standard drug concentrations and smart-pump technology reduce continuous-medication-infusion errors in pediatric patients. Pediatrics. 2005;116: e21-5.

Annexure

2

Drugs for Emergent Conditions

Arohi Gupta, Abhijeet Saha

ACETAMINOPHEN

Route of administration: PO, PR, IV.

Dose: 15 mg/kg/dose (PO/PR) in four to six divided doses (max daily dose: 90 mg/kg/day or 4 g, whichever is less); IV: administer the dose undiluted over 15 min.

Precautions: No anti-inflammatory activity. Use with caution in patients with known G6PD deficiency and liver disease and adjust dose in renal failure.

Adverse effects: Nausea, vomiting, pruritus, agitation. Rare risk of serious skin reactions (e.g. SJS, TEN) has been reported.

Availability: Chewable tablets: 80, 160 mg; Tablets: 325, 500, 650 mg; Drops: 100 mg/mL; Oral suspension: 24 mg/mL; Capsules with powder for oral solution: 80, 160 mg; Suppositories: 80, 120, 325, 650 mg.

ACYCLOVIR

Route of administration: IV, PO, Topical.

Dose:

Immunocompetent

- Neonatal (*HSV and HSV encephalitis*; birth–3 mo): Initial IV therapy (duration of therapy: 14–21 days): <30-wk postmenstrual age: 40 mg/kg/24 h ÷ Q12 h; IV ≥30-wk postmenstrual age: 60 mg/kg/24 h ÷ Q8 h IV; oral therapy for HSV suppression and neurodevelopment following treatment with IV acyclovir for 14–21 days: 300 mg/m^2/dose Q8 h PO × 6 mo.
- *HSV encephalitis* (duration of therapy: 14–21 days): Birth–3 mo: use above IV dosage; 3 mo–12 y: 60 mg/kg/24 h ÷ Q8 h IV; ≥12 y: 30 mg/kg/24 h ÷ Q8 h IV.
- *Zoster*: IV (all ages): 30 mg/kg/24 h or 1500 mg/m^2/24 h ÷ Q8 h × 7–10 days
- *Varicella*: IV (≥2 y): 30 mg/kg/24 h or 1500 mg/m^2/24 h ÷ Q8 h × 7–10 days; PO (≥2 y): 80 mg/kg/24 h ÷ QID × 5 days (begin treatment at earliest signs/symptoms); max. dose: 3200 mg/24 h.
- *Mucocutaneous HSV (including genital ≥12 y)*: Initial infection: IV: 15 mg/kg/24 h or 750 mg/m^2/24 h ÷ Q8 h × 5- 7 days; PO: 1000–1200 mg/24 h ÷ 3–5 doses/24 h × 7–10 days. For pediatric dosing, use 40–80 mg/kg/24 h ÷ Q6–8 h × 5–10 days (max pediatric dose: 1000 mg/24 h). Recurrence (≥ 12 y): PO: 1000 mg/24 h ÷ 5 doses/24 h × 5 days, or 1600 mg/24 h ÷ Q12 h × 5 days, or 2400 mg/24 h ÷ Q8 h × 2 days. Chronic suppressive therapy (≥ 12 y): PO: 800 mg/24 h ÷ Q12 h for up to 1 year.

Immunocompromised

- *HSV*: IV (all ages): 750–1500 mg/m^2/24 h ÷ Q8 h × 7–14 days PO (≥2 y): 1000 mg/24 h ÷ 3–5 times/24 h × 7–14 days; max dose for child: 80 mg/kg/24 h HSV prophylaxis: IV (all ages): 750 mg/m^2/24 h ÷ Q8 h during risk period. PO (≥2 y): 600–1000 mg/24 h ÷ 3–5 times/24 h during risk period; max dose for child: 80 mg/kg/24 h.
- *Varicella or zoster*: IV (all ages): 1500 mg/m^2/24 h ÷ Q8 h × 7–10 days PO: Infant and child: 20 mg/kg/dose (max 800 mg) Q6 h × 7–10 days; Adolescent and adult: 20 mg/kg/dose (max 800 mg) 5 times daily × 7–10 days.

Precautions: Dosage adjustment required with renal dysfunction and patient should be adequately hydrated.

Adverse effects: Nephrotoxicity, headache, vertigo, GI upset, encephalopathy, GI tract irritation, hepatitis, rash, urticaria, arthralgia, fever, and adverse hematologic effects.

Availability: Injection: 500 mg, 1 g; Capsules: 200 mg; Tablets: 400 mg, 800 mg; Oral suspension: 40 mg/mL; Topical ointment: 5%.

ALBUTEROL

Route of administration: PO, inhalation.

Dose: PO: children (age 2–6 years): Initial dose 0.1 mg/kg/dose given TID (do not exceed 2 mg TID initially). May increase dose gradually to 0.2 mg/kg/dose given TID (not to exceed 12 mg/day); children (6–14 years): initial dose 2 mg given TID to QID. May cautiously increase to a maximum daily dose of 24 mg/day; inhalation: MDI (90 µg/puff): children younger than 12 years: one to two inhalations four times/day; children older than 12 years: one to two inhalations given four to six times daily. PO: *Rotahaler*: older than 4 years: 200 µg every 4 to 6 hours; may increase to 400 µg/dose. *Nebulizer*: 0.15 mg/kg (0.03 mL/kg of 0.5% solution) (maximum single dose: 5 mg or 1 mL of 0.5% solution) every 20 minutes for three doses (may use standard doses of 0.5 mL for <30 kg and 1 mL for >30 kg), then q1–6h. Continuous nebulization 0.5 mg/kg/hour.

Adverse effects: Tachycardia, tremors, palpitations, changes in blood sugar level, hypokalemia.

Availability: Tablets: 2, 4 mg, Extended-release tablets: 4, 8 mg, Oral syrup: 0.4 mg/mL Metered-dose aerosol: each actuation delivers 90 µg of albuterol capsules containing powder for oral inhalation: 200 µg; Solution for nebulization: 0.5% (5 mg/mL) concentrate.

ASPIRIN

Route of administration: PO, PR.

Dose: *Fever/analgesia*: 10 to 15 mg/kg/dose every 4 to 6 hours, max 4 g/day. *Rheumatoid arthritis*: 60 to 90 mg/kg/day initial dose in four divided doses (max dose 4 g/day). *Kawasaki disease*: 80 to 100 mg/kg/day divided every 6 hours until fever resolves, then 3 to 5 mg/kg/day.

Precautions: Avoid use in patients with varicella or influenza and during presumed outbreaks of influenza because of a possible associated risk of Reye syndrome. Use with caution in bleeding disorders or when using concomitantly with other medications that carry a risk of bleeding.

Adverse effects: GI upset, GI bleeding, tinnitus, reduced platelet function, bronchospasm.

Availability: Tablets: 75, 81, 165, 325, 500 mg; Suppositories: 300, 600 mg.

ATENOLOL

Route of administration: PO.

Dose: Initial: 0.8 to 1 mg/kg/day PO daily; maintenance: 0.8 to 2 mg/kg/day PO daily.

Precautions: IV preparation not used in children.

Adverse effects: Hypotension, heart block, headache, wheezing.

Availability: Tablets: 25, 50, 100 mg Injection: 0.5 mg per mL.

CAPTOPRIL

Route of administration: PO.

Dose: *Hypertension*: neonate: 0.01 to 0.1 mg/kg/dose; older infants and children: 0.15 to 0.5 mg/kg/dose (max 12.5 mg initial dose). Twofold increments in the dosage can be made after an observation period of 1 to 2 hours if the initial doses are ineffective. Maintenance doses may be given every 8 to 12 hours.

Precautions: Pronounced hypotension may be observed when captopril is administered in conjunction with diuretics or other antihypertensive drugs. Hyperkalemia may occur when used with potassium-sparing diuretics or potassium supplementation. Dosages should be reduced in patients with impaired renal function. Do not use in patients with bilateral renal artery stenosis or unilateral renal artery stenosis with a solitary kidney as renal blood flow may be severely impaired.

Adverse effects: Excessive lowering of BP, cough, proteinuria, neutropenia, rash, altered taste perception, angioedema.

Availability: Tablets: 12.5, 25, 50, 100 mg.

CARBAMAZEPINE

Route of administration: PO.

Dose: Initial:5 to 10 mg/kg/day in three to four divided doses, increasing every 5 to 7 days as needed. Usual maintenance: 15 to 35 mg/kg/day in three to four divided doses for immediate-release products and in two divided doses for extended-release products (max 1,200 mg/day).

Precautions: Major drug interactions may occur with other medications metabolized via the 3A3/4 and 2C19 enzyme pathways. Carbamazepine induces its own metabolism approximately 14 days after starting therapy; therefore, a dose increase may be required at this time. Serum trough concentrations of carbamazepine (therapeutic 4 to 12 mg/dL) and any other concomitant anticonvulsants should be monitored.

Adverse effects: Hepatotoxicity, ataxia, transient leukopenia, aplastic anemia, GI upset, constipation, rash, Stevens-Johnson syndrome.

Availability: Tablets: 100 mg (chewable), 200-mg tablets, extended-release: 100, 200, 400 mg capsules, extended-release: 200, 300 mg; Oral suspension: 20 mg/mL.

CEFIXIME

Route of administration: PO

Dose: Age older than 6 months: 8 mg/kg/day in one to two divided doses (max 400 mg/day); gonorrhea: 400 mg PO as a single dose.

Adverse effects: Nausea, vomiting, diarrhea.

Availability: Oral suspension: 20 mg/mL Tablets: 200, 400 mg.

CEFOTAXIME

Route of administration: IV, IM.

Dose: Age younger than 1 week: 100 mg/kg/day in two divided doses; age 1 to 4 weeks: 150 mg/kg/day in three divided doses; age 1 month to 12 years: 50 to 200 mg per kg/day in four to six equally divided doses (max 12 g/day).

Precautions. Use with caution in penicillin-allergic patients and in the presence of renal impairment (reduce dosage). Probenecid increases serum cefotaxime levels.

Adverse effects: Allergy, neutropenia, thrombocytopenia, eosinophilia, elevated blood urine nitrogen (BUN), creatinine, and liver enzymes.

Availability: Injection: 1-, 2-g vials.

CEFTRIAXONE

Route of administration: IV, IM

Dose: Usual dose: 50 to 100 mg/kg/day in one or two divided doses. *Bacterial meningitis*: Initial dosage should be 100 mg/kg as a single dose followed by 100 mg/kg/day in two divided doses (max 2,000 mg/dose). *Uncomplicated gonorrhea*: 125 mg IM single dose; use 250 mg IM single dose if concomitant PID (max 4 g/day). Chancroid: 250 mg IM single dose.

Adverse effects: Neutropenia, thrombocytopenia, eosinophilia, allergy, elevated blood urine nitrogen (BUN), creatinine, and liver enzymes, biliary sludging/cholelithiasis; avoid use in neonates with hyperbilirubinemia because ceftriaxone has been shown to displace bilirubin from albumin-binding sites, possibly leading to kernicterus.

Availability: Injection: 250-, 500-mg vials; 1-, 2-g vials.

CETIRIZINE

Route of administration: PO

Dose: 2 to 5 years: 2.5 to 5 mg/day in one to two divided doses. Older than 5 years: 5 to 10 mg/day in one to two divided doses.

Adverse effects: Drowsiness, GI distress, paresthesias, cough, bronchospasm.

Availability: Tablets: 5, 10 mg; Oral solution: 1 mg/mL.

CHARCOAL, ACTIVATED

Route of administration: PO

Dose: 1 g/kg (or approximately 5 to 10 times the amount of poison ingested), max 100 g/dose. Multiple doses should be considered for ingestions that are extended-release preparations or undergo enterohepatic circulation.

Precautions: Do not administer concurrently with syrup of ipecac or dairy products. Adequate airway protection is essential.

Adverse effects: Use sorbitol containing suspensions as initial dose with caution, generally not recommended in children. Sorbitol acts as a cathartic. Plain charcoal suspensions should be used for subsequent doses. Careful monitoring of fluid and electrolyte status is essential in patients receiving sorbitol. Vomiting, constipation, or diarrhea may occur.

Availability: Loose powder for suspension, mix in 6 to 8 oz of water; Oral suspension in aqueous or sorbitol solution:

many strengths such as 15 g in 75 mL or 120 mL, 30 g in 120 mL, or 50 g in 250 mL.

CHLORAL HYDRATE

Route of administration: PO, PR.

Dose: *Hypnosis*: 25 to 50 mg/kg/dose; may be repeated once at half the initial dose (max 1 g/dose).

Procedural sedation: 50 to 100 mg/kg/dose; may be repeated once at 25 to 75 mg/kg/dose for inadequate sedation (total max 1 g infants, 2 g children). Administer capsule with full glass of water or fruit juice. Dilute chloral hydrate syrup in water or fruit juice before administration.

Adverse effects: CNS depression, vomiting, abdominal pain.

CIPROFLOXACIN

Route of administration: PO, IV.

Dose: 20 to 30 mg/kg/day in two divided doses (max 800 mg/day IV, 1,500 mg/day PO); *P. aeruginosa*: 30 mg IV/kg/day IV divided q12h (max 1,200 mg/day).

Precautions: Currently not approved for use in younger children.

Adverse effects: Tendonitis, headache, rash, photosensitivity, GI distress, interstitial nephritis.

Availability: Oral suspension 50, 100 mg/mL; Tablets: 100, 250, 500, 750 mg; Injection: 200–400 mg premixed infusions/vials.

CLONAZEPAM

Route of administration: PO.

Dose: Initial: 0.01 to 0.03 mg/kg/day in two to three divided doses, increase slowly; Maintenance: 0.1 to 0.2 mg/kg/day in two to three divided doses.

Adverse effects: Sedation, hypotension, nausea, vomiting, anorexia.

Availability: Tablets: 0.5, 1, 2 mg.

CLONIDINE

Route of administration: PO, topical, epidural.

Dose: *Hypertension*: Initial:0.005 to 0.01 mg/kg/day PO divided q8–12h; maintenance: 0.005 to 0.025 mg/kg/day PO divided q6h (max 0.9 mg/day); *ADHD*: initial: 0.05 mg/day, increase every 3 to 7 days to 0.003 to 0.008 mg/kg/day PO divided TID-QID (max 0.4 mg/day).

Adverse effects: Hypotension, sedation, rash, GI upset.

Availability: Tablets: 0.1, 0.2 mg; Transdermal patches: 0.1, 0.2, 0.3 mg; Injection: 100 µg/mL.

DESMOPRESSIN

Route of administration: Intranasal, SC, IV.

Dose: *Acute hemophilia, von Willebrand*: 0.3 µg/kg IV over 30 minutes or high dose nasal spray; *Enuresis/diabetes insipidus*: LOW-DOSE nasal spray.

Note: Do not use in patients younger than 2 years old.

Adverse effects: Facial flushing, headache, hypertension, water retention, hyponatremic seizures.

Availability: Injection 4 µg/mL; Intranasal 100 µg/mL or 1.5 mg/mL; Tablet 0.1 mg, 0.2 mg; Tablet sublingual 60, 120, and 240 µg.

DEXAMETHASONE

Route of administration: PO, IM, IV.

Dose: *Dependent on disease*: usual range is 0.024 to 1 mg/kg/day. *Croup*: 0.6 mg/kg/dose (usual max 12 mg/dose); *Inflammation*: 0.5 to 2 mg/kg/day divided q6–8h; *Bacterial meningitis*: 0.6 mg/kg/day IV in four divided doses; *Epidural abscess/cerebral edema*: 2 mg/kg IV load (max 100 mg) followed by 1 to 2 mg/kg/day in four divided doses for 24 hours.

Adverse effects: Hyperglycemia, sodium and water retention, hypokalemia, hypertension, leukocytosis, behavioral disturbances, peptic ulcer.

Availability: Injection: 4, 8, 10, 16, 20, 24 mg/mL; Tablets: various strengths ranging from 0.25 to 6 mg/tablet.

DIAZEPAM

Route of administration: PO, IV, PR.

Dose: *Status epilepticus*: 0.05 to 0.3 mg/kg/dose IV over 3 to 5 minutes every 15 minutes to a cumulative maximum total dose of 0.75 mg/kg or 10 mg, whichever is less. *Epilepsy*: 0.1 to 0.8 mg/kg/day PO divided q6–8h; sedation:1 to 2.5 mg/dose PO, TID-QID. Alternatively, initial dosages of 0.1 to 0.3 mg/kg/day PO in two to three divided doses may be used; PR: 0.5 mg/kg (max 20 mg/dose), then 0.25 mg/kg in 10 minutes if needed.

Precautions: When given IV for status epilepticus, dose may be repeated at 15-minute intervals to a maximum total of 0.75 mg/kg or 10 mg, whichever is less.

Adverse effects: Sedation, cardiorespiratory depression, hypotension.

Availability: Injection: 5 mg/mL; Tablets: 2, 5, 10 mg; Oral solution: 1,5 mg/mL; Rectal gel: 2.5, 5, 10, 20 mg.

DIAZOXIDE

Route of administration: IV, PO.

Dose: *Hypertensive crisis*: 1 to 3 mg/kg/dose (max: 150 mg) given by rapid IV injection: over 10 to 30 seconds. Dose may be repeated in 5 to 15 minutes, if necessary (max 10 to 15 mg/kg/day); hyperinsulinemic hypoglycemia (PO): newborns/ infants: initial dosage of 10 mg/kg/day PO in two to three divided doses; maintenance: 8 to 15 mg/kg/day PO in two to three divided doses. Children and adults: initial dosage of 3 mg/kg/day PO in two to three divided doses; maintenance: 3 to 8 mg/kg/day PO in two to three divided doses.

Precautions: Severe orthostatic hypotension may occur after IV administration.

Adverse effects: Hyperglycemia, tachycardia, salt and water retention, nausea, vomiting.

Availability: Injection: 15 mg/mL; Oral capsules: 50 mg; Oral suspension: 50 mg/mL.

DIGOXIN

Route of administration: PO, IV.

Dose:

Digoxin digitalizing and maintenance doses

Age	TDD		Daily maintenance	
	PO	IV/IM	PO	IV/IM
Premature neonate	20	15	5	3–4
Full-term neonate	30	20	8–10	6–8
1 mo <2 y	40–50	30–40	10–12	7.5–9
2–10 y	30–40	20–30	8–10	6–8
>10 y and <100 kg	10–15	8–12	2.5–5	2–3

Initial: 1/2 TDD, then 1/4 TDD Q8–18 h × 2 doses; obtain electrocardiogram (ECG) 6 h after dose to assess for toxicity.

Maintenance: <10 y: Give maintenance dose ÷ BID ≥10 y: Give maintenance dose once daily.

Precautions: Contraindicated in patients with ventricular dysrhythmias. Use with caution in renal failure, calcium channel blockers (may result in heart block), and adenosine [enhanced depressant effects on sinoatrial (SA) and atrioventricular (AV) nodes]. Decreased serum potassium and magnesium or increased magnesium and calcium may increase risk for digoxin toxicity.

Adverse effects: Nausea, vomiting, weakness, worsening of preexisting heart failure, arrhythmias.

Availability: Injection: Lanoxin 100 µg/mL; Lanoxin and generics: 250 µg/mL (2 mL); Tabs: 125, 250 µg; Oral solution: 50 µg/mL (60 mL).

DIGOXIN IMMUNE FAB

Route of administration: IV.

Dose: Initial: Determine the TBL (total body load) of digoxin: Divide the TBL by 0.5 to get the initial number of vials to treat empirically. If the amount of digoxin ingested is known, multiply by 0.8 to determine TBL and infuse over 5 minutes.

Adverse effects: Anaphylaxis, hypotension, chills, wheezing, hypokalemia, arrhythmias.

Availability: Powder for injection: vial 38 mg.

DIHYDROERGOTAMINE

Route of administration: IV, IM, SC, Intranasal.

Dose: *Migraine headache*: 0.5 mg intranasal, may repeat in 15 minutes if necessary up to a total 4 mg. 1 mg if giving via IM/SC/IV injection, may repeat up to a total of 3 mg for IM/SC or 2 mg for IV. Maximum for all routes is 6 mg/week.

Adverse effects: Nausea, vomiting, paresthesias, cramping, subarachnoid hemorrhage, ergot poisoning.

Note: Do not use in renal dysfunction, cardiac disease or if a triptan has been used in the past 24 hours. Many dangerous drug interactions may occur.

Availability: Injection 1 mg/mL; nasal spray 4 mg/mL.

DOXYCYCLINE

Route of administration: PO, IV.

Dose: *Acute pelvic inflammatory disease/chlamydial infections*: 100 mg BID; *Anthrax, other severe susceptible infections*: 2 to 5 mg/kg/day in two divided doses (max 200 mg/day).

Precautions: Due to teeth staining, limit use to patients older than 8 years of age and weighing more than 45 kg. Rocky Mountain spotted fever and anthrax should be treated with doxycycline, regardless of age.

Adverse effects: GI distress, photosensitivity, pseudotumor cerebri.

Availability: Capsules: 50, 100 mg; Tablets: 100 mg; Powder for oral suspension: 5 mg/mL when reconstituted Syrup, suspension: 10 mg/mL; Injection: 100 mg/vial.

ENOXAPARIN

Route of administration: SC.

Dose: Adjust dose based on anti-Xa levels. Deep vein thrombosis (DVT) treatment: younger than 2 months: 1.5 mg/kg/dose SC BD; older than 2 months: 1 mg/kg/dose SC BD; DVT prophylaxis: younger than 2 months: 0.75 mg/kg/dose SC BD; older than 2 months: 0.5 mg/kg/dose SC BD.

Precautions: Do not use in patients with active hemorrhage or risk of GI bleeding.

Adverse effects: Hemorrhage, edema, local irritation.

Availability: Injection 100 mg/mL.

FLUTICASONE

Route of administration: Oral inhalation, nasal spray

Dose: Oral inhalation (MDI) depends on disease severity and previous steroid requirements. Nasal spray: 1 squirt to each nostril daily.

Adverse effects: Dry, itchy mouth and throat, hoarseness, epistaxis (nasal spray).

Note: Use spacer device. Instruct patient to use bronchodilator prior to fluticasone dose.

Availability: Oral inhalation: 44, 110, 220 µg/actuation; Nasal spray: 50 µg/spray.

FUROSEMIDE

Route of administration: IV.

Dose: IV: Initial: 1 mg/kg over 1 to 2 minutes (max initial dose: 40 mg); subsequent: if no response in 20 to 30 minutes, a repeat dose of 1 to 2 mg/kg may be given. Continuous infusion: 0.05 to 0.1 mg/kg/hour, usual max 6 mg/kg/day; oral: 1 to 2 mg/kg/dose every 6 hours.

Precautions: Hypokalemia in a patient on digoxin may result in the development of life-threatening arrhythmias.

Adverse effects: Hypokalemia, hypocalcemia, metabolic alkalosis, hypotension.

Availability: Injection: 10 mg/mL; Tablet: 20, 40, 80 mg; Oral solution: 8, 10 mg/mL.

HALOPERIDOL

Route of administration: PO, IM.

Dose: Age older than 3 years: initial dose: 0.01 to 0.03 mg/kg/day in two to three divided doses. Acute agitation: 0.025 to 0.075 mg/kg/dose q6h. Usual maintenance: 0.05 to 0.15 mg/kg/day in two to three divided doses (max 6 mg/day).

Adverse effects: Dystonic reactions, tardive dyskinesia, hypotension, rash.

Availability: Injection (lactate salt): 5 mg/mL; Tablets: 0.5, 1, 2, 5, 10, 20 mg; Oral solution: 2 mg/mL.

HYDROCORTISONE

Route of administration: PO, IM, IV.

Dose: *Acute adrenal insufficiency*: 1 to 2 mg/kg IV initial dose, followed by 3 to 5 mg/kg/day in four divided doses; *Status asthmaticus*: 4 to 8 mg/kg IV initial dose followed by 2 to 4 mg/kg/day in four to six divided doses; *Shock*: 50 mg/kg IV initial dose followed by 50 to 75 mg/kg/day in four to six divided doses for 2 days (max 2 g/dose).

Adverse effects: Hypokalemia, hyperglycemia, sodium and water retention, hypertension, leukocytosis, behavioral disturbances.

Availability: Injection: 100, 250, 500 mg, and 1 g/vial; Tablets: 20 mg; Oral suspension: 2 mg/mL.

HYDROXOCOBALAMIN

Route of administration: IV.

Dose: *Cyanide toxicity*: 70 mg/kg IV over 15 minutes (max 5 g/dose), may repeat dose.

Precautions: Will interfere with colorimetric tests, such as bilirubin and co-oximetry.

Adverse effects: Headache, hypertension, discoloration of skin.

Availability: Injection: 5-g kit.

HYDROXYCHLOROQUINE

Route of administration: PO.

Dose: *Malaria prophylaxis*: 5 mg/kg (base) once/week; malaria treatment: 10 mg/kg (base) load, then 5 mg/kg (base) daily; *Rheumatoid arthritis*: 3 to 6 mg/kg/day in a single daily dose (max 400 mg/day).

Precautions: This drug should be given with extreme caution to children and to any patients with potential G6PD deficiency.

Adverse effects: Headache, rash, corneal deposits, drowsiness, visual disturbances, retinopathy, discoloration of skin and mucous membranes, alopecia, blood dyscrasias, behavioral changes.

Availability: Tablets: 200 mg hydroxychloroquine sulfate (equivalent to 155 mg of hydroxychloroquine base).

IBUPROFEN

Route of administration: PO.

Dose: *Fever*: 10 mg/kg/dose every 6 to 8 hours (max 1,200 mg/day); *Inflammatory diseases*: 30 to 50 mg/kg/day in three or four divided doses (max 3,200 mg/day); *Analgesia*: 4 to 10 mg/kg/dose every 6 to 8 hours (max 1,200 mg/day).

Precautions: Avoid in patients with aspirin hypersensitivity and bleeding disorders. Administer doses with food or milk.

Adverse effects: GI upset, bleeding, headache, fluid retention, acute renal failure.

Availability: Tablets: 200, 300, 400, 600 mg; Chewable tablets: 50, 100 mg; Oral suspension: 20 mg/mL; Oral drops: 40 mg/mL.

IPRATROPIUM BROMIDE

Route of administration: Oral inhalation, nasal inhalation.

Dose: Nebulization: *Acute asthma*: weight less than 10 kg: 0.25 mg every 20 minutes for three doses, then q4–6h if needed; weight more than 10 kg: 0.5 mg every 20 minutes for three doses, then q4–6h if needed;*MDI*: 3 to 12 years: 1 to 2 puffs TID (max 6 puffs/24 hours); older than 12 years: 2 puffs QID (max 12 puffs/24 hours); nasal spray: 2 sprays each nostril two to four times/day.

Adverse effects: Pharyngitis, blurred vision, nervousness, dyspnea, dizziness.

Availability: Metered-dose aerosol: 18 μg/spray; Solution for nebulization: 0.02% (0.5 mg/2.5 mL); Nasal spray: 0.03%, 0.06%.

MEROPENEM

Route of administration: IV.

Dose: 60 to 120 mg/kg/day divided every 8 hours, use higher dose in meningitis (max 6 g/day).

Adverse effects: Hypotension, seizures, nausea, vomiting, neutropenia, transient elevation of liver enzymes.

Availability: Injection: 500 mg, 1 g.

METHYLENE BLUE

Route of administration: IV.

Dose: *Methemoglobinemia*: 1 to 2 mg/kg/dose (infuse over 5 minutes); may repeat after 1 hour, if needed.

Adverse effects: Hypertension, discoloration of urine and feces, nausea, vomiting, abdominal pain, excessive formation of methemoglobin, cyanosis.

Availability: Injection: 10 mg/mL.

METOCLOPRAMIDE

Route of administration: PO, IV.

Dose: 0.1 to 0.2 mg/kg/dose PO/IV every 6 hours, max 10 mg/dose. Higher doses of 1 mg/kg/dose (max 50 mg/dose) may be used for acetaminophen overdose or chemotherapy-induced nausea and vomiting. Prophylactic diphenhydramine may be beneficial in decreasing extrapyramidal side effects seen with higher doses.

Adverse effects: Dystonic reactions, hypertension, bradycardia, agitation, hallucinations, constipation, diarrhea.

Availability: Injection: 5 mg/mL; Solution: 1, 10 mg/mL; Tablets: 5, 10 mg.

METRONIDAZOLE

Route of administration: PO, IV.

Dose: *Antibiotic-associated pseudomembranous colitis*: 20 to 35 mg/kg/day in four divided doses. *Amebiasis*: 35 to 50 mg/kg/day PO in three divided doses for 5 to 10 days (max 750 mg TID). *Giardiasis*: 15 mg/kg/day PO in three divided doses for 5 days (max 250 mg TID). *Helicobacter pylori infection*: 15 to 20 mg/kg/day in two divided doses for 4 weeks (max 1 to 1.5 g/day). *Trichomonas vaginalis*: 15 mg/kg/day PO in three divided doses for 7 days (max 1 g/day); usual adult dose: 500 mg PO BID for 7 days or a single dose of 2 g. IV: 30 mg/kg/day divided every 6 hours; IV doses should be administered over 1 hour (max 4 g/day).

Precautions: Disulfiram-like reaction may occur with ingestion of alcohol. Palatability is poor and compliance may be an issue.

Adverse effects: Metallic taste, GI distress, peripheral neuropathy.

Availability: Tablets: 250, 500 mg; Injection: 5 mg/mL

MORPHINE SULFATE

Route of administration: PO, IM, IV, SC.

Dose: Oral: 0.1 to 0.5 mg/kg/dose PO q4–6h as needed Initial (SC, IM, IV): younger than 6 months: 0.05 mg/kg/dose IV every 2 to 4 hours as needed; older than 6 months: 0.1 mg/kg every 2 to 6 hours as needed (usual max 10 mg/dose). Initial IV infusion: 0.01 to 0.04 mg/kg/hour (postoperative pain) or 0.04 to 0.07 mg/kg/hour (sickle cell or cancer pain). For neonates, use an initial rate of 0.01 mg/kg/hour. Maximum initial dose: 2 mg/hour.

Precautions: IV morphine should be administered slowly (over 4 to 5 minutes) while monitoring respiratory rate, BP, and heart rate.

Adverse effects: Bradycardia, respiratory depression, apnea, hypotension, rash, allergic reaction.

Availability: Oral solution: 2, 4, 20 mg/mL; Tablets: 15, 30 mg; Sustained release tablets: 15, 30, 60 mg; Injection: Multiple concentrations ranging from 2 to 15 mg/mL.

NIFEDIPINE

Route of administration: PO.

Dose: Hypertensive emergencies (child): Clinical experience is limited but doses in the range of 0.25 to 0.5 mg/kg/dose have been used (max 10 mg/dose).

Note: Rapid reduction of BP occurs when administered sublingually or intrabuccally by puncturing or chewing the liquid-filled capsule and expressing the liquid into the mouth.

Precautions: Additive or synergistic hypotension occurs with other antihypertensives.

Adverse effects: Hypotension, worsening of heart failure, dizziness, flushing, peripheral edema.

Availability: Capsules: 10, 20 mg; Extended-release tablets: 30, 60, 90 mg.

NORETHINDRONE

Route of administration: PO.

Dose: Amenorrhea, uterine bleeding: 2.5 to 10 mg/day norethindrone acetate, 5 to 20 mg/day of norethindrone.

Precautions: Contraindicated in patients with history of thromboembolic disorders.

Adverse effects: Breakthrough bleeding, edema, weight loss or gain, mental depression.

Availability: Tablets: 5 mg norethindrone, 5 mg norethindrone acetate.

OCTREOTIDE

Route of administration: IV, SC.

Dose: *Diarrhea*: 1 to 10 μg/kg/dose every 12 hours; *GI hemorrhage*: initial: 1 to 2 μg/kg, max 50 μg/dose, followed by a continuous infusion 1 to 2 μg/kg/hour, max 50 μg/hour; sulfonylurea overdose: 1 to 2 μg/kg, max 50 μg/dose.

Adverse effects: Hyper/hypotension, palpitations, anxiety, headache, fever, rash, hyper/hypoglycemia.

Availability: Injection: 0.05, 0.1, 0.2, 0.5, 1 mg/mL Depot injection: 10, 20, 30 mg.

OMEPRAZOLE

Route of administration: PO

Dose: 0.6 to 1 mg/kg/dose daily, may increase to 3.3 mg/kg/day divided BID; usual adult: 20 mg/dose.

Precautions: Possible drug interactions with other medications metabolized via the CYP3A3/4 enzyme pathway.

Adverse effects: GI distress, tachycardia, bradycardia, insomnia, anxiety, rash, myalgias, tinnitus.

Availability: Capsules, delayed release: 10, 20, 40 mg.

ONDANSETRON

Route of administration: PO, IV, IM.

Dose: *Nononcology nausea and vomiting*: 0.15 mg/kg/dose PO/IV/IM every 8 hours as needed. Age-based dosing:

6 months to 1 year: 2 mg; 1 to 12 years:4 mg; >12 years: 8 mg/dose; *Chemotherapy associated nausea and vomiting*: 0.45 mg/kg/day IV/PO divided every 8 to 24 hours.

Adverse effects: Headache, dizziness, seizures, tachycardia, bradycardia, rash, fever.

Availability: Injection: 2 mg/mL; Solution: 0.8 mg/mL; Tablet: 4, 8 mg Tablet, orally dissolving: 4, 8 mg.

PANTOPRAZOLE

Route of administration: IV, PO.

Dose: 0.5 to 1 mg/kg/day given IV/PO q12–24h, 0.1 mg/kg/hour for continuous infusion.

Precautions: *Vessel irritant*: dilute to 4 mg/mL for intermittent infusion, 0.8 mg/mL for continuous infusion.

Adverse effects: Phlebitis, GI distress, myalgia, arthralgia diarrhea.

Availability: Injection: 40 mg/vial; Tablets: 20,40 mg; Oral suspension (compounded): 2 mg/mL.

PHENOBARBITAL

Route of administration: PO, IM, IV.

Dose: Initial: 10 to 20 mg/kg; Subsequent infants and children: 3 to 6 mg/kg/day in two divided doses.

Precautions: Administer by IV route at a rate no faster than 1 mg/kg/minute. Serum concentrations should be monitored.

Adverse effects: Cardiorespiratory depression, sedation, ataxia, paradoxical excitation, hypotension.

Availability: Injection: 30, 60, 65, 130 mg/mL; Tablets: 8, 15, 30, 60, 100 mg;Oral elixir: 3, 4 mg/mL.

PHENTOLAMINE

Route of administration: IM, IV.

Dose: *Hypertensive crisis*: 0.05 to 0.1 mg/kg/dose, do not exceed 5 mg/dose; Vasoconstrictor infiltration: Infants: 2.5 to 5 mg diluted in 10 mL of NS. Children and adolescents: 5 to 10 mg diluted in 10 mL of NS.

Precautions: Must be on CV monitor for intravenous/intramuscular doses.

Adverse effects: Hypotension, cardiac arrhythmias.

Availability: Injection: 5 mg/mL.

PHYTONADIONE (VITAMIN K)

Route of administration: Subcutaneous, IM, IV, PO.

Dose: *Life-threatening bleeding*: Infants and children: 5 mg/dose IV, *Non-life-threatening serious bleeding*: Infants and children: 0.5 to 2.5 mg SC or IV.

Precautions: Subcutaneous administration strongly preferred when possible due to serious infusion reactions occurring with IV administration. Dilute in 5 to 10 mL of NS for IV administration, give no faster than 1 mg/minute.

Adverse effects: Anaphylactoid reactions, hypotension.

Availability: Injection: 2, 10 mg/mL Tablet: 5 mg.

PIPERACILLIN/TAZOBACTAM

Route of administration: IV.

Dose: Dose is based on piperacillin component. Usual 200 to 300 mg/kg/day divided every 6 hours. Cystic fibrosis: 300 to 500 mg/kg/day divided every 6 hours. Max 18 g/day as piperacillin.

Adverse effects: Allergic reactions, interstitial nephritis, nausea, vomiting, diarrhea, seizures.

Availability: Injection: 2.25, 3.375, 4.5 g.

POLYETHYLENE GLYCOL

Route of administration: PO.

Dose: *Disimpaction*: 1 to 1.5 g/kg/day (max 100 g/day) PO daily for 3 days. *Constipation*: <10 kg: 4.25 g/day, 10 to 30 kg: 8.5 g/day, >30 kg: 17 g/day.

Adverse effects: Diarrhea, electrolyte imbalance with overdose.

Availability: Powder for suspension.

POLYSTYRENE SULFONATE, SODIUM

Route of administration: PO, PR.

Dose: 1 g/kg/dose (max 60 g/dose); 1 g of resin binds approximately 1 mEq of potassium. Administer powder orally as a suspension in water. Dilute each 1 g of powder to at least 4 mL. If administering via NG tube, dilute suspension 1:1 with tap water to aid in delivery. If administered rectally, give as a retention enema. PR administration is generally less effective than PO administration. Enema should be retained for at least 30 minutes.

Precautions: Monitor serum electrolytes. Each gram of resin contains approximately 4 mEq of sodium. Resin delivers 1 mEq of sodium for each 1 mEq of potassium removed. Resin may also bind other cations (e.g. calcium, magnesium).

Availability: Suspension: 0.25 g sodium polystyrene sulfonate/1 mL.

POTASSIUM CHLORIDE

Route of administration: PO, IV.

Dose: *Oral, hypokalemia*: 1 to 2 mEq/kg/day; IV dosing and infusion use 0.5 mEq/kg/dose (max 40 mEq) infused over 2 hours at 0.1 mEq/mL for peripheral line, 0.2 mEq/mL for central line infusion.

Precautions: Ensure adequate monitoring (laboratory, urine output, and cardiorespiratory). Use caution in patients with renal dysfunction.

Adverse effects: Arrhythmias, GI erosion, rash.

Availability: Capsules 8, 10 mEq; Liquid 20 mEq/15 mL, 40 mEq/15 mL; Capsules extended release 8, 10, 20 mEq; Powder for reconstitution 20, 25 mEq; Injection 2 mEq/mL concentrated; 10, 20, 30, and 40 mEq mixed in 100 mL NS.

PREDNISOLONE

Route of administration: PO.

Dose: *Acute asthma*: 1–2 mg/kg 1 dose, then 2 mg/kg/day in two divided doses; anti-inflammatory: 0.5 to 2 mg/kg/day in divided doses. Max 80 mg/dose.

Precautions: Every-other-day therapy is advised once dosage is established to minimize adrenal suppression and growth retardation.

Adverse effects: Hypotension and vasodilation may occur with rapid IV injection. Electrolyte abnormalities, mood disturbances, infection.

Availability: Oral solution: 3 mg/mL; Tablets: 5 mg; Oral disintegrating tablets: 15 mg, 30 mg.

PROCAINAMIDE

Route of administration: PO, IM, IV.

Dose: PO: 15 to 50 mg/kg/day in four to eight divided doses (for prompt-release products); once stabilized, therapy can be changed to sustained-release product at same total daily dosage but administered in four divided doses; IV: Initial loading dose of 3 to 7 mg/kg/dose (max 100 mg/dose) diluted and given slowly over 5 minutes, may be repeated after 10 to 30 minutes; continuous IV infusion: 20 to 80 μg/kg/minute (0.02 to 0.08 mg/kg/minute); maximum total daily dose: 2 to 4 g PO or IM, or 1 to 2 g IV.

Precautions: IV administration may cause hypotension if given too rapidly or in excessive doses. Dosage adjustment is recommended for patients with reduced renal function. Avoid using in patients with myasthenia gravis or second- or third-degree heart block.

Adverse effects: Mental confusion, myocardial depression, cardiac arrhythmias, lupus-like syndrome, nausea, vomiting.

Availability: Injection: 100, 500 mg/mL; Capsules/tablets: 250, 375, 500 mg Tablets, extended-release: 250, 500, 750 mg; 1 g: Twice-daily extended-release: 500 mg, 1 g.

PROPRANOLOL

Route of administration: PO, IV.

Dose: IV: *Acute antiarrhythmic*: 0.01 to 0.1 mg/kg/dose given slowly (max 1 mg/dose) every 6 to 8 hours as needed; PO: *Hypertension*: usual starting dose 0.5 to 1 mg/kg/day in four divided doses; maintenance dose 1 to 5 mg/kg/day in two to four divided doses (max 240 mg/day); *Migraine prophylaxis*: 0.6 to 1.5 mg/kg/day in three divided doses, max 4 mg/kg/day.

Precautions: IV injection should be given slowly over 10 minutes. Use with extreme caution, if at all, in patients with asthma, diabetes, or CHF.

Adverse effects: Myocardial depression, hypoglycemia, nausea, vomiting.

Availability: Injection: 1 mg/mL; Tablets: 10, 20, 40, 60, 80 mg; Oral solution: 4, 8, 80 mg/mL.

PYRIDOSTIGMINE

Route of administration: PO, IM, IV.

Dose: PO: *Myasthenia gravis*: usual starting dose 1 mg/kg/dose every four hours; IV/IM: 0.05 to 0.15 mg/kg/dose (max 10 mg/dose). *Reversal of NMBA*: 0.1 to 0.25 mg/kg/dose IV (max 20 mg/dose).

Precautions: Must use atropine or glycopyrrolate for secretion control when reversing NMBAs.

Adverse effects: Increased respiratory secretions, nausea, vomiting, cramping, diarrhea.

Availability: Tablets 60 mg; Injection: 5 mg/mL Syrup: 12 mg/mL.

RABIES IMMUNE GLOBULIN

Route of administration: IM, infiltration around wound.

Dose: 20 units/kg administered at the same time as rabies vaccine, but in a different site. Use one-half the dose to infiltrate the wound site unless the wound involves mucous membranes.

Adverse effects: Local soreness, muscle stiffness at injection site, fever.

Availability: Injection: 150 units/mL.

RABIES VIRUS VACCINE

Route of administration: IM.

Dose: *Postexposure prophylaxis*: Five doses of 1 mL each administered on days 0, 3, 7, 14, and 28. Low risk patients do not require day 28 dose. The first dose should be administered at the same time as the immunoglobulin, but in a different muscle.

Adverse effects: Local pain and erythema, fever, encephalomyelitis, peripheral neuropathy.

Availability: Injection: 2.5 U/mL.

RANITIDINE

Route of administration: IV, PO.

Dose: IV: 1 mg/kg/dose IV every 8 hours (max 50 mg/dose); continuous infusion: 0.15 mg/kg/hour; oral: 2 mg/kg/dose PO every 12 hours (max 150 mg/dose). Higher dosages may be necessary in pathologic hypersecretory conditions.

Adverse effects: Dizziness, headache, bradycardia, rash, thrombocytopenia.

Availability: Injection: 25 mg/mL; Oral liquid: 15 mg/mL; Tablets: 75, 150, 300 mg.

RASBURICASE

Route of administration: IV.

Dose: IV: 0.15 to 0.2 mg/kg/dose IV rounded to the nearest vial size.

Note: Do NOT use alkaline hydration prior to rasburicase (use hydration without sodium bicarbonate). Allopurinol should not be given simultaneously with rasburicase.

Adverse effects: Dizziness, headache, nausea, severe hemolysis (G6PD).

Availability: Injection: 1.5, 7.5 mg.

RIFAMPIN/RIFAMPICIN

Route of administration: PO.

Dose: *Prophylaxis against H. influenzae type b*: age younger than 1 month: 10 mg/kg/day as a single daily dose for 4 days; age 1 month to 12 years: 20 mg/kg/day as a single daily dose for 4 days (max 600 mg); *Prophylaxis against Neisseria meningitidis*: age younger than 1 month: 10 mg/kg/day in two divided doses for 2 days; age 1 month 12 years: 20 mg/kg/day in two divided doses for 2 days (max 1,200 mg); *Tuberculosis*: age older than 1 week: 10 to 20 mg/kg/day (maximum daily dose: 600 mg).

Precautions: When using rifampin in conjunction with isoniazid, limit rifampin dose to 15 mg/kg daily and isoniazid to 10 mg/kg daily to minimize risk of hepatotoxicity.

Adverse effects: Hepatotoxicity, GI disturbances, flulike syndrome, red-orange discoloration of urine, feces, sweat, and tears. Discoloration of contact lenses may also occur.

Availability: Capsules: 150, 300 mg.

RISPERIDONE

Route of administration: PO, IM.

Dose: Oral: range is 0.5 mg/day titrated up to a max of 6 mg/day; IM 12.5 to 25 mg every two weeks.

Adverse effects: Prolonged QTc, arrhythmias, blood dyscrasias, neuroleptic malignant syndrome (NMS), dystonias, hyperglycemia, orthostatic hypotension, suicidal ideation.

Availability: Tablet: 0.25, 0.5, 1, 2, 3, 4 mg; Orally disintegrating tablet: 0.25, 0.5, 1, 2, 3, 4 mg Oral solution: 1 mg/mL; Injection: 12.5, 25, 37.5, 50 mg with administration pack.

SUMATRIPTAN

Route of administration: SC, PO, intranasal.

Dose: Limited information suggests SC doses of 3 mg for children 6 years of age or older weighing 22 to 30 kg or 6 mg in children weighing more than 30 kg are safe and effective. Alternatively, a dose of 0.06 mg/kg SC has been used. Currently, only adult dosing is available for the oral and intranasal preparations.

Precautions: Use with caution in patients with preexisting coronary, hepatic, or renal disease or epilepsy.

Adverse effects: Flushing, pain, and/or edema at the injection site, chest tightness, and atypical nervous system effects such as tingling, numbness, feelings of warmth, heat, burning, cold or pressure, dizziness, or drowsiness.

Availability: Injection: 12 mg/mL.

TERBUTALINE

Route of administration: PO, IV, SC.

Dose: PO: 0.05 mg/kg/dose three times/day, max 7.5 mg/day SC: status asthmaticus load: 10 µg/kg for 1 dose followed by continuous IV infusion,alternatively 0.003 to 0.005 mg/kg/dose (3 to 5 µg/kg/dose) to a maximum single dose of 0.25 mg; may repeat once after 15 to 20 minutes. IV: status asthmaticus: load: 10 µg/kg for 1 dose, followed by a continuous infusion of 0.4 µg/kg/minute. Titrate as needed to maintain aeration and heart rate less than 200. Max dose 6 µg/kg/minute.

Precautions: Manufacturer does not recommend use in children younger than 12 years of age.

Adverse effects: Tachycardia, nervousness, tremor, palpitations, alterations in blood glucose, hypokalemia.

Availability: Tablets: 2.5, 5 mg; Injection: 1 mg/mL.

TETANUS IMMUNE GLOBULIN

Route of administration: IM only (do NOT administer IV).

Dose: Postexposure prophylaxis: 250 units IM × 1 dose; treatment: therapeutic dose: 3,000 to 6,000 units IM × 1 dose.

Note: The need for TIG is dependent on previous immunization history.

Precautions: Allergic reactions are possible (epinephrine should be immediately available).

Adverse effects: Pain at injection site, myalgias, fever, flu like symptoms, allergic reactions.

Availability: Injection: 250 units/vial.

VANCOMYCIN

Route of administration: IV, PO.

Dose: IV: Age 1 to 2 months: 10 mg/kg/dose every 12 hours; age older than 2 months: 40 to 60 mg/kg/day in three to four divided doses. Use higher doses for CNS infections. PO, for treatment of antibiotic-associated pseudomembranous colitis only: 10 mg/kg/dose every 6 hours (max 2 g/day).

Precautions: Administer IV over 60 minutes to minimize risk of "red-man's syndrome" (hypotension and rash). PO route should not be used for treatment of systemic infections. Monitor trough levels.

Adverse effects: Ototoxicity and nephrotoxicity, thrombophlebitis, hypotension, rash.

Availability: Capsules: 125, 250 mg; Injection: 500 mg, 1, 2 g/vial; Powder for oral solution: 1, 10 g.

VARICELLA-ZOSTER IMMUNE GLOBULIN

Route of administration: IM, IV.

Dose: 125 units for every 10 kg of weight (min dose 125 units, max 625 units).

Notes: Give within 96 hours of exposure. May diminish efficacy of live vaccines, ensure administration of varicella vaccine if needed prior to or at the same time as the administration of VariZIG.

Precautions: Watch for signs of varicella for 28 days post-administration.

Adverse effects: Site reaction, fever, anaphylaxis, pulmonary edema, renal dysfunction.

Availability: Injection 125 units/vial.

VECURONIUM

Route of administration: IV.

Dose: Maintenance of paralysis postintubation: 0.1 mg/kg/dose every 1 hour or more frequently as needed to maintain paralysis; continuous infusion: 0.05 to 0.07 mg/kg/hour. RSI: 0.3 mg/kg IV for 1 dose.

Precautions: A higher dose is needed to obtain rapid onset needed for RSI therefore, paralysis may persist for more than 2 hours post dose.

Adverse effects: Respiratory arrest, hyper/hypotension, arrhythmias.

Availability: Injection: 10-mg vial.

VERAPAMIL

Route of administration: IV.

Dose: *Supraventricular tachycardia*: age 1 to 16 years: 0.1 to 0.3 mg/kg over 2 minutes (max dose: 5 mg). May repeat dose once after 30 minutes if adequate response is not achieved. Repeat dose in children 2 to 15 years of age should not exceed 10 mg.

Precautions: Because of the risk of severe hypotensive responses, use with extreme caution. Use with continuous EKG monitoring in all children.

Adverse effects: Hypotension, bradycardia, tachycardia, dizziness, headache, nausea. Hypotension or bradycardia caused by verapamil may be reversed by administration of calcium salts or adrenergic agents. Atropine may counteract the bradycardia.

Availability: Injection: 2.5 mg/mL.

WARFARIN

Route of administration: PO.

Dose: Load on day 1: 0.2 mg/kg × 1 dose (max 10 mg/dose); Maintenance: Dosing is based on INR. Usual maintenance is 0.1 mg/kg/day but is highly variable.

Precautions: The potential for many serious drug interactions exist.

Adverse effects: Hemorrhage, fever, skin lesions, anorexia.

Availability: Tablet: 1, 2, 2.5, 4, 5, 7.5, 10 mg.

ZINC SULFATE

Route of administration: PO.

Dose: 0.5 to 1 mg elemental zinc/kg/day in 1 to 3 divided doses, normal adult dose 25 to 50 mg elemental zinc (110 to 220 mg zinc sulfate) PO daily-TID.

Precautions: Clinical response often takes several weeks, up to two months.

Adverse effects: GI distress.

Availability: Capsule 220 mg (50 mg elemental zinc); liquid can be compounded.

Annexure

3

Antiarrhythmic Drugs

Utkarsh Kohli, Srikant Das

Vaughn-Williams classification	Mechanism of action	Drug	Recommended pediatric dose	Indications	Contraindications	Side effects	Monitoring
IA	Na^+ channel blockade (moderate). Moderate ↓ in phase 0 slope and peak of AP, ↑ AP duration, ↑ ERP. Mild cardiac antimuscarinic effect	Quinidine[1-3]	**Oral** Quinidine sulfate (immediate release): Usual dose: 30 mg/kg/day in divided doses every 6 hours; more frequent dosing may be required due to the ↑ clearance seen in pediatric patients; range: 15 to 60 mg/kg/day; maximum adult daily dose: 2,400 mg/day **IV** Not recommended; use with extreme caution: Quinidine gluconate: 2 to 10 mg/kg/dose every 3 to 6 hours as needed	SVT, AFib, AF, VT, Brugada syndrome, early repolarization syndrome, idiopathic ventricular fibrillation	• Hypersensitivity • Thrombocytopenia • Myasthenia gravis • Heart block >1° • Idioventricular conduction delays • Concurrent use of quinolone antibiotics which prolong QTc • Concurrent use of cisapride, amprenavir, ritonavir • May↑ ventricular response rate in patients with AFib or AF; control AV conduction before initiating. • Hemolysis may occur in patients with G6PD deficiency • Use with caution in patients with ↓ LVEF (may precipitate heart failure) • ↓ dosage with hepatic impairment • May cause digoxin toxicity; adjust digoxin dose.	• Diarrhea, nausea and vomiting (33–50%) • *Cinchonism* (may include tinnitus, high-frequency hearing loss, deafness, vertigo, blurred vision, diplopia, photophobia, headache, confusion, and delirium; usually associated with chronic toxicity but may occur after brief exposure to a moderate dose) • Thrombocytopenia • ↑in sinus node dysfunction, QT ↑ and TdP, syncope • Fever • Hepatitis • Angioneurotic edema • **Rare but important or life-threatening**: Acute psychosis, depression, exfoliative dermatitis, ↑ CPK, lupus-like syndrome, lymphadenopathy, optic neuritis, pneumonitis, Sjogren's syndrome, photosensitivity, uveitis, vasculitis, visual field loss	**Discontinue use** • QRS ↑ to 130% of its pretreatment duration • QTc interval ↑ to 130% of its pretreatment duration and is >500 msec • P waves disappear • Significant tachycardia, symptomatic bradycardia, or hypotension • Monitor patients for 2 to 3 days once the appropriate dose has been achieved • CBC with differential, platelet count, liver and renal function test and serum concentrations should be routinely performed during long-term administration • IV use: Continuously monitor BP and ECG (for ↑ QRS duration and ↑ QTc interval) and periodically monitor blood glucose for hypoglycemia with IV use • ***Serum therapeutic concentration: 2 to 5 μg/mL***

Contd...

Contd...

Vaughn-Williams classification	*Mechanism of action*	*Drug*	*Recommended pediatric dose*	*Indications*	*Contraindications*	*Side effects*	*Monitoring*
IA	Na^+ channel blockade (moderate). Moderate ↓ in phase 0 slope and peak of AP, ↑ AP duration, ↑ ERP, may ↓ myocardial contractility. Direct depressant action on SA and AV nodes Extracardiac effects: Ganglion-blocking properties	Procainamide[2-4]	**Neonates: IV:** Loading dose 7 to 10 mg/kg infused over 60 minutes followed by a continuous IV infusion of 20 to 80 µg/kg/minute. **Infants and children: IV:** Loading dose: 10 to 15 mg/kg over 30 to 60 minutes; in adults, maximum dose range: 1000 to 1500 mg. Continuous IV infusion: 20 to 80 µg/kg/minute; maximum daily dose: 2000 mg/24 hours	SVT, AFib, AF, VT	• Hypersensitivity to procainamide, procaine, other ester-type local anesthetics • Complete heart block, 2° AV block or various types of hemiblock (without a functional artificial pacemaker) • SLE • TdP • Myasthenia gravis • Severe heart failure (↓ dose) • Renal failure (↓ dose) • Shock • May ↑ ventricular response rate in patients with Afib or AF; control AV conduction before initiating	• CVS:↑ QTc, TdP, syncope, hypotension (rapid infusion) • GI: Diarrhea, dysgeusia, nausea, vomiting (up to 10%) • Positive ANA titer (100% with long-term administration). Not an indication to stop treatment, lupus like syndrome (⅓ on long-term procainamide therapy) • Skin Rash • Fever • Hepatitis (<5%) • Agranulocytosis (<1%) **Rare but important or life-threatening:** Cerebellar ataxia, demyelinating disease, disorientation, hallucination, hemolytic anemia, mania, myopathy, pancreatitis, peripheral neuropathy	• Monitor ECG and BP; stop the infusion if hypotension occurs or QRS complex ↑ by >50% of baseline • Weekly CBC during the first 3 months of therapy and periodically thereafter • ↓ dose if 1° heart block occurs. • Discontinue if ANA positivity • Decrease dose with renal function ↓ • Monitor serum drug concentration (procainamide and NAPA) especially in patients with hepatic impairment, renal failure, or those receiving a higher maintenance dose. Draw 6 to 12 hours after start of IV infusion; half-life is 2.5 to 5 hours in adults • ***Serum therapeutic concentration: Procainamide: 4 to 10 µg/mL. Sum of procainamide and N-acetyl procainamide: 10 to 30 µg/mL.↑ risk of toxicity with plasma concentrations greater than 8 µg/mL or NAPA concentrations greater than 20 µg/mL***

Contd...

Contd...

Vaughn-Williams classification	*Mechanism of action*	*Drug*	*Recommended pediatric dose*	*Indications*	*Contraindications*	*Side effects*	*Monitoring*
IA	Na^+ channel blockade (moderate). Moderate ↓ in phase 0 slope and peak of AP, ↑ AP duration, ↑ ERP, negative inotropic effect, potent cardiac antimuscarinic effect, peripheral vasoconstrictive effect	Disopyramide[2,3,5]	**Immediate release: Oral: Infants:** 10 to 30 mg/kg/day in divided doses every 6 hours. **Children 1 to 4 years:** 10 to 20 mg/kg/day in divided doses every 6 hours; **Children >4 to 12 years:** 10 to 15 mg/kg/day in divided doses every 6 hours; **Children >12 and Adolescents ≤18 years:** 6 to 15 mg/kg/day in divided doses every 6 hours; adult maximum daily dose: 1,600 mg/day	SVT, AFib, AF, VT, HOCM	• Hypersensitivity • Cardiogenic shock (negative inotropic effect) • Preexisting 2°- or 3° heart block (except in patients with a functioning artificial pacemaker) • Congenital LQTS • Glaucoma • Urinary retention • Myasthenia gravis • Use with caution or avoid in patients LV dysfunction or history of HF; may precipitate or exacerbate condition. • ↓ dosage in renal and hepatic failure	• Hypotension, cardiac failure, syncope, dizziness • ↑ serum cholesterol, ↑ serum triglycerides • Weight gain, abdominal distention, anorexia, bloating, constipation, diarrhea, flatulence, nausea, vomiting • Dry mouth, urinary frequency, hesitancy, retention and urgency • Myalgia • Blurred vision, xerophthalmia, • Dry throat • Dyspnea **Rare but important or life-threatening:** Agranulocytosis, cholestatic jaundice, gynecomastia, hepatotoxicity, hypoglycemia, ↑ blood urea nitrogen, ↑ serum creatinine, ↑ serum transaminases, insomnia, paresthesia, peripheral neuropathy, psychosis, thrombocytopenia	• Patient should be hospitalized during the initial treatment and dose initiated at the lower end of dose range with cardiac monitoring. • ↑ in QTc >25% over baseline should result in cessation or ↓ in disopyramide dosing. • Monitor: BP, ECG (important in hepatic or renal disease, heart disease, or others with increased risk of adverse effects), urinary retention, CNS anticholinergic effects (confusion, agitation, hallucinations, etc.), drug serum concentrations; serum potassium, glucose • ***Serum therapeutic concentration: 2 to 5 µg/mL***
IB	Na^+channel blockade (weak). Small ↓ in phase 0 slope; ↓ AP duration; ↓ in ERP	Lidocaine[2,3,6]	**Loading dose:** 1 mg/kg/dose; follow by continuous IV infusion; may repeat bolus if delay between initial bolus and start of infusion is >15 minutes. **Continuous IV infusion:** 20 to 50 µg/kg/minute ; do not exceed 20 µg/kg/minute in patients with shock, hepatic disease, cardiac arrest, or CHF	VT, digitalis toxicity	• Hypersensitivity to amide type local anesthetics • WPW syndrome • Severe degrees of SA, AV or intraventricular block • Use with caution in hepatic dysfunction or pseudocholinesterase deficiency • ↓ dose in heart failure	• Bradycardia, cardiac arrhythmias, shock, flushing, heart block, hypotension • Local thrombophlebitis • Methemoglobinemia • Seizures, agitation, hallucinations • Anxiety, • Nausea, vomiting • Tremor, weakness • Anaphylaxis • Tinnitus • Bronchospasm	• Continuous ECG monitoring during administration • ***Serum therapeutic concentration: 1.5 to 5 µg/mL***

Contd...

Contd...

Vaughn-Williams classification	*Mechanism of action*	*Drug*	*Recommended pediatric dose*	*Indications*	*Contraindications*	*Side effects*	*Monitoring*
IB	Na^+ channel blockade (weak). Small ↓ in phase 0 slope; ↓ AP duration; ↓ in ERP	Mexiletine[2,3,7]	**Oral:** Initial: 6 to 8 mg/kg/day in 2 or 3 divided doses for 2 to 3 days, then increase to 2 to 5 mg/kg/dose every 8 to 12 hours; continue to increase by 1 to 2 mg/kg/dose every 2 to 3 days until desired effect; monitor serum concentrations. Maximum daily dose: 15 mg/kg/day or 1,200 mg/day whichever is less. Based on experience in adult patients, do not exceed the maximum single adult doses of: 400 mg every 8 hours, or 450 mg every 12 hours	VT, digitalis toxicity, LQTS types 2 and 3	• Cardiogenic shock • 2°- or 3° AV block (except in patients with a functioning artificial pacemaker) • If significant hematologic changes occur, discontinue therapy (blood counts usually return to normal within a month of discontinuation) • Drug reactions with eosinophilia and systemic symptoms (DRESS): Discontinue if DRESS is suspected. Symptoms of DRESS include eosinophilia, fever, rash, and/or lymphadenopathy in association with other organ involvement, such as hepatitis, nephritis, hematologic abnormalities, myocarditis, or myositis, sometimes resembling an acute viral infection. • Carefully monitor patients who develop abnormal LFTs or who have signs/symptoms of liver dysfunction. If persistent or worsening elevation of hepatic enzymes occurs, consider discontinuing therapy	• Proarrhythmic effect • CNS side effects: Ataxia, confusion depression, dizziness, headache, insomnia, numbness (fingers or toes), nervousness, paresthesia, unsteady gait, tremor, weakness, nystagmus, seizures (rare) • Skin rash • Abdominal pain, constipation, diarrhea, gastrointestinal distress, nausea, vomiting • Blurred vision **Rare but important or life-threatening:** • Alopecia, exfoliative dermatitis, hepatic necrosis, hepatitis, impotence, lupus-like syndrome (drug-induced), pancreatitis (rare), psychosis, pulmonary fibrosis, sinoatrial arrest, Stevens-Johnson syndrome, thrombocytopenia, urinary retention	Monitor: Liver enzymes, CBC, ECG and HR • ***Serum therapeutic serum concentration: Children and Adolescents: 0.75 to 2 μg/mL; infants: 0.5 to 2 μg/mL***

Contd...

Contd...

Vaughn-Williams classification	*Mechanism of action*	*Drug*	*Recommended pediatric dose*	*Indications*	*Contraindications*	*Side effects*	*Monitoring*
IB	Na^+ channel blockade (weak). Small ↓ in phase 0 slope; ↓ AP duration; ↓ in ERP.	Phenytoin[2,3,8]		VT, digitalis toxicity	• Hypersensitivity • Concurrent use of delavirdine • History of hepatotoxicity attributable to phenytoin • Sinus bradycardia, SA block, 2°- or 3° AV block	• Proarrhythmia, conduction abnormalities • Circulatory shock, hypotension • Ataxia, cerebral atrophy (↑ serum levels and/or long-term use), cerebral dysfunction (↑ serum levels and/or long-term use), confusion, dizziness, drowsiness, headache, insomnia, nervousness, paresthesia, peripheral neuropathy (associated with chronic treatment), slurred speech, suicidal ideation, twitching, vertigo • Bullous dermatitis, exfoliative dermatitis, morbilliform rash, scarlatiniform rash • ↓ T4, ↑ GGT, vitamin D ↓ (chronic treatment), constipation, dysgeusia, gingival hyperplasia, nausea, vomiting, megaloblastic anemia, pseudolymphoma, purpuric dermatitis, acute hepatic failure, ↑ serum alkaline phosphatase, injection site reaction ("purple glove syndrome"), osteomalacia, nystagmus, drug fever	• **Monitor:** CBC with differential, liver function, suicidality, bone growth or BMD and vitamin D status (chronic use; particularly pediatric patients) • **Timing of serum samples**: Peak serum concentrations may occur 4–8 hours after ingestion of an oral dose due to slow absorption. Half-life is about 24 hours in adults; in pediatric patients, the apparent half-life is age-dependent (longer in neonates). Steady-state concentrations are reached in 5–10 days • ***Serum therapeutic concentration: Total phenytoin: Neonates: 8–15 µg/mL; pediatric patients ≥1 month and adults: 10–20 µg/mL***

Contd...

Contd...

Vaughn-Williams classification	Mechanism of action	Drug	Recommended pediatric dose	Indications	Contraindications	Side effects	Monitoring
IC	Na^+ channel blockade (strong). Marked ↓ in phase 0 slope, no effect on AP duration or ERP. Local anesthetic and moderate negative inotropic effects	Flecainide[2,39]	**Neonates** **BSA-directed dosing:** **Initial: Oral:** 70 to 100 mg/m²/day divided every 12 hours. Titrated based on response and serum concentrations **Weight-directed dosing: Oral:** 2 mg/kg/day divided every 12 hours; titrate to clinical response, monitor serum concentration; usual dose range in infants and children is 3 to 6 mg/kg/day. Doses >8 mg/kg/day have been associated with ↑ proarrhythmic effects in children **Pediatric:** **BSA-directed dosing:** **Infants ≤6 months:** **Oral:** Initial: 50 mg/m²/day divided every 8 to 12 hours; may titrate dose at 4-day intervals; maximum daily dose: 200 mg/m²/day; **Infants >6 months, Children, and Adolescents: Oral:** Initial: 100 mg/m²/day divided every 8 to 12 hours; may titrate dose at 4-day intervals; maximum daily dose: 200 mg/m²/day **Weight-based dosing: Limited data available; dosing regimens variable: Infants, Children, and Adolescents: Oral:** Initial 1 to 3 mg/kg/day divided every 8 hours; may titrate dose at 4-day intervals; usual maintenance range: 3 to 6 mg/kg/day	SVT, AFib, AF, VT, PVCs, EAT, PJRT, JT, LQTS type 3, CPVT	• Hypersensitivity to flecainide • Pre-existing 2°–or 3° AV block or with right bundle branch block when associated with a left hemiblock • Cardiogenic shock • Concurrent use of ritonavir • **Structural heart disease** • Use is not recommended in patients with chronic AFib due to an ↑ risk of life-threatening ventricular arrhythmias, When treating AF 1:1 AV conduction may occur; pre-emptive negative chronotropic therapy (e.g. digoxin, beta-blockers) may lower the risk • Dose-related ↑ in PR and QRS intervals • Use with extreme caution in patients with sick sinus syndrome; treatment with flecainide may result in sinus bradycardia, sinus pause, or sinus arrest • Avoid use in patients with HF; may precipitate or exacerbate HF, ↑ the risk of proarrhythmia, and contribute to an ↑ risk of mortality • Use with caution in patients with significant hepatic impairment. Careful monitoring during initiation of therapy	• Edema, palpitations, sinus node dysfunction, syncope, tachycardia, anxiety • Ataxia, depression, dizziness • Fatigue, fever, headache, hypoesthesia, insomnia, malaise, nervousness, paresis, somnolence, tinnitus, vertigo, rash • Abdominal pain, anorexia, constipation, diarrhea, nausea • Paresthesias, tremor, weakness, blurred vision, diplopia, visual disturbances • Dyspnea **Rare but important or life-threatening:** Alopecia, altered pacing threshold, amnesia, angina, bronchospasm, CHF, corneal deposits, depersonalization, euphoria, exfoliative dermatitis, metallic taste, neuropathy, pancytopenia	• **Monitor:** ECG, BP, pulse • Periodic serum concentrations after at least 5 doses when doses are started or changed or when dietary changes due to maturation or concurrent illness occur • Liver enzymes • Clearance may be decreased in patients following strict vegetarian diets due to urinary pH ≥8 • Milk may interfere with the absorption of flecainide. Dose ↓ should be considered when milk is removed from the diet • Patients with permanent pacemakers or temporary pacing wires; can increase endocardial pacing thresholds and suppress ventricular escape rhythms. The pacing threshold in patients with pacemakers should be determined at baseline, 1 week after initiation and at regular intervals thereafter • Monitor QRS width and PR interval. PR ↑ >50% and QRS ↑ >20% may indicate toxicity • **Serum *therapeutic trough: 0.2 to 1 μg/mL Pediatric patients may respond at the lower end of the recommended therapeutic range (0.2 to 0.5 μg/mL) but up to 0.8 μg/mL may be required. Note: Hemolysis during blood sampling may cause a falsely elevated flecainide concentration***

Contd...

Contd...

Vaughn-Williams classification	*Mechanism of action*	*Drug*	*Recommended pediatric dose*	*Indications*	*Contraindications*	*Side effects*	*Monitoring*
					Dose titration should occur only after steady state has been achieved (≥4 days after initiation). Frequent plasma level monitoring is required in patients with severe hepatic impairment; if unavailable, use is not recommended		
IC	Na^+ channel blockade (strong). Marked ↓ in phase 0 slope, no effect on AP duration or ERP, local anesthetic and a weak β-blocker effect	Propafenone[2,3,10]	Adult dose: 450–900 mg/day in three divided doses	SVT, Atrial fibrillation, atrial flutter, VT, PVCs, EAT, PJRT, JT	• Hypersensitivity to propafenone • SA or AV nodal dysfunction • Brugada syndrome • Cardiogenic shock • HF • Bronchospastic disorders or COPD • MI within past 3 months • Severe hepatic impairment • Myasthenia gravis • Concurrent use with ritonavir • Agranulocytosis within the first 2 months of therapy. Normalizes by 14 days upon discontinuation • CNS effects: dizziness, fatigue, blurred vision; caution patients about performing dangerous tasks (e.g. driving, operating machinery) • Positive ANA titers: Discontinue if symptomatic and positive ANA titers • Hepatotoxicity	• CNS (common): Unusual taste, dizziness, nausea, vomiting • CVS: Cardiac arrhythmia (2% to 10%), angina pectoris, cardiac failure, 1° AV block, widened QRS complex, syncope, hypotension -Fatigue, headache, ataxia, insomnia, anxiety, drowsiness • Skin rash, diaphoresis • Constipation, diarrhea, dyspepsia, abdominal pain, anorexia, xerostomia, flatulence -Weakness, arthralgia, tremor • Blurred vision • Dyspnea	• ECG, BP, pulse (particularly at initiation of therapy)

Contd...

Contd...

Vaughn-Williams classification	Mechanism of action	Drug	Recommended pediatric dose	Indications	Contraindications	Side effects	Monitoring
II	β-blockade. Block sympathetic activity, ↓ conduction, ↓ heart rate, ↓ myocardial contractility, BP, and myocardial oxygen demand, ↓ portal pressure by producing splanchnic vasoconstriction (β_2 effect)	Propranolol[2,3,11]	**Neonates: Oral: Immediate release formulation:** Initial: 0.5 to 1 mg/kg/dose for 1 dose; then 1 mg/kg/dose every 6 to 8 hours. **Older Children: Oral: Immediate release formulation:** Initial: 0.5 to 1 mg/kg/day in divided doses every 6 to 8 hours; titrate dosage upward every 3 to 5 days; usual daily dose: 2 to 4 mg/kg/day; higher doses may be needed; maximum daily dose: 16 mg/kg/day or 60 mg/day; **IV:** 0.01 to 0.15 mg/kg/dose slow IV over 10 minutes; may repeat every 6 to 8 hours as needed; maximum dose is age-dependent: Infants: 1 mg/dose children and adolescents: 3 mg/dose	Sinus tachycardia, AFib, AF, VT, SVT, PVCs, EAT, PJRT, LQTS	• Hypersensitivity • Uncompensated HF (unless the HF is due to tachyarrhythmias being treated with propranolol) • Cardiogenic shock • Severe sinus bradycardia • Sick sinus syndrome; or heart block greater than 1° • Bronchial asthma • Premature infants with corrected age <5 weeks; infants weighing <2 kg; heart rate <80 bpm; blood pressure <50/30 mm Hg • Pheochromocytoma • Cor pulmonale • Allergic rhinitis during pollen season • Hypotension • Metabolic acidosis • Vasospastic angina • Severe peripheral arterial circulatory disturbance **Use with caution in** • Patients with a history of anaphylaxis • Bronchospastic disease • Patients prone to hypoglycemia • Compensated heart failure • Myasthenia gravis • Psoriasis • Renal impairment • Thyrotoxicosis • β-blocker therapy should not be withdrawn abruptly (particularly in patients with CAD), but gradually	• **CVS**: Angina pectoris, AV conduction disturbance, bradycardia, cardiac failure, cardiogenic shock, hypotension, syncope • **CNS**: Agitation, amnesia, carpal tunnel syndrome, catatonia, cognitive dysfunction, confusion, dizziness, drowsiness, fatigue, hypersomnia, irritability, lethargy, nightmares, paresthesia, psychosis, sleep disorder, vertigo • **Dermatologic**: Changes in nails, contact dermatitis, dermal ulcer, eczematous rash, erosive lichen planus, hyperkeratosis, pruritus, skin rash • **Endocrine and Metabolic**: Hyperglycemia, hyperkalemia, hyperlipidemia, hypoglycemia • **GI**: Abdominal pain, anorexia, constipation, ↓ appetite, diarrhea, stomach discomfort • **GU**: Oliguria, proteinuria • **Hematologic and oncologic**: Thrombocytopenia • **Hepatic:** ↑ serum alkaline phosphatase, ↑ serum transaminases • **Neuromuscular and skeletal**: Arthropathy, oculomucocutaneous syndrome, polyarthritis • **Ophthalmic**: Conjunctival hyperemia, decreased visual acuity, mydriasis • **Renal:** ↑ BUN, interstitial nephritis (rare) • **Respiratory:** Bronchiolitis, bronchitis, bronchospasm, dyspnea, pulmonary edema, wheezing	• CVS concerns: Monitor HR and BP after propranolol initiation or ↑ in dose; discontinue treatment if severe or symptomatic bradycardia or hypotension occurs. • ↓ in BP caused by propranolol may ↑ risk of stroke in PHACE syndrome patients with cerebrovascular anomalies. • Hypoglycemia: May potentiate hypoglycemia and/or mask signs and symptoms. Withhold the dose in infants or children who are not feeding regularly or who are vomiting; discontinue therapy and seek immediate treatment if hypoglycemia occurs. • Monitor ECG, BP, HR with IV administration; HR and BP with oral administration • ***Serum therapeutic concentration: 50 to 100 ng/mL at the end of dosing interval***

Contd...

Contd...

Vaughn-Williams classification	*Mechanism of action*	*Drug*	*Recommended pediatric dose*	*Indications*	*Contraindications*	*Side effects*	*Monitoring*
					tapered to avoid acute tachycardia, hypertension, and/or ischemia • Chronic β-blocker therapy should not be routinely withdrawn prior to major surgery		
II	β-blockade. Block sympathetic activity, ↓ conduction, ↓ heart rate, myocardial contractility, blood pressure, and myocardial oxygen demand. β_1 selective	Atenolol[2,3,12]	**SVT:** Usual range: 0.3 to 1 mg/kg/day either once daily or in divided doses every 12 hours; titration of the dose to >1.4 mg/kg/day did not show additional treatment successes and potentially ↑ the risk of adverse effects	Sinus tachycardia, AFib, AF, VT, SVT, PVCs, EAT, PJRT	• Same as propranolol • Limited data suggests that atenolol may have a shorter half-life and faster clearance in patients with Marfan syndrome. Higher doses (2 mg/kg/day divided every 12 hours) have been used in patients with Marfan syndrome to ↓ aortic root growth rate and prevent aortic dissection or rupture	Similar to other β-blockers	BP, HR, ECG, fluid intake and output, daily weight and respiratory rate
II	β-blockade. Block sympathetic activity, ↓ conduction, ↓ heart rate, myocardial contractility, blood pressure, and myocardial oxygen demand. β_1 selective	Metoprolol[2,3,13]	**Immediate-release tablets (metoprolol tartrate): Children and Adolescents ≤17 years: Oral:** Initial: 0.5 to 1 mg/kg/dose (maximum initial dose: 25 mg/dose) twice daily; maximum daily dose: 6 mg/kg/day or 200 mg/day, whichever is less **Extended-release sprinkle capsules or tablets (metoprolol succinate): Children ≥6 years and Adolescents: Oral:** Initial: 1 mg/kg/dose once daily (maximum initial dose: 50 mg/dose); maximum daily dose: 2 mg/kg/day or 200 mg/day, whichever is less	Sinus tachycardia, AFib, AF, VT, SVT, PVCs, EAT, PJRT	Similar to propranolol and atenolol	Similar to other β-blockers	Oral: BP, HR and rhythm

Contd...

Contd...

Vaughn-Williams classification	Mechanism of action	Drug	Recommended pediatric dose	Indications	Contraindications	Side effects	Monitoring
II	β-blockade. Block sympathetic activity, ↓ conduction, ↓ heart rate, myocardial contractility, blood pressure, and myocardial oxygen demand	Nadolol[2,3,14]	**Infants ≥3 months, Children, and Adolescents:** Oral: Initial: 0.5 to 1 mg/kg once daily; increase dose gradually to a maximum of 2.5 mg/kg/day; CPVT maximum tolerated dose	Sinus tachycardia, AFib, AF, VT, SVT, PVCs, EAT, PJRT, LQTS, CPVT	Similar to other β-blockers	Similar to other β-blockers	BP, HR, fluid intake and output and weight
II	β-blockade. Block sympathetic activity, ↓ conduction, ↓ heart rate, myocardial contractility, blood pressure, and myocardial oxygen demand	Esmolol[2,3,15]	**Children and Adolescents: Initial IV bolus:** 100 to 500 µg/kg over 1 minute followed by a continuous IV infusion: initial rate: 25 to 100 µg/kg/minute, titrate in 25 to 50 µg/kg/minute increments; usual maintenance dose: 50 to 500 µg/kg/minute; doses up to 1,000 µg/kg/minute	Sinus tachycardia, AFib, AF, VT, SVT, PVCs, EAT, PJRT	Same as other β-blockers	• Similar to other β-blockers • Skin necrosis if extravasation	BP, ECG, HR, respiratory rate, IV site; serum potassium (especially with renal impairment)
II	Ultrashort acting β1-blocker. Block sympathetic activity, ↓ rate and conduction, ↑ refractory period, ↓ spontaneous firing of ectopic pacemakers. More potent negative chronotropic and less potent negative inotropic effect that esmolol.	Landiolol Hydrochloride[16] (approved in EU and Japan)	• Not intended for use in chronic settings • Short-term heart rate control, the recommended starting dosage is 0.1 to 0.2 mg/kg IV which provides a bradycardic effect for 5 to 20 min; if inadequate effect ↑ to 0.2 or 0.3 mg/kg. The maximum recommended dosage is 100 mg /day divided into 5 to 15 doses/day • When rapid (within 2 to 4 min) onset of bradycardic effect is required, the infusion should be initiated with a loading dose of 100 µg/kg for 1 min, followed by a maintenance dose of 10 to 40 µg/kg/min	Sinus tachycardia, AFib, AF, VT, SVT, PVCs, EAT, PJRT	Similar to other β-blockers	Similar to other β-blockers	BP, ECG, HR, respiratory rate and IV site

Contd...

Contd...

Vaughn-Williams classification	*Mechanism of action*	*Drug*	*Recommended pediatric dose*	*Indications*	*Contraindications*	*Side effects*	*Monitoring*
			• When rapid onset of bradycardic effect is not required, starting the infusion with the maintenance dose without the loading dose will provide the effect within 10 to 20 min. The maintenance dose may be increased up to 80 µg/kg/min if the efficacy is not sufficient and the cardiovascular status of the patient requires and allows such an increase. The maximum recommended daily dose is 8064 mg/day.				
III	K^+ channel blockade. Delay repolarization (phase 3) and thereby ↑ AP duration and ERP. Has an effect across all 4 classes	Amiodarone[2,3,17]	**Neonatal Oral:** **Loading dose:** 10 to 20 mg/kg/day in 2 divided doses for 7 to 10 days; dosage should then be reduced to 5 to 10 mg/kg/day once daily. **IV Dosing based on µg/kg/minute:** Initial: 5 µg/kg/minute; ↑ incrementally as clinically needed; usual required dose: 10 µg/kg/minute; range: 5 to 15 µg/kg/minute **Dosing based on mg/kg/day:** Initial: 10 mg/kg/day; ↑ incrementally as clinically needed; range: 10 to 20 mg/kg/day	SVT, AFib, AF, VT, PVCs, JT, PJRT, EAT	• Hypersensitivity to amiodarone • Sick sinus syndrome • AV block • Cardiogenic shock • Symptomatic bradycardia • Hepatitis, pulmonary interstitial abnormalities, thyroid dysfunction • Iodine hypersensitivity	• Bradycardia, 2°- or 3° AV block • ↑ QT, cardiac arrhythmias • Ataxia • Dizziness • Fatigue • Paresthesias • Headache • Photosensitivity • Hypo or hyperthyroidism • Abdominal pain, anorexia, abnormal salivation, constipation, diarrhea, dysgeusia, nausea, vomiting • Thrombocytopenia • Tremor • Liver dysfunction, ↑ SGOT and SGPT • Blurred vision, optic neuritis, corneal deposits • Pneumonitis, pulmonary fibrosis • Fever	• HR and rhythm, BP, ECG • Chest X-ray • PFT • Thyroid function tests • Serum glucose, electrolytes (especially potassium and magnesium), triglycerides, liver enzymes • Ophthalmologic • Monitor pacing or defibrillation thresholds in patients with ICDs at initiation of therapy and periodically during treatment • Monitor infusion site • ***Serum therapeutic concentration: Chronic oral dosing: 1 to 2.5 mg/L (parent); desmethyl metabolite (active) is present in equal concentration to parent drug; serum concentrations may not be of great value for predicting toxicity and efficacy; toxicity may occur even at therapeutic concentrations***

Contd...

Contd...

Vaughn-Williams classification	Mechanism of action	Drug	Recommended pediatric dose	Indications	Contraindications	Side effects	Monitoring
			Children **Oral:** Loading dose: 10 to 15 mg/kg/day in 1 to 2 divided doses/day for 4 to 14 days or until adequate control of arrhythmia or prominent adverse effects occur; dosage should then be reduced to 5 mg/kg/day given once daily; if arrhythmia does not recur, reduce to lowest effective dosage possible; usual daily minimal dose: 2.5 mg/kg/day; maintenance doses may be given for 5 of 7 days/week. **Dosing based on µg/kg/minute:** Initial: 5 µg/kg/minute; ↑ incrementally as clinically needed; usual required dose: 10 µg/kg/minute; range: 5 to 15 µg/kg/minute; maximum daily dose: 2200 mg/day **Dosing based on mg/kg/day:** Initial: 10 mg/kg/day; ↑ incrementally as clinically needed; range: 10 to 20 mg/kg/day; maximum daily dose: 2,200 mg/day				
III	K^+ channel blockade. Delayed repolarization (phase 3) and thereby ↑ AP duration and ERP. β_1- and β_2-receptor blocking activity. ↑ of atrial muscle, ventricular muscle, and	Sotalol[2,3,18]	**Neonates: Initial:** 2 mg/kg/day divided every 8 hours; if needed, ↑ dosage gradually by 1 to 2 mg/kg/day increments; allow at least 3 days between dosage ↑ to achieve new steady-state and to monitor clinical response, HR,	SVT, AFib, AF, VT, PVCs, JT, PJRT, EAT	• Anaphylactic reactions • Bradycardia and hypotension • Proarrhythmic effects • Bronchospastic conditions • Conduction abnormality (sick sinus syndrome) • Dyselectrolytemia	• CVS: angina pectoris, bradycardia, edema, hypotension, proarrhythmia, QTc prolongation • CNS: Anxiety, depression, dizziness, fatigue, headache, insomnia, paresthesia	• Obtain ECG 2 to 4 hours after each dose • QTc ≥500 msec during initiation period: ↓ dose, ↑ the dosing interval, or discontinue sotalol • QTc ≥520 msec (or JT interval ≥430 msec if the QRS >100 msec) during maintenance therapy:

Contd...

Contd...

Vaughn-Williams classification	*Mechanism of action*	*Drug*	*Recommended pediatric dose*	*Indications*	*Contraindications*	*Side effects*	*Monitoring*
	atrioventricular accessory pathways in both the antegrade and retrograde directions. Sotalol is a racemic mixture of *d*- and *l*-sotalol; both isomers have similar Class III antiarrhythmic effects while the l-isomer is responsible for virtually all of the β-blocking activity. The Class III effects are seen only at oral doses ≥160 mg/day.		and QTc intervals, maximum: 10 mg/kg/day. **Infants and Children 1 month to 6 years:** 6 mg/kg/day divided every 8 hours. **Children >6 years and Adolescents:** 4 mg/kg/day divided every 8 hours not to exceed adult doses.		• Heart failure • Myasthenia gravis • Post myocardial infarction • Peripheral vascular disease and Raynaud disease • Pheochromocytoma (α-blockade is required before β-blockade) • Renal impairment • May mask symptoms of hyperthyroidism	• Dermatologic: Diaphoresis, hyperhidrosis and skin rash • Endocrine and metabolic: Weight changes • GI: Abdominal distension, abdominal pain, ↓ appetite, diarrhea, nausea and vomiting • GU: Sexual disorder • Hematologic and oncologic: Hemorrhage • Musculoskeletal pain • Visual disturbance • Asthma • Fever • Alopecia, eosinophilia, ↑ liver enzymes, leukopenia, paralysis, phlebitis, pruritus, pulmonary edema, photosensitivity, thrombocytopenia	↓ dose and carefully monitor QTc until <520 msec. If QTc interval ≥520 msec on the lowest maintenance dose, discontinue sotalol • QTc ≥550 msec: ↓ dose or discontinue sotalol • To minimize the risk of drug-induced arrhythmia, initiate or reinitiate sotalol in a facility that can provide and continuous ECG monitoring. Do not initiate sotalol therapy if the baseline QTc is longer than 450 msec • Calculate creatinine clearance to determine appropriate dosing
III	A non-iodinated antiarrhythmic agent structurally related to amiodarone exhibiting properties of all 4 antiarrhythmic classes. Dronedarone inhibits Na^+ and K^+ channels resulting in ↑ in AP and ERP of the myocardial tissue without reverse-use dependent effects; ↓ AV conduction and sinus node function through inhibition	Drone-darone[2,3,19]	**Adults:** 400 mg twice a day	Atrial arrhythmias	• Hypersensitivity • Permanent AF • Symptomatic HF • Liver or lung toxicity related to previous amiodarone use • 2°- or 3° AV block or sick sinus syndrome • Concomitant use of CYP3A4 inhibitors • Severe hepatic impairment • Pregnancy • Breastfeeding • QTc>500 msec, PR>280 msec • QTc prolonging drugs • Prior to initiation of dronedarone, class I or III antiarrhythmics must be stopped	**>10%** • Prolonged QTc • ↑ serum creatinine **1–10%** • Bradycardia (3%) • Allergic dermatitis, eczema, pruritus, skin rash • Diarrhea, nausea, abdominal pain, dyspepsia, vomiting • Weakness **<1%** • Acute hepatic failure • Anaphylaxis • Angioedema • Cardiac failure • Dysgeusia • ↑BUN • Interstitial pulmonary fibrosis • Vasculitis • Photosensitivity	• **Monitoring Parameters**: ECG (at least every 3 months), BP, HR and rhythm throughout therapy; assess patient for signs of lethargy, edema of the hands or feet; monitor serum electrolytes, especially potassium and magnesium; serum liver enzymes and bilirubin (periodically, especially during the first 6 months of therapy) • Monitor pacing or defibrillation thresholds with initiation of dronedarone and during treatment.

Contd...

Contd...

Vaughn-Williams classification	*Mechanism of action*	*Drug*	*Recommended pediatric dose*	*Indications*	*Contraindications*	*Side effects*	*Monitoring*
	Ca^{2+} channels and β_1-receptor blocking activity. Dronedarone also inhibits α_1-receptor mediated ↑ in BP.						
III	Inhibits HERG channels, suggesting the selective inhibition of the rapid component of the delayed rectifier K^+ current. A pure K^+ channel blocker with a minimal negative inotropic effect in contrast to amiodarone which has negative inotropic effect via β-blocking action. ↓ the defibrillation threshold	Nifekalant[20]	Adults: 0.19 ± 0.14 mg/kg/hour	JT, atrial arrhythmias		Proarrhythmia (TdP)	Continuous ECG monitoring
IV	Block L-type Ca^{2+} channels; most effective at SA and AV nodes; ↓ rate and conduction	Verapamil[2,3,21]	**IV: Infants:** May result in cardiac arrest and hypotension therefore the use is relatively contraindicated. If used, it should only be with expert consultation and continuous ECG monitoring with IV Ca^{2+} at the bedside: 0.1 to 0.2 mg/kg/dose (usual: 0.75 to 2 mg/dose) may repeat dose after at least 30 minutes if inadequate response **Children and**	SVT, AFib, AF	• Hypersensitivity • Severe LV dysfunction • Hypotension or cardiogenic shock • Sick sinus syndrome • 2°- or 3° AV block • AF or AFib and an accessory bypass tract • DMD • Myasthenia gravis • Hepatic failure • HOCM • ↑ ICP • Renal impairment	• CVS: Angina pectoris, AV block, bradycardia, HF, hypotension, MI, syncope • CNS: Confusion, dizziness, drowsiness, fatigue, headache • Dermatologic: Alopecia, diaphoresis, erythema multiforme, urticaria, Stevens-Johnson syndrome • Endocrine and Metabolic: Galactorrhea, gynecomastia, spotty menstruation • GI: Abdominal distress, constipation, diarrhea, nausea, gingival hyperplasia, xerostomia	Monitor BP and HR; periodic liver function tests; ECG, especially with renal and/or hepatic impairment

Contd...

Contd...

Vaughn-Williams classification	*Mechanism of action*	*Drug*	*Recommended pediatric dose*	*Indications*	*Contraindications*	*Side effects*	*Monitoring*
			Adolescents 1 to 15 years: 0.1 to 0.3 mg/kg/dose (usual dose: 2 to 5 mg/dose); maximum dose: 5 mg/dose; may repeat dose in 15 to 30 minutes if inadequate response; maximum dose for second dose: 10 mg/dose **Adolescents ≥16 years:** 0.1 to 0.3 mg/kg/dose; maximum dose: 5 mg/dose **Oral:** **Children and Adolescents:** **Immediate release:** 2 to 8 mg/kg/day in 3 divided doses; maximum daily dose: 480 mg/day			• GU: Impotence • Hematologic and Oncologic: Bruise, purpuric vasculitis • Hepatic: ↑ liver enzymes • Blurred vision • Tinnitus • Polyuria • Dyspnea, flu-like symptoms, pulmonary edema	
IV	Block L-type Ca^{2+} channels; most effective at SA and AV nodes; ↓ rate and conduction. Coronary vasodilation	Diltiazem[2,3,22]	**Infants ≥6 months, Children, and Adolescents: IV:** Initial bolus: 0.25 mg/kg over 5 minutes (maximum dose: 20 mg/dose [average adult dose]) followed by a continuous IV infusion 0.05 to 0.15 mg/kg/hour. In adult patients, infusions >24 hours are not recommended. **Oral:** Immediate-release formulations: Initial: 1.5 to 2 mg/kg/day in 3 to 4 divided doses; ↑ gradually, at 1- to 2-day intervals until optimum response is obtained; usual maximum daily dose: 3.5 mg/kg/day	Sinus tachycardia, SVT, verapamil sensitive intrafascicular VT, AFib, AF	Same as verapamil	• Same as verapamil • Endocrine and metabolic: Gout	BP, HR, renal function, liver enzymes, heart function (e.g. echocardiogram); continuous ECG with IV therapy

Contd...

Contd...

Vaughn-Williams classification	Mechanism of action	Drug	Recommended pediatric dose	Indications	Contraindications	Side effects	Monitoring
	A1 receptor antagonist. ↓ SA nodal automaticity and ↓ AV nodal conduction	Adenosine[3,23]	**Neonatal: Rapid IV** Initial dose: 0.05 to 0.1 mg/kg; if not effective within 1 to 2 minutes, increase dose by 0.05 to 0.1 mg/kg increments every 1 to 2 minutes to a maximum single dose of 0.3 mg/kg or until termination of SVT **Infants, Children, and Adolescents <50 kg: Initial dose:** 0.05 to 0.1 mg/kg via peripheral or central line; maximum initial dose: 6 mg/dose; if not effective within 1 to 2 minutes, increase dose by 0.05 to 0.1 mg/kg increments every 1 to 2 minutes to a maximum single dose of 0.3 mg/kg or 12 mg, whichever is lower or until termination of SVT **Children and Adolescents ≥50 kg: Initial:** 6 mg via peripheral line, if not effective within 1 to 2 minutes, 12 mg may be given; may repeat 12 mg bolus if needed. -Administer over 1 to 2 seconds at peripheral IV site closest to the patient's heart. Follow each bolus with NS flush (Infants and Children 5 to 10 mL; adults 20 mL)	SVT, PJRT, RVOT VT, verapamil sensitive intrafascicular VT	• Initial dose of adenosine should be ↓ to 3 mg if 1) The patient is receiving carbamazepine or dipyridamole 2) Has a transplanted heart 3) If adenosine is administered via a central line • Can precipitate Afib/AF in patients with SVT and WPW • Avoid use in patients with cardiovascular instability • Avoid use in patients with high grade AV block or sinus node dysfunction • Hypersensitivity • Hypertension and hypotension may be exacerbated with continuous adenosine infusion • Seizures may be exacerbated by adenosine administration. The risk may be ↑ with concurrent use of aminophylline • Avoid use with wide-complex tachycardia. May degenerate into ventricular fibrillation • Use with extreme caution in patients with heart transplant. Can cause prolonged sinus arrest • Use with extreme caution in patients with pulmonary arterial hypertension. Can precipitate acute pulmonary edema	• CVS: AV block, cardiac arrhythmias, chest pain, chest pressure, depression of ST segment on ECG, hypotension • CNS: Apprehension, dizziness, headache, nervousness, numbness, paresthesia • Dermatologic: Diaphoresis, facial flushing • GI: Nausea, GI distress • Neuromuscular: Neck and upper extremity discomfort • Respiratory: Dyspnea and hyperventilation **Rare but important or life-threatening:** AF, blurred vision, bradycardia, bronchospasm, cardiac arrest, ↑ ICP, injection site reaction, MI, ventricular arrhythmias, hypotension	Continuous ECG, BP, HR and respiratory monitoring

Contd...

Contd...

Vaughn-Williams classification	*Mechanism of action*	*Drug*	*Recommended pediatric dose*	*Indications*	*Contraindications*	*Side effects*	*Monitoring*
					• Avoid use in patients with bronchospasm and bronchoconstriction (Asthma) • Caffeine and theophylline antagonize the activity of adenosine • Carbamazepine and dipyridamole potentiate the effect of adenosine		
	Vagotonic effect, ↓ AV nodal conduction	Digoxin[2,3,24-26]	• Individualized dosage due to substantial individual variation • Must take into account renal function • Doses should be based on lean body weight. When changing from oral solution to IV therapy, dosage should be reduced by 20% to 25% **Term neonates:** Oral: Initial digitalizing dose: 20 to 40 µg/kg divided every 8 hours for 2 to 3 doses followed by maintenance dose: 8 to 10 µg/kg/day divided every 12 hours **Infants, Children, and Adolescents:** Initial (digitalizing dose): IV: 10 to 12 µg/kg/dose every 8 hours for 3 doses; Oral: 13 to 17 µg/kg/dose every 8 hours for 3 doses. Maintenance: Oral: 8 to 10 µg/kg/day divided once or twice daily; use twice daily dosing in infants and young children	SVT, EAT, JT	• Dosage adjustment is necessary in renal failure • Avoid extravasation due to vesicant effect • Avoid in patients with WPW • Use with caution in patients with acute coronary ischemia • Patients with thiamine deficiency related cardiomyopathy may not respond adequately • Ensure normal electrolytes • Relatively contraindicated in HOCM • Use with caution in patients with myocarditis • Hypo and hyperthyroidism	• ***Digoxin toxicity:*** Anorexia, nausea, vomiting, visual changes and cardiac arrhythmias; usually associated with levels >2 ng/mL. ↑ risk with low body weight, renal impairment, hypokalemia, hypomagnesemia and hypercalcemia • CVS: Accelerated junctional rhythm, asystole, atrial tach with or without AV block, facial edema, PR prolongation, PVCCs, ST segment depression, VT or ventricular fibrillation • CNS: Apathy, anxiety, confusion, delirium, depression, dizziness, fever, hallucinations, headache, mental disturbance • Dermatologic: Rash, pruritus, urticaria, angioedema • GI: Abdominal pain, anorexia, diarrhea, nausea and vomiting • Neuromuscular and skeletal: Weakness • Ophthalmic: Visual disturbance (blurred or yellow vision) • Respiratory: Laryngeal edema	• HR and rhythm, periodic ECG; follow serum potassium, magnesium, and calcium closely • Digoxin serum concentrations should be drawn at least 6 to 8 hours after the previous dose, regardless of route of administration (optimally 12 to 24 hours after a dose) • Serum digoxin concentrations may decrease in response to exercise due to increased skeletal muscle uptake; a period of rest (e.g. ~2 hours) after exercise may be necessary prior to drawing blood for serum digoxin concentrations • **Toxic concentration: >2 ng/mL** • Serum digoxin concentration should be interpreted with caution in neonates and infants as digoxin like immunoreactive substance can be detected in plasma of infants who are not on digoxin

Contd...

Contd...

Vaughn-Williams classification	Mechanism of action	Drug	Recommended pediatric dose	Indications	Contraindications	Side effects	Monitoring
						Rare but life threatening: Asymmetric chorea, gynecomastia, thrombocytopenia, palpitation, eosinophilia, sexual dysfunction, diaphoresis	
	Selective and specific inhibition of the hyperpolarization-activated cyclic nucleotide-gated (HCN) channels within the sinoatrial (SA) node resulting in disruption of I_f ion current flow ↑ diastolic depolarization, ↓ firing in the SA node, and ultimately ↓ HR. No effects on myocardial contractility or relaxation, ventricular repolarization and conduction apart. Partial inhibition of the retinal I_h current may explain visual disturbances	Ivabradine[2,27]	**Adults:** Oral: Initial: 5 mg twice daily; maintenance: 7.5 mg twice daily	Inappropriate sinus tachycardia, JT	• Acute decompensated HF (BP<90/50 mm Hg) • Sick sinus syndrome • Sinoatrial block • 3° heart block • Resting heart rate < 60 bpm prior to treatment • Severe hepatic impairment • Pacemaker dependence • Concomitant use of strong CYP3A4 inhibitors • Prolonged QTc • Acute MI • Concomitant use of verapamil and diltiazem • Pregnancy • Breastfeeding • Use ↑ the risk of AFib. Discontinue if AFib develops	**1–10%** • CVS: Bradycardia, hypertension and AFib • CNS: Phosphene (transient visual abnormalities) **<1%** • Angioedema • Diplopia • Erythema • Hypotension • Pruritus • Skin rash • Syncope • Torsades de pointes • Urticaria • Ventricular arrhythmias • Vertigo • Visual impairment **Frequency unknown** • Heart block, sinoatrial arrest	

Contd...

Contd...

Vaughn-Williams classification	*Mechanism of action*	*Drug*	*Recommended pediatric dose*	*Indications*	*Contraindications*	*Side effects*	*Monitoring*
	Acts on myocardium by ↓ rate of SA node impulse formation and ↑ conduction time. Magnesium is necessary for the movement of calcium, sodium, and potassium in and out of cells, as well as stabilizing excitable membranes	Magnesium sulfate[2,28]	**IV/IO:** 25 to 50 mg/kg/dose, administer as a bolus, if pulse administer over 10 to 20 minutes; maximum dose: 2,000 mg/dose	TdP	Dosage ↓ required in renal dysfunction, severe heart block, myocardial damage and hypersensitivity	• Flushing, hypotension, vasodilation • CNS depression • Respiratory depression • Nausea, vomiting, lethargy, drowsiness, flushing • Loss of DTRs • Bradycardia, ↑ PR, ↑ QRS	Monitor HR, BP, RR and neurological status
	Stimulates β_1- and β_2-receptors resulting in ↑ heart rate and contractility, vasodilation of peripheral vasculature	Iso-proterenol[2,29]	Continuous IV infusion: 0.05 to 0.5 µg/kg/minute; titrate to effect; doses as high as 2 µg/kg/minute may be needed	TdP (drug-or bradycardia induced, LQTS type 2), Brugada storm	Pre-existing HF, ischemic heart disease	• Flushing, hypotension, cardiac arrhythmias, hypertension • Dizziness, headache • Diaphoresis, nausea, vomiting • Hypokalemia • Tremor, weakness • Blurred vision • Dyspnea	Continuous ECG monitoring

(HR: heart rate; BP: blood pressure; AP: action potential; ERP: effective refractory period; LVEF: left ventricular ejection fraction; SVT: supraventricular tachycardia; VT: ventricular tachycardia; Afib: atrial fibrillation; AF: atrial flutter; CPK: creatine phosphokinase; SLE: systemic lupus erythematosus; TdP: torsades de pointes; HOCM: hypertrophic obstructive cardiomyopathy; LQTS: long QT syndrome; BMD: bone mineral density; CBC: complete blood count; COPD: chronic obstructive pulmonary disease; HF: heart failure; ECG: electrocardiogram.)

REFERENCES

1. Available from: *https://www.accessdata.fda.gov/drugsatfda_docs/label/ 2010/089338s036lbl.pdf*
2. Available from: *https://online.lexi.com*
3. Katzung BG, editor. Basic and Clinical Pharmacology, 14th edition. New York, USA: Mgraw-Hill Education; 2017.
4. Available from: *https://dailymed.nlm.nih.gov/dailymed/drugInfo.cfm?setid= 17e47845-daad-434c-a784-6d3875b0d704*
5. Available from: *https://www.pfizer.com/files/products/uspi_norpace.pdf*
6. Available from: *https://www.accessdata.fda.gov/drugsatfda_docs/label/2010/006488s074lbl.pdf*
7. Available from: *https://docs.boehringer-ingelheim.com/Prescribing%20Information/PIs/Mexitil%20Caps/Mexitil.pdf*
8. Available from: *https://www.accessdata.fda.gov/drugsatfda_docs/label/2009/084349s060lbl.pdf*
9. Available from: *https://gp2u.com.au/static/pdf/T/TAMBOCOR-PI.pdf*
10. Available from: *https://www.accessdata.fda.gov/drugsatfda_docs/label/2013/019151s012lbl.pdf*
11. Available from: *https://www.accessdata.fda.gov/drugsatfda_docs/label/2011/016418s080,016762s017,017683s008lbl.pdf*
12. Available from: *https://www.accessdata.fda.gov/drugsatfda_docs/label/2011/018240s031lbl.pdf*
13. Available from: *https://www.accessdata.fda.gov/drugsatfda_docs/label/2008/017963s062,018704s021lbl.pdf*
14. Available from: *https://www.accessdata.fda.gov/drugsatfda_docs/label/2008/018063s060lbl.pdf*
15. Available from: *https://www.accessdata.fda.gov/drugsatfda_docs/label/2016/205703s000lbl.pdf*
16. Syed YY. Landiolol: A review in tachyarrhythmias. Drugs. 2018;78:377-88.
17. Available from: *https://www.accessdata.fda.gov/drugsatfda_docs/label/2016/018972s051lbl.pdf*
18. Available from: *https://www.accessdata.fda.gov/drugsatfda_docs/label/2011/021151s010lbl.pdf*
19. Available from: *https://www.accessdata.fda.gov/drugsatfda_docs/label/2009/022425lbl.pdf*
20. Ohashi J, Yasuda S, Miyazaki S, *et al*. Prevention of life-threatening ventricular tachyarrhythmia by a novel and pure class-III agent, nifekalant hydrochloride. J Cardiovasc Pharmacol. 2006;48:274-9.
21. Available from: *https://www.accessdata.fda.gov/drugsatfda_docs/label/2009/018817s021lbl.pdf*
22. Available from: *https://www.accessdata.fda.gov/drugsatfda_docs/label/2010/020062s040lbl.pdf*
23. Available from: *https://www.accessdata.fda.gov/drugsatfda_docs/label/2011/019937s026lbl.pdf*
24. Moffett BS, Garner A, Zapata T, *et al*. Serum digoxin concentrations and clinical signs and symptoms of digoxin toxicity in the paediatric population. Cardiol Young. 2016;26: 493-8.
25. Kurugol Z, Ozyurek R, Levent E, *et al*. The influence of feeding regimens on endogenous digoxin-like immunoreactive substance concentrations in infants. Acta Paediatr. 1996;85: 753-4.
26. Available from: *https://www.accessdata.fda.gov/drugsatfda_docs/label/2011/020405s006lbl.pdf*
27. Available from: *https://www.accessdata.fda.gov/drugsatfda_docs/label/2015/206143Orig1s000lbl.pdf*
28. Available from: *https://www.accessdata.fda.gov/drugsatfda_docs/label/2013/020309s028lbl.pdf*
29. Available from: *https://www.accessdata.fda.gov/drugsatfda_docs/label/2013/010515s031lbl.pdf*

Annexure

4

Reference Laboratory Values

Peeyush Jain, Preeti Jain

Laboratory results of analytes are interpreted on the basis of *Reference Range* for the test, which are also called as *Reference Values* or *Normal Values*. Reference range is defined as *limiting values within which a specific percentage (usually 95%) of apparently healthy individuals' result would fall*—usually between the 2.5th and 97.5th centiles of the test result distribution in the reference population. These are essentially based on the test results for a large group of healthy population.

The process of determining reference values or range for any biochemical or pathological test is a complex, lengthy as well as a costly proposition. There is an appreciable variability in these values between populations differing in terms of age, gender, ethnicity, geographical distribution or lifestyles. Establishing reference values for pediatric population is especially challenging as the reference values across pediatric age groups are not easily available for all tests.

The reference values should never be considered as sacrosanct. For some analytes, the reference values are laboratory/method dependent and hence, the test results tend to vary between different labs. It is advisable that the reference range of the concerned laboratory performing the test may be considered is such cases.

Various analytes and their reference laboratory values as applicable to the age groups mentioned therein, are given in the following tables. The information provided has been updated as far as possible; some values however have been retained from the previous edition. Most of the reference values have been given in the *Units* which are commonly being used. The conversion factor (for multiplication) has also been provided to enable conversion to other units (SI/ Conventional).

A. Hematology: Coagulation profile

Analyte or Procedure	*Specimen*	*Reference values*
Activated partial thromboplastin time (APTT) (sec)	Plasma (citrate)	25–35 Infants <90
Bleeding time (Ivy) (min)		Normal 2–7
Clotting time Lee-White, 37°C (min)	Whole blood	Glass tubes 5–8 (5–15 min at RT) Silicone tubes about 30 min prolonged
D-dimer (µg/mL)	Plasma Cord blood Adult	<3.40 ≤0.40
Factor I, see *Fibrinogen*		
Factor II (U/mL)	Plasma (citrate)	0.5–1.5 or 60–150% of normal

Contd...

Contd...

Analyte or Procedure	*Specimen*	*Reference values*
Factor IV, see *Calcium*		
Factor V (U/mL)		0.5–2.0 or 60–150% of normal
Factor VII		65–135% of normal
Factor VIII		60–145% of normal
Factor VIII antigen		50–200% of normal
Factor IX		60–140% of normal
Factor X		60–130% of normal
Factor XI		65–135% of normal
Factor XII		65–150% of normal
Factor XII (fibrin stabilizing factor, FSF) (U/mL)	Whole blood (citrate, oxalate)	Minimal hemostatic level 0.02–0.05 1–2% of normal
Fibrin degradation products (D-dimer) (μg/L)	Plasma (citrate)	Adults 68–494 Mean 207
Fibrinogen (mg/dL)	Whole blood (sodium citrate)	Newborn: 125–300 Adult: 200–400
Prothrombin time (PT) One-stage (Quick) (sec)	Whole blood (sodium citrate)	In general, 11–15 (varies with type of thromboplastin) Newborn prolonged by 2–3
Thrombin time (sec)	Whole blood (sodium citrate)	Control time ± 2 when control is 9–13

B. Hematology: Blood counts

Analyte or Procedure	*Specimen*	*Age*	*Reference values*
Erythrocyte count (RBC count) (millions of cells/mm^3)	Whole blood (ethylenediaminetetraacetic acid)	Cord blood 1–3 days (cap) 1 wk 2 wk 1 mo 2 mo 3–6 mo 0.5–2 yrs 2–6 yrs 6–12 yrs 12–18 yrs, M	3.9–5.5 4.0–6.6 3.9–6.3 3.6–6.2 3.0–5.4 2.7–4.9 3.1–4.5 3.7–5.3 3.9–5.3 4.0–5.2 4.5–5.3
Red cell distribution width (RDW) (%)		0–6 mo 7 mo–2 yrs 3–6 yrs >7 yrs	13.0–18.0 11.5–16.0 11.5–15.0 11.5–14.0
Hematocrit (HCT, Hct) % of packed red cells	Whole blood (ethylenediaminetetraacetic acid)	1 day (cap) 2 days 3 days 2 mo 6–12 yrs 12–18 yrs, M F	48–69% 48–75% 44–72% 28–42% 35–45% 37–49% 36–46%

Contd...

Contd...

Analyte or Procedure	*Specimen*	*Age*	*Reference values*
Hemoglobin (Hb) (g/dL) Conversion Factor 0.155 to mmol/L	Whole blood (ethylenediaminetetraacetic acid)	1–3 days (cap) 2 mo 6–12 yrs 12–18 yrs, M F	14.5–22.5 9.0–14.0 11.5–15.5 13.0–16.0 12.0–16.0
Hemoglobin (Hb) electrophoresis (%)	Whole blood (heparin, ethylenediaminetetraacetic acid, citrate)		HbA > 95 HbA2 1.5–3.5 HbF < 2
Hemoglobin F (%)	Whole blood (ethylenediaminetetraacetic acid)	1 day 5 day 3 wk 6–9 wk 3–4 mo 6 mo Adult	63–92 65–88 55–85 31–75 <2–59 <2–9 <2
Erythrocyte sedimentation rate (ESR) Westergren, modified (mm/hr)	Whole blood (ethylenediaminetetraacetic acid)	Child Adult M F	0–13 0–9 0–20
Leukocyte count (WBC) (× 1,000 cells/mm^3)	Whole blood (ethylenediaminetetraacetic acid)	0–30 days 1–23 mo 2–9 yrs 10–17 yrs Adult	9.1–34.0 6.0–14.0 4.0–12.0 4.0–10.5 4.0–10.0
Leukocyte differential (% (cells/mm^3))	Whole blood (ethylenediaminetetraacetic acid)	Myelocytes Neutrophils (bands) Neutrophils (segs) Lymphocytes Monocytes Eosinophils Basophils	0 (0) 3–5 (150–400) 54–62 (3000–5800) 25–33 (1500–3000) 3–7 (285–500) 1–3 (50–250) 0–0.75 (15–50)
Mean corpuscular hemoglobulin (MCH) (pg/cell) Conversion Factor 0.0155 to fmol/L	Whole blood (ethylenediaminetetraacetic acid)	0–30 days 1–23 mo 2–9 yrs 10–17 yrs >18 yrs	33–39 24–30 25–31 26–32 27–31
Mean corpuscular hemoglobin Conc. (MCHC) % Hb/cell or g Hb/dL RBC Conversion Factor 0.0155 to mmol Hb/L RBC	Whole blood (ethylenediaminetetraacetic acid)		32–36
Mean corpuscular volume (MCV) μm^3 Conversion Factor 1 to fL	Whole blood (ethylenediaminetetraacetic acid)	0–30 days 1–23 mo 2–9 yrs 10–17 yrs >18 yrs	99–115 72–88 76–90 78–95 78–100

Contd...

Contd...

Analyte or Procedure	*Specimen*	*Age*	*Reference values*
Platelet count (Thrombocyte count) (× 10^3/mm^3)	Whole blood (ethylenediaminetetraacetic acid)	Newborn 84–478 Adult 150–400	(after 1 wk, same as Adults)
Reticulocyte count % (× 10^6 cells/µL)	Whole blood	0–2 days 3–4 days >4 days	3.0–7.0 (0.14–0.22) 1.0–3.0 (0.04–0.11) 0.5–1.5 (0.02–0.08)
C. Biochemistry			
Analyte or Procedure	*Specimen*	*Age*	*Reference values*
Acetone (mg/dL)			0.3–2.0
ACTH Hormone (pg/mL) Conversion Factor 0.22 to pmol/L	Plasma	Cord Newborn Adult (morning)	50–570 10–185 <120
Alanine aminotransferase (ALT, SGPT) U/L	Serum	0–5 days 1–19 yrs	6–50 5–45
Albumin (g/dL)	Plasma	Premature 1 day Full term <6 day <5 yrs 5–19 yrs 3–5 yrs 6–8 yrs 9–19 yrs	1.8–3.0 2.5–3.4 3.9–5.0 4.0–5.3 1.5–21.5 1.5–37.8 1.5–169.6
Albumin Micro (mg/dL)	Urine	Random Timed 24 hrs	0–3.7 <20 µg/min <30 mg/24 h
Aldolase (U/L)	Serum	10–24 mo 25 mo–16 yr	10–40 5–20
Ammonia nitrogen (µg N/dL) Conversion Factor 0.714 to µmol N/L	Plasma (Hep) Urine (24 hrs)	Newborn 0–2 wks >1 month Infant Adult	90–150 80–130 30–70 560–2900 140–1500
Amylase (U/L)	Serum, Plasma		30–100
Anti-Streptolysin–O titer (ASO titer) (Todd units) Upper limit of normal	Serum	2–5 yrs 6–9 yrs 10–12 yrs	120–160 240 320
Alpha 1 Antitrypsin (mg/dL) Conversion Factor 0.01 to g/L	Serum	0–5 days 1–9 yrs 9–19 yrs	143–440 147–245 152–317
Aspartate aminotransferase (AST, SGOT) (U/L)	Serum	0–5 days 1–9 yrs 10–19 yrs	35–140 15–55 5–45

Contd...

Contd...

Analyte or Procedure	*Specimen*	*Age*	*Reference values*	
Bilirubin total (mg/dL)	Serum, Plasma		Premature	Full-term
Conversion Factor 71.1 to µmol/L		Cord blood	<2.0	<2.0
		0–1 day	<8.0	<6.0
		1–2 days	<12.0	<8.0
		2–5 days	<16.0	<12.0
		>5 days	<20.0	<10
Bilirubin conjugated (mg/dL) Conversion Factor 71.1 to µmol/L	Serum		0–0.2	
C-reactive protein (mg/L) Conversion Factor 0.1 to mg/dL	Serum	0–14 days 15 days–3 yrs >3 yrs	0.3–6 0.1–1 0.1–6	
Calcium, ionized (Ca) (mg/dL)	Serum, Plasma	Cord blood	5.0–6.0	
Conversion Factor 0.25 to mmol/L	Whole blood (heparin)	Newborn,		
		3–24 hrs	4.3–5.1	
		24–48 hrs	4.0–4.7	
		Thereafter	4.8–4.9	
Calcium, total (mg/dL)	Serum	Cord blood	9.0–11.5	
Conversion Factor 0.25 to mmol/L		Newborn, 3–24 hrs	9.0–10.6	
		24–48 hrs	7.0–12.0	
		4–7 days	9.0–10.9	
		Child	8.8–10.8	
		Thereafter	8.4–10.2	
Ceruloplasmin (mg/L) Conversion Factor 0.001 to g/L	Plasma	Cord <2 months 2 months–1 yr 1–14 yrs	52–330 74–240 135–390 210–400	
Chloride (mmol/L) Conversion Factor 1 to mEq/L	Serum, Plasma (heparin)	Cord blood Newborn Thereafter	96–104 97–110 98–106	
Cholesterol (mg/dL) Conversion Factor 0.026 to mmol/L	Serum	15 days–1 yrs 1–15 yrs	64–230 110–210	
Creatine kinase (U/L)	Serum	Cord blood 5–8 hrs 24–33 hrs 72–100 hrs Adult	70–380 210–1,175 130–1,200 85–725 5–130	
Creatine kinase Isoenzymes	Serum		% MB	%BB
		Cord blood	0.3–3.1	0.3–10.5
		5–8 hrs	1.7–7.9	3.6–13.4
		24–33 hrs	1.8–5.0	2.3–8.6
		72–100 hrs	1.4–5.4 5	1–13.3
		Adult	0–2%	0

Contd...

Contd...

Analyte or Procedure	*Specimen*	*Age*	*Reference values*
Creatinine (Kinetic, or enzymatic) (mg/dL)	Serum, Plasma	Cord blood	0.6–1.2
Conversion Factor 88.4 to μmol/L		Newborn	0.3–1.0
		Infant	0.2–0.4
		Child	0.3–0.7
		Adolescent	0.5–1.0
Creatinine clearance (endogenous) (mL/min/1.73 m^2)	Serum, Plasma and Urine	Newborn	40–65
		<40 yrs, M	97–137
		F	88–128
Ferritin (ng/mL)	Serum	Newborn	25–200
Conversion Factor 1 to μg/L		1 mo	200–600
		2–5 mo	50–200
		6 mo–15 yrs	7–140
Glucose (mg/dL)	Serum	Cord blood	45–96
Conversion Factor 0.055 to mmol/L		Premature	20–60
		Newborn 1 day	40–60
		>1 day	50–90
		Child	60–100
	CSF		50–70% of serum glucose
	Urine (24 hrs)		<500 mg/24h
	Urine (random)		<30 mg/dL
Glucose, 2 hr postprandial	Serum		<120 mg/dL
Conversion Factor 0.055 to mmol/L			
Glucose tolerance test (GTT) (mg/dL)			Normal Range / Diabetic
Child: To give glucose1.75 g/kg of ideal			
Weight up to maximum of 75 g	Serum	Fasting	70–105 / >126
Conversion Factor 0.055 to mmol/L		60 min	120–170 / >200
		90 min	100–140 / >200
		120 min	70–120 / >200
Glycohemoglobin hemoglobin A_{1c}	Whole blood (heparin)	1–5 yrs	2.1–7.7
(% of total Hb)		5–16 yrs	3.0–6.2
Iron (μg/dL)	Serum	Infant	22–184
Iron-binding capacity, total (TIBC)	Serum	Thereafter	100–400
(μg/dL)		Children	250–400
% Saturation			>16%
Ketone bodies, qualitative	Serum		Negative
Ketone bodies, quantitative	Whole blood	1–12 mo	0.1–1.5
(mmol/L)		1–7 yrs	0.15–2.0
		7–15 yrs	<0.1–0.5

Contd...

Contd...

Analyte or Procedure	*Specimen*	*Age*	*Reference values*	
Lactate (mmol/L)	Plasma (venous)		0.2–2.0	
Conversion Factor 0.99 to mg/dL	Plasma (arterial)		0.3–0.8	
	CSF		0.6–2.2	
	Whole blood		0.2–1.7	
Lactate dehydrogenase (U/L)	Serum	2–12 yrs	180–360	
		12–60 yrs	125–220	
Lead (µg/dL)	Whole blood (heparin)	Child	<10	
Conversion Factor 0.048 to µmol/L		Adult	<40	
		Toxic	100	
Lipase (U/L)	Serum	0–19 yrs	4–39	
Magnesium (mg/dL)	Plasma (heparin)	0–6 days	1.2–2.6	
Conversion Factor 0.41 to mmol/L		7 d–2 yrs	1.6–2.6	
		2–14 yrs	1.5–2.3	
Methemoglobin (MetHb) (g/dL)	Whole blood		0.06–0.24	
(% of total Hb)			0.78 ± 0.37	
Myoglobin (ng/mL)	Serum		6–85	
Methylmalonic acid (µmol/L)	Serum		0.03–0.26	
Osmolality (mOsm/kg H_2O)	Serum/Plasma		275–295	
	Urine		300–1000	
Phenylalanine (mg/dL)	Serum	Premature	2.0–7.5	
		Newborn	1.2–3.4	
		Thereafter	0.8–1.8	
Phosphorus, inorganic (mg/dL)	Serum	0–14 days	5.6–10.5	
Conversion Factor 0.32 to mmol/L		15 days–1 yr	4.8–8.4	
		1–3 yrs	4.3–6.8	
		3–5 yrs	4.4–6	
		6–10 yrs	4.4–5.7	
		11–15 yrs M	3.8–5.9	
		F	3.6–5.6	
Phosphatase, acid prostatic (RIA) (ng/mL)	Serum		<3.0	
Phosphatase, alkaline	Serum	1–9 yrs	145–420	
(U/L)		10–11 yrs	130–560	
			Male	Female
		12–13 yrs	200–495	105–420
		14–15 yrs	130–525	70–230
		16–19 yrs	65–260	50–130
Potassium (mmol/L)	Serum	<2 mo	3.0–7.0	
Conversion Factor 1.0 to mEq/L		2–12 mo	3.5–6.0	
		>12 mo	3.5–5.0	

Contd...

Contd...

Analyte or Procedure	*Specimen*	*Age*	*Reference values*
Protein, total (g/dL)	Serum	Premature	4.3–7.6
Conversion Factor 10 to g/L		Newborn	4.6–7.4
		1–7 yrs	6.1–7.9
		8–12 yrs	6.4–8.1
		13–19 yrs	6.6–8.2
(mg/dL)	CSF	>1 month	15–45
	Urine		30–140 mg/24 hrs
Pyruvate (mmol/L) Conversion Factor 0.114 to µmol/L	Whole blood		0.076 ± 0.026
Sodium (mEq/L)	Serum, Plasma	Newborn	134–146
Conversion factor 1.0 to mmol/L		Infant	139–146
		Child	138–145
		Thereafter	136–146
Thyroid stimulating hormone	Serum	Birth–3 days	1.0–20.0
(TSH)(mIU/L)		3–30 days	0.5–6.5
Conversion Factor 1.0 to µIU/mL		1–5 mo	0.5–6.0
		6 mo–18 yrs	0.5–4.5
Thyrotropin releasing hormone (hTRH) (pg/mL) Conversion Factor 2.76 to pmol//L	Plasma		5–60
Thyroxine (T4), Total (µg/dL)	Serum	0–3 days	8.0–20.0
Conversion Factor 12.9 to nmol/L		3–30 days	5.0–15.0
		1 mo–1 yr	6.0–14.0
		1–5 yrs	4.5–11.0
		6–18 yrs	4.5–10
Thyroxine (T4), Free (ng/dL)	Serum	0–3 days	2.0–5.0
Conversion Factor 12.9 to pmol/L		3–30 days	0.9–2.2
		1 mo–1 yr	0.7–2.0
Triiodothyronine, Total (ng/dL)	Serum	0–3 days	60–300
Conversion Factor 0.015 to nmol/L		4 days–1 yr	90–260
		1–6 yrs	90–240
		7–11 yrs	90–230
		12–18 yrs	100–210
Triiodothyronine, Free (pg/dL)	Serum	Cord blood	20–240
Conversion Factor 0.015 to pmol/L		1–3 days	200–610
		6 wks	240–560
		Adult	230–660
Transferrin (siderophilin) (mg/dL)	Serum	2 m–1 yr	110–320
Conversion Factor 0.01 to gm/L		1–19 yrs	220–340

Contd...

Contd...

Analyte or Procedure	*Specimen*	*Age*	*Reference values*
Urea (mg/dL)	Serum, Plasma	Cord blood	21–40
Conversion Factor 0.357 to mmol/L		Premature (1 wk)	3–25
		Newborn	3–12
		Infant/child	5–18
		Thereafter	7–18
Uric acid (mg/dL)	Serum	1–5 yrs	1.7–5.8
Conversion Factor 59.48 to µmol/L		6–11 yrs	2.2–6.6
		12–19 yrs M	3.0–7.7
		F	2.7–5.7
Urinalysis	Urine	Specific gravity	1.001–1.035
		pH	4–9
		Protein	Neg
		Glucose	Neg
		Ketone	Neg
		Bilirubin	Neg
		Urobilinogen	<2.0
		WBC	0–4/HPF

Index

Page numbers followed by *b* refer to box, *f* refer to figure, *fc* refer to flow chart, and *t* refer to table.

A

B

C

E

F

G

J

K

L

M

Q

R

S

T

U

V

W

X

Y

Z